T0127987

Clinical
Naturopathy 3e

An evidence-based guide to practice

Clinical Naturopathy 3e

An evidence-based guide to practice

Jerome Sarris & Jon Wardle

ELSEVIER

ELSEVIER

Elsevier Australia. ACN 001 002 357
(a division of Reed International Books Australia Pty Ltd)
Tower 1, 475 Victoria Avenue, Chatswood, NSW 2067

ISBN: 978-0-7295-4302-6

National Library of Australia Cataloguing-in-Publication Data

A catalogue record for this book is available from the National Library of Australia

Head of Content: Larissa Norrie
Content Project Manager: Fariha Nadeem
Edited and Proofread by Leanne Peters, Letterati Publishing Services
Cover by Alice Weston
Internal design: Lisa Petroff
Index by Innodata Indexing
Typeset by Toppan Best-set Premedia Limited
Printed in Singapore by Markono Print Media Pte Ltd

Last digit is the print number: 9 8 7 6 5 4 3 2

Contents

Preface

As we look back on the past decade since the first edition in 2010, a lot has evolved in the field of Naturopathy. Not only has research in the therapies and practices employed by naturopaths grown considerably, more and more studies now also emphasise the value of 'whole practice' naturopathy—or the application of naturopathic approaches to healing. Naturopaths are increasingly being recognised as research leaders, with successful applications to highly competitive conventional funding schemes such as the National Health and Medical Research Council (NHMRC) in Australia or the National Institutes of Health in the United States. Naturopathy is recognised as one of the major traditional systems of medicine by the World Health Organization, and the profession has made remarkable strides globally through initiatives such as the World Naturopathic Federation.

This third edition aims to retain much of what is familiar and well-loved from previous editions, updated with the most recent research as well as some new content that reflects the evolution of naturopathic practice. We hope to have captured this evolution, but no doubt the text will still need to evolve further in future editions to keep pace with contemporary practice. As discussed in the preface of the previous editions, we do recognise that the field should not sacrifice the core philosophical tenants that place it as a unique healing system in the pursuit of 'evidence-based medicine'. This third edition is still focused on reconnecting more with the fundamentals of naturopathy, as well as pushing the scientific boundaries even further.

Patients rarely fit into textbook examples, and individualisation of treatment is integral to naturopathic philosophy. Feedback from students and practitioners noted that case studies in the first edition tended to funnel readers towards predetermined outcomes, and often obscured the flexibility of options presented in the chapter material. As such, the case studies were omitted in the second edition and in this edition. However, we are pleased to have assisted recently in the creation of *Clinical Naturopathy: Case Studies*, which allowed a collection of clinically-relevant cases to be enshrined, as well unshackle these case studies from the constraints of fitting into discrete textbook chapters so that they could more truly reflect the inter-systems approaches to diagnosis and treatment seen in naturopathic practice.

We respect that the practise of naturopathic medicine is complex and individualised, and thus acknowledge that this text does not provide a definitive 'how-to' guide. As with all previous and subsequent editions, the purpose of this text is to articulate evidence-based clinical practice (principles, treatment protocols and interventions) in a reader-friendly format for practitioners, academics and students. We have aimed to develop a resource that is comprehensive enough to serve as a robust resource reference, but compact enough to be carried around as desired and to be a useful tool to be used in practice. It is a book we hope will be thumbed through extensively, rather than one that spends most of its life on a shelf.

A strength of this text that we have maintained is that it explores the key principles and philosophies used in modern naturopathy for treating a range of conditions. The essence of this is detailed in the 'key treatment protocols' section in each chapter. An additional strength is the critical evaluation of the current evidence of both diagnostic and practice methods, and naturopathic interventions (whether they come from the conventional or complementary sphere). This differentiates *Clinical Naturopathy: An Evidence-Based Guide to Practice* from some other publications that, while informative, often do not provide an evidence-based, referenced analysis of the treatment protocols underpinning the therapeutic use of naturopathic interventions.

Of course, we do acknowledge some limitations. First, it is recognised that it is not possible to detail all diseases and disorders that are encountered in clinical practice. As any naturopathic clinician will know, people are treated, not diseases, and each person manifests a unique combination of variations of signs and symptoms rather than an isolated textbook-diagnosed disease. Regardless, categorisation by major diseases and illnesses provides a useful framework with which to discuss naturopathic treatment protocols and interventions. The protocols and principles discussed in each chapter will in many cases be clinically relevant to the treatment of various other conditions where similar underlying causes exist. To assist readers we have made some of the major links of these between chapters overt, but we also acknowledge that there are far more than has been detailed.

As this is meant to be a clinical reference, rather than a purely academic tome or research publication, detailed analysis of each and every trial has not been entered into. However, all treatments have been duly referenced and readers, as always, are encouraged to explore these further. A selection of relevant further reading has been listed by individual contributors for those who wish to undertake additional investigation of the chapter content. It can also be noted that we focus primarily on the major evidence from clinical trials over that of *in vivo* or *in vitro* studies. Traditional evidence is also discussed when relevant. It will be apparent to readers that not every method, diagnostic technique or intervention included in this book has solid clinical evidence, and some herbal medicines or nutrients rely largely on traditional evidence. However, we feel as though it would be remiss to ignore those treatments and practices based on traditional evidence that form core parts of modern naturopathic practice in strict deference to modern scientific evidence.

Research in the naturopathic medicine field is still slowly advancing. Much of the research on complementary medicines is being led by naturopaths themselves—with the World Naturopathic Federation identifying over 2000 peer-reviewed medical research publications authored by naturopaths. The number of naturopathic 'whole practice' trials has increased from six studies with a total 692 patients showing the effectiveness of naturopathic 'whole practice' care at the time of our second edition to 33 trials with a total of 9859 patients at the time of publication of this edition. There is much work remaining, but the momentum and trajectory of naturopathic research is very promising.

The future direction of naturopathy and its components more broadly appears positive, with mainstream acceptance—including government regulation or degree education—evolving in countries such as Australia, Brazil, Canada, Germany, India, Mexico, Spain, South Africa, the United Kingdom and the United States. To maintain the development of the profession and to enable more effective healers, education is paramount. *Clinical Naturopathy: An Evidence-Based Guide to Practice*, 3rd edition is developed to be at the forefront of naturopathic education in the 21st century. This book is designed for naturopaths, allied health or conventional medical practitioners, researchers and anyone with an interest in the principles, practices and treatments of naturopathic medicine. We are pleased with this third edition and the fantastic contributions from the leaders in our field, and feel honoured that this may in part contribute to shaping better healthcare.

Jerome Sarris and Jon Wardle

Acknowledgements

To the special ladies in my life. The young to the old, past, present, and future.
You are my greatest teachers.

For Kath and Molly, who inspire me in ways they don't even know

We would like to thank the contributors who assisted the third edition of *Clinical Naturopathy* into a unique contribution to the field. We would also like to thank those practitioners and students who so willingly provided feedback that has helped with this current edition. Thanks are also extended to the talented and supportive Elsevier staff for their assistance throughout the development of the manuscript. Finally, as usual we would like to acknowledge all of the students, practitioners and academics who strive to evolve and enhance their knowledge of the art and science of naturopathy for the easing of human suffering and the betterment of humanity.

About the editors

Jerome Sarris, ND (ACNM), MHSc HMed (UNE), Adv Dip Acu (ACNM), Dip Nutri (ACNM), PhD (UQ) is an NHMRC Clinical Research Fellow and Professor of Integrative Mental Health, and Deputy Director and Research Director of NICM Health Research Institute at Western Sydney University, Westmead. He also holds an honorary Principal Research Fellow appointment at Melbourne University, Department of Psychiatry. Jerome moved from clinical practice as a naturopath, nutritionist, and acupuncturist to academic work, and completed a doctorate at The University of Queensland in the field of psychiatry. He undertook his postdoctoral training at The University of Melbourne, Department of Psychiatry; the Centre for Human Psychopharmacology, Swinburne University of Technology; and the Depression Clinical & Research Program at Harvard Medical School (Massachusetts General Hospital). He has a particular interest in anxiety and mood disorder research pertaining to nutraceutical psychopharmacology, in integrative medicine, lifestyle medicine and psychotropic plant medicine (in particular on kava and medicinal cannabis). Jerome has over 165 publications and has published in many eminent medical journals including *Lancet Psychiatry*, *American Journal of Psychiatry*, *JAMA Psychiatry*, and *World Psychiatry*. Jerome was a founding Vice Chair of the International Network of Integrative Mental Health & an Executive Committee Member of the International Society for Nutritional Psychiatry. He has been awarded the NHAA most notable contribution to herbal medicine research award, and the ANS Dr Tini Gruner Educator of the year in the field of Naturopathy.

Jon Wardle, ND (ACNM), MPH (UQ), LLM (Melb.), PhD (UQ) is Associate Professor of Public Health at the Faculty of Health, University of Technology Sydney and is also a National Health and Medical Research Council Translating Research into Practice Fellow. Jon also heads the Regulatory, Policy and Legislative Stream at the Australian Research Centre in Complementary and Integrative Medicine, University of Technology Sydney. Jon has visiting positions at the Schools of Medicine at the Chinese University of Hong Kong, Oxford University and Boston University. Jon is Secretary General of the World Naturopathic Federation, and has served in this position since the Federation's inception. Jon is convenor of the Public Health Association of Australia's special interest group on traditional and complementary medicine and serves on the Policy Committee of the American Public Health Association's integrative health section. Jon maintains a naturopathic practice at Herbs on the Hill, Brisbane. Jon is on the editorial board of several journals, including serving as editor-in-chief of *Advances in Integrative Medicine* and the *International Journal of Naturopathic Medicine*. Jon lectures internationally on complementary medicine and public health; has worked with numerous governments on primary care, public health and traditional medicine; has published over 120 peer-review research publications; and writes several popular Australian health columns, in addition to his academic publishing endeavours.

Contributors

Leslie Axelrod ND, LAc
Professor of Clinical Sciences, Southwest College of Naturopathic Medicine, Tempe, Arizona, United States

Diana Bowman ND, MHSc (Herbal Medicine), BHSc (Naturopathy), Dip Health Science (Naturopathy), Dip Teaching, PhD Candidate
Lecturer, Endeavour College of Natural Medicine, Brisbane, Queensland, Australia
Board Director, Naturopaths and Herbalists Association of Australia

Michelle Boyd ND, MHSc (Herbal Medicine), GradCertHEd, FNHAA
Lecturer, Faculty of Naturopathy, Endeavour College of Natural Health, Brisbane, Queensland, Australia
Private Practitioner, Queensland, Australia

David Casteleijn ND, MHSc (Herbal Medicine), Academic, PhD Candidate
Naturopath, HerbsontheHill, Brisbane, Queensland, Australia

Greg Connolly ND, BHSc (Naturopathy), PhD
Senior Lecturer, Southern School of Natural Therapies, Victoria, Australia

Kieran Cooley ND, BSc
Director of Research, Department of Research and Clinical Epidemiology, Canadian College of Naturopathic Medicine, Toronto, Ontario, Canada
Adjunct Faculty, Transitional Doctorate Department, Pacific College of Oriental Medicine, Chicago, Illinois, United States
Research Fellow, The Australian Research Centre in Complementary and Integrative Medicine (ARCCIM), Faculty of Health, University of Technology Sydney, Sydney, New South Wales, Australia

Phillip Cottingham ND, BHSc (CompMed), PostGradDip (HlthSci), GradDip (HerbMed), DipHom, DipMass
Principal, Wellpark College of Natural Therapies, Auckland, New Zealand

Gary Deed MBBS, DipHerbMed, FACNEM
Chair, RACGP Diabetes Network of the Faculty of Specific Interests
Editorial Board Member, Endocrinology Today
Integrative Medical Practitioner, Queensland, Australia

Stephanie Gadsden ND, BHSc (Naturopathy), GradCert (Mental Health Science)
Co-founding Director, Merge Health Pty Ltd, Surrey Hills, Victoria, Australia
Graduate Psychology Student, University of Melbourne, Victoria, Australia
Wellness Consultant, Waterman Business Centre, Chadstone, Victoria, Australia

Neville Hartley ND, AdvDipHSc (Nat), BHSc, MPhil (BioMed)
Senior Learning Facilitator, Naturopathy and Western Herbal Medicine, Torrens University, Brisbane, Queensland, Australia

Jason Hawrelak ND, BNat (Hons), PhD, FNHAA, MASN, FACN
Senior Lecturer, College of Health and Medicine, University of Tasmania, Hobart, Tasmania, Australia
Visiting Research Fellow, Australian Research Centre for Complementary and Integrative Medicine, University of Technology Sydney, Sydney, New South Wales, Australia
Chief Research Officer, Probiotic Advisor, Hobart, Tasmania, Australia
Private Practitioner, Goulds Natural Medicine, Hobart, Tasmania

Rhoslyn Humphreys ND, BSc (Hons), BNat, PGDPM, AdvDipNutr, AdvDipYoga, MATMS
Private Practitioner, Home Clinic, Manly, New South Wales

Christina Kure ND, BAppSci, BHSc, PhD
Research Manager, Cardiothoracic Surgery and Transplantation, The Alfred, Victoria, Australia
Adjunct Lecturer, Department of Medicine, Central Clinical School, Monash University, Victoria, Australia

James Lake MD
Clinical Assistant Professor, Department of Psychiatry, University of Arizona College of Medicine, Tucson, Arizona, United States
Adjunct Fellow, National Institute of Complementary Medicine, Health Research Institute, Western Sydney University, Sydney, New South Wales, Australia

Matthew Leach ND, RN, BN, BN (Hons), DipClinNutr, PhD
Senior Research Fellow, Department of Rural Health, University of South Australia, Adelaide, South Australia, Australia

Bradley Leech ND, BHSc (Hons), Adv Dip Ayur, PhD Candidate
Nutritionist, Ayurvedic Herbalist, New South Wales
Lecturer, Clinic Supervisor, Endeavour College of Natural Health, Sydney, New South Wales

Karen Martin ND, BTeach (Adult), MDistEd
Director and Naturopath, Well2, South Australia, Australia

Erica Oberg ND, MPH
Private Practitioner, La Jolla, California, United States

Paul Orrock ND, GradCertHEd DO, PhD MAppSc (Research)
Senior Lecturer, Coordinator of osteopathic programme (Bachelor of Clinical Sciences and Master of Osteopathic Medicine), School of Health and Human Sciences, Southern Cross University, Lismore, New South Wales, Australia

Daniel Roytas ND, MHSc (Nutrition), BHSc (Naturopathy), DipRM, MANTA
Senior Lecturer, Nutritional Medicine, Torrens University, Brisbane, Queensland, Australia
Principle Clinician and Owner, Ultima Healthcare, Fortitude Valley, Queensland, Australia

Ses Salmond ND, PhD, BA, DBM, DNutr, DHom, DRM
Fellow and Life Member, Naturopaths and Herbalists Association of Australia (NHAA)
Director and Private Practitioner, Arkana Therapy Centre, New South Wales, Australia
Clinical Sciences, Leichhardt Women's Community Health Centre, New South Wales, Australia
Clinical Sciences, Liverpool Women's Health Centre, New South Wales, Australia

Jerome Sarris ND, MHSc HMed, AdvDipAcu, Dip Nutri, PhD
NHMRC Clinical Research Fellow
Professor of Integrative Mental Health
Deputy Director and Research Director of NICM, Health Research Institute at Western Sydney University, Westmead, New South Wales, Australia

Janet Schloss ND, PGCNut, ADipHSc, PhD
Office of Research, Endeavour College of Natural Health, Brisbane, Queensland, Australia
Fellow, ARRICM, The University of Sydney, Sydney, New South Wales, Australia

Niikee Schoendorfer ND, MHSc, BHSc, PhD
Research Fellow, Discipline Medical Education, University of Queensland, Queensland, Australia

Justin Sinclair ND, MHerbMed, BHSc, DBM, DRM, Dip Nut, FNHAA, MATMS, PhD Candidate
Research Fellow, NICM Health Research Institute, Western Sydney University, New South Wales, Australia
Sessional Lecturer, Endeavour College of Natural Health, Sydney, New South Wales, Australia

Amie Steel ND, MPH, PhD
Senior Research Fellow, Australian Research Centre in Complementary and Integrative Medicine, Faculty of Health, University of Technology Sydney, Sydney, Australia

Jon Wardle ND, MPH, LLM, PhD
Associate Professor, Public Health, Faculty of Health, University of Technology Sydney, Sydney, New South Wales, Australia
National Health and Medical Research Council Translating Research into Practice Fellow

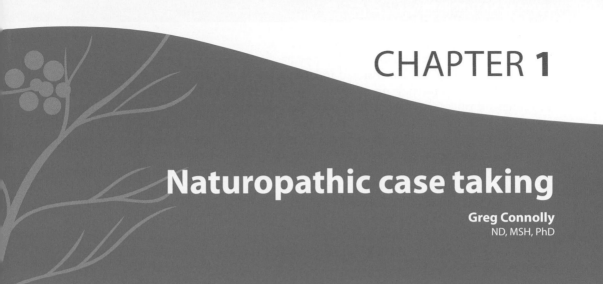

CHAPTER 1

Naturopathic case taking

Greg Connolly
ND, MSH, PhD

OVERVIEW OF NATUROPATHIC PHILOSOPHY AND PRINCIPLES

For naturopaths, the 'patient-centred approach' to case taking emphasises rapport, empathy and authenticity as a vital part of the healing process. This approach is based not just on current accepted health practices but also on the philosophy and principles that have underpinned naturopathy since its beginnings. This chapter examines how to establish and maintain a therapeutic relationship with patients through the process of a holistic consultation. It also presents a model of holistic case taking that provides both patient and naturopath with the knowledge and insight needed for healing and wellness.

Historical precursors

Having a philosophy by which to practise gives a clearer understanding of what constitutes good health, how illness is caused, what the role of the practitioner should be and the type of treatments that should be given.[1] Naturopathy has a loosely defined set of principles that have arisen from three interrelated philosophical sources. The first main source is the *historical precursors* of eclectic healthcare practices that formed naturopathy in the 19th and 20th centuries.[2] Allied to this are two other essential philosophical concepts intertwined with the historical development of naturopathy: *vitalism*[3,4] and *holism*.[5]

The tenets of naturopathic philosophy have developed from its chequered historical background, which includes the traditions of Hippocratic health, herbal medicine, homeopathy, nature cure, hydrotherapy, dietetics and manipulative therapies.[6] The historical precursors of naturopathy emphasise the responsibility of the patient in: following a healthy lifestyle with a balance of work, recreation, exercise, meditation and rest; eating healthily; getting fresh air, water and sunshine; regularly detoxifying and cleansing; experiencing healthy emotions within healthy relationships; leading an ethical life; and living in a healthy environment. These views highlight the fact that each patient is unique and, in light of this, naturopathic treatments for each patient are tailored to addressing the individual factors that cause their ill health. An essential part of a holistic consultation is the education of the patient to promote healthy living, self-care, preventive medicine and the unique factors affecting their vitality.

In modern times naturopathic philosophy has borrowed from the social movements of the 1960s and 1970s that fostered independence from authoritative structures and challenged the dependency upon technology and drugs for healthcare. These social movements emphasised a holistic approach to the environment and ecology with a yearning for healthcare that was natural and promoted self-reliance harking back to late 19th-century principles of nature care philosophy.[7] Naturopathy also borrowed from other counterculture movements and began to be suffused with New Age themes of transpersonal and humanistic psychology, spirituality, metaphysics and new science paradigms.[8] Since the 1980s naturopathy has increasingly used scientific research to increase understanding of body systems and validate treatments.[9,10]

From this variety of sources, naturopathy has consolidated a number of core principles. These principles have had many diverse adherents and an eclectic variety of blended philosophies. Over the course of the 20th century naturopathy began to be increasingly defined by its modalities and methods and less attention was paid to its underlying principles. This issue began to be addressed in the 1980s, particularly in the United States under the auspices of the American Association of Naturopathic Physicians, which sought to consolidate a number of core principles from the eclectic variety of naturopathic modalities.[11] These principles were further promulgated internationally through landmark naturopathic educational texts such as Pizzorno and Murray's *A Textbook of Natural Medicine*[12] and conferences such as the 2007 Foundations of Naturopathic Medicines Project.[13] The aim was to promote key concepts within naturopathy that are agreed upon and are flexible enough to accommodate a broad range of styles in naturopathic practice.[14]

These key concepts are now the de facto definition of internationally accepted principles to guide naturopathic practitioners in the care of their patients:

- the healing power of nature (*vis medicatrix naturae*)
- identify and treat the cause (*tolle causum*)
- first do no harm (*primum non nocere*)
- doctor as teacher (*docere*)
- treat the whole person
- prevention.

Vis medicatrix naturae sees the role of the practitioner as finding the cause (*tolle causum*) of the disturbance of vital force. The practitioner must then do no harm (*primum non nocere*) by using gentle, safe and non-invasive treatments from nature to restore the vital force, and to use preventative medicine by teaching (*docere*—doctor as teacher) the principles of good health to treat the whole person in body, mind and spirit.[15]

The above six principles rest upon those two essential tenets of the naturopathic understanding of health: vitalism and holism.

Vitalism

A fundamental belief of naturopathy is that ill health begins with a loss of vitality. Health is positive vitality and not just an absence of medical findings of disease. Health is restored by raising the vitality of the patient, which initiates the regenerative capacity for self-healing. The vital force is diminished by a range of physical, mental, emotional, spiritual and environmental factors.[16]

Vitalism is the belief that living things depend on the action of a special energy or force that guides the processes of metabolism, growth, reproduction, adaptation and

Modifying effects on health and vitality
• Constitutional strength—familial, genetic, congenital
• Diet—excess and deficiency
• Exposure to fresh air, clean water, sunlight and nature
• Lifestyle—work, education, exercise, rest and recreation
• Injury or disease
• Toxaemia—external (such as pollution, pesticides and drugs) and internal (such as metabolic by-products and cell waste)
• Health of organs of detoxification—liver, kidney and lymph
• Health of organs of elimination—bowel, gallbladder, bladder, respiratory, skin
• Emotions and relationships
• Exposure to culture and creativity
• Philosophy, religion and an ethical life
• Community, environment and ecology
• Social, economic and political factors

interaction.[17] This vital force is capable of interactions with material matter, such as a person's biochemistry, and these interactions of the vital force are necessary for life to exist. The vital force is non-material and occurs only in living things. It is the guiding force that accounts not only for the maintenance of life but for the development and activities of living organisms such as the progression from seed to plant, or the development of an embryo to a living being.[18]

The vital force is seen to be different from all the other forces recognised by physics and chemistry. And, most importantly, living organisms are more than just the effects of physics and chemistry. Vitalists agree with the value of biochemistry and physics in physiology but claim that such sciences will never fully comprehend the nature of life. Conversely, vitalism is not the same as a traditional religious view of life. Vitalists do not necessarily attribute the vital force to a creator, a god or a supernatural being, although vitalism can be compatible with such views. This is considered a 'strong' interpretation of vitalism. Naturopaths use a 'moderate' form of vitalism: *vis medicatrix naturae*, or the healing power of nature.[1]

Vis medicatrix naturae defines health as good vitality where the vital force flows energetically through a person's being, sustaining and replenishing us, whereas ill health is a disturbance of vital energy.[3] While naturopaths agree with modern pathology about the concepts of disease (cellular dysfunction, genetics, accidents, toxins and microbes), naturopathic philosophy further believes that a person's vital force determines their susceptibility to illness, the amount of treatment necessary, the vigour of treatment and the speed of recovery.[19] Those with poor vitality will succumb more quickly, require more treatment, need gentler treatments and take longer to recover.[20]

Vitality and disease

Vitalistic theory merges with naturopathy in the understanding of how disease progresses (Table 1.1). The *acute* stages of disease have active, heightened responses to challenges within the body systems. When the vital force is strong it reacts to an acute crisis by mobilising forces within the body to 'throw off' the disease.[17] The effect on vitality is usually only temporary as the body reacts with pain, redness, heat and swelling. If this stage is not dealt with appropriately where suppressive medicines are used, the vital force is weakened and acute illnesses begin to become *subacute*. This is where there is less activity, less pain and less reaction within the body, accompanied by a lingering loss of vitality, mild toxicity and

Table 1.1
Stages of disease

Stage	Acute	Subacute	Chronic	Degenerative
Symptoms	Pain, heat, redness, swelling, high activity, discharges, sensitivities	Lowered activity, relapsing symptoms	Persistent symptoms, constant discomfort, accumulation of cellular debris	Overwhelmed with toxicity, cellular destruction, physical and mental decay
Toxicity	Toxic discharges	Toxic absorption	Toxic encumbrance	Toxic necrosis
Vitality	Temporarily weak vitality	Variable vitality, ill at ease, feeling 'not quite right', sluggish	Poor vitality, malaise, susceptible to other physical or mental distress	Very low vitality, pernicious disruption of life processes at all levels

sluggishness. The patient begins to feel more persistently 'not quite right' but nothing will show up on medical tests and, in the absence of disease, the patient will be declared 'healthy' in biomedical terms. If the patient continues without addressing their health and lifestyle in a holistic way they can begin to experience *chronic* diseases where there are long-term, persistent health problems. This is highlighted by weakened vitality, poor immune responses, toxicity and metabolic sluggishness, and the relationships between systems both within and outside the patient become dysfunctional. The final stage of disease is *destructive* where there is tissue breakdown, cellular dysfunction, low vitality and high toxicity.[21]

In traditional naturopathic theory the above concepts emphasise the connections between lowered vitality and ill health. Traditional naturopathic philosophy also emphasises that the return of vitality through naturopathic treatment will bring about healing. The stages of this healing are succinctly summarised by Dr Constantine Hering, a 19th-century doctor, and these principles of healing are known as Hering's law of cure.[21,22]

Hering's law of cure

- Healing begins on the inside in the vital organs first, from the most important organs to the least important organs. The outer surfaces are healed last.
- Healing begins from the middle of the body out to the extremities.
- Healing begins from the top and goes down the body.
- Retracing—healing begins on the most recent problems back to the original problems.
- Healing crisis—as retracing and healing take place the body will re-experience any prior illness where the vital force was inappropriately treated. In re-experiencing the symptoms the patient will awaken their vitality and have an inner sense that the cleansing is 'doing them good'. A healing crisis is usually of a brief duration.

Holism

Another essential tenet of naturopathy developed from its eclectic history is the importance of a holistic perspective to explore, understand and treat the patient. Holism comes from the Greek word *holos*, meaning whole.[23,24] The concept of holism has a more formal description in general philosophy and has three main beliefs.[25] First, it is important to consider an organism as a whole. The best way to study the behaviour of a complex system is to treat it as a whole and not merely to analyse the structure and behaviour of its component parts. It is the principles governing the behaviour of the whole system rather than its parts that best elucidate an understanding of the system.

Second, every system within the organism loses some of its characteristics when any of its components undergo change. The component parts of a system will lose their nature, function, significance and even their existence when removed from their interconnection with the rest of the systems that support them. An organism is said to differ from a mere mechanism by reason of its interdependence with nature and its parts in the whole. For instance, any changes that occur in the nervous system can cause changes in other systems such as the musculoskeletal and digestive systems, as well as affecting cognition and mood. Or, more widely, any changes that occur in social relationships have an effect on the nervous system and vice versa.

Third, the important characteristics of an organism do not occur at the physical and chemical levels but at a higher level where there is a holistic integration of systems within the whole being. There are important interrelations that define the systems and these may be completely missed in a 'parts-only' perspective. These interrelations are completely independent of the parts. For instance, the digestive tract is functional only when its blood supply, nerve supply, enzymes and hormones are integrated and unified by complex interrelationships.

In naturopathic healthcare, holism is the understanding that a person's health functions as a whole, unified, complex system in balance. When any one part of their human experience suffers, a person's entire sense of being may suffer.

PATIENT-CENTRED APPROACH TO HOLISTIC CONSULTATION

One of the most difficult duties as a human being is to listen to the voices of those who suffer ... listening is hard but fundamentally a moral act.

Frank 1995[26]

A holistic consultation and treatment of the whole person includes emotional, mental, spiritual, physical and environmental factors; it aims to promote wellbeing through the whole person rather than just the symptomatic relief of a disease. To best enhance this holistic consultative process, a patient-centred approach is used. This is where the emphasis is on patient autonomy; the patient and practitioner are in an equal relationship that values and respects the wants and needs of the patient.[27] The role of the practitioner is to develop a therapeutic relationship of rapport, empathy and authenticity to serve the patient's choices and engender the healing process.

An essential component of developing a therapeutic relationship with the patient is the ability to listen.[28]

Naturopaths must never forget that each patient is an individual with their own unique story of illness and treatment. The patient needs to be allowed to tell that story and in turn the naturopathic practitioner needs to listen with sensitive, authentic attention and empathy. This disciplined type of therapeutic listening bonds the patient and practitioner and enhances the effectiveness of treatment.[29] When patients feel listened to, they open up and declare hidden information that can be clinically significant to the type of treatment given and to how well that treatment works.

If a naturopath does not holistically enquire into the causes of a patient's presenting complaint and merely follows a protocol—in the case of an insomnia prescription, for example—they may be, at the very least, clinically ineffective in treating insomnia or, worse, prolonging the patient's suffering and increasing their risk of self-harm.

A practitioner also needs to be aware that a holistic consultation is not a routine event for the patient. It is dense with meaning and can represent a turning point for them.[30] Fully listening to a patient's concerns in a patient-centred holistic consultation helps the naturopath to explore and understand what is at stake and why it matters so much.[31] With this knowledge it is then possible to provide appropriate and effective treatment. Establishing rapport, empathy and authenticity in a patient-centred, holistic consultation also enhances the practitioner's ongoing ability to assess recovery and to achieve the patient-centred aim of independent self-care.[32]

This therapeutic relationship depends upon the practitioner being proficient in consulting skills, communication skills and counselling skills. This chapter now focuses on consulting skills and the reader should consult the Further Reading section at the end of this chapter for texts discussing communication skills and counselling skills.

It should also be noted that some patients present to clinics with little or no prior understanding of what the naturopathic consultation involves. Some preliminary steps can be taken to facilitate a better understanding for the patient. Initially, a practitioner's website can provide explanatory details of naturopathic philosophy, treatment modalities and the consulting process. This can be reinforced with brochures provided in the reception area of the clinic. As the holistic consultation begins, the practitioner can sensitively enquire as to the patient's level of understanding of naturopathy and what their expectations about the consultation are.

Phases of the holistic consultation

Adapting the Nelson-Jones[33] model, there are five phases to the holistic patient-centred consultation.

1. *Explore* the range of problems.
2. *Understand* each problem.
3. Determine the *goals*.
4. Provide *treatments*.
5. Consolidate the patient's *independence*.

In a brief acute case of a minor condition, such as a minor head cold, these five phases can be completed over a single session. In a complex case with multiple pathologies and myriad personal issues, the phases discussed below can occur and recur over a long period of time and completion may entail many sessions.

Explore

The task here is to establish rapport with the patient and to help the patient reveal, identify and describe their problems. The naturopath can facilitate this by providing a structure for the interview and by fostering an ambience where the patient's views are valued. The naturopath's empathy with the patient will sensitise the practitioner to the tone, pace, depth and breadth of their enquiry into the patient's health issues. The enquiry should be patient-centred, where the patient sets the parameters of what they feel comfortable discussing while the naturopath maintains a heightened awareness of the clinical significance of what they are saying—or indeed not saying. The patient in this process has an opportunity to share their thoughts and feelings and for the naturopath to join with them in identifying the problem areas in their health from a holistic perspective.

Understand

Understanding the problems involves a focused attempt to gather more specific details of the problems experienced by the patient. The naturopath's facilitation skills will help the patient accurately focus on symptoms while also using the naturopath's clinical skills in physical examination, body sign observations, reviewing medical reports and completing a systems history to gain and impart a holistic overview. The knowledge gained from this helps the patient to acknowledge areas of strength and weakness in their health and to develop new insights and perceptions that will help them relate to their health issues holistically. It is also appropriate in this phase to seek referrals for further diagnosis where necessary from biomedical or allied health professionals.

Set goals

The next step is to work with the patient to negotiate goals and strategies to achieve positive outcomes for their health. The naturopath needs to discuss with the patient the types of modalities that can be used and which treatments are expected to be efficacious. It is appropriate at this juncture to give a prognosis of what can be reasonably achieved within a specified time. The patient then has an opportunity to ask questions, discuss costs and be in an active position to make an informed choice in setting goals and deciding on the best treatment options. The patient should be encouraged to acknowledge their active participation in their health improvement. They can also discuss with the naturopath their preferences for various modalities, and the naturopath can highlight what the patient can expect as their health improves.

Treatment

The task now is to assist the patient in gaining better vitality, building health resources and skills and lessening health deficits. The patient's role is to acquire self-help skills. Active encouragement is crucial in developing and maintaining the patient's self-motivation. Encourage the patient to acquire books, internet resources and community resources and to undertake courses to further self-support the recovery. The issues of compliance, or how well the patient can follow a treatment plan, can be discussed with the patient in a supportive way by identifying any possible difficulties. The treatment plan may need to be modified or strategies developed to ensure the patient gains the full benefit of their treatment program.

Potential barriers to treatment need to be anticipated, assessed and discussed, with contingencies put in place within the treatment plan to account for these. For example, if the treatment goal is weight loss and exercise is suggested as a primary treatment strategy, then the attitude of the patient towards exercise needs to be assessed. If those potential barriers are anticipated, plans can be suggested that overcome them and improve compliance, such as by exercising with a friend rather than alone.

Also in this phase the need for 'follow-up' is assessed. The patient may require further appointments to refine the processes of exploring, understanding, goal setting and treating their health issues. At this point, referrals to other practitioners for treatment may also be necessary where it can be seen that this would be beneficial.

Independence

The final step in the patient-centred therapeutic process is to consolidate the patient's independence. The task is to ensure the patient has the necessary self-help skills and is prepared for the naturopath's helping role to end. At this stage, both the naturopath and the patient review the progress and goal achievements. The naturopath can assist the patient to plan independent control of their health. The patient should be encouraged to share their thoughts on their own progress, as well as any exit issues, such as their readiness for self-management. The patient can now consolidate all their learning and is ready to implement self-help skills in daily life.

From novice to experienced naturopath

Novice naturopaths tend to use learned protocols that give treatment programs for a disease or syndrome.

Advanced beginners soon find that the 'one-size-fits-all' approach, besides being contradictory to naturopathic philosophy, is problematic and begin to adapt and vary the protocols to each patient.

Competent naturopaths begin to develop their own independent strategies for patients.

Professional naturopaths develop treatments based on traditional learning, evidence-based practice and their intuition in selecting treatments that best align with a patient's individual holistic causes of ill health.

Experienced naturopaths are immersed in an intuitive proficiency where they: understand tradition and evidence; can listen carefully and sensitively to the patient's issues; adapt readily and easily to the patient's personality; motivate and educate the patient; are aware of the nuances in patient rapport, red flags and need for referrals; and are calm, gentle and understanding in the face of uncertainty and suffering.

Adapted from Boon et al. 2006[34]

Structure and technique of case taking

Basic case-taking skills take one to two years to develop and a diligent naturopath over the years will be constantly improving and refining techniques.[35] It may be overwhelming in the first few cases for novice practitioners, especially if the case is complex. At times a patient may be difficult, angry or demanding and a practitioner needs to have insight and strategies for dealing with this (see Further Reading at the end of this chapter, which highlights useful texts discussing these issues).

Novice practitioners may wish to begin any case, no matter how chronic or complex, by starting with a good case history of one key ailment that bothers the patient. This is designated as the 'presenting complaint'.[36] For example, if the patient has five health issues to discuss, negotiate with the patient what is most important to them to work on first.

The case-taking process

- *Location*. Ask about the nature of the problem. Get an idea of the physical, emotional, spiritual and environmental dimensions of the problem. Note if it affects a certain location of the anatomy or a physiological system. Be aware that certain conditions have multiple locations, such as arthritis or systemic lupus erythematosus (SLE).
- *Onset*. Ask about the factors that seemed to initiate or trigger the problem. In a holistic manner, enquire as to what was occurring for the patient before and at the start of the problem. When did the problem first start?
- *Course*. Ask whether the problem seems to be constant (there all the time with minimal variation), fluctuating (there all the time but varies in presentation and intensity) or intermittent (it stops and starts or happens occasionally). The treatment of headaches, for example, could be quite different if they are constant or fluctuating, or happen twice a week or twice a year.

- *Duration*. Ask when the problem first started if it has been constant or fluctuating, and also how long an episode of the problem endures if it is intermittent.
- *Sensation/quality*. Ask the patient to describe in their own words how they experience their symptoms via the five senses of feeling (e.g. ache, burn, numb, pinch, stab, throb, hot, cold, itch, anxious, sad, dizzy, nauseous, twisting, wrenching or tingling), sight (such as colour, consistency, texture or shape), sound (e.g. crepitation, rattling, gasping, rumbling or buzzing), odour (e.g. fetid, ketosis, fishy, yeasty or sharp) and taste (such as bitter, salty, rancid, bloody or metallic). Note that a loss of any sensation is also clinically significant.
- *Intensity*. Ask about how mild, moderate or severe the problem is. Be aware that different personalities may under-report or over-report the severity. You can get the patient to give it a score out of 10 to make a useful comparison on follow-up visits.
- *Modulating factors*. What makes it better or worse? Time of day, week, season or year; situation, such as in bed, at work, in hot weather; certain activities triggering it; or certain emotional or spiritual crises.
- *Radiates*. Does the problem shift, extend or move around one location or between other locations?
- *Concomitants*. When the problem occurs, is there any other part of the person that seems to be affected? Examples are irritability with hot flushes, loss of appetite with depression, and headaches with existential crises.
- *Past history*. In an acute case this can be a previous history of this presenting complaint. It can also include a general past history of all health issues.
- *Family history*. As above, this can be a family history of the presenting complaint as well as a general history of all health issues in the family.
- *Medications*. Include all medical, naturopathic, Chinese medicine and other health modalities, including self-prescribed supplements. It often occurs that the presenting complaint is directly linked to a side effect or interaction of medications.
- *Diet*. Discuss a typical day's diet. For a more comprehensive approach the naturopath can give the patient a diet diary to record their diet and symptoms over a one- or two-week period and review this in a follow-up appointment.
- *Observation of body signs and relevant physical examinations* (refer to Chapter 2 on diagnosis).
- *Timeline*. The information gathered can also be represented in the format of a timeline that illustrates the sequence of events.

This single-issue case-taking process can take 20–45 minutes for novice practitioners in the early days of training or practice. It is always important not to spend an overly long time in getting the case details. There also has to be sufficient time for: explaining the holistic diagnosis and naturopathic understanding of why this problem is occurring; treatment goals; prognosis; remedy preparation and label instructions; doing the account; and booking the patient for the next appointment. Bear in mind that the patient is likely to be unwell, tired, in pain or may have restless children in tow and it is a strain on the patient to have them there for one or two hours while trying to pack too much into the first session. It is more appropriate to use the second and third appointments to gather further information. Psychologists, for example, may spend at least the first 5 to 10 sessions getting a general background and then may spend the next year or more listening to the patient's life narrative on a once-a-week basis.

Holistic review

As part of a holistic consultation it is essential to enquire into a broad range of factors. This is where the consultation moves beyond the presenting complaint.[37] It encompasses a review of the patient's:

- general past history
- family history
- lifestyle history
- psychological history
- physiological systems.

This can be done in any order that seems most comfortable between practitioner and patient. A holistic assessment is made of the patient's vitality and symptoms by exploring the physical, mental, social and spiritual factors that affect them. A simple model of holistic assessment is first to explore the factors affecting the patient's constitutional strength, which are the physical and mental attributes they are born with. This includes genetics, temperament and the inherent strengths and weaknesses of different physiological systems. Second, factors that occur over time are considered. These include the family and culture that the patient grew up with and the socioeconomic status and environment they live in. They also include the types of diseases or traumas the patient has had, the diets and lifestyle they have followed and the patterns of adaptive behaviour they have adopted. Third, a holistic assessment needs to consider important, dramatic events that have overwhelmed an otherwise healthy person, such as severe stress, trauma or toxicity. Fourth, the factors that trigger disturbances to vitality such as stress, injury, infection, toxicity, allergens and drugs need to be considered. Finally, a holistic assessment of the factors that sustain ongoing health issues, such as psychological, social, economic, environmental and ecological factors, is made.

Galland[38] cautions that care must be taken in holistic assessments. Careful listening to the patient is required, as the range of possibilities is extensive. The assessment needs to be comprehensive as there can be multiple factors that reinforce each other; the practitioner needs to constantly reassess patients who have complex symptoms to avoid misdiagnosis. Practitioners also need to be flexible as the same symptom in two different people, such as joint pain, may have different triggers; conversely, the same trigger, such as hot weather, may induce headache in one person and asthma in another.

General past history

- General level of vitality and health in infancy, childhood, teens, twenties and subsequent decades; the effect on vitality of life stages such as puberty, education, relationships, marriage, pregnancy, parenting, work, menopause/andropause, retiring
- Immunisations, vaccinations, reactions
- Allergies, intolerances
- Childhood illnesses, either minor but persistent, or major; episodes requiring medical supervision, hospitalisation, surgery, medication
- Major illnesses, accidents, genetic issues, hospitalisations, disabilities
- Past use of medications

Family history
- Major diseases, syndromes and level of vitality that affect family members
- Causes of mortality in the family
- Familial, hereditary, genetic issues

Lifestyle history
- Exercise, fitness, coordination, mobility, flexibility, strength, stamina, aerobic capacity
- Recreation, entertainment, rest, holidays
- Alcohol consumption, coffee/tea consumption, smoking, recreational drug use
- Daily exposure to toxins, pollutants, chemicals
- Education
- Work conditions (exposure to toxins; stress, injury)
- Home conditions
- Social, economic, financial and political conditions
- Health issues with class, race, religion or gender
- Travel
- Military service

Psychological history
- Life satisfaction; relationships; connectedness to friends, family, colleagues, community, society
- Reactions to stress, grief, trauma; coping mechanisms; resilience, vulnerability
- Moods, perceptions, sensitivities, motivation, will, intensity, personal characteristics, attachments, obsessions
- Attitudes, optimism
- Mental capacities, performance, confidence, procrastinations, decision-making ability
- Speech, gesture, posture, thinking, feeling, behaviour
- Creativity, arts, music, dance, theatre, hobbies, collecting
- Religion, spirituality, philosophy, self-discovery, ethics, purpose of existence, world view, meditation, revelation, prayer, metaphysics
- Spiritual and cultural issues in healthcare

Physiological systems
In each of these sections, if there are relevant symptoms to discuss, then follow the format as given regarding the presenting complaint, such as location, duration, onset, course, sensation and so forth:

- *general*: fatigue, pallor, fever, chills, sweats; proneness to infection; allergies, intolerances; weight, posture, build; age, stage of life; gender
- *gastrointestinal*: problems with mouth, gums, tongue, oesophagus, swallowing, reflux, eructation, stomach pain, gastritis, ulcers, bloating, fullness, appetite, nausea, vomiting, cramping, flatulence, stool (frequency, consistency, colour, odour, blood), haemorrhoids, fissures; infections (viral, bacterial, fungal, protozoal); polyps, tumours
- *hepatic-biliary*: jaundice, cirrhosis, gallstones, abnormal liver function tests, bile duct inflammation or obstruction, right shoulder or flank pain, ascites

- *respiratory*: pain; difficulty or obstruction in breathing; wheezing, shortness of breath; cough; sputum; smoking; asthma
- *head/neurological*: headaches, migraines, dizziness, fainting, epilepsy, head trauma, confusion, memory loss; eyes (vision, discharge, pain, redness, change in appearance of eye such as unequal pupils, cataracts, glaucoma)
- *ear, nose, throat*: pain, hearing problems, sense of smell, sense of taste, sinus, rhinitis, allergens, discharges, change in voice, gums, teeth, lips, tongue, tonsils, adenoids, mouth ulcers
- *cardiovascular*: chest pain; palpitations, arrhythmias; oedema; dyspnoea; blood pressure; cholesterol; anaemia; blood disorders; claudication; varicosities; circulation—cold hands/feet; bruising; bleeding
- *lymph nodes*: sore, swollen, infected
- *endocrine*: pituitary/hypothalamus; thyroid (hyper and hypo symptoms); thymus; pancreas (pancreatitis, diabetes, hypoglycaemia); adrenal (Addison's disease, fatigue, immune, oedema); ovary/testes
- *female*: breast—pain, tender, lumps, change in appearance, galactorrhoea; menses—menarche, hormonal contraceptives, frequency, duration, volume, colour, consistency, pain, premenstrual tension; libido, sexual function, pain, itch, discharge, infections, Pap smears, surgery, investigations, uterine, ovarian, fallopian, cervical, vaginal; polycystic ovarian syndrome, endometriosis; fertility, pregnancies, births; menopause, hot flushes, headaches, mood, vaginal dryness, weight gain
- *males*: infection, discharge, lesions, sexual dysfunction (libido, erection, ejaculation), pain, infertility, testes, prostate (benign prostate hyperplasia, prostatitis, cancer), varicocele, phimosis, balanitis
- *genitourinary*: frequency, volume, colour, odour, infections, blood, urgency, incontinence, pain (flank, suprapubic, urethral), rigors; dribbling, hesitancy; calculi; kidneys, ureters, bladder, urethra; abnormal urinary test results; renal effects on sodium, blood pressure, acid–base balance, fluid retention
- *peripheral neurological*: weakness, abnormal sensation, numbness, coordination, loco motor, paralysis, tremor
- *musculoskeletal*: bone deformities, ligament, tendon, muscle, joints, discs, inflammation, pain, swelling, redness, hot, cold, stiffness, crepitation, range of motion, functional loss
- *Skin, hair, nails*: rash, itch, eruption, discharge, flaking, erosive, pitting, peeling, lumps, cysts, change in colour, texture, shape; hair loss, dandruff.

In chronic, complex cases with multiple symptoms and pathologies it may take two or three sessions to get a complete and accurate history. As a novice practitioner gains more experience, all the details of complex cases can be gained in one to two sessions.

POSOLOGY

Posology is the determination of the appropriate dosage of remedies for the patient. In general terms if a patient has good vitality they can handle the rigour of more remedies at higher doses and more aggressive treatment regimens of exercise and detoxification if required. For those patients with moderate vitality their treatment is modified with milder doses of tonics and supplements in an effort to strengthen vitality and prevent relapses occurring. Patients with weakened vitality are best administered treatments that offer gentle relief of symptoms and the mildest of programs to support the affected systems. This is done through toning, building and adaptogenic remedies.

These general guidelines for dosages and range of remedies are modified by the *pace*, *intensity*, *location* and *natural history* of the illness. First, vary the treatment according to the pace of the symptoms. The dosage and range of remedies will vary according to the symptoms being slow and sluggish as compared with symptoms that are rapid in onset. Second, the intensity of the symptoms dictates that a higher dose is required for symptoms of a florid, aggressive nature with a potential for pathological sequelae. The naturopath may also have to factor in that some patients are particularly stressed by the symptoms and demand more urgent treatment programs than is necessarily required. Third, the location of the illness may change the posology because symptoms in the eye, for example, are more sensitive than in the heel of the foot. Fourth, treatments will vary according to the natural history of an illness where dosages change between the onset, middle and resolution of an illness.

SIGNPOSTS FOR RECOVERY

Patients always ask 'When will I get better?'. Prognosis is the forecast of the course of a disease. With illnesses that are familiar, such as a head cold, it is relatively predictable how long it takes for symptoms to resolve with treatment. As a novice practitioner progresses through their career and experiences a wider range of patients, the ability to give an accurate prognosis of a variety of health problems improves. However, there are always instances when it is very difficult to predict how a patient's illness will respond to treatment and over what period of time. In instances of difficulty with predicting how long a patient will take to recover it is better to approach the issue from another angle. That is, rather than trying to give the patient a definitive time frame of amelioration of the illness it is better to give estimations of what signposts or stages the patient is expected to experience and leave the issue of duration open-ended. This prevents the frustration a patient may experience when told they should be better by a certain date but they are not.

The first signpost for recovery is that the condition has stabilised and is no longer deteriorating. Second, the intensity of symptoms begins reducing. Third, the symptoms are no longer constant. Fourth, the symptoms no longer fluctuate. Fifth, there are longer periods of intermittence and, if they do return, the symptoms are milder and of shorter duration. And finally there is remission or cure. The patient is asked to watch for these stages as signs of improvement. Discuss with the patient the fact that it is often too difficult to give an exact time estimation as to how long each stage of recovery will take.

To assist in prognostic skills the following practice tips will be useful. For a known disease or syndrome there is excellent information in pathology texts and medical journals that indicates the natural history of a disease—that is, how a disease behaves and over what period of time. Second, check the naturopathic information from academic notes, texts, journals and seminars on the action of naturopathic remedies and how long these remedies take to reduce symptoms. Also enquire further from senior naturopathic colleagues, mentors and academic staff who can give information about how this disease normally behaves and how it responds to the proposed treatments. Third, having established a good knowledge of how the disease behaves and the efficacy of the treatments, make an assessment of the patient's capabilities and compliance with following the treatment plan. This is where a holistic understanding of the patient's vitality, preferences for modalities and personal circumstances will help in judging when the patient will improve.

CASE TAKING: THE RETURN VISIT

Novice practitioners can sometimes feel confusion as to what they are supposed to say or do in the return visit. For 'follow-up' of acute, minor cases, use the guidelines below. For follow-up of complex, chronic cases see the Case Taking: Advanced section opposite.

At the end of the first session

The return visit is made easier for novice practitioners if they get into the habit of making notes at the end of the initial visit as a reminder of what needs to be done at the next session. At the end of the 'first visit history form', make a box with the heading 'Follow-up'. In this box write down any items the practitioner promised the patient to look into. Also in this box write down the patient's symptoms to review in follow-up; for example, check temperature, mucus (colour, consistency), sneezing and fatigue to compare with the first session to gauge the treatment response. Also write in this box any other issues that the practitioner or the patient wants to explore in the second session because they did not get time in the first session.

What to do in the second session

Before the patient arrives the practitioner needs to re-familiarise themselves with the patient's case. This can include the patient's personal and social anecdotes of things that they were going to be doing during the week, such as family functions, outings with friends, work issues or relationship issues. To quickly re-establish rapport the practitioner can remind themselves of how the patient was feeling in the first session.

An important feature of the follow-up session is to review the patient's symptoms. This enables the practitioner to make comparisons of the patient's progress and to gauge the effectiveness of the treatment program. Make new notes on what changes have occurred in signs and symptoms since the previous visit. It may be necessary to repeat any physical examinations that were done in the first session, such as vitals. The practitioner needs to enquire how the patient managed with the remedies and lifestyle advice and check whether the patient has been taking the remedies in the manner prescribed.

If acute symptoms have resolved, then remind the patient about holistic, preventive measures to maintain good health to avoid the symptoms reoccurring. If acute symptoms have not resolved, then explore the reasons for this. Confirm that the original diagnosis and naturopathic understanding were correct. This may require referrals to other health professionals for further diagnostic assessment and testing. Check antecedents, triggers and mediators as discussed earlier. For example, the patient may still be under the same stresses at work, or their diet may need further support. Check materia medica selection and posology and that the patient knows how to take the remedies properly; check patient compliance or any difficulties with taking the remedies, managing the diet or following exercise programs. Check information on the expected prognosis and natural history of the condition. That is, how long does a particular condition normally take to clear up? For example, some sinus conditions take a few weeks to heal and there may be little change in the first week. Often the reason for lack of improvement is obvious and it is easy to make adjustments to the treatment program or support the patient with ways to achieve their health goals. At other times, there are cases that, even with the best intentions of the practitioner and the patient, are not responding very well. It is appropriate here to seek the patient's permission to discuss their case with colleagues or a mentor with experience in similar cases. It can happen that the practitioner needs to refer the patient to another modality that might have more success with that particular condition. For example, with persistent back pain the patient can be referred to remedial massage, chiropractic, physiotherapy or osteopathy.

The second visit also allows the opportunity to discuss if there are any other different issues or symptoms not mentioned in the first visit. First, ask the patient if there are other concerns they have that they wish to talk about. This needs to be done every session. It may take some patients many repeated sessions to gain the trust to discuss sensitive issues like a past history of bulimia, sexual abuse or a worrisome ailment they feel embarrassed about. The practitioner can also initiate discussion on any issues that are apparent; for example, if the patient looks pale or jaundiced or their thyroid looks swollen, or has signs of body systems under stress that were not part of the initial discussions.

The second session allows completion of any further history that may have not been obtained in the first session or going into issues in more depth if that seems appropriate. At the end of the second session the practitioner always has to remember to draw up a 'Follow-up' box on the end of the history forms so they know what needs to be done in the third session. This needs to be done for every subsequent session.

CASE TAKING: ADVANCED

Getting the details of chronic complex cases requires careful attention. As previously stated getting these details could take a number of sessions for novice practitioners. The written data obtained need to be accurate, comprehensive and easily recoverable. The practitioner should be able to quickly find any data on any question from any session because all the data are put into specific locations in the history form.

The case history requires the patient's words verbatim if possible. However, this does not mean that every word is written in the order that the patient has said it. Patients tend to talk by random association where one thing reminds them of something else and will jump from topic to topic and back again. The skill is allowing this to occur to obtain rich information but also to do three other things simultaneously. The first is to write or type fluently key words or phrases while maintaining eye contact and rapport. The second is to write in such a way that the practitioner does not end up with line after line of the patient's words on a blank sheet in a disorganised fashion. After six or seven sessions there will be 10 to 20 pages of notes and it is very embarrassing when it takes five minutes to check some detail the patient has asked about. Instead, the history forms should have predefined sections where the patient's verbatim data can go. If the answers and details about, say, body systems are put in predefined sections on the history form under the heading 'Body systems', the information can be located in a matter of seconds. For example, information on coughing goes under 'Respiratory'; information on depression goes under 'Mind'. In later sessions when the practitioner wants to compare coughs or depressive symptoms the information is easy to find. Also, by following a format for history taking the practitioner can see the gaps in the history form. This then is a reminder to get the relevant information for those sections that have been missed. For example, there may be a blank space on the history form under 'Circulation' and this will prompt the practitioner to complete this part of the history.

Third, the art of patient interviews is to gauge when to gently direct or turn the patient's conversation towards information that the practitioner wishes to gain. If the practitioner is too directive the patient will learn only to briefly answer in a perfunctory way and to wait for the next question. This static style is quite mechanical and only emphasises to the patient that the practitioner's questions are more important than the patient's needs. This could stifle much rich information about the patient's personal thoughts, symptoms and motivations that can be discovered by a spontaneous, free-flowing conversation. On the other hand, if the practitioner is too non-directive the patient may digress into sessions of repetitive minutiae on one symptom or random generalisations that do not articulate context or specificity; the conversation could be extended into blander areas to avoid enquiry into sensitive issues.

After taking a couple of sessions to obtain a complete case history a practitioner's subsequent sessions now involve tracking and reviewing symptoms and response to treatment. This can be done on a simple spreadsheet by asking specific questions in each category and recording it in a summary table (such as Table 1.2). Every month the practitioner checks these symptoms and adds or subtracts other symptoms that come and go.

Case study

John is an 84-year-old male. He is a very friendly and cheerful man of slim build and, considering the range of health issues he has, he is mobile and independent and pursues hobbies in music and literature. He has health issues with diabetes, asthma, insomnia, stress, headaches, elevated cholesterol, palpitations, skin rash, sinusitis, depression, reflux and diarrhoea. Other issues can come and go, and these are recorded in a similar fashion by adding more bottom rows (Table 1.2). All symptoms are chronic; some are constant, some fluctuate and some are intermittent.

Table 1.2
Case history summary table

Symptoms	February	March	April
Diabetes	Stable (6–7 on rising)	Same	
Asthma	Stable (same)	Same	
Insomnia	> 8/10; herbs good	> 9/10	
Stress	> 8/10; herbs good	Same	
Headache	> 4/10; occurs 2/7—mild	> 8/10	
Cholesterol	No data this month	Total 5.8; LDL 2.6; Tryg 2.6	
Palpitation	> 8/10 for magnesium	Same	
Skin rash	> 4/10—shrunk 1 cm	< 2/10; increased 2 cm; hot weather	
Sinusitis	> generally; but worse in last two days	Clear	
Depression	> 8/10 with herbs	All good	
Reflux	Same—still occurs after meals	Same	
Diarrhoea	Variable—no incontinence this month	Same	

This simple method keeps track of the patient's 12 or more symptoms and pathologies. Within each session the treatment program can be reviewed and adjusted to address the patient's changing circumstances. If clarification or comparison of the past history of the patient's symptoms is required it can be readily accessed in the written history form in good detail. Discussion can then be directed to what symptoms bother the patient the most and to jointly decide whether or not to treat particular symptoms, given that the patient in the case study above is already on multiple medications. Therefore the patient's wishes and values are respected and the patient feels secure in the knowledge that all his issues are being addressed in a holistic way.

KEY POINTS

- Time is needed for a thorough case taking, and this process evolves over several consultations.
- The case-taking skills of clinicians also evolve over time, culminating in the ability to perceptively assess the health of the client in less time, while accurately recording key information. The therapeutic connection is strongly maintained during this process.
- A clearly defined case-taking process is required, in addition to the confidential and secure maintenance of record keeping.

FURTHER READING

Cava R. Dealing with difficult people. Sydney: Pan Macmillan; 2002.

Egan G, Reese RJ. The skilled helper: a problem management approach to healing. 11th ed. Boston: Cengage Learning; 2019.

Geldard D, Geldard K, Foo RY. Basic personal counselling: a training manual for counsellors. 8th ed. South Melbourne: Cengage Learning; 2017.

Ivey AE, Ivey MB, Zalaquett CP. Intentional interviewing and counselling: facilitating client development in a multicultural society. 9th ed. Boston: Cengage Learning; 2018.

Judd F, Weissman M, Hodgins G, et al. Interpersonal counselling in general practice. Aust Fam Physician 2004;33(5):332.

Murtagh JE, Rosenblatt J, Coleman J, et al. General practice. 7th ed. North Ryde: McGraw-Hill Australia; 2018. Chapter 4 Communication skills. Chapter 5 Counselling skills. Chapter 6 Difficult, demanding and trying patients.

Robertson K. Active listening: more than just paying attention. Aust Fam Physician 2005;34(12):1053.

Stone L. Navigating through the swampy lowlands: dealing with the patient when the diagnosis is unclear. Aust Fam Physician 2006;35(12):991.

REFERENCES

1. Coulter ID, Willis M. The rise and rise of complementary and alternative medicine: a sociological perspective. Med J Aust 2004;180:587.
2. Pizzorno JE, Snider P. Naturopathic medicine. In: Micozzi M, editor. Fundamentals of complementary and integrative medicine. 3rd ed. St Louis: Saunders Elsevier; 2006. p. 221–55.
3. Kaptchuck TJ. Vitalism. In: Micozzi M, editor. Fundamentals of complementary and integrative medicine. 3rd ed. St Louis: Saunders Elsevier; 2006. p. 53–63.
4. Bradley R. Philosophy of natural medicine. In: Pizzorno JE, Murray MT, editors. Textbook of natural medicine. 2nd ed. Edinburgh: Churchill Livingstone; 1999. p. 42–4.
5. Di Stefano V. Holism and complementary medicine: origin and principles. Sydney: Allen & Unwin; 2006. [Chapter 4].
6. Cody G. History of naturopathic medicine. In: Pizzorno JE, Murray MT, editors. Textbook of natural medicine. 2nd ed. Edinburgh: Churchill Livingstone; 1999. p. 41–9.
7. Schneirov M, Geczik J. Alternative health care and the challenges of institutionalization. Health 2002;6(2):201–20.
8. Baer HA, Coulter ID. Introduction—taking stock of integrative medicine; broadening biomedicine or co-option of complementary and alternative medicine? Health Sociol Rev 2008;17(4):332.
9. Braun L, Cohen M. Herbs and natural supplements: an evidence based guide. 3rd ed. Marrickville: Elsevier Churchill Livingstone; 2010.
10. Ernst E. The clinical researcher. J Complement Med 2004;3(1):44–5.
11. Myers S, Hunter A, Snider P, et al. Naturopathic medicine ch 3. In: Robson T, editor. An introduction to complementary medicine. Crows Nest NSW: Allen & Unwin; 2003. p. 48–66.
12. Pizzorno JE, Murray MT, editors. A textbook of natural medicine. Seattle: John Bastyr College Publications; 1985–1996.
13. Foundations project. The Healing Power of Nature: The Foundations of Naturopathic Medicine and the Ecology of Healing: Primary Care for the Twenty First Century. Online. Available: http://www.foundationsproject.com/documents/Chapters_Outline.pdf 29 Mar 2013.
14. Bradley R. Philosophy of natural medicine. In: Pizzorno JE, Murray MT, editors. Textbook of natural medicine. 2nd ed. Edinburgh: Churchill Livingstone; 1999. p. 41.
15. Pizzorno JE, Snider P. Naturopathic medicine. In: Micozzi M, editor. Fundamentals of complementary and integrative medicine. 3rd ed. St Louis: Saunders Elsevier; 2006. p. 236–8.
16. Di Stefano V. Holism and complementary medicine: origin and principles. Sydney: Allen & Unwin; 2006. p. 107–8.
17. Kirschner M, et al. Molecular vitalism. Cell 2000;100(1):87.
18. Bechtel W, et al. Vitalism. Concise routledge encyclopedia of philosophy. London: Routledge; 2000. p. 919.

19. Turner RN. The foundations of health. Naturopathic medicine, England: Thorsons Publishing Group; 1990. p. 17–27.

20. Jacka J. A philosophy of healing. Melbourne: Inkata Press; 1997. p. 36–8.

21. Jensen B, editor. Iridology: the science and practice in the healing arts, vol. 2. Escondido: Bernard Jensen Publisher; 1982. p. 181–3.

22. Models for the study of whole systems. In Bell IR, Koithan M, editors. Integr Cancer Ther 2006;5(4):295.

23. Dunne R, Watkins J. Complementary medicine—some definitions. J R Soc Health 1997;117(5):287–91.

24. Moore B, editor. The Australian Oxford dictionary. 2nd ed. South Melbourne: Oxford University Press; 2004. p. 598.

25. Wentzel J. Holism. In: Van Huyssteen W, et al, editors. Encyclopedia of science and religion. 2nd ed. New York: Thomson Gale Macmillan Reference; 2003. p. 412–14.

26. Frank A. The wounded story teller: body, illness and ethics. Chicago: University of Chicago Press; 1995. p. 25.

27. Emmanuel E, Emmanuel K. Four models of the physician–patient relationship. JAMA 1992;267(16): 2225–6.

28. Connelly J. Narrative possibilities: using mindfulness in clinical practice. Perspect Biol Med 2005;48(1):84.

29. Charon R. The ethicality of narrative medicine. In: Hurwitz B, Greenhalgh T, Skultans V, editors. Narrative research in health and illness. Massachusetts: Blackwell Publishing; 2004. p. 30.

30. Mattingly C. Performance Narratives in the clinical world. In: Hurwitz B, Greenhalgh T, Skultans V, editors. Narrative research in health and illness. Massachusetts: Blackwell Publishing; 2004. p. 73.

31. Berlinger N. After harm: medical harm and the ethics of forgiveness. Baltimore: Johns Hopkins University Press; 2005. p. 3.

32. Kumar P, Clarke M, editors. Kumar & Clark clinical medicine. Edinburgh, New York: WB Saunders; 2005. p. 8.

33. Nelson-Jones R. Practical counselling and helping skills. 2nd ed. Marrickville: Holt Rhinehart Wilson/Harcourt Brace Jovanovich Group (Australia); 1988. p. 92.

34. Murtagh JE. General practice. 3rd ed. North Ryde: McGraw-Hill Australia; 2006. [chapters 4–5].

35. Boon NA, et al, editors. Davidson's principles and practice of medicine. 20th ed. Philadelphia: Churchill Livingstone Elsevier; 2006. p. 6.

36. Bates B. A guide to physical examination and history taking. Philadelphia: J.B. Lippincott Company; 1995.

37. Seidel H. Mosby's guide to physical examination. St Louis: Mosby Elsevier; 2006. p. 9–22.

38. Galland L. Patient-centered care: antecedents, triggers, and mediators. Altern Ther Health Med 2006;12(4):62.

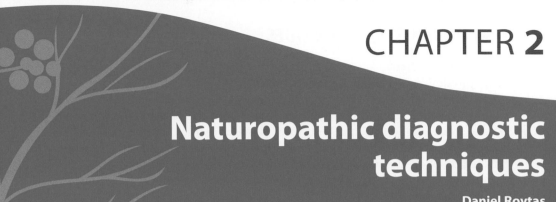

CHAPTER 2

Naturopathic diagnostic techniques

Daniel Roytas
ND, MHumNut

Niikee Schoendorfer
ND, MHSc, PhD

OVERVIEW

An important aspect of naturopathic clinical practice is the use of diagnostic techniques to ascertain the patient's state of health or disease. Naturopathy makes use of orthodox medical diagnostic techniques involving pathology testing and clinical examination but also uses a combination of several other modalities such as a broader physical examination to incorporate traditional theories, dietary assessment and other pathology testing techniques not currently endorsed by mainstream medicine.

The diagnostic process should flow from an extensive case history and physical examination to a differential diagnosis that lists possible alternatives for the presentations within the patient. An awareness of different types of pathology that may lead to particular signs and symptoms will assist the naturopath to narrow down the list of possibilities and select the most likely hypothesis.[1]

Further investigations, including pertinent biochemical evaluations, should then be performed to point to a more definitive diagnosis. This diagnosis, along with any other health issues that may have presented during the investigation, should all be used to address a patient from a holistic perspective and develop an adequate management plan. Clinical methods of diagnosis are best used in combination, and when interpreted alone possess definite disadvantages. Physical signs in conjunction with dietary and biochemical methods may provide a clearer picture of the physiology or pathophysiology at play in each individual.

This chapter provides an overview of a variety of physical examination techniques such as anthropometric data, body signs and symptoms and gastrointestinal palpation. Further exploration continues into dietary assessment methods and biochemical evaluations via a variety of pathology testing methods, both standard and specialised functional (including use of genomic technologies). Some of these types of assays have robust scientific bases, while others that have not been so extensively studied have been included as an overview of available popular techniques. A section on factors that affect nutritional status has also been included as a tool to assist with identifying potential confounding variables that should also be taken into consideration when assessing a patient's overall nutritional profile.

CLINICAL DIAGNOSTIC TECHNIQUES

Physical examination

The use of physical examination should be systematic and precisely recorded while relating particular signs to standardised definitions. Assessment of a patient begins as soon as the consultation starts. A person's disposition, facial complexion and expression, body size and shape, mobility, gait and posture, as well as the way they conduct or hold themselves, may provide important clues in relation to their mental and physical states.[1] A general inspection of the whole body may reveal external evidence of a disease; for example, obesity, wasting, arthritis, abnormal stature or development, presence of pain, jaundice, pallor or cyanosis.[2]

Warm, sweaty palms on the initial handshake may indicate an overactive thyroid due to increased circulation with blood vessel dilation. In contrast, an underactive thyroid may cause the hands to be cool and dry in texture.[3] People with alcohol dependence may attempt to conceal their addiction; however, certain signs may provide indicators such as plethoric faces, rhinophymic noses and alcoholic aroma. Smokers may also be revealed by their scent or nicotine-stained fingers. A person's facial expression may portray psychiatric illness such as depression, while conversation may alert to an anxiety disorder. Where trained personnel are available, appropriate gynaecological and other standard primary care examinations should also be performed as deemed necessary.

In developing countries, malnutrition with subsequent wasting and loss of weight is a relatively common occurrence; however, when these signs appear in more developed populations, naturopaths should be alerted to potential underlying pathological conditions such as diabetes, thyrotoxicosis, malabsorption syndromes or chronic infections.[4]

Physical body signs and symptoms may be important aids in identifying nutritional dysfunction, though care should also be taken during case taking as particular signs may not be specific and may relate to non-biological factors (such as injury or excessive sun exposure). Signs may also differ between populations and may also vary over time periods within a population.[5] Any findings suggesting an abnormality should be considered a clue rather than a diagnosis. A complete physical examination should be undertaken as part of every initial consultation. This will not only assist with identifying red flags, but also help to establish baseline measurements so that the effect of a treatment can be more thoroughly assessed at subsequent consultations.

Anthropometric data

To begin a regular physical examination, a person's anthropometric data—including height, weight, waist and hip measures, as well as skin fold or bioelectrical impedance analysis (BIA) to give an estimation of body fat percentages and lean mass—can be collected. Next, a methodical inspection of the hands and nails, skin colour and texture, hair, face and mouth, including the tongue, eyes, irises and sclera, should be conducted, concluding with gastrointestinal palpation.

Height and weight should be determined to assess if a person is over- or under-weight. Waist-to-hip ratio (WHR) is the most useful predictor of cardiovascular disease mortality, while body mass index—BMI = weight (kg)/height (m^2)—may be a better predictor of increased mortality from raised blood pressure (Table 2.1).[6]

Some form of body composition analysis, whether via skin fold or BIA, should also be performed to determine lean mass or protein sufficiency. Protein insufficiency may have widespread ramifications as outlined in the section on nutritional assessment on page 24.

Table 2.1
Data that predict increased mortality from cardiovascular disease and raised blood pressure

Females	Males
WHR > 0.8	WHR > 0.9
Waist circumference of > 88 cm	Waist circumference > 102 cm
BMI > 25	BMI > 30

Source: World Health Organization 1973[5]

Bioelectrical impedance analysis

BIA measures the impedance or opposition to the flow of an electric current (usually 50 kHz) through the body fluids contained mainly in the lean and fat tissue. This is generally low in lean tissue, where intracellular fluid and electrolytes are primarily contained, but high in fat tissue. In practice, a small constant current is passed between electrodes spanning the body and the voltage drop between electrodes provides a measure of impedance. The resulting impedance reading is proportional to the total body water volume. Prediction equations are used to convert impedance to a corresponding estimate of total body water.[7] Lean body mass is then calculated from this estimate using an assumed hydration fraction for lean tissue. Fat mass may then be calculated by subtracting lean mass from total body weight. More recently validation studies have been performed on its use in calculating body composition utilising the variety of available equations.[8,9] It should be noted that the evidence base surrounding this method only relates to the use of this technology for calculating body composition such as fat mass and fat-free mass.

Gastrointestinal palpation

The use of gastrointestinal palpation should be performed only by practitioners trained in this skill and when deemed appropriate through the case-taking process. In addition to its more generalised conventional application, it may also be a beneficial technique to alert a practitioner to an underlying digestive dysfunction in a naturopathic consult.

Palpation of the abdominal area may reveal various underlying organ pathologies of the liver, gall bladder, spleen, kidneys and gastrointestinal tract (Figure 2.1a):

- muscle guarding may indicate pain—voluntary guarding may occur in people who are cold, tense or ticklish, and relaxation techniques may reduce this type
- tenderness or rigidity may also be indicative of underlying pathology in the palpated area,[10] such as rectal sheath sensitivity, which may indicate dysbiosis
- the liver may be enlarged; this may indicate toxicity or dysfunctions causing hepatomegaly
- the spleen may be enlarged, signifying immune system up-regulation or trauma.

Palpation may also locate a mass. If so, it must be distinguished from a normally palpable structure or enlarged organ and note must be taken of its location, size, shape, tenderness, consistency, surface, mobility, pulsatility and tenderness. Gastrointestinal palpation may also be used in conjunction with other abdominal physical examinations, such as auscultation (outlined overleaf) and percussion, to elicit required information. An example of this is that a fluid wave indicates ascites, which may occur with heart failure, portal hypertension, cirrhosis of the liver, hepatitis, pancreatitis and cancer.[10]

The abdomen should be viewed for any intestinal bloating or asymmetry prior to palpating each organ individually. On palpation look for any tenderness or muscular guarding, which may indicate potential issues in that region. When palpating, keep one hand flat; this will be in contact with the abdomen and the other on top to apply pressure for palpation. Initially, gentle pressure should be applied, then pressure more deeply.

Palpation should begin in the upper middle region below the ribcage where the stomach is located. To the right along the line of the ribs is the gallbladder and further to the right is the liver. Across on the far left of the stomach, the spleen is located somewhat deeper than the previous organs. If the person is rolled onto their right side the pancreas may be felt if deep pressure is placed from near the side moving towards the midline and slightly upwards. Next to the area around the umbilicus is the small intestines, while slightly above and towards the right is the duodenum. Distal to the small intestine is the ascending colon, with the appendix situated below the latter. The jejunum is located to the left of the small intestine; continuing in this direction the descending colon with the sigmoid is found below. From this position moving medially, above the pubic bone, is the rectal sheath (Figure 2.1).

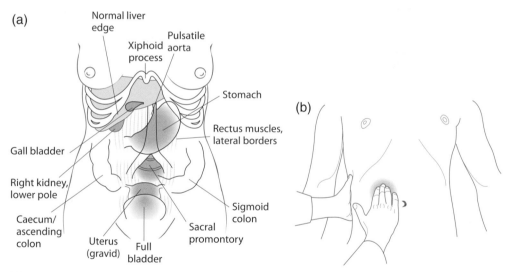

Figure 2.1a

Normally palpable abdominal structures

Source: Adapted from Jarvis 2007[10]

Figure 2.1b

Palpating the liver

Auscultation

Undertaking of a comprehensive clinical examination, especially during an initial investigation, is an integral part of the consultation process that should be adopted as standard practice by complementary medicine practitioners. A thorough clinical examination can provide clinicians with critical information and insights into a patient's overall health and detect changes in a health condition. Information obtained through physical examination can guide a practitioner to formulate specific treatment protocols but, more importantly, may uncover undiagnosed pathologies, which could warrant referral to another healthcare professional.

Auscultation is an important investigatory technique employed in the assessment of the cardiovascular and respiratory systems. Auscultation is arguably the most difficult physical examination technique to perform. Therefore, practitioners should utilise this technique frequently in clinical practice to maintain this skill to a high standard.

Note: The following is a brief overview of the cardiac and respiratory auscultation process and clinicians should refer to texts on the clinical examination process in the Further Reading section for more information.

Cardiovascular auscultation

Prior to auscultation, clinicians should perform the necessary palpation and visual inspections to detect secondary changes resulting from vascular disease. These include inspecting the quality of the femoral and carotid pulses and jugular venous pulsations, identifying the presence of cyanosis in the lips and nail beds and assessing capillary refill. Patients should be positioned lying face-up on an examination table, standing, squatting or sitting down. Clinicians may wish to auscultate a patient in a variety of these positions as various positions may accentuate murmurs. To minimise patient discomfort the stethoscope should be warmed up between the hands before beginning.[11,12]

Cardiac auscultation should be performed in four locations on a patient's chest in this order:

1. aortic area (second intercostal space along the right sternal border)[11,12]
2. pulmonic area (second intercostal space along the left sternal border)[12]
3. tricuspid area (fifth intercostal space along the left sternal border)[12]
4. mitral area (fifth intercostal space near the midclavicular line).[12]

At each location, clinicians should listen for these sounds using the diaphragm and the bell of the stethoscope.

Normal heart sounds

S1 (first heart sound) is produced by closure of the mitral and tricuspid valves. This sound may be increased in mitral valve stenosis and decreased in mitral regurgitation.[11,12]

S2 (second heart sound) is produced by closure of the aortic and pulmonic valve. Upon inspiration, the increase in right ventricular stroke volume results in what is commonly heard as two distinct sounds, also referred to as splitting. The first S2 sound may be increased in systemic hypertension and decreased in aortic stenosis.[11,12]

Extra heart sounds

S3 (third heart sound) is produced by ventricular filling during diastole. This sound is commonly heard in children and young adults. It is abnormal to hear this sound in individuals aged over 40 years and may indicate mitral regurgitation or advanced heart failure. This sound is best heard with the bell of the stethoscope.

S4 (fourth heart sound) is produced during forceful atrial contraction, which forces blood into a ventricle that cannot expand further. This sound is rarely audible in the young but commonly heard in older adults. This sound may indicate heart failure or ischaemic heart disease.

Respiratory auscultation

Prior to auscultation of the lungs, clinicians should observe the patient and identify any abnormalities associated with respiration, including cyanosis, symmetrical lung expansion and use of accessory muscles to assist with inspiration. Other examination methods should also be employed such as palpation (to check for tactile fremitus) and percussion.[13]

Clinicians should auscultate a patient's lungs, using the stethoscope at various locations on the rib cage, both posteriorly and anteriorly. This examination is aimed at assessing the quality of breath sounds and identifying the presence of any abnormal sounds (adventitious sounds, see Table 2.2).[13] A normal breath sound (vesicular breath sound) is associated with healthy lung tissue, primarily audible during inspiration and heard as a relatively smooth, soft sound.

Table 2.2
Characteristics of adventitious sounds

Sound	Description	Possible causes
Crackles (rales)	Intermittent, scratchy, bubbly noises Heard predominantly on inspiration Produced by reopening of airways closed on previous expiration	Bronchiolitis, pulmonary oedema Pneumonia
Wheezes	Continuous, high-pitched, musical sound	Asthma, bronchiolitis, foreign body
Rhonchi	Continuous, low-pitched, non-musical sound	Pneumonia, cystic fibrosis
Stridor	High-pitched, harsh, blowing sound Heard predominantly on inspiration	Croup, laryngomalacia, subglottic stenosis, allergic reaction, vocal cord dysfunction

Source: John Hopkins Hospital KA & Megan Tschudy 2011[14]

During auscultation of the lungs, clinicians may identify consolidated lung tissue, which is caused by the presence of fluid, inflammatory cells or masses. The quality of sounds is transmitted much better through consolidated lung tissue and can be identified by asking the patient to say the vowel 'E'. The patient should repeat this vowel each time the clinician listens to a different area of the lung.[13] When the stethoscope is placed over an area of consolidated tissue, the sound will change from an 'E' to a nasal 'A' sound.[13] The identification of altered transmission sounds through means of auscultation should warrant further investigation and referral when necessary.

Nutritional assessment

Clinical signs due to insufficient nutrition may occur primarily due to underlying changes in metabolic processes.[15] Optimal nutrition is indispensible for proper physiological functioning, where adequate intakes need to be considered with factors such as impaired digestion and absorption. Excessive losses may result from chronic haemorrhage or catabolic states, as well as from the use of certain medications such as diuretics or corticosteroids.[16] At any time a need is elevated, the risk of developing a deficiency is increased. Adequate macro- and micronutrients are crucial for growth and maintenance of tissues, preventing cell damage and mutation,[17] as well as immune system function[18] and may decrease the likelihood of chronic disease development. It is considered by some investigators that an underlying condition linked to nutritional status may cause undefined or subsyndromal symptoms such as irritability, insomnia, lethargy and difficulty in concentrating.[19] If tissue stores become depleted, various clinical manifestations become apparent and, if left untreated, progress to deficiency disease states.

For example, protein deficiency can affect the status of many other nutrients, namely type II nutrients such as phosphorus, potassium, sodium, chlorine, water, nitrogen, sulfur, zinc and magnesium, as well as the essential amino acids. Deficiency of any one of these nutrients may result in cessation of growth, increased catabolism and, eventually, loss of all tissue components.[20] These nutrients are required to be absorbed in approximately the same ratios as occur in the body. Secondary deficiencies may manifest if supplements that do not contain all of the necessary nutrients for tissue synthesis are given. It is possible to unbalance the diet and cause a greater level of malnutrition via the dilution of any potentially existing marginal levels of these nutrients.[21] The *Oxford Textbook of Medicine* states:

> *These types of deficiency states have always posed problems for clinicians because of the difficulty in making a diagnosis, the non-specificity of weight loss and the lack of confirmatory tests. This has led these nutrients to be largely ignored and their importance to be grossly underestimated. As a group, their deficiency is responsible for malnutrition in half the world's children and to the unrecognised problems of ill health in many others.[20]*

These interactions may be bidirectional. For example, protein deficiency can significantly affect vitamin A metabolism and, in turn, its deficiency can influence protein metabolism. Protein insufficiency principally affects vitamin A status via mechanisms such as impeding intestinal absorption, release from the liver and blood transport. In light of this, protein deficiency can lead to a secondary deficiency of this vitamin, despite an adequate intake. Vitamin A deficiency, on the other hand, can also influence the metabolism of proteins by lowering the plasma levels of retinol-binding protein, impairing nitrogen balance and decreasing the synthesis of other specific proteins such as enzymes and hormones.[22]

Validity of direct micronutrient analyses

Assessment of mineral status has traditionally included body signs and symptoms, although in recent times it has relied on the quantification of mineral element concentrations in a variety of components and cells in the blood. This strategy is based on the assumption that circulating mineral concentrations reflect organ and tissue mineral contents. Although methods such as these have been used, it has not been a sensitive approach for evaluating the total body nutritional status of mineral elements.[23]

The term *acute phase response* is used to describe a short-term metabolic change, encompassing increased plasma levels of particular proteins and decreased levels of others. These responses not only occur in tissue injury such as infection, burns, tissue infarction and a variety of idiopathic inflammatory states but also have been documented in pregnancy, during the first few days in a neonate's life and in neoplastic states.[24] Several frequently used indicators of micronutrient status are affected by the acute phase response and may not effectively reflect micronutrient status. During an acute phase response, there can be a redistribution of micronutrients without actual alterations in the total body content of the micronutrient, resulting in commonly used serum indicators producing inaccurate measurements. On the other hand, requirements or losses may be amplified during this time and also occasionally in combination with impaired assimilation, inevitably resulting in an alteration in body stores.[25]

Micronutrients are also disseminated among circulating, storage and tissue pools, depending on the chemical nature of their environment. Physiological stress, intercompartmental fluid shifts, acid–base balance and recent dietary intake can all influence a nutrient's existence within a particular pool. Serum levels of iron,[26] zinc[27] and selenium[28] have been demonstrated to decrease in the presence of an acute phase reaction, while serum copper increases, regardless of tissue stores.[27] These same minerals are also affected by hypoproteinaemia during malnutrition as this alters the circulating levels of their respective protein carriers. More recently, vitamin D has also been demonstrated to be a negative acute phase reactant and as such the commonly utilised serum measure of 25OHD may be invalid in the presence of inflammation.[29] Plasma levels of vitamins A, C, E and B6 have also been shown to be altered during an acute phase response.[30] In these instances a measure of an acute phase protein such as C-reactive protein (CRP) would be useful in identifying the presence of an acute phase response.[26]

Furthermore, levels of micronutrients may also be modified during the haemodilution at certain stages of pregnancy or surgery and have been shown to be influenced by exercise, with the most evident changes occurring throughout the inflammatory processes of infection[31] or trauma. Nutrient levels in both plasma and serum may also appear to be sufficient, even when there is verification of functional impairment due to the serum concentrations of some nutrients, such as calcium, vitamin A and zinc, being strongly homeostatically regulated,[32,33] therefore providing little information on total body status. In cases such as these, alternative biochemical indicators may be needed, such as the assay of intracellular enzymes or other metabolites known to be dependent upon an adequate supply of a micronutrient.[34]

Functional laboratory tests assess the extent of functional impairments during a specific nutrient deficiency and as such have greater biological implication than commonly used static laboratory tests. Functional biochemical tests may involve measuring an abnormal metabolic product in blood or urine samples caused by the overflow of an intermediary by-product. This is due to a lack of a nutrient-dependent enzyme. For some nutrients, reduction in the activity of enzymes that require a nutrient as a coenzyme or prosthetic group can also be assayed[35] (Table 2.3). Here the underlying assumption is that loss of such functions is biologically more important than the levels of a mineral element in circulation or in a tissue or organ. In light of this concept, various functional parameters may serve as diagnostic tests to verify the adequacy of a variety of vitamins and minerals to permit cells, tissues, organs, anatomical systems and the individual to optimally carry out nutrient-dependent biological functions.[23]

Nutrient status assessment

Assessment of the majority of vitamins and trace elements in urine is of limited value as most are not under homeostatic regulation. Excretion may be a direct measure of intake as opposed to active retention even in cases of whole body deficiency. Large dosages of supplements at any given time can lead to high levels of excretion.[37] Urine specimens may be used to assess recent dietary intake of some trace elements such as chromium, iodine and selenium, as well as protein and the water-soluble B and C vitamins, if renal function is normal. This type of assessment is invalid in cases where metabolites are not excreted in proportion to amounts consumed, absorbed and metabolised, such as vitamins A, D, E and K.[35]

In relation to the minerals for which the kidneys are not involved in maintaining homeostasis, measurement of urinary excretion rates does not provide useful information

Table 2.3
Assessment methods for specific nutrients*

Nutrient	Assay	Confounding variables
Vitamin A	Retinol-binding protein: transthyretin (prealbumin)	Vitamin A is strongly homeostatically regulated[36] Acute phase response will decrease levels irrespective of tissue status[37] Protein–energy malnutrition may affect the binding of retinol[38] Ratio < 036 → marginal deficiency[38]
B1	Red cell thiamine pyrophosphate	
B2	Erythrocyte glutathione reductase activity coefficient	Severe tissue deficiency may reduce apoenzyme activity → falsely elevated activity coefficient[39] Decreased values may exist with a negative nitrogen balance[35]
B6	Urinary kynurenate or xanthurenate + PLP coenzyme	Interferences in the tryptophan pathway → increased metabolic flux by corticoids and oestrogens Bacterial endotoxins, viral infections, protein intake, exercise, lean body mass and pregnancy → increased metabolite excretion[36] No single marker adequately reflects status; a combination may be the best approach[37]
B12	Methylmalonic acid in serum	
Folic acid	Red cell folate	
Vitamin C	Leucocyte vitamin C	Complex methodology → issues with accuracy and precision[40] Acute disease → increased uptake by leucocytes[34]
Vitamin D	25-hydroxy vitamin D	Initial chromatographic sample clean-up is essential for accurate results[41] Presence of inflammation will decrease levels irrespective of tissue status, due to acute phase response[29] Oral contraceptive use → increased levels due to oestrogen increasing levels of vitamin D-binding protein[35]
Vitamin E	Plasma α-tocopherol:cholesterol ratio	Acute phase inflammatory response decreases circulating levels[42] Ratio < 2.2 μmol α-tocopherol/mmol cholesterol is associated with deficiency
Magnesium	Red cell magnesium	
Calcium	Osteocalcin	Serum calcium is strongly homeostatically regulated Alcohol intake and vitamin D status[35]
Zinc	Plasma zinc	Acute phase response lowers circulating levels irrespective of body status[26]
Selenium	Red cell glutathione peroxidase	Deficiencies of iron, vitamin B12 or essential fatty acids, exposure to pro-oxidants, toxins or heavy metals[43]
Iodine	Thyroglobulin	High variability between methods and laboratories[44] Administration of thyroid hormone decreases levels[45] Values increased in thyroid cancer, pregnancy, thyroiditis, thyrotoxicosis[45]
Iron	Soluble transferrin receptor:ferritin ratio	Any change in erythropoiesis such as folate or B12 deficiency increases transferrin receptor, while inflammation increases ferritin; therefore, a ratio may be more ideal Receptor values > 8.5 mg/L and ferritin < 12 mg/L is indicative of deficiency[46]

*The best readily available assessment methods to determine status, as well as factors that may affect results.

on dietary intake or mineral status. In contrast, excretion rates of iodine for which the kidneys have a prominent role in homeostasis provide a useful biomarker of dietary intake of this mineral.[47] In circumstances such as infections, after trauma, with the use of antibiotics or other medications, as well as in conditions that produce negative balance, increases in urinary excretion may occur regardless of depletion of body nutrient stores.[35]

Dietary assessment

In naturopathic practice, dietary assessment forms an integral part of the diagnostic process. While signs and symptoms and blood tests (discussed previously and to follow) may reveal nutritional deficiencies, dietary assessment may reveal patterns of macro- or micronutrient intake. In general, dietary analysis involves recording the patient's dietary habits and making an assessment of which nutrients are in excess or deficiency. In addition, recording the patient's dietary habits can allow the clinician to observe the preferred eating patterns of the patient and allow them to individually tailor a dietary prescription that can improve compliance. In brief, the typical Western diet can be high in refined carbohydrates and saturated fats while low in lean protein, complex carbohydrates and fibre as well as micronutrients (such as B vitamins, vitamin C, zinc, magnesium and calcium), essential fatty acids and other beneficial phytochemicals. After an assessment is made, general dietary advice and a more complex individualised nutritional program can be instituted.

Dietary assessment methods may be controversial as they require a patient's recall of either their usual or their actual diet and may be influenced by the patient not consuming a representative diet during the assessment period, along with variations in perceived quantities also having the potential to occur. Retrospective methods such as 24-hour recall, semi-quantitative food frequency questionnaires and diet histories all have the disadvantage of assessing memory, which may limit the quality of information presented. Factors that have been documented to affect recall accuracy include food consumption patterns, gender, age, weight status and even mood.[48]

Other methods such as three- to seven-day food diaries and weighed food records may be better alternatives. This information is documented at the actual time the food is consumed. The information gained from such exercises may be analysed by various software programs to provide a more detailed assessment of actual nutrient intakes.[49] Various commercial programs are available. Alternatively, food table information databases are accessible on the internet for various nations including Australia,[50] the United States,[51] Canada[52] and Europe.[53] These methods may also be subject to the bias of variations in a patient's change of dietary choices during the assessment period, as well as deviations in perceived quantities for the former method. Although weighed records may be the most accurate, this process is extremely labour intensive and may have issues with compliance. Digestion and absorption may also affect the accuracy of intake estimates on body status.[37]

Prior to undertaking such an investigation, patients should be assured that they will not be judged on their food diaries and that the more accurate the information they provide, the better they can be assisted to improve their overall health. Again, these types of methods should be used as another piece to the complex physiological puzzle.

STANDARD MEDICAL PATHOLOGY TESTING

Blood analysis

Analysing blood cells may be a useful tool to confirm a suspected dysfunction or deficiency. This may also play an important role in monitoring the efficacy of a treatment program and to highlight improvements in a patient's condition. Particular reference ranges for specific assays may be laboratory, age and gender specific; therefore, it is best to consult national standards for their appropriate values.

Full blood count

The full blood count is a pathology test that is readily available to clinicians through several pathology laboratories, providing clinicians with essential information regarding a patient's health status. Interpretation of the full blood count is an important skill that clinicians must be versed in, not only to identify states of disease such as anaemia, allergy, infection and inflammatory disorders but also to gauge the efficacy of a specific therapy. Furthermore, the results of such a test may provide clinicians with insight into potential nutrient deficiencies contributing to a patient's ill health. The full blood count provides information about three cellular components: white cells, red cells and platelets (Table 2.4).

Table 2.4
Nutrient supplement suggestions for abnormal full blood count parameters

Marker	Condition	Nutrient required
Red blood cells		
Mean corpuscular volume	Macrocytic anaemia	Folate, B12, cobalt, B group vitamins[54,55]
	Microcytic anaemia	Iron[54]
Haemoglobin	Anaemia	Iron, B12, isoleucine[56,57]
White blood cells		
Basophils	Basophilia	L-histidine,[58] quercetin[59]
Leucocytes	Leucopenia	Zinc[60]
Lymphocytes	Lymphopenia	Zinc, arginine,[61] vitamin A[62]

Urinalysis

Dipstick urinalysis is a simple standardised method of urine analysis involving dipping a plastic strip, with a series of pads that change colour according to specific chemical reactions, into a sample of urine. Results are then read off this strip by comparing it with a chart that shows levels of substances in the urine, depending on any colour change that may have occurred. A variety of substances, including protein, glucose, bilirubin, blood and pH, may be investigated at one time. Despite being simple, fast and easy to use, many dipsticks may not be completely accurate and therefore may provide false positive results.[63]

No test can replace a good case-taking technique

It is advisable for clinicians to undertake the necessary questioning, physical examination and other naturopathic diagnostic techniques prior to ordering functional pathology tests. Functional testing is designed to complement the overall naturopathic case-taking process and should not be used as the sole investigatory method in clinical diagnoses. Furthermore, clinicians should exercise due diligence when ordering any test. The choice of test should be based upon individual findings on a case-by-case basis. A haphazard, non-selective approach should be avoided.

FUNCTIONAL PATHOLOGY TESTING

Functional pathology is a method of specialty investigation that may be used in conjunction with other naturopathic diagnostic techniques to assist healthcare professionals in gathering information to make informed clinical diagnoses. These tools may assist healthcare professionals in gathering information, hence informing clinical diagnoses. These tests differ from routine pathology tests in that they may provide a detailed assessment of an individual's biochemical, hormonal, nutritional and metabolic status. Clinicians generally employ these methods for early detection and intervention of potential underlying pathological processes otherwise not identified via previous medical investigations. These tests may also be useful in determining baseline measures, so that the efficacy of treatment interventions, such as dietary, nutritional and herbal medicine, may be assessed.

Caution regarding choice of techniques

Many 'new' diagnostic techniques are often commercial or proprietary in nature, incurring significant costs. Although some may be based on a sound theory, practice or evidence base, others may often exaggerate or over-extrapolate diagnostic ability or have no diagnostic usefulness. Practitioners need to apply critical analysis to their choice of diagnostic tools.

To date, evidence supporting the practice, quality and safety of functional pathology is lacking. While an emphasis on demonstrating the clinical efficacy of diagnostic tests exists, the methods used for evaluation are complicated, which may inform the lack of current evidence.[64] In light of this, results obtained from functional pathology tests should be interpreted with caution until further scientific validation has occurred.

A comprehensive range of functional pathology tests are readily available. The following provides a brief overview of some of the more commonly prescribed tests.

Organic acid assays

Organic acid assays provide a unique chemical profile of cellular health. This test is a useful tool in detecting abnormalities in macronutrient, micronutrient, vitamin, sterol, mitochondrial and nucleic acid metabolism.[65] Key intermediate metabolic markers of cellular physiology are quantified to assess compromised energy production, detoxification, intestinal microbial activity, neurotransmitter metabolism and nutrient deficiencies. Clinically, these markers may offer valuable information into possible causative factors of dysfunctional cellular physiology, physical and mental performance, as well as overall health status.[66] Organic acid assays should be considered in patients presenting with fatigue, mood disorders, headaches, muscular pain and digestive problems to identify potential metabolic dysfunction.[67]

This test involves analysing accumulated organic acids in a sample of urine by gas chromatography and mass spectrometry.[68] Abnormal levels of organic acids may be due to drug effects, inherited acquired enzyme deficiencies or toxic exposure. Furthermore, results may provide clinicians with valuable information to identify potential factors contributing to abnormal parameters, such as nutrient insufficiencies, metabolic dysfunction and microbial overgrowth.[69]

Abnormalities in various organic acids provide insight into diseases possibly caused or complicated by toxin accumulation or vitamin insufficiency.[67] For example, a commonly ordered organic acid test known as methylmalonic acid is indicative of a functional B12 deficiency.[70] Elevated levels of citric acid are indicative of amino acid deficiencies, while elevations in succinic acid excretion suggest deficiencies of CoQ10 and riboflavin. Fatty acid peroxidation results in elevated levels of adipic and suberic acid levels and may indicate the presence of diabetes.[71] In this circumstance, supplementation of carnitine and riboflavin should be considered.[72]

Mauve factor 'malvaria' (pyrroluria)

Malvaria or mauve factor is often mistakenly referred to as kryptopyrrole (KP) or pyrroluria.[73] This is due to studies incorrectly classifying mauve and KP as the same substance, owing to similarities in the chemical structure. Mauve factor or hydroxy-haemopyrrolin-2-one (HPL) is produced through the hydroxylactam of haemopyrrole and not kryptopyrrole.[74] Therefore, the terms pyrroluria or kryptopyrrole should technically not be used interchangeably to refer to mauve factor or malvaria.

Low-level HPL production and accumulation occurs in all humans as a by-product of altered haemoglobin synthesis, haemoglobin breakdown and dietary intake. Nutrient deficiencies, toxic exposure, intestinal dysbiosis, intestinal hyperpermiability, oxidative stress, emotional stress and genetic predispositions are attributed to elevated HPL concentrations.[75] Although elevations in HPL were originally proposed to only be present in patients with schizophrenia,[76] more recent studies have found elevated levels in a wide range of cognitive, affective and neurobehavioural disorders. Such disorders include Down syndrome,[77] autism, epilepsy,[78] attention deficit hyperactivity disorder (ADHD), depression[79] and anxiety.[80] The normal HPL concentrations vary between laboratories, ranging from 2–25 µg/dL to 8–20 µg/dL. As a general rule, levels over twice the upper normal limit are classified as highly elevated.[81]

Elevated levels of aluminium, lead, iron, arachidonic acid to eicosapentanoic acid (EPA) ratio and omega-3 to omega-6 fatty acid ratio are typically observed in patients with pyrroluria. HPL irreversibly binds to various nutrients including pyridoxine, zinc and magnesium, and results in increased urinary excretion of these nutrients.[82] Early studies found supplementation of B3[76,83] reduces mauve factor urine excretion and relieves symptoms. More recent studies achieved superior clinical results through oral B6 (400–3000 mg/day) and zinc (160 mg/day) supplementation.[84] White flecks in the nails are detectable in 60% of patients with malvaria,[79] and usually resolve with high-dose zinc supplementation.[84] Biotin supplementation may also be necessary to assist in normal haem production as HPL can bind to haem and render it inert.[85] As increased HPL concentrations may also affect methylation pathways, clinicians should consider methionine or SAMe in patients who are undermethylating and B3, B12 and folate in patients who are overmethylating.[86] Vitamin C supplementation should also be considered, as insufficiency of this vitamin is linked to elevated urinary pyrrole concentrations.[87]

While this particular form of pathology testing has been used to assist in the diagnosis of mental disorders, it is still relatively unknown and seldom used by medical practitioners. Individuals experiencing conditions such as Down syndrome,[77] autism, epilepsy,[78] ADHD, depression[79] or anxiety[80] should be screened for mauve factor as they may benefit from supplementation of B6 and zinc.[84] Other investigations such as neurotransmitter profiles, allergy testing and heavy metal tests may also be used in conjunction with mauve factor assays to improve clinical outcomes.[77] A large body of evidence exists surrounding the presence of nutritional deficiencies in individuals with mental illness; however, no double-blind randomised controlled trials have been undertaken to assess the effects of supplementation in malvaria. Therefore, clinicians should not rely solely on supplement therapy in managing this condition but include it as one component in a comprehensive treatment regimen.

Comprehensive stool analysis

Comprehensive stool analysis (CSA) may provide an overview of the components of digestion, absorption, intestinal function and microbial flora, as well as identifying the presence of any pathogenic bacteria, yeasts or parasites. These assays can be extremely useful as intestinal dysfunction may play a crucial role in the underlying cause of many health conditions (refer further to the section on the gastrointestinal system—Chapters 4–6).

CSA is commonly used in cases of chronic gastrointestinal disorders. While there is data to support various aspects of stool analysis in disease, CSA as a whole practice is yet to be thoroughly investigated. Scientifically proven aspects of the CSA include the presence of parasites, protozoa and trematodes, which may cause a range of gastro-intestinal disorders including diarrhoea.[88] Occult blood in the stool may indicate mucosal damage from the live feeding of parasites,[89] Crohn's disease[90] or gastrointestinal cancer.[91] Low levels of short-chain fatty acids, as a result of insufficient functional microbiota, may indicate a concomitant impairment in digestive and immune function.[92] Little data exists supporting the clinical relevance of identifying undigested plant tissues and meat fibres as present within a stool sample.

Stool analysis has potential practical diagnostic value[93]; however, further studies are required if a relationship between abnormal CSA markers and disease risk is to be established.[94] There is some evidence demonstrating associations between the human microbiome and specific diseases; however, the generalisability of these test results to population groups is complicated.[95] Furthermore, because laboratories can employ different analytical and data interpretation techniques, clinicians should interpret test results with care[93] and consider a range of markers to inform a diagnosis, as opposed to one definitive assay.

Immunoglobulin G food intolerance test

Food intolerances have been implicated in the presentation of various conditions such as irritable bowel syndrome[96] and migraines.[97] To date, the gold standard for diagnosing food reactions remains the double-blind, placebo-controlled food challenge[98]; however, this method is costly, time consuming and demanding on the patient. Blood tests measuring immunoglobulin G (IgG) serum antibodies were developed as an alternative investigatory method based on early evidence where patients with food sensitivities had significant elevations in food-specific IgG antibodies.[99,100]

There is much conflicting evidence regarding the efficacy, reliability and clinical appli-cability of food-specific IgG assays. Studies examining food elimination, based on these investigations, found promising results in the symptomatic management of irritable bowel disease[96] and migraine.[97] However, another study utilising similar methodologies found this method to be ineffective in preventing migraine.[101] Furthermore, IgG food antibodies have been identified in apparently healthy individuals,[102] which may explain why IgG testing is unable to accurately distinguish between people with or without intolerances.[103]

Due to the conflicting available literature, several international bodies have made recommendations against the use of IgG testing to diagnose food intolerances until a consensus over the validity of such examinations is reached.[104–107] Therefore, it is advisable that clinicians consider conducting food challenges in patients with chronic symptoms before eliminating foods based purely on IgG food intolerance tests.[108] Results of IgG assays should be interpreted with caution.[108]

FODMAPs

FODMAPs (fermentable oligosaccharides, disaccharides, monosaccharides and polyols) is an acronym used to classify a collection of dietary short-chain carbohydrates and sugar alcohols.[109] In functional gastrointestinal disorders such as irritable bowel syndrome, visceral hypersensitivity and abnormal motility responses result in the malabsorption of short-chain carbohydrates.[109] The impeded diffusion of these carbohydrates across the brush border results in rapid fermentation by bacteria in the small and proximal large intestine. This fermentation generates production of hydrogen and carbon dioxide gas, which induces the symptoms of pain, bloating and abdominal distension. Hydrogen in the gastrointestinal tract diffuses readily into splanchnic venous circulation, where it is eventually transported to the lungs and excreted in the breath.[110]

Diagnosis of food intolerances through functional testing is often not possible; however, hydrogen breath tests are a useful method of identifying which specific sugars act as FODMAPs within an individual.[111] Not all FODMAPs trigger symptoms in sensitive individuals and therefore different challenge substances are used.[111] Typically, only one challenge substance is used per day.[112] For example, an oral load of lactulose may be used as a challenge substance as the human small intestine does not possess the hydrolases required to digest it.[112] Therefore, it must be fermented by bacteria. In individuals with FODMAP sensitivities, methanogens, sulfate-reducing bacteria and acetogens are unable to efficiently utilise hydrogen and, therefore, the hydrogen must be excreted in the breath.[111]

Hydrogen breath testing has been proposed as a diagnostic test for functional digestive diseases such as FODMAPs and small intestinal bacterial overgrowth (SIBO).[113] There is currently much conflicting evidence in regards to the validity and accuracy of this test in the diagnosis of functional digestive diseases. For example, the prevalence of sorbitol, fructose and lactose is similar in patients with FODMAPs and SIBO compared to healthy controls. This suggests carbohydrate malabsorption may be a normal physiological occurrence and not indicative of disease. Therefore, clinicians should interpret the findings of these tests with caution.[114,115]

The detection of high amounts of breath hydrogen after a challenge phase indicates that the person may require a low-FODMAP diet.[110,111] Due to the chemical structure of fructans and galacto-oligosaccharides, these substances are always malabsorbed and fermented by gut bacteria. While this process produces flatulence in healthy people, it is likely to initiate symptoms in those with irritable bowel syndrome.[110,111] The other FODMAPs, such as fructose and sorbitol, will only produce symptoms in those who malabsorb them and can be tested using the breath test. Mannitol is not generally used as a challenge substance because it is rarely found in the diet and can be identified as a trigger by eliminating and rechallenging.[111] Clinicians should consider restricting foods in patients eliciting a response to any of the challenge substances (Table 2.5).

Table 2.5
Food sources of FODMAPs

FODMAP	Richest food sources
Fructo-oligosaccharides (fructans)	Wheat, rye, onion, garlic, artichoke
Galacto-oligosaccharides (GOS)	Legumes
Lactose	Milk and dairy products
Fructose	Honey, apple, pear, watermelon, mango
Sorbitol	Apple, pear, stone fruit, sugar-free sweets
Mannitol	Mushroom, cauliflower, sugar-free sweets

Source: Barrett & Gibson 2012[111]

Salivary hormones

Salivary testing to measure levels of hormones such as cortisol and the sex steroid hormones has many advantages, both scientific and practical, over serum testing (see Chapter 18 on stress and fatigue). The non-protein bound or unbound fractions of these hormones are measured, as opposed to the total levels, which are quantitated in serum measures. As these steroid hormones are predominantly bound to specific protein carriers, it is the free hormones that are considered to best reflect a person's hormonally related symptoms.[116] Conversely, saliva levels of dehydroepiandrosterone (DHEA), thyroxine and cortisone may be of little value due to changes in their concentrations dependent upon salivary flow rate, enzymatic production or degradation by the salivary glands themselves, as well as contamination by plasma exudates, respectively.[117]

Hair

Hair analysis is a valuable and representative method to detect and monitor heavy metal exposure[118] or the ingestion of drugs, although its usefulness in identifying nutrient status remains controversial. It has been proposed that a hair mineral analysis is an accurate method of assessing a patient's whole blood mineral concentration. However, there are only a limited number of studies establishing hair mineral concentrations as a marker of intracellular mineral content. Despite its many advantages such as its non-invasive manner, a number of pitfalls exist in using hair in nutritional assessment, including the wide variability in levels reported in healthy people; this may be due to methods of sampling and sample preparation, as well as alterations caused by shampoos, hair treatments and other forms of environmental contamination that may make mineral content inconsistent throughout the length of the hair strand.[119] Furthermore, results of measuring metal concentrations in hair, even under ideal circumstances, may not correlate with those obtained in blood pathology.[120] Some evidence exists indicating an association between hair mineral concentrations and red blood cell concentrations. It is important to highlight that this data is preliminary and further research is required before a clear association can be established.[121,122]

NUTRIGENETIC AND GENOMIC TECHNOLOGIES

From the advent of the mapping of the human genome, many subsequent 'omic' technologies have been born. Nutritional genomics studies the relationship between diet and genes from the perspective of how diets may affect gene function (*nutrigenomics*) and how variations or variants in genetic make-up may influence how particular diets (or nutrient supplements) affect an individual (*nutrigenetics*). The use of genomic technology to assess how plant-based medicines (*herbomics*) may be affected by people's individual genetics is also being assessed.[123] In essence, these new technologies may be a method of delivering personalised nutritional/herbal advice in order to negate potential genetic predispositions to particular disease states and to tailor individualised prescriptions.[124]

The identification of single-nucleotide polymorphisms (SNPs) have led this revolution, although its steady adoption into clinical practice has been marred by the current cost and the time necessary to accrue and understand the relevance of available population SNP data that has been steadily collected from many observational studies. The significance of a variety of variants in clinical disease is progressing and suitable diagnostic tests are being developed. In relation to nutrigenetics, the next step is the elucidation of the most appropriate diets and other treatments given how an individual's genetic profile may present.[124]

Epigenetics examines alterations that do not modulate the deoxyribonucleic acid (DNA) sequence itself, rather gene expression via chromatin structure, histone codes and DNA methylation patterns. Genes generally possess two copies or alleles—one maternal and one paternal. When both of these are active the system may be less inclined towards dysfunction; if one is 'turned off' ordinary function may be altered much more readily. Through identifying potential epigenetic modifications, early diagnosis and preventative treatments may take the place of treating diseases once symptoms become apparent.[125] Nutrigenomics, with reference to the effect of the diet on gene expression, is being increasingly recognised as important due to the likelihood of the development of disease increasing in proportion to DNA damage. This damage can be minimised by optimising nutritional status and concomitant ability for the body to continue to repair and replicate DNA adequately.[126] The evidence is overwhelming that a number of micronutrients are required as enzyme cofactors or structural components necessary for synthesis and repair, as well as for preventing oxidation and methylation of DNA. Deficiencies of these may present the same level of damage to the genome caused by significant environmental exposures such as chemical carcinogens and radiation.[127] The most noteworthy of nutrients appearing to confer the most protective benefits include vitamin E, calcium, folate, retinol and nicotinic acid, while riboflavin, pantothenic acid and biotin in high quantities may cause more damage to the genome.[128]

A variety of other nutritional components and botanicals have been demonstrated to modulate gene expression via their interactions with the genome. The way in which a variety of compounds such as soy protein[129] and fatty acids,[130] as well as a number of nutrient[131,132] and herbal[133,134] compounds, modulate gene expression has been extensively studied. The metabolic effects of the molecular interactions of the genome with substances such as resveratrol,[135] phyto-oestrogens[129] and curcumin[136] has allowed amounting scientific rationale into the efficacy of such products in maintaining health.

Both translation and post-translational modification of ribonucleic acid (RNA) to proteins may also be influenced by dietary intakes. This constitutes the proteome of the organism, which fluctuates depending on cell type and its functional state. *Proteomics* or the study of such proteomes may be useful in categorising atypical protein structures and how these subsequently affect biology in response to diet. *Metabolomics* is the newest of the 'omic' technologies whereby changes in small molecular weight compounds within cells are mapped in response to dietary treatments. It is hoped that their analysis may elucidate the potential mechanisms by which dietary components may regulate metabolic processes.[137]

It is a potential oversight to assume that all individuals respond in a similar manner to their dietary and supplement intake. As more information about genetic and genomic variations comes to the fore, a personalised approach to nutrition based on nutrient–gene interactions will become a priority to properly target health interventions. At present, the clinical applicability of nutrigenomics and herbomics is limited. Despite the marked drop in costs associated with genotyping in recent years, the number of markers now available per gene makes the genotyping of all markers expensive. Further nutrigenomic and herbomic research must also be undertaken to establish a more comprehensive database of gene–nutrient and gene–herb associations.

Table 2.6 lists a selection of clinically important polymorphisms and their relevance.

Liver detoxification tests

The liver is a metabolically complex organ involved primarily in detoxifying endotoxic and exotoxic chemicals, commonly known as xenobiotics. The metabolism of xenobiotics occurs through the induction of the phase I and II enyzmatic pathways. Phase I enzymes such as cytochrome P450 (CYP450) are involved in hydrolysis, reduction and oxidation reactions. Phase II detoxification involves conjugation reactions known as glutathione and amino acid conjugation, glucoronidation, sulfation, acetylation and methylation. After exposure to phase I metabolism, xenobiotics are biotransformed in to water-soluble metabolites and become substrates for phase II enzyme reactions.[162]

Liver detoxification assays challenge phase I through low-level doses of caffeine. Caffeine is used as the substrate due to being an accepted substance to accurately assess cytochrome P1A2 (CYP1A2) induction, an iso-enzyme of CYP450.[163] Phase II is challenged through low-level doses of paracetamol as its major metabolites are sulfate, glucoronide and glutathione conjugates[164] while aspirin is used to assess glycine conjugation.[165] As metabolites from these three compounds are present in saliva and urine,[163–165] specimens are collected and then analysed to assess hepatic conversion and clearance from the body.

Results of this test indicate the efficiency of both phase I and II reactions, providing clinicians with valuable information for implementing comprehensive treatment strategies. High phase I activity results in increased free radical production, while reduced activity indicates impaired enzyme activity. Similarly, impaired phase II activity may result in a range of maladies including chemical sensitivity.[162] Therefore, regulation of both phases is required for efficient detoxification to occur. Interpretation of results, however, should be conducted with caution, as abnormal markers may represent normal physiological processes.

Factors such as sex, age, genetics, BMI and insulin production[166] have been shown to affect enzymatic activity, hence affecting results. Interestingly, 10–20% of the population are genetically predisposed to have under-functioning phase I pathways.[167] Additionally, premenopausal versus postmenopausal women have 30–40% increases in cytochrome P3A4 activity due to the hormonal fluctuations in progesterone.[168] Clinicians should be aware that such factors may influence test results and account for this prior to arriving at a differential diagnosis.

Liver detoxification profiles are based around the notion that xenobiotics undergo phase I and then phase II detoxification; however, new evidence reports some chemicals are actually metabolised in reverse.[169] Therefore, clinicians should undertake a

Table 2.6
Selection of clinically important polymorphisms and their relevance

System	Gene (polymorphism)	Risk allele	Relevance
Cardiovascular disease— dyslipidaemia	Cholesterol esther transfer protein (Taq1B)	B1B1	Lower HDL-c levels due to increased transfer of cholesterol to LDL-c via increased CETP[138]
	Hepatic lipase (−514C/T)	T	Lower HDL-c levels due to increased gene expression[139]
	Paraoxonase arylesterase (192R)	G	Increased lipoprotein oxidation[140]
	NADPH oxidase (CYBA)	C	Increased ROS in endothelium via increased enzyme activity[141]
Cardiovascular disease— hypertension	Angiotensinogen (M235T)	C	Increased blood pressure through vasoconstriction[142]
	Angiotensin II receptor (A1166C)	C	Increased receptor function via sensitivity to hormone stimulation[143]
	Endothelial nitric oxide synthase (G894T)	T	Endothelial dysfunction and vasoconstriction via decreased nitric oxide production[144]
Central nervous system	5-hydroxytryptamine transporter gene (5-HTTLPR)	Short (SS)	Increased risk of major depressive disorder following stressful events Also closely linked with conditions such as suicidal behaviour, psychoses, personality disorders and aggressive-impulsive traits[145]
	Centaurin-gamma-2 (AGAP1)	G	Strong association with schizophrenia and autism[146]
	Voltage-gated L-type calcium channel ion pores (CACNA1C rs1006737)	A	Affects neurotransmitter release from neurons, associated with both schizophrenia and bipolar disorder[147]
	Phosphatidylinositol binding clathrin assembly protein (PICALM rs3851179)	G	Increased susceptibility to Alzheimer's disease[148]
Metabolic	Adiponectin (+276G/T)	C	Decreased levels with increased insulin resistance and body weight[149]
	Adrenergic receptor beta 2 (Gln27Glu)	G	Decreased lipolysis and increased fat mass via decreased receptor function[150]
	Adrenergic receptor beta 3 (Trp64Arg)	C	Increased resistance to weight loss and insulin via decreased receptor function[151]
	Fatty acid–binding protein 2 (Ala54Thr)	A	Increased absorption of dietary fats and reduced insulin sensitivity via increased activity[152]
	Melanocortin 4 receptor (rs17782313)	A	Increased risk of obesity via decreased regulation of feeding behaviour[153]
	Fat mass and obesity gene (FTO rs9939609)	A	Increased risk of overweight and diabetes via inability to control food intake[154]
	Leptin receptors (Gln223Arg) and (Lys109Arg)	G	Increased risk of obesity and rebound weight gain via decreased leptin receptor levels[155]
Antioxidants	Glutathione peroxidase (Pro198Leu)	T	Increased risk of oxidative damage via reduced enzyme activity[156]
	Catalase (262C/T)	T	Increased cellular oxidative stress via reduced catalase activity[157]
	Manganese superoxide dismutase (rs4880)	C	Increased free radical production via reduced enzyme activity[158]
Inflammation	Tumor necrosis factor alpha (−308G/A)	A	Increased TNF-α production[159]
	C-reactive protein-1 (0169171C/T) and 2 (0143294C/T)	T G	Increased risk of inflammation via increased CRP production[160]
	Cyclo-oxygenase 2 (−899G/C or −765G/C)	G	Increased risk of chronic inflammation via increased promoter activity[161]

comprehensive case history and use information from a variety of investigatory methods rather than relying on the results of one particular test.

Genetic polymorphisms of drug metabolising enzymes (DMES)

Clinicians should also be aware of the potential role genetic polymorphisms play in hepatic metabolic processes, which have the potential to influence drug metabolism and affect the results of functional liver tests.[170] The metabolism of the majority of drugs and xenobiotics are attributed to just over one dozen enzymes, all of which belong to the CYP 1, 2 and 3 family.[171] For example, polymorphisms of the CYP2D6 gene are one major factor for determining what type of 'metaboliser' an individual is—extensive, intermediate or ultra-rapid. Therefore, heritable genetic variations in the genes responsible for producing these hepatic enzymes can significantly influence the rate and efficiency at which drugs and xenobiotics are metabolised.[171] Genetic polymorphisms are the result of copy number variation, single nucleotide polymorphisms and gene amplification and deletion.[172] Table 2.7 lists a selection of gene polymorphisms that affect how specific nutrients and herbs are used.

Clinicians should also consider other non-genetic host factors that can influence the activity of metabolic enzymes. For example, inflammation may cause decreased activity of CYP1A2, CYP2A6 and CYP3A4/5 and increase activity of CYP2E1.[186,187] Cholestasis may decreases CYP1A2 activity and diseases such as diabetes, obesity and liver disease may increase CYP2E1 activity.[188,189] Age may increase activity of CYP1A2, CYP3A4/5, CYP2A6, CYP2B6, CYP2C8 and CYP2C9[190]; however, the exact effects of gender over variations in enzymatic activity is still relatively unknown.

FACTORS AFFECTING NUTRITIONAL STATUS

A variety of factors may influence nutritional status other than dietary insufficiency and therefore should be taken into account if a particular deficiency is suspected or a specific condition is present. Some conditions may increase the need for a particular nutrient, while others may interfere with its absorption or excretion.

Examples of these include omega-3 essential fatty acid status being affected by excessive omega-6 due to their competition for the enzyme delta-6-desaturase, or the antagonism between zinc and copper.[191] A variety of genetic polymorphisms that may affect the absorption of a nutrient or its bioavailability on a number of different levels depending on the position of the amino acid replacement on the nucleotide base within the DNA strand also exist.[192–194]

Conditions causing potential nutrient deficiencies

Vitamin A
- Pre-existing conditions such as abetalipoproteinaemia, carcinoid syndrome, chronic infections, cystic fibrosis, disseminated tuberculosis, hypothyroidism,[45] liver disease or a systemic inflammatory response,[34] as well as diseases that cause fat malabsorption, including impaired pancreatic and/or biliary secretions such as Crohn's and coeliac disease, radiation enteritis, ileal resection or damage[195]
- Zinc deficiency impairs the absorption, transport and metabolism of vitamin A[196]
- Protein deficiency can markedly affect vitamin A nutriture and, in turn, vitamin A deficiency can also influence protein metabolism[22]
- Pre-term infants are generally considered to be at risk because their plasma retinol concentrations are usually low[27]

Table 2.7
Selection of gene polymorphisms that affect the utilisation or efficacy of specific nutrients and herbs

Nutrient/ herb	Gene/ polymorphism	Condition	Study methodology	Results	Clinical comment
B2[173]	*MTHFR* 677C→T rs1801133	Elevated homocysteine and cardiovascular risk	Participants ($n = 128$) with elevated homocysteine received 1.6 mg/day of B2 per day for 12 weeks	Homocysteine concentrations decreased by 22% after B2, in individuals with the *MTHFR* 677 TT genotype	B2 may be more effective in people who carry *MTHFR* 677 T alleles compared with the C alleles
Folate[174]	*MTHFR* 677C→T rs1801133	Colon cancer	The relationship between plasma folate, *MTHFR* 677C→T and colon cancer was assessed in healthy and colon cancer participants ($n = 526$)	*MTHFR* 677 CC genotype is associated with half the risk of colon cancer
Low folate and excessive alcohol intake negates this protective effect	Folate supplementation is warranted in deficient individuals carrying the *MTHFR* 677 C allele rather than the T allele
B12 and folic acid[175]	*MTHFR* 677C→T rs1801133	Depression and anxiety	The relationship between plasma B12, folic acid, *MTHFR* 677C→T, anxiety and depression was assessed in healthy and psychiatric outpatients ($n = 90$)	Those with anxiety and/or depression carrying the *MTHFR* 677 TT genotype have significantly lower levels of B12 and folic acid compared with the CC genotype carriers	B12 and folic acid supplementation may be indicated in TT carriers with depression and/or anxiety to assist with monoamine production and methylation reactions
Vitamin K[176]	*GGCX* rs699664	Osteoporosis	Bone mineral density (BMD) scans and DNA samples were obtained from postmenopausal women ($n = 500$)	Vitamin K activity and BMD is significantly reduced in individuals with the *GGCX* 325-Arg compared with *GGCX* 325-Gln	Supplementation of vitamin K may overcome the negative effects associated with the *GGCX* 325-Arg polymorphism
Vitamin E[177]	*SCARB1* rs675	Vitamin E deficiency	Participants ($n = 212$) were analysed for lipoprotein turnover and vitamin E plasma and tissue levels	Women with the T allele had significantly lower γ-tocopherol concentrations than those carrying the homozygous A allele	In deficient states, women carrying the T allele may be more responsive to vitamin E supplementation
B12[178]	*TCN2* TC776C→G rs1801198	Hyperhomocystein-aemia	Participants' ($n = 359$) serum plasma levels were screened to determine the relationship between plasma B12, holo-trans cobalamin and homocysteine levels carrying the TC 776 gene	Carriers of the TC 776 GG genotype have significantly lower mean serum holo-trans cobalamin concentrations than those with the TC 776 CC genotype	Less vitamin B12 is available for cellular uptake and metabolism in individuals with a homozygous G allele
Supplementation may be beneficial
Vitamin C[179]	*SLC23A1* rs4257763 and rs6596473	Vitamin C absorption	The relationship between participants' ($n = 1046$) serum blood samples and SNPs was evaluated	Carriers of the G allele were associated with lower fasting serum ascorbic acid levels than those carrying the A allele of the *SLC23A1* gene	Vitamin C supplementation may be more effective in people who carry the *SLC32A1* G allele compared with the A allele

(cont.)

Table 2.7
Selection of gene polymorphisms that affect the utilisation or efficacy of specific nutrients and herbs (continued)

Nutrient/ herb	Gene/ polymorphism	Condition	Study methodology	Results	Clinical comment
Calcium (Ca)/ magnesium (Mg)[180]	*TRPM7 Thr1482 Ile1482* rs8042919	Colorectal neoplasia	The association of Ca and Mg intake and colorectal cancer was assessed in participants (n = 2204) with and without colorectal adenoma	Compared with those with the *TRPM7 Thr1482*, people who have the *TRPM7 Ile1482* were found to have a significantly (60%) greater risk of colorectal denoma with a high Ca:Mg intake	Mg supplementation may reduce the risk of colorectal cancer in people with the *TRPM7 Ile1482* polymorphism
Choline[181]	*PEMT*744 G→C rs12325817	Choline deficiency	Participants (n = 57) were fed low-choline diets for 42 days DNA SNPs were tested for allelic association for the susceptibility of developing choline deficiency	78% of participants carrying the C allele of *PEMT*744 developed choline deficiency over those carrying the G allele	SNPs in the *PEMT* gene affect the dietary requirement of choline C allele carriers may require supplementation
EPA[182]	*FABP2*	Hypertriglyceridaemia	2 g of pure EPA was administered to participants (n = 46) with hypertriglyceridaemia for eight weeks	Levels of plasma EPA and omega-3 fatty acids were more responsive to supplementation in participants with the *FABP2* compared with the A allele	EPA and omega-3 fatty acid levels are more likely to increase after supplementation in carriers of the *FABP2* gene
Kava[183]	*SLC6A1* rs2601126 and rs2697153	Generalised anxiety disorder (GAD)	The effect of kava (120/240 mg of kavalactones) versus placebo in participants with GAD (n = 75) was assessed over six weeks	The anxiolytic response to kava was more significant in carriers of GABA transporter rs2601126 T and rs2697153 A alleles	Kava's ability to reduce anxiety in GAD is potentially modified by polymorphisms of the GABA transporter gene
Silymarin[184]	*TNF* G-308A rs 1800629	Hepatotoxicity	Participants (n = 77) with chronic hydrogen sulfide exposure received 140 mg of silymarin, 3 × per day for 30 days	Decrease in ALT and AST in high TNF-α producers (A allele) treated with silymarin is significantly lower than low TNF-α producers	An increased dose of silymarin in high TNF-α producers to obtain therapeutic effects might be needed
Tianqi Jiangtang[185]	*TPMT* rs1142345	Diabetes	Pre-diabetic participants (n = 194) were treated with Tianqi Jiangtang, 1.6g 3 × per day for 12 months	Hypoglycaemic responses were 2.8 times greater in carriers of the A allele compared with the G allele	An increased risk of diabetes was observed in G allele carriers This herbal prescription may only be warranted in carriers of the A allele

SNP = single nucleotide polymorphism; rs = reference sequence; A/G/C/T = alleles; MTHFR = methyltetrahydrofolate-reductase; GGCX = gamma-glutamyl carboxylase; SCARB1 = scavenger receptor class B type I; TCN2 = transcobalamin II; GC = group-specific component vitamin D binding protein; SLC23A1 = solute carrier family 23; TRPM7 = transient receptor potential cation channel; PEMT = phosphatidylethanolamine N-methyltransferase; FABP2 = fatty acid-binding protein 2; SLC6A1 = solute carrier family 6; TNF = tumour necrosis factor; TPMT = thiopurine methyltransferase; EPA = eicosapentanoic acid; ALT = alanine aminotransferase; AST = aspartate aminotransferase

Vitamin B1

- Chronic alcoholism, gastric bypass surgery and gastrointestinal disorders[197]
- Thiaminases that degrade thiamine are present in raw fish, fish paste and betel nut[197]
- Antithiamine factors are also found in caffeic acid, tannic acid and salicylic acid, as well as blueberries, black currants, red cabbage, beetroot and brussels sprouts[198]

Vitamin B2

- Alcoholism,[199] diabetes mellitus, thyroid and adrenal insufficiency, liver disease and gastrointestinal or biliary obstruction[35]
- Several metals form chelates or complexes that may affect their bioavailability, such as copper, zinc, iron, tryptophan, vitamins B3 and C, as well as caffeine and saccharin[200]
- Protein–energy malnutrition leads to increased urinary losses[201]
- Exercise increases requirements[201]

Vitamin B3

- Alcoholism, Crohn's disease and anorexia[201]

Vitamin B6

- Alcoholism, asthma, carpal tunnel syndrome, gestational diabetes, lactation, malabsorption, malnutrition, neonatal seizures, normal pregnancies, occupational exposure to hydrazine compounds, pellagra, pre-eclamptic oedema, renal dialysis, uraemia,[45] liver disease, oestrogen therapy, rheumatoid arthritis, HIV[202]
- B6 antagonists in foods such as some varieties of mushrooms, flaxseed meal, jack beans and mimosa, possibly via a systemic effect rather than interfering with its absorption[203]
- B2 deficiency[204]

Vitamin B12

- Inadequate peptic digestion and gastric acid,[205] pancreatic insufficiency[195] or alcoholism may result in deficiency due to inadequate ingestion and absorption, as well as enhanced utilisation and excretion[206]
- Bacterial overgrowth,[207] tropical or non-tropical sprue, Crohn's disease and inflammatory bowel disease may cause decreased levels[45]
- Absorption through receptor sites in the ileum occurs in alkaline pH in the presence of calcium[35]
- Diabetes, leucocytosis, hepatitis, cirrhosis, obesity and protein–energy malnutrition may cause increased levels[45]

Folate

- Hyperthyroidism, pregnancy, haemolytic anaemia, need for intensive care or any other sustained metabolic drain may increase folate need up to six- to eightfold[208]
- Malabsorption of folate secondary to an infection with *Giardia lamblia* and bacterial overgrowth[35]
- Achlorhydria, oral contraceptive agents,[203] oral oestrogen and antacids[209]
- Conditions of increased cellular turnover such as cancer
- B12 deficiency may induce a secondary folate deficiency by reducing the activity of the enzyme methionine synthase, which activates folate[35]

Biotin
- Achlorhydria and alcoholism[210]
- Biotinases that degrade biotin are found in raw egg white 'avidin'[210]

Vitamin C
- Alcoholism, anaemia, cancer, haemodialysis, hyperthyroidism, malabsorption, rheumatoid disease[45] and women using the oral contraceptive pill, while acute infection and stress may increase urinary excretion[35]
- Deficiency can occur secondary to some disease states such as liver disease, cancer, gastrointestinal disorders and cigarette smoking, as well as environmental exposure[35]
- Aspirin usage[211]
- Excess iron and copper[203]
- Pregnancy also lowers serum levels due to haemodilution and active transfer to the fetus, especially during the last trimester[35]

Vitamin D
- Nephrotic syndrome, advanced renal failure, chronic liver diseases and severe small-bowel disease, Fanconi syndrome, vitamin D-dependent rickets type I, neonatal hypocalcaemia, osteomalacia, osteoporosis, renal osteodystrophy[212]
- Bowel resection, coeliac disease, inflammatory bowel disease, malabsorption, pancreatic insufficiency, thyrotoxicosis[45]
- Magnesium deficiency, which may be due to both the decrease in parathyroid hormone (PTH) secretion and a renal resistance to PTH[213]
- Lack of exposure to ultraviolet light combined with a bad diet[214]

Vitamin E
- Fat malabsorption syndromes such as coeliac disease, cystic fibrosis and chronic cholestatic liver disease,[215] chronic pancreatitis, pancreatic carcinoma and chronic cholestasis,[45] gastric surgery and alcoholism[201]
- Abetalipoproteinaemia, which involves a defect in chylomicron synthesis, hyperthyroidism, cirrhosis of the liver, hereditary spherocytosis and β-thalassaemia, as well as associated with conditions such as bronchopulmonary dysplasia and retrolental fibroplasia[212]
- Protein–energy malnutrition,[216] premature[217] and low-birthweight infants[218] and children with cystic fibrosis are often found to have a vitamin E deficiency, which may also occur in children with chronic cholestasis[219]
- Obstructive liver disease may increase levels[45]
- Increased values occur in primary hyperparathyroidism associated with hypophosphataemia, vitamin D-dependent rickets type II or sarcoidosis[213]

Vitamin K
- Chronic fat malabsorption, liver disease, primary biliary cirrhosis, cancer, surgery and chronic alcoholism,[27] Crohn's disease, ulcerative colitis, chronic gastrointestinal diseases or resection,[220] obstructive jaundice, pancreatic disease, diarrhoea in infants, haemorrhagic disease of the newborn, hypoprothrombinaemia[45]

- Subjects treated with antibiotics for extended periods, as approximately half of vitamin K intake is provided by bacterial synthesis in the jejunum and ileum[27]
- Ingestion of supraphysiological doses of vitamins A and E[221] may inhibit by competitive mechanisms

Magnesium

- Cardiovascular disease, myocardial infarction, toxaemia of pregnancy, hypertension or post-surgical complications, excessive vomiting and/or diarrhoea and burns, protein malnutrition, malabsorption syndromes, endocrine disorders such as diabetes mellitus, parathyroid disease, hyperparathyroidism with hypercalcaemia, hyperthyroidism and hyperaldosteronism,[191,222] as well as with alcoholism, chronic glomerulonephritis, haemodialysis, pancreatitis, severe loss of body fluids as in diarrhoea, sweating and laxative abuse[45]
- Pregnancy and lactation[45]
- High levels of carbohydrates and ethanol[223]
- Diets high in caffeine, calcium, protein,[224] although intakes of protein < 30 g/day may also reduce magnesium absorption[35]
- High dietary fibre, phytate, oxalate and phosphate intakes reduce magnesium absorption by binding cations[225]
- Potassium depletion[195] and hypophosphataemia stimulates magnesium excretion[226]
- Magnesium also shares a common renal reabsorption pathway with sodium and increased sodium results in magnesuria[221]
- May be increased in Addison's disease, adrenocortical insufficiency, severe diabetic acidosis, multiple myeloma, overuse of antacids, renal insufficiency, systemic lupus erythematosus, tissue trauma,[195] increased PTH,[191] hypocalcaemia, fluid depletion and hypothyroidism (which inhibits magnesium excretion)[222]

Calcium

- Hypoparathyroidism,[27] hypomagnesaemia,[218] phosphate supplementation and impaired vitamin D synthesis are also associated with depression of serum calcium levels[17]
- Acute pancreatitis malabsorption is associated with gastrointestinal diseases such as Crohn's and coeliac disease, intestinal resection or bypass and patients with renal failure caused by the reduced synthesis of 1,25-dihydroxyvitamin D[173]
- Calcium absorption may also be decreased with age, diabetes, chronic renal failure, nontropical sprue and primary biliary cirrhosis[27]; low-protein diets can also affect calcium absorption[214] and cause decrease in bone mineral density[227]
- Diets high in protein increase the urinary excretion of calcium, which is not compensated by increased calcium absorption[228]; caffeine and sodium also increase urinary losses, while high phosphorus intakes reduce urinary losses although increases faecal losses, which may negate any effects on calcium balance[191]
- Calcium absorption in the intestine also may be inhibited by the presence of oxalate, which is found in a variety of vegetables such as spinach, beets, celery, eggplant, greens, okra and squash, as well as fruits such as strawberries, blackberries, blueberries, gooseberries and currants, nuts such as pecans and peanuts, and beverages such as tea, Ovaltine and cocoa; oxalate chelates calcium and increases faecal excretion of the complex[191]

- Divalent cations such as magnesium and calcium compete for intestinal absorption whenever an excess of either is in the gastrointestinal tract, while diets high in phosphorus relative to calcium have also been shown to impair calcium balance[191]
- Hyperparathyroidism is the most common cause of hypercalcaemia[27]
- Elevated serum levels occur in association with hyperthyroidism, sarcoidosis and also when large parts of the body are immobilised, as well as in vitamin D intoxication and in patients with kidney stones, usually due to excessive absorption[35]

Zinc

- Malabsorption syndromes such as Crohn's disease, short bowel syndrome and cystic fibrosis.[218] Increased urinary losses occur in alcohol, cirrhosis, infections, diabetes mellitus, renal tubular diseases, anorexia, starvation, catabolism such as burns, dialysis, pregnancy, oral contraceptives and hypoalbuminaemia[201]
- Disease processes such as infection, surgery, pancreatic insufficiency and alcoholism may sometimes alter zinc absorption in humans[229]
- Gastric acid secretion inhibition, phytate such as in soy protein, fibre in wheat and cornflour, tea, coffee, cheeses and cow's milk, calcium supplements and pregnancy[230]
- As albumin appears to be the major portal carrier for newly absorbed zinc, changes in the systemic level of albumin such as inflammation or protein deficiency may also alter zinc balance,[230] while high levels of protein intake enhance urinary excretion[228]
- Inorganic iron in pharmacological doses may increase zinc uptake, while other studies suggest haem iron has the same effect[230]

Iron

- Lead poisoning may also be associated with iron deficiency as absorption of lead may be increased in iron deficiency, since lead and iron share a common absorptive mechanism whose activity is enhanced in iron deficiency[231]
- Copper and vitamin A deficiencies can diminish iron status,[232] while intermediate to high levels of manganese interfere with iron metabolism as shown by decreased haemoglobin concentrations and reversal by dietary iron supplementation[233]
- High levels of zinc also decrease iron bioavailability, but it is not entirely clear whether this is a direct effect or is mediated indirectly through the copper effect on iron metabolism[233]; a ratio of 3:1 iron to zinc is desirable to prevent competitive interference[234]
- Ascorbic acid enhances the absorption of non-haem iron from foods consumed at the same meal, while absorption of haem iron is not affected by vitamin C intake[232]

Selenium

- Catabolic states and deficiency over time may occur with increased oxidative stress and a concurrent inadequate dietary intake[17]
- Premature infants are found to have lower plasma concentrations of selenium and glutathione peroxidase than full-term infants. To compound this problem, other commonly used supplements such as iron, calcium and phosphate may impair selenium absorption. These infants also have an increased need because of the high risk of oxidative diseases, such as bronchopulmonary dysplasia and retinopathy[16]
- Other groups prone to a low status include low-birthweight neonates, alcoholics, patients with Down syndrome or acquired immune deficiency disease, as well as those with malabsorption syndromes such as coeliac disease and cystic fibrosis[35]

- Iron deficiency may be affecting selenium absorption or increasing selenium use in the body. Another possibility is that iron or an iron-containing protein may be needed for glutathione peroxidase activity[191]

Iodine
- Secondary iodine deficiency may develop in the presence of a number of diseases of the thyroid gland, pituitary or hypothalamus[35]
- Goitrogens, which inhibit iodine activity, occur naturally in foods such as cabbage, broccoli, turnips and cauliflower, as well as soybeans and bacterial products of *Escherichia coli* in drinking water[235]
- In populations with a high intake of cassava, the thiocyanate present may act as a goitrogen and impair the uptake of iodine by the thyroid gland[27]
- Iodide forms of iodine in large doses have the potential to block the synthesis of thyroid hormone, usually temporarily, after which hormone synthesis resumes[236]

Essential fatty acids
- Malabsorption, obesity-related bypass surgery, alcoholism, malignancy, biliary disease and multiple sclerosis, while surgery and trauma patients need increases up to fivefold[201]

CHOOSING DIAGNOSTIC METHODS

There is a vast array of diagnostic tools and techniques available to clinicians; these are best used in combination. When interpreted alone many have explicit shortcomings due to the lack of available evidence of efficacy. Each person's needs should be evaluated and investigations adjusted accordingly, always keeping in mind what level of evidence is available, as well as the relative strengths and weaknesses of each. It is essential to always be mindful of the costs (Table 2.8) associated with pathology testing and only make use of these if necessary to investigate a particular condition or dysfunction, if the results will determine the mode of treatment. If a particular test will have no bearing on the management plan, it is unnecessary to have these carried out. It is likely that patients have already had a test, if not a number of them, performed by their general practitioners and in these cases it is beneficial to seek the results.

It is always important to consider biological individuality, where diagnostic tools and treatments should be tailored to suit individual needs and not have individuals fit into specific predetermined treatment protocols. Naturopaths should also always be clear to patients as to whether diagnostic techniques are 'orthodox' or 'naturopathic' practices.

Consider cost
While modern technology may provide added diagnostic techniques that may be valuable, they may also be expensive. Naturopaths should be judicious regarding which tests they advise their patients to undertake to avoid overburdening their patients financially personally, or if publicly subsidised to ensure limited public funds are diverted to those who need them most. Naturopathic diagnosis should always be founded on solid case-taking skills. While tests are invaluable in specific scenarios, in many cases a thorough case history and physical examination will elicit the same information as many diagnostic tests.

Table 2.8
Review of the major evidence

Technique	Evidence	Comment	Evidence rating
Anthropometric data	Established public health application	Has a valuable place in clinical assessment	4–5
Body signs and symptoms	Semi-established public health applications	Some controlled studies with mixed results	3–4
Palpation	Established traditional use in orthodox medicine	Semi-established public health applications	3–4
Dietary assessment	Controlled studies with mixed results	Strength varies depending on method	3–4
Pathology testing	Several robust controlled studies, established public health application	Strength depending on method and adequacy for particular investigation	4–5
Bioelectrical impedance for body composition	Several studies have established the validity of a variety of equations utilised based on study population	Has a place in clinical assessment with the consideration of underlying pathology	4

Evidence rating: 1 = poor (no clinical studies, mainly anecdotal), 2 = average (open studies, some traditional evidence), 3 = moderate (some controlled studies with mixed results, established traditional use), 4 = good (controlled studies with mainly positive results, semi-established public health applications), 5 = strong (several robust controlled studies, established public health application)

KEY POINTS

- Naturopathic practice often uses a variety of 'evidence-based clinical' and 'traditional' techniques.
- Consider the levels of evidence and limitations to methods.
- Only use extra, costly diagnostic tools if it is likely that the technique will positively benefit the diagnosis and treatment of the patient.
- Individualise the use of diagnostic techniques for different patients and health conditions.
- Use diagnostic techniques holistically, professionally and sensitively.

FURTHER READING

Fenech M, et al. Nutrigenetics and nutrigenomics: viewpoints on the current status and applications in nutrition research and practice. J Nutrigenet Nutrigenomics 2011;4:69–89.

Hughes HK, Kahl L. The Harriet Lane handbook. 21st ed. USA: Elsevier; 2017.

Lord RS, Bralley JA. Laboratory evaluations for integrative and functional medicine. Canada: Metametrix Institute; 2008.

Royal College of Pathologists of Australasia. RCPA Manual; 2018. Online. Available: https://www.rcpa.edu.au/Manuals/RCPA-Manual.

Sim S, Kacevska M, Ingleman-Sundberg M. Pharmacogenomics of drug-metabolizing enzymes: a recent update on clinical implications and endogenous effects. Pharmacogenomics J 2013;13:1–11.

Walls R, Hockberger R, Gausche-Hill M. Rosen's emergency medicine. 9th ed. USA: Elsevier; 2017.

REFERENCES

1. Model D. Making sense of clinical examination of the adult patient. New York: Oxford University Press; 2006.
2. Olgilvie C, Evans CC. Symptoms and signs in clinical medicine; an introduction to medical diagnostics. 12th ed. Oxford: Butterworth–Heinemann; 1997.
3. Welsby PD. Clinical history taking and examination. New York: Churchill Livingstone; 1995.
4. Toghill P. First impressions. In: Toghill PJ, editor. Examining patients: an introduction to clinical medicine. London: Edward Arnold; 1995.

5. World Health Organization. Clinical assessment of nutritional status. AJPH 1973;63(Suppl.):18–27.

6. Welborn T, Satvinder S, Dhaliwal S, et al. Waist–hip ratio is the dominant risk factor predicting cardiovascular death in Australia. Med J Aust 2003;179(11):580–5.

7. Sun SS, Chumlea WC, Heymsfield SB, et al. Development of bioelectrical impedance analysis prediction equations for body composition with the use of a multicomponent model for use in epidemiologic surveys.[see comment]. Am J Clin Nutr 2003;77(2):331–40.

8. Boneva-Asiova Z, Boyanov MA. Body composition analysis by leg-to-leg bioelectrical impedance and dual-energy X-ray absorptiometry in non-obese and obese individuals. Diabetes Obes Metab 2008;10(11):1012–18.

9. Jaffrin MY, Morel H. Body fluid volumes measurements by impedance: a review of bioimpedance spectroscopy (BIS) and bioimpedance analysis (BIA) methods. Med Eng Phys 2008;30(10):1257–69.

10. Jarvis C. Physical examination and health assessment. St Louis: Elsevier Saunders; 2007.

11. Goldman L, Schafer AI. Goldman's cecil medicine. USA: Elsevier; 2012.

12. Marx JA, Hockberger RS, Walls RM, et al, editors. Rosen's emergency medicine. USA: Elsevier; 2009.

13. Weingberger SE, Cockrill BA, Mandel J. Principles of pulmonary medicine. 5th ed. USA: Elsevier; 2008.

14. John Hopkins Hospital KA, Megan Tschudy. The Harriet Lane handbook. 19th ed. USA: Mosby; 2011.

15. Mertz W. Metabolism and metabolic effects of trace elements. Trace elements in nutrition of children, vol. 8. New York: Raven press; 1985. p. 107–17.

16. Salmenpera L. Detecting subclinical deficiency of essential trace elements in children with special reference to zinc and selenium. Clin Biochem 1997;30(2):115–20.

17. Prelack K, Sheridan RL. Micronutrient supplementation in the critically ill patient: strategies for clinical practice. J Trauma 2001;51(3):601–20.

18. Chandra RK, Sarchielli P. Immunocompetence methodology immunity. In: Fidanza F, editor. Nutritional status assessment—a manual for population studies. London: Chapman & Hall; 1991. p. 425–41.

19. Holmes S. Undernutrition in hospital patients. Nurs Stand 2003;17(19):45–52.

20. Golden M. Severe malnutrition. In: Weatherall D, Ledingham J, Warrell D, editors. Oxford textbook of medicine, vol. 1. 3rd ed. 1995. p. 1279–80.

21. Golden MH. Malnutrition. In: Guandalini S, editor. Textbook of pediatric gastroenterology and nutrition. London: Taylor & Francis; 2004. p. 489–525.

22. Mejia L. Vitamin A-nutrient interrelationships. In: Bauernfeind J, editor. Vitamin A deficiency and its control. Orlando: Academic Press; 1986.

23. Lukaski HC, Penland JG. Functional changes appropriate for determining mineral element requirements. J Nutr 1996;126(9S):2354S.

24. Kushner I. The phenomenon of the acute phase response. C-reactive protein and the plasma protein response to tissue injury. Ann N Y Acad Sci 1982;389:39–48.

25. Wieringa FT, Dijkhuizen MA, West CE, et al. Estimation of the effect of the acute phase response on indicators of micronutrient status in indonesian infants. J Nutr 2002;132(10):3061–6.

26. Shenkin A. Trace elements and inflammatory response: implications for nutritional support. Nutrition 1995; 11(1 Suppl.):100–5.

27. Sauberlich HE. Laboratory tests for the assessment of nutritional status. 2nd ed. USA: CRC Press; 1999.

28. Maehira F, Miyagi I, Eguchi Y. Selenium regulates transcription factor NF-kappa B activation during the acute phase reaction. Clin Chim Acta 2003;334(1–2):163–71.

29. Waldron J, Ashby H, Cornes M. Vitamin D: a negative acute phase reactant. J Clin Pathol 2013;66(7):120–2.

30. Louw JA, Werbeck A, Louw ME, et al. Blood vitamin concentrations during the acute-phase response. Crit Care Med 1992;20(7):934–41.

31. Tomkins A. Assessing micronutrient status in the presence of inflammation. J Nutr 2003;133(5 Suppl. 2):1649S–55S.

32. Ruz M, Cavan KR, Bettger WJ, et al. Development of a dietary model for the study of mild zinc deficiency in humans and evaluation of some biochemical and functional indices of zinc status. Am J Clin Nutr 1991;53(5): 1295–303.

33. Hambidge M. Biomarkers of trace mineral intake and status. J Nutr 2003;133(Suppl. 3):948S–55S.

34. Fell G, Talwar D. Assessment of status. Curr Opin Clin Nutr Metab Care 1998;1(6):491–7.

35. Gibson R. Principles of nutritional assessment. 2nd ed. USA: Oxford University Press; 2005.

36. Bates C. Vitamin analysis. Ann Clin Biochem 1997;34: 599–626.

37. Shenkin A, Baines M, Fell GS, et al. Vitamins and trace elements. In: Burtis C, Ashwood E, Bruns D, editors. Tietz textbook of clinical chemistry and molecular diagnostics. 4th ed. Missouri: Elsevier Saunders; 2006.

38. Rosales FJ, Chau KK, Haskell MH, et al. Determination of a Cut-Off value for the molar ratio of Retinol-Binding protein to transthyretin (RBP:TTR) in Bangladeshi patients with low hepatic vitamin a stores. J Nutr 2002;132(12):3687–92.

39. Shenkin A. The key role of micronutrients. Clin Nutr 2006;25(1):1–13.

40. Bates C, Schrijver J, Speek A, et al. Vitamin C. In: Fidanza F, editor. Nutritional status assessment—a manual for population studies. London: Chapman & Hall; 1991. p. 309–19.

41. Maiani G, Raguzzini A, Mobarhan S, et al. Vitamin A. Int J Vitam Nutr Res 1993;63(4):252–7.

42. Talwar D, Ha T, Scott H, et al. Effect of inflammation on measures of antioxidant status in patients with non-small cell lung cancer. Am J Clin Nutr 1997;66(5):1283–5.

43. Ganther HE. Selenium and glutathione peroxidase in health and disease: a review. In: Prasad AS, Oberleas D, editors. Trace elements in human health and disease, vol. 2. New York: Academic Press; 1976.

44. Spencer CA, Wang CC. Thyroglobulin measurement. Techniques, clinical benefits, and pitfalls. Endocrinol Metab Clin North Am 1995;24(4):841–63.

45. Van Leeuwen A, Kranpitz T, Smith L. Davis's comprehensive handbook of laboratory and diagnostic tests with nursing implications. 2nd ed. Philadelphia: FA Davis Company; 2006.

46. Skikne BS, Flowers CH, Cook JD. Serum transferrin receptor: a quantitative measure of tissue iron deficiency. Blood 1990;75(9):1870–6.

47. Sweetman L. Qualitative and quantitative analysis of organic acids in physiologic fluids for diagnosis of the organic acidurias. In: Nyhan W, editor. Abnormalities in amino acid metabolism in clinical medicine. Norwalk: Appleton-Century-Crofts; 1984. p. 419–53.

48. Krall EA, Dwyer JT, Coleman KA. Factors influencing accuracy of dietary recall. Nutr Res 1988;8(7):829–41.

49. Nelson M. Methods and validity of dietary assessment. In: Garrow JS, James WPT, Ralph A, editors. Human nutrition and dietetics. Edinburgh: Churchill Livingstone; 2000. p. 311–31.

50. Food Standards Australia New Zealand. NUTTAB data base. Online. Available: http://www.foodstandards.gov.au/monitoringandsurveillance/nuttab2006 1 Nov 2013.

51. Agricultural Research Service. USDA Nutrient Database. Online. Available: http://www.nal.usda.gov/fnic/foodcomp/search/ 1 Nov 2013.

52. Health Canada. The Canadian Nutrient File. Online. Available: http://www.hc-sc.gc.ca/fn-an/nutrition/fiche-nutri-data/index-eng.php 1 Nov 2013.

53. European Food Information Resource Network. Food Composition Databases. Online. Available: http://www.eurofir.net/public.asp?id=8778 1 Nov 2013.

54. Irwin JJ, Kirchner JT. Anemia in children. Am Fam Physician 2001;64(8):1379–86.

55. Barceloux DG. Cobalt. J Toxicol Clin Toxicol 1999;37(2):201–6.

56. Kaemmerer H, Fratz S, Braun SL, et al. Erythrocyte indexes, iron metabolism, and hyperhomocysteinemia in adults with cyanotic congenital cardiac disease. Am J Cardiol 2004;94(6):825–8.

57. Olde Damink SW, Jalan R, Deutz NE, et al. Isoleucine infusion during 'simulated' upper gastrointestinal bleeding improves liver and muscle protein synthesis in cirrhotic patients. Hepatology 2007;45(3):560–8.

58. Kriengsinyos W, Rafii M, Wykes LJ, et al. Long-term effects of histidine depletion on whole-body protein metabolism in healthy adults. J Nutr 2002;132(11):3340–8.

59. Trnovsky J, Letourneau R, Haggag E, et al. Quercetin-induced expression of rat mast cell protease II and accumulation of secretory granules in rat basophilic leukemia cells. Biochem Pharmacol 1993;46(12):2315–26.

60. Taylor CG, Giesbrecht JA. Dietary zinc deficiency and expression of T lymphocyte signal transduction proteins. Can J Physiol Pharmacol 2000;78(10):823–8.

61. Provinciali M, Montenovo A, Di Stefano G, et al. Effect of zinc or zinc plus arginine supplementation on antibody titre and lymphocyte subsets after influenza vaccination in elderly subjects: a randomized controlled trial. Age Ageing 1998;27(6):715–22.

62. Kramer TR, Udomkesmalee E, Dhanamitta S, et al. Lymphocyte responsiveness of children supplemented with vitamin A and zinc. Am J Clin Nutr 1993;58(4):566–70.

63. Talley NJ, O'Connor S. Clinical examination. 4th ed. New Delhi: JP Brothers; 2003.

64. Doust JA. Evaluation of the Clinical Effectiveness of Tests. Pathology 2013;45.

65. Gallagher R, Pollard L, Scott A, et al. Laboratory analysis of organic acids, 2018 update: a technical standard of the American College of Medical Genetics and Genomics. Genet Med 2018;Epub ahead of print.

66. Newman M, Gordon S, Suen R. Urinary organic acid analysis: a powerful clinical tool, potentially muddled by poor testing methods. Seattle: US BioTek Laboratories; 2004.

67. Lord RS, Bralley JA. Clinical applications of urinary organic acids. Part I: detoxification markers. Altern Med Rev 2008;13(3):205–15.

68. Johnson DW. Contemporary clinical usage of LC/MS: analysis of biologically important carboxylic acids. Clin Biochem 2005;38(4):351–61.

69. Kumps A, Duez P, Mardens Y. Metabolic, nutritional, iatrogenic, and artifactual sources of urinary organic acids: a comprehensive table. Clin Chem 2002;48(5):708–17.

70. Obeid R, Geisel J, Herrmann W. Comparison of two methods for measuring methylmalonic acid as a marker for vitamin B12 deficiency. Diagnosis 2015;2(1):667–72.

71. Inouye M, Mio T, Sumino K. Dicarboxylic acids as markers of fatty acid peroxidation in diabetes. Atherosclerosis 2000; 148(1):197–202.

72. Peters V, Garbade SF, Langhans CD, et al. Qualitative urinary organic acid analysis: methodological approaches and performance. J Inherit Metab Dis 2008;31(6):690–6.

73. O'Reilly PO, Hughes G, Russell RT, et al. The mauve factor: an evaluation. Dis Nerv Syst 1965;26(9):562–8.

74. Sohler A, Beck R, Noval JJ. Mauve factor re-identified as 2,4-dimethyl-3-ethylpyrrole and its sedative effect on the CNS. Nature 1970;228(5278):1318–20.

75. Mirikova N. Clinical tests of pyrroles: usefulness and association with other biochemical markers. Clin Med Rev Case Rep 2015;2(2).

76. Hoffer A, Osmond H. The association between schizophrenia and two objective tests. Can Med Assoc J 1962;87:641–6.

77. Jackson JA, Riordan HD, Neathery S. Vitamin, blood lead, and urine pyrrole levels in Down syndrome. Am Clin Lab 1990;8–9.

78. Isaacson IIR, Moran MM, Hall A. Autism: a retrospective outcome study of nutrient therapy. J Appl Nutr 1996; 110–18.

79. Cutler P. Pyridoxine and trace element therapy in selected clinical cases. J Orthomolec Psychiatr 1974;89–95.

80. Huszak I, Durko I, Karsai K. Experimental data to the pathogenesis of cryptopyrrole excretion in schizophrenia, I. Acta Physiol Acad Sci Hung 1972;42(1):79–86.

81. McGinnis WR, Audhya T, Walsh WJ, et al. Discerning the mauve factor, part 1. Altern Ther Health Med 2008;14(2):40–50.

82. Mirikova N. Clinical tests of pyrroles: usefulness and association with other biochemical markers. Clin Med Rev Case Rep 2015;2(2).

83. Hoffer A. The presence of malvaria in some mentally retarded children. Am J Ment Defic 1963;67:730–2.

84. Pfeiffer CC, Jenney EH. Letter: fingernail white spots: possible zinc deficiency. JAMA 1974;228(2):157.

85. Ames BN, Atamna H, Killilea DW. Mineral and vitamin deficiencies can accelerate the mitochondrial decay of aging. Mol Aspects Med 2005;26(4–5):363–78.

86. Stuckey R, Walsh W, Lambert B. The effectiveness of targeted nutrient therapy in treatment of mental illness. ACNEM 2010;29(8):3–8.

87. Mirikova N. Clinical tests of pyrroles: usefulness and association with other biochemical markers. Clin Med Rev Case Rep 2015;2(2).

88. Zaglool DA, Khodari YA, Gazzaz ZJ, et al. Prevalence of intestinal parasites among patients of Al-Noor specialist Hospital, Makkah, Saudi Arabia. Oman Med J 2011;26(3):182–5.

89. Amin OM. Evaluation of a new system for the fixation, concentration, and staining of intestinal parasites in fecal specimens, with critical observations on the trichrome stain. J Microbiol Methods 2000;39(2):127–32.

90. Vilela EG, Torres HO, Martins FP, et al. Evaluation of inflammatory activity in Crohn's disease and ulcerative colitis. World J Gastroenterol 2012;18(9):872–81.

91. Hol L, van Leerdam ME, van Ballegooijen M, et al. Screening for colorectal cancer: randomised trial comparing guaiac-based and immunochemical faecal occult blood testing and flexible sigmoidoscopy. Gut 2010;59(1):62–8.

92. Topping DL, Clifton PM. Short-chain fatty acids and human colonic function: roles of resistant starch and nonstarch polysaccharides. Physiol Rev 2001;81(3):1031–64.

93. Steffer KJ, Santa Ana CA, Cole JA, et al. The practical value of comprehensive stool analysis in detecting the cause of idiopathic chronic diarrhea. Gastroenterol Clin North Am 2012;41(3):539–60.

94. Kristin Y. Characteristics associated with comprehensive stool analysis findings in adult integrative medicine patients. Kansas: University of Kansas; 2011.

95. Duvallet C, Gibbons S, Gurry T, et al. Meta-analysis of gut microbiome studies identifies disease-specific and shared responses. Nat Commun 2017;8(1).

96. Atkinson W, Sheldon TA, Shaath N, et al. Food elimination based on IgG antibodies in irritable bowel syndrome: a randomised controlled trial. Gut 2004;53(10):1459–64.

97. Alpay K, Ertas M, Orhan EK, et al. Diet restriction in migraine, based on IgG against foods: a clinical double-blind, randomised, cross-over trial. Cephalalgia 2010;30(7):829–37.

98. Chafen JJ, Newberry SJ, Riedl MA, et al. Diagnosing and managing common food allergies: a systematic review. JAMA 2010;303(18):1848–56.

99. Host A, Husby S, Gjesing B, et al. Prospective estimation of IgG, IgG subclass and IgE antibodies to dietary proteins in infants with cow milk allergy. Levels of antibodies to whole milk protein, BLG and ovalbumin in relation to repeated milk challenge and clinical course of cow milk allergy. Allergy 1992;47(3):218–29.

100. Zar S, Benson MJ, Kumar D. Food-specific serum IgG4 and IgE titers to common food antigens in irritable bowel syndrome. Am J Gastroenterol 2005;100(7):1550–7.

101. Mitchell N, Hewitt CE, Jayakody S, et al. Randomised controlled trial of food elimination diet based on IgG antibodies for the prevention of migraine like headaches. Nutr J 2011;10:85.

102. Teuber SS, Porch-Curren C. Unproved diagnostic and therapeutic approaches to food allergy and intolerance. Curr Opin Allergy Clin Immunol 2003;3(3):217–21.

103. Hochwallner H, Schulmeister U, Swoboda I, et al. Patients suffering from non-IgE-mediated cow's milk protein intolerance cannot be diagnosed based on IgG subclass or IgA responses to milk allergens. Allergy 2011;66(9):1201–7.

104. Carr S, Chan E, Lavine E, et al. CSACI Position statement on the testing of food-specific IgG. Allergy Asthma Clin Immunol. 2012;8(1):12.

105. Stapel SO, Asero R, Ballmer-Weber BK, et al. Testing for IgG4 against foods is not recommended as a diagnostic tool: EAACI Task Force Report. Allergy 2008;63(7):793–6.

106. Bock SA. AAAAI support of the EAACI Position Paper on IgG4. J Allergy Clin Immunol 2010;125(6):1410.

107. Lomer M. Review article: the aetiology, diagnosis, mechanisms and clinical evidence for food intolerance. Aliment Pharmacol Ther 2015;41(3):262–75.

108. Zeng Q, Dong S-Y, Wu LX. Variable food-specific IgG antibody levels in healthy and symptomatic Chinese adults. PLOS ONE 2013;8(1).

109. Gibson PR, Shepherd SJ. Evidence-based dietary management of functional gastrointestinal symptoms: the FODMAP approach. J Gastroenterol Hepatol 2010;25(2):252–8.

110. Ong DK, Mitchell SB, Barrett JS, et al. Manipulation of dietary short chain carbohydrates alters the pattern of gas production and genesis of symptoms in irritable bowel syndrome. J Gastroenterol Hepatol 2010;25(8):1366–73.

111. Barrett JS, Gibson PR. Fermentable oligosaccharides, disaccharides, monosaccharides and polyols (FODMAPs) and nonallergic food intolerance: FODMAPs or food chemicals? Therap Adv Gastroenterol 2012;5(4):261–8.

112. Teitelbaum JE, Ubhrani D. Triple sugar screen breath hydrogen test for sugar intolerance in children with functional abdominal symptoms. Indian J Gastroenterol 2010;29(5):196–200.

113. Paterson W, Camilleri M, Simren M, et al. Breath testing consensus guidelines for SIBO. Am J Gastroenterol 2017;112:1888–9.

114. Yao C, Tuck C. The clinical value of breath hydrogen testing. J Gastroenterol Hepatol 2017;32(1):20–2.

115. Pimentel M. Breath testing for small intestinal bacterial overgrowth: should we bother? Am J Gastroenterol 2016;111(3):307–8.

116. Lac G. Saliva assays in clinical and research biology. Pathol Biol (Paris) 2001;49(8):660–7.

117. Vining RF, McGinley RA. The measurement of hormones in saliva: possibilities and pitfalls. J Steroid Biochem 1987;27(1–3):81–94.

118. Jenkins DW Toxic trace metals in mammalian hair and nails. In: Agency UEP, ed. Vol Number 6001/4–79–0491979.

119. Haddy T, Czajka-Narins D, Sky-Peck H, et al. Minerals in hair, serum and urine of healthy and anemic black children. Public Health Rep 1991;106(5):557–63.

120. Rivlin RS. Misuse of hair analysis for nutritional assessment. Am J Med 1983;75(3):489–93.

121. Sahin C, Pala C, Kaynar L, et al. Measurement of hair iron concentration as a marker of body iron content. Biomed Rep 2015;3(3):383–7.

122. Kim J, Yoo S, Jeong M, et al. Hair zinc levels and the efficacy of oral zinc supplementation in children with atopic dermatitis. Acta Derm Venereol 2014;94:558–62.

123. Sarris J, Ng C, Schweitzer I. 'Omic' genetic technologies for herbal medicines in psychiatry. Phytother Res 2012;26(4):522–7.

124. Subbiah R. Nutrigenetics and nutraceuticals: the next wave riding on personalized medicine. Transl Res 2007;149:55–61.

125. Kussmann M, Krause L, Siffert W. Nutrigenomics: where are we with genetic and epigenetic markers for disposition and susceptibility? Nutr Rev 2010;68(Suppl. 1):S38–47.

126. Ames BN. Low micronutrient intake may accelerate the degenerative diseases of aging through allocation of scarce micronutrients by triage. Proc Natl Acad Sci USA 2006;103(47):17589–94.

127. Fenech M. Genome health nutrigenomics and nutrigenetics—diagnosis and nutritional treatment of genome damage on an individual basis. Food Chem Toxicol 2007;46:1365–70.

128. Fenech M. The genome health clinic and genome health nutrigenomics concepts: diagnosos and nutritional treatment of genome and epigenome damage on an individual basis. Mutagenesis 2005;20(4):255–69.

129. Huang WX, Wood C, L'Abbe MR, et al. Soy protein isolate increases hepatic thyroid hormone receptor content and inhibits its binding to target genes in rats. J Nutr 2005;135(7):1631–5.

130. Kitajka K, Sinclair AJ, Weisinger RS, et al. Effects of dietary omega-3 polyunsaturated fatty acids on brain gene expression. Proc Natl Acad Sci USA 2004;101:10931–6.

131. Mezei O, Li Y, Mullen E, et al. Dietary isoflavone supplementation modulates lipid metabolism via PPAR alpha-dependent and -independent mechanisms. Physiol Genomics 2006;26(1):8–14.

132. Vissac-Sabatier C, Bignon YJ, Bernard-Gallon DJ. Effects of the phytoestrogens genistein and daidzein on BRCA2 tumor suppressor gene expression in breast cell lines. Nutr Cancer 2003;45(2):247–55.

133. Shay NF, Banz WJ. Regulation of gene transcription by botanicals: novel regulatory mechanisms. Annu Rev Nutr 2005;25:297–315.

134. Rimbach G, Wolffram S, Watanabe C, et al. Effect of Ginkgo biloba (EGb 761 (R)) on differential gene expression. Pharmacopsychiatry 2003;36:S95–9.

135. Marambaud P, Zhao HT, Davies P. Resveratrol promotes clearance of Alzheimer's disease amyloid-beta peptides. J Biol Chem 2005;280(45):37377–82.

136. Peshel D, Koerting R, Nass N. Curcumin induces changes in expression of genes involved in cholesterol homeostasis. J Nutr Biochem 2006.

137. Milner J. Chapter 2—Nutrigenomics and nutrigenetics. In: Heber D, Blackburn G, Go V, et al, editors. Nutritional oncology. 2nd ed. Burlington: Academic Press; 2006. p. 15–24.

138. Boekholdt S. Cholesterol ester transfer protein Taq1B variant, HDL cholesterol levels, CV risk and efficacy of pravastatin treatment: individual patient meta-analysis of 13677 subjects. Circulation 2005;111(3):278–87.

139. Jansen H. Common C-to-T substitution at position-480 of the hepatic lipase promoter associated with a lowered lipase activity in coronary artery disease patients. Arterioscler Thromb Vasc Biol 1997;17:2837–42.

140. Mackness B, Durrington P, McElduff P, et al. Low paraoxonase activity predicts coronary events in the Caerphilly Prospective Study. Circulation 2003;107:2775–9.

141. San Jose G. NADPH oxidase CYBA polymorphisms, oxidative stress and cardiovascular diseases. Clin Sci 2008;114:173–82.

142. Norat T, Bowman R, Luben R, et al. Blood pressure and interactions between the angiotensin polymorphism AGT M235T and sodium intake: a cross-sectional study. Am J Clin Nutr 2008;88(2):392–7.

143. Fung M. Early inflammatory and metabolic changes in association with AGTR1 polymorphisms in prehypertensive subjects. Am J Hypertens 2011;24(2):225–33.

144. Casas J. Endothelial nitric oxide synthase gene polymorphisms and cardiovascular disease: a HUGE review. Am J Epidemiol 2006;164(10):921–35.

145. Daniele A, Divella R, Paradiso A, et al. Serotonin transporter polymorphism in major depressive disorder (MDD), psychiatric disorders, and in MDD in response to stressful life events: causes and treatment with antidepressant. In Vivo 2011;25(6):895–901.

146. Wassink T, Piven J, Vieland V, et al. Evaluation of the chromosome 2q37.3 gene CENTG2 as an autism susceptibility gene. Am J Med Genet B Neuropsychiatr Genet 2005;136B(1):36–44.

147. Moskvina V, Craddock N, Holmans P, et al. Gene-wide analyses of genome-wide association data sets: evidence for multiple common risk alleles for schizophrenia and bipolar disorder and for overlap in genetic risk. Mol Psychiatry 2009;14(3):252–60.

148. Liu G, Zhang S, Cai Z, et al. PICALM Gene rs3851179 Polymorphism contributes to Alzheimer's disease in an Asian population. Neuromolecular Med 2013;15(2):384–8.

149. Shin M. The association of SNP276G>T at adiponectin gene with circulating adiponectin and insulin resistance in response to mild weight loss. Int J Obesity 2008;30:1702–8.

150. Arner P, Hoffstedr J. Aderenoceptor genes in human obesity. J Intern Med 1999;245:667–72.

151. Hoffstedr J. Polymorphism of the human beta3-adrenoceptor gene forms a well-conserved haplotype that is associated with moderate obesity and altered receptor function. Diabetes 1999;48(1):203–5.

152. Weiss E. FABP2 Ala54Thr genotype is associated with glucoregulatory function and lipid oxidation after a high fat meal in sedentary nondiabetic men and women. Am J Clin Nutr 2007;85:102–8.

153. Qi L. The common obesity variant near MC4R gene is associated with higher intakes of total energy and dietary fat, weight change and diabetes risk in women. Hum Mol Genet 2008;17:3502–8.

154. Tanofsky-Kraff M. The FTO gene rs9939609 obesity-risk allele and loss of control over eating. Am J Clin Nutr 2009;90(6):1483–8.

155. Sun Q, Cornelis MC, Kraft P, et al. Genome-wide association study identifies polymorphisms in LEPR as determinants of plasma soluble leptin receptor levels. Hum Mol Genet 2010;19(9):1846–55.

156. Tang TS, Prior SL, Li KW, et al. Association between the rs1050450 glutathione peroxidase-1 (C>T) gene variant and peripheral neuropathy in two independent samples of subjects with diabetes mellitus. Nutr Metab Cardiovasc Dis 2012;22(5):417–25.

157. Nadif R. Association of CAT polymorphisms with catalase activity and exposure to environmental oxidative stimuli. Free Radic Res 2005;39(12):1345–50.

158. Bastaki M, Huen K, Manzanillo P, et al. Genotype-activity relationship for Mn-superoxide dismutase, glutathione peroxidase 1 and catalase in humans. Pharmacogenet Genomics 2006;16(4):279–86.

159. Giannoudis P. The genetic predisposition to adverse outcome after trauma. J Bone Joint Surg Br 2007;89B(10):1273–9.

160. Hage F, Szalai A. The role of C-reactive protein polymorphisms in inflammation and cardiovascular risk. Curr Atheroscler Rep 2009;11:124–30.

161. Panguluri R. COX-2 gene promoter haplotypes and prostate cancer risk. Carcinogenesis 2004;25(6):961–6.

162. Xu C, Li CY, Kong AN. Induction of phase I, II and III drug metabolism/transport by xenobiotics. Arch Pharm Res 2005;28(3):249–68.

163. Perera V, Gross AS, McLachlan AJ. Measurement of CYP1A2 activity: a focus on caffeine as a probe. Curr Drug Metab 2012;13(5):667–78.

164. Prescott LF, Critchley JA, Balali-Mood M, et al. Effects of microsomal enzyme induction on paracetamol metabolism in man. Br J Clin Pharmacol 1981;12(2):149–53.

165. Campbell L, Wilson HK, Samuel AM, et al. Interactions of m-xylene and aspirin metabolism in man. Br J Ind Med 1988;45(2):127–32.

166. Rannug A, Alexandrie AK, Persson I, et al. Genetic polymorphism of cytochromes P450 1A1, 2D6 and 2E1: regulation and toxicological significance. J Occup Environ Med 1995;37(1):25–36.

167. Liska DJ. The detoxification enzyme systems. Altern Med Rev 1998;3(3):187–98.

168. Gustavson LE, Benet LZ. Menopause: pharmacodynamics and pharmacokinetics. Exp Gerontol 1994;29(3–4):437–44.

169. Udayan Apte PK. Detoxification functions of the liver. In: Monga SPS, editor. Molecular pathology of liver diseases. New York: Springer Publications; 2011. p. 147–63.

170. Lin JH. Pharmacokinetic and pharmacodynamic variability: a daunting challenge in drug therapy. Curr Drug Metab 2007;8:109–36.

171. Zanger UM, Schwab M. Cytochrome P450 enzymes in drug metabolism: regulation of gene expression, enzyme activities, and impact of genetic variation. Pharmacol Ther 2013;138:103–41.

172. Sim S, Kacevska M, Ingleman-Sundberg M. Pharmacogenomics of drug-metabolizing enzymes: a recent update on clinical implications and endogenous effects. Pharmacogenomics J 2013;13:1–11.

173. McNulty H, Dowey LR, Strain JJ, et al. Riboflavin lowers homocysteine in individuals homozygous for the MTHFR 677C–T polymorphism. Circulation 2006;113:74–80.

174. Ma J, Stampfer MJ, Giovannucci E, et al. Methylenetetrahydrofolate reductase polymorphism, dietary interactions and risk of colorectal cancer. Cancer Res 1997;57:1098–102.

175. Fathy H, Abd El-Mawella SM, Abdou H, et al. Methyltetrahydrofolate reductase polymorphism, folic acid, and B12 in a sample of patients with depressive and anxiety symptoms. MECPsych 2011;18(2):118–25.

176. Kinoshita H, Nakagawa K, Narusawa K, et al. A functional single nucleotide polymorphism in the vitamin-K-dependent gamma-glutamyl carboxylase gene (Arg325Gln) is associated with bone mineral density in elderly Japanese Women. Bone 2007;40(2):451–6.

177. Borel P, Moussa M, Reboul E, et al. Human plasma levels of vitamin E and carotenoids are associated with genetic polymorphisms in genes involved in lipid metabolism. J Nutr 2007;137(12):2653–9.

178. Castel-Dunwoody KM, Von Kauwell GPA, Shelnutt KP, et al. Transcobalamin 776C 3 G polymorphism negatively affects vitamin. Am J Clin Nutr 2005;81:1436–41.

179. Cahill LE, El-Sohemy A. Vitamin C transporter gene polymorphisms, dietary vitamin C and serum ascorbic acid. J Nutrigenet Nutrigenomics 2009;2(6):292–301.

180. Dai Q, Shrubsole MJ, Ness RM, et al. The relation of magnesium and calcium intakes and a genetic polymorphism in the magnesium transporter to colorectal neoplasia risk. Am J Clin Nutr 2007;86(3):743–51.

181. Da Costa K-A, Kozyreva OG, Song J, et al. Common genetic polymorphisms affect the human requirement for the nutrient choline. FASEB J 2006;20(9):1336–44.

182. Pishva H, Amini M, Eshraghian MR, et al. Effects of EPA supplementation on plasma fatty acids composition in hypertriglyceridemic subjects with FABP2 and PPARα genotypes. J Diabetes Metab Disord 2012;11(1):25.

183. Sarris J, Stough C, Bousman CA, et al. Kava in the treatment of generalized anxiety disorder: a double-blind, randomized, placebo-controlled study. J Clin Psychopharmacol 2013;33(5):1–6.

184. Mandegary A, Saeedi A, Eftekhari A, et al. Hepatoprotective effect of silymarin in individuals chronically exposed to hydrogen sulfide; modulating influence of TNF-α cytokine genetic polymorphism. Daru 2013;21(1):28.

185. Li X, Lian F-M, Guo D, et al. The rs1142345 in TPMT affects the therapeutic effect of traditional hypoglycemic herbs in prediabetes. Evidence-based Complementary and Alternative Medicine. eCAM 2013;327629.

186. Slaviero KA, Clarke SJ, Rivory LP. Inflammatory response: an unrecognised source of variability in the pharmacokinetics and pharmacodynamics of cancer chemotherapy. Lancet Oncol 2003;4(4):224–32.

187. Aitken AE, Richardson TA, Morgan ET. Regulation of drug-metabolizing enzymes and transporters in inflammation. Annu Rev Pharmacol Toxicol 2006;46:123–49.

188. Caro AA, Cederbaum AI. Oxidative stress, toxicology, and pharmacology of CYP2E1. Annu Rev Pharmacol Toxicol 2004;44:27–42.

189. Aubert J, Begriche K, Knockaert L, et al. Increased expression of cytochrome P450 2E1 in nonalcoholic fatty liver disease: mechanisms and pathophysiological role. Clin Res Hepatol Gastroenterol 2011;35(10):630–7.

190. Yang JC, Lin CJ. CYP2C19 genotypes in the pharmacokinetics/pharmacodynamics of proton pump inhibitor-based therapy of Helicobacter pylori infection. Expert Opin Drug Metab Toxicol 2010;6(1):29–41.

191. Gropper S, Smith J, Groff J. Advanced nutrition and human metabolism. 5th ed. Belmont, USA: Wadsworth/Thompson Learning; 2009.

192. Zeisel SH. Genetic polymorphisms in methyl-group metabolism and epigenetics: lessons from humans and mouse models. Brain Res 2008;1237:5–11.

193. Yates Z, Lucock M. Interaction between common folate polymorphisms and B-vitamin nutritional status modulates homocysteine and risk for a thrombotic event. Mol Genet Metab 2003;79(3):201–13.

194. Whitehead VM. Acquired and inherited disorders of cobalamin and folate in children. Br J Haematol 2006;134(2):125–36.

195. Heimburger D, Shils M, McLaren D. Clinical manifestations of nutrient deficiencies and toxicities: a resume. Modern Nutrition in Health and Disease. 10th ed. USA: Lippincott Williams & Wilkins; 2006.

196. Solomons NW, Russell RM. The interaction of vitamin A and zinc: implications for human nutrition. Am J Clin Nutr 1980;33(9):2031–40.

197. Butterworth RF. Maternal thiamine deficiency: still a problem in some world communities. Am J Clin Nutr 2001;74(6):712–13.

198. Hilker DM, Somogyi JC. Antithiamins of plant origin: their chemical nature and mode of action. Ann N Y Acad Sci 1982;378(Thiamin: Twenty Years of Progress):137–45.

199. Pinto J, Huang Y, Rivilin R. Mechanisms underlying the differential effects of ethanol on the bioavailability of riboflavin and flavin adenine dinucleotide. J Clin Invest 1987;79(5):1343–8.

200. Rivlin R. Riboflavin. Present knowledge in nutrition. Washington: ILSI Press; 1996. p. 167–73.

201. Ryan AS, Goldsmith LA. Nutrition and the skin. Clin Dermatol 1996;14(4):389–406.

202. Rall L, Meydani SN. Vitamin B6 and immune competence. Nutr Rev 1993;51(8):217.

203. Sauberlich HE. Bioavailability of vitamins. Prog Food Nutr Sci 1985;9:1–33.

204. Leklem J. Vitamin B6. Present knowledge in nutrition. Washington: ILSI Press; 1996. p. 175–83.

205. Ralph C. Subtle and atypical cobalamin deficiency states. Am J Hematol 1990;34(1):108–14.

206. Kanazawa S, Herbert V. Total corrinoid, cobalamin and cobalamin analogue levels may be normal in serum despite cobalamin in liver depletion in patients with alcoholism. Lab Invest 1985;53:108–10.

207. Cooke W, Cox E, Fone D, et al. The clinical and metabolic significance of Jejunal diverticula. Gut 1963;4(2):115–31.

208. Herbert V. Making sense of laboratory tests of folate status: folate requirements to sustain normality. Am J Hematol 1987;26(2):199–207.

209. Thongprasom K, Youngnak P. Folate and vitamin B12 levels in patients with oral lichen planus, stomatitis or glossitis. Southeast Asian J Trop Med Public Health 2001;32(3):643–7.

210. Bonjour JP. Biotin in man's nutrition and therapy—a review. Int J Vitam Nutr Res 1977;47:107–18.

211. Basu T. The influence of drugs with particular reference to aspirin on the bioavailability of vitamin C. In: Counsell J, Hornig D, editors. Vitamin C. London: Applied Science Publishers; 1981. p. 273–81.

212. Rader DJ, Brewer HB Jr. Abetalipoproteinemia: new insights into lipoprotein assembly and vitamin E metabolism from a rare genetic disease. JAMA 1993;270(7):865–9.

213. De Leenheer AP, Nelis HJ, Lambert WE, et al. Chromatography of fat-soluble vitamins in clinical chemistry. J Chromatogr 1988;429:3–58.

214. Kalra V, Grover J, Ahuja GK, et al. Deficiency and associated neurological deficits in children with protein–energy malnutrition. J Trop Pediatr 1998;44(5):291–5.

215. Kelly FJ, Rodgers W, Handel J, et al. Time course of vitamin E repletion in the premature infant. Br J Nutr 1990;63(3):631–8.

216. Bieri JG, Evarts RP. Tocopherols and polyunsaturated fatty acids in human tissues. Am J Clin Nutr 1975;28(7):717–20.

217. Sokol R, Butler-Simon N, Heubi J, et al. Vitamin E deficiency neuropathy in children with fat malabsorption studies in cystic fibrosis and chronic cholestasis. Ann N Y Acad Sci 1989;570(Vitamin E: Biochemistry and Health Implications):156–69.

218. Fatemi S, Ryzen E, Flores J, et al. Effect of experimental human magnesium depletion on parathyroid hormone secretion and 1,25-dihydroxyvitamin D metabolism. J Clin Endocrinol Metab 1991;73(5):1067–72.

219. Krasinski SD, Russell RM, Furie BC, et al. The prevalence of vitamin K deficiency in chronic gastrointestinal disorders. Am J Clin Nutr 1985;41(3):639–43.

220. Olson R. The function and metabolism of vitamin K. Annu Rev Nutr 1984;4:281–337.

221. Ryzen E. Magnesium homeostasis in critically ill patients. Magnesium 1989;8(3–4):201–12.

222. Whang R, Hampton EM, Whang DD. Magnesium homeostasis and clinical disorders of magnesium deficiency. Ann Pharmacother 1994;28(2):220–6.

223. Kesteloot H, Joossens JV. The relationship between dietary intake and urinary excretion of sodium, potassium, calcium and magnesium: Belgian Interuniversity Research on Nutrition and Health. J Hum Hypertens 1990;4:527–33.

224. Rude RK. Magnesium deficiency: a cause of heterogenous disease in humans. J Bone Miner Res 1998;13(4):749–58.

225. Maclean AR, Renwick C. Audit of pre-operative starvation. Anaesthesia 1993;48(2):164–6.

226. Kerstetter JE, O'Brien KO, Insogna KL. Dietary protein affects intestinal calcium absorption. Am J Clin Nutr 1998;68(4):859–65.

227. Hannan MT, Tucker KL, Dawson-Hughes B, et al. Effect of dietary protein on bone loss in elderly men and women: the Framingham osteoporosis study. J Bone Miner Res 2000;15(12):2504–12.

228. Mahalko JR, Sandstead HH, Johnson LK, et al. Effect of a moderate increase in dietary protein on the retention and excretion of Ca, Cu, Fe, Mg, P, and Zn by adult males. Am J Clin Nutr 1983;37(1):8–14.

229. Pironi L, Miglioli M, Cornia GL, et al. Urinary zinc excretion in Crohn's disease. Dig Dis Sci 1987;32(4):358–62.

230. Cousins RJ. Zinc. Present knowledge in nutrition. Washington: ILSI Press; 1996. p. 293–306.

231. Smith H. Diagnosis in paediatric haematology. New York: Churchill Livingstone; 1996.

232. Lynch SR. Interaction of iron with other nutrients. Nutr Rev 1997;55(4):102–10.

233. O'Dell B. Bioavailability of and interactions among trace elements. Trace Elements in Nutrition of Children, vol. 8. New York: Raven Press; 1985. p. 41–55.

234. Rushton DH. Nutritional factors and hair loss. Clin Exp Dermatol 2002;27(5):400–8.

235. Gaitan E. Goitrogens in food and water. Annu Rev Nutr 1990;10:21–39.

236. Wolff J, Chaikoff IL. Plasma inorganic iodide as a homeostatic regulator of thyroic function. J Biol Chem 1948;174(2):555–64.

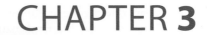

CHAPTER **3**

Wellness, lifestyle and preventive medicine

Erica Oberg
ND, MPH

OVERVIEW

The origins of 'wellness' in naturopathic medicine stem from the 19th century European tradition of health spas, nature cure and the hygiene movement. German healers such as Father Sebastian Kniepp and Henry Lindlar practised 'drugless healing' and promoted water therapies, walking barefoot in the forest and clean living in both bodily and mental practices. Benedict Lust, a student of Father Kniepp, learned these concepts and brought them to the United States in 1901, establishing the American School of Naturopathy in New York, the first institution of naturopathic medicine. Wellness sits at the centre of naturopathic practice philosophy. The Principles of Naturopathic Medicine,[1] the philosophical foundations of modern naturopathic practice, include *prevention and wellness* and the concept of the *Vis,* the innate vitality within a person. Naturopathic philosophy recognises that the health of any person in any disease state can be enhanced and quality of life improved with attention to the underlying factors that promote health and wellness.

The therapeutic order

1. *Re-establish the basis for health.* Remove obstacles to cure (i.e. establishing a healthy 'regimen').
2. *Stimulate the healing power of nature.* Use low-force methods to stimulate the body's innate ability to heal itself.
3. *Tonify weakened systems.* Strengthen the immune system, decrease toxic load, *normalise* inflammatory function, optimise metabolic function, balance regulatory systems and enhance regeneration.
4. *Correct structural integrity.* Use therapeutic exercise, massage, hydrotherapy and spinal manipulation to optimise physical function.
5. *Prescribe specific natural substances for pathology.* Use nutraceuticals and herbs to promote or return to health.
6. *Prescribe pharmacological substances for pathology.* Use pharmacological drugs to return to health.
7. *Prescribe surgery, suppressive drugs, radiation and chemotherapy.* Use aggressive therapies to attempt to maintain health.

Source: Zeff et al. 2006[2]

Naturopathic medicine philosophy uses the therapeutic order—a hierarchy of therapeutic interventions. This lends naturopathic medicine to wellness and health promotion particularly well, as focus remains initially on low-level and preventive interventions first.

THE PHILOSOPHY OF WELLNESS

The World Health Organization (WHO) defines *health* in its constitution as 'a state of complete physical, mental, and social well being and not merely the absence of disease or infirmity'.[3] This definition aligns with the broader concept of health held in naturopathic practice and the intent behind prioritising wellness and stimulating the *Vis*. Over the past 50 years healthcare has increasingly focused on disease and pharmaceutical intervention, with decreasing prioritisation of health or prevention. Even further forgotten are concepts of wellness or vitality. Today, a short list of chronic diseases are responsible for a large part of the disease burden in Europe. Of the six WHO regions, the European region is the most affected by non-communicable diseases (diabetes, cardiovascular diseases, cancer, chronic respiratory diseases and mental disorders). These conditions account for an estimated 86% of the deaths and 77% of the disease burden in Europe.[4] Re-iterating this perspective, a joint statement from the American Cancer Society, American Diabetes Association and American Heart Association calls for:

> … *a concerted effort to increase application of public health and clinical interventions of known efficacy to reduce prevalence of tobacco use, poor diet, and insufficient physical activity—the major risk factors for these diseases—and to increase utilization of screening tests for their early detection could substantially reduce the human and economic cost of these diseases.*[5]

There is a clear need for a cultural shift in healthcare as a whole and naturopathic medicine can be considered an example of what wellness-oriented healthcare looks like. Achieving wellness is a dynamic process that reflects a person's inherent constitutional and environmental differences and potential through stimulation of the vital force. Naturopathic clinicians place high prioritisation on this and incorporate concepts of wellness into every clinical encounter[6]; it is not a separate consideration in the presence of disease or illness.

The concept of wellness per se as a balanced state of physical, social, emotional, intellectual and spiritual health emerged in the 1950s. Figure 3.1 (on the following page) illustrates the holistic way in which wellness can be considered. Through attention to all of the domains, promotion of wellness is integrated into diagnosis of the pathophysiology of presenting illness and the evaluation and management of the clinical encounter. Figure 3.2 extends this model and demonstrates how the application of the domains of wellness are incorporated into specific clinical recommendations and personal practices. As indicated in this figure, while pharmacotherapy often has a central role in prescriptions, it is just one element. This chapter investigates the domains of wellness and the specific implementation of health promotion and prevention in naturopathic practice. These principles of wellness serve as the foundation to naturopathic approaches to disease-based healthcare as well as standing independently as strategies to enhance individual vitality and quality of life.

Social wellness

Maslow's hierarchy of needs (Figure 3.3), first proposed in 1943, posits that human potential is realised systematically.[7] Humans are motivated to meet basic survival needs

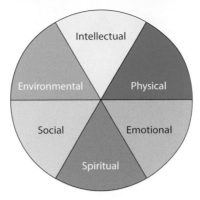

Figure 3.1
Conceptual model of holistic wellness

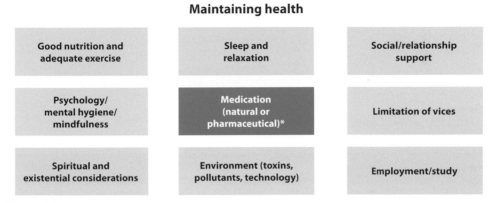

Figure 3.2
Key elements underpinning wellness and the maintenance of health

* Used judiciously if required

first, and until these needs are met, 'higher' levels of development are unattainable. Social wellness meets our hierarchy of needs fairly low on the pyramid. The sense of belonging, being loved and having our basic safety secured are inherent to social wellness.

For many of our patients, unaddressed chronic stress associated with dissatisfaction with economic status or an unhealthy relationship are unappreciated contributors to their overall disease risk. Locus of control, the sense that one has choice and control in their life, is particularly significant. Working in an environment in which one is 'micromanaged' or otherwise unable to take control of their own situation is not only a measurable stressor that may lead to other risk factors such as depression but also a risk factor to cardiovascular disease itself. Naturopathic approaches to wellness and health promotion attend to the social determinants of health and psychosocial risk factors commensurate with the known risk these factors contribute to health status. Without addressing these foundations of health, higher levels of needs (and wellness) cannot be achieved. Sometimes, the best medicine may be connecting someone to social services for housing assistance or encouraging them to speak up in a situation in which they feel no control.

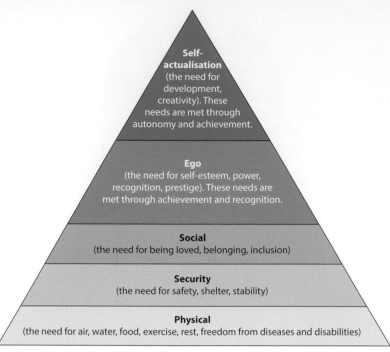

Figure 3.3
Maslow's hierarchy of needs

INTERHEART study

The INTERHEART study was a case-control study involving more than 30 000 people in 52 countries. The study sought to determine the relationship between lifestyle factors (smoking, history of hypertension or diabetes, waist–hip ratio, dietary patterns, physical activity, consumption of alcohol, blood lipoproteins and psychosocial factors) and cardiovascular events.[8] Hypertension and heart attacks were associated with chronic stress. The magnitude of risk is equivalent to traditional cardiovascular disease risk factors like smoking, obesity and diabetes; there is a nearly 50% increase risk of having a heart attack after several periods of recent general stress and a twofold increase for permanent or chronic stress.[9] Overall, people who experienced a myocardial infarction during the study had a significantly higher prevalence of all four stress factors.[9]

The results of INTERHEART provide a clear case for the importance of psychosocial determinants of health. In INTERHEART, psychosocial stress was assessed by four simple questions about stress at work and at home, financial stress, and major life events in the past year. Additional questions assessed locus of control and presence of depression. For example, the occurrence of major adverse life events were assessed by asking participants whether they had experienced life events such as: marital separation or divorce; loss of job or retirement; loss of crop or business failure; violence; major intra-family conflict; major personal injury or illness; death or major illness of a close family member; death of a spouse; or other major stress.[9]

Physical wellness

The domain of physical health is where clinicians classically think of health promotion, and for good reason. Lifestyle factors—specifically tobacco use, alcohol use, diet and physical activity—are the leading causes of death.[10] Solutions to emergent public health crises such as the obesity epidemic rest in identifying ways in which we can encourage individuals to adopt more healthful lifestyle behaviours.

Healthful dietary patterns

The evidence supporting a relationship between unhealthy diet and mortality was demonstrated as early as 1981 in a landmark epidemiological study by Doll and Peto.[11] They calculated that 35% of cancer deaths may be due to unhealthy diet, which was soon corroborated by others.[12] In the mid 2000s, Mokdad et al. famously estimated the actual causes of death attributable to diet and physical inactivity at 15.2%.[10] Epidemiological studies examining healthful eating patterns add evidence; for example, a study of a 350 000-person American cohort found that a diet highest in whole grains, fruits and vegetables and low in discretionary fat was associated with a significant all-cause mortality risk reduction.[13] Among an Australian cohort of elderly adults, adherence to a Mediterranean-type dietary pattern or a healthful diet (as defined by the highest quintile of the Recommended Foods Score) had lower all-cause mortality.[14] Globally, a number of regions (termed Blue Zones) have investigated to find lessons in patterns of longevity and wellness. While these communities are scattered across the globe, there are commonalities which are similar to the domains of wellness previously discussed. These range from common lifestyle factors such as regular activity, a plant-based diet and moderate alcohol consumption to behavioral and cultural patterns such as strong social connections, a slower pace, and a sense of purpose and belonging in the community.[15]

WHO estimates that dietary factors represent five of the seven underlying causes for non-communicable-disease deaths (the remaining two factors being physical inactivity and tobacco use).[4] Healthful diet is critical and promotion of healthful eating is one of the ways naturopaths exert influence on both chronic disease and the prevention of future disease. Yet, at the population level, dietary recommendations of recent years seem to have lost the forest for the trees. Recommendations to consume x per cent of polyunsaturated fats and y per cent of unrefined carbohydrates are lost on most individuals who have neither nutrition degrees nor a desire to think of their plate in terms of macronutrient ratios. Fad diets that emphasise single food sources or extreme dietary patterns (i.e. a 700 kcal 'HCG diet') are not only unsuccessful for weight loss, they may be harmful. One of the best ways we can help our patients understand and implement healthier eating behaviours is to educate them in the dietary patterns known to promote health and reduce risk of chronic disease.

The Mediterranean diet is perhaps the best studied and generally healthful dietary pattern globally. It has been summarised in a food pyramid (Figure 3.4). The characteristics of a Mediterranean diet include[17]:

- high consumption of fruits, vegetables, bread and other cereals, potatoes, beans, nuts, seeds and garlic
- olive oil as the major dietary fat, providing monounsaturated fat
- dairy products, fish and poultry are consumed in low to moderate amounts, and little red meat is eaten
- eggs are consumed in moderation from zero to four times a week
- wine is consumed in low to moderate amounts; one to two drinks per day with meals.

Adhering to a Mediterranean diet is associated with a lower risk of all-cause mortality, mortality from coronary heart disease, cardiovascular diseases and cancer.[18–21] *Not* following this low-risk pattern was associated with a population attributable risk of 60% of all deaths, 64% of deaths from coronary heart disease, 61% from cardiovascular

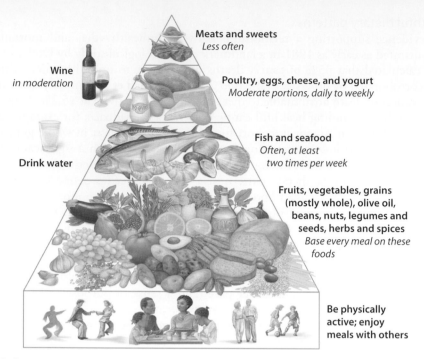

Figure 3.4
Mediterranean diet pyramid

Source: Oldways 1999[16] (© 2009 Oldways Preservation & Exchange Trust)

diseases and 60% from cancer.[20] This is consistent with other prospective studies in which adopting comprehensive healthful dietary patterns was associated with a 56% reduced mortality.[22]

Dietary quality

While rarely discussed in the epidemiology of protective dietary patterns, dietary quality, not simply macronutrient ratio, contributes to the overall health promotion and risk reduction of a healthful diet. This is most clearly illustrated in the research examining glycaemic index and glycaemic load versus total carbohydrate intake. Glycaemic index and glycaemic load are standardised measures of how quickly a carbohydrate will raise blood sugar after ingestion. It is a function of the total available carbohydrate in the food (total carbohydrate—fibre), not simply the grams of carbohydrate itself. Less processed food, such as fruit, vegetables and unrefined grains, have lower glycaemic loads than the same weight of carbohydrates from highly refined sources such as flour, sugar or fruit juice. This is especially relevant to Indigenous Australians and Torres Strait Islanders, who consume high glycaemic index diets and have high risk of chronic disease.[23] Low glycaemic index diets (not low-carbohydrate diets) also have demonstrated benefit for weight loss and metabolic syndrome,[24,25] diabetes[26] and lipid profiles.[27]

Another domain of dietary quality, albeit a controversial one, is organic food. Meta-analysis comparing conventionally grown produce to organically grown produce received substantial press coverage, with headlines emphasising the lack of micro-nutrient superiority of organic produce.[28] While this was among the findings (although other studies have found otherwise),[29–31] the headlines missed the critical point: organic produce has significantly lower residues of herbicides and pesticides, substances known to have negative impacts of human health. Consumption of organic food may also lower the risk of exposure to antibiotic-resistant bacteria.[28]

Caloric restriction and fasting

There has been a recent surge in evidence supporting the value of therapeutic fasting and caloric restriction in human health. Historically, these dietary practices have been well represented in naturopathic practice, yet had fallen out of favour under criticism from biomedicine in the past 50 years. The early animal research in fasting demonstrated consistent and strong impact on longevity. Subsequently, human studies have explored a number of patterns and strategies to realistically achieve a significantly reduced caloric intake. Extending the overnight fast is perhaps one of the most realistic strategies, and studies show a benefit for cancer and all-cause mortality with fasting for 13 hours overnight.[32] Fasting and caloric reduction is helpful for more than just weight loss. Although it is well established that obesity increases all-cause mortality by 30%,[33] the benefits towards overall health and wellness occur independent of BMI. Eating less than 30% of your calories in the evening is beneficial, and every 2-hour increase in the duration (up to 13 hours) reduces inflammatory markers such as CRP and insulin.[34] For all of these reasons, a return to naturopathic fasting may have a public health impact.

Naturopathic approaches to diet address both dietary quality and macronutrient balance. Table 3.1 illustrates the components of a naturopathic diet, as derived from a formal Delphi process involving North American naturopathic doctors.[26] This approach was subsequently applied in a prospective outcomes study in which patients with diabetes were taught to follow a naturopathic approach through individualised counselling and group visits. Participants' dietary patterns significantly improved, as did glycaemic control. Interestingly, even though physical activity recommendations were not made, participants spontaneously increased physical activity, suggesting that a holistic approach to health promotion can be beneficial across multiple domains.

Physical activity

The science of physical activity and exercise can help naturopaths finetune lifestyle recommendations to maximise health potential. Diet, without physical activity, or vice versa, is insufficient for weight loss, chronic disease reversal or optimal wellbeing. When matched calorie to calorie, dietary caloric restriction or increasing caloric expenditure through physical activity will result in equivalent weight loss.[51] However, important differences exist. First, for most people, a larger caloric deficit can be accomplished through dietary restriction than with increasing caloric expenditure with exercise. Therefore, we see numerous trials of diet versus exercise demonstrating superior weight loss and metabolic improvements in the diet arms.[52,53]

Importantly, physical activity leads to improvements in fitness and cardiometabolic risk reduction even in the absence of weight loss, a phenomenon largely attributed to improvements in visceral fat loss. There is an increasing body of literature demonstrating the importance of body composition over weight loss alone.[54–56] From a naturopathic perspective, 'fitness over fatness' resonates with a holistic perspective in which the total health of the individual is prioritised over individual risk factors.

Table 3.1
Summary of key concepts in a naturopathic diet

Dietary principle	Specific recommendation	Rationale
Macronutrient balance	20–40% carbohydrate, 25–45% protein, 15–35% fat	This is a lower carbohydrate diet that is still diverse, well balanced and achievable in practice[35,36]
Low glycaemic index (GI)	Select low GI carbohydrates by paying attention to fibre and whole foods	Low-GI foods have a reduced post-prandial glycaemic spike and subsequently keep insulin lower[24,25,27]
Micronutrient density	Select foods that provide maximal micronutrient intake per calorie	Because health-oriented diets are often low-calorie, it is important to maximise nutrition, especially dietary antioxidant intake[37–40]
Functional foods	Based on individual needs, select foods that have function beyond calorie or nutrients	For example, including oats in the diet will lower cholesterol and allow emphasis on food rather than medication[41–44]
Understand quality of foods	Learn to select healthy fats Make conscious choices about organic, wild and local foods	Some fats, like omega-3 fatty acids, have beneficial effects on glycaemic control, whereas trans-fatty acids and saturated fat increase cardiovascular risk[28–31,45]
Understand personal eating behaviour	Understand emotional and situational eating habits to avoid overeating	Several eating patterns have been linked to overeating; empowerment over negative habits creates change and leads to self-efficacy across self-care skills[46–48]
Cultivate healthful attitudes towards food	Understand food nourishes more than the physical body	For example, children who eat meals with family at a table have lower rates of obesity[49,50]

For example, among study participants who exercised, for every metabolic equivalent (MET) improvement in fitness an associated 7%, 22% and 12% lower risk resulted in developing hypertension, metabolic syndrome and hypercholesterolaemia, respectively. Every unit increase in percentage of body fat was associated with a 4%, 10% and 5% increased risk of developing the cardiovascular risk factors.[57] Even among people with diabetes, exercise leads to improvements in cardiometabolic fitness (and decreased disease risk) independent of weight loss. As illustrated in Figure 3.5, men in the low-fitness group had a 1.9-fold risk for impaired fasting glucose and a 3.7-fold risk for diabetes compared with those in the high-fitness group.[58]

A final perspective on physical activity in naturopathic health promotion is that, for most patients, increases in physical activity, however small, are beneficial for disease prevention, chronic disease management and promotion of wellness including improved mood[59,60] and energy.[61] Table 3.2 summarises some of the key benefits of different types of physical activity and can be used to individualise recommendations. Individualised activity goals, with appropriate attention to avoidance of over-training, should be incorporated into every patient encounter. Encouraging patients to be more active may be the best prescription we can make.

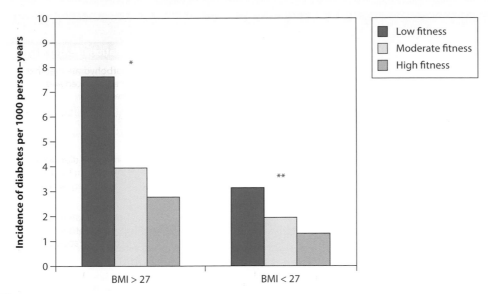

Figure 3.5
Metabolic fitness versus body weight and the incidence of diabetes
* $p = 0.005$; ** $p = 0.001$

Table 3.2
Benefits of different types of exercise

Type of exercise	Specific benefits
Strength/resistance training	Improves insulin sensitivity Increases lean muscle Prevents age-related declines Safer for people at high cardiovascular risk Reduces blood pressure Improves bone mineral density Useful for weight loss
Aerobic	Improves overall glycaemic control Improves mood Improves lipids / cardiovascular risk profile Intense aerobic activity effective for weight loss Improves cognitive function
Balance training	Reduces risk of fall Improves core strength and stability Improves mobility and healing post-surgery/injury
Swimming or water aerobics	Minimal impact on joints—minimises pain Great for beginning activity or for overweight
Yoga	Develops mind–body awareness, relaxation Helps balance and strength
General physical activity	Benefits glycaemic control beyond weight loss alone Reduces the risk of diabetes, cancer and heart disease Reduces stress

---

Diabetes prevention program

The landmark Diabetes Prevention Program trial randomised 3234 non-diabetic people with impaired glucose tolerance to three groups: metformin, placebo or lifestyle modification.[62] Lifestyle modification focused primarily on exercise; it targeted a goal of 7% weight loss and 150 minutes of exercise per week. At the end of the three-year study period 74% of participants in the lifestyle arm achieved these exercise goals. Comparison between the three groups found that the lifestyle intervention reduced the incidence of diabetes by 58% compared with the metformin arm, which reduced incidence by 31%. The number needed to treat (NNT) to prevent one case of diabetes with lifestyle change was 6.9; to do the same with metformin, the number NNT was 13.9.

Emotional wellness

As witnessed in other biomedical fields, the mental health field has experienced a similar trend away from holistic, wellness-oriented care. Even the very terminology of 'mental health' takes the emphasis away from the emotional epicentre of the 'dis-ease' addressed by the field (i.e. depression, grief, anxiety). For example, psychiatry primarily focuses on pharmaceutical treatment and brief appointments addressing medication adjustment while spending less time on psychotherapy.[63] Naturopathic approaches to emotional wellbeing and mental health can incorporate natural medications; however, naturopaths typically focus on holistic dimensions and often promote emotional and mental health through encouraging patients to engage in other domains of wellness such as physical activity. Additionally emotional dis-ease can impact physical health (e.g. irritable bowel syndrome, sleep disorders, disordered eating, 'psychosomatic' illness). A naturopathic approach addresses the symptoms of these somatic complaints concurrent with addressing the underlying cause of emotional distress.

A large body of literature demonstrates the effectiveness of physical activity on mood in a range of populations.[64–66] Evidence regarding the underlying mechanisms of this benefit has elucidated several potential pathways. Neurogenesis, the generation of new synapses, occurs in the hippocampus following physical activity; neurogenesis is known to be suppressed in association with both depression and obesity.[67] Physical activity also increases the neurotransmitter serotonin (the pharmacological basis for numerous antidepressant medications) and the number of dopamine receptors in the brain, a key component of reward/motivational circuitry.[68]

Another perspective on promoting emotional wellbeing can be found in ancient texts of Ayurveda and yogic spiritual practices concerning the 'heart chakra'.[69] The English language reflects a cultural appreciation for the role of the 'heart' in emotional health; we speak of 'broken hearts' and 'heartaches' and use symbology of the heart to express the concept of love. Western science has made inroads to explaining the heart as our emotional epicentre. Some of the best examples of this research, and its practical application to improving emotional wellness, are done by the HeartMath Institute in California. HeartMath is a therapeutic approach to changing reactions to stressors. It is a series of techniques that helps people focus on their emotional responses to stress. Many colloquialisms illustrate the emotional responses to stress. We all know what it feels like to 'get our blood pumping' when we are angry; that is an example of an emotional response to stress causing high blood pressure. It is thought that the expression 'seeing red' relates to blood vessels dilating in the eyes in response to really high blood pressure. HeartMath applies a concept called *rhythm coherence* based on the premise that modern life stressors influence the coherence of heart rhythms, and that the coherence itself can be influenced by intentionally and sincerely focusing on positive feelings. In general, the techniques help focus on remembering positive experiences (and how the mind–body feel in those situations) and then cultivating the ability to 'interrupt' yourself when negative feelings begin. There are many specific exercises used to teach patients to develop this pattern. HeartMath focuses attention on the heart, uses heart-centred breathing (described as extending the exhalation longer than the inhalation) and other mind–body exercises such as 'freeze-frame'.[70] People who practise HeartMath principles generally experience blood pressure reductions of approximately 10 points.[70]

Mental and cognitive wellness

Mental (intellectual) stress is a modern phenomenon. Most doctors can recall the stress of medical school, the impacts of which have well-documented effects on health.[71,72] High-pressure work environments are not limited to healthcare and are increasingly common. Similar to psychosocial stressors in general, intellectual stress is primarily driven by qualitative factors, such as the degree of control one has, the degree of emotional involvement and the overall 'intellectual demand'. It appears these factors have a greater impact on physical health among women, although men are not immune.[73] Studies of job burnout, especially common among healthcare workers and professional athletes, have described the cardiovascular and neuroendocrine implications.[74] When experiencing burnout, individuals are in a state of increased sympathetic tone that affects the vasculature and experience lowered post-stress vagal rebound to the heart along with lowered arterial baroreflex sensitivity.[74] While external stressors cannot always be changed, the response to a stressor can be modified. Indeed, patients (and doctors) can be taught concrete skills to improve their ability to respond to stressors in a more healthful way, thereby reducing the physiological impact of stress[74] (for more detail, see Chapter 18 on stress and fatigue).

Technology stress

Australian governmental recommendations state that children and young people should not spend more than two hours a day using electronic media for entertainment (e.g. computer games, the internet, television), particularly during daylight hours.[75] Excess media use has measureable impacts on health. Psychology literature now describes several distinct phenomena and psychological dysfunctions related to technology.[75] Overuse of technology and its psychological sequelae are described in the psychology literature as causing 'digital fog' and 'data smog', 'frazzing' (frantic ineffectual multitasking) and 'techno-stress'. This may also result in a potential 'online compulsive disorder'.

Developing coping skills to decrease reactivity to stressors is sometimes termed mindfulness.[76] The physiological effects are called the relaxation response.[77] In general, it is the intentional cultivation of awareness of the mind–body connection. The mind–body connection is an internal focus that turns attention to the inner state of being. Taken to a deeper level, this inner focus is called meditation. This is not an easy or automatic thing to do, as evidenced by thousands of years of religious and spiritual literature from monks and shamans discussing the challenge of achieving a meditative state. Almost all trials of mind–body techniques have shown positive, if sometimes small, benefits compared with usual care over relatively short time periods (mean study durations of eight weeks).[78,79] Recent studies suggest that the use of mindfulness-based training decreases stress-related neuroendocrine parameters, enhances psychological state and improves behavioural choices such as eating behaviours.[46,80,81]

Applications of mindfulness-based meditation practice are being designed and introduced into therapeutic regimens for a wide variety of illnesses and pathologies including posttraumatic stress disorder, substance/alcohol abuse, intractable pain, stress, panic disorder, generalised anxiety disorder, binge eating and, more recently, obesity and associated non-healthful choices. These techniques also have beneficial 'side effects' in other dimensions. The majority of clinical trials have found non-specific or generic benefits on measures of mood, wellbeing and quality of life.[82] Figure 14.1 in Chapter 14 on anxiety illustrates the technique of mindfulness meditation.

Spiritual wellness

At the centre of spiritual wellness is the existential quest for meaning and purpose in our lives. It relates to finding harmony and peace within one's self and within our relationships with others. Spirituality also includes ways in which daily activities can be approached—with compassion, altruism, mindfulness and love. Spiritual wellness is a highly individualised pursuit; each person must explore their own sense of meaning and purpose and find practices that foster spirituality within their own lives.

For some, a spiritual practice is synonymous with time in nature. *Biophilia*, a term coined by Wilson in the 1980s' ecopsychology movement, describes 'the connections that human beings subconsciously seek with the rest of life'.[83] This movement modernised the 'nature cure' philosophy in the traditional writings of the European naturopaths of the 18th century. Eco-psychologists express concern for the mental health and developmental implications of modern society and how far we have strayed from nature.[84] The therapeutic benefits of natural elements on human health were recently summarised in a meta-analysis. The analysis included 38 studies investigating nature-assisted therapy. Included studies ranged from evaluations of wilderness adventure programs to walking in gardens to non-specific exposure to nature. Results of prospective studies demonstrate moderate effect sizes in outcomes including mood, depression, motivation, wellbeing and capacity for attention.[85]

Separate from the small but growing trend to acknowledge the healing power of nature in healthcare, promotion of spiritual wellness has largely been separated from healthcare over the past century, instead relegated to religious institutions and leaders. While religion is a *part* of some people's spirituality, it is not the same and is inclusive of much more. Spirituality may include meditation, prayer, affirmation or other spiritual practices that connect one to a sense of a greater power. Bringing spirituality back into healthcare is a topic of discussion in nursing; 'spirituality interventions' are beginning to be described in the literature and have even been the subject of a Cochrane review.[86,87] For many healthcare providers, respectfully and delicately asking patients if they have a spiritual practice may be an appropriate entré to begin to incorporate spiritual wellness into holistic care.

Environment and wellness

The benefits of exposure to nature provide a segue into the health promotion domain of 'environment'. The natural world is fairly unanimously considered a salugenic environment. As mentioned previously, early leaders in wellness (and naturopathic philosophy) placed high emphasis on the healing power of nature; conceptual models of the relationship between wellbeing and environmental factors summarise this (Figure 3.6). However, there are increasing concerns about the sustainability and accessibility of the natural environment as human impact and urbanisation touch a growing percentage of the planet. A discussion of the role of the environment within the topics of health promotion, prevention and wellness would be incomplete without addressing concerns about the impact of pollutants and toxins in the environment and their impact on human health.

The bioaccumulation of persistent organic chemicals and toxicants poses a serious threat to physical health. Indoor air pollution is an established contributor and trigger for asthma.[89,90] Numerous cancers are linked to environmental pollutants as initiators of oncogenic processes if not directly associated with exposure.[91] Environmental toxicants such as persistent organic pollutants, phthalates, bisphenol A and contemporary-use pesticides are known endocrine disruptors and have been linked to precocious puberty among girls.[92,93] Unfortunately, exposure is nearly ubiquitous. In the United States the Environmental Protection Agency sponsors research investigating more than 40 persistent pesticides and organic pollutants, including herbicides (atrazine), insecticides (organophosphorus, carbamate, pyrethrin and organochlorine), phthalate esters

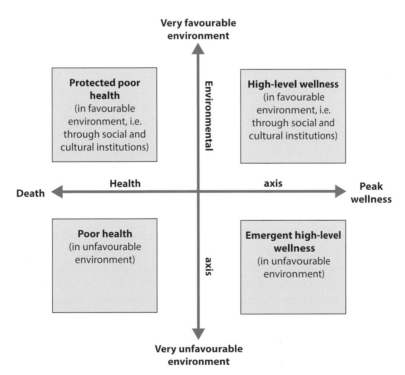

Figure 3.6
Dunn's 'health grid' illustrating the relationship between environment and wellness
Source: Miller 1959[88]

(butylbenzyl, di-n-butyl), phenols, polychlorinated biphenyls and polycyclic aromatic hydrocarbons, all of which are common in the environment. The bioburden of exposure based on population-based sampling, according to the most recent research, found 100% of sampled children had detectable levels of 3,5,6-trichloro-2-pyridinol (TCP), a known carcinogen, with reproductive and developmental toxicity, neurotoxicity and acute toxicity.[94]

Remediation strategies to reduce the bioburden of these toxicants and the numerous others that we encounter on a daily basis are beyond the scope of this discussion. These are areas in which future research and healthcare interventions will be needed. From the perspective of prevention and health promotion, the best practice is to minimise exposure. For the naturopath, this means understanding the sources of potential toxicants and educating patients on the risks of exposure and strategies to reduce it. The science of environmental health is complex and the popular media confounds this. Helping patients sort through the relative risks of exposures and the impact of exposure at different times across the lifecycle (e.g. in utero, during childhood development) is important so that informed decisions can be made. For example, the non-profit Environmental Working Group publishes the annual *Dirty Dozen: Clean fifteen shopper's guide to organic produce* to help consumers prioritise consumption.[95]

PUBLIC HEALTH PERSPECTIVE

Health behaviours are modifiable, yet data from the National Ambulatory Medical Care Survey reveal that only 15.7% of office visits to primary care providers include health counselling on diet, physical activity or stress reduction.[96] Although considerable debate exists regarding how best to deliver health promotion (i.e. workplace versus community versus clinical), the magnitude of the chronic disease burden warrants investment in health promotion in *every* setting. Thus, we must ask, how do we do this effectively?

Although recommendations for increasing physical activity and eating a healthful diet are available ubiquitously through every possible type of communication medium, the committed adoption of lifestyle changes remains a hurdle for both individuals and society at large. From a public health perspective, health promotion strategies are needed from every sector of the community, yet our focus here is on the role of clinicians (for more information on the naturopathic interface with public health see the Further Reading list).

Much research supports individually tailored recommendations and the application of multi-approach solutions simultaneously in an integrated fashion.[97] There is substantive evidence from clinical trials that a moderate exercise regimen, change of diet and eating patterns, or use of stress reduction techniques on their own, have modest but clinically significant efficacy in reducing metabolic parameters such as body fat, HbA_{1c} (in people with type 2 diabetes), blood pressure and cardiovascular risk-related blood lipids (e.g. triglycerides, total cholesterol, HDL/LDL profile), as well as stress hormone levels and inflammatory markers.[62,98–100] However, there is evidence that multi-component approaches, typical of a holistic naturopathic approach, further improve health outcomes.[97] For example, both exercise and mindfulness practice improve psychological wellbeing and stress-related physiological parameters, which may contribute both directly and indirectly to obesity. Naturopathic health promotion counselling is a more intensive model, typically done face to face and is reiterated in almost every clinical encounter.[6] The holistic approach taken by naturopaths may affect meaningful, longer term health behaviour change.

Public health considerations

- Lifestyle modification programs have been estimated to be highly cost-effective, at $1880 per quality-adjusted life year ($42 000 per quality-adjusted life year is the Australian threshold for cost-effectiveness[101]).
- Wellbeing is associated with lower costs and lower healthcare utilisation. For every point of increased wellness (on a validated scale), there is a 2% lower likelihood for hospital admission or emergency department visits. People with low wellbeing scores had 2.7 times greater annual medical costs than people with high wellbeing.[102]
- Naturopathic care for low back pain, a source of significant morbidity and cost, was found to be highly cost-effective, saving US$1096 in additional medical costs and US$1212 in societal costs (lost productivity). The return on investment for including naturopathic care for low back pain in a healthcare plan was 7.9%.[103]
- In the American state of Washington, laws mandate insurance reimbursement for naturopaths; as such the State provides an example of what healthcare fully inclusive of naturopathic doctors could become. Research of healthcare costs in Washington found that users of complementary and alternative medicine (CAM) with low back pain, fibromyalgia or menopausal symptoms had significantly lower average expenditures compared with non-CAM users ($3797 versus $4153). The largest reductions in costs were among patients with the highest disease burden. Patients with the poorest health cost an average of $1420 less annually if they were CAM users compared with those who were under the exclusive care of conventional providers.[104]

Prevention and health promotion in practice

The prevention and reversal of chronic disease must be improved if developed countries are to maintain the gains in life expectancy and disease prevention that have been seen over the previous century. As stated previously, chronic diseases are the leading causes of death in most developed countries. The underlying unhealthy behaviours are also estimated as the cause of the four leading non-communicable-disease-related deaths globally.[105] Among indigenous people, the impact of chronic disease is even greater.

Prevention is best understood when we add precision to our language. Primary prevention refers to screening programs aimed at early detection of disease before it becomes symptomatic, such as routine Cervical Screening Test for detecting human papillomavirus (HPV) or colonoscopy screening to detect polyps and pre-cancerous lesions prior to it progressing to cervical or colon cancer, respectively. Secondary prevention refers to preventive strategies aimed at preventing recurrence. For example, cardiac rehabilitation programs following myocardial infarction aim to prevent second cardiovascular events. There is another level of prevention, termed primordial prevention, that best describes the type of prevention naturopaths typically think about—a focus on health promotion and wellness that can prevent many future diseases.

AUSDRISK

In April 2007 the Council of Australian Governments (COAG) announced the Prevention of Type 2 Diabetes Program to help slow the growth in this disease. The centrepiece of this effort was the development and implementation of AUSDRISK, a self-administered diabetes risk assessment tool with good sensitivity (74%) and specificity (67.7%).[106] This well-designed, evidence-based program screens patients and, upon identification, refers high-risk individuals to subsidised lifestyle modification programs. This intervention strategy has the potential to have a significant impact on the Australian people, and the AUSDRISK tool has been promoted (and general practitioners are reimbursed for its use). Though the strategy has since become increasingly integrated, uptake remains unknown. The most recent study of general practitioners was conducted in 2011 and found 68% awareness but only 14% implementation.[107]

One of the well-described barriers to delivering health behaviour change interventions in primary care settings is the lack of an integrated screening and intervention approach that can cut across multiple risk factors and help clinicians and patients to address these risks in an efficient and productive manner.[108] Health promotion and wellness are strongly emphasised in the clinical practices of naturopathic medicine. Pilot data from retrospective studies suggest that the inclusion of diet, physical activity and stress reduction counselling are nearly ubiquitous in patient encounters; among hypertensive patients, 97.6% received dietary counselling, reiterated over 54.8% of all visits and 68.2% received counselling to increase physical activity, reiterated over 33% of all visits.[109] Among patients with diabetes, 100% received dietary recommendations, reinforced at 46% of visits, 94% received physical activity counselling, reiterated at 38% of visits, and 69% received counselling on stress reduction (including optimising sleep), with follow-up at 13% of visits.[6]

This is another opportunity for an expanded role for naturopaths, specifically in underserved areas (e.g. rural Australia) where there is high use and strong need for additional naturopathic services.[110] Health promotion counselling with simplified messages about nutrition, physical activity, stress reduction and avoidance of tobacco and excessive alcohol are becoming more prevalent, but true behavioural change accomplished through individualised one-on-one health promotion counselling using proven techniques such as motivational interviewing, stages of change-appropriate messaging and concrete, specific problem solving are required. Naturopathic medicine does this particularly well. Of course, naturopaths can contribute to wellness and health promotion in many ways outside the clinic. Table 3.3 illustrates additional non-clinical domains of health promotion.

Practising what we preach

A growing body of research demonstrates that healthy healthcare workers have healthier patients. The link between personal health practices and healthcare delivery is consistent; providers who get preventive screenings on time are more likely to recommend screenings to their patients.[111,112] For female doctors, being up to date on mammogram and Pap testing predicted provision of those services to their patients. Doctors who are physically active, regularly use sunscreen or follow healthy dietary patterns recommend those behaviours to their patients are at higher rates than their inactive, unhealthy colleagues.[113] Furthermore, providers report difficulty counselling patients on behaviours that they struggle with themselves.[114]

Table 3.3
Additional non-clinical domains of health promotion

Clinical	Community	Corporate	Personal
• Encourage age-appropriate preventive screenings • Target and transform known risk factors • Screen for depression, anxiety, isolation	• Promote safe environments and healthy food supplies • Connect people to community, especially older adults • Use technology and social media to extend community in rural/isolated settings • Volunteer/disseminate knowledge as a health educator	• Promote healthy food supplies, health-promoting culture • Bring screenings into the workplace • Encourage flex time for family and health practices • Reward preventive health behaviors	• Practice your own health promotion • Sleep • Watch risk factors • Get screenings • Connect to community

Staying positive

Complementary and alternative medicine has been associated with engaging in positive health behaviours and self-care in both interventional research and epidemiology.[6,26,115–117] Naturopaths are well trained in the science of health promotion and the art of the therapeutic relationship. By attending to one's own health, clinicians can further enhance the effectiveness of health promotion counselling and contribute to reducing the chronic disease epidemic facing the Western world.

KEY POINTS

- Health promotion is the foundation of naturopathic clinical practice, emphasising wellness, lifestyle and prevention.
- A holistic approach to health promotion seeks to achieve a balanced state of social, physical, emotional, intellectual and spiritual wellbeing.
- Social wellness is rooted in the social determinants of health, which are conceptualised in Maslow's hierarchy of needs.
- Physical wellness includes attention to nutrition and physical activity; naturopathic approaches to nutrition focus on macronutrient intake, dietary quality, eating patterns and the cultivation of lifelong healthful attitudes towards food.
- Naturopathic approaches to emotional wellbeing include acknowledgement of the interplay between mental health and personal health behaviours. The naturopathic approach acknowledges the folk wisdom as well as the science of the 'heart' in wellness.
- To promote intellectual wellness, the stressors of daily life must be addressed, taking responsibility both to change factors under our control and to learn proven stress-reducing strategies such as mindfulness to increase our resilience in the face of stressors we cannot control.
- Spiritual wellness rests in finding meaning and purpose in our lives, harmony and peace within one's self and within our relationships with others.
- From a public health perspective, naturopaths are expertly trained in health promotion and a growing body of positive research supports the role of naturopaths as agents of change towards reversing the public health epidemic of unhealthy lifestyle that is plaguing our modern era.

FURTHER READING

Egger G, Binns A, Rôssner S, et al, editors. Lifestyle medicine: lifestyle, the environment and preventive medicine in health and disease. 3rd ed. London: Academic Press; 2017.

Milani RV, Franklin NC. The role of technology in healthy living medicine. Prog Cardiovasc Dis 2017;59(5):487–91.

Murphy J, Oliver G, Ng C, et al. The development and pilot-testing of the 'Healthy Body Healthy Mind (HBHM)': an integrative lifestyle program for patients with serious mental illness and co-morbid metabolic syndrome. Front Psychiatry 2019;6 March. doi: 10.3389/fpsyt.2019.00091.

Shah AK, Becicka R, Talen MR, et al. Integrative medicine and mood, emotions and mental health. Prim Care 2017;44(2):281–304.

Wardle J, Oberg EB. The intersecting paradigms of naturopathic medicine and public health: opportunities for naturopathic medicine. J Altern Complement Med 2011;17(11):1079–84.

REFERENCES

1. Fleming SA, Gutknecht NC. Naturopathy and the primary care practice. Prim Care 2009;37(1):119–36.
2. Zeff J, Snider P, Myers SP. A hierarchy of healing: the therapeutic order. In: Pizzorno J, Murray MT, editors. Textbook of natural medicine, vol. 1. 3rd ed. St Louis: Churchill Livingstone Elsevier; 2006. p. 27–39.
3. WHO. Constitution of the World Health Organization. Preamble. Vol signed on 22 July 1946. New York; 1947.

4. World Health Organization. Global strategy on diet, physical activity and health. Geneva, Switzerland: WHO; 2004.

5. Eyre H, Kahn R, Robertson RM, et al. Preventing cancer, cardiovascular disease, and diabetes: a common agenda for the American Cancer Society, the American Diabetes Association, and the American Heart Association. Circulation 2004;109(25):3244–55.

6. Bradley R, Oberg EB. Naturopathic medicine and type 2 diabetes: a retrospective analysis from an academic clinic. Altern Med Rev 2006;11(1):30–9.

7. Maslow AH. A theory of human motivation. Psychol Rev 1943;50(4):370–96.

8. Yusuf S, Hawken S, Ounpuu S, et al. Effect of potentially modifiable risk factors associated with myocardial infarction in 52 countries (the INTERHEART study): case-control study. Lancet 2004;364(9438):937–52.

9. Rosengren A, Hawken S, Ounpuu S, et al. Association of psychosocial risk factors with risk of acute myocardial infarction in 11119 cases and 13648 controls from 52 countries (the INTERHEART study): case-control study. Lancet 2004;364(9438):953–62.

10. Mokdad AH, Marks JS, Stroup DF, et al. Actual causes of death in the United States, 2000. JAMA 2004;291(10):1238–45.

11. Doll R, Peto R. The causes of cancer: quantitative estimates of avoidable risks of cancer in the United States today. J Natl Cancer Inst 1981;66(6):1191–308.

12. Willett WC. Diet, nutrition, and avoidable cancer. Environ Health Perspect 1995;103(Suppl. 8):165–70.

13. Kant AK, Leitzmann MF, Park Y, et al. Patterns of recommended dietary behaviors predict subsequent risk of mortality in a large cohort of men and women in the United States. J Nutr 2009;139(7):1374–80.

14. McNaughton SA, Bates CJ, Mishra GD. Diet quality is associated with all-cause mortality in adults aged 65 years and older. J Nutr 2012;142(2):320–5.

15. Buettner D, Skemp S. Blue Zones: lessons from the world's longest lived. Am J Lifestyle Med 2016;10(5):318–21. doi:10.1177/1559827616637066. eCollection 2016 Sep-Oct.

16. Oldways Preservation Trust. Mediterranean Diet Pyramid. Online; 1999. Available: http://oldwayspt.org/resources/ heritage-pyramids/mediterranean-pyramid/overview. [Accessed 9 April 2013].

17. Willett WC. The Mediterranean diet: science and practice. Public Health Nutr 2006;9(1A):105–10.

18. Dilis V, Katsoulis M, Lagiou P, et al. Mediterranean diet and CHD: the Greek European Prospective Investigation into Cancer and Nutrition cohort. Br J Nutr 2012;108(4):699–709.

19. Fung TT, Rexrode KM, Mantzoros CS, et al. Mediterranean diet and incidence of and mortality from coronary heart disease and stroke in women. Circulation 2009;119(8):1093–100.

20. Knoops KT, de Groot LC, Kromhout D, et al. Mediterranean diet, lifestyle factors, and 10-year mortality in elderly European men and women: the HALE project. JAMA 2004;292(12):1433–9.

21. de Lorgeril M, Salen P, Martin JL, et al. Mediterranean diet, traditional risk factors, and the rate of cardiovascular complications after myocardial infarction: final report of the Lyon Diet Heart Study. Circulation 1999;99(6):779–85.

22. Iestra JA, Kromhout D, van der Schouw YT, et al. Effect size estimates of lifestyle and dietary changes on all-cause mortality in coronary artery disease patients: a systematic review. Circulation 2005;112(6):924–34.

23. Louie JC, Gwynn J, Turner N, et al. Dietary glycemic index and glycemic load among Indigenous and non-Indigenous children aged 10–12 years. Nutrition 2012;28(7–8):e14–22.

24. Ebbeling CB, Swain JF, Feldman HA, et al. Effects of dietary composition on energy expenditure during weight-loss maintenance. JAMA 2012;307(24):2627–34.

25. Pereira MA, Swain J, Goldfine AB, et al. Effects of a low-glycemic load diet on resting energy expenditure and heart disease risk factors during weight loss. JAMA 2004;292(20):2482–90.

26. Oberg EB, Bradley RB, Allen J, et al. Evaluation of a naturopathic nutrition program for type 2 diabetes. Complement Ther Clin Pract 2011;doi:10.1016/j. ctcp.2011.02.00.

27. Thomas DE, Elliott EJ, Baur L. Low glycaemic index or low glycaemic load diets for overweight and obesity. Cochrane Database Syst Rev 2007;(3):CD005105.

28. Smith-Spangler C, Brandeau ML, Hunter GE, et al. Are organic foods safer or healthier than conventional alternatives? A systematic review. Ann Intern Med 2012;157(5):348–66.

29. Lu C, Toepel K, Irish R, et al. Organic diets significantly lower children's dietary exposure to organophosphorus pesticides. Environ Health Perspect 2006;114(2):260–3.

30. Palupi E, Jayanegara A, Ploeger A, et al. Comparison of nutritional quality between conventional and organic dairy products: a meta-analysis. J Sci Food Agric 2012;92(14):2774–81.

31. Hunter D, Foster M, McArthur JO, et al. Evaluation of the micronutrient composition of plant foods produced by organic and conventional agricultural methods. Crit Rev Food Sci Nutr 2011;51(6):571–82.

32. Marinac CR, Nelson SH, Breen CI, et al. Prolonged nightly fasting and breast cancer prognosis. JAMA Oncol 2016;2(8):1049–55. doi:10.1001/jamaoncol.2016.0164.

33. Kramer CK, Zinman B, Retnakaran R. Are metabolically healthy overweight and obesity benign conditions? A systematic review and meta-analysis. Ann Intern Med 2013;159(11):758–69.

34. Marinac CR, Sears DD, Natarajan L, et al. Frequency and circadian timing of eating may influence biomarkers of inflammation and insulin resistance associated with breast cancer risk. PLoS ONE 2015;10(8):e0136240. doi:10.1371/journal.pone.0136240. eCollection 2015.

35. Sargrad KR, Homko C, Mozzoli M, et al. Effect of high protein vs high carbohydrate intake on insulin sensitivity, body weight, hemoglobin A1c, and blood pressure in patients with type 2 diabetes mellitus. J Am Diet Assoc 2005;105(4):573–80.

36. Miyashita Y, Koide N, Ohtsuka M, et al. Beneficial effect of low carbohydrate in low calorie diets on visceral fat reduction in type 2 diabetic patients with obesity. Diabetes Res Clin Pract 2004;65(3):235–41.

37. Zino S, Skeaff M, Williams S, et al. Randomised controlled trial of effect of fruit and vegetable consumption on plasma concentrations of lipids and antioxidants. BMJ 1997;314(7097):1787–91.

38. Schroder H. Protective mechanisms of the Mediterranean diet in obesity and type 2 diabetes. J Nutr Biochem 2007;18(3):149–60.

39. Russo GL. Ins and outs of dietary phytochemicals in cancer chemoprevention. Biochem Pharmacol 2007;74:533–44.

40. Liu RH. Health benefits of fruit and vegetables are from additive and synergistic combinations of phytochemicals. Am J Clin Nutr 2003;78(3 Suppl.):517S–520S.

41. Sumner MD, Elliott-Eller M, Weidner G, et al. Effects of pomegranate juice consumption on myocardial perfusion

in patients with coronary heart disease. Am J Cardiol 2005;96(6):810–14.

42. Kerckhoffs DA, Brouns F, Hornstra G, et al. Effects on the human serum lipoprotein profile of beta-glucan, soy protein and isoflavones, plant sterols and stanols, garlic and tocotrienols. J Nutr 2002;132(9):2494–505.

43. Department of Health and Human Services USFaDA. Food labeling: health claims; oats and coronary heart disease. Fed Regist 1997;62:3484–601.

44. Riccardi G, Capaldo B, Vaccaro O. Functional foods in the management of obesity and type 2 diabetes. Curr Opin Clin Nutr Metab Care 2005;8(6):630–5.

45. Nettleton JA, Katz R. Omega-3 long-chain polyunsaturated fatty acids in type 2 diabetes: a review. J Am Diet Assoc 2005;105(3):428–40.

46. Kristeller JL, Wolever RQ. Mindfulness-based eating awareness training for treating binge eating disorder: the conceptual foundation. Eat Disord 2011;19(1):49–61.

47. Oberg EB, Pagano G, Kesten D, et al. How one eats may be more important than what one eats: eating styles correlate with glycemic control more strongly than macronutrient intake. Composing Effective Patient Care: American Association of Naturopathic Physicians, vol. 5. Phoenix: Raintree Publishing; 2011.

48. Scherwitz L, Kesten D. Seven eating styles linked to overeating, overweight, and obesity. Explore (NY) 2005;1(5):342–59.

49. Neumark-Sztainer D, Wall M, Story M, et al. Are family meal patterns associated with disordered eating behaviors among adolescents? J Adolesc Health 2004;35(5):350–9.

50. Mannucci E, Tesi F, Ricca V, et al. Eating behavior in obese patients with and without type 2 diabetes mellitus. Int J Obes Relat Metab Disord 2002;26(6):848–53.

51. Ross R, Freeman JA, Janssen I. Exercise alone is an effective strategy for reducing obesity and related comorbidities. Exerc Sport Sci Rev 2000;28(4):165–70.

52. Foster-Schubert KE, Alfano CM, Duggan CR, et al. Effect of diet and exercise, alone or combined, on weight and body composition in overweight-to-obese postmenopausal women. Obesity (Silver Spring) 2012;20(8):1628–38.

53. Abbenhardt C, McTiernan A, Alfano CM, et al. Effects of individual and combined dietary weight loss and exercise interventions in postmenopausal women on adiponectin and leptin levels. J Intern Med 2013;25.

54. Duncan GE, Anton SD, Sydeman SJ, et al. Prescribing exercise at varied levels of intensity and frequency: a randomized trial. Arch Intern Med 2005;165(20):2362–9.

55. Chambliss HO. Exercise duration and intensity in a weight-loss program. Clin J Sport Med 2005;15(2):113–15.

56. Sato Y, Nagasaki M, Nakai N, et al. Physical exercise improves glucose metabolism in lifestyle-related diseases. Exp Biol Med (Maywood) 2003;228(10):1208–12.

57. Lee DC, Sui X, Church TS, et al. Changes in fitness and fatness on the development of cardiovascular disease risk factors hypertension, metabolic syndrome, and hypercholesterolemia. J Am Coll Cardiol 2012;59(7):665–72.

58. Wei M, Gibbons LW, Mitchell TL, et al. The association between cardiorespiratory fitness and impaired fasting glucose and type 2 diabetes mellitus in men. Ann Intern Med 1999;130(2):89–96.

59. Patten SB, Williams JV, Lavorato DH, et al. Recreational physical activity ameliorates some of the negative impact of major depression on health-related quality of life. Front Psychiatry 2013;4:22.

60. Danielsson L, Noras AM, Waern M, et al. Exercise in the treatment of major depression: a systematic review

61. Friedberg F. Does graded activity increase activity? A case study of chronic fatigue syndrome. J Behav Ther Exp Psychiatry 2002;33(3–4):203–15.

62. Knowler WC, Barrett-Connor E, Fowler SE, et al. Reduction in the incidence of type 2 diabetes with lifestyle intervention or metformin. N Engl J Med 2002;346(6):393–403.

63. Mojtabai R, Olfson M. National trends in psychotherapy by office-based psychiatrists. Arch Gen Psychiatry 2008;65(8):962–70.

64. Mishra SI, Scherer RW, Snyder C, et al. Exercise interventions on health-related quality of life for people with cancer during active treatment. Cochrane Database Syst Rev 2012;(8):CD008465.

65. Larun L, Nordheim LV, Ekeland E, et al. Exercise in prevention and treatment of anxiety and depression among children and young people. Cochrane Database Syst Rev 2006;(3):CD004691.

66. Mather AS, Rodriguez C, Guthrie MF, et al. Effects of exercise on depressive symptoms in older adults with poorly responsive depressive disorder: randomised controlled trial. Br J Psychiatry 2002;180:411–15.

67. Fabricatore AN, Wadden TA, Higginbotham AJ, et al. Intentional weight loss and changes in symptoms of depression: a systematic review and meta-analysis. Int J Obes (Lond) 2011;35(11):1363–76.

68. Olsen CM. Natural rewards, neuroplasticity, and non-drug addictions. Neuropharmacology 2011;61(7):1109–22.

69. Khalsa SB. Yoga as a therapeutic intervention: a bibliometric analysis of published research studies. Indian J Physiol Pharmacol 2004;48(3):269–85.

70. Tiller WA, McCraty R, Atkinson M. Cardiac coherence: a new, noninvasive measure of autonomic nervous system order. Altern Ther Health Med 1996;2(1):52–65.

71. Barrett B, Marchand L, Scheder J, et al. What complementary and alternative medicine practitioners say about health and health care. Ann Fam Med 2004;2(3):253–9.

72. Kushnir T, Cohen AH. Job structure and burnout among primary care pediatricians. Work 2006;27(1):67–74.

73. Rivera-Torres P, Araque-Padilla RA, Montero-Simo MJ. Job stress across gender: the importance of emotional and intellectual demands and social support in women. Int J Environ Res Public Health 2013;10(1):375–89.

74. Cursoux P, Lehucher-Michel MP, Marchetti H, et al. Burnout syndrome: a 'true' cardiovascular risk factor. Presse Med 2012;41(11):1056–63.

75. Department of Health. Austalia's Physical Activity recommendations for children. Online; 2007. Available: http://www.health.gov.au/internet/main/publishing.nsf/content/health-pubhlth-strateg-active-recommend.htm. [Accessed 1 November 2013].

76. Kabat-Zinn J. Full catastrophe living: using the wisdom of your body and mind to face stress, pain, and illness. New York, NY: Delta Trade Paperbacks; 1991.

77. Lazar SW, Bush G, Gollub RL, et al. Functional brain mapping of the relaxation response and meditation. Neuroreport 2000;11(7):1581–5.

78. Sampalli T, Berlasso E, Fox R, et al. A controlled study of the effect of a mindfulness-based stress reduction technique in women with multiple chemical sensitivity, chronic fatigue syndrome, and fibromyalgia. J Multidiscip Healthc 2009;2:53–9.

79. Astin JA, Shapiro SL, Eisenberg DM, et al. Mind-body medicine: state of the science, implications for practice. J Am Board Fam Pract 2003;16(2):131–47.

grading the quality of evidence. Physiother Theory Pract 2013;PMID: 23521569.

80. Ludwig DS, Kabat-Zinn J. Mindfulness in medicine. JAMA 2008;300(11):1350–2.

81. Marchand WR. Mindfulness-based stress reduction, mindfulness-based cognitive therapy, and Zen meditation for depression, anxiety, pain, and psychological distress. J Psychiatr Pract 2012;18(4):233–52.

82. Merkes M. Mindfulness-based stress reduction for people with chronic diseases. Aust J Prim Health 2010;16(3):200–10.

83. Wilson E. Biophilia. The human bond with other species. Cambridge, MA: Harvard University Press; 1984.

84. Walsh R. Lifestyle and mental health. Am Psychol 2011;66(7):579–92.

85. Annerstedt M, Währborg P. Nature-assisted therapy: systematic review of controlled and observational studies. Scand J Public Health 2011;39:371.

86. Tuck I. A critical review of a spirituality intervention. West J Nurs Res 2012;34(6):712–35.

87. Candy B, Jones L, Varagunam M, et al. Spiritual and religious interventions for well-being of adults in the terminal phase of disease. Cochrane Database Syst Rev 2012;(5):CD007544.

88. Miller HL. What high-level wellness means. Can J Public Health 1959;50(11):447–57.

89. Takaro TK, Krieger JW, Song L. Effect of environmental interventions to reduce exposure to asthma triggers in homes of low-income children in Seattle. J Expo Anal Environ Epidemiol 2004;14 Suppl 1:S133–43.

90. Richardson G, Eick S, Jones R. How is the indoor environment related to asthma?: literature review. J Adv Nurs 2005;52(3):328–39.

91. Anand P, Kunnumakara AB, Sundaram C, et al. Cancer is a preventable disease that requires major lifestyle changes. Pharm Res 2008;25(9):2097–116.

92. Meeker JD. Exposure to environmental endocrine disruptors and child development. Arch Pediatr Adolesc Med 2012;166(10):952–8.

93. Deng F, Tao FB, Liu DY, et al. Effects of growth environments and two environmental endocrine disruptors on children with idiopathic precocious puberty. Eur J Endocrinol 2012;166(5):803–9.

94. Morgan MK, Sheldon LS, Croghan CW, et al. Exposures of preschool children to chlorpyrifos and its degradation product 3,5,6-trichloro-2-pyridinol in their everyday environments. J Expo Anal Environ Epidemiol 2005; 15(4):297–309.

95. Environmental Working Group. Shopper's Guide to Pesticides in Produce; 2013. http://www.ewg.org/foodnews/summary/ [Accessed 12 April 2013].

96. Ma J, Urizar GG Jr, Alehegn T, et al. Diet and physical activity counseling during ambulatory care visits in the United States. Prev Med 2004;39(4):815–22.

97. Daubenmier JJ, Weidner G, Sumner MD, et al. The contribution of changes in diet, exercise, and stress management to changes in coronary risk in women and men in the multisite cardiac lifestyle intervention program. Ann Behav Med 2007;33(1):57–68.

98. Toobert DJ, Strycker LA, Barrera M, et al. Seven-year follow-up of a multiple-health-behavior diabetes intervention. Am J Health Behav 2010;34(6):680–94.

99. Ornish D, Scherwitz LW, Billings JH, et al. Intensive lifestyle changes for reversal of coronary heart disease. JAMA 1998;280(23):2001–7.

100. O'Hara BJ, Phongsavan P, Eakin EG, et al. Effectiveness of Australia's Get Healthy Information and Coaching Service®: maintenance of self-reported anthropometric and behavioural changes after program completion. BMC Public Health 2013;13:175.

101. Dalziel K, Segal L. Time to give nutrition interventions a higher profile: cost-effectiveness of 10 nutrition interventions. Health Promot Int 2007;22(4):271–83.

102. Harrison PL, Pope JE, Coberley CR, et al. Evaluation of the relationship between individual well-being and future health care utilization and cost. Popul Health Manag 2012;15(6):325–30.

103. Herman PM, Szczurko O, Cooley K, et al. Cost-effectiveness of naturopathic care for chronic low back pain. Altern Ther Health Med 2008;14(2):32–9.

104. Lind BK, Lafferty WE, Tyree PT, et al. Comparison of health care expenditures among insured users and nonusers of complementary and alternative medicine in Washington State: a cost minimization analysis. J Altern Complement Med 2010;16(4):411–17.

105. Danaei G, Ding EL, Mozaffarian D, et al. The preventable causes of death in the United States: comparative risk assessment of dietary, lifestyle, and metabolic risk factors. PLoS Med 2009;6(4):e1000058.

106. Chen L, Magliano DJ, Balkau B, et al. AUSDRISK: an Australian Type 2 Diabetes Risk Assessment Tool based on demographic, lifestyle and simple anthropometric measures. Med J Aust 2010;192(4):197–202.

107. Wong KC, Brown AM, Li SC. AUSDRISK—application in general practice. Aust Fam Physician 2011;40(7): 524–6.

108. Goldstein MG, Whitlock EP, DePue J. Multiple behavioral risk factor interventions in primary care. Summary of research evidence. Am J Prev Med 2004;27(2 Suppl.):61–79.

109. Bradley R, Kozura E, Buckle H, et al. Description of clinical risk factor changes during naturopathic care for type 2 diabetes. J Altern Complement Med 2009;15(6):633–8.

110. Wardle JL, Adams J, Lui CW. A qualitative study of naturopathy in rural practice: a focus upon naturopaths' experiences and perceptions of rural patients and demands for their services. BMC Health Serv Res 2010;10:185.

111. Frank E, Segura C, Shen H, et al. Predictors of Canadian physicians' prevention counseling practices. Can J Public Health 2010;101(5):390–5.

112. Frank E, Dresner Y, Shani M, et al. The association between physicians' and patients' preventive health practices. CMAJ 2013;185(8):649–53.

113. Oberg EB, Frank E. Personal health practices efficiently and effectively influence patient health practices. J R Coll Physicians Edinb 2009;39(4):290–1.

114. Vickers KS, Kircher KJ, Smith MD, et al. Health behavior counseling in primary care: provider-reported rate and confidence. Fam Med 2007;39(10):730–5.

115. Nahin RL, Dahlhamer JM, Taylor BL, et al. Health behaviors and risk factors in those who use complementary and alternative medicine. BMC Public Health 2007;7:217.

116. Hawk C, Ndetan H, Evans MW Jr. Potential role of complementary and alternative health care providers in chronic disease prevention and health promotion: an analysis of National Health Interview Survey data. Prev Med 2012;54(1):18–22.

117. Bradley RD, Kozura EV, Oberg EB, et al. Observed changes in risk during naturopathic treatment of hypertension. Evid Based Complement Alternat Med 2010;doi:10.1093/ecam/nep219.

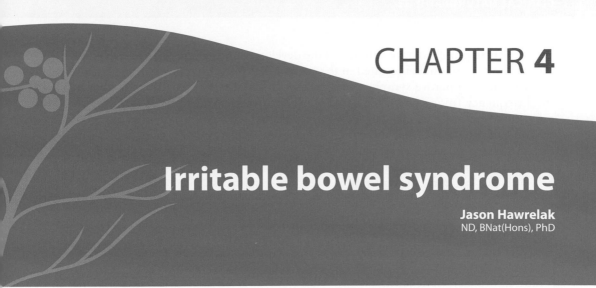

CHAPTER 4

Irritable bowel syndrome

Jason Hawrelak
ND, BNat(Hons), PhD

OVERVIEW

Irritable bowel syndrome (IBS) is a functional gastrointestinal disorder characterised by altered bowel habit and abdominal pain.[1] It is a chronic disorder of unclear aetiology.[2] Research, however, has brought to light a number of possible aetiological factors.

IBS is believed to be the most common gastrointestinal disorder in Western countries. Its prevalence is estimated to be 7–15% in Western European, North American and Australian populations, with a higher incidence in women.[3]

Possible aetiological factors
• *Enhanced visceral perception*. Patients with IBS have been found to have increased visceral sensation and visceral hyperalgesia compared with healthy controls.[4,5]
• *Low-grade inflammation*. IBS patients show no identifiable inflammation on routine colonic biopsies. However, some do show increased expression of inflammatory markers (increased enterochromaffin and mast cell numbers, increased intraepithelial T-lymphocytes and increased mucosal interleukin-1β messenger RNA), suggesting low-grade inflammation is present. This mild mucosal inflammation is thought to cause local disruptions to neuromuscular function.[5,6]
• *Altered gastrointestinal tract (GIT) motility*. People diagnosed with constipation-predominant IBS (C-IBS) have been found to have significant delays in overall colonic transit time and decreased numbers of fast and propagated colonic contractions compared with healthy controls.[7] There also appears to be impaired transit of intestinal gas.[8] Conversely, people with diarrhoea-predominant IBS (D-IBS) have increased occurrences of high amplitude colonic contractions and rapid colonic transit time.[9]
• *Altered GIT microbiota (dysbiosis)*. Colonic fermentation studies have found patients with IBS produce significantly more colonic hydrogen than healthy controls,[10] as well as having altered faecal short-chain fatty acid profiles.[11] Additional studies have found the GIT microbiota of IBS patients to differ from that of healthy controls, most notably lower faecal concentrations of bifidobacteria and lactobacilli and higher concentrations of Enterobacteriaceae.[12–14] Other studies have found a greater occurrence of small intestinal bacterial overgrowth in IBS patients.[15]

Diagnosis

The diagnosis of IBS is considered one of exclusion and requires the absence of any other GIT pathology. In addition there is an absence of any reproducible or accepted biological marker that can be used in diagnosing IBS. There is no simple diagnostic test either.[16] These problems have stimulated the development of symptom-based diagnostic criteria—an approach that resulted in the current diagnostic criteria for IBS—the Rome IV criteria.[17] Supportive symptoms that are not part of the criteria include abnormal stool frequency (more than three bowel movements per day or fewer than three bowel movements per week), abnormal stool form (lumpy/hard stools or loose/watery stools), straining at defecation, faecal urgency, feeling of incomplete bowel evacuation, bloating or the passage of mucus.[17] Patients with IBS can be further classified according to their predominant bowel pattern into one of four subtypes. It should be remembered, however, that patients can transition between these subtypes.

Rome IV diagnostic criteria for IBS

Recurrent abdominal pain, on average, at least one day per week in the last three months, associated with two or more of the following criteria:

- related to defecation
- associated with a change in frequency of stool
- associated with a change in the form (appearance) of stool.

Source: Lacy et al. 2016[17]

DIFFERENTIAL DIAGNOSIS

D-IBS and M-IBS

Dietary causes: lactose, sorbitol (and other sugar alcohols), fructose, excess alcohol, caffeine, gas-producing foods (i.e. oligosaccharide-rich foods), gluten sensitivity

Infections: *Giardia* spp., *Amoeba* spp., *Blastocystis* spp., *Dientamoeba fragilis*, small-intestinal bacterial overgrowth, human immunodeficiency virus (HIV)

Inflammatory bowel diseases: ulcerative colitis, Crohn's disease, microscopic colitis, collagenous colitis, lymphocytic colitis

Adverse drug reaction: antibiotics, proton-pump inhibitors, chemotherapy, non-steroidal anti-inflammatory drugs, ACE inhibitors, beta-blockers

Malabsorption: coeliac disease

Other: ovarian cancer, endometriosis, colorectal cancer, ischaemic colitis, hyperthyroidism, carcinoid

C-IBS

Neurological: multiple sclerosis, Parkinson's disease, spinal cord injuries

Drug toxicity: antidepressants, opiates, calcium-channel blockers, clonidine

Endocrine: hypothyroidism, diabetes, hypercalcaemia

Other: colorectal cancer, ovarian cancer, endometriosis, diverticular disease, bowel obstruction, coeliac disease

Sources: Lucak 2004,[18] Biesiekierski et al. 2011,[19] Jimenez-Gonzalez et al. 2012,[20] Barratt et al. 2011,[21] Pimentel et al. 2000[22] and Ozdil et al. 2011[23]

RISK FACTORS

Several factors that appear to play a role in initiating and maintaining IBS have been identified. These factors include a genetic predisposition, a history of enteric infections, antibiotic use, a history of stressful life events and concurrent anxiety and/or depressive disorders.

IBS subtyping by predominant stool pattern
1. Constipation-predominant IBS (C-IBS): hard or lumpy stools[a] ≥ 25% and loose water stools[b] < 25% of bowel movements.[c]
2. Diarrhoea-predominant IBS (D-IBS): loose (mushy) or watery stools[b] ≥ 25% and hard lumpy stools[a] < 25% of bowel movements.[c]
3. Mixed IBS (M-IBS): hard or lumpy stools[a] ≥ 25% and loose (mushy) watery stools[b] ≥ 25% of bowel movements.[c]
4. Unsubtyped IBS: insufficient abnormality of stool consistency to meet criteria for C-IBS, D-IBS or M-IBS

[a]Bristol stool form scale 1–2 (separate hard lumps like nuts [difficult to pass] or sausage shaped but lumpy).
[b]Bristol stool form scale 6–7 (fluffy pieces with ragged edges, a mushy stool or watery, no solid pieces, entirely liquid).
[c]In the absence of use of antidiarrhoeals or laxatives.
Source: Lacy et al. 2016[17]

- It is believed that a genetic disposition may contribute to the development of IBS in some patients.[24] This predisposition may not be disease-specific but more related to alterations in the responsiveness of the central nervous system to stimuli.
- Studies have shown a relationship between acute gastrointestinal infections (viral, protozoal and bacterial) and the onset of IBS symptoms—a condition termed postinfectious IBS.[25–28] It has been postulated that long-lasting alterations in mucosal function and structure may be responsible for postinfective IBS. These alterations include increased intestinal permeability, low-grade lymphocytic infiltration and increases in other inflammatory components, such as enterochromaffin and mast cells. This can result in both visceral hypersensitivity and dysmotility. Bacterial endotoxins are believed to play a causative role in the development of post-infectious IBS.[29]
- A number of studies have found an association between antibiotic use and increased frequency of IBS symptoms.[30–32] This association is thought to be mediated via antibiotic-induced alterations in the GIT microbiota and enhanced visceral sensitivity.[33]
- Stressful and traumatic life events are frequently reported to precede the initial onset of IBS symptoms and symptom flare-ups in patients already suffering from IBS.[34,35] Additionally, IBS has consistently been found to have a high degree of psychiatric comorbidities, such as dysthymia, depression, panic disorder and generalised anxiety disorder.[36,37]

CONVENTIONAL TREATMENT

Many agents are currently used for treating IBS and no one agent has proven particularly effective and/or free from side effects. Key classes of medications used to treat IBS include antispasmodics and antidepressants, with laxatives, 5-hydroxytryptamine type 4 receptor agonists (such as tegaserod) and guanylate cyclase-C agonists (linaclotide) used in C-IBS and antidiarrhoeals (loperamide) and 5-hydroxytryptamine-3 receptor antagonists (alosetron) in D-IBS.[15,38] Antibiotics have recently been trialled to treat IBS. Therapeutic gains (the difference in treatment response between placebo and active therapy) have often been minimal with these agents[39,40] and adverse events are sometimes severe.[41,42]

KEY TREATMENT PROTOCOLS

Optimise GIT microbiota

The microbiota of the GIT represents an ecosystem of the highest complexity. Over 1000 different species have been isolated from the GIT to date, with each individual harbouring at least 160 different species.[43] The adult human GIT is estimated to contain 10^{15} viable microorganisms, which is 10 times the number of eukaryotic cells found within the entire human body.[44] Some researchers have called this microbial population the 'microbe' organ—an organ that is similar in size to the liver (1–1.5 kg in weight).[45] Indeed, this 'microbe' organ is now recognised as rivalling the liver in the number of biochemical transformations and reactions in which it participates.[46]

> ### Naturopathic Treatment Aims
>
> - Optimise GIT microbiota.
> - Support the nervous system.
> - Promote normalisation of bowel patterns.
> - Manage GIT symptoms.
> - Decrease gut inflammation and diminish visceral hypersensitivity.
> - Support liver function.
> - Manage adverse food reactions.

The microbiota plays many critical roles in the body; thus, there are many areas of host health that can be compromised when the microbiota is altered. The GIT microbiota is involved in modulating the immune system, synthesising vitamins (B group and K), enhancing GIT motility and function, digestion and nutrient absorption, inhibiting pathogens (colonisation resistance), metabolising plant compounds (e.g. phyto-oestrogens, glycosides and other polyphenols) and producing short-chain fatty acids and polyamines.[47–49]

The colon is the most heavily colonised area of the GIT and this microbial ecosystem is believed to play the greatest role in human health. The colonic microbiota is composed almost entirely of anaerobic bacteria. The dominant genera in most individuals are *Bacteroides* and *Faecalibacterium*, and more rarely *Bifidobacterium*, although this varies considerably between individuals, with dietary factors and medication use able to cause significant alterations in the proportion of these microbe populations. Other numerically dominant anaerobes include *Eubacterium*, *Blautia*, *Roseburia* and *Ruminococcus*.[43,50] Existing in smaller proportions are coliforms, methanogens, enterococci and dissimilatory sulfate-reducing bacteria. These important groups of bacteria have been divided into species that have the capacity to exert either beneficial or harmful effects on the host, as outlined in Figure 4.1.[49] When the beneficial species are present in insufficient numbers or when concentrations of potentially harmful bacteria are relatively high, then dysbiosis is said to result. Dysbiosis is a state in which the microbiota produces harmful effects through one or more of the following factors: qualitative and quantitative changes in the intestinal flora itself; changes in their metabolic activities; and changes in their local distribution.[51]

After publication of an open-label case series in 2000,[22] in which antibiotic treatment significantly improved gastrointestinal symptoms in some patients with IBS, the idea that small intestinal bacterial overgrowth (SIBO) was *the* cause of IBS has grown considerably. The results of recent meta-analyses have questioned this theory, however. A 2009 meta-analysis examining the presence of SIBO in IBS found that the majority of IBS patients did not have SIBO.[53] Even using the most inclusive definition of SIBO found that its prevalence in IBS subjects was only 38% (versus 12% of healthy controls). So while the evidence suggests that SIBO is more prevalent in IBS patients, the majority of patients diagnosed with IBS do not suffer from SIBO. This conclusion is also supported by the results of a 2012 meta-analysis of clinical trials using rifaximin (a non-absorbable antibiotic) in the treatment of IBS.[39] The analysis did find rifaximin more efficacious than placebo for reducing global IBS symptoms and bloating. However, therapeutic gains were very modest, with antibiotic treatment improving symptoms by less than

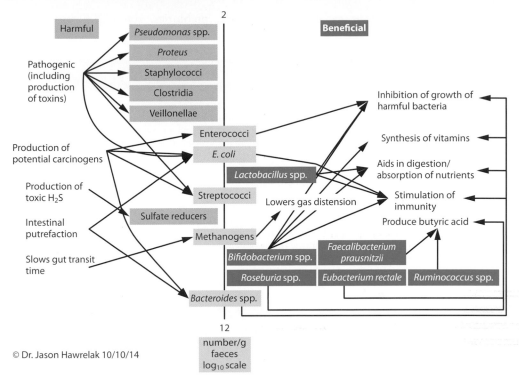

© Dr. Jason Hawrelak 10/10/14

Figure 4.1
The predominant microbiota of the colon, categorised into health-promoting and potentially harmful groups
Source: Adapted from Roberfroid et al. 2010[52] and Gibson & Roberfroid 1995[49]

10% (relative to placebo) and 10 subjects needed to be treated with antibiotics for one to benefit from the treatment. So where does this leave the role of SIBO in IBS? As SIBO is more prevalent in IBS patients than healthy controls and SIBO treatment does appear to relieve symptoms in *some* IBS patients, ascertaining if individual patients are suffering from SIBO is important in determining the optimal approach to addressing their GIT symptoms. Unfortunately, the diagnosis of SIBO is far from straightforward.[54] The current gold standard (jejuna aspirate and culture) is highly invasive and is only able to examine the proximal small bowel. The most commonly discussed diagnostic method (the lactulose breath test) is non-invasive and is theoretically able to identify SIBO of the distal small bowel but is of questionable efficacy—particularly in patients with IBS.[55] Hence it is often not recommended in this patient group.[56] The glucose breath test is currently the non-invasive test of choice,[57] but even this test has problems, such as an inability to accurately assess SIBO of the distal small bowel. The lactulose breath test, while being of questionable accuracy in the assessment of SIBO, does have a role in determining methane-producer status, particularly in C-IBS patients, where production of excess methane by methanogens in the microbiota can result in slowed intestinal transit time.[58,59]

In the naturopathic treatment of IBS, dysbiosis is viewed as one of the most important aetiological factors. Hence, treatments aimed at addressing this imbalance are seen as crucial to managing this condition. Treatments aimed at improving the GIT ecosystem can be divided into four categories: probiotics, prebiotics, symbiotics and herbal antimicrobials.

Accurately assessing the GIT microbiota

A number of tools are currently being offered to practitioners as ways of assessing the GIT ecosystem. These can be broadly broken down into techniques that rely on culture and those that are independent of culture, such as techniques based on 16S ribosomal RNA. Methods that rely on microorganism culturing will have issues with accuracy due to the problems inherent in maintaining viable faecal organisms after collection to be later grown out in the lab. Time spent in storage and transport, exposure to different temperatures (e.g. refrigeration, ambient air temperatures, hot delivery vehicles) and exposure to oxygen all have the capacity to significantly alter microorganism populations before they arrive at the lab for culturing. Culture-independent methods do not share these challenges, as microbes are killed at the time of collection; thereby an accurate picture of the ecosystem is maintained to be later analysed. Culture-independent techniques utilising 16S ribosomal RNA technology are currently considered the gold standard method to accurately assess the GIT microbiota. Perhaps the biggest issue with culture, however, is its inability to grow the majority of species found in the human GIT. This is obviously a substantial limitation because culturing techniques, independent of the factors discussed above, will not be able to detect most species in the GIT, including many species that play pivotal roles in human health.[60]

Dysbiosis in systemic disorders

Intestinal dysbiosis appears to play a contributing role to systemic disorders in addition to gastrointestinal conditions, with research highlighting the potential aetiological role of dysbiosis in obesity,[61] non-alcoholic fatty liver disease,[62] rheumatoid arthritis,[63] allergic diseases,[64] depression and anxiety,[65] Parkinson's disease,[66] multiple sclerosis,[67] Alzheimer's disease,[68] and chronic fatigue syndrome.[69]

Probiotics

The term 'probiotic' is derived from Greek and literally means 'for life'. The current World Health Organization definition of probiotics is 'live microorganisms which when administered in adequate amounts confer a health benefit on the host'.[70] Probiotic organisms can be found in fermented foods (such as yoghurt), as well as supplements. The microorganisms found in these products are typically, although not exclusively, lactobacilli and bifidobacteria. With research in the field of faecal bacteriotherapy blossoming, probiotic products derived from faeces, containing a multitude of bacterial strains, may become commercially available in the near future.[71]

Probiotics have a long history of successful use in treating IBS. In fact the first case series detailing the efficacy of a ***Lactobacillus acidophilus*** supplement in IBS was published in 1955.[72] A recent systematic review and meta-analysis of randomised controlled trials found probiotic use to be associated with improvements in global IBS symptoms compared with placebo and reductions in abdominal pain.[73] It is well known, however, that efficacy in this condition, as it is in all conditions, is strain dependent. Commercially available probiotic strains that have shown efficacy in treating IBS include ***Bifidobacterium animalis* DN-173 010**,[74] ***Bifidobacterium infantis* 35624**,[75,76] ***Lactobacillus fermentum* PCC**,[77,78] ***Lactobacillus plantarum* 299v**[79,80] and ***Bacillus coagulans* GBI-30 6086**,[81] as well as the proprietary multistrain probiotic combinations **Lab4**[82] (containing two strains of *Lactobacillus acidophilus* and two strains of *Bifidobacterium* in defined ratios) and **VSL#3** (containing one strain of *Streptococcus thermophilus*, three strains of *Bifidobacterium* and four strains of *Lactobacillus* in defined ratios).[83] Commercially available strains found to be ineffective in the management of IBS include ***Lactobacillus acidophilus* NCFM**[84] and ***Lactobacillus rhamnosus* GG** (in isolation).[85,86] See Table 4.5 for a summary of research for IBS.

To achieve the desired therapeutic results, it is imperative to prescribe the precise probiotic strains that have demonstrated therapeutic and clinical efficacy in the condition in question. Strains that work in one condition will not necessarily be effective in other conditions. For example, *Lactobacillus rhamnosus* GG appears to be effective in preventing antibiotic-associated side effects[87] but not of any demonstrable benefit in urinary tract infections.[88] Table 4.1 outlines the most appropriate probiotic strains to use for specific gastrointestinal disease conditions, as determined by human trials.

Probiotic organisms can be delivered through a variety of mechanisms: fermented foods (such as yoghurt), capsules, tablets and powders. Each method has its advantages and disadvantages, which are listed in Table 4.2.

Prebiotics

A prebiotic is defined as 'a substrate that is selectively utilised by host microorganisms conferring a health benefit'.[147] For food ingredients to be classified as gastrointestinal prebiotics, they must:

- be neither digested nor absorbed in the stomach or small intestine[148]
- act as a selective food source for one or a limited number of potentially beneficial indigenous bacteria in the large intestine[148]
- change the colonic microbiota towards a healthier composition[148]
- induce luminal or systemic changes that improve the health of the host.[149]

Most emphasis to date has been on finding and trialling food sources that are used by lactic acid-producing bacteria. This is due to the health-promoting properties of these organisms.[148] The best known lactic acid-producing bacteria belong to the genera *Lactobacillus* and *Bifidobacterium*. Commonly used prebiotics include **lactulose, fructooligosaccharides** (FOS), **galactooligosaccharides** (GOS) and **partially hydrolysed guar gum** (PHGG). The most appropriate prebiotics to use for specific health conditions are highlighted in Table 4.3.

One trial has been performed investigating the efficacy of FOS in IBS, with disappointing results.[163] However, the dose of FOS used in the study (20 g/day in a single dose) is known to cause significant gastrointestinal side effects even in healthy subjects (such as bloating, distension, borborygmi and increased flatulence).[164] Therefore it is not surprising that FOS failed to reduce these same GIT symptoms in trial participants. Other prebiotics appear to hold more promise in treating IBS, such as GOS and PHGG (Table 4.3).[155,156]

Prebiotics versus colonic foods

A number of other substances are frequently referred to as prebiotics. Many of these, however, fail to meet the criteria outlined above. Slippery elm, psyllium husks and pectin would more accurately be described as colonic foods rather than prebiotics as they appear to lack the selectivity of fermentation that is required of prebiotics.[165–167] Other substances, such as polydextrose and larch arabinogalactans, have been shown to increase the growth of beneficial bacteria in human trials.[168,169] However, they have thus far been the subject of inadequate research to determine if they meet all of the prebiotic requirements.

Table 4.1
Most appropriate probiotic strains for specific disease conditions

Condition		Evidence level	Most appropriate probiotic strains	Reference
Abdominal pain (functional)		I	*Lactobacillus rhamnosus* GG	89
Amoebiasis (amoebic dysentery)		II	*Saccharomyces cerevisiae* var *boulardii* Biocodex	90
Antibiotic use		I	*Lactobacillus rhamnosus* GG	91
		I	*Saccharomyces cerevisiae* var *boulardii* Biocodex	92
		II	*Lactobacillus acidophilus* strains CUL-60 and CUL-21, *Bifidobacterium lactis* CUL-34, and *Bifidobacterium bifidum* CUL-20 (Lab4)	93
		II	*Lactobacillus plantarum* 299v	94
		II	*Lactobacillus reuteri* DSM 17938	95
		II	*Lactobacillus rhamnosus* GG, *Lactobacillus acidophilus* LA5, and *Bifidobacterium lactis* Bb12	96
Bacterial gastroenteritis	*Clostridium difficile*	II	*Lactobacillus plantarum* 299v	97
		II	*Saccharomyces cerevisiae* var *boulardii* Biocodex	98
		III	*Lactobacillus rhamnosus* GG	99
	Vancomycin-resistant enterococci	II	*Lactobacillus rhamnosus* GG	100
Chemotherapy-induced diarrhoea		III	*Lactobacillus rhamnosus* GG	101
Collagenous colitis		II	*Lactobacillus acidophilus* LA5 and *Bifidobacterium lactis* Bb12	102
Constipation		II	*Bifidobacterium animalis* DN-173 010	103
		II	*Bifidobacterium lactis* Bb12	104
		II	*Lactobacillus casei* Shirota	105
Crohn's disease		III	*Saccharomyces cerevisiae* var *boulardii* Biocodex	106
Diverticular disease		III	*Escherichia coli* Nissle 1917	107
Gastrointestinal candidiasis		II	*Lactobacillus rhamnosus* GG	108
Gastro-oesophageal reflux		II	*Lactobacillus reuteri* MM53	109
Giardia infection		II	*Saccharomyces cerevisiae* var *boulardii* Biocodex	110,111
Helicobacter pylori infection		II	*Lactobacillus reuteri* DSM 17938	112
		III	*Lactobacillus acidophilus* LA5 and *Bifidobacterium lactis* Bb12	113
		III	*Lactobacillus casei* Shirota	114
		III	*Saccharomyces cerevisiae* var *boulardii* Biocodex	115
		III	*Lactobacillus acidophilus* NAS	116
HIV/AIDS-associated diarrhoea		II	*Lactobacillus rhamnosus* GR-1 and *Lactobacillus reuteri* RC-14	117

Table 4.1
Most appropriate probiotic strains for specific disease conditions (continued)

Condition		Evidence level	Most appropriate probiotic strains	Reference
Infantile colic		III	*Lactobacillus reuteri* MM53	118
Intestinal dysbiosis		II	*Bifidobacterium lactis* Bb12	119
		II	*Bifidobacterium lactis* HN019	120
		II	*Lactobacillus casei* Shirota	121
		III	*Lactobacillus rhamnosus* GG	122
Intestinal transit time—slow transit		II	*Bifidobacterium lactis* HN019	123
		III	*Bifidobacterium animalis* DN-173 010	124
Irritable bowel syndrome		II	*Bifidobacterium animalis* DN-173 010	74
		II	*Bifidobacterium infantis* 35624	76
		II	*Lactobacillus acidophilus* strains CUL-60 and CUL-21, *Bifidobacterium lactis* CUL-34, and *Bifidobacterium bifidum* CUL-20 (Lab4)	82
		II	*Lactobacillus fermentum* VRI-003 (PCC)	77,78
		II	*Lactobacillus plantarum* 299v	79,80
		II	VSL#3	83,125
Lactose intolerance		II	*Lactobacillus acidophilus* LA5	126
		II	*Lactobacillus acidophilus* NCFM	127
Nosocomial diarrhoea		I	*Lactobacillus rhamnosus* GG	128
Radiation-induced diarrhoea		II	VSL#3	129
Small intestinal bacterial overgrowth		III	*Lactobacillus casei* Shirota	130
Small intestinal damage		II	*Saccharomyces cerevisiae* var *boulardii* Biocodex	110
Traveller's diarrhoea—prevention		II	*Lactobacillus acidophilus* LA5 and *Bifidobacterium lactis* Bb12	131
		II	*Lactobacillus rhamnosus* GG	132
		II	*Saccharomyces cerevisiae* var *boulardii* Biocodex	133
Ulcerative colitis	Inducing remission	II	*Escherichia coli* Nissle 1917	134
		II	VSL#3	135
	Maintaining remission	II	*Escherichia coli* Nissle 1917	136
		III	*Lactobacillus rhamnosus* GG	137
		III	VSL#3	138
	Preventing pouchitis	II	VSL#3	139
		III	*Lactobacillus rhamnosus* GG	140
Viral gastroenteritis	Prevention	II	*Bifidobacterium lactis* Bb12	141
		II	*Lactobacillus rhamnosus* GG	142
	Treatment	I	*Lactobacillus rhamnosus* GG	143
		II	*Lactobacillus reuteri* DSM 17938	144
		II	VSL#3	145

Table 4.2
Ways of delivering probiotics and their advantages and disadvantages

Delivery system	Advantages	Disadvantages
Fermented foods	Affordable and accessible Easily incorporated into daily lifestyle Additional nutritional benefits Enhanced bacterial survival through upper GIT (100 × less can be given per dose if given in a dairy base)[146] Effective in upper GIT	May contain dairy proteins or lactose Unsuitable when travelling Unsuitable for vegans (if dairy based)
Capsules	Ease of administration No binders	Not therapeutic for upper GIT unless opened or chewed May contain allergenic excipients Higher cost
Tablets	Ease of administration Effective in upper GIT (if chewed)	May contain allergenic binders and excipients such as gluten Higher cost
Powders	Effective in upper GIT Dosage easily adjusted May be incorporated into food and drinks No binders	May contain allergenic excipients Higher cost
Oil based	Ease of administration Effective in upper GIT Dosage can be easily modified May be incorporated into food or drinks No binders or fillers Tend to be stable at room termperature	Higher cost

Table 4.3
Prebiotics for disease conditions

Disease conditions	Prebiotic
Atopic eczema: prevention in formula-fed infants	GOS and FOS (0.8 g/100 mL formula)[150]
Constipation	Lactulose (10–40 g/day)[151] GOS (9 g/day)[152] FOS (10 g/day)[153] PHGG (5 g/day)[154]
IBS	GOS (3.5 g/day)[155] PHGG (5 g/day)[156]
Improved stress response	GOS (5.5 g/day)[157]
Lowered immunity: decreased rates of infection	FOS (2 g/day in infants)[158]
Metabolic syndrome	GOS (2.65 g/day)[159]
Poor calcium absorption	FOS (8 g/day)[160]
Prevention of traveller's diarrhoea	GOS (2.65 g/day)[161]
Prevention of urinary tract infections	Lactulose (20 g/day)[162]

Synbiotics

Synbiotics are products that contain both probiotic and prebiotic agents.[170] The combination is thought to enhance the survival of the probiotic bacteria through the upper GIT, improve implantation of the probiotic in the colon and have a stimulating effect on the growth and/or activities of both the exogenously provided probiotic strains and the endogenous inhabitants of the bowel.[171] Synbiotics are a promising treatment avenue in C-IBS, with two recently published open-label trials finding a synbiotic preparation (containing a daily dose of 5×10^9 CFU ***Bifidobacterium longum* W11** and 2.5 g FOS) to significantly decrease abdominal pain and bloating in patients with C-IBS, as well as increasing stool frequency.[172,173]

Herbal antimicrobials

For patients who test positive for SIBO on breath testing, the use of antimicrobial herbs may prove necessary in an effort to decrease the bacterial load in the small bowel.

Few clinical trials have been done investigating phytotherapeutic agents in SIBO. In fact, there is only a single trial to date. This open-label trial compared a number of commercially available herbal combination formulas to the standard treatment (the antibiotic rifaximin). The herbal preparations were found to be equally efficacious in reducing the bacterial load in the small bowel.[174]

Herbal medicines with potent in-vitro antimicrobial activity that are frequently used in the treatment of SIBO include: *Allium sativum*,[175] *Punica granatum*,[176] *Syzygium aromaticum*,[177] *Thymus vulgaris*,[178] *Origanum vulgare*,[179] and berberine-rich herbs (e.g. *Coptis chinensis*, *Phellodendron amurense* and *Hydrastis canadensis*).[180]

Support the nervous system

Given that IBS is often associated with anxiety and depression disorders[181] and the link between perceived stress levels and IBS symptom severity,[182] support for the nervous system is also an important component of naturopathic management. Mood has also been shown to affect bowel habit, with depression significantly slowing gastrointestinal transit time and anxiety significantly speeding it.[183]

Both nervines and adaptogens have a role to play in treating IBS. Depending upon patient presentation, **thymoleptics** (*Hypericum perforatum*, *Albizia julibrissin*, *Crocus sativus*, *Sceletium tortuosum* or *Leonurus cardiaca*) or **anxiolytics** (*Passiflora incarnata*, *Valeriana officinalis*, *Piper methysticum*, *Eschscholzia californica* or *Lavandula angustifolia*) can be used alongside **trophorestoratives** (e.g. *Verbena officinalis* or green seed *Avena sativa*). If patients are currently experiencing conditions of high stress, **adaptogens** will also play an important role in management. If fatigue is part of the patient presentation, stimulating **adaptogens** such as *Rhodiola rosea*, *Panax ginseng* and *Eleutherococcus senticosus* may be the best choices. If anxiety or overstimulation is present, less stimulating **adaptogens** may be more appropriate (e.g. *Withania somnifera*, *Schisandra chinensis* or *Ganoderma lucidum*). For a discussion of non-herbal nervous system support, please refer to Chapter 3 on wellness and Chapters 14–17 on the nervous system).

Preliminary evidence is also supporting a role for prebiotics like FOS and GOS in the modulation of the stress response and improving mood. GOS at a dose of 5.5 g/day has been found to positively influence the hypothalamic–pituitary–adrenal (HPA) axis, significantly decreasing the salivary cortisol awakening response after three weeks of ingestion, and at 7 g/day in IBS patients, significantly reduced anxiety scores. Whereas a combination of FOS and GOS in animal models of chronic stress has been shown to attenuate stress-induced corticosterone release, decrease the number of stress-induced bowel movements and reduce depression- and anxiety-like behaviour.[184–186]

Promote normalisation of bowel pattern

C-IBS

The presentation of C-IBS is associated with infrequent bowel movements and hard, lumpy stools. Interventions aimed at increasing stool frequency and softening the stools are therefore well indicated. The three main tools used to address this issue are fibre, fluid and exercise, with probiotics also playing a potential role.

Dietary fibre

Epidemiological studies have consistently found correlations between dietary fibre intake and improved bowel function.[187,188] As the amount of dietary fibre in the diet is increased, mean gastrointestinal transit time decreases, stool frequency increases and stools become softer and easier to pass.[187] Clinical trials of fibre supplementation have also consistently found increased bowel movement frequency and improved stool consistency.[189]

One specific dietary fibre that has shown beneficial effects in normalising bowel pattern in patients with C-IBS is partially hydrolysed guar gum (PHGG). In an open-label trial, four weeks' supplementation with PHGG resulted in a 34% increase in the number of daily evacuations, a 73% decrease in laxative use and an improvement in Bristol stool scale (all $P < 0.05$ versus baseline). Bloating scores and feeling of incomplete evacuation also significantly improved (both $P < 0.01$).[190]

Another open-label trial evaluated a novel prebiotic-fibre combination, composed of powdered lactulose (3 g twice daily [bid]), *Ulmus fulva* (7 g bid), oat bran (2 g bid) and *Glycyrrhiza glabra* (1.5 g bid) in patients with C-IBS. After three weeks' treatment, subjects experienced a 20% increase in bowel movement frequency ($p = 0.016$) and significant reductions in straining ($p < 0.0001$), abdominal pain ($p = 0.032$), bloating ($p = 0.034$) and global IBS symptom severity ($p = 0.0005$), as well as improvements in stool consistency ($p < 0.0001$).[191]

How does dietary fibre work?

There appear to be at least five ways by which dietary fibre consumption improves laxation. First, plant cell walls that resist microfloral degradation are able to exert a physical bulking effect by retaining water within their cellular structure. This increased bulk stimulates colonic movement. Second, the vast majority of consumed dietary fibre is extensively broken down and metabolised by the colonic microbiota. This stimulates microbial growth, leading to an increase in microbial products and microbes themselves in faeces—again leading to an increase in faecal bulk. Third, the increase in faecal bulk speeds up the faeces' rate of passage through the bowel. As transit time decreases, the efficiency with which the bacteria grow improves—further bulking the stools. Shortened transit time also leads to reduced water absorption by the colon and, hence, moister stools. Fourth, fermentation of dietary fibre by the colonic microbiota results in the production of hydrogen, methane and carbon dioxide gas. When trapped within the gut contents they further add to stool bulk.[192] Lastly, other end-products of fermentation (short-chain fatty acids, particularly acetate) enhance muscular contraction in the colon.[193,194]

A recent systematic review and meta-analysis found fibre to significantly improve global IBS symptoms and IBS-related constipation. However, fibre supplementation was found to significantly worsen abdominal pain. When soluble fibre was examined in isolation, it was found to induce a greater reduction in global IBS symptoms and to improve constipation in C-IBS subjects. Conversely, insoluble fibre supplementation was found to have no significant effect upon global IBS symptoms, although it did improve constipation. The authors concluded that fibre supplementation appears to be of benefit in improving global IBS symptoms and particularly constipation; it does not, however, improve IBS-related abdominal pain.[195]

The findings from this systematic review suggest that sources of soluble fibre would be more appropriate therapeutic tools than sources of insoluble fibre in the treatment of C-IBS. Good sources of supplemental soluble fibre include ground flaxseeds,[196] slippery elm powder,[197] psyllium husks,[198] oat bran[199] and pectin.[200]

Fluid intake

Ensuring the intake of adequate fluid is also a vital, although under-researched, therapeutic tool. Positive associations have been observed between bowel movement frequency and fluid intake in epidemiological research.[188] Stool frequency and stool weight have also been found to be significantly decreased during enforced periods of low fluid intake in prospective human research.[201] Adequate fluid intake is usually described as 2100–2600 mL daily, although this would need to be increased in warmer climates.[202]

Exercise

Epidemiological research has found an association between level of physical activity and frequency of bowel habit, with lower levels of physical activity being linked with impaired bowel habit.[203] This link between physical activity levels and bowel health is widely known among the general populace, with even Roald Dahl remarking in his *Revolting Rhymes*[204]:

> *An early morning stroll is good for people on the whole.*
> *It makes your appetite improve,*
> *It also helps your bowels to move.*

In support of this connection, prospective human research has found that daily moderate exercise is capable of significantly accelerating gastrointestinal transit time, which should equate to softer, easier-to-pass stools.[205] Additionally, a recently published, randomised controlled trial found daily exercise to significantly improve constipation-related symptoms in IBS subjects.[206]

Probiotics

Two probiotic strains have shown the capacity to significantly speed whole-gut transit time: ***Bifidobacterium lactis* HN019** and ***Bifidobacterium animalis* DN-173 010**. Strain HN019 was found to significantly decrease transit time from a mean of 49.2 hours to 21.0 hours after two weeks of supplementation.[123] In subjects with a gut transit time of more than 40 hours, two weeks' administration of *Bifidobacterium animalis* strain DN-173 010 was found to decrease gut transit time by 47% (from 61.6 hours to 32.9 hours compared with baseline).[124]

D-IBS

Solidify stools and decrease bowel movement frequency

If anxiety plays a pivotal role in bowel symptoms, and particularly in increased stool frequency, then supporting the nervous system with anxiolytics, nervous system trophorestoratives, adaptogens and thymoleptics (as discussed earlier) is well indicated.

Herbal antidiarrhoeal agents will have a more direct effect in the bowel. Herbal antidiarrhoeal agents can be divided into those that are tannin based and those that are not. Tannin-based agents include ***Quercus robor***, ***Polygonum bistorta***, ***Geranium maculatum***, ***Croton lechlerii*** and ***Agrimonia eupatoria***. In Western herbal medicine, two of the few non-tannin based antidiarrhoeal agents currently in use are nutmeg (***Myristica fragrans***) and black pepper (***Piper nigrum***)—although black pepper can be too 'spicy' for some patients with D-IBS. The benefit of using non-tannin antidiarrhoeals is that they can be mixed together with alkaloid-containing herbs without causing precipitation.

The prebiotic fibre PHGG can also play a role in normalising bowel patterns in patients with D-IBS. In one open-label trial, after 24 weeks' supplementation (at 5 g/day) bowel evacuation frequency went from an extreme of 35 movements/week down to 9 per week, while another trial found PHGG supplementation (5 g/day) to acutely suppress the diarrhoea induced by the ingestion of large doses of osmotic sugar polyols.[207,208]

Another agent capable of slowing colonic transit time is **melatonin**. A recent trial found administration of 3 mg melatonin per day over an eight-week period to significantly slow colonic transit time from 27.4 to 37.4 hours.[209]

What is a 'normal' bowel pattern?

This question should really be broken up into two questions: what is a 'normal' bowel habit and what is a 'healthy' or 'optimal' bowel habit? A 'normal' bowel habit has been defined by conventional medicine as between three bowel movements per day to three bowel movements per week. These frequencies are based on epidemiological studies conducted on Western populations that have found the vast majority of individuals to have a bowel frequency within this range, with the most common frequency being once daily.[210,211] Constipation is thus defined as less than three bowel movements per week.[212]

Naturopaths would generally not consider patients who experience three bowel movements per week to have a 'normal' bowel habit. Naturopath Henry Lindlahr stated in his 1919 classic *Natural therapeutics* that 'normally a person should have a copious movement of the bowels once in 24 hours—twice is better'.[213] Studies looking at non-Western populations eating traditional fibre-rich diets found defecation frequencies to average two or three times daily.[214] Other studies looking at vegans eating high-fibre diets (about 47 g fibre daily) have found a mean bowel movement frequency of 1.5 times per day or more.[188,189] From these data we can gather that individuals consuming a high-fibre, plant-based diet pass stools more frequently than individuals consuming the typical low-fibre, Western diet (about 11–16 g fibre daily).[215] Optimal bowel frequency should be considered to be one, two or three movements daily. Naturopaths generally consider patients as being constipated if they experience less than one bowel movement daily.

In terms of consistency, the most common stool passed by typical Western populations is well formed (sausage or snake-like) with either cracks on its surface or a smooth and soft surface (types 3 and 4 in Figure 4.2).[216] Populations consuming a predominantly plant-based, high-fibre diet, on the other hand, have softer, bulkier stools that tend to be less formed and more 'mushy' (type 5). These stools are associated with shorter gastrointestinal transit times, whereas harder stools are associated with longer transit times.[187] So, what is the perfect bowel movement? Optimal stool form should vary between well-formed, sausage-like stools with cracks on its surface (type 3) through to softer blobs with clear-cut edges (type 5). In addition, there should be little-to-no straining at stool, little urgency and a feeling of complete evacuation after the event.[217]

Bowel habit: men versus women

Studies have consistently found men to have an increased frequency of daily bowel movements, to produce a greater quantity of faeces daily, to have shorter gastrointestinal transit times and to have softer, less-formed faeces than women.[187,188,216] Stool form and bowel movement frequency also appears to vary in women according to the menstrual cycle. During the luteal phase of the cycle, gastrointestinal transit time significantly slows, resulting in more formed, harder stools.[187]

What stimulates the bowels to move?

Colonic motility is the key factor determining the whens and whys of bowel movements. The greatest stimulant of colonic contractile activity is morning awakening. Colonic motility is greatly reduced and sometimes even completely abolished during sleep. Upon awakening, contractile activity increases briskly.[219] Not surprisingly, population studies have found that the vast majority of bowel movements occur between 6 and 9 am.[216] The other main stimulus of colonic motility is eating—referred to as the *colonic motor response to eating* or the *gastrocolonic reflex*. Within minutes of consuming the first mouthful of food, colonic contractile activity begins, and lasts for at least three hours.[219] In Western populations, a second peak of defecation frequency has been observed at 6–7 pm, the time at which the largest meal of the day is typically consumed.[216]

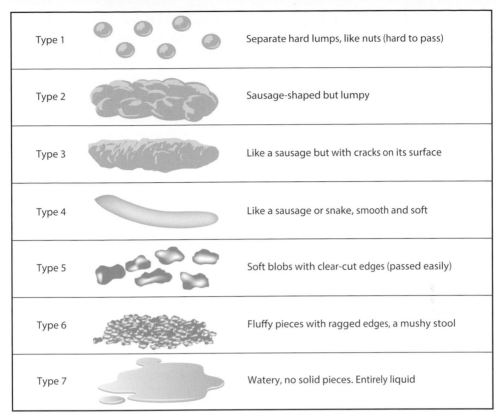

Type 1		Separate hard lumps, like nuts (hard to pass)
Type 2		Sausage-shaped but lumpy
Type 3		Like a sausage but with cracks on its surface
Type 4		Like a sausage or snake, smooth and soft
Type 5		Soft blobs with clear-cut edges (passed easily)
Type 6		Fluffy pieces with ragged edges, a mushy stool
Type 7		Watery, no solid pieces. Entirely liquid

Figure 4.2
The Bristol stool form scale
Source: Lewis & Heaton 1997[218]

Manage GIT symptoms

Although it is a benign disorder, IBS is associated with significant impairments in quality of life.[220] Recent research has found that three gastrointestinal symptoms (straining at stool, abdominal pain and abdominal bloating) have the greatest negative impact upon quality of life among IBS sufferers.[221] Providing relief from these symptoms should therefore be at the forefront of naturopathic management of this condition.

Straining at stool is usually addressed with the agents and interventions discussed in the Promote normalisation of bowel pattern section earlier. Occasionally, however, laxative herbs are needed at the onset of treatment in C-IBS patients. Sometimes gentle **laxatives** like *Glycyrrhiza glabra* are adequate. In more severe cases of constipation, the anthraquinone-containing laxatives can be used: *Senna* spp., *Rhamnus purshiana*, *Rumex crispus* or *Juglans cinerea*. The use of these agents can result in griping abdominal pain; concurrent administration of carminatives and antispasmodics is therefore highly recommended. If anthraquinone-containing laxatives are used, the aim should be to use them for a short-term period only.

Abdominal pain and bloating can be addressed using a combination of **carminatives** and antispasmodics. Useful carminatives include *Mentha piperita*, *Mentha spicata*,

Carum carvi, Foeniculum vulgare, Citrus reticulata, Coriandrum sativum, Elettaria cardamomum, Origanum vulgare and *Anethum graveolens*. Commonly prescribed GIT antispasmodics include *Matricaria recutita, Viburnum opulus, Dioscorea villosa, Melissa officinalis* and *Zingiber officinale*.

Decrease gut inflammation and diminish visceral hypersensitivity

Patients with IBS have been shown to have increased visceral sensation and may suffer from mild colonic mucosal inflammation.[3,4] Ingestion of gastrointestinal **anti-inflammatories** such as *Curcuma longa, Boswellia serrata, Glycyrrhiza glabra* and *Matricaria recutita* may help decrease this inflammation. Recent research has found a combination of peppermint (*Mentha piperita*) and caraway (*Carum carvi*) essential oils effective in decreasing visceral hypersensitivity in an animal model of IBS.[222] A proprietary herbal preparation (Iberogast) has also been found to decrease visceral hypersensitivity in an animal model.[223] Iberogast is an ethanolic extract containing *Iberis amara, Angelica archangelica, Silybum marianum, Carum carvi, Glycyrrhiza glabra, Chelidonium majus, Matricaria recutita, Melissa officinalis* and *Mentha piperita*. Melatonin is another agent that has shown the capacity to diminish visceral hypersensitivity.[224] An additional strategy that can be used to decrease visceral hypersensitivity is to increase the concentration of the short-chain fatty acid butyrate in the colonic lumen. This can be done through the supplementation of enteric-coated, slow-release butyrate as a supplement or by 'feeding' the butyrate-producing microbes in the colon. The latter can be achieved though the ingestion of PHGG and foods or supplements rich in resistant starch.[225–228]

Recent research has also found a link between local exposure to endotoxins (the major component of the cell wall from gram-negative bacteria) and decreased visceral sensory and pain thresholds.[229] This research suggests that treatments that can reduce the population of gram-negative bacteria in the human GIT may improve visceral hypersensitivity. Interventions capable of decreasing gram-negative microbe population numbers along the GIT include prebiotics (GOS,[230] lactulose[231] and FOS[232]) and some probiotic strains (see the intestinal dysbiosis section in Table 4.1), as well as the ingestion of green tea (300 mg catechins/day)[233] and brown rice.[234]

Support liver function

Poor liver function is viewed by some practitioners as an important contributing factor in IBS.[235] Liver congestion has also long been seen by naturopaths as a common cause of constipation[213] and bile salts are well-known laxative agents.[236] Accordingly, patients with IBS, and C-IBS more specifically, can sometimes receive benefit from ingesting **cholagogues** (*Cynara scolymus, Curcuma longa, Taraxacum officinale radix, Chelidonium majus, Berberis vulgaris* or *Juglans cinerea*). See Chapter 7 for information on liver function and detoxification.

In support of the use of cholagogues in IBS, and C-IBS in particular, two clinical trials have been conducted on herbal cholagogues, with both trials finding evidence of therapeutic effectiveness. In a post-marketing surveillance study *Cynara scolymus* extract was found to significantly decrease abdominal pain, bloating, flatulence and constipation in subjects with IBS over a six-week period.[237] In an open-label trial, two different doses of turmeric extract (*Curcuma longa*) were examined to assess their effects on IBS symptoms.[238] Both extracts were found over an eight-week period to significantly reduce abdominal pain/discomfort scores from baseline. Additionally, bowel pattern was found to normalise. There were, however, no significant differences between the high- and low-dose groups.

Manage diverse food reactions

Adverse food reactions have long been discussed as potential causes of gastrointestinal symptoms in at least some patients with IBS.[239] Research suggests that some of these reactions may be mediated by immune mechanisms (IgE- or IgG-related).[240] Gluten sensitivity[241] and/or intolerance to fermentable foodstuffs (FODMAPs)[242] can also play a role in some IBS patients. See Chapter 6 for more detail.

INTEGRATIVE MEDICAL CONSIDERATIONS

In many ways, IBS is a clinical diagnosis—a diagnosis is based on the presence of typical signs and symptoms (see the Rome IV criteria for current diagnostic criteria). Specificity of using the Rome criteria for diagnosing IBS has been found to be about 98% in the absence of 'alarm features'. Hence further investigations are typically not required to confirm the diagnosis and exclude organic disease. If 'alarm features' are present, however, referral for further investigation is recommended. 'Alarm features' include the presence of blood in the stools, weight loss, fever and family history of colon cancer.[4] Any change in bowel pattern in people older than 45 years of age is also an 'alarm feature' requiring further investigation.[243]

Traditional Chinese medicine

Initial research suggested that acupuncture may have a role to play in managing IBS.[244] However, follow-up research using more rigorous designs has not backed this up[245,246] and a recent systematic review of randomised controlled trials failed to find acupuncture more effective than sham acupuncture in managing IBS symptoms.[247] The results of a recent systematic review of herbal medicines in IBS found Chinese herbal medicine formulas effective in relieving IBS symptoms, while being very well tolerated. Unfortunately many of the trials were of poor quality, preventing firm conclusions about efficacy from being drawn.[248]

Hypnotherapy

The use of hypnotherapy has shown some degree of efficacy in treating IBS, with a number of studies demonstrating efficacy of gut-directed hypnotherapy.[249–251] The benefits appear to be long-lasting in some patients.[252] Additionally, a recent systematic review found gut-directed hypnotherapy superior to standard medical care in children with IBS.[253]

Traditional herbal medicine

Western herbalists have always been eclectic, using herbs from many different locations and herbal traditions. Western herbalists have also, until recently, been intimately involved with making the medicines they use. Today, industry supplies herbal medicines to the bulk of practitioners, meaning that very few herbalists have a close connection to the plant medicines they currently use in practice. This situation has also indirectly limited the materia medica most practitioners can practise with. Only those herbs that are commercially profitable become available to use; the others become 'lost'. There is, however, a renaissance of sorts occurring today, with practitioners reconnecting with the herbs they use as medicines, with a growing number of herbalists returning to making their own medicines.

A number of herbs with specific actions very helpful to GIT disorders have been 'lost' to modern practitioners. Some of these and their actions are listed in Table 4.4.

Table 4.4
Rediscovering our herbal roots

| Herb | Uses in traditional systems of medicine | | | Supportive evidence (in vitro, animal and human research) |
	Western	Traditional Chinese medicine	Ayurvedic	
Black pepper (*Piper nigrum*)	Digestive stimulant Carminative Antiemetic Circulatory stimulant[254]	Vomiting Diarrhoea Abdominal pain[255]	Indigestion Colic Diarrhoea Cold extremities Adjuvant use[256]	Stimulates gastric acid secretion[257] Enhances bile flow[258] Improves functioning of digestive enzymes[259] Slows gastrointestinal transit[260] and exhibits antisecretory action[261]
Caraway (*Carum carvi*)	Carminative Gastrointestinal anti-spasmodic[262]	–	Digestive complaints[256]	Human trials have found a combination of caraway and peppermint essential oils effective in alleviating the symptoms of functional dyspepsia, such as abdominal pain and the sensation of fullness and heaviness after meals[263,264]
Nutmeg (*Myristica fragrans*)	Nausea Vomiting Abdominal pain Flatulence Diarrhoea[265]	Abdominal pain and distension Vomiting Chronic diarrhoea[255]	Diarrhoea Excessive intestinal gas Insomnia[256]	Slows gastrointestinal transit and possesses antisecretory activity[266] Exhibits antidepressant-like activity[267] and anxiolytic activity[268]
Oregano (*Origanum vulgare*)	Diaphoretic Emmenagogue Respiratory tract infections Anorexia[259,267]	–	–	Essential oil displays potent antimicrobial activity against a range of pathogens[269,270] Essential oil effective in eradicating intestinal protozoal infections[271]
Pomegranate (*Punica granatum*)	Diarrheoa Intestinal worms Stopping bleeding[254]	Intestinal worms Diarrhoea and dysentery Stopping bleeding[255]	Diarrhoea and dysentery Intestinal parasites[272]	Rich in antioxidants[273] Potent antimicrobial activity against a range of pathogenic bacteria and protozoa[274,275] Slows gastrointestinal transit and prevents intestinal fluid accumulation[276] Decreases intestinal inflammation[277]

Table 4.4
Rediscovering our herbal roots (continued)

Herb	Uses in traditional systems of medicine			Supportive evidence (in vitro, animal and human research)
	Western	**Traditional Chinese medicine**	**Ayurvedic**	
Saffron (*Crocus sativus*)	Antispasmodic Thymoleptic Indigestion Cognition enhancer[267]	Invigorates the blood Dispels stasis Unblocks the menses Lifts the spirits[255]	Depression Dysmenorrhoea Impotence Asthma[278]	Similarly effective as pharmaceutical antidepressants in the treatment of mild-to-moderate depression[279,280] Similarly effective as donepezil in the treatment of mild-to-moderate Alzheimer's disease[281] In combination with *Apium graveolens* seed and *Pimpinella anisum* seed was effective in treating dysmenorrhoea[282]

CLINICAL SUMMARY

IBS is a commonly encountered condition in naturopathic practice, typically diagnosed on clinical findings such as the presence of typical signs and symptoms. Be aware of alarm features, which indicate the need for referral and/or further investigation. Additional diagnostic investigations may be needed to rule out other potential diagnoses and to help tailor the treatment approach for individual patients (Figure 4.3). In respect to prescribing probiotic preparations, it is important to note that within each species of bacteria there is a multitude of strains. Some probiotic strains are resilient and strong, with a demonstrated capacity to survive passage through the upper GIT and inhibit pathogenic bacteria, whereas others are weak and cannot even survive transit through the stomach. It is vital to note that just because one strain of bacteria in a given species has a proven action or characteristic, it does not mean that another strain will too, even if they are closely related. Strains of bacteria within the same species can have significantly different actions, properties and characteristics, as these are all essentially strain-specific qualities.[283] In conclusion, IBS is a treatable condition, and although it may be recurrent in the advent of specific stressors, it can be managed with an integrative approach.

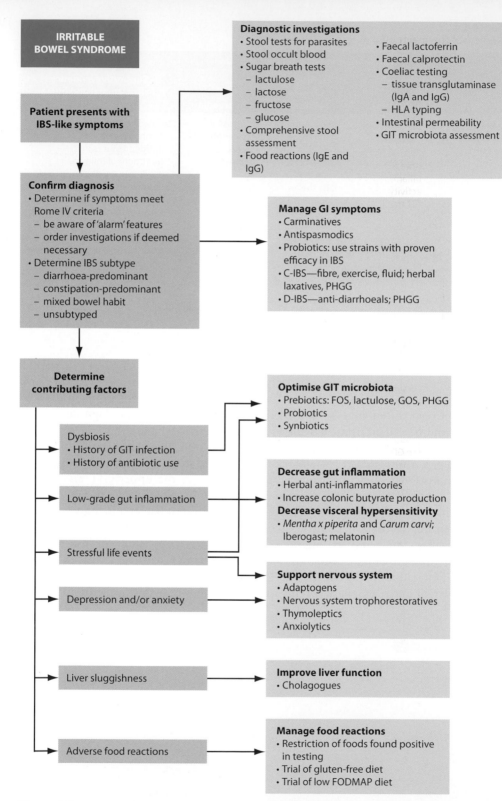

Figure 4.3
Naturopathic treatment decision tree—IBS

Table 4.5
Review of the major evidence

Intervention	Mechanisms of action	Key literature	Summary of results	Comment
Probiotics	Probiotics may help restore balance to the GIT ecosystem, decrease visceral hypersensitivity, have anti-inflammatory activity and alter GIT transit	Meta-analysis: McFarland & Dublin 2008[73] RCTs: Agrawal et al. 2009[74] Whorwell et al. 2006[76] Ducrotte et al. 2012[284] Williams et al. 2008[82]	Probiotic use was associated with improvement in global IBS symptoms compared with placebo [pooled relative risk 0.77, 95% CI = 0.62–0.94] Probiotic use was also associated with less abdominal pain compared with placebo [RRpooled = 0.78 (0.69–0.88), 95% CI 0.45–0.81]	Probiotics as a whole appear effective in treating IBS, but some probiotic strains were not found to be effective; efficacy is a strain-specific attribute Strains with demonstrated efficacy include: *Lactobacillus plantarum* 299v, *Bifidobacterium animalis* DN-173 010, *Bifidobacterium infantis* 35624, and the Lab4 combination (*Lactobacillus acidophilus* strains CUL-60 and CUL-21, *Bifidobacterium lactis* CUL-34 and *Bifidobacterium bifidum* CUL-20)
Galactooligo-saccharides (GOS) (3.5–7.0 g/day)	GOS supplementation may decrease gas (hydrogen) production in the GIT, as well as beneficially altering the GIT ecosystem[285]	RCT: Silk et al. 2009[155]	When subjects took 3.5 g/day, significant improvements were observed in stool consistency ($p < 0.05$), flatulence ($p < 0.05$), bloating ($p < 0.05$) and overall IBS symptom scores ($p < 0.05$) compared with placebo When subjects took 7.0 g/day, significant improvements observed in subjective assessment of global IBS symptom score ($p < 0.05$) and anxiety scores ($p < 0.05$) compared with placebo controls	The lower dose of GOS (3.5 g/day) appears to be more effective than the higher dose in reducing IBS symptoms The higher dose was also associated with a significant increase in bloating scores relative to baseline at the end of the four-week intervention period

Table 4.5
Review of the major evidence (continued)

Intervention	Mechanisms of action	Key literature	Summary of results	Comment
Peppermint (*Mentha piperita*) essential oil (typical dose 0.2 mL three times a day [tds])	Peppermint essential oil displays marked antispasmodic activity, most likely through the interference of the movement of calcium across the cell membrane of colonocytes[286]	RCT: Kline et al. 2001[287]	Significant reduction in severity of abdominal pain ($p < 0.03$) and significant improvement in global IBS symptoms ($p < 0.001$) compared with placebo	This is one of 10 trials with results in favour of peppermint essential oil in treating IBS. Not all trials have been positive, however. Two trials utilising a crossover design with an inadequate washout period did not show favourable results. The apparent lack of efficacy in these latter two studies is most likely due to poor study design
Padma lax—a tableted combination of herbs, heavy kaolin, sodium bicarbonate and sodium sulfate	This herbal combination contained herbal bitters, carminatives and anthraquinone-containing laxatives	RCT: Sallon et al. 2002[288]	Significant increase in stool frequency ($p = 0.002$) and a significant improvement in gastroenterologist-rated constipation severity ($p = 0.0001$) compared with placebo; significant reduction in presence of moderate to severe pain ($p = 0.05$) and effect of pain on daily activities ($p = 0.002$) compared with placebo	Despite the fact that some herbal authorities do not recommend the prescription of anthraquinone-containing herbs in IBS, these results clearly demonstrate that they can be efficacious in increasing stool frequency and reducing abdominal pain
Carmint—an aqueous-ethanolic extract of *Melissa officinalis*, *Mentha spicata* and *Coriandrum sativum* (30 drops tds)	The three medicinal plants in this formula are traditionally considered antispasmodics and carminatives	RCT: Vejdani et al. 2006[289]	Significantly decreased the severity ($p = 0.016$) and frequency ($p = 0.001$) of abdominal pain/discomfort and the severity ($p = 0.02$) and frequency of bloating ($p = 0.002$) compared with placebo	Significant differences in abdominal pain and bloating severity in favour of Carmint were noted from the beginning of the second week of treatment
Flaxseeds (ground) (dose gradually increased from 6 g/day depending on response)	Bulking laxative	RCT: Tarpila et al. 2003[290]	Constipation ($p = 0.05$), bloating ($p = 0.001$) and pain scores ($p = 0.001$) were improved significantly more in the flax group than the psyllium group	Ground flax was found to be significantly better than psyllium husks in the treatment of C-IBS; gastrointestinal symptoms improved further over an additional three-month open-label phase

Table 4.5
Review of the major evidence (continued)

Intervention	Mechanisms of action	Key literature	Summary of results	Comment
Partially hydrolised guar gum (PHGG) (typical dose 5 g/day)	GIT anti-inflammatory effects; beneficial modification of the GIT microbiota; modulation of GIT transit time	Systematic review: Hawrelak & Whitten, 2016[156]	All clinical trials conducted to date have produced positive findings, including improvements in overall IBS symptoms, and bowel pattern, as well as mood and quality of life	Despite the positive research to date, firm conclusions are hampered by the relatively small numbers of participants in most trials and lack of methodological rigour in trials to date
Melatonin (typical dose 3 mg taken at bedtime)	Melatonin decreases visceral hypersensitivity, modifies GI transit time, and has healing and anti-inflammatory effects in the colon[224]	Meta-analysis: Mozaffari et al., 2010[224]	All RCTs to date have demonstrated positive results, with studies consistently finding improved overall IBS symptom scores and reductions in abdominal pain	The findings of this systematic review were supportive of melatonin use in IBS. However, to date, trial sizes have all been small, with no trial examining more than 40 subjects

KEY POINTS

- Dysbiosis appears to be a key aetiological factor in IBS and treatments aimed at addressing this imbalance (probiotics, prebiotics, synbiotics and, if appropriate, herbal anti-microbials) have shown great promise in its treatment.
- In some patients, stress will be *the* key contributing factor to their IBS symptoms. Avoid the temptation to focus solely on the GIT to the neglect of the nervous system.
- Although addressing aetiological factors is important in the long term, providing relief of gastrointestinal symptoms (such as abdominal pain and bloating) needs to be done in the short term to ensure the patient will come back.

FURTHER READING

Chey WD, Kurlander J, Eswaran S. Irritable bowel syndrome: a clinical review. JAMA 2015;313(9):949–58.

Hawrelak JA, Myers SP. The causes of intestinal dysbiosis: a review. Altern Med Rev 2004;9(2):180–97.

Lacy BE, Mearin F, Chang L, et al. Bowel disorders. Gastroenterology 2016;150(6):1393–407.e5. doi:10.1053/j.gastro.2016.02.031.

Liu H-N, Wu H, Chen Y-Z, et al. Altered molecular signature of intestinal microbiota in irritable bowel syndrome patients compared with healthy controls: a systematic review and meta-analysis. Dig Liver Dis 2017;49(4):331–7.

Schumann D, Klose P, Lauche R, et al. Low fermentable, oligo-, di-, mono-saccharides and polyol diet in the treatment of irritable bowel syndrome: a systematic review and meta-analysis. Nutrition 2018;45:24–31.

REFERENCES

1. American Gastroenterology, A. Irritable Bowel Syndrome: a technical review for practice guideline development. Gastroenterology 2002;112:2120–37.

2. Mayer EA. Emerging disease model for functional gastrointestinal disorders. Am J Med 1999;107(5A): 12S–19S.

3. Quigley EMM, et al. Irritable bowel syndrome: a global perspective. World Gastroenterology Organisation Global Guideline; 2009. p. 1–20.

4. Delvaux M. Role of visceral sensitivity in the pathophysiology of irritable bowel syndrome. Gut 2002;51(Suppl. 1):i67–71.

5. Camilleri M, Heading RC, Thompson WG. Consensus report: clinical perspectives, mechanisms, diagnosis and management of irritable bowel syndrome. Aliment Pharmacol Ther 2002;16:1407–30.

6. Bercik P, Verdu EF, Collins SM. Is irritable bowel syndrome a low-grade inflammatory bowel disease? Gastroenterol Clin North Am 2005;34:235–45.

7. Coulie B. Role of GI motor abnormalities in irritable bowel syndrome. Acta Gastroenterol Belg 2001;64(3):276–80.

8. Serra J, Azpiroz F, Malagelada J. Mechanisms of intestinal gas retention in humans: impaired propulsion versus obstructed evacuation. Am J Physiol Gastrointest Liver Physiol 2001;281(1):G138–43.

9. Chey WY, et al. Colonic motility abnormality in patients with irritable bowel syndrome exhibiting abdominal pain and diarrhea. Am J Gastroenterol 2001;96(5):1499–506.

10. King TS, Elia M, Hunter JO. Abnormal colonic fermentation in irritable bowel syndrome. Lancet 1998;352:1187–9.

11. Treem WR, et al. Fecal short-chain fatty acids in patients with diarrhea-predominant irritable bowel syndrome: in vitro studies of carbohydrate fermentation. J Pediatr Gastroenterol Nutr 1996;23:280–6.

12. Balsari A, et al. The fecal microbial population in the irritable bowel syndrome. Microbiologica 1982;5:185–94.

13. Si JM, et al. Intestinal microecology and quality of life in irritable bowel syndrome patients. World J Gastroenterol 2005;10:1802–5.

14. Malinen E, et al. Analysis of the fecal microbiota of irritable bowel syndrome patients and healthy controls with real-time PCR. Am J Gastroenterol 2005;100:373–82.

15. Ford AC, Spiegel BM, Talley NJ, et al. Small intestinal bacterial overgrowth in irritable bowel syndrome: systematic review and meta-analysis. Clin Gastroenterol Hepatol 2009;7(12):1279–86. S1542-3565(09)00660-0 [pii].

16. Hammer J, Talley NJ. Diagnostic criteria for the irritable bowel syndrome. Am J Med 1999;107(5A):5S–11S.

17. Lacy BE, Mearin F, Chang L, et al. Bowel disorders. Gastroenterology 2016;150(6):1393–407.e5. doi:10.1053/j.gastro.2016.02.031.

18. Lucak S. Diagnosing irritable bowel syndrome: what's too much, what's enough? Medgenmed 2004;6(1):17.

19. Biesiekierski JR, et al. Gluten causes gastrointestinal symptoms in subjects without celiac disease: a double-blind randomized placebo-controlled trial. Am J Gastroenterol 2011;106(3):508–14, quiz 515.

20. Jimenez-Gonzalez D, et al. Blastocystis infection is associated with irritable bowel syndrome in a Mexican patient population. Parasitol Res 2012;110(3):1269–75.

21. Barratt JLN, et al. A review of Dientamoeba fragilis carriage in humans: several reasons why this organism should be considered in the diagnosis of gastrointestinal illness. Gut Microbes 2011;2(1):3–12.

22. Pimentel M, Chow EJ, Lin HC. Eradication of small intestinal bacterial overgrowth reduces symptoms of irritable bowel syndrome. Am J Gastroenterol 2000;95(12):3503–6.

23. Ozdil K, et al. The frequency of microscopic and focal active colitis in patients with irritable bowel syndrome. BMC Gastroenterol 2011;11:96.

24. Morris-Yates AD, et al. Evidence of a genetic contribution to self reported symptoms of irritable bowel syndrome. Gastroenterology 1995;108:A652.

25. Wensaas KA, et al. Irritable bowel syndrome and chronic fatigue 3 years after acute giardiasis: historic cohort study. Gut 2012;61(2):214–19.

26. Marshall JK, et al. Postinfectious irritable bowel syndrome after a food-borne outbreak of acute gastroenteritis attributed to a viral pathogen. Clin Gastroenterol Hepatol 2007;5(4):457–60.

27. Zanini B, et al. Incidence of post-infectious irritable bowel syndrome and functional intestinal disorders following a water-borne viral gastroenteritis outbreak. Am J Gastroenterol 2012;107(6):891–9.

28. Thabane M, et al. An outbreak of acute bacterial gastroenteritis is associated with an increased incidence of irritable bowel syndrome in children. Am J Gastroenterol 2010;105(4):933–9.

29. Spiller R, Campbell E. Post-infectious irritable bowel syndrome. Curr Opin Gastroenterol 2006;22(1):13–17.

30. Mendall MA, Kumar D. Antibiotic use, childhood affluence and irritable bowel syndrome. Eur J Gastroenterol Hepatol 1998;10(1):59–62.

31. Maxwell PR, et al. Antibiotics increase functional abdominal symptoms. Am J Gastroenterol 2002;97(1):104–8.

32. Villarreal AA, et al. Use of broad-spectrum antibiotics and the development of irritable bowel syndrome. WMJ 2012;111(1):17–20.

33. Verdú EF, et al. Specific probiotic therapy attenuates antibiotic induced visceral hypersensitivity in mice. Gut 2006;55(2):182–90.

34. Bennett EJ, et al. Level of chronic stress predicts clinical outcome in irritable bowel syndrome. Gut 1998;43:256–61.

35. Whitehead WE, et al. Symptoms of psychological distress associated with irritable bowel syndrome. Gastroenterology 1998;95:709–14.

36. Masand PS, et al. Major depression and irritable bowel syndrome: is there a relationship? J Clin Psychiatry 1995;56(8):363–7.

37. Kabra N, Nadkarni A. Prevalence of depression and anxiety in irritable bowel syndrome: a clinic based study from India. Indian J Psychiatry 2013;55(1):77–80.

38. Occhipinti K, Smith JW. Irritable bowel syndrome: a review and update. Clin Colon Rectal Surg 2012;25(1):46–52.

39. Menees SB, et al. The efficacy and safety of rifaximin for the irritable bowel syndrome: a systematic review and meta-analysis. Am J Gastroenterol 2012;107(1):28–35, quiz 36.

40. Schoenfeld P. Efficacy of current drug therapies in irritable bowel syndrome: what works and does not work. Gastroenterol Clin North Am 2005;34(2):319–35.

41. Wysowski DK, et al. Post-marketing reports of QT prolongation and ventricular arrhythmia in association with cisapride and Food and Drug Administration regulatory actions. Am J Gastroenterol 2001;96(6):1698–703.

42. DiBaise JK. Tegaserod-associated ischemic colitis. Pharmacotherapy 2005;25:620–5.

43. Qin J, Li R, Raes J, et al. A human gut microbial gene catalogue established by metagenomic sequencing. Nature 2010;464(7285):59–65.

44. Savage DC. Microbial ecology of the gastrointestinal tract. Annu Rev Microbiol 1997;31:107–33.

45. Bengmark S. Probiotics and prebiotics in prevention and treatment of gastrointestinal diseases. Gastroenterol Int 1998;11(Suppl. 1):4–7.

46. Macfarlane GT, Macfarlane S. Human colonic microbiota: ecology, physiology and metabolic potential of intestinal bacteria. Scand J Gastroenterol 1997;32(Suppl. 222):3–9.

47. Holzapfel WH, et al. Overview of gut flora and probiotics. Int J Food Microbiol 1998;41(2):85–101.

48. Noack J, et al. Dietary guar gum and pectin stimulate intestinal microbial polyamine synthesis in rats. J Nutr 1998;128:1385–91.

49. Gibson GR, Roberfroid MB. Dietary modulation of the human colonic microbiota: introducing the concept of prebiotics. J Nutr 1995;125:1401–12.

50. Louis P, Scott KP, Duncan SH, et al. Understanding the effects of diet on bacterial metabolism in the large intestine. J Appl Microbiol 2007;102(5):1197–208. doi:10.1111/j.1365-2672.2007.03322.x.

51. Hawrelak JA, Myers SP. Intestinal dysbiosis: a review of the literature. Altern Med Rev 2004;9(2):180–97.

52. Roberfroid M, Gibson GR, Hoyles L, et al. Prebiotic effects: metabolic and health benefits. Br J Nutr 2010;104(Suppl. 2):S1–63. doi:10.1017/S0007114510003363.

53. Ford AC, et al. Small intestinal bacterial overgrowth in irritable bowel syndrome: systematic review and meta-analysis. Clin Gastroenterol Hepatol 2009;7(12):1279–86.

54. Khoshini R, et al. A systematic review of diagnostic tests for small intestinal bacterial overgrowth. Dig Dis Sci 2008;53(6):1443–54.

55. Yu D, Cheeseman F, Vanner S. Combined oro-caecal scintigraphy and lactulose hydrogen breath testing demonstrate that breath testing detects oro-caecal transit, not small intestinal bacterial overgrowth in patients with IBS. Gut 2011;60(3):334–40.

56. Rana SV, et al. Comparison of lactulose and glucose breath test for diagnosis of small intestinal bacterial overgrowth in patients with irritable bowel syndrome. Digestion 2012;85(3):243–7.

57. Gasbarrini A, et al. Methodology and indications of H2-breath testing in gastrointestinal diseases: the Rome Consensus Conference. Aliment Pharmacol Ther 2009;29(Suppl. 1):1–49.

58. Rezaie A, Buresi M, Lembo A, et al. Hydrogen and methane-based breath testing in gastrointestinal disorders: the North American consensus. Am J Gastroenterol 2017;112(5):775–84. doi:10.1038/ajg.2017.46.

59. Kunkel D, Basseri RJ, Makhani MD, et al. Methane on breath testing is associated with constipation: a systematic review and meta-analysis. Dig Dis Sci 2011;56(6):1612–18. doi:10.1007/s10620-011-1590-5.

60. Blaut M, Clavel T. Metabolic diversity of the intestinal microbiota: implications for health and disease. J Nutr 2007;137(3):751S–5S.

61. Gibson GR. Dietary modulation of the human gut microflora using prebiotics. Br J Nutr 1998;80(Suppl. 2):S209–12.

62. Henao-Mejia J, et al. Inflammasome-mediated dysbiosis regulates progression of NAFLD and obesity. Nature 2012;482(7384):179–85.

63. Scher JU, Abramson SB. The microbiome and rheumatoid arthritis. Nat Rev Rheumatol 2011;7(10):569–78.

64. Hörmannsperger G, Clavel T, Haller D. Gut matters: Microbe-host interactions in allergic diseases. J Allergy Clin Immunol 2012;129(6):1452–9.

65. Foster JA, McVey Neufeld K-A. Gut–brain axis: how the microbiome influences anxiety and depression. Trends Neurosci 2013;36(5):305–12.

66. Unger MM, Spiegel J, Dillmann K-U, et al. Short chain fatty acids and gut microbiota differ between patients with Parkinson's disease and age-matched controls. Parkinsonism Relat Disord 2016;32:66–72.

67. Miyake S, Kim S, Suda W, et al. Dysbiosis in the gut microbiota of patients with multiple sclerosis, with a striking depletion of species belonging to clostridia XIVa and IV clusters. PLoS ONE 2015;10(9):e0137429.

68. Cattaneo A, Cattane N, Galluzzi S, et al. Association of brain amyloidosis with pro-inflammatory gut bacterial taxa and peripheral inflammation markers in cognitively impaired elderly. Neurobiol Aging 2017;49:60–8.

69. Giloteaux L, Goodrich JK, Walters WA, et al. Reduced diversity and altered composition of the gut microbiome in individuals with myalgic encephalomyelitis/chronic fatigue syndrome. Microbiome 2016;4(1):30.

70. Food, O. Agriculture, and C. World Health Organization Expert. Evaluation of health and nutritional properties of powder milk and live lactic acid bacteria; 2001.

71. Petrof E, et al. Stool substitute transplant therapy for the eradication of Clostridium difficile infection: 'RePOOPulating' the gut. Microbiome 2013;1(1):1–12.

72. Winkelstein A. Lactobacillus acidophilus tablets in the therapy of various intestinal disorders: a preliminary report. Am Pract Dig Treat 1955;6:1022–5.

73. McFarland LV, Dublin S. Meta-analysis of probiotics for the treatment of irritable bowel syndrome. World J Gastroenterol 2008;14(17):2650–61.

74. Agrawal A, et al. Clinical trial: the effects of a fermented milk product containing Bifidobacterium lactis DN-173 010 on abdominal distension and gastrointestinal transit in irritable bowel syndrome with constipation. Aliment Pharmacol Ther 2009;29(1):104–14.

75. O'Mahony L, et al. Lactobacillus and Bifidobacterium in irritable bowel syndrome: symptom responses and relationship to cytokine profiles. Gastroenterology 2005;128:541–51.

76. Whorwell PJ, et al. Efficacy of an Encapsulated Probiotic Bifidobacterium infantis 35624 in Women with Irritable Bowel Syndrome. Am J Gastroenterol 2006;101(7):1581–90.

77. Amansec S, et al. Lactobacillus fermentum PCCT relieves the symptoms of medically diagnosed irritable bowel syndrome (unpublished); 2005.

78. Conway PL. Probiotic bacterium: Lactobacillus fermentum. U.S. Patent Application 12/384, 336.

79. Nobaek S, et al. Alteration of intestinal microflora is associated with reduction in abdominal bloating and pain in patients with irritable bowel syndrome. Am J Gastroenterol 2000;95(5):1231–8.

80. Niedzielin K, Kordecki H, Birkenfeld B. A controlled, double-blind, randomized study on the efficacy of Lactobacillus plantarum 299V in patients with irritable bowel syndrome. Eur J Gastroenterol Hepatol 2001;13:1143–7.

81. Hun L. Original research: bacillus coagulans significantly improved abdominal pain and bloating in patients with IBS. Postgrad Med 2009;121(2):119–24.

82. Williams EA, et al. Clinical trial: a multi-strain probiotic preparation significantly reduces symptoms of irritable bowel syndrome in a double-blind placebo-controlled study. Aliment Pharmacol Ther 2008;29(1):97–103.

83. Kim HJ, et al. A randomized controlled trial of a probiotic, VSL#3, on gut transit and symptoms in diarrhea-predominant irritable bowel syndrome. Aliment Pharmacol Ther 2003;17(7):895–904.

84. Newcomer AD, et al. Response of patients with irritable bowel syndrome and lactase deficiency using unfermented acidophilus milk. Am J Clin Nutr 1983;38(2):257–63.

85. O'Sullivan MA, O'Morain CA. Bacterial supplementation in the irritable bowel syndrome: a randomised double-blind placebo-controlled crossover study. Dig Liver Dis 2000;32(4):294–301.

86. Bausserman M, Michail S. The use of Lactbacillus GG in irritable bowel syndrome in children: a double-blind randomized control trial. J Pediatr 2005;147:197–201.

87. Arvola T, et al. Prophylactic Lactobacillus GG reduces antibiotic-associated diarrhea in children with respiratory infections: a randomized study. Pediatrics 1999;104(5):1–4.

88. Kontiokari T, et al. Randomised trial of cranberry-lingonberry juice and Lactobacillus GG drink for the prevention of urinary tract infections in women. BMJ 2001;322:1571.

89. Horvath A, Dziechciarz P, Szajewska H. Meta-analysis: Lactobacillus rhamnosus GG for abdominal pain-related functional gastrointestinal disorders in childhood. Aliment Pharmacol Ther 2011;33(12):1302–10.

90. Mansour-Ghanaei F, et al. Efficacy of saccharomyces boulardii with antibiotics in acute amoebiasis. World J Gastroenterol 2003;9(8):1832–3.

91. Szajewska H, Ruszczynski M, Radzikowski A. Probiotics in the prevention of antibiotic-associated diarrhea in children: a meta-analysis of randomized controlled trials. J Pediatr 2010;149(3):367–72.

92. Szajewska H, Mrukowicz J. Meta-analysis: non-pathogenic yeast Saccharomyces boulardii in the prevention of antibiotic-associated diarrhoea. Aliment Pharmacol Ther 2005;22(5):365–72.

93. Plummer SF, et al. Effects of probiotics on the composition of the intestinal microbiota following antibiotic therapy. Int J Antimicrob Agents 2005;26(1):69–74.

94. Lonnermark E, et al. Intake of Lactobacillus plantarum reduces certain gastrointestinal symptoms during treatment with antibiotics. J Clin Gastroenterol 2010;44:106–12.

95. Lionetti E, et al. Lactobacillus reuteri therapy to reduce side-effects during anti-Helicobacter pylori treatment in children: a randomized placebo controlled trial. Aliment Pharmacol Ther 2006;24:1461–8.

96. Wenus C, et al. Prevention of antibiotic-associated diarrhoea by a fermented probiotic milk drink. Eur J Clin Nutr 2008;62:299–301.

97. Klarin B, et al. Lactobacillus plantarum 299v reduces colonisation of Clostridium difficile in critically ill patients treated with antibiotics. Acta Anaesthesiol Scand 2008;52(8):1096–102.

98. Surawicz CM, McFarland LV, Greenberg RN. The search for a better treatment for recurrent Clostridium difficile disease: use of high-dose vancomycin combined with Saccharomyces boulardii. Clin Infect Dis 2000;31(4):1012–17.

99. Bennett RG, et al. Treatment of relapsing Clostridium difficile diarrhea with Lactobacillus GG. Nutr Today 1996;31:35S–9S.

100. Manley KJ, et al. Probiotic treatment of vancomycin-resistant enterococci: a randomised controlled trial. Med J Aust 2007;186:454–7.

101. Osterlund P, et al. Lactobacillus supplementation for diarrhoea related to chemotherapy of colorectal cancer: a randomised study. Br J Cancer 2007;97(8):1028–34.

102. Wildt S, et al. Probiotic treatment of collagenous colitis: a randomized, double-blind, placebo-controlled trial with Lactobacillus acidophilus and Bifidobacterium animalis subsp. Lactis. Inflamm Bowel Dis 2006;12(5):395–401.

103. Yang YX, et al. Effect of a fermented milk containing Bifidobacterium lactis DN-173010 on Chinese constipated women. World J Gastroenterol 2008;14(40):6237–43.

104. Pitkala KH, et al. Fermented cereal with specific bifidobacteria normalizes bowel movements in elderly nursing home residents. A randomized, controlled trial. J Nutr Health Aging 2007;11:305–11.

105. Koebnick C, et al. Probiotic beverage containing Lactobacillus casei Shirota improves gastrointestinal symptoms in patients with chronic constipation. Can J Gastroenterol 2003;17:655–9.

106. Guslandi M, et al. Saccharomyces boulardii in maintenance treatment of Crohn's disease. Dig Dis Sci 2000;45(7):1462–4.

107. Fric P, Zavoral M. The effect of non-pathogenic Escherichia coli in symptomatic uncomplicated diverticular disease of the colon. Eur J Gastroenterol Hepatol 2003;15(3):313–15.

108. Manzoni P, et al. Oral supplementation with Lactobacillus casei subspecies rhamnosus prevents enteric colonization by Candida species in preterm neonates: a randomized study. Clin Infect Dis 2006;42(12):1735–42.

109. Indrio F, et al. Lactobacillus reuteri accelerates gastric emptying and improves regurgitation in infants. Eur J Clin Invest 2011;41(4):417–22.

110. Guillot CC, et al. Effects of Saccharomyces boulardii in children with chronic diarrhea, especially cases due to giardiasis. Rev Mex Pueric Pediatr 1995;2(12):1–5.

111. Besirbellioglu BA, et al. Saccharomyces boulardii and infection due to Giardia lamblia. Scand J Infect Dis 2006;38(6–7):479–81.

112. Saggioro A, et al. Helicobacter pylori eradication with Lactobacillus reuteri. A double-blind placebo-controlled trial. Dig Liver Dis 2005;37S:S88.

113. Wang KY, et al. Effects of ingesting Lactobacillus— and Bifidobacterium-containing yogurt in subjects with colonized Helicobacter pylori. Am J Clin Nutr 2004;80:737–41.

114. Sahagun-Flores JE, et al. Eradication of Helicobacter pylori: triple treatment scheme plus Lactobacillus vs. triple treatment alone. Cir Cir 2007;75(5):333–6.

115. Gotteland M, et al. Effect of regular ingestion of Saccharomyces boulardii plus inulin or Lactobacillus acidophilus LB in children colonized by Helicobacter pylori. Acta Paediatr 2005;94(12):1747–51.

116. Mrda Z, et al. Therapy of Helicobacter pylori infection using Lactobacillus acidophilus [Croatian]. Med Pregl 1998;51:343–5.

117. Anukam KC, et al. Yogurt containing probiotic Lactobacillus rhamnosus GR-1 and L. reuteri RC-14 helps resolve moderate diarrhea and increases CD4 count in HIV-AIDS patients. J Clin Gastroenterol 2008;42: 239–43.

118. Savino F, et al. Lactobacillus reuteri (American Type Culture Collection Strain 55730) versus simethicone in the treatment of infantile colic: a prospective randomized study. Pediatrics 2007;119:e124–30.

119. Mohan R, et al. Effects of Bifidobacterium lactis Bb12 supplementation on intestinal microbiota of preterm infants: a double-blind, placebo-controlled, randomized study. J Clin Microbiol 2006;44(11):4025–31.

120. Ahmed M, et al. Impact of consumption of different levels of Bifidobacterium lactis HN019 on the intestinal microflora of elderly human subjects. J Nutr Health Aging 2007;11:26–31.

121. Spanhaak S, Havenaar R, Schaafsma G. The effect of consumption of milk fermented by Lactobacillus casei

strain Shirota on the intestinal microflora and immune parameters in humans. Eur J Clin Nutr 1998;52(12):899–907.

122. Benno Y, et al. Effects of Lactobacillus GG yoghurt on human intestinal microecology in Japanese subjects. Nutr Today 1996;31:9S–12S.

123. Waller PA, et al. Dose-response effect of Bifidobacterium lactis HN019 on whole gut transit time and functional gastrointestinal symptoms in adults. Scand J Gastroenterol 2011;46(9):1057–64.

124. Meance CC, Turchet P, Raimondi A, et al. Séverine, a fermented milk with a bifidobacterium probiotic strain DN-173 010 shortened oro-fecal gut transit time in elderly. Microb Ecol Health Dis 2001;13(4):217–22.

125. Kim HJ, et al. A randomized controlled trial of a probiotic combination VSL#3 and placebo in irritable bowel syndrome with bloating. Neurogastroenterol Motil 2005;17:1–10.

126. Lin MY, Savaiano D, Harlander S. Influence of nonfermented dairy products containing bacterial starter cultures on lactose maldigestion in humans. J Dairy Sci 1991;74(1):87–95.

127. Montes RG, et al. Effects of milks inoculated with Lactobacillus acidophilus or a yoghurt starter culture in lactose-maldigesting children. J Dairy Sci 1995;78:1657–64.

128. Szajewska H, Wanke M, Patro B. Meta-analysis: the effects of Lactobacillus rhamnosus GG supplementation for the prevention of healthcare-associated diarrhoea in children. Aliment Pharmacol Ther 2011;34(9):1079–87.

129. Delia P, et al. Use of probiotics for prevention of radiation-induced diarrhea. World J Gastroenterol 2007;13:912–15.

130. Barrett JS, et al. Probiotic effects on intestinal fermentation patterns in patients with irritable bowel syndrome. World J Gastroenterol 2008;14(32):5020–4.

131. Black F, et al. Prophylactic efficacy of Lactobacilli on travellers' diarrhea. J Travel Med 1989;7:333–5.

132. Hilton E, et al. Efficacy of Lactobacillus GG as a diarrheal preventive in travelers. J Travel Med 1997;4:41–3.

133. Kollaritsch H, et al. Prevention of traveller's diarrhea: comparison of different nonantibiotic preparations. Travel Med Int 1989;9–17.

134. Rembacken BJ, et al. Non-pathogenic Escherichia coli versus mesalazine for the treatment of ulcerative colitis: a randomized trial. Lancet 1999;354(9179):635–9.

135. Sood A, et al. The probiotic preparation, VSL#3 induces remission in patients with mild-to-moderately active ulcerative colitis. Clin Gastroenterol Hepatol 2009;7:1202–9.

136. Kruis W, et al. Maintaining remission of ulcerative colitis with the probiotic Escherichia coli Nissle 1917 is as effective as with standard mesalazine. Gut 2004;53(11):1617–23.

137. Zocco MA, et al. Efficacy of Lactobacillus GG in maintaining remission of ulcerative colitis. Aliment Pharmacol Ther 2006;23(11):1567–74.

138. Venturi A, et al. Impact on the composition of the faecal flora by a new probiotic preparation: preliminary data on maintenance treatment of patients with ulcerative colitis. Aliment Pharmacol Ther 1999;13(8):1103–8.

139. Mimura T, et al. Once daily high dose probiotic therapy (VSL#3) for maintaining remission in recurrent or refractory pouchitis. Gut 2004;53(1):108–14.

140. Gosselink MP, et al. Delay of the first onset of pouchitis by oral intake of the probiotic strain Lactobacillus rhamnosus GG. Dis Colon Rectum 2005;47:876–84.

141. Saavedra JM, et al. Feeding of Bifidobacterium bifidum and Streptococcus thermophilus to infants in hospital for prevention of diarrhoea and shedding of rotavirus. Lancet 1994;344:1046–9.

142. Szajewska H, et al. Efficacy of Lactobacillus GG in prevention of nosocomial diarrhea in infants. J Pediatr 2001;138(3):361–5.

143. Szajewska H, et al. Meta-analysis: Lactobacillus GG for treating acute diarrhoea in children. Aliment Pharmacol Ther 2007;25:871–81.

144. Shornikova AV, et al. Bacteriotherapy with Lactobacillus reuteri in rotavirus gastroenteritis. Pediatr Infect Dis 1997;16:1103–7.

145. Dubey AP, et al. Use of VSL#3 in the treatment of rotavirus diarrhea in children. J Clin Gastroenterol 2008;42:S126–9.

146. Saxelin M, Ahokas M, Salminen S. Dose response on the faecal colonisation of Lactobacillus strain GG administered in two different formulations. Microb Ecol Health Dis 1993;6(3):119–22.

147. Gibson GR, Hutkins R, Sanders ME, et al. Expert consensus document: the International Scientific Association for Probiotics and Prebiotics (ISAPP) consensus statement on the definition and scope of prebiotics. Nat Rev Gastroenterol Hepatol 2017;14(8):491–502.

148. Collins MD, Gibson GR. Probiotics, prebiotics, and synbiotics: approaches for modulating the microbial ecology of the gut. Am J Clin Nutr 1999;69(Suppl.): 1052S–7S.

149. Gibson GR. Dietary modulation of the human gut microflora using prebiotics. Br J Nutr 1998;80(Suppl. 2):S209–12.

150. Arslanoglu S, et al. Early dietary intervention with a mixture of prebiotic oligosaccharides reduces the incidence of allergic manifestations and infections during the first two years of life. J Nutr 2010;138:1091–5.

151. Bass P, Dennis S. The laxative effects of lactulose in normal and constipated subjects. J Clin Gastroenterol 1981;3(Suppl. 1):23–8.

152. Teuri U, Korpela R. Galacto-oligosaccharides relieve constipation in elderly people. Ann Nutr Metab 1998;42:319–27.

153. Chen H-L, et al. Effects of fructooligosaccharide on bowel function and indicators of nutritional status in constipated elderly men. Nutr Res 2000;20(12):1725–33.

154. Polymeros D, Beintaris I, Gaglia A, et al. Partially hydrolyzed guar gum accelerates colonic transit time and improves symptoms in adults with chronic constipation. Dig Dis Sci 2014;59(9):2207–14.

155. Silk DB, et al. Clinical trial: the effects of a trans-galactooligosaccharide prebiotic on faecal microbiota and symptoms in irritable bowel syndrome. Aliment Pharmacol Ther 2009;29:508–18.

156. Hawrelak J, Whitten DL. Does partially hydrolysed guar gum have a role to play in the treatment of irritable bowel syndrome: a systematic review. J Clin Gastroenterol 2016;50(Suppl. 2):S200.

157. Schmidt K, Cowen PJ, Harmer CJ, et al. Prebiotic intake reduces the waking cortisol response and alters emotional bias in healthy volunteers. Psychopharmacology (Berl) 2015;232(10):1793–801.

158. Waligora-Dupriet AJ, et al. Effect of oligofructose supplementation on gut microflora and well-being in young children attending a day care centre. Int J Food Microbiol 2007;113:108–13.

159. Vulevic J, et al. A mixture of trans-galactooligosaccharides reduces markers of metabolic syndrome and modulates the fecal microbiota and immune function of overweight adults. J Nutr 2013;143(3):324–31.

160. van den Heuvel E, et al. Oligofructose stimulates calcium absorption in adolescents. Am J Clin Nutr 1999;69(3):544–8.

161. Drakoularakou A, et al. A double-blind, placebo-controlled, randomized human study assessing the capacity of a novel galacto-oligosaccharide mixture in reducing travellers' diarrhoea. Eur J Clin Nutr 2009;64:146–52.

162. McCutcheon J, Fulton JD. Lowered prevalence of infection with lactulose therapy in patients in long-term hospital care. J Hosp Infect 1989;13(1):81–6.

163. Olesen M, Gudmand-Hoyer E. Efficacy, safety, and tolerability of fructooligosaccharides in the treatment of irritable bowel syndrome. Am J Clin Nutr 2000;72(6):1570–5.

164. Bouhnik Y, et al. Short-chain fructo-oligosaccharide administration dose-dependently increases fecal bifidobacteria in healthy humans. J Nutr 1999;129:113–16.

165. Salyers AA, Leedle JAZ. Carbohydrate metabolism in the human colon. In: Hentges DJ, editor. Human intestinal microflora in health and disease. New York: Academic Press; 1983. p. 129–46.

166. Bernalier A, Dore J, Durand M. Biochemistry of fermentation. In: Gibson GR, Roberfroid M, editors. Colonic microbiota, nutrition and health. Dordrecht: Kluwer Academic Publishers; 1999. p. 37–54.

167. Gibson SAW, Conway PL. Recovery of a probiotic organism from human faeces after oral dosing. In: Gibson SAW, editor. Human health: the contribution of microorganisms. London: Springer-Verlag; 1994. p. 119–21.

168. Robinson RR, Feirtag J, Slavin JL. Effects of dietary arabinogalactan on gastrointestinal and blood parameters in healthy human subjects. J Am Coll Nutr 2001;20(4):279–85.

169. Jie Z, et al. Studies on the effects of polydextrose intake on physiologic functions in Chinese people. Am J Clin Nutr 2000;72:1503–9.

170. Schrezenmeir J, de Vrese M. Probiotics, prebiotics, and synbiotics-approaching a definition. Am J Clin Nutr 2001;73(2):361–4.

171. Casiraghi MC, et al. Effects of a synbiotic milk product on human intestinal ecosystem. J Appl Microbiol 2007;103(2):499–506.

172. Colecchia A, et al. Effects of a symbiotic preparation on the clinical manifestations of irritable bowel syndrome, constipation-variant. Results of an open, uncontrolled multicenter study. Minerva Gastroenterol Dietol 2006;52:349–58.

173. Dughera L, et al. Effects of symbiotic preparations on constipated irritable bowel syndrome symptoms. Acta Biomed 2007;78(2):111–16.

174. Chedid V, Dhalla S, Clarke JO, et al. Herbal therapy is equivalent to rifaximin for the treatment of small intestinal bacterial overgrowth. Glob Adv Health Med 2014;3(3):16–24. doi:10.7453/gahmj.2014.019.

175. Filocamo A, Nueno-Palop C, Bisignano C, et al. Effect of garlic powder on the growth of commensal bacteria from the gastrointestinal tract. Phytomedicine 2012;19(8–9):707–11. doi:10.1016/j.phymed.2012.02.018.

176. Pai V, Chanu TR, Chakraborty R, et al. Evaluation of the antimicrobial activity of Punica granatum peel against the enteric pathogens: an in vitro study. Asian J Plant Sci Res 2011;1(2):57–62.

177. Nzeako BC, Al-Kharousi ZS, Al-Mahrooqi Z. Antimicrobial activities of clove and thyme extracts. Sultan Qaboos Univ Med J 2006;6(1):33–9.

178. Dorman HJD, Deans SG. Antimicrobial agents from plants: antibacterial activity of plant volatile oils. J Appl Microbiol 2000;88(2):308–16. doi:10.1046/j.1365-2672.2000.00969.x.

179. Chaudhry NM, Saeed S, Tariq P. Antibacterial effects of oregano (Origanum vulgare) against gram negative bacilli. Pak J Bot 2007;39(2):609–13.

180. Peng L, Kang S, Yin Z, et al. Antibacterial activity and mechanism of berberine against Streptococcus agalactiae. Int J Clin Exp Pathol 2015;8(5):5217–23.

181. Thijssen AY, et al. Dysfunctional cognitions, anxiety and depression in irritable bowel syndrome. J Clin Gastroenterol 2010;44(10):e236–41. doi:10.1097/MCG.0b013e3181eed5d8.

182. Blanchard EB, et al. The role of stress in symptom exacerbation among IBS patients. J Psychosom Res 2008;64(2):119–28.

183. Gorard DA, et al. Intestinal transit in anxiety and depression. Gut 1996;39(4):551–5.

184. Silk DB, Davis A, Vulevic J, et al. Clinical trial: the effects of a trans-galactooligosaccharide prebiotic on faecal microbiota and symptoms in irritable bowel syndrome. Aliment Pharmacol Ther 2009;29:508–18.

185. Schmidt K, Cowen PJ, Harmer CJ, et al. Prebiotic intake reduces the waking cortisol response and alters emotional bias in healthy volunteers. Psychopharmacology (Berl) 2015;232(10):1793–801.

186. Burokas A, Arboleya S, Moloney RD, et al. Targeting the microbiota-gut-brain axis: prebiotics have anxiolytic and antidepressant-like effects and reverse the impact of chronic stress in mice. Biol Psychiatry 2017;doi:10.1016/j.biopsych.2016.12.031.

187. Davies GJ, et al. Bowel function measurements of individuals with different eating patterns. Gut 1986;27(2):164–9.

188. Sanjoaquin MA, et al. Nutrition and lifestyle in relation to bowel movement frequency: a cross-sectional study of 20,630 men and women in EPIC-Oxford. Public Health Nutr 2004;7(1):77–83.

189. Tramonte SM, et al. The treatment of chronic constipation in adults: a systematic review. J Gen Intern Med 1997;12(1):15–24.

190. Russo L, Andreozzi P, Zito F, et al. Partially hydrolyzed guar gum in the treatment of irritable bowel syndrome with constipation: effects of gender, age, and body mass index. Saudi J Gastroenterol 2015;21(2):104–10.

191. Hawrelak JA, Myers SP. Effects of two natural medicine formulations on irritable bowel syndrome symptoms: a pilot study. J Altern Complement Med 2010;16(10):1065–71.

192. Cummings JH. The effect of dietary fiber on fecal weight and composition, in CRC Handbook of Dietary Fibre. In: Spiller GA, editor. Human nutrition. Boca Raton: CRC Press; 2001. p. 183–252.

193. Cherbut C, et al. Effects of short-chain fatty acids on gastrointestinal motility. Scand J Gastroenterol 1997;32(Suppl. 222):58–61.

194. Topping DL. Short-chain fatty acids produced by intestinal bacteria. Asia Pac J Clin Nutr 1996;5(Suppl.):15–19.

195. Bijkerk CJ, et al. Systematic review: the role of different types of fibre in the treatment of irritable bowel syndrome. Aliment Pharmacol Ther 2004;19:245–51.

196. Cunnane SC, et al. High a-linolenic acid flaxseed (Linum usitatissimum): some nutritional properties in humans. Br J Nutr 1993;69:443–53.

197. van Wyk BE, Wink M. Medicinal Plants of the World. Pretoria: Briza Publications; 2004.

198. Sierra M, et al. Therapeutic effects of psyllium in type 2 diabetic patients. Eur J Clin Nutr 2002;56:830–42.

199. Knudsen KEB, Johansen HN. Mode of action of oat bran in the gastrointestinal tract. Eur J Clin Nutr 1995;49(Suppl. 3):S163–9.

200. Southgate DA. Dietary fiber parts of food plants and algae, in CRC Handbook of Dietary Fibre. In: Spiller GA, editor. Human nutrition. Boca Raton: CRC Press; 2001. p. 11–13.

201. Klauser AG, et al. Low fluid intake lowers stool output in healthy male volunteers. Z Gastroenterol 1990;28:606–9.

202. National H, C. Medical Research. Nutrient Reference Values for Australia and New Zealand; 2006.

203. Everhart JE, et al. A longitudinal survey of self-reported bowel habits in the United States. Dig Dis Sci 1989;34:1153–62.

204. Dahl R. Revolting rhymes. London: Puffin Books; 1995.

205. Oettle GJ. Effect of moderate exercise on bowel habit. Gut 1991;32:941–4.

206. Daley AJ, et al. The effects of exercise upon symptoms and quality of life in patients diagnosed with irritable bowel syndrome: a randomised controlled trial. Int J Sports Med 2008;29:778–82.

207. Giaccari S, Grasso G, Tronci S, et al. Partially hydrolyzed guar gum: a fiber as coadjuvant in the irritable colon syndrome. Clin Ter 2001;152(1):21–5.

208. Nakamura S, Hongo R, Moji K, et al. Suppressive effect of partially hydrolyzed guar gum on transitory diarrhea induced by ingestion of maltitol and lactitol in healthy humans. Eur J Clin Nutr 2007;61(9):1086–93.

209. Lu W-Z, et al. The effects of melatonin on colonic transit time in normal controls and IBS patients. Dig Dis Sci 2009;54(5):1087–93.

210. Heaton KW, et al. Defecation frequency and timing, and stool form in the general population: a prospective study. Gut 2009;33:818–24.

211. Bassoti G, et al. An extended assessment of bowel habits in a general population. World J Gastroenterol 2004;10:713–16.

212. Longstreth GF, et al. Functional bowel disorders. Gastroenterology 2006;130:1480–91.

213. Lindlahr H. Natural therapeutics: volume 2 practice. Essex UK: CW Daniel Company Ltd; 1981. p. 136–8.

214. Walker ARP. Nutritionally related disorders/diseases in Africans. Highlights of half a century of research with special reference to unexpected phenomena, in Dietary Fibre. In: Kritchevsky D, Bonfield C, editors. Health and Disease. New York: Plenum Press; 1997. p. 1–14.

215. Jones JM. Consumption of dietary fibre 1992–2000, in CRC Handbook of Dietary Fibre. In: Spiller GA, editor. Human nutrition. Boca Raton: CRC Press; 2001. p. 553–66.

216. Heaton KW, et al. Irritable bowel syndrome in a British urban community. Gastroenterology 1992;102(6):1962–7.

217. Heaton KW, Ghosh S, Braddon FEM. How bad are the symptoms and bowel dysfunction of patients with the irritable bowel syndrome? A prospective, controlled study with emphasis on stool form. Gut 1991;32:73–9.

218. Lewis SJ, Heaton KW. Stool form scale as a useful guide to intestinal transit time. Scand J Gastroenterol 1997;32(9):920–4.

219. Bassoti G, Germani U, Moelli A. Human colonic motility: physiological aspects. Int J Colorectal Dis 1995;10:173–80.

220. Gralnek IM, Hays RD, Kilbourne A. The impact of irritable bowel syndrome on health-related quality of life. Gastroenterology 2000;119(3):654–60.

221. Spiegel B, et al. Predictors of patient-assessed illness severity in irritable bowel syndrome. Am J Gastroenterol 2008;103(10):2536–43.

222. Adam B, et al. A combination of peppermint oil and caraway oil attenuates the post-inflammatory visceral hyperalgesia in a rat model. Scand J Gastroenterol 2006;41(2):155–60.

223. Muller MH, et al. STW 5 (Iberogast) reduces afferent sensitivity in the rat small intestine. Phytomedicine 2006;13(Suppl. 5):100–6.

224. Mozaffari S, Rahimi R, Abdollahi M. Implications of melatonin therapy in irritable bowel syndrome: a systematic review. Curr Pharm Des 2010;16(33):3646–55.

225. Vanhoutvin SALW, Troost FJ, Kilkens TOC, et al. The effects of butyrate enemas on visceral perception in healthy volunteers. Neurogastroenterol Motil 2009;21(9):952–e76.

226. Tarnowski W, Borycka-Kiciak K, Kiciak A, et al. Outcome of treatment with butyric acid In irritable bowel syndrome—preliminary report. Gastroenterol Prakt 2011;1:43–8.

227. Ohashi Y, Sumitani K, Tokunaga M, et al. Consumption of partially hydrolysed guar gum stimulates Bifidobacteria and butyrate-producing bacteria in the human large intestine. Benef Microbes 2015;6(4):451–5.

228. Kelly J, Ryan S, McKinnon H, et al. Dietary supplementation with a type 3 resistant starch induces butyrate producing bacteria within the gut microbiota of human volunteers. Appetite 2015;91:438.

229. Benson S, et al. Acute experimental endotoxemia induces visceral hypersensitivity and altered pain evaluation in healthy humans. Pain 2012;153(4):794–9.

230. Vulevic J, et al. Modulation of the fecal microflora profile and immune function by a novel trans-galactooligosaccharide mixture (B-GOS) in healthy elderly volunteers. Am J Clin Nutr 2008;88:1438–46.

231. Ballongue J, Schumann C, Quignon P. Effects of lactulose and lactitol on colonic microflora and enzymatic activity. Scand J Gastroenterol 1997;(Suppl. 222):41–4.

232. Gibson GR, et al. Selective stimulation of bifidobacteria in the human colon by oligofructose and inulin. Gastroenterology 1995;108:975–82.

233. Goto K, et al. The influence of tea catechins on fecal flora of elderly residents in long-term care facilities. Ann Long-Term Care 1998;6:43–8.

234. Benno Y, et al. Effect of rice fiber on human fecal microflora. Microbiol Immunol 1989;33(5):435–40.

235. Bone K. Phytotherapy and irritable bowel syndrome. British J Phytotherapy 1997;4(4):190–8.

236. Bretagne JF, et al. Increased cell loss in the human jejunum induced by laxatives (ricinoleic acid, dioctyl sodium sulphosuccinate, magnesium sulphate, bile salts). Gut 1981;22(264):269.

237. Walker AF, Middleton RW, Petrowicz O. Artichoke leaf extract reduces symptoms of irritable bowel syndrome in a post-marketing surveillance study. Phytother Res 2001;15(1):58–61.

238. Bundy R, et al. Turmeric extract may improve irritable bowel syndrome symptomology in otherwise healthy adults: a pilot study. J Altern Complement Med 2004;10(6):1015–18.

239. Petitpierre M, Gumowski P, Girard JP. Irritable bowel syndrome and hypersensitivity to food. Ann Allergy 1985;54(6):538–40.

240. Park MI, Camilleri M. Is there a role of food allergy in irritable bowel syndrome and functional dyspepsia? A systematic review. Neurogastroenterol Motil 2006;18(8):595–607.

241. Verdu EF. Editorial: can gluten contribute to irritable bowel syndrome[quest]. Am J Gastroenterol 2011;106(3):516–18.

242. Staudacher HM, et al. Comparison of symptom response following advice for a diet low in fermentable carbohydrates (FODMAPs) versus standard dietary advice in patients with irritable bowel syndrome. J Hum Nutr Diet 2011;24(5):487–95.

243. Jones J, et al. British Society of Gastroenterology guidelines for management of the irritable bowel syndrome. Gut 2000;47(Suppl. 2):ii1–19.

244. Chan J, Carr I, Mayberry JF. The role of acupuncture in the treatment of irritable bowel syndrome: a pilot study. Hepatogastroenterology 1997;44(17):1328–30.

245. Forbes A, et al. Acupuncture for irritable bowel syndrome: a blinded placebo-controlled trial. World J Gastroenterol 2005;11(26):4040–4.

246. Schneider A, et al. Acupuncture treatment in irritable bowel syndrome. Gut 2006;55:649–54.

247. Lim B, et al. Acupuncture for treatment of irritable bowel syndrome. Cochrane Database Syst Rev 2006;(4):CD005111.

248. Shi J, et al. Effectiveness and safety of herbal medicines in the treatment of irritable bowel syndrome: a systematic review. World J Gastroenterol 2008;14(3):454–62.

249. Moser G, et al. Long-term success of GUT-directed group hypnosis for patients with refractory irritable bowel syndrome: a randomized controlled trial. Am J Gastroenterol 2013;108:602–9.

250. Lindfors P, et al. Effects of gut-directed hypnotherapy on IBS in different clinical settings—results from two randomized, controlled trials. Am J Gastroenterol 2012;107(2):276–85.

251. Vlieger AM, et al. Long-term follow-up of gut-directed hypnotherapy vs. standard care in children with functional abdominal pain or irritable bowel syndrome. Am J Gastroenterol 2012;107(4):627–31.

252. Lindfors P, et al. Long-term effects of hypnotherapy in patients with refractory irritable bowel syndrome. Scand J Gastroenterol 2012;47(4):414–21.

253. Rutten JM, et al. Gut-directed hypnotherapy for functional abdominal pain or irritable bowel syndrome in children: a systematic review. Arch Dis Child 2013;98(3):252–7.

254. Felter HW, Lloyd JU. King's American dispensatory. 19th ed. Cincinnati: The Ohio Valley Company; 1905.

255. Bensky D, Clavey S, Stoger E. Chinese herbal medicine materia medica. 3rd ed. Seattle: Eastlands Press; 2004.

256. Khare CP. Indian herbal remedies: rational Western therapy, Ayurvedic and other traditional usage, botany. Berlin: Springer; 2004.

257. Ononiwu IM, Ibeneme CE, Ebong OO. Effects of piperine on gastric acid secretion in albino rats. Afr J Med Med Sci 2002;31(4):293–5.

258. Ganesh Bhat B, Chandrasekhara N. Effect of black pepper and piperine on bile secretion and composition in rats. Nahrung 1987;31(9):913–16.

259. Platel K, Srinivasan K. Influence of dietary spices and their active principles on pancreatic digestive enzymes in albino rats. Nahrung 2000;44(1):42–6.

260. Izzo AA, et al. Effect of vanilloid drugs on gastrointestinal transit in mice. Br J Pharmacol 2001;132(7):1411–16.

261. Bajad S, et al. Antidiarrhoeal activity of piperine in mice. Planta Med 2001;67(3):284–7.

262. Weiss RF. Herbal medicine. Beaconsfield: AB Arcanum; 1988.

263. May B, et al. Efficacy of a fixed peppermint oil/caraway oil combination in non-ulcer dyspepsia. Arzneimittelforschung 1996;46:1149–53.

264. Madisch A, et al. Treatment of functional dyspepsia with a fixed peppermint oil and caraway oil combination preparation as compared with cisapride. A multicenter, reference-controlled double-blind equivalence study. Arzneimittelforschung 1999;49:925–32.

265. Felter HW. The eclectic materia medica, pharmacology and therapeutics. Cincinnati: John K Scudderl; 1922. p. 25.

266. Bennett A, et al. The biological activity of eugenol, a major constituent of nutmeg (Myristica fragrans): studies on prostaglandins, the intestine and other tissues. Phytother Res 1988;2(3):124–30.

267. Dhingra D, Sharma A. Antidepressant-like activity of n-hexane extract of nutmeg (Myristica fragrans) seeds in mice. J Med Food 2006;9(1):84–9.

268. Sonavane GS, et al. Anxiogenic activity of Myristica fragrans seeds. Pharmacol Biochem Behav 2002;71(1–2):239–44.

269. Penalver P, et al. Antimicrobial activity of five essential oils against origin strains of the Enterobacteriaceae family. APMIS 2005;113(1):1–6.

270. Dorman HJD, Deans SG. Antimicrobial agents from plants: antibacterial activity of plant volatile oils. J Appl Microbiol 2000;88(2):308–16.

271. Force M, Sparks WS, Ronzio RA. Inhibition of enteric parasites by emulsified oil of oregano in vivo. Phytother Res 2000;14:213–14.

272. Tiwari S. Punica granatum—A 'Swiss Army Knife' in the field of ethnomedicines. J Nat Prod 2012;5:4.

273. Chidambara Murthy KN, Jayaprakasha GK, Singh RP. Studies on antioxidant activity of pomegranate (Punica granatum) peel extract using in vivo models. J Agric Food Chem 2002;50(17):4791–5.

274. Pai V, et al. Evaluation of the antimicrobial activity of Punica granatum peel against the enteric pathogens: an in vitro study. Asian J Plant Sci Res 2011;1(2):57–62.

275. Calzada F, Yépez-Mulia L, Aguilar A. In vitro susceptibility of Entamoeba histolytica and Giardia lamblia to plants used in Mexican traditional medicine for the treatment of gastrointestinal disorders. J Ethnopharmacol 2006;108(3):367–70.

276. Qnais EY, et al. Antidiarrheal activity of the aqueous extract of Punica granatum (Pomegranate) Peels. Pharm Biol 2007;45(9):715–20.

277. Singh K, Jaggi AS, Singh N. Exploring the ameliorative potential of Punica granatum in dextran sulfate sodium induced ulcerative colitis in mice. Phytother Res 2009;23(11):1565–74.

278. Frawley D, Lad V. The yoga of herbs. Twin Lakes: Lotus Press; 1986.

279. Akhondzadeh S, et al. Crocus sativus L. in the treatment of mild to moderate depression: a double-blind, randomized and placebo-controlled trial. Phytother Res 2005;19(2):148–51.

280. Noorbala AA, et al. Hydro-alcoholic extract of Crocus sativus L. versus fluoxetine in the treatment of mild to moderate depression: a double-blind, randomized pilot trial. J Ethnopharmacol 2005;97(2):281–4.

281. Akhondzadeh S, et al. A 22-week, multicenter, randomized, double-blind controlled trial of Crocus sativus in the treatment of mild-to-moderate Alzheimer's disease. Psychopharmacology (Berl) 2010;207(4):637–43.

282. Nahid K, et al. The effect of an Iranian herbal drug on primary dysmenorrhea: a clinical controlled trial. J Midwifery Womens Health 2009;54:401–4.

283. Guarner F, et al. Probiotics and prebiotics. World Gastroenterology Organisation Global Guideline; 2011.

284. Ducrotte P, Sawant P, Jayanthi V. Clinical trial: Lactobacillus plantarum 299v (DSM 9843) improves symptoms of irritable bowel syndrome. World J Gastroenterol 2012;18(30):4012–18.

285. Bouhnik Y, et al. Administration of transgalacto-oligosaccharides increases fecal bifidobacteria and modifies colonic fermentation metabolism in healthy humans. J Nutr 1997;127(3):444–8.

286. Grigoleit HG, Grigoleit P. Pharmacology and preclinical pharmacokinetics of peppermint oil. Phytomedicine 2005;12(8):612–16.

287. Kline RM, et al. Enteric-coated, pH-dependent peppermint oil capsules for the treatment of irritable bowel syndrome in children. J Pediatr 2001;138(1):125–8.

288. Sallon S, et al. A novel treatment for constipation-predominant irritable bowel syndrome using Padma © Lax, a Tibetan herbal formula. Digestion 2002;65(3):161–71.

289. Vejdani R, et al. The efficacy of an herbal medicine, Carmint, on the relief of abdominal pain and bloating in patients with irritable bowel syndrome: a pilot study. Dig Dis Sci 2006;51(8):1501–7.

290. Tarpila S, Tarpila A, Gröhn P, et al. Efficacy of ground flaxseed on constipation in patients with irritable bowel syndrome. Curr Top Nutraceutical Res 2004;2: 119–25.

CHAPTER 5

Gastro-oesophageal reflux disease

Jason Hawrelak
ND, BNat(Hons), PhD

OVERVIEW

Gastro-oesophageal reflux disease (GORD) is commonly encountered in clinical practice. Recent research has estimated the prevalence at 10–20% in Western nations.[1] GORD has been defined as 'a condition which develops when the reflux of stomach contents causes troublesome symptoms and/or complications'.[2] Signs and symptoms of GORD result primarily from the recurrent reflux of gastric contents into the oesophagus (Figure 5.1) and can include a burning sensation in the retrosternal area, regurgitation, epigastric pain, dysphagia, sleep disturbances, laryngitis and a chronic cough.[2–4] The pathogenesis of GORD is complex and multifactorial with a number of mechanisms appearing to be involved (Figure 5.2).

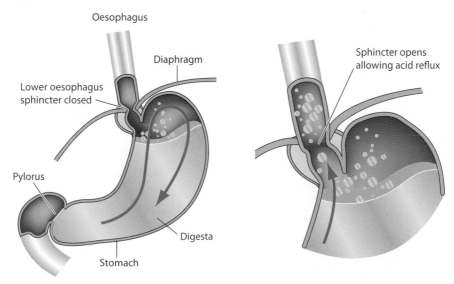

Figure 5.1
Acid reflux into the oesophagus in GORD

Factors involved with GORD

- *Lower oesophageal sphincter incompetence*. The role of the lower oesophageal sphincter (LOS) is to allow the passage of food into the stomach while preventing the reflux of gastric contents back into the oesophagus. Patients with GORD have been found to suffer from frequent transient LOS relaxations and decreased LOS resting pressure compared with healthy controls.[5,6]

- *Poor oesophageal acid clearance*. Patients with GORD have been found to have less oesophageal peristaltic activity. This results in a reduced capacity to clear reflux contents from the oesophagus.[7] Contact between the refluxed gastric contents and the oesophageal mucosa results in inflammation. This inflammation has been found to further reduce oesophageal peristalsis, further impairing acid clearance, and causing a worsening of reflux symptoms—a vicious circle.[8]

- *Slow gastric emptying*. Delayed gastric emptying (particularly of the proximal stomach) has been correlated with increased severity and frequency of reflux episodes in GORD patients.[9] Delayed gastric emptying of ingesta has been postulated to contribute to GORD symptoms via two mechanisms: by increasing the length of time refluxate is available in the stomach; and increasing gastric distension, which has been found to increase the rate of transient LOS relaxations.[10]

- *Impaired saliva flow*. Salivary secretion plays an important role in the clearance of regurgitated gastric contents in the oesophagus. GORD patients have been found to suffer from impaired salivary gland function and reduced saliva production.[11]

- *Hiatal hernia*. Hiatal hernias have been found to be relatively common in patients suffering from GORD.[12] They appear to promote LOS incompetence via a decrease in LOS resting pressure,[13,14] and their presence is associated with increased severity of reflux.[15]

- *Oxidative stress*. Research has shown that mucosal damage in oesophagitis is mediated, at least in part, by oxygen-derived free radicals.[16] Animal research has also found considerable levels of oxidative stress in the oesophageal mucosa after reflux episodes. This research also noted a significant mucosa protective effect from antioxidant supplementation.[17]

- *Food allergy and intolerance*. Gastro-oesophageal reflux in infants and toddlers is frequently linked to a dairy allergy.[18] Patients with coeliac disease have also been found to have a high prevalence of gastro-oesophageal reflux. Although the exact mechanism of how gluten exposure leads to GORD is not known, gluten-free diets have been found to significantly reduce GORD symptoms and effectively prevent their recurrence in these patients.[19]

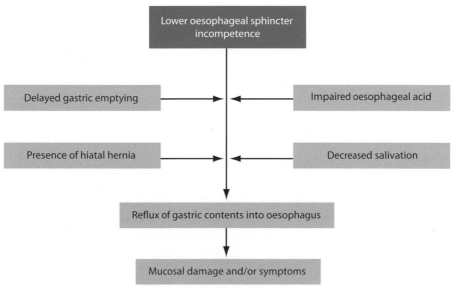

Figure 5.2
The key aetiological factors involved in GORD

Diagnosis

A diagnosis of GORD is typically made clinically, based on the presence of the classic symptoms—a burning feeling rising from the stomach or lower chest up towards the neck (heartburn) and/or the effortless return of stomach contents into the pharynx (regurgitation). The diagnosis is usually confirmed by its good response to therapy. In conventional medicine, this equates to antacids, proton-pump inhibitors (PPIs) or histamine type 2 receptor antagonists (H$_2$RAs). In naturopathic medicine, this could equate to a short trial of antacids but more probably a trial of gastrointestinal demulcents. If the patient presents with the classic symptom picture and responds to demulcent therapy, that confirms the diagnosis. If alarm signs and symptoms are present (e.g. weight loss, dysphagia, an epigastric mass upon examination, anaemia or signs of internal bleeding), then patients should be referred for further investigation (endoscopy). If the patient presents with the classic symptoms of GORD but does not respond to treatment (within six weeks), then referral for further investigations is also recommended.[20,21]

The clinical presentation of GORD is usually classic; however, patients sometimes present uncharacteristically with non-specific symptoms of epigastric pain, atypical chest pain, dyspepsia, dysphagia or odynophagia which may be indicative of GORD or other disorders.

DIFFERENTIAL DIAGNOSIS

- Epigastric pain: cholelithiasis, choledocholithiasis, acute viral hepatitis, alcoholic hepatitis, peptic ulcer disease, gastritis, acute pancreatitis, pyelonephritis, nephrolithiasis, shingles or mesenteric ischaemia

- Atypical chest pain: angina, myocardial infarction or diffuse oesophageal spasm

- Dyspepsia: peptic ulcer disease, gastritis, gastric cancer, cholelithiasis, chronic pancreatitis, pancreatic cancer, NSAID-induced dyspepsia, functional dyspepsia or eosinophilic oesophagitis

- Dysphagia: oesophageal obstruction, foreign body ingestion, paraoesophageal hernia, oesophageal adenocarcinoma, radiation-induced stricture or achalasia

- Odynophagia: infectious oesophagitis (*Candida*, herpes simplex, cytomegalovirus or HIV), pill oesophagitis or radiation-induced oesophageal injury

Source: Cappell 2005,[3] Moonen & Boeckxstaens 2014[22] and Kia & Hirano 2015[23]

RISK FACTORS

A number of risk factors that appear to contribute to the initiation and maintenance of GORD symptoms have been identified. These usually involve lifestyle factors, although genetic influences and medications can also contribute to the disorder.

- *Dietary factors.* Imbibed foods, beverages and substances capable of precipitating reflux episodes include coffee and other caffeinated beverages, alcoholic beverages, chocolate, meals high in fat and, potentially, peppermint essential oil (e.g. peppermint lollies).[24] These substances are capable of increasing acid secretion (alcohol, coffee), reducing LOS pressure (alcohol, chocolate, coffee, fatty meals), causing transient LOS relaxations (alcohol, peppermint essential oil), slowing gastric emptying (alcohol, fatty foods) and/or impairing oesophageal motility (alcohol). Agents that can trigger pain by irritating an already inflamed oesophageal mucosa include tomato and citrus juice, soft drinks and spicy foods. From a naturopathic perspective, eating meals too quickly, consuming too-large meals, consuming fluids with meals, eating close to bedtime and chewing food inadequately are other potential contributing factors to GORD.

- *High BMI*. Research has found a clear association between reflux symptoms and the presence of overweight or obesity.[25]
- *Smoking*. Tobacco smokers report higher rates of reflux symptoms than non-smokers do.[26] This is thought to be caused by smoking-induced decreases in resting LOS pressure. Coughing or even deep inhalation can cause acute increases in intra-abdominal pressure capable of overpowering their feeble LOS.[27]
- *Psychological stress*. A significant proportion of subjects with GORD have been found to suffer from psychological distress[28] and stress appears to increase sensitivity to heartburn pain in some GORD sufferers.[29]
- *Genetic disposition*. A genetic predisposition may contribute to the development of GORD in some patients, with one study estimating that genetic influences comprise almost 30% of attributable risk for GORD.[30]
- *Pregnancy*. GORD symptoms are reported by 40–85% of women during pregnancy.[31]
- *Medications*. Nitrates, calcium channel blockers, NSAIDs, theophylline, morphine, meperidone, diazepam, barbiturates and sildenafil are all capable of decreasing LOS pressure.[3,32]

CONVENTIONAL TREATMENT

Conventional treatment aims to reduce the symptoms of GORD and reduce oesophageal damage through the use of antisecretory therapies such as PPIs or H_2RAs. Although these agents have been found to be effective in reducing the oesophageal symptoms of GORD and, to a lesser extent, extraoesophageal symptoms,[20] their use is also associated with significant side effects and risks. Common adverse events of antisecretory therapies include diarrhoea, nausea, abdominal pain and headaches.[33] Longer term use of antisecretory drugs is associated with increased risk of gastroenteritis,[34] pneumonia,[35] spinal fracture,[36] small intestinal bacterial overgrowth,[37] dementia,[38] and vitamin and mineral malabsorption.[39,40] The surgical procedure laparoscopic fundoplication is also sometimes advocated for treating GORD. This procedure, however, carries a small, but significant, risk of life-threatening complications.[41]

KEY TREATMENT PROTOCOLS

The naturopathic protocols adopted to treat GORD usually focus on dietary and lifestyle modifications, in addition to botanical treatments. After relieving symptoms, the aim is to initially identify any factors that contribute to GORD and remove these triggers. If inflammation, ulceration or poor motility/sphincter tone is present, herbal or nutritional prescription may be of benefit.

> **Naturopathic Treatment Aims**
>
> - Relieve symptoms.
> - Treat the cause—eliminate/minimise exacerbating factors to support the nervous system
>   - address dietary factors
>   - address lifestyle factors.
> - Decrease oesophageal inflammation and promote oesophageal healing.
> - Tone the lower oesophageal sphincter.
> - Speed gastric emptying.
> - Prevent oesophageal cancer.
> - Promote antioxidant defences.

Relieve symptoms

Relief of heartburn is paramount in managing GORD. Gastrointestinal demulcents are typically very effective in providing prompt relief of heartburn symptoms (usually within minutes of ingestion). Effective demulcents include *Althaea officinalis radix*, *Ulmus fulva cortex* and *Glycyrrhiza glabra*. Gastrointestinal demulcents are most effective when administered in powdered form—mixed into a little water or apple juice to form a slurry or gruel. Tablets and capsules will be significantly less effective. Demulcents can be used 'on demand' or taken after meals and/or before bed for a preventative effect. Honey also has a history of being used as a demulcent in GORD.

Preliminary research utilising **D-limonene** (1000 mg every second day) has shown promising results, with 86% of subjects in one small trial experiencing complete relief of GORD symptoms after 14 days of treatment compared with 29% of placebo-treated controls.[42] Its mechanism of action is unknown, but D-limonene may coat the oesophageal mucosa, protecting the underlying tissue from gastric acid exposure. It may also speed gastric emptying.[43]

Eliminate exacerbating factors to support the nervous system

Dietary factors

The naturopathic axiom *tolle causum* ('treat the cause') is particularly relevant to managing GORD. While herbal demulcents can relieve heartburn symptoms effectively and promptly, their use, in some respects, is only palliative if patients continue to indulge in dietary factors known to exacerbate their condition. Avoidance of food and drinks known to precipitate reflux episodes (e.g. chocolate, alcoholic beverages, caffeinated beverages, carbonated beverages and fatty foods) is an important therapeutic strategy that can produce excellent clinical outcomes. These foods can precipitate reflux episodes by reducing the LOS resting pressure, causing transient relaxations of the LOS, impairing oesophageal motility and/or slowing gastric emptying.[44–51] Despite the fact that these substances contribute significantly to the main physiological causes of reflux episodes, there is a paucity of research that has examined the efficacy of avoidance of these dietary triggers in managing GORD.[24]

Other recommendations, such as taking time when eating, consuming smaller meals, avoiding fluid consumption with meals (both should decrease gastric distension) and chewing food adequately, are traditional naturopathic recommendations.[52] Chewing food as thoroughly as possible is a traditional recommendation that may result in improved salivary gland function over time and, hence, improved oesophageal acid clearance. Changing the evening meal time to earlier in the evening (at least three hours before bedtime) can also be helpful.[53]

In infants and toddlers with GORD, a dairy-free diet should be implemented. If they are formula-fed, the mother should be encouraged to relactate. The use of an extensively hydrolysed whey formula is the next best option. Goat's milk formulas should be avoided because goat's milk shares a significant amount of cross-reactivity with cow milk proteins,[54] as can soy in some patients.[55] There have also been a number of studies demonstrating the efficacy of **carob bean powder** (*Ceratonia siliqua*) as a formula additive.[56,57] Carob powder has been found to significantly decrease the severity and frequency of vomiting in infants with GORD, as well as increasing weight gain.[56] If the infant is exclusively breastfed, then the mother should be placed on a dairy-free diet, as small, but clinically significant, amounts of dairy proteins do appear in the breast milk.

Coeliac disease sufferers are significantly more prone to GORD symptoms.[58] These symptoms typically improve rapidly (within three months) after beginning a strict gluten-free diet. Given the frequency in which GORD symptoms occur in undiagnosed coeliac sufferers, it would be prudent to screen GORD sufferers for coeliac disease, particularly if they present with other clinical manifestations of the disease, have a family history of it or respond poorly to initial therapy.[59]

Based on the results from one small trial that found administration of a large daily dose of fructooligosaccharides (~20 g/day) to result in an increase in the number of transient lower oesophageal sphincter relaxations, reflux episodes and a worsening of GORD symptoms in patients with GORD,[60] and presumably the efficacy of a low FODMAP diet in some patients with IBS,[61] a low-FODMAP diet has recently been advocated as a treatment approach to GORD.

A small, open-label trial recently evaluated the impact of a diet low in FODMAPs on reflux symptoms in subjects with GORD. After an average of seven weeks, subjects following the diet experienced a significant reduction in total reflux episodes and significantly less heartburn and regurgitation symptoms. However, they also experienced an increase in nausea and epigastric pain. Given these results, it may be worthwhile considering the implementation of a low-FODMAP diet in some GORD patients, especially those that do not respond to the recommendations detailed above.[62]

The low-FODMAP diet may best be reserved as a last resort where elimination of other dietary triggers has failed, as it eliminates many healthy foods (many fruits, vegetables and legumes) and may have negative repercussions on the GIT microbiota.[63,64]

Lifestyle factors

In addition to the dietary factors just discussed, lifestyle factors such as obesity and smoking should be addressed. Weight loss has been shown in some research to result in reduced reflux episodes and should be encouraged in all overweight and obese patients.[65] Cessation of smoking could be recommended for a number of compelling reasons, not the least of which is its effect on oesophageal reflux. Short-term studies (of 24–48 hours' duration) have not consistently found a reduction in reflux episodes after smoking cessation.[66,67] However, no longer term studies have yet been performed and, in light of smoking's well-known adverse effects, GORD patients who smoke should be encouraged to quit. **Herbal thymoleptics**, **anxiolytics** and **adaptogens** can play an important supportive role in this process by reducing the impact of nervous dysfunction on GORD (see Chapters 14–17 on the nervous system).

Raising the head of the bed is another easy-to-implement lifestyle intervention that has demonstrated beneficial effects in GORD.[24] This recommendation is based on the theory that acidic stomach contents will be more likely to reflux when patients are lying flat. Research has, so far, mostly supported this theory, with intervention trials finding reduced frequency of reflux episodes, shorter reflux episodes and fewer reflux symptoms when bedheads were raised (one trial raised the head by 28 cm).[68]

Interestingly, **bedtime posture** has been found to influence GORD symptoms. Lying GORD patients on their right side after a meal increased the number of transient LOS relaxations and reflux episodes, as well as distended the proximal stomach when compared with lying patients on their left side.[69]

Decrease oesophageal inflammation and promote oesophageal healing

The reduction of oesophageal inflammation and the promotion of oesophageal healing will help reduce the vicious circle of GORD. As previously discussed, inflammation is a common occurrence in GORD. Demulcents (as discussed earlier), anti-inflammatory and vulnerary herbs may soothe the tissue and enhance healing. Useful anti-inflammatory phytomedicines for the digestive system include **Filipendula ulmaria**, **Curcuma longa**, **Glycyrrhiza glabra** and **Matricaria recutita**, while vulnerary herbal medicines traditionally used to help heal the upper gastrointestinal tract include **Althaea officinalis**, **Ulmus fulva**, **Calendula officinalis**, **Symphytum officinale** and **Aloe barbadensis**. Given that alcohol is a common reflux exacerbating factor, teas or tablets/capsules are the preferred methods of administration.

The results of a recent open-label trial have suggested a role for the anti-inflammatory compound **curcumin** (from *Curcuma longa*) in treating GORD. Fourteen typical GORD patients who were dependent on PPIs or H_2RAs were started on curcumin therapy (2 g/day). After two weeks their conventional medications were withdrawn. Eleven subjects were completely asymptomatic over the two-month follow-up period. Of the three non-responders, one was able to have complete symptom relief on a lower dose of PPI therapy than previously used.[70]

What about hypochlorhydria and digestive bitters?

A common naturopathic theory is that GORD is actually caused by hypochlorhydria—too little gastric acid. This theory is based on the idea that sufficient gastric acid in the stomach functions as a signal informing the LOS to remain tightly closed. When there is insufficient gastric acid, the LOS allows the reflux of the gastric contents into the oesophagus where it causes damage and inflammation. Another theory is that insufficient digestion causes fermentation, which creates increased intragastric pressure and the subsequent opening of the LOS.

At this point in time, however, there is little hard evidence to support either theory. Research has, in fact, found the amount of gastric acid produced by GORD sufferers to be greater than, or at least equal to, that produced by healthy controls.[71,72]

Given the theoretical causative role of hypochlorhydria in GORD, it is not surprising that bitters has been suggested as a potential therapeutic substance. Bitter herbs tend to be viewed as increasing gastric acid output via taste receptors on the tongue. Independent of this effect on gastric acid output, bitters, such as *Gentiana lutea*, produce a number of effects that are potentially beneficial in GORD.

Bitters increase saliva secretion,[73] speed gastric emptying[74] and exhibit mucosal protective activity.[75] Caution should be used in their application, however, as any increase in gastric acidity could significantly aggravate GORD symptoms.

Similarly, caution should be exercised when considering supplementation with betaine hydrochloride (HCL), both in light of the scant evidence in support of its use and also based on the capacity of more acidic refluxate to cause worsening damage to the oesophageal mucosa (a situation previously clinically observed in patients taking supplementary HCL in an effort to manage their heartburn symptoms).

Melatonin has shown promise as a novel oesophageal mucosa protector, with animal research finding pretreatment with melatonin protects the mucosa from gastric acid and pepsin-induced oesophageal injury and improves oesophageal mucosa blood flow.[76] Other research has found melatonin to display free-radical scavenging properties and local anti-inflammatory effects in the oesophageal mucosa, thereby protecting against reflux oesophagitis.[77] Preliminary human research has also found melatonin capable of healing even severe oesophageal ulcerations.[78]

Given the role of free radicals in reflux-induced oesophageal inflammation,[79] the promotion of antioxidant defences is a worthwhile, but as yet under-researched, therapeutic approach. Animal research has, however, found antioxidant supplementation (quercetin, α-tocopherol and lycopene) to attenuate the severity of reflux oesophagitis.[80,81]

Incorporating **brightly coloured fruits**, **vegetables**, **legumes** and **whole grains** into the diet should be encouraged (see the food nutrient chart in Appendix 4).

Animal research has also found benefit in favourably altering the omega-3 and omega-6 dietary ratio. Increasing the relative amount of omega-3 fats consumed resulted in a significant decrease in experimental oesophageal mucosal inflammation and a reduction in oxidative damage.[82]

Phytotherapy in GORD
Aside from the use of carminative herbs in dyspepsia and IBS, phytotherapy in most other digestive conditions including GORD is under-researched.
Currently, most evidentiary support is based on traditional use and in vitro studies. This remains a potential area of research. This is starting to change, however, with some recent research exploring the impact of herbal preparations in GORD treatment.
In a six-week randomised controlled trial, an extract of myrtle berries (1000 mg/day; aqueous freeze-dried *Myrtillus communis* berry) was compared to the proton pump inhibitor omeprazole (20 mg/day), or the combination. All treatment groups reported significant reductions in both reflux and dyspeptic scores from baseline, with no significant differences found between the groups—suggesting equivalency between omeprazole and the myrtle berry extract.[83]

Tone the lower oesophageal sphincter

A traditional naturopathic focus of treating GORD is to improve the tone of the smooth muscle of the LOS, thereby enhancing its capacity to hold gastrointestinal contents in the stomach. Poor LOS tone may be potentially improved by the use of tannin-rich herbs, which provide astringency and increased tissue tone, in addition to reducing inflammation.[84] Hydrolysable tannin constituents (higher molecular weight tannins) primarily affect astringency. Botanicals that contain these tannins include ***Geranium maculatum***, ***Achillea millefolium***, ***Calendula officinalis***, ***Hamamelis virginiana*** and ***Agrimonia eupatorium***.[85] Naturopaths should be aware that long-term use or high doses of tannins may impede digestion by binding to digestive enzymes. One suggested approach is to co-prescribe a herbal medicine with a bitter principle to stimulate digestion and to provide an adjuvant anti-inflammatory effect. However, to complicate matters, the use of bitters should be monitored carefully as this may worsen some people's GORD.[86]

The only agent so far demonstrated to significantly improve the functioning of the LOS is melatonin. In an open-label trial, administration of melatonin (3 mg nightly) was found to significantly improve LOS pressure after four weeks' administration and to normalise it by eight weeks. This coincided with the complete elimination of heartburn symptoms in all melatonin-treated subjects and epigastric pain in 83% of subjects.[87]

Speed gastric emptying

To speed gastric emptying, avoidance of food and drinks that slow gastric emptying is recommended, such as high-fat meals and alcohol.[88,89] The probiotic strain ***Lactobacillus reuteri*** **MM53** is also capable of accelerating gastric emptying.[90] Certain bitter herbal medicines may also assist in this process; however, this intervention may cause aggravation in some as highlighted above. Other herbal agents shown to speed gastric emptying time in human trials include ginger *Zingiber officinale* and the Indian spice mix garam masala.[91,92]

Prevent oesophageal cancer and promote antioxidant defences

One of the more serious complications of GORD is the development of Barrett's oesophagus, a metaplastic change of the lining of the oesophagus that is associated with an increased risk of oesophageal adenocarcinoma.[93] Preventing the development of Barrett's oesophagus and preventing the change of Barrett's oesophagus to adeno-carcinoma should be major naturopathic treatment aims. Preventing reflux episodes, reducing oesophageal inflammation and promoting mucosal healing using the strategies discussed above will be part of this approach. Reducing oxidative stress is an additional approach to this issue, as research has found patients with Barrett's oesophagus have lower plasma concentrations of antioxidants (selenium, vitamin C, β-cryptoxanthine and xanthophyll) than GORD patients without Barrett's oesophagus.[94] Additionally, a recent Australian study found high intakes of beta-carotene to be inversely associated with risk of dysplastic Barrett's oesophagus and a high intake of vitamin E and a high overall antioxidant intake to be inversely associated with risk of oesophageal adeno-carcinoma.[95] GORD patients should be encouraged to increase their consumption of antioxidant-rich fruits and vegetables, legumes and wholegrain products on a daily basis.

Beta-carotene supplementation also shows promise in treating Barrett's oesophagus. A small open-label study administered beta-carotene (25 mg/day) to subjects with Barrett's oesophagus for a period of six months. GORD symptoms significantly reduced from baseline by the end of the trial (62% decrease; $p < 0.05$), but, more importantly, the length of the Barrett's oesophageal segment significantly reduced (from a mean of 2.4 to 1.1 cm; $p < 0.05$). In 33% of subjects, there was a complete disappearance of Barrett's oesophagus.[96]

Epidemiological research has found an inverse relationship between dietary intake of **zinc** and incidence of oesophageal adenocarcinoma[97]; animal models have found zinc deficiency to be a significant contributing factor to developing Barrett's oesophagus.[98] In light of this research, zinc supplementation may also be warranted in GORD sufferers in an attempt to prevent the development of Barrett's oesophagus (see Chapter 32 on cancer for overarching protocols and interventions).

INTEGRATIVE MEDICAL CONSIDERATIONS

Acupuncture

In a randomised trial, the efficacy of acupuncture was compared with doubling the dose of a PPI in patients unresponsive to the standard dose of a PPI. Subjects were randomised to receive either 10 acupuncture sessions over a four-week period in combi-nation with their original PPI or the same PPI at double the daily dose. At the end of a four-week treatment period, subjects in the acupuncture group had significant decreases in daytime heartburn, night-time heartburn, acid regurgitation and dysphagia compared with baseline versus no significant change in the double-dose PPI group.[99] In subjects unresponsive to initial naturopathic therapy, referral to a traditional Chinese medicine practitioner may be warranted.

Other gastrointestinal conditions

There are a number of less common gastrointestinal conditions. These are listed in Table 5.1.

Table 5.1
Other gastrointestinal conditions

Condition	Signs and symptoms[100]	Protocols	Complementary and alternative medicine treatments[86,101,102]
Colorectal polyps	Typically asymptomatic	Eliminate dietary and lifestyle risk factors Ensure optimal intake of antioxidants Establish healthy colonic milieu	Lifestyle: eliminate smoking and alcohol use[103]; increase physical activity levels[104] Dietary change: encourage consumption of a diet rich in colourful fruits, vegetables, whole grains and legumes[105,106] Nutrients: calcium,[107] N-acetylcysteine,[108] antioxidant vitamins,[109] selenium[110] Prebiotics: lactulose[109] Probiotics: *Lactobacillus casei* Shirota[111]
Dyspepsia	GIT discomfort (especially after meals), bloating and wind, nausea or vomiting	Regulate GIT motility Enhance digestion Provide antiemesis Soothe tissue Reduce intestinal gas	Lifestyle: stress reduction Dietary change: avoid food triggers; reduce greasy foods; avoid alcohol, over-eating, rushed eating Herbal carminatives such as *Matricaria recutita, Mentha piperita, Melissa officinalis, Cinnamomum zeylanicum, Carum carvi* Herbal antiemetics such as *Zingiber officinale, Mentha piperita, Citrus reticulata* Herbal bitters such as *Cynara scolymus, Gentiana lutea, Centaurium erythraea* Digestive enzymes such as amylase, protases, lipases, HCl Combination phytotherapy product containing *Iberis amara*[112]
Gastritis	Similar symptoms to ulceration conditions, may be initiated by alcohol, stress, medications or bacteria overgrowth such as *Helicobacter pylori*	Reduce pain Reduce inflammation Heal GIT tissue Eradicate *Helicobacter pylori*	Lifestyle: stress reduction Dietary change: avoid food triggers; reduce greasy foods; avoid alcohol, over-eating, rushed eating Herbal anti-inflammatories, vulneraries and demulcents such as *Glycyrrhiza glabra, Althaea officinalis, Symphytum officinale, Ulmus fulva, Achillea* spp., cabbage leaf soup, cabbage juice, sauerkraut, melatonin[113] Herbal antimicrobials with demonstrated anti-*Helicobacter pylori* activity such as berberine-containing herbs, propolis, *Origanum vulgare, Cinnamomum zeylanicum, Thymus vulgaris*[114–119] Probiotics (see Table 4.1 in Chapter 4 on irritable bowel syndrome)
Malabsorption	Bloating and wind, undigested food in the stool, diarrhoea, weight loss over time, nutrient deficiencies	Enhance digestion Supplement nutrients Regulate stool Reduce symptoms	Lifestyle: stress reduction Dietary change: avoid food triggers; reduce greasy foods; avoid alcohol, over-eating, rushed eating Herbal digestives (bitters, aromatics—see above) Digestive enzymes Nutrients: broad-spectrum vitamin/mineral supplement Probiotic: *Saccharomyces cerevisiae* variety *boulardii* (Biocodex)[120]

Table 5.1
Other gastrointestinal conditions (continued)

Condition	Signs and symptoms[100]	Protocols	Complementary and alternative medicine treatments[86,101,102]
Ulceration	GIT pain relieved by food, worse with hunger signal, relief from antacids/antiulcer drugs, potential blood in stool (melaena)	Stop bleeding and pain Reduce inflammation Heal GIT tissue Eradicate *Helicobacter pylori*	Lifestyle: stress reduction Dietary change: avoid food triggers, avoid alcohol, instil good eating patterns Plant demulcents/anti-inflammatories/vulneraries (see above) Wound-healing nutrients: zinc, vitamin C, folate, glutamine, melatonin,[113] mastic gum[121] Herbal antimicrobials with demonstrated anti-*Helicobacter pylori* activity (see above) Probiotics (see Table 4.1 in Chapter 4 on irritable bowel syndrome)

CLINICAL SUMMARY

Lifestyle and dietary factors often play pivotal roles in the pathogenesis of GORD. Avoidance of food and drinks known to precipitate reflux episodes (chocolate, alcoholic beverages, caffeinated beverages, carbonated beverages and fatty foods) is an important therapeutic strategy that typically produces excellent clinical outcomes. In overweight patients, encouraging loss of weight will be an important therapeutic approach.

Newer research suggests that both psychological stress and inflammation play additional roles in the pathogenesis of GORD, as does oxidative stress. These underlying issues will also need to be addressed through lifestyle, dietary and herbal interventions (Figure 5.3).

Lesser-known herbs for GORD-related coughs

Sanguinaria canadensis (blood root)

A North American native, blood root is slow growing and rich in alkaloids. It is prescribed only in small doses, as it is emetic in larger doses. Blood root is one of the strongest stimulating expectorants, useful in dry, tickly, unproductive coughs and when the respiratory tract is congested with tenacious, thick, hard-to-expel mucus. Its acrid taste is due to its alkaloid content (principally sanguinarine), which is also responsible for its expectorant activity. After ingestion, blood root alkaloids irritate the vagus nerve along the GIT, resulting in the secretion of water and thin mucus in the upper GIT and reflexively in the respiratory tract. This can soothe a dry, irritated mucosa or dislodge thick, tenacious mucus from the respiratory tract. This ability to soothe an irritated oesophageal mucosa is what makes it useful in GORD-related coughs.

Ophiopogon japonicus (mondo grass)

Mondo grass is a Chinese herb, traditionally classified as a 'yin' tonic. It is sweet in taste, cooling and moistening in nature and makes a thick, rich, excellent-tasting tincture. In addition to its respiratory demulcent activity, it is also a relaxing nervine, making it a specific for dry, tickly coughs that keep a patient awake at night.

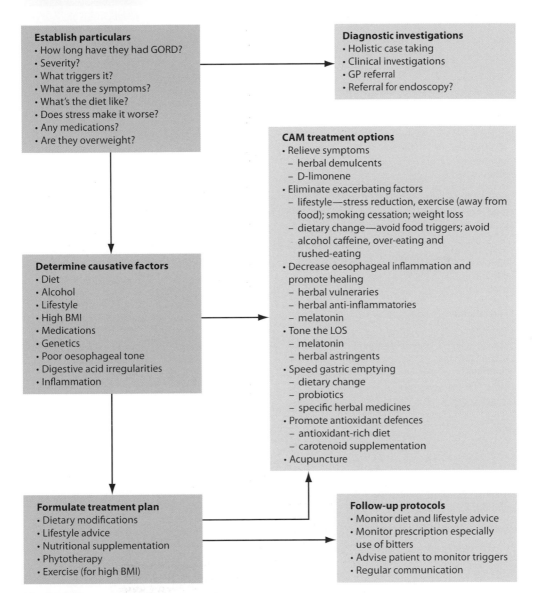

Figure 5.3
Naturopathic treatment decision tree—GORD

Table 5.2
Review of the major evidence

Intervention	Mechanisms of action	Key literature	Summary of results	Comment
Weight loss	Decreased upward pressure on the LOS	RCT: Singh et al. 2013[122] Cohort: Ness-Jensen et al. 2013[123]	In overweight and obese subjects, weight loss results in a significant decrease in the overall prevalence of GORD and a reduction in GORD symptoms	Weight loss is an effective treatment option for high-BMI patients with GORD
Dietary supplement containing melatonin (6 mg), L-tryptophan (200 mg), vitamin B6 (25 mg), folic acid (10 mg), vitamin B12 (50 µg), methionine (100 mg) and betaine (100 mg)	Melatonin improves the functioning of the LOS	RCT: Pereira 2006[124]	All patients (100%) in the dietary supplement group reported complete relief of GORD symptoms at 40 days versus 65.7% in the omeprazole group ($p < 0.05$) Complete relief was noted after seven days' treatment with the supplement	These are very promising results, particularly for a formula that does not appear on the surface to have a 'gut' focus. It is now known, however, that a substantial amount of melatonin is produced along the GIT (~500 times more than in the pineal gland) and that there are melatonin receptors along the GIT as well[125]
Myrtle berry extract (*Myrtus communis*; 1000 mg/day)	Myrtle berries are rich in tannins and polyphenols, so are believed to tone the oesophgeal sphincter and provide oxidative support	RCT: Zohalinezhad et al. 2016[83]	The myrtle berry extract appeared to be similarly effective as omeprazole in the reduction of GORD symptoms	One of the few studies to investigate botanical medicines in the treatment of GORD. This study evaluated a tannin- and polyphenol-rich herb that has long been used to treat GORD symptoms with excellent results
Melatonin (3 mg/day taken at bedtime)	Improves tone of the LOS	RCT: Kandil et al. 2010[87]	Heartburn eliminated in 100% of melatonin-treated subjects by week 8 and epigastric pain in 83% of subjects. Lower oesophageal pH increased from 2.3 at baseline to 6.7 after eight weeks melatonin treatment LOS pressure improved only in the melatonin and the combined treatment groups	Melatonin is the only substance clearly shown to improve the functioning of the LOS, thereby rectifying the predominant underlying issue in GORD—LOS incompetence More research is needed to ascertain if the improvement in LOS functioning persists after discontinuation of melatonin supplementation

Table 5.2
Review of the major evidence (continued)

Intervention	Mechanisms of action	Key literature	Summary of results	Comment
Lactobacillus reuteri MM53 (1×10^8 CFU/ day)	Accelerates gastric emptying	RCT: Indrio et al. 2011[90]	Regurgitation frequency significantly reduced in probiotic group (one versus four episodes daily; $p < 0.001$); gastric emptying significantly accelerated in probiotic group ($p = 0.01$)	Positive results in paediatric GORD This promising study needs to be followed up with research in different population groups (e.g. adults)
D-limonene (1000 mg every second day)	D-limonene may coat the oesophageal mucosa protecting the underlying tissue from gastric acid exposure and/or it may speed gastric emptying[43]	RCT: Wilkens 2002[42]	86% of subjects in the D-limonene group experienced complete relief of their GORD symptoms by day 14 versus only 29% of controls	This small study is part of a patent application and has not been published in peer-reviewed literature Replication of the trial with a larger patient cohort and a more standardised treatment regimen is needed

KEY POINTS

- GORD is typically diagnosed based on the presence of classic symptoms (heartburn and/or regurgitation) but can also present with extraoesophageal manifestations such as a chronic cough or laryngitis as the main presenting complaint.
- Be aware of the alarm features that require immediate referral.
- In GORD, the cause is often diet- or lifestyle-related; unless these underlying issues are dealt with, treatment is only palliative.
- GORD symptoms usually respond quickly to gastrointestinal demulcents.
- In regards to demulcents, powders or teas are the preferred methods of application—tablets and capsules will be least effective.

FURTHER READING

Baille N. Indigestion: antacids, bitters, digestive enzymes; when to use what? Aust J Med Herbalism 2002;14(4):151–7.

Mehdi S, Hossein K-B, Mehrdad K, et al. Medicinal plants for management of gastroesophageal reflux disease: a review of animal and human studies. J Altern Complementary Med 2017;23(2):82–95.

Ness-Jensen E, Hveem K, El-Serag H, et al. Lifestyle intervention in gastroesophageal reflux disease. Clin Gastroenterol Hepatol 2016;14(2):175–82.

Sethi S, Richter JE. Diet and gastroesophageal reflux disease: role in pathogenesis and management. Curr Opin Gastroenterol 2017;33(2):107–11.

REFERENCES

1. Dent J, et al. Epidemiology of gastroesophageal reflux disease: a systematic review. Gut 2005;54(5):710–17.

2. Vakil N, et al. The Montreal definition and classification of gastroesophageal reflux disease: a global evidence-based consensus. Am J Gastroenterol 2006;101:1900–20.

3. Cappell MS. Clinical presentation, diagnosis, and management of gastroesophageal reflux disease. Med Clin North Am 2005;89(2):243–91.

4. Moore JM, Vaezi MF. Extraesophageal manifestations of gastro-oesophageal reflux disease: real or imagined? Curr Opin Gastroenterol 2010;26(4):389–94. 10.1097/MOG.0b013e32833adc8d.

5. Cadiot G, et al. Multivariate analysis of pathophysiological factors in reflux oesophagitis. Gut 1997;40(2):167–74.

6. Dent J, et al. Mechanisms of lower oesophageal sphincter incompetence in patients with symptomatic gastrocsophageal reflux. Gut 1988;29(8):1020–8.

7. Anggiansah A, et al. Oesophageal motor responses to gastroesophageal reflux in healthy controls and reflux patients. Gut 1997;41(5):600–5.

8. Stanciu C, Bennett JR. Oesophageal acid clearing: one factor in the production of reflux oesophagitis. Gut 1974;15(11):852–7.

9. Stacher G, et al. Gastric emptying: a contributory factor in gastro-oesophageal reflux activity? Gut 2000;47:661–6.

10. Holloway RH, et al. Gastric distention: a mechanism for postprandial gastroesophageal reflux. Gastroenterology 1985;89(4):779–84.

11. Urita Y, et al. Salivary gland scintigraphy in gastro-esophageal reflux disease. Inflammopharmacology 2007;15:141–5.

12. Van Niewenhove YV, et al. Clinical relevance of laparoscopically diagnosed hiatal hernia. Surg Endosc 2009;23:1093–8.

13. Van Herwaarden MA, Samsom M, Smout AJ. Excess gastroesophageal reflux in patients with hiatus hernia is caused by mechanisms other than transient LES relaxations. Gastroenterology 2000;119(6):1439–46.

14. Kahrilla PJ, et al. The effect of hiatus hernia on gastro-oesophageal junction pressure. Gut 1999;44:476–82.

15. Jones MP, et al. Hiatal hernia size is the dominant determinant of esophagitis presence and severity in gastroesophageal reflux disease. Am J Gastroenterol 2001;96(6):1711–17.

16. Kim YJ, Kim EH, Hahm KB. Oxidative stress in inflammation-based gastrointestinal tract diseases: challenges and opportunities. J Gastroenterol Hepatol 2012;27(6):1004–10.

17. Oh TY, et al. Oxidative stress is more important than acid in the pathogenesis of reflux oesophagitis in rats. Gut 2001;49:364–71.

18. Salvatore S, Vandenplas Y. Gastroesophageal reflux and cow milk allergy: is there a link? Pediatrics 2002;110(5):972–84.

19. Usai P, et al. Effect of gluten-free diet on preventing recurrence of gastroesophageal reflux disease-related symptoms in adult celiac patients with nonerosive reflux disease. J Gastroenterol Hepatol 2009;23:1369–72.

20. American Gastroenterological Association. American Gastroenterological Association Institute technical review on the managment of gastroesophageal reflux disease. Gastroenterology 2008;135(4):1392–413.

21. DeVault KR, Castell DO. Updated guidelines for the diagnosis and treatment of gastroesophageal reflux disease. Am J Gastroenterol 2005;100(1):190–200.

22. Moonen A, Boeckxstaens G. Current diagnosis and management of achalasia. J Clin Gastroenterol 2014;48(6):484–90.

23. Kia L, Hirano I. Distinguishing GERD from eosinophilic oesophagitis: concepts and controversies. Nat Rev Gastroenterol Hepatol 2015;12(7):379–86.

24. Kaltenbach T, Crockett S, Gerson LB. Are lifestyle measures effective in patients with gastroesophageal reflux disease? Arch Intern Med 2006;166(9):965–71.

25. Hampel H, Abraham NS, El-Serag HB. Meta-analysis: obesity and the risk for gastroesophageal reflux disease and its complications. Ann Intern Med 2005;143(3):199–211.

26. Watanabe Y, et al. Cigarette smoking and alcohol consumption associated with gastro-oesophageal reflux disease in Japanese men. Scand J Gastroenterol 2003;38:807–11.

27. Kahrilas PJ, Gupta RR. Mechanisms of acid reflux associated with cigarette smoking. Gut 1990;31(1):4–10.

28. Rey E, et al. Influence of psychological distress on characteristics of symptoms in patients with GERD: the role of IBS comorbidity. Dig Dis Sci 2009;54(2):321–7.

29. Bradley LA, et al. The relationship between stress and symptoms of gastroesophageal reflux: the influence of psychological factors. Am J Gastroenterol 1993;88:11–19.

30. Cameron AJ, et al. Gastroesophageal reflux disease in monozygotic and dizygotic twins. Gastroenterology 2002;122:55–9.

31. Ali RAR, Egan LJ. Gastroesophageal reflux disease in pregnancy. Best Pract Res Clin Gastroenterol 2007;1(5):793–806.

32. Castell DO, et al. Review article: the pathophysiology of gastro-oesophageal reflux disease—oesophageal manifestations. Aliment Pharmacol Ther 2004;20(Suppl. 9):14–25.

33. Davies M, Wilton LV, Shakir SAW. Safety profile of esomeprazole: results of a prescription monitoring study of 11 595 patients in England. Drug Saf 2008;31(4):313–23.

34. Canani RB, et al. Therapy with gastric acidity inhibitors increases the risk of acute gastroenteritis and community-acquired pneumonia in children. Pediatrics 2006;117(5):817–20.

35. Gulmez SE, et al. Use of proton pump inhibitors and the risk of community-acquired pneumonia. Arch Intern Med 2007;167(9):950–5.

36. Elaine WY, et al. Acid-suppressive medications and risk of bone loss and fracture in older adults. Calcif Tissue Int 2008;83(4):251.

37. Lombardo L, et al. Increased incidence of small intestinal bacterial overgrowth during proton pump inhibitor therapy. Clin Gastroenterol Hepatol 2010;8(6):504–8.

38. Gomm W, von Holt K, Thome F. Association of proton pump inhibitors with risk of dementia: a pharmacoepidemiological claims data analysis. JAMA Neurol 2016;73(4):410–16.

39. Ruscin JM, Page RL, Valuck RJ. Vitamin B(12) deficiency associated with histamine(2)-receptor antagonists and a proton pump inhibitor. Ann Pharmacother 2002;36:812–16.

40. Kuipers MT, Thang HD, Arntzenius AB. Hypomagnesaemia due to use of proton pump inhibitors—a review. Neth J Med 2009;67(5):169–72.

41. Rantanen TK, Salo JA, Sipponen JT. Fatal and life-threatening complications in antireflux surgery: analysis of 5502 operations. Br J Surg 1999;86(12):1573–7.

42. Wilkens JSJ. Method for treating gastrointestinal disorders, U Patent, Editor. US; 2002.

43. Sun J. D-Limonene: safety and clinical applications. Altern Med Rev 2007;12(3):259–64.

44. Shukla A, et al. Ingestion of a carbonated beverage decreases lower esophageal sphincter pressure and increases frequency of transient lower esophageal sphincter relaxation in normal subjects. Indian J Gastroenterol 2012;31(3):121–4.

45. Stacher G, et al. Slow gastric emptying induced by high fat content of meal accelerated by cisapride administered rectally. Dig Dis Sci 1991;36(9):1259–65.

46. Bujanda L. The effects of alcohol consumption upon the gastrointestinal tract. Am J Gastroenterol 2000;95(12):3374–82.

47. Thomas FB, et al. Inhibitory effect of coffee on lower esophageal sphincter pressure. Gastroenterology 1980;79(6):1262–6.

48. Wright L, Castell D. The adverse effect of chocolate on lower esophageal sphincter pressure. Am J Dig Dis 1975;20(8):703–7.

49. Lohsiriwat S, Puengna N, Leelakusolvong S. Effect of caffeine on lower esophageal sphincter pressure in Thai healthy volunteers. Dis Esophagus 2006;19(3):183–8.

50. Hamoui N, et al. Response of the lower esophageal sphincter to gastric distention by carbonated beverages. J Gastrointest Surg 2006;10(6):870–7.

51. Stacher G, et al. Fat preload delays gastric emptying: reversal by cisapride. Br J Clin Pharmacol 1990;30(6):839–45.

52. Benjamin H. Everybody's guide to nature cure. Vol. 2nd. 1961; p. 292–9.

53. Duroux P, et al. Early dinner reduces nocturnal gastric acidity. Gut 1989;30:1063–7.

54. Bellioni-Businco B, et al. Allergenicity of goat's milk in children with cow's milk allergy. J Allergy Clin Immunol 1999;103(6):1191–4.

55. Rozenfeld P, et al. Detection and identification of a soy protein component that cross-reacts with caseins from cow's milk. Clin Exp Immunol 2002;130(1):49–58.

56. Vivatvakin B, Buachum V. Effect of carob bean on gastric emptying time in Thai infants. Asia Pac J Clin Nutr 2003;12(2):193–7.

57. Wenzl TG, et al. Effects of thickened feeding on gastroesophageal reflux in infants: a placebo-controlled crossover study using intraluminal impedance. Pediatrics 2003;111:355–9.

58. Nachman F, et al. Gastroesophageal reflux symptoms in patients with celiac disease and the effects of a gluten-free diet. Clin Gastroenterol Hepatol 2011;9(3):214–19.

59. Leffler DA, Kelly CP. Celiac disease and gastroesophageal reflux disease: yet another presentation for a clinical chameleon. Clin Gastroenterol Hepatol 2011;9(3):192–3.

60. Piche T, et al. Colonic fermentation influences lower esophageal sphincter function in gastroesophageal reflux disease. Gastroenterology 2003;124(4):894–902.

61. Staudacher HM, et al. Comparison of symptom response following advice for a diet low in fermentable carbohydrates (FODMAPs) versus standard dietary advice in patients with irritable bowel syndrome. J Hum Nutr Diet 2011;24(5):487–95.

62. Kristianslund CH, Hatlebakk JG, Hausken T, et al. Effect of a FODMAP-restricted diet on gastroesophageal reflux disease. Clin Nutr 2014;33(1):S50.

63. Staudacher HM, et al. Fermentable carbohydrate restriction reduces luminal bifidobacteria and gastrointestinal symptoms in patients with irritable bowel syndrome. J Nutr 2012;142(8):1510–18.

64. Halmos EP, Christophersen CT, Bird AR, et al. Diets that differ in their FODMAP content alter the colonic luminal microenvironment. Gut 2015;64:93–100.

65. Fraser-Moodie CA, et al. Weight loss has an independent beneficial effect on symptoms of gastro-oesophageal reflux in patients who are overweight. Scand J Gastroenterol 1999;34:337–40.

66. Schindlbeck NE, Heinrich C, Dendorfer A. Influence of smoking and esophageal intubation on esophageal pH-metry. Gastroenterology 1987;92(6):1994–7.

67. Kadakia SC, et al. Effect of cigarette smoking on gastroesophageal reflux measured by 24-h ambulatory esophageal pH monitoring. Am J Gastroenterol 1995;90(10):1785–90.

68. Stanciu C, Bennett JR. Effects of posture on gastro-oesophageal reflux. Digestion 1977;15:104–9.

69. Loots C, et al. Effect of lateral positioning on gastroesophageal reflux (GER) and underlying mechanisms in GER disease (GERD) patients and healthy controls. Neurogastroenterol Motil 2013;25(3):222–31.

70. Park JH, Conteas CN. W1074 curcumin, a possible alternative treatment for gastroesophageal reflux. Gastroenterology 2010;138(5, Suppl. 1):S-646.

71. Gardner JD, et al. Meal-stimulated gastric acid secretion and integrated gastric acidity in gastro-oesophageal reflux disease. Aliment Pharmacol Ther 2003;17(7):945–53.

72. Collen MJ, Johnson DA, Sheridan MJ. Basal acid output and gastric acid hypersecretion in gastroesophageal reflux disease. Correlation with ranitidine therapy. Dig Dis Sci 1994;39(2):410–17.

73. Borgia M, et al. Pharmacological activity of an herbal extract: controlled clinical study. Curr Ther Res 1981;29:525–36.

74. Metugriachuk Y, et al. Effect of a phyto-compound on delayed gastric emptying in functional dyspepsia: a randomized-controlled study. J Dig Dis 2008;9:204–7.

75. Niiho Y, et al. Gastroprotecive effects of bitter principles isolated from gentain root and swertia herb on experimentally-induced gastric lesions in rats. J Nat Med 2006;60:82–8.

76. Konturek SJ, et al. Protective influence of melatonin against acute esophageal lesions involves prostaglandins, nitric oxide and sensory nerves. J Physiol Pharmacol 2007;58(2):361–77.

77. Lahiri S, et al. Melatonin protects against experimental reflux esophagitis. J Pineal Res 2009;46(2):207–13.

78. de Oliveira Torres JD, de Souza Pereira R. Which is the best choice for gastroesophageal disorders: melatonin or proton pump inhibitors? World J Gastrointest Pharmacol Ther 2010;1(5):102–6.

79. Yoshida N. Inflammation and oxidative stress in gastroesophageal reflux disease. J Clin Biochem Nutr 2007;40(1):13–23.

80. Rao CV, Vijayakumar M. Effect of quercetin, flavonoids and alpha-tocopherol, an antioxidant vitamin, on experimental reflux oesophagitis in rats. Eur J Pharmacol 2008;589(1–3):233–8.

81. Giri AK, Rawat JK, Singh M, et al. Effect of lycopene against gastroesophageal reflux disease in experimental animals. BMC Complement Altern Med 2015;15:110.

82. Zhuang ZH, Xie JJ, Wei JJ, et al. The effect of n-3/n-6 polyunsaturated fatty acids on acute reflux esophagitis in rats. Lipids Health Dis 2016;15:172.

83. Zohalinezhad ME, Hosseini-Asl MK, Akrami R, et al. Myrtus communis L. freeze-dried aqueous extract versus omeprazol in gastrointestinal reflux disease: a double-blind randomized controlled clinical trial. J Evid Based Complementary Altern Med 2016;21(1):23–9. doi:10.1177/2156587215589403.

84. Pengelly A. The constituents of medicinal plants, vol. 2. Glebe NSW: Fast Books; 1997.

85. Bone K. A clinical guide to blending liquid herbs: herbal formulations for the individual patient. St Louis: Churchill Livingstone; 2003.

86. Baille N. Indigestion: antacids, bitters, digestive enzymes: when to use what? Aust J Med Herb 2002;14(4):151–7.

87. Kandil TS, et al. The potential therapeutic effect of melatonin in Gastro-Esophageal Reflux Disease. BMC Gastroenterol 2010;10:7.

88. Sidery MB, Macdonald LA, Blackshaw PE. Superior mesenteric artery blood flow and gastric emptying in humans and the differential effects of high fat and high carbohydrate meals. Gut 1994;35(2):186–90.

89. Mushambi MC, et al. Effect of alcohol on gastric emptying in volunteers. Br J Anaesth 1993;71(5):674–6.

90. Indrio F, et al. Lactobacillus reuteri accelerates gastric emptying and improves regurgitation in infants. Eur J Clin Invest 2011;41(4):417–22.

91. Hu ML, Rayner CK, Wu KL, et al. Effect of ginger on gastric motility and symptoms of functional dyspepsia. World J Gastroenterol 2011;17(1):105–10. doi:10.3748/wjg.v17.i1.105.

92. Kochhar KP, Bijlani RL, Sachdeva U, et al. Gastro-intestinal effects of Indian spice mixture (Garam Masala). Trop Gastroenterol 1999;20(4):170–4.

93. Shaheen N, Ransohoff DF. Gastroesophageal reflux, Barrett esophagus and esophageal cancer. J Am Med Assoc 2002;287:1972–81.

94. Clements DM, et al. A study to determine plasma antioxidant concentrations in patients with Barrett's oesophagus. J Clin Pathol 2005;58(5):490–2.

95. Ibiebele TI, et al. Dietary antioxidants and risk of Barrett's esophagus and adenocarcinoma of the esophagus in an Australian population. Int J Cancer 2013;133(1):214–24.

96. Dutta SK, et al. Barrett's esophagus and beta-carotene therapy: symptomatic improvement in GERD and enhanced HSP70 expression in esophageal mucosa. Asian Pac J Cancer Prev 2012;13(12):6011–16.

97. Chen H, et al. Nutrient intakes and adenocarcinoma of the esophagus and distal stomach. Nutr Cancer 2002;42(1):33–40.

98. Guy NC, et al. A novel dietary-realted model of esophagitis and Barrett's esophagus, a premalignant lesion. Nutr Cancer 2007;59(2):217–27.

99. Dickman R, et al. Clinical trial: acupuncture vs. doubling the proton pump inhibitor dose in refractory heartburn. Aliment Pharmacol Ther 2007;26:1333–44.

100. Kumar P, Clark ME. Clinical medicine. London: W.B. Saunders; 2002.

101. Mills S, Bone K. Principles and practice of phytotherapy. 2nd ed. London: Churchill Livingstone; 2013.

102. Blumenthal M. The ABC clinical guide to herbs. Austin: American Botanical Council; 2004.

103. Sanjoaquin MA, et al. Nutrition, lifestyle and colorectal cancer incidence: a prospective investigation of 10 998 vegetarians and non-vegetarians in the United Kingdom. Br J Cancer 2004;90(1):118–21.

104. Kono S, et al. Physical activity, dietary habits and adenomatous polyps of the sigmoid colon: a study of self-defense officials in Japan. J Clin Epidemiol 1991;44(11):1255–61.

105. Witte JS, et al. Relation of vegetable, fruit, and grain consumption to colorectal adenomatous polyps. Am J Epidemiol 1996;144(11):1015–25.

106. Michels KB, et al. Fruit and Vegetable Consumption and Colorectal Adenomas in the Nurses' Health Study. Cancer Res 2006;66(7):3942–53.

107. Weingarten MA, Zalmanovici A, Yaphe J. Dietary calcium supplementation for preventing colorectal cancer and adenomatous polyps. Cochrane Database Syst Rev 2008;(1):CD003548.

108. Estensen RD, et al. N-Acetylcysteine suppression of the proliferative index in the colon of patients with previous adenomatous colonic polyps. Cancer Lett 1999;147(1–2):109–14.

109. Ponz de Leon M, Roncucci L. Chemoprevention of colorectal tumors: role of lactulose and of other agents. Scand J Gastroenterol 1997;33(Suppl. 222):72–5.

110. Reid ME, et al. Selenium supplementation and colorectal adenomas: an analysis of the nutritional prevention of cancer trial. Int J Cancer 2006;118(7):1777–81.

111. Ishikawa H, et al. Randomized trial of dietary fiber and Lactobacillus casei administration for prevention of colorectal tumors. Int J Cancer 2005;116(5):762–7.

112. Melzer J, et al. Meta-analysis: phytotherapy of functional dyspepsia with the herbal drug preparation STW 5 (Iberogast). Aliment Pharmacol Ther 2004;20(11–12):1279–87.

113. Ganguly K, et al. Melatonin promotes angiogenesis during protection and healing of indomethacin-induced gastric ulcer: role of matrix metaloproteinase-2. J Pineal Res 2010;49(2):130–40.

114. Tabak M, Armon R, Neeman I. Cinnamon extracts' inhibitory effect on Helicobacter pylori. J Ethnopharmacol 1999;67:269–77.

115. Tabak M, et al. In vitro inhibition of Helicobacter pylori by extracts of thyme. J Appl Bacteriol 1996;80:667–72.

116. Chung JG, et al. Inhibitory actions of berberine on growth and arylamine N-acetyltransferase activity in strains of Helicobacter pylori from peptic ulcer patients. Int J Toxicol 1999;18(1):35–40.

117. Nostro A, et al. Effects of combining extracts (from Propolis or Zingiber officinale) with clarithromycin on Helicobacter pylori. Phytother Res 2006;20:187–90.

118. Stamatis G, et al. In vitro anti-Helicobacter pylori activity of Greek herbal medicines. J Ethnopharmacol 2003;88(3):175–9.

119. Salem EM, Yar T, Bamosa AO, et al. Comparative study of Nigella sativa and triple therapy in eradication of Helicobacter Pylori in patients with non-ulcer dyspepsia. Saudi J Gastroenterol 2010;16(3):207–14. doi:10.4103/1319-3767.65201.

120. Buts J-P, Keyser N. Effects of Saccharomyces boulardii on intestinal mucosa. Dig Dis Sci 2006;51(8):1485–92.

121. Al-Habbal MJ, Al-Habbal Z, Huwez FU. A double-blind controlled clinical trial of mastic and placebo in the treatment of duodenal ulcer. J Clin Exp Pharm Physiol 1984;11:541–4.

122. Singh M, et al. Weight loss can lead to resolution of gastroesophageal reflux disease symptoms: a prospective intervention trial. Obesity (Silver Spring) 2013;21(2):284–90.

123. Ness-Jensen E, et al. Weight loss and reduction in gastroesophageal reflux. A prospective population-based cohort study: the HUNT study. Am J Gastroenterol 2013;108(3):376–82.

124. Pereira RS. Regression of gastroesophageal reflux disease symptoms using dietary supplementation with melatonin, vitamins and amino acids: comparison with omeprazole. J Pineal Res 2006;41(3):195–200.

125. Konturek SJ, et al. Role of melatonin in upper gastrointestinal tract. J Physiol Pharmacol 2007;58(Suppl. 6):23–52.

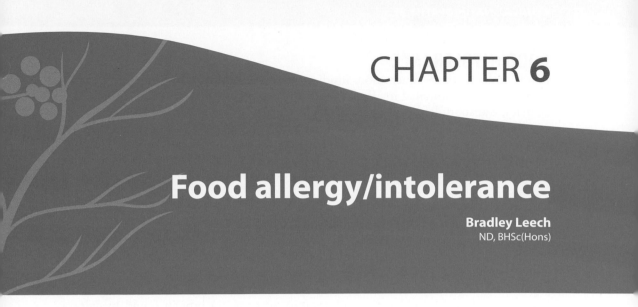

CHAPTER 6

Food allergy/intolerance

Bradley Leech
ND, BHSc(Hons)

OVERVIEW

Food reactions can be divided into immune-mediated (hypersensitivities) and non-immune-mediated (toxic, metabolic, pharmacologic or aversive).[1] Toxic food reactions are rare and usually involve food toxins that may be naturally present in food or a consequence of food processing, contaminants or additives, such as aflatoxin found in contaminated grains and peanuts. In the modern world, reactions are rare due to diet variety and food-processing standards. They are dose-dependent reactions and have the same effect on everybody. Reactions that involve immune activation are mediated by immunoglobulins, especially immunoglobulin E (IgE) but can also involve IgG, IgA, IgM and T-cells. Immune-mediated food reactions can be categorised as either IgE mediated (such as in the case of anaphylaxis to peanuts) and non-IgE-mediated (which include conditions like T-cell-mediated coeliac disease).[2] Non-immune-mediated food hypersensitivity reactions are often termed 'food intolerances' or 'food sensitivities'.

FOOD ALLERGY

While it is acknowledged there is no universally accepted definition of food allergy, the National Institute of Allergy and Infectious Diseases in the United States define it as an 'adverse health effect arising from a specific immune response that occurs reproducibly on exposure to a given food'.[3] The prevalence of IgE-mediated food allergy is reported to be highest in Australia, with a staggering 10% of infants diagnosed with one or more food allergy, whereas other Western countries have a suggested prevalence of 1–5%.[1] Most severe food allergies are IgE-mediated. IgE is associated with receptors on mast cells, fixed cells in the mucosa and skin, and basophils in the blood; conjugation with an allergen leads to cell granulation and the subsequent release of inflammatory mediators. Vasodilation, exudation, smooth muscle contraction and mucus secretion (largely due to histamine) are common consequences.[4] The greatest concern about an IgE-mediated food allergy is the chance that it will culminate in anaphylaxis. Common food culprits include fish, eggs, cow's milk and peanuts. It is usually a reaction to the protein component of the food such as casein in milk; if the patient is reacting to another food component, such as lactose, it is more likely to be a food intolerance.[2]

FOOD INTOLERANCE

Food intolerances are much more insidious and often cause delayed symptoms. Food intolerances are estimated to affect 15–20% of the population, involving enzyme deficiencies, transport defects or pharmacological effects, or are idiosyncratic in nature and are generally thought to be non-immune activated.[5] Common food intolerances to be aware of in clinical practice include salicylates, casein, amines, caffeine, sulphite, aspartame, MSG, food colouring, yeast and sugar alcohols. The following is an outline of three common food intolerances: lactose, fructose and gluten intolerance.

Lactose intolerance

Lactose intolerance is due to the inability of the body to produce enough of the enzyme lactase to break down the lactose in dairy-based products. If lactose is undigested, it will pass through to the large colon where it is acted on by colonic flora causing pain, bloating and osmotic diarrhoea. Lactose is a disaccharide and is metabolised by β-galactosidase (lactase is a subclass of this) to glucose and galactose. Distinguishing between other dairy intolerances is important as casein, a protein found in dairy, is highly allergenic and may also contribute to symptoms. Lactose maldigestion affects up to 20% of Caucasians, but the incidence in some ethnic groups is significantly higher, with reports suggesting that nearly 100% of Asians experience some degree of lactase deficiency.[6] A recent study reported the incidence of lactose malabsorption and lactose intolerance in children with gastrointestinal diseases.[7] Irritable bowel syndrome (IBS) was reported to have the highest incidence of lactose intolerance (65.2%) and the highest combined lactose malabsorption and lactose intolerance (47.8%) compared to other gastrointestinal diseases.

Fructose intolerance

Fructose is a six-carbon monosaccharide that is naturally found in fruit and honey or synthetically added by food manufacturers as high-fructose corn syrup. Fructose can also be ingested as the disaccharide sucrose (glucose + fructose) or in polymerised forms such as oligosaccharides and polysaccharides. Another form of dietary fructose is the galacto-oligosaccharides (fructose + glucose + galactose), usually present as raffinose.[8] Additional substances also poorly absorbed and readily fermented are:

- sugar alcohols (sorbitol, xylitol, mannitol and maltitol), which occur naturally in some fruits; they are also added as humectants and artificial sweeteners
- polydextrose and isomalt, used as food additives, which behave in a similar way.

Fructose intolerance may be a primary or secondary condition. Hereditary fructose intolerance is a rare autosomal recessive disorder that is due to a deficiency of the liver enzyme fructose-1,6-biphosphate aldolase.[9,10] It is particularly dangerous and can result in vomiting, failure to thrive, hypoglycaemia and liver failure with jaundice and bleeding in children.[9] Secondary fructose intolerance is quite different and much more common. It is usually due to abnormalities in the expression of GLUT5,[11] with recent research suggesting that it affects around 30% of the population and is in 45% of individuals with a functional gastrointestinal disorder.[12,13] If fructose is not absorbed in the small intestine, it reaches the distal end of the small intestine and the colon where it is fermented by colonic flora to produce hydrogen and carbon dioxide.[11] Fructose is fermented especially quickly, so there is not enough time for gas to be further metabolised or absorbed, increasing intraluminal pressure and producing an osmotic effect. As a result, fructose intolerance is associated with bloating, flatulence, fullness, diarrhoea and tiredness.[13]

Gluten intolerance

Gluten is a collective term used to describe a family of proteins found in grains like wheat, rye, barley and spelt. Adverse reactions after the consumption of gluten-containing products can be the result of numerous individual components found within gluten foods. The most serious of these is coeliac disease, where gliadin (a protein found within gluten) is responsible for the cascade of events leading to the cellular destruction of the intestinal lining.[14] However, less serious yet estimated to be more prevalent than coeliac disease is non-coeliac gluten sensitivity (NCGS).[14] NCGS is diagnosed in patients when coeliac disease and wheat allergy have been eliminated yet the patient experiences symptoms after gluten consumption and symptoms dissipate upon the removal of gluten from the diet.[15] Mechanisms in which gluten may cause symptoms include inducing intestinal permeability, altering the microbiome and promoting the release of inflammatory cytokines.[16,17]

DIFFERENTIAL DIAGNOSIS

- Gastrointestinal disorders such as gastro-oesophageal reflux disease, *Helicobacter pylori* gastritis, peptic ulcer disease, coeliac disease, parasitic infection, inflammatory bowel disease (Crohn's disease and ulcerative colitis), diverticulitis and chronic appendicitis
- Functional disorders such as functional abdominal pain, functional abdominal pain syndrome, IBS, functional dyspepsia and abdominal migraine
- Hepatobiliary disorders such as cholelithiasis, choledochal cyst, hepatitis, liver abscess and recurrent pancreatitis
- Genitourinary conditions such as urinary tract infection, hydronephrosis, urolithiasis, dysmenorrhoea and pelvic inflammatory disease

Source: Vlieger & Benninga 2009[18]

RISK FACTORS

Genetic and epigenetic factors

It appears that genetic predisposition is a strong determining factor in allergic disease. There is an 11–13% risk of developing allergies if there is no parental history, a 20–30% risk if the patient has one allergic parent and 40–60% risk if both parents are allergic.[19] A study involving monozygotic and dizygotic twins demonstrates that both genetic and environmental factors are important in the sensitisation to food and aeroallergens.[20] Early research suggests that genetic mutations/single nucleotide polymorphisms (SNPs) may influence food intolerances and food allergies. A genetic mutation of diamine oxidase gene, the enzyme responsible for the breakdown and metabolism of histamine, may play a role in histamine-mediated food intolerances.[21] Whereas an SNP affecting vitamin D-binding protein which results in vitamin D insufficiency is associated with persistent food allergy in infancy.[22] Another SNP, FOXO3, has been suggested to be responsible for adverse effects after the consumption of wasabi, mustard, and raw and cooked tomatoes.[23] Genetic mutations/SNPs have been associated with migraines[24] and allergic rhinitis.[25]

Increased intestinal permeability

The mucosal barrier in the small intestine is composed of epithelial cells held together by an array of structures; the most significant are the tight junctions. Many factors, including dietary intake, strenuous exercise, psychological stress, chemical exposure, nutrient deficiencies and medications, appear to increase intestinal permeability.[26] If the intestinal integrity is compromised, proteins, pathogens and antigens may pass through the intestinal wall stimulating inflammation and causing immune dysregulation.[26] One study has demonstrated that patients with food allergies and food intolerances have increased intestinal permeability and that the more significant the permeability, the more severe the allergy or intolerance.[27] Food intolerances have been observed by naturopaths, nutritionists and Western herbal medicine practitioners to be the condition most indicative of intestinal permeability in clinical practice.[28]

Environmental and lifestyle factors

Factors such as eating habits, meal frequency, lack of exercise, poor sleep and use of analgesic medication are often thought to increase the likelihood of food sensitivities or increase the intensity of symptoms in some individuals. However, one study found no difference between these factors in a group of adults with abdominal discomfort, self-attributed to food intolerance, and a placebo group.[29] Other environmental factors such as skin barrier dysfunction, dysbiosis, food processing, vitamin D status, chemical exposure and therapeutic drugs (antibiotics) are suggested to influence the development of food allergies/intolerances.[30] Stress may be an added risk factor for the development of food sensitivities. Stress (physical, biochemical, psychological) induces intestinal permeability, intestinal inflammation and dysbiosis, increasing the likelihood of food sensitivities.[31]

CONVENTIONAL TREATMENT

There is no particular conventional medical treatment available for IgG-mediated food allergies or food intolerances. However, in the case of lactose intolerance, lactase supplementation can be used to alleviate symptoms. Preliminary research supports the use of oral xylose isomerase in the treatment of fructose malabsorption.[32] Patients with IgE-mediated food allergies are often prescribed epinephrine and antihistamines.[33] Once the offending foods have been identified, strict dietary avoidance is usually recommended for food intolerances and allergies. Specific oral tolerance induction (SOTI), a process where oral exposure to a specific allergen is increased over time, has been shown to be safe and effective at treating persistent food allergies.[34] However, more research is needed to determine the best protocol.

KEY TREATMENT PROTOCOLS

The first protocol is to assess and isolate the food causing the intolerance/allergy. A range of questions should be asked, such as the following.

- *How long after you eat the suspect foods do you get symptoms?* This is called the latency period. If it is immediate or very soon after, it is more likely to be an IgE-mediated allergic response.
- *How severe are the symptoms?* If they are immediate and very severe, it is quite possibly an IgE-mediated allergy.
- *Do the symptoms change in severity and get stronger after repeated exposure?* If this is the case it is more likely to be a food intolerance.

- *How long do the symptoms last?* If they last many days after exposure, then it is unlikely to be an IgE-mediated allergy.
- *Are the symptoms easy and clear to define or more vague?*
- *Are the symptoms present without the offending food?*

Identify and remove offending foods and substances

A food/symptom diary is often useful in identifying potential allergens or intolerances. Identify and remove offending foods and substances (Table 6.1). There are various ways to identify problematic foods and substances, depending on what foods are suspected. A **de-challenge re-challenge diet** is ideal to assess this (Figure 6.1), but never if IgE allergic reactions are expected. Below is a summary of tests that are useful in identifying food allergies and intolerances.

> **Naturopathic Treatment Aims**
>
> - Identify and remove offending foods and substances.
> - Design an appropriate, healthy diet.
> - Reduce inflammation.
> - Repair intestinal permeability.
> - Modulate the immune system.
> - Ensure healthy gastrointestinal function.

- *IgE radioallergosorbent test (RAST).* This test measures IgE antibodies in the blood for specific antigens. IgE testing is considered the gold standard for conventional medical practitioners.[35]
- *IgG radioallergosorbent test (RAST).* This test measures IgG4 antibodies for specific antigens. It is very sensitive and useful for identifying food intolerances. Various studies have found positive results,[36–38] including a recent systematic review that found IgG tests show promise and report clinically relevant results.[35]
- *Food avoidance and challenge.* These diets are useful for identifying food intolerances but are unsafe for many allergies (Figure 6.1).
- *Hydrogen/methane breath test.* These tests are useful for identifying lactose and fructose malabsorption. They involve drinking a test substance such as fructose or lactose and then having regular hydrogen or methane breath tests over a two- to three-hour period. If the sugar isn't absorbed, excessive hydrogen or methane is exhaled in the breath.[11]
- *Lactulose/mannitol test.* This test is frequently used in clinical practice to measure intestinal permeability. The test involves the consumption of lactulose and mannitol in a water solution upon rising, followed by the collection of urine for four to six hours. The principle behind this test is that mannitol (a monosaccharide) is absorbed passively in the small intestine whereas lactulose (a disaccharide) remains within the intestines. Increased intestinal permeability will result in a higher ratio of lactulose to mannitol.[39]
- *Serum zonulin.* Another marker of intestinal permeability which correlates with the lactulose/mannitol test is serum zonulin.[40] Zonulin is released within the intestines and causes tight junction proteins to disassemble resulting in intestinal permeability.[41]

Once a food has been identified, it must be removed from the diet (Figure 6.1). In the case of IgG-triggered reactions, most of these foods need to be avoided only for a period of time until the reason for their existence is rectified. They can be due to myriad causes such as increased intestinal permeability, immune dysregulation and poor digestive function. Foods that provoke an IgE reaction, however, need to be thoroughly avoided as inclusion in the diet may invoke a dangerous reaction.

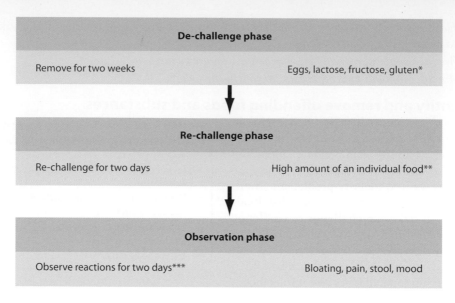

De-challenge phase

Remove for two weeks   Eggs, lactose, fructose, gluten*

Re-challenge phase

Re-challenge for two days   High amount of an individual food**

Observation phase

Observe reactions for two days***   Bloating, pain, stool, mood

*   Example foods
** Stop eating any foods found to cause reactions
*** Have two days' break between new challenge foods
Note: After two-day observation phase, new food can be 're-challenged'.

Figure 6.1
De-challenge re-challenge diet

Design an appropriate healthy diet

Maintenance of a healthy diet is crucial. This includes good-quality sources of protein, wholegrains, fresh fruit and vegetables that are well tolerated (see Chapter 3 on wellness). Many people who have suffered from long-term food allergies or hypersensitivities may have self-restricted their diet, potentially leading to various nutrient deficiencies. This is a perilous situation and one that needs addressing immediately if present. Deficiencies of protein, calcium, zinc, iron, vitamin B12 and magnesium are common, and a diet should always be designed with this in mind (see Appendix 4 for nutritional chart). Problematic foods must be avoided and the patient needs to be offered as many alternatives as possible in order to increase compliance and treatment success. When removing major food groups for an extended period of time, the emphasis needs to be placed on meeting the recommended dietary intake (RDI) of macro/micronutrients. For patients with lactose intolerance, the severity of symptoms depends on how much lactase is being produced by the small intestine. Most people with lactose intolerance can tolerate up to 7 g of lactose and in some cases 500 mL of milk.[6] This is important when designing a diet for a lactose-intolerant patient; however, caution is advised as secondary casein intolerance may be present. It is also essential to understand hexose transport in the gastrointestinal tract in order to design a diet for fructose-intolerant patients.

GLUT5 is a fructose transporter that is responsible for moving fructose across the brush border; it has a low capacity but is present along the whole length of the small intestine.[11] It is this mechanism that is often deficient in fructose intolerance. Glucose enhances the absorption of fructose by its co-presence in the small intestine. GLUT2 (a low-affinity transporter that will carry glucose, fructose and galactose, found on the basolateral membrane) is shunted into the brush border to facilitate the diffusion of glucose.[11,42] This, in turn, means that higher luminal concentrations of glucose are taken up by the cells via an active process, which in turn activates a system that can more efficiently take up all hexoses including fructose.[11,42] This becomes very important when designing a diet for fructose intolerance because foods with an amount of glucose equal to or higher than the amount of fructose can be included. Hence it is only foods with higher fructose than glucose that are avoided.

Dairy foods to avoid in lactose intolerance

- Milk—cow's, sheep's, goat's—more than $\frac{1}{2}$ a cup at any serving
- Yoghurt—more than 100 g a serving ($\frac{1}{2}$ an average tub)
- Ice-cream
- Cream cheese
- Cheese, especially soft cheese—mature, hard cheeses such as parmesan are usually tolerated

---

Reduce inflammation

Food hypersensitivities may lead to inflammation of the wall of the small intestine. While the small intestine can in most cases repair this damage, it does not have the opportunity to do so if problematic foods remain in the diet due to persistent inflammatory activity.[1] These foods cause an increase in local immune system activation, which further damages the intestinal mucosa, potentially leading to more food sensitivities. Inflammation also increases intestinal permeability, therefore increasing the amount of food antigens and lipopolysaccharides that can cross the bowel wall and provoke an immune response.[26]

There are several nutrients, herbs and therapeutic agents that may reduce inflammation in the gastrointestinal tract. These include **glutamine**, fish oils, **vitamin D**, *Urtica dioica*, *Curcuma longa and* probiotics.

Glutamine appears to down-regulate inflammatory mediators in the gastrointestinal system by stimulating the protective stress response in intestinal cells.[43] The anti-inflammatory effects of fish oil have been touted for some time now and these also appear to be relevant to the digestive system. Although no clinical trials have investigated the effects of fish oil in food intolerance/allergy, randomised controlled trials have demonstrated anti-inflammatory effects in other conditions such as systemic lupus erythematosus.[44]

High-fructose foods to avoid (fructose higher than glucose)

- Fruits—apple, coconut (also coconut milk and cream), grape, guava, honeydew melon, mango, nashi fruit, paw paw/papaya, pear, quince, star fruit, tomato and watermelon; all fruit juice, fruit juice concentrate, dried fruit and tinned fruit
- Vegetables—Lebanese cucumber, sweet potatoes
- Other—tomato sauce, tomato paste, chutney, relish, plum sauce, sweet and sour sauce, barbecue sauce, high-fructose corn syrup, fructose, honey and fortified wines; insulin and fructo-oligosaccharides should also be avoided
- Fructan-containing foods—vegetables such as artichokes, asparagus, garlic, green beans, leek, onions, spring onion and shallots, and wheat (many breakfast cereals, bread, biscuits, crackers, cakes, pies, pastas, pizzas and some noodles)

Sources: Varney et al. 2017,[45] Fedewa & Rao 2014[46]

Supplementation of vitamin D has many actions in which it influences the inflammatory cascade. **Vitamin D** downregulates gene expression within the inflammatory activation process[47] and reduces inflammatory markers: C-reactive protein (CRP), erythrocyte sedimentation rate (ESR) and tumour necrosis factor alpha (TNF-α).[48–50] It also increases antioxidant capacity[48,50] and can regulate blood sugar.[51] The vitamin D receptors (VDR) expressed in the intestines also play a significant role in modulating inflammation.[52] Prescribing the correct dose of vitamin D for the right duration of time is essential for clinical outcomes and is calculated based on the patient's 25OH vitamin D level. Many studies use large weekly doses of vitamin D; however, smaller daily doses ranging from 1000–10 000 IU are generally accepted. A recent study has shown that 40 000 IU of vitamin D taken once a week for eight weeks significantly increased serum vitamin D and reduced intestinal inflammation,[53] whereas another study using 2000 IU/day of vitamin D also resulted in a significant reduction of inflammation after three months.[54]

Saccharomyces boulardii, a yeast commonly classified as a probiotic, has both anti-inflammatory and microbiome modulating actions, *Saccharomyces boulardii* may be beneficial in the treatment of food intolerances. Although no clinical trials are available, dosage for other gastrointestinal and inflammatory conditions range from 100–200 mg three times daily.[55,56]

Urtica dioica is a traditional treatment for inflammation and allergy. Recent research suggests the phenolic acids and flavonol glycosides present in the aerial parts of *Urtica dioica* have anti-inflammatory properties and supports intestinal integrity.[57] Lipophilic extracts of *Urtica dioica* are suggested to be more effective than tinctures (water, methanol, ethanol) in the treatment of inflammatory conditions.[58]

Curcuma longa and in particular its chief constituent, curcumin, inhibit multiple inflammatory mediators such as NFKB, cyclo-oxygenase-2 (COX-2), LOX and inducible nitric oxide synthase (iNOS).[59] Clinical trials of *Curcuma longa*'s anti-inflammatory effects in allergy are lacking; however, animal studies provide promising results.[60,61]

Recent research suggests that inflammation mediated by TNF-α may cause an increase in intestinal permeability. *Curcuma longa* has been shown to inhibit TNF-α and may be considered a useful adjunct treatment.[92]

Repair intestinal permeability

Repairing the integrity of the gastrointestinal wall is an essential aspect in the management of food intolerances as damage leads to further inflammation and immune dysregulation. The first and most important step in the treatment of increased intestinal permeability is the removal of dietary and environmental triggers. Such recommendations include the removal of alcohol, gluten and other trigger foods while limiting saturated fats and arachidonic acid.[26,62–64] The overuse of medications such as antibiotics, aspirin, non-steroidal anti-inflammatory drugs and methotrexate can induce intestinal permeability and warrant review.[65–67] Preliminary research also suggests reducing acoustic stress, intense exercise, acute psychological stress and glyphosate exposure may be beneficial in the treatment of increased intestinal permeability.[68–71] While treating digestive health, especially intestinal permeability it is advised to limit exercise to below two hours per session at 60% VO$_2$max for the period of time required to modulate digestive health.[71]

Glutamine, **zinc**, **vitamin D**, **probiotics**, *Aloe barbadensis* Miller and **N-acetyl glucosamine** may help to heal a damaged intestinal wall. Glutamine has been shown to decrease intestinal permeability. One study has demonstrated that glutamine taken at

0.25–0.9 g/kg^{-1} of fat-free mass significantly reduces exercise-induced intestinal permeability.[72] Another study showed that supplementing with 0.5 g/kg ideal body weight/day of glutamine significantly reduced intestinal permeability after two months.[73]

Low zinc concentrations have been associated in children with food allergies.[74] One clinical trial has shown that zinc carnosine at 37.5 mg (8.34 mg elemental zinc) taken for two weeks reduced exercise-induced intestinal permeability by 70%.[75] These results highlight the role zinc plays in supporting intestinal integrity. Vitamin D taken at 2000 IU for three months significantly increased 25OH vitamin D and as a consequence was associated with improvement in intestinal integrity.[54]

Various strains of probiotics have been shown to modulate many aspects surrounding intestinal integrity. First, *Saccharomyces boulardii* has been shown to reduce intestinal permeability when supplemented at 200 mg three times a day for three months.[76] Furthermore, multi-strain probiotics also reduce intestinal permeability and are especially warranted in the treatment of exercise-induced intestinal permeability.[77,78] Preliminary research suggests *Escherichia coli* Nissle 1917 may be a promising probiotic in the management of increased intestinal permeability and consequently food intolerances.[79]

Modulate immune function

Food intolerances/allergies provoke an inappropriate immune response to food antigens, commonly referred to as oral tolerance.[1] Therefore, modulating and retraining the immune system is an important aspect of treating food intolerances/allergies. **Probiotics**, **vitamin D**, **quercetin** and other flavonoids may help modulate the immune system.

Clinical trials have shown that probiotics such as *Lactobacillus paracasei* LP-33 and *Lactobacillus rhamnosus* GG are effective in the treatment of allergic conditions.[80,81] Supplementing *Lactobacillus rhamnosus* GG alongside extensively hydrolysed casein promotes tolerance in infants with cow's milk allergy, possibly due to the change in the microbiome and synthesis of butyrate.[82] Supporting the synthesis of butyrate should be considered; however, caution is advised as many of the prebiotic foods bacteria use may also be the triggers for food intolerances.

A recent systematic review identified no association between vitamin D status and the presence of food allergies in children.[83] However, many other studies provide a clear justification for the use of vitamin D in modulating the immune system and treating food intolerances/allergies.[84,85]

Although no clinical trials are available, quercetin has immune-modulating actions, improving the balance of Th1/Th2 (T-helper cells).[86] Animal studies suggest that quercetin may be used to suppress peanut-induced anaphylaxsis.[87] However, this is recognised as a serious condition requiring medical management.

INTEGRATIVE MEDICAL CONSIDERATIONS

Very few integrative medical therapies can be considered at this present time. Therapies such as homeopathy and kinesiology are often used by patients with food allergies or intolerances; however, there is no current research to support this use. A small amount of research supports the use of traditional Chinese medicine in treating food allergies. A Chinese herbal medicine formula (FAHF-2) has been studied; however, the correct dose and duration requires further research.[88]

CLINICAL SUMMARY

Patients with long-term gastrointestinal complaints have frequently tried many treatments and dietary interventions with limited or no success. It is very important to thoroughly investigate these patients to determine if intolerances and/or allergies are present and treat accordingly if appropriate. It is also crucial to correct the three major contributing factors in the development and exacerbation of food intolerances: inflammation, intestinal integrity and immune dysfunction. The ultimate goal, if possible, is to reintroduce foods in the future in order to remove the chance of further complications from a restricted diet (Figure 6.2).

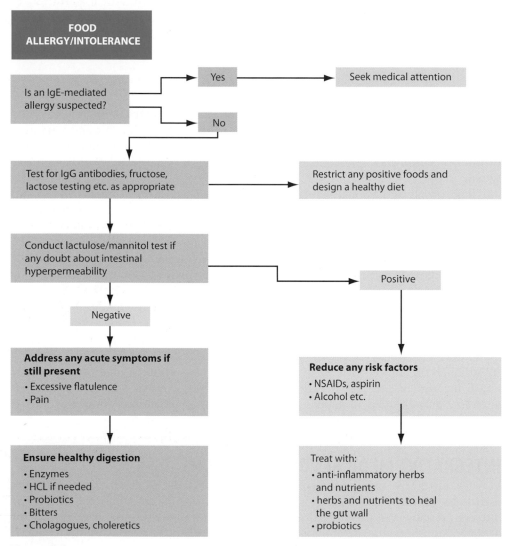

Figure 6.2
Naturopathic treatment decision tree—food allergy/intolerance

Table 6.1
Review of the major evidence*

Intervention	Key literature	Summary of results	Comment
Comparison between a low FODMAPs diet and traditional dietary advice for the treatment of IBS	Bohn et al. 2015[89]	Both intervention groups showed significant results at reducing IBS severity. No significant difference was seen between the two groups	Combining elements from the FODMAPs diet and traditional recommendations may provide synergistic outcomes
Compared food and yeast-specific IgG and IgG4 antibodies in subjects with and without IBS	Ligaarden et al. 2012[90]	No significant differences in food antibodies between subjects with IBS and controls	Presence of food and yeast IgG and IgG4 antibodies in the blood
Gluten-free diet in subjects with non-coeliac gluten sensitivity or coeliac disease	Caio et al. 2014[36]	After six months of a gluten-free diet, 93.2% of patients with non-coeliac gluten sensitivity had a disappearance of IgG class anti-gliadin antibodies	A strict compliance to a gluten-free diet reduces IgG antibodies in subjects with non-coeliac gluten sensitivity
Exclusion diets based on IgG results in subjects with either Crohn's disease or ulcerative colitis	Wang et al. 2018[38]	Disease relapse was seen in 12.5% of the study group and 25% in the control group	Food elimination diets based on IgG results may increase remission rates among subjects with Crohn's disease
Exclusion diets based on IgG results in subjects with ulcerative colitis	Jian et al. 2018[37]	IgG antibodies where elevated in 70% of subjects with ulcerative colitis. The foods most frequently positive for IgG antibodies were egg (60.0%), wheat (38.1%), milk (32.0%), corn (30.0%), and tomato (25.8%)	Food elimination diets based on IgG antibodies may be effective for reducing symptoms and improving quality of life in subjects with ulcerative colitis after six months
Fructose-reduced diet in subjects with IBS	Berg et al. 2013[91]	After following a fructose-reduced diet for four weeks, subjects with IBS reported improvements in abdominal pain, abdominal discomfort and bloating	Adherence to a low-fructose diet may improve symptoms in people with IBS regardless of fructose breath test results

*No *Mechanisms of action* column added, as the effects of dietary modulation is covered in the above protocols.

KEY POINTS

- It is essential to differentiate between different types of allergy and/or intolerance.
- Testing is frequently required and is a valuable clinical tool.
- Diets need to be designed to take into account potential nutrient deficiencies.
- It is essential to identify underlying causes such as inflammation or intestinal permeability.
- It should be the goal of practitioners to re-introduce foods if possible.

FURTHER READING

Czaja-Bulsa G. Non-coeliac gluten sensitivity—a new disease with gluten intolerance. Clin Nutr 2015;34(2):189–94.

Dolan R, Chey WD, Eswaran S. The role of diet in the management of irritable bowel syndrome: a focus on FODMAPs. Expert Rev Gastroenterol Hepatol 2018;12(6):607–15.

Lomer MC. Review article: the aetiology, diagnosis, mechanisms and clinical evidence for food intolerance. Aliment Pharmacol Ther 2015;41(3):262–75.

Renz H, Allen KJ, Sicherer SH, et al. Food allergy. Nat Rev Dis Primers 2018;4:17098.

Acknowledgment: The author would like to acknowledge Jane Frawley who authored a previous version of this chapter.

REFERENCES

1. Renz H, Allen KJ, Sicherer SH, et al. Food allergy. Nat Rev Dis Primers 2018;4:17098.

2. Nowak-Wegrzyn A, Szajewska H, Lack G. Food allergy and the gut. Nat Rev Gastroenterol Hepatol 2017;14(4):241–57.

3. Boyce JA, Assa'ad A, Burks AW, et al. Guidelines for the diagnosis and management of food allergy in the United States: summary of the NIAID-sponsored expert panel report. J Allergy Clin Immunol 2010;126(6): 1105–18.

4. Hamad A, Burks W. Oral tolerance and allergy. Semin Immunol 2017;30:28–35.

5. Lomer MC. Review article: the aetiology, diagnosis, mechanisms and clinical evidence for food intolerance. Aliment Pharmacol Ther 2015;41(3):262–75.

6. Vandenplas Y. Lactose intolerance. Asia Pac J Clin Nutr 2015;24(Suppl. 1):S9–13.

7. Pawlowska K, Umlawska W, Iwanczak B. Prevalence of lactose malabsorption and lactose intolerance in pediatric patients with selected gastrointestinal diseases. Adv Clin Exp Med 2015;24(5):863–71.

8. Mehta M, Beg M. Fructose intolerance: cause or cure of chronic functional constipation. Glob Pediatr Health 2018;5:2333794x18761460.

9. Wong D. Hereditary fructose intolerance. Mol Genet Metab 2005;85(3):165–7.

10. Yasawy MI, Folsch UR, Schmidt WE, et al. Adult hereditary fructose intolerance. World J Gastroenterol 2009;15(19):2412–13.

11. Ebert K, Witt H. Fructose malabsorption. Mol Cell Pediatr 2016;3(1):10.

12. Gibson PR, Shepherd SJ. Personal view: food for thought—western lifestyle and susceptibility to Crohn's disease. The FODMAP Hypothesis. Aliment Pharmacol Ther 2005;21(12):1399–409.

13. Wilder-Smith CH, Materna A, Wermelinger C, et al. Fructose and lactose intolerance and malabsorption testing: the relationship with symptoms in functional gastrointestinal disorders. Aliment Pharmacol Ther 2013;37(11):1074–83.

14. Lebwohl B, Ludvigsson JF, Green PH. Celiac disease and non-celiac gluten sensitivity. BMJ 2015;351:H4347.

15. Czaja-Bulsa G. Non-celiac gluten sensitivity—a new disease with gluten intolerance. Clin Nutr 2015;34(2):189–94.

16. de Punder K, Pruimboom L. The dietary intake of wheat and other cereal grains and their role in inflammation. Nutrients 2013;5(3):771–87.

17. Daulatzai MA. Non-celiac gluten sensitivity triggers gut dysbiosis, neuroinflammation, gut-brain axis dysfunction, and vulnerability for dementia. CNS Neurol Disord Drug Targets 2015;14(1):110–31.

18. Vlieger AM, Benninga MA. Chronic abdominal pain. Complementary Therapies in Paediatric Gastroenterology: Prevalence, Safety and Efficacy. 2009:61.

19. Samartín S, Marcos A, Chandra RK. Food hypersensitivity. Nutr Res 2001;21(3):473–97.

20. Liu X, Zhang S, Tsai HJ, et al. Genetic and environmental contributions to allergen sensitization in a Chinese twin study. Clin Exp Allergy 2009;39(7):991–8.

21. Manzotti G, Breda D, Di Gioacchino M, et al. Serum diamine oxidase activity in patients with histamine intolerance. Int J Immunopathol Pharmacol 2016;29(1):105–11.

22. Koplin JJ, Suaini NH, Vuillermin P, et al. Polymorphisms affecting vitamin d-binding protein modify the relationship between serum vitamin D (25[OH]D3) and food allergy. J Allergy Clin Immunol 2016;137(2):500–6, E504.

23. Marlow G, Han DY, Triggs CM, et al. Food intolerance: associations with the RS12212067 polymorphism of FOXO3 in Crohn's disease patients in New Zealand. J Nutrigenet Nutrigenomics 2015;8(2):70–80.

24. Garcia-Martin E, Martinez C, Serrador M, et al. Diamine oxidase RS10156191 and RS2052129 variants are associated with the risk for migraine. Headache 2015;55(2):276–86.

25. Meza-Velazquez R, Lopez-Marquez F, Espinosa-Padilla S, et al. Association between two polymorphisms of histamine-metabolising enzymes and the severity of allergic rhinitis in a group of Mexican children. Allergol Immunopathol (Madr) 2016;44(5):433–8.

26. Bischoff SC, Barbara G, Buurman W, et al. Intestinal permeability—a new target for disease prevention and therapy. BMC Gastroenterol 2014;14:189.

27. Ventura MT, Polimeno L, Amoruso AC, et al. Intestinal permeability in patients with adverse reactions to food. Dig Liver Dis 2006;38(10):732–6.

28. Leech B, Schloss J, Steel A. Investigation into complementary and integrative medicine practitioners' clinical experience of intestinal permeability: a cross-sectional survey. Complement Ther Clin Pract 2018;31:200–9.

29. Lind R, Olafsson S, Hjelland I, et al. Lifestyle of patients with self-reported food hypersensitivity differ little from controls. Gastroenterol Nurs 2008;31(6): 401–10.

30. Yu JE, Mallapaty A, Miller RL. It's not just the food you eat: environmental factors in the development of food allergies. Environ Res 2018;165:118–24.

31. Schreier HM, Wright RJ. Stress and food allergy: mechanistic considerations. Ann Allergy Asthma Immunol 2014;112(4):296–301.

32. Komericki P, Akkilic-Materna M, Strimitzer T, et al. Oral xylose isomerase decreases breath hydrogen excretion and improves gastrointestinal symptoms in fructose

malabsorption—a double-blind, placebo-controlled study. Aliment Pharmacol Ther 2012;36(10):980–7.

33. Abrams EM, Sicherer SH. Diagnosis and management of food allergy. CMAJ 2016;188(15):1087–93.

34. Luyt D, Bravin K, Luyt J. Implementing specific oral tolerance induction to milk into routine clinical practice: experience from first 50 patients. J Asthma Allergy 2014;7:1–9.

35. Mullin GE, Swift KM, Lipski L, et al. Rampertab SD. Testing for food reactions: the good, the bad, and the ugly. Nutr Clin Pract 2010;25(2):192–8.

36. Caio G, Volta U, Tovoli F, et al. Effect of gluten free diet on immune response to gliadin in patients with non-celiac gluten sensitivity. BMC Gastroenterol 2014;14:26.

37. Jian L, Anqi H, Gang L, et al. Food exclusion based on IgG antibodies alleviates symptoms in ulcerative colitis: a prospective study. Inflamm Bowel Dis 2018.

38. Wang G, Ren J, Li G, et al. The utility of food antigen test in the diagnosis of Crohn's disease and remission maintenance after exclusive enteral nutrition. Clin Res Hepatol Gastroenterol 2018;42(2):145–52.

39. Galipeau HJ, Verdu EF. The complex task of measuring intestinal permeability in basic and clinical science. Neurogastroenterol Motil 2016;28(7):957–65.

40. Lin R, Zhou L, Zhang J, et al. Abnormal intestinal permeability and microbiota in patients with autoimmune hepatitis. Int J Clin Exp Pathol 2015;8(5):5153–60.

41. Sturgeon C, Fasano A. Zonulin, a regulator of epithelial and endothelial barrier functions, and its involvement in chronic inflammatory diseases. Tissue Barriers 2016;4(4): E1251384.

42. Putkonen L, Yao CK, Gibson PR. Fructose malabsorption syndrome. Curr Opin Clin Nutr Metab Care 2013;16(4):473–7.

43. Kim MH, Kim H. The roles of glutamine in the intestine and its implication in intestinal diseases. Int J Mol Sci 2017;18(5).

44. Arriens C, Hynan LS, Lerman RH, et al. Placebo-controlled randomized clinical trial of fish oil's impact on fatigue, quality of life, and disease activity in systemic lupus erythematosus. Nutr J 2015;14:82.

45. Varney J, Barrett J, Scarlata K, et al. FODMAPs: food composition, defining cutoff values and international application. J Gastroenterol Hepatol 2017;32(Suppl. 1):53–61.

46. Fedewa A, Rao SS. Dietary fructose intolerance, fructan intolerance and FODMAPs. Curr Gastroenterol Rep 2014;16(1):370.

47. Haddad Kashani H, Seyed Hosseini E, Nikzad H, et al. The effects of vitamin D supplementation on signaling pathway of inflammation and oxidative stress in diabetic hemodialysis: a randomized, double-blind, placebo-controlled trial. Front Pharmacol 2018;9:50.

48. Akbari M, Ostadmohammadi V, Lankarani KB, et al. The effects of vitamin D supplementation on biomarkers of inflammation and oxidative stress among women with polycystic ovary syndrome: a systematic review and meta-analysis of randomized controlled trials. Horm Metab Res 2018;50(4):271–9.

49. Mousa A, Naderpoor N, Teede H, et al. Supplementation for improvement of chronic low-grade inflammation in patients with type 2 diabetes: a systematic review and meta-analysis of randomized controlled trials. Nutr Rev 2018;76(5):380–94.

50. Mansournia MA, Ostadmohammadi V, Doosti-Irani A, et al. The effects of vitamin D supplementation on biomarkers of inflammation and oxidative stress in diabetic patients: a systematic review and meta-analysis of randomized controlled trials. Horm Metab Res 2018;50(6):429–40.

51. Asemi Z, Hashemi T, Karamali M, et al. Effects of vitamin D supplementation on glucose metabolism, lipid concentrations, inflammation, and oxidative stress in gestational diabetes: a double-blind randomized controlled clinical trial. Am J Clin Nutr 2013;98(6):1425–32.

52. He L, Liu T, Shi Y, et al. Gut epithelial vitamin D receptor regulates microbiota-dependent mucosal inflammation by suppressing intestinal epithelial cell apoptosis. Endocrinology 2018;159(2):967–79.

53. Garg M, Hendy P, Ding JN, et al. The effect of vitamin D on intestinal inflammation and faecal microbiota in patients with ulcerative colitis. J Crohns Colitis 2018;21(8):963–72.

54. Raftery T, Martineau AR, Greiller CL, et al. Effects of vitamin D supplementation on intestinal permeability, cathelicidin and disease markers in Crohn's disease: results from a randomised double-blind placebo-controlled study. United European Gastroenterol J 2015;3(3): 294–302.

55. Bafutto M, Almeida JR, Leite NV, et al. Treatment of diarrhea-predominant irritable bowel syndrome with mesalazine and/or Saccharomyces boulardii. Arq Gastroenterol 2013;50(4):304–9.

56. Villar-Garcia J, Guerri-Fernandez R, Moya A, et al. Impact of probiotic Saccharomyces boulardii on the gut microbiome composition in HIV-treated patients: a double-blind, randomised, placebo-controlled trial. PLoS ONE 2017;12(4):E0173802.

57. Franciskovic M, Gonzalez-Perez R, Orcic D, et al. Chemical composition and immuno-modulatory effects of Urtica dioica L. (stinging nettle) extracts. Phytother Res 2017;31(8):1183–91.

58. Johnson TA, Sohn J, Inman WD, et al. Lipophilic stinging nettle extracts possess potent anti-inflammatory activity, are not cytotoxic and may be superior to traditional tinctures for treating inflammatory disorders. Phytomedicine 2013;20(2):143–7.

59. Kumar G, Mittal S, Sak K, et al. Molecular mechanisms underlying chemopreventive potential of curcumin: current challenges and future perspectives. Life Sci 2016;148:313–28.

60. Kinney SR, Carlson L, Ser-Dolansky J, et al. Curcumin ingestion inhibits mastocytosis and suppresses intestinal anaphylaxis in a murine model of food allergy. PLoS ONE 2015;10(7):E0132467.

61. Shin HS, See HJ, Jung SY, et al. Turmeric (Curcuma longa) attenuates food allergy symptoms by regulating type 1/type 2 helper T cells (TH1/TH2) balance in a mouse model of food allergy. J Ethnopharmacol 2015;175:21–9.

62. Elamin E, Masclee A, Troost F, et al. Ethanol impairs intestinal barrier function in humans through mitogen activated protein kinase signaling: a combined in vivo and in vitro approach. PLoS ONE 2014;9(9):E107421.

63. Lyte JM, Gabler NK, Hollis JH. Postprandial serum endotoxin in healthy humans is modulated by dietary fat in a randomized, controlled, cross-over study. Lipids Health Dis 2016;15(1):186.

64. Vincentini O, Quaranta MG, Viora M, et al. Docosahexaenoic acid modulates in vitro the inflammation of celiac disease in intestinal epithelial cells via the inhibition of CPLA2. Clin Nutr 2011;30(4):541–6.

65. Tulstrup MV, Christensen EG, Carvalho V, et al. Antibiotic treatment affects intestinal permeability and gut microbial composition in Wistar rats dependent on antibiotic class. PLoS ONE 2015;10(12):E0144854.

66. Sequeira IR, Lentle RG, Kruger MC, et al. Assessment of the effect of intestinal permeability probes (lactulose and mannitol) and other liquids on digesta residence times in various segments of the gut determined by wireless motility capsule: a randomised controlled trial. PLOS ONE 2015;10(12):E0143690.

67. Meng Y, Zhang Y, Liu M, et al. Evaluating intestinal permeability by measuring plasma endotoxin and diamine oxidase in children with acute lymphoblastic leukemia treated with high-dose methotrexate. Anticancer Agents Med Chem 2016;16(3):387–92.

68. Miranda S, Roux ME. Acoustic stress induces long term severe intestinal inflammation in the mouse. Toxicol Lett 2017;280:1–9.

69. Vanuytsel T, van Wanrooy S, Vanheel H, et al. Psychological stress and corticotropin-releasing hormone increase intestinal permeability in humans by a mast cell-dependent mechanism. Gut 2014;63(8):1293–9.

70. Samsel A, Seneff S. Glyphosate, pathways to modern diseases II: celiac sprue and gluten intolerance. Interdiscip Toxicol 2013;6(4):159–84.

71. Costa RJS, Snipe RMJ, Kitic CM, et al. Systematic review: exercise-induced gastrointestinal syndrome-implications for health and intestinal disease. Aliment Pharmacol Ther 2017;46(3):246–65.

72. Pugh JN, Sage S, Hutson M, et al. Glutamine supplementation reduces markers of intestinal permeability during running in the heat in a dose-dependent manner. Eur J Appl Physiol 2017;117(12):2569–77.

73. Benjamin J, Makharia G, Ahuja V, et al. Glutamine and whey protein improve intestinal permeability and morphology in patients with Crohn's disease: a randomized controlled trial. Dig Dis Sci 2012;57(4):1000–12.

74. Kamer B, Wasowicz W, Pyziak K, et al. Pasowska R. Role of selenium and zinc in the pathogenesis of food allergy in infants and young children. Arch Med Sci 2012;8(6):1083–8.

75. Davison G, Marchbank T, March DS, et al. Zinc carnosine works with bovine colostrum in truncating heavy exercise-induced increase in gut permeability in healthy volunteers. Am J Clin Nutr 2016;104(2):526–36.

76. Garcia Vilela E, De Lourdes De Abreu Ferrari M, Oswaldo Da Gama Torres H, et al. Influence of Saccharomyces boulardii on the intestinal permeability of patients with Crohn's disease in remission. Scand J Gastroenterol 2008;43(7):842–8.

77. Lamprecht M, Bogner S, Schippinger G, et al. Probiotic supplementation affects markers of intestinal barrier, oxidation, and inflammation in trained men; a randomized, double-blinded, placebo-controlled trial. J Int Soc Sports Nutr 2012;9(1):45.

78. Shing CM, Peake JM, Lim CL, et al. Effects of probiotics supplementation on gastrointestinal permeability, inflammation and exercise performance in the heat. Eur J Appl Physiol 2014;114(1):93–103.

79. Secher T, Kassem S, Benamar M, et al. Oral administration of the probiotic strain Escherichia coli Nissle 1917 reduces susceptibility to neuroinflammation and repairs experimental autoimmune encephalomyelitis-induced intestinal barrier dysfunction. Front Immunol 2017;8:1096.

80. Costa DJ, Marteau P, Amouyal M, et al. Efficacy and safety of the probiotic Lactobacillus paracasei LP-33 in allergic rhinitis: a double-blind, randomized, placebo-controlled trial (GA2LEN study). Eur J Clin Nutr 2014;68(5):602–7.

81. Nermes M, Kantele JM, Atosuo TJ, et al. Interaction of orally administered Lactobacillus rhamnosus GG with skin and gut microbiota and humoral immunity in infants with atopic dermatitis. Clin Exp Allergy 2011;41(3):370–7.

82. Berni Canani R, Sangwan N, Stefka AT, et al. Lactobacillus rhamnosus GG-supplemented formula expands butyrate-producing bacterial strains in food allergic infants. ISME J 2016;10(3):742–50.

83. Willits EK, Wang Z, Jin J, et al. Vitamin D and food allergies in children: a systematic review and meta-analysis. Allergy Asthma Proc 2017;38(3):21–8.

84. Mirzakhani H, Al-Garawi A, Weiss ST, et al. Vitamin D and the development of allergic disease: how important is it? Clin Exp Allergy 2015;45(1):114–25.

85. Suaini NH, Zhang Y, Vuillermin PJ, et al. Immune modulation by vitamin D and its relevance to food allergy. Nutrients 2015;7(8):6088–108.

86. Mlcek J, Jurikova T, Skrovankova S, et al. Quercetin and its anti-allergic immune response. Molecules 2016; 21(5).

87. Shishehbor F, Behroo L, Ghafouriyan Broujerdnia M, et al. Quercetin effectively quells peanut-induced anaphylactic reactions in the peanut sensitized rats. Iran J Allergy Asthma Immunol 2010;9(1):27–34.

88. Wang J, Jones SM, Pongracic JA, et al. Safety, clinical, and immunologic efficacy of a Chinese herbal medicine (food allergy herbal formula-2) for food allergy. J Allergy Clin Immunol 2015;136(4):962–70, E961.

89. Bohn L, Storsrud S, Liljebo T, et al. Diet low in FODMAPs reduces symptoms of irritable bowel syndrome as well as traditional dietary advice: a randomized controlled trial. Gastroenterology 2015;149(6):1399–407, E1392.

90. Ligaarden SC, Lydersen S, Farup PG. IgG and IgG4 antibodies in subjects with irritable bowel syndrome: a case control study in the general population. BMC Gastroenterol 2012;12:166.

91. Berg LK, Fagerli E, Martinussen M, et al. Effect of fructose-reduced diet in patients with irritable bowel syndrome, and its correlation to a standard fructose breath test. Scand J Gastroenterol 2013;48(8):936–43.

92. Tian S, Guo R, Wei S, et al. Curcumin protects against the intestinal ischemia-reperfusion injury: involvement of the tight junction protein ZO-1 and TNF-alpha related mechanism. Korean J Physiol Pharmacol 2016;20(2):147–52.

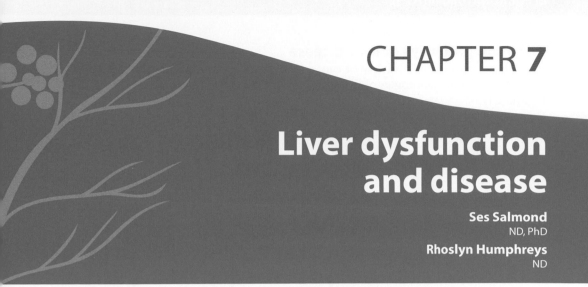

CHAPTER 7

Liver dysfunction and disease

Ses Salmond
ND, PhD

Rhoslyn Humphreys
ND

OVERVIEW

It is important to understand the functions of the liver, the systemic implications of liver disease and the importance of also treating the liver as an adjunct to other conditions, such as metabolic syndrome and hormone dysregulation.

The liver is involved in the metabolism of carbohydrates, proteins and fats. It converts simple carbohydrates in the form of fructose and galactose to glucose and then converts glucose to glycogen for storage. If carbohydrate intake exceeds requirements sugars are converted to triglycerides (TG), contributing to dyslipidaemia.[1]

Protein metabolism in the liver is responsible for the synthesis of non-essential amino acids and functional proteins such as: fibrinogen and prothrombin for clotting; transferrins and lipoproteins for transport of iron and cholesterol, respectively; albumin for maintaining oncotic pressure; and globulins for immune function. Amino acids are also important for maintaining blood pH. If protein metabolism in the liver is disturbed this can lead to: bleeding disorders such as oesophageal varices and excess bruising; ascites due to low albumin and reduced oncotic pressure; impaired immune function; anaemia and fatigue as seen in non-alcoholic fatty liver disease (NAFLD), alcoholic liver disease (ALD) and hepatitis C virus (HCV) infection.

The liver is also involved in the production and regulation of triglycerides, phospholipids, lipoproteins and cholesterol. It metabolises fats by lipolysis and transforms fatty acids via β-oxidation to acetyl-CoA, the substrate for energy production via the Krebs cycle.[1] The liver stores fat-soluble vitamins (A, D, E, K) and other vitamins and minerals (B12, Zn, Fe, Cu, Mg). The liver converts carotene to vitamin A, folate to 5-methyl tetrahydrofolic acid and vitamin D to 25-hydroxycholecalciferol.

The liver synthesises bile, which emulsifies lipids and fat-soluble vitamins in the intestines to aid digestion and prevent cholesterol precipitation in the gallbladder. Bile synthesis and excretion is also a mechanism for reducing excess cholesterol. Another major role of the liver is the metabolism and detoxification of: alcohol; synthetic and natural drugs; steroidal hormones such as the corticosteroids, testosterone, progesterone and oestrogen; non-steroidal hormones such as thyroid hormones; and insulin and growth hormones. It also converts ammonia to urea.[1]

Common pathways of liver disease

Liver diseases can have a variety of causes but can progress through similar pathology, therefore different aetiologies of liver disease can have common treatments, as shown in Figure 7.1.

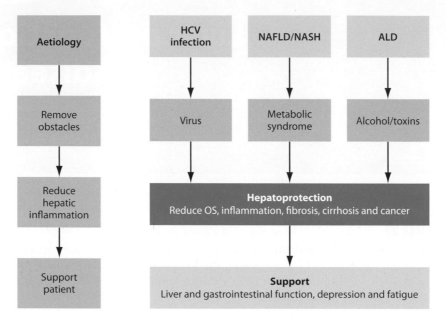

HCV = hepatitis C virus; NAFLD = non-alcoholic fatty liver disease;
NASH = non-alcoholic steatohepatitis; ALD = alcoholic liver disease

Figure 7.1
Common pathology and treatment in liver diseases

Aetiologies
- Viral infection—hepatitis (A, B, C, D, E)
- NAFLD/non-alcoholic steatohepatitis (NASH), dysregulated free fatty acid (FFA) metabolism and accumulation due to obesity, insulin resistance and metabolic syndrome
- ALD, accumulation of toxins due to excess alcohol consumption

Common pathology
- *Hepatitis (B and C).* Increased oxidative stress as a direct consequence of the virus and indirectly as a result of the immune response.
- *NAFLD and NASH.* Increased oxidative stress as a result of FFA accumulation and lipid peroxidation, exacerbated by increased inflammatory cytokines from adipose tissue, damages the liver.
- *ALD.* Increased oxidative stress as a result of toxins.

Common treatment—reduction of hepatic inflammation

Oxidative stress in liver disease accelerates inflammation, fibrosis and necrosis, creating additional oxidative stress, which causes further damage to proteins, DNA, lipids and sensitises redox-regulated necrotic cell signalling pathways, affecting gene expression[2] and causing mitochondrial dysfunction and pathology.[3] Increased oxidative stress leads to reduced liver function and can progress through fibrosis to cirrhosis and possibly cancer.

Liver disease can lead to metabolic syndrome with dysglycaemia or dyslipidaemia and increases in the frequency of comorbidities.[4]

Treatment based on reducing oxidative stress, inflammation, regulating digestive dysfunction and supporting fatigue will assist in the treatment of most chronic liver diseases.

Common comorbidities

- Metabolic syndrome
- Cardiovascular disease
- Depression and fatigue
- Hormonal dysregulation
- Dyspepsia

NON-ALCOHOLIC FATTY LIVER DISEASE

NAFLD is the hepatic manifestation of metabolic syndrome.[5-7] The Asia-Pacific Guidelines on NAFLD recommend that the term NAFLD is retained for cases of fatty liver associated with the metabolic complications of over-nutrition, usually with central obesity and overweight.[8] NAFLD is the most common liver disease worldwide in adults and children.[9] NAFLD usually occurs in the fourth or fifth decade of life and is predominantly asymptomatic. NAFLD may progress from simple steatosis to steatohepatitis, advanced fibrosis and cirrhosis. An estimated 20–35% of the general population has steatosis, 10% developing more progressive NASH, which is associated with increased risk of cardiovascular and liver-related mortality.[10]

The prevalence of NAFLD is higher among the obese and patients with type 2 diabetes. In fact in a cohort of NAFLD patients, 50% had diabetes, 44% had hypertension and 12% had previous vascular disease.[11] The environmental factors involved in NAFLD and metabolic syndrome are diet, physical activity and gut microflora. Metabolic syndrome with dysglycaemia, dyslipidaemia and obesity results in an increase in the level of FFAs from the breakdown of adipose tissue and from the metabolism of excess dietary carbohydrates (hyperlipidaemia); this dysregulation leads to lipotoxicity in the liver, causing oxidative stress and liver inflammation.[10]

Signs and symptoms
<ul><li>Fatigue[7] and depression[12]</li><li>Right upper quadrant pain or discomfort or fullness, possibly due to stretching of the hepatic capsule and hepatomegaly[9]</li><li>Metabolic syndrome[7]—type 2 diabetes mellitus, insulin resistance (IR), hyperlipidaemia and obesity</li><li>Acanthosis nigricans,[9] a cutaneous manifestation of IR, was found in 12% of NAFLD patients. This regional hyperpigmentation is typically found in adults around the neck, over knuckles, elbows and knees and offers the clinician and patients a physical clue as to the presence of IR.[13]</li></ul>

Pathophysiology

The hallmark of NAFLD is the deposition of excess FFAs within hepatocytes and is associated with the loss of insulin sensitivity.[14] There are theories as to whether the fat accumulation in the hepatocytes occurs first or IR; the literature is moving towards the theory that IR occurs first.[7,10]

Hepatic FFAs' concentration is increased by the following.[15,16]

- Obesity and IR cause excess FFAs in the liver from adipose tissue—60%.
- IR increases *de novo* lipogenesis (DNL) from excess dietary carbohydrates—25%.
- Poor diet increases dietary fatty acids—15%.
- Lipotoxicity, oxidative stress and mitochondrial damage results in decreased hepatic β-oxidation of FFAs.[17]
- Steatosis reduces very low density lipoprotein (VLDL) synthesis, export and clearance of FFAs.

Excess FFAs accumulate in the liver, leading to macrovesicular steatosis and lipid-induced cellular injury, worsening hepatic IR and reducing hepatic function; this contributes to a vicious cycle.[7,10] Both IR and obesity are pro-inflammatory conditions, resulting in high oxidative stress exacerbated by the aldehyde by-products of lipid peroxidation, which increase the production of pro-inflammatory cytokines and recruit inflammatory cells into the liver.[10]

In summary, the pathophysiology of NAFLD is complex and includes IR, disrupted lipid, protein and carbohydrate homoeostasis, oxidative stress, FFA-mediated lipotoxicity, defects in mitochondrial function, endoplasmic reticulum stress, cytokine mediated toxicity, inflammation and fibrosis.[17]

Diagnosis

A diagnosis of NAFLD requires confirmation of hepatic steatosis, with the additional exclusion of excessive intake of alcohol. The alternative causes for fatty liver (genetic, viral, metabolic, drug) must be excluded before a diagnosis of NAFLD can be made.[10]

Clinically, elevated liver transaminases, gamma glutamyl-transpeptidase (GGT), hypertriglyceridaemia, ferritin[9] and numerous weight-loss and weight-gain cycles would alert the practitioner to a possible NAFLD diagnosis. Serum ferritin is elevated in 20–50% of NAFLD patients and the raised transferrin saturation (> 55%) occurs in 5–10% of patients; both may reflect hepatic steatosis and fibrosis due to oxidative stress and inflammation. Hypertriglyceridaemia is often present in more than 50% of NAFLD patients.[9] Refer to Appendix 5 for more information on laboratory reference values.

An ultrasound of the liver, computed tomography and magnetic resonance imaging will detect moderate to severe steatosis (> 30% steatosis). A liver biopsy may be necessary to quantify the degree and stage of hepatic steatosis and fibrosis. The presence of more than 5% of steatotic hepatocytes in a section of liver tissue from a liver biopsy is the accepted minimum standard for a histological diagnosis of NAFLD.[18]

DIFFERENTIAL DIAGNOSIS—NAFLD

- Non-alcoholic steatosis
- ALD[7]
- HCV
- Wilson's disease[7]
- Cardiovascular disease
- Gallbladder disease
- Irritable bowel syndrome

Risk factors

Practitioners should be aware of the existence of conditions that commonly co-occur with NAFLD. The presence of NAFLD is an independent risk factor for coronary artery disease.[19] The hepatic metabolism of methionine is perturbed in NASH,[20] which may provide a reason for the increased coronary artery risk in this population. Recently polycystic ovarian syndrome was proposed as the ovarian manifestation of metabolic syndrome.[21]

Risk factors for mortality in NAFLD patients are the presence of cirrhosis, impaired fasting glycaemia or diabetes.[22]

NAFLD: at-risk groups	
• Histological NASH on diagnosis[22]	• Older age[22]
• Metabolic syndrome[4,5]	• Smokers[23]
• Major health conditions (especially cardiovascular disease)[19,20]	

Conventional treatment

A 2017 attempted network Cochrane meta-analysis looking at the pharmacological interventions for non-alcohol related fatty liver disease concluded that due to the very low quality evidence, the effectiveness of pharmacological treatments for people with NAFLD, including those with steatohepatitis, are uncertain.[24] Although there is no pharmacological agent approved for treating NAFLD, vitamin E (in patients without type 2 diabetes mellitus) and thiazolidinedione pioglitazone (in patients with and without type 2 diabetes mellitus) have shown the most consistent results in randomised controlled trials.[25] However, a recent systematic review of the use of thiazolidinediones (peroxisome proliferator activator receptor-γ agonists) in NAFLD concluded that while they modestly improve fibrosis and hepatocellular ballooning, it is at the cost of significant weight gain. In seven randomised trials the average weight gain was 4.4 kg (CI, 2.6–5.2 kg).[26] There is an increased cardiovascular risk with rosiglitazone. Other side effects are fluid retention and osteoporosis. The evidence that insulin-sensitising drugs are able to modify the natural history of NAFLD is not currently available.[27]

Key treatment protocols

The first goal is to address the metabolic syndrome picture and reverse the lipotoxicity and insulin resistance via lifestyle interventions[25,28] using diet and exercise.

At the same time it is important to protect the liver from oxidative stress and subsequent inflammation and fibrosis, as well as supporting liver function and healing. Supporting the digestive system will reduce the dyspeptic symptoms of NAFLD thereby improving client wellbeing and nutrient status. Two of the major symptoms of NAFLD are fatigue and depression so in order to motivate the client to make positive lifestyle choices the treatment protocol needs to address these issues.

Naturopathic Treatment Aims

- Encourage beneficial dietary and lifestyle changes.
- Treat the underlying metabolic causes:
  - modulate fatty acid pathways
  - regulate blood glucose
  - reduce weight.
- Reduce hepatic inflammation:
  - reduce oxidative stress.
- Reduce systemic inflammation.
- Reduce the likelihood of fibrosis.
- Support liver function.
- Support digestive function.
- Support mood and energy levels.

Encourage beneficial dietary and lifestyle changes

Dietary and lifestyle advice

Identifying and removing potential liver stresses is one of the first steps in instigating beneficial lifestyle changes, such as alcohol moderation and smoking cessation. The 2016 European Association for the Study of the Liver (EASL), European Association for the Study of Diabetes (EASD) and European Association for the Study of Obesity (EASO) clinical guidelines for the management of NAFLD state that lifestyle correction is mandatory in all patients. The EASL-EASD-EASO guidelines plus other studies recommend the Mediterranean diet and state that it can achieve benefits even without calorie restriction and weight loss.[29-31] The diet needs to be low in carbohydrates and particularly low in high-fructose corn syrup as fructose is lipogenic and stimulates triglyceride synthesis.[32] Where there is a high-fructose diet, especially with soft drink consumption, all the signs relating to NAFLD are present: increased blood glucose, triglyceride, alanine aminotransferase (ALT), cholesterol, weight and hepatic steatosis. In NASH patients high fructose ingestion was associated with hepatic insulin resistance and higher fibrosis.[33] High-fructose diets increase hepatic reactive oxygen species (ROS) and macrophage aggregation, resulting in TGF-beta-1 signalled collagen deposition and hepatic fibrosis.[34] This potentially leads to decreased copper absorption and a resulting deficiency.[33,35]

The diet should also be high in protein, fibre, good fats, antioxidants and anti-inflammatory foods such as lean meat and fresh vegetables to regulate blood glucose levels and support antioxidant status, bowel and liver function. High-protein diets prevent and reverse steatosis independently of fat and carbohydrate intake more efficiently than a 20% reduction in energy intake.[36] The effect appears to result from small, synergistic increases in lipid and branched-chain amino acids (BCAA) catabolism, and a decrease in cell stress. Similarly, low-carbohydrate diets are useful in reducing circulating insulin levels and decreased intrahepatic triglycerides (IHTG) due to enhanced lipolysis and fatty acid oxidation.[37] Studies involving low-carbohydrate diets with less than 50 g/day of carbohydrate saw a reduction in insulin sensitivity and decreased endogenous glucose production rate—more than an isocaloric low-fat diet—and encouraged hepatic and visceral fat loss. Attention to nutrition status is important as malnutrition accounts for more than 60% of patients with severe liver failure and negatively affects clinical outcomes in terms of survival and complications.[38]

Exercise or physical activity

Exercise of sufficient duration and intensity will reduce adipose tissue therefore reducing a source of adipose-derived FFAs; it also enhances insulin sensitivity. Exercise will increase muscle mass, adiponectin and the biogenesis of mitochondria. **Endurance exercise** uses muscles that use triglycerides for energy rather than carbohydrates and therefore there is an overall decrease of FFAs and an increase in the β-oxidation of FFAs in NAFLD.[16,27,39,40]

There is emerging and growing evidence for the effectiveness of increasing physical activity reducing hepatic fat content,[27] regardless of whether it is resistance based or aerobic or combined with diet and weight loss. Therefore it is important to find some form of exercise that is physically possible for the patient. **Resistance exercise** independent of weight loss is also associated with significant reduction in hepatic fat[40] and may improve insulin sensitivity more than aerobic exercise alone.[39] Resistance exercise may be more accessible to some patients than aerobic exercise and may achieve better compliance than diet; therefore, it is a more sustainable treatment option.[40,41]

Aerobic exercise training and dietary restriction can positively affect NAFLD when weight loss approximating 4–9% of body weight is achieved; an inverse correlation between NAFLD and physical activity or fitness levels has also been demonstrated.[16,27,39] Weight loss, irrespective of diet, reduces aminotransferases in obese women with NAFLD[42] and 7–10% weight loss coincided with significant histological improvement of liver disease.[43] Therefore a combination of exercise, diet and weight loss is synergistic in the amelioration of liver disease in NAFLD.[44]

A systematic review with meta-analysis concluded that exercise is efficacious in modifying liver fat in adults. Interventions ranged from 2–24 weeks in duration and prescribed exercise on two to six days per week at intensities between 45% and 85% of VO_{2peak}.[27] The review could not report an improvement in ALT due to many ALT measures being normal at baseline and because studies with positive results were excluded due to lack of a control group. In a study that lacked a control group a near 50% reduction in ALT was achieved in patients who complied with the prescribed exercise regimen, indicating reduced liver inflammation.[45] The exercise regimen consisted of aerobic exercise for 30 minutes per day at a heart rate of 60–70% of maximal for at least five days a week for three months.

In rodents regular exercise reduced DNL, increased β-oxidation and increased the removal and clearance of FFAs via VLDL. Sedentary behaviour, on the other hand, resulted in the reduced oxidation of fatty acids and mitochondrial activity with the up-regulation of fatty acid synthesis.[16,27]

Kistler et al. suggest that intensity of exercise may be more important than duration or total volume of exercise in the treatment of NAFLD, with vigorous activity associated with significantly lower odds of fibrosis.[46] The suggested mechanisms for the benefits of vigorous exercise over moderate are that vigorous exercise increases adiponectin and AMP-activated protein kinase (AMP-kinase) in the liver, which increases fatty acid oxidation, decreases glucose production, regulates mitochondrial biogenesis and reduces inflammation and fibrosis.[46,47] Decrease in adiponectin plays a significant role in metabolic disorders such as obesity, type 2 diabetes, coronary heart disease and metabolic syndrome due to its insulin sensitising, anti-inflammatory and anti-atherogenic properties.[48] Decreases in adiponectin and increases in leptin in metabolic syndrome and obesity are linked to fibrosis in NAFLD.[49] Coker et al.[50] found that exercise training with calorie restriction achieved better results in visceral fat loss, weight loss and improvements in insulin resistance than calorie restriction alone.

Treat the underlying metabolic causes

Modulate fatty acid pathways and regulate blood glucose

In obese individuals it is important to reduce adipose tissue as a source of FFAs as well as to control insulin resistance that results in excess lipolysis of adipose tissue. Also, controlling insulin resistance will help decrease rates of DNL from carbohydrate metabolism. Exercise can reduce adipose tissue, and improvements in insulin resistance combined with a diet containing low carbohydrates and healthy fats are essential to improving NAFLD. Strong evidence exists for **omega-3 fatty acids**[51] reducing hepatic fat content in children with NAFLD. **Vitamin E (natural)**[52,53] as a fat-soluble antioxidant is also useful in reducing lipid peroxidation in NAFLD.

Whole ***Curcuma longa*** oleoresin up-regulated the expression of genes related to glycolysis, β-oxidation and cholesterol metabolism in obese diabetic KKAy mice and down-regulated the gluconeogenesis related genes (see Chapter 19 on diabetes for more information).[54] In a recent trial, participants received an amorphous dispersion curcumin formulation (500 mg/day equivalent to 70 mg curcumin) or matched placebo for a period of eight weeks. Curcumin achieved a significant reduction in liver fat content (78.9% improvement in the curcumin versus 27.5% improvement in the placebo group). There were also significant reductions in cholesterol, triglycerides, body mass index, glucose and glycated haemoglobin, and liver inflammation.[55] Berberine is a plant alkaloid with several pharmacological activities, including antimicrobial, antidiabetic, hypoglycemic, hypocholesterolemic, anti-tumoral, immunomodulatory properties, anti-inflammatory and antioxidant.[56–59] Berberine improves mitochondrial function[56] and inhibits hepatic lipogenesis.[57]

Reduce hepatic inflammation

The inflammatory process causes oxidative stress and vice versa, driving liver disease progression. Therefore a key treatment goal in NAFLD is to reduce hepatic inflammation and oxidative stress by using hepatoprotective herbal medicines with specific hepatic anti-inflammatory and antioxidant activity. Hepatoprotection is defined as more than just antioxidant and anti-inflammatory effects; it also includes several non-mutually exclusive biological activities including antifibrotic, antiviral and immunomodulatory functions.[60]

One of the ways that oxidative stress damage can be reduced is through hormesis. It is postulated that hormesis is a mechanism by which phytochemical adaptogens such as *Astragalus membranaceus* and antioxidant-rich plants such as *Silybum marianum* strengthen mitochondria by improving the β-oxidation of FFAs, increasing energy and stamina.[61] In calorie restriction, exercise and hormesis, increased ROS up-regulates adaptive responses. This results in a net reduction in ROS due to the stimulation of antioxidant defences and detoxification.[62] This adaptation or preconditioning of the mitochondria has been named 'mitochondrial hormesis' or 'mitohormesis'.[62–64] These hormetic pathways, activated by phytochemicals, include the sirtuin-FOXO pathway, the NF-kappa B pathway and the Nrf-2/ARE pathway.[61] Surh[65] terms this exogenous form of hormesis 'xenohormesis'.[61,66] Bitter foods such as dandelion coffee, rocket and radicchio also have a hormetic effect as well as stimulate digestion and aid dyspepsia.

Silymarin (an active constituent of *Silybum marianum*) protects cells against oxidative stress by stabilising cell membranes, radical scavenging, chelating iron and supporting endogenous antioxidants such as glutathione.[67] *Silybum marianum* also has anti-inflammatory[68,69] and antifibrotic[70,71] effects through the reduction of inflammatory cytokines and TNF-α as well as hypoglycaemic, choleretic and cholagogic actions. The latter two actions help remove fat from the liver through the fatty acid metabolism pathways, thereby preventing deposition of fat in the liver.

Curcuma longa interrupts insulin signalling, which stimulates hepatic stellate cell activation (a key element in fibrogenesis), suppresses the gene expression of type I collagen and also increases the *de novo* synthesis of glutathione, thereby exerting anti-inflammatory, antioxidant, antidiabetic and antifibrotic effects.[72] The antioxidant and anti-inflammatory actions of **baicalin** and *Scutellaria baicalensis* make it a very useful clinical tool in NAFLD[73] and ALD[74] management.

Baicalin, the active ingredient in *Scutellaria baicalensis*, has been shown to reduce dyslipidaemia and hepatic lipid accumulation, improve hepatic steatosis and reduce visceral fat mass in vivo.[73]

Glycyrrhiza glabra has an anti-inflammatory effect in NAFLD by lowering elevated ALT and aspartate aminotransferase (AST) in a randomised, double-blind, placebo-controlled clinical trial.[75] The biologically active metabolite of **glycyrrhizin** (18 beta-glycyrrhetinic acid [GA]) prevented FFA-induced lipid accumulation and toxicity by stabilising the lysosomal membranes, inhibiting cathepsin B activity and inhibiting mitochondrial cytochrome *c* release.[76] Another preparation of GA (**carbenoxolone**, 3-hemisuccinate of glycyrrhetinic acid) inhibited pro-inflammatory cytokine expression, inhibited FFA-induced ROS formation and reversed FFA-induced mitochondrial membrane depolarisation in HepG2 cells. GA also prevented the development of fatty liver by inhibiting the sterol regulatory element binding protein 1c (SREBP-1c) expression and activity via antiapoptotic mechanisms and the inhibition of inflammatory cytokines and ROS formation in the liver.[77]

Grapeseed extract improved markers of inflammation and glycaemia in obese type 2 diabetes mellitus patients[78] and reduced ALT and improved grade of steatosis in NAFLD patients.[79] (See Chapter 19 on diabetes and Chapters 11–13 on the cardiovascular system for more information.)

Both **omega-3**[51] and **vitamin E (natural)**[52] have shown some effectiveness in reducing inflammation in NAFLD and/or NASH. Deficiencies in vitamin E lead to an increased risk of developing advanced inflammation (6.5-fold) and lower riboflavin intake is associated with increased risk of advanced steatosis (6.2-fold) compared with those chronic hepatitis C patients with adequate intakes.[80]

Accumulation of lipids in the hepatocyte impairs the metabolic capacity of the mitochondria, leading to a buildup of reduced electron transport chain substrates and lipid peroxidation, leading to increased ROS.[81] Therefore stimulation of mitochondrial function through **L-carnitine**,[82,83] **alpha lipoic acid**[84] and **coenzyme Q10**[85] may be effective in NAFLD and other liver conditions associated with mitochondrial dysfunction. **Melatonin** (5 mg) and **tryptophan** (500 mg) twice daily for four weeks reduced the plasma levels of pro-inflammatory cytokines in NASH.[86]

Support liver function

Herbs that support liver function such as *Silybum marianum*, *Berberis aristata*,[87] *Cynara scolymus*,[88] *Curcuma longa*[54] and *Schisandra chinensis* also help support the production and elimination of bile that promotes the elimination of cholesterol, which lowers FFAs (see Table 7.1 and Figure 7.2).[89] See the following liver detoxification section for herbs and nutrients specific to supporting detoxification. **SAMe**[90] supports methylation and has shown some effectiveness in NAFLD and NASH. **N-acetylcysteine** (600 mg/day) reduced ALT in NAFLD patients and improved liver function through supporting glutathione production.[91]

Reduced dietary protein intake is an independent predictor of complications in cirrhosis.[117,118] In those with liver cirrhosis with low serum albumin or globulin, extra **protein**, approximately 1.0–1.2 g of protein per kilogram of body weight,[119] is required to assist the liver to synthesise proteins. Compromised liver function will also result in reduced protein synthesis, possibly resulting in signs such as prolonged prothrombin time due to reduced synthesis of clotting factors. The provision of a night-time feed to cirrhotic patients led to a body protein increment of about 2 kg of lean tissue sustained over 12 months.[120]

Support liver detoxification

A protocol to enhance liver detoxification is an adjunct treatment to all acute and chronic inflammatory conditions and conditions associated with hormone imbalance through the removal of exogenous and endogenous toxins that may cause oxidative stress, drive inflammation and act as carcinogens.

Liver detoxification refers to the phase I, phase II and phase III enzymes in the liver. Phase I enzymes activate both toxins and drugs, potentially increasing the effects of both. Phase II enzymes conjugate the metabolites of phase I, making them more water soluble and available for excretion, thereby reducing toxic metabolites and the need for therapeutic drugs.[121] Phase III involves the mobilisation of the products of phase II from the intracellular environment to the extracellular environment for excretion as bile, urine, sweat and via the lungs. Toxic compounds such as 2,3,7,8-tetrachlorodibenzo-*p*-dioxin (TCDD), polycyclic aromatics and beta-naphthoflavone induce both phase I and phase II activity.[122] Conversely, therapeutic interventions tend to inhibit phase I and induce phase II, protecting the body from a buildup of the toxic metabolites of phase I (Table 7.1 and Figure 7.2).

Table 7.1
Required nutrients, inducers and inhibitors of phase I and phase II[92]

	Required nutrients	Induced by	Inhibited by
Phase I	B2, B3, B6, B9, B12 Branched-chain amino acids Glutathione Bioflavonoids Phospholipids	Tobacco[93] Omeprazole Ethanol *Hypericum perforatum* (hyperforin)[94] Caffeine (CYP1A2)[95] High-protein diet[96] Charcoal-broiled food[93] Flavonoids[97] *Rosmarinus officinalis*[98]	Grapefruit juice[99] Oranges[99,100] Legumes Quinidine Erythromycin Fluvoxamine *Carum carvi*[101] Brassica family[102] Bioflavonoids[94] *Cuminum cyminum*[101] *Taraxacum officinale* *Allium sativum*[103,104] *Schisandra chinensis*[105] *Glycyrrhiza glabra*[106] *Withania somnifera* *Curcuma longa* *Foeniculum vulgare*[107] *Cynara scolymus* *Silybum marianum*[108]
Phase II	Acetylation: B5 Methylation: B6, B9, B12, SAMe and betaine Conjugation: amino acids Glucuronidation: taurine and glucoronic acid Glutathione: glutamate, cysteine and glycine Sulfation: glutathione, cysteine and methionine	Caffeine[109] *Cymbopogon citratus* (citral) *Salvia officinalis* *Camellia sinensis* *Thymus vulgare* *Zingiber officinale*[110] Brassica family[111] Bioflavonoids[94] *Cuminum cyminum*[101] *Taraxacum officinale* *Allium sativum*[103,104] *Schisandra chinensis*[112,113] *Humulus lupus*[114] *Glycyrrhiza glabra*[115] *Rosmarinus officinalis*[116] *Withania somnifera* *Curcuma longa* *Silybum marianum*[113] N-acetylcysteine	Deficiencies in selenium, zinc, B1, B2, molybdenum Low-protein diet, NSAIDs, aspirin

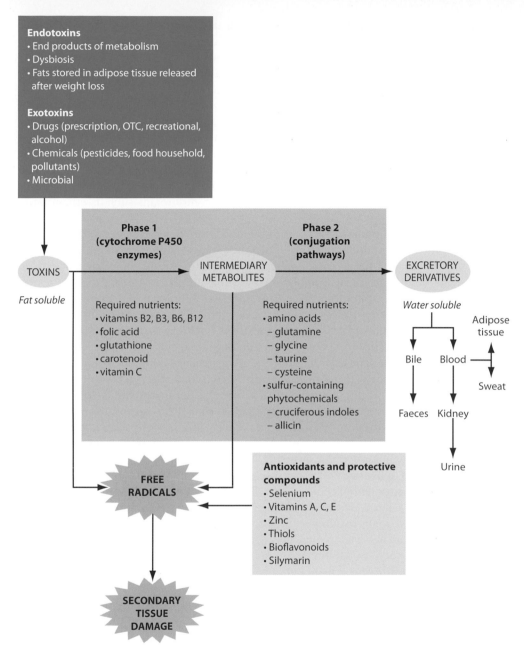

Figure 7.2
Biochemical and nutritional factors affecting liver metabolism

A detoxification protocol requires, first of all, a healthy diet and good digestive function to reduce the intake and maximise the output of toxins. This should be combined with lifestyle changes such as exercise and relaxation and be supported by foods, nutrients and herbs that optimise liver function by balancing phase I and phase II enzyme activity and providing antioxidants' protection.

A **healthy diet** (see Chapter 3 on wellness) is essential in effective detoxification. A diet high in fibre and water will promote the elimination of waste products and reduce the enterohepatic circulation of toxins. Enterohepatic circulation involves reabsorbing substances through the gastrointestinal tract rather than excreting them. This can be particularly problematic with the reabsorption of hormones excreted via the bile, such as oestrogen, leading to hormone imbalances. **Probiotics** and **prebiotics** can help gastro-intestinal tract function and reduce the formation of endotoxins such as ethanol and lipopolysaccharide (LPS).[123]

Foods containing **flavonoids** (e.g. kaempferol, diosmetin, theaflavin and biochanin A) can inhibit the metabolic activation of procarcinogens by phase I enzymes and some dietary flavonoids (e.g. naringenin, quercetin, biochanin A and prenylchalcones) can stimulate the detoxification of carcinogens by inducing phase II enzymes.[94] A review cautions that a number of studies have demonstrated inhibition and induction effects on drug bioavailability by flavonoids, raising concerns about the safe use of flavonoid supplements that are not subject to legal regulations.[97] *Allium sativum* can be beneficial through an inhibitory effect on phase I[124] and an induction effect on phase II[103] enzymes as well as increasing the synthesis of endogenous antioxidants and glutathione via Nrf2/ARE[104] and is therefore very useful in detoxification and easily accessible as a food. Another food example is the phytochemical phenethyl isothiocyanate, a constituent of **cruciferous vegetables** that can modulate cytochrome P450 composition in human liver at concentrations that can be achieved by dietary intake.[102] This can antagonise the carcinogenicity of chemicals that rely on the CYP1 family for their bioactivation such as heterocyclic amines and polycyclic aromatic hydrocarbons.[102]

Teas can be used to hydrate and to gently cleanse the body, with various herbal teas and dandelion root coffee potential choices. Also the use of **culinary herbs and spices** such as turmeric, cumin, fenugreek, rosemary and sage is a great way to introduce a variety of herbs into the diet. Diets low in **protein** may predispose patients to lowered liver detoxification, as key amino acids are involved in these liver processes.[36,119] Increasing crude protein intake will also help to improve availability of amino acid precursors for conjugation.

Fasting is also known to enhance the detoxification process,[125] in part because the main source of energy is hydrolysed fatty acid tissue from adipose tissue stores, where many toxins are stored.[126] However, due prudence needs to be displayed, as fasting may liberate toxins faster than they can be eliminated (because in part the adequate substrates from phase II detoxification may be missing or compromised) and may potentially endanger the patient.

Hydrotherapy is thought to increase filtration through the liver by encouraging blood circulation, in addition to aiding excretion through sweating.[126] Sauna therapy has also been used to encourage elimination through the skin, with substantial elimination and significant clinical improvement thought possible through this mechanism.[125,127] **Sauna** exposure of 5–15 minutes per day is safe and effective in enhancing detoxification, though caution is advised in patients with recent myocardial infarction or other serious cardiovascular complications, and patients need to be advised that eliminating toxins through the skin may initially irritate (though ultimately improve) conditions such as atopic dermatitis.[128] Many nutrients, particularly trace elements such as zinc, copper, iron and chromium as well as electrolytes, may be lost through sweating and may need monitoring or replacement.

Some herbs have a history of use for detoxification and are used in traditional herbal medicine for their role in supporting liver function including ***Silybum marianum***, ***Cynara scolymus***, ***Bupleurum falcatum***, ***Schisandra chinensis***, ***Peumus boldo*** and ***Taraxacum officinale***. Herbs such as *Silybum marianum* and *Schisandra chinensis* can increase levels of Nrf2 either by stimulating its release or inhibiting its proteolytic breakdown. Activated Nrf2 translocates into the nucleus where it interacts with small MAF family proteins bound to the antioxidant response element (ARE), allowing transcription of target genes including those that regulate antioxidant and phase II enzymes.[113]

Exercise will also promote hepatic biotransformation processes.[129,130]

Detoxification is also an area in which unproven and often ineffective remedies are aggressively marketed, both to practitioners and to patients, implying careful consideration before their use in clinical practice.[131] Therefore, while detoxification regimens may provide a clinically valuable adjuvant to treatment, naturopathic practitioners should be sure to focus on more relevant primary treatment aims in the clinical setting. More extreme detoxification methods can be very dangerous and should be avoided. While it is true that many traditional methods may fall into this category, it should also be acknowledged that these traditions were born of a time when environmental toxic burdens were far lower and would have resulted in fewer side effects and lower risk.

Support digestive function

Dyspeptic symptoms associated with NAFLD include burping, bloating, reflux, flatulence and indigestion with intolerances to fatty foods. Common herbal medicines used to stimulate secretion of bile and pancreatic enzymes are ***Gentiana lutea*** and ***Cynara scolymus***. Bitter foods such as dandelion coffee, rocket, radicchio, watercress, radish, cauliflower and the rest of the Brassicaceae family also stimulate digestion. Cholagogues aid digestion and carminatives reduce spasm and wind. Dysbiosis plays a role in the pathogenesis of liver disease through inflammation and damage to the epithelial cells of the intestines. This damage can then expose the liver to intestinally derived toxins such as ethanol and lipopolysaccharides (LPS), which drive inflammation in the liver.[123]

Probiotics, **prebiotics** and **increased dietary fibre** can be used to help restore intestinal flora balance and function to the gastrointestinal tract. They can be useful in reducing the enterohepatic reabsorption of toxins from the gastrointestinal tract. The inclusion of a range of probiotics such as ***Lactobacillus bulgaricus*** and ***Streptococcus thermophilus*** reduce hepatic necroinflammation in NAFLD patients.[132] ***Bifidobacterium longum*** with FOS and lifestyle modification significantly reduced tumour necrosis factor alpha (TNF-α), C-reactive protein (CRP), serum AST levels, HOMA-IR, serum endotoxin, steatosis and NASH activity score[133] (see Chapters 4–6 on the gastrointestinal system for more detail).

Support mood and energy levels

A number of epidemiological studies have found links between chronic liver diseases such as NAFLD and hepatitis B and C with depression.[144,145] Weinstein et al. suggest that NAFLD and HCV patients have a higher prevalence of depression than the wider population.[12]

Probiotics

Dysbiosis of the gut microbiota affects the pathogenesis and progression of NAFLD and NASH.[134–137] Gut microbiota-mediated inflammation of the intestinal mucosa leads to compromised intestinal permeability and impairment in mucosal immune function.[138] Compromised intestinal permeability means that bacterial products such as lipopolysaccharide (LPS) and toxins are carried to the liver via the portal circulation and can trigger an immune response, oxidative stress, inflammation, fibrosis and promote insulin resistance, obesity and metabolic syndrome.[139–142] A specific mechanism of injury that can occur in NAFLD is the microbiota converting choline into methylamines; this reduced availability of choline reduces the export of VLDL from the liver and increases fat accumulation and ROS.[135,140]

Evidence suggests that diet and lifestyle factors which are known to exacerbate NAFLD may do this by changing the gut microbiota.[140,141] Poor diets, which are low in fibre and high in fats and sugars, reduce gut motility and that affects the microbiota and intestinal permeability which further degrades gut motility. A high-fat diet increases inflammatory microbiota and causes an increase in bile acids, which then increase intestinal permeability.[7] A high-fructose diet increases bacteria that can extract energy from complex polysaccharides resulting in an increase of free fatty acids reaching the liver, with consequent hepatic lipogenesis.[140] Changes to diet within a few days lead to a change in microbiota; however, if the diet reverts so do the microbiota. Therefore, changes to diet need to be sustainable, containing plenty of plant food and fermented foods.

The use of probiotics improves the pathology of NAFLD in animal models, and to some extent in human models probiotics led to decreases in liver fat and serum ALT and lipid levels and improvements in inflammation, liver fibrosis, oxidative stress and insulin resistance.[140,142,143] In an animal intervention, the authors concluded that probiotics can improve intestinal integrity, ameliorate dysbiosis, improve liver pathology and reduce gut endotoxemia and the consequent inflammatory response by the Kupffer cells in the liver.[137] A review of the literature concluded that probiotics could ameliorate hepatic steatosis via reduction in inflammation; reduce endotoxemia by inhibiting epithelial invasion, maintaining intestinal barrier integrity and the production of antimicrobial peptides; and enhance insulin sensitivity.[135]

Depression and mood disorders are often seen in obesity and diabetes mellitus, two of the major metabolic pictures seen in NAFLD. While mood disorders are not always present, they are relevant to some sufferers of chronic liver disease and symptoms must be supported. (See also Chapter 15 on depression and Chapter 18 on stress and fatigue.)

Integrative medical considerations

After a thorough naturopathic consultation, it may become apparent that the patient has a number of risk factors and symptoms that suggest the presence of NAFLD. If this diagnosis is not confirmed at the time of their initial consultation, a referral to a general practitioner in the first instance would be worthwhile for further investigation.

Refer for liver ultrasound or further medical care if there are signs of:

- severe fluctuations in weight (loss and gain)
- elevated GGT
- elevated ALT
- raised triglycerides
- raised ferritin.

Clinical summary

Refer to the naturopathic treatment decision tree (Figure 7.3) regarding clinical decisions in the treatment and management of liver disease. From the thorough case history taking and observation of the clinical signs and symptoms of liver disease, a potential diagnosis of NAFLD may be apparent. It would be useful to confirm the diagnosis of NAFLD with a general practitioner, who may refer the patient for biochemical tests and liver ultrasound or liver biopsy if indicated. An individualised treatment plan considering causation, age, sex, culture, current dietary and lifestyle factors and family and social history should be discussed with the patient. This treatment plan would address the underlying causes (alcohol, viral infection, metabolic syndrome), support liver and digestive function, reduce inflammation and oxidative stress, address obstacles to healing and encourage beneficial dietary and lifestyle changes.

OTHER LIVER AND BILIARY DISEASES

Hepatitis

According to the World Health Organisation (WHO), an estimated 71 million people have chronic hepatitis C infection.[146] Chronic hepatitis C can lead to hepatic fibrosis, cirrhosis and hepatocellular carcinoma. It is the leading cause of liver transplantation in Australia.[147] Estimates indicate that 25 per cent of those infected with hepatitis C will clear the virus, with 75 per cent having chronic infection.[148] Clinical symptoms of chronic hepatitis C include fatigue,[149] right upper quadrant pain or discomfort, nausea, malaise, anorexia, pruritus, weight loss, arthralgia, musculoskeletal pain, night sweats and dry eyes (sicca syndrome). Extrahepatic manifestations of chronic hepatitis C are: mixed cryoglobulinaemia, glomerulonephritis, porphyria cutanea tarda, low-grade malignant lymphoma, autoimmune thyroiditis, Sjögren's syndrome, lichen planus, aplastic anaemia, polyarteritis nodosa, erythema nodosum, idiopathic pulmonary fibrosis and diabetes mellitus.[150] The pathophysiology of chronic hepatitis C is multifactorial and the key players are the hepatitis C virus directly, the immune response to HCV infection and oxidative stress.

DIFFERENTIAL DIAGNOSIS

- Chronic fatigue syndrome
- Fibromyalgia
- NAFLD
- NASH
- Autoimmune hepatitis

Risk factors[151]

Modifiable risk factors include:

- intravenous drug and tobacco use
- blood transfusions
- tattoos
- needle-stick injuries
- steatosis
- insulin resistance, type 2 diabetes
- body mass index (BMI) over 25.

Non-modifiable risk factors include:

- age at acquisition of HCV infection
- age and necrosis stage at liver biopsy
- gender (male)
- duration of infection
- ALT levels ranging from 1.5–5 times the upper limit of normal (ULN), ALT > 70 IU/L and genetics (immune function and interferon sensitivity).

Conventional treatment

- Since 2013/2014 direct acting antivirals (DAAs) have become the gold standard of treatment for CHC, leading to sustained viral response (SVR) in 91% of CHC patients in 12 weeks.[152] However, treatment response does depend on the HCV genotype, the presence or otherwise of cirrhosis and whether the patient is treatment naïve or treatment experienced.[152–156]
- Overall, the adverse events associated with DAAs are mild: nausea, fatigue and anaemia. However, Sofosbuvir (NS5B polymerase inhibitor) is contraindicated in patients with severe renal impairment (it is metabolised through the kidneys).[157–159]
- There is also some controversy as to whether the direct-acting antivirals increase the incidence or recurrence[160,161] of hepatocellular carcinomas or not[162–164] particularly in patients with cirrhosis.

Within the hepatitis C population, one subtype of the virus (HCV genotype 3) is difficult to treat despite the advances in the new direct-acting antivirals for the other hepatitis C genotypes (1, 2, 4, 5 and 6) so the complementary medicine treatment of this subtype still has relevance.[152–155]

Key treatment protocols

- From a naturopathic clinical perspective, the goal of supporting treatment of chronic hepatitis C is to reduce oxidative stress caused by the hepatitis C virus (proteins) and the inflammatory mediators produced by the ineffectual immune response to the virus and thereby reduce disease progression in the form of inflammation, fibrosis, cirrhosis and potentially cancer.
- Encourage beneficial dietary and lifestyle changes. (See the NAFLD section earlier in this chapter and Chapter 3 on wellness.)
- Antiviral and immune support. An immediate, strong and persistent CD4+ T-cell response[166,167] and a vigorous multispecific cytotoxic T lymphocyte response[167–170] against multiple HCV epitopes coupled with a predominant T helper 1 cytokine profile is more likely to encourage viral clearance in response to acute HCV infection.[171] Herbal medicines such as **Astragalus membranaceus**,[172] **Echinacea spp.**[173] and **Phyllanthus amarus**[174] which influence the Th1–Th2 balance may assist in both acute and chronic hepatitis C infection. **Zinc** and **vitamin E** are particularly important for an effective immune response. **Intravenous silibinin** has shown direct anti-HCV activity in chronic hepatitis C patients who were previous non-responders to standard therapy[175] and to prevent HCV re-infection after liver transplantation.[176]
- The treatment strategies to reduce hepatic inflammation and oxidative stress, support liver function and digestive function and alleviate depression and fatigue are outlined in the NAFLD treatment protocol section.

- Use of specific nutraceuticals. Studies have shown that 2 g **L-carnitine** taken concurrently with interferon and ribavirin for 12 months helped chronic hepatitis C patients clear the hepatitis C virus and reduced fatty liver and fibrosis by 70%.[177] The sustained virological response was also greater in the L-carnitine group (46%) compared with the interferon and ribavirin group (39%). A total 800 IU **vitamin D3** per day given at the same time as pegylated interferon and ribavirin helped liver transplant patients with chronic hepatitis C achieve greater rates of SVR.[178] Between 50% and 73% of chronic hepatitis C patients were deficient in vitamin D3.[179,180] Correcting vitamin D deficiency before antiviral therapy is recommended[178] as low vitamin D is linked to severe liver fibrosis and low levels of SVR on interferon-based therapy.[180]

Cholecystitis

Cholelithiasis is the medical term for the presence of gallstones in the gallbladder. An estimated 14–20% of Australians will develop gallstones in their lifetime. There are three main types of gallstones: cholesterol stones—70% cholesterol crystals; black pigment stones—calcium bilirubinate present in haemolytic disorders; and brown pigment stones—linked to bacterial or helminthic infection in the biliary tree.[181]

In respect to aetiology and pathophysiology, hypersecretion of cholesterol and the hyposecretion of bile acids and phosphatidylcholine (lecithin)[182,183] causes the bile to contain more cholesterol than the bile salts and phospholipids can solubilise. Chemical components of bile precipitate in the gallbladder and occasionally in the bile duct[181] to form microscopic cholesterol-rich vesicles.[183] Pathogenic development of these cholesterol-rich vesicles into macroscopic gallstones has been linked to hypomotility and excess biliary mucin excretion,[184] which is linked to hepatic cholesterol hypersecretion and a cycle of lithogenesis. Gallstones are asymptomatic in 60–80% of cases and, of those, only 10–20% will develop symptoms. Gallstone-associated pain can increase the risk of complications such as acute cholecystitis, cholangitis and pancreatitis.

Cholecystitis can be classified as acute or chronic. Acute cholecystitis is indicated if the pain lasts longer than 12 hours, and may be due to gallstone impaction in the cystic duct. The clinical presentations include fever, upper abdominal pain with marked tenderness and guarding in the right upper quadrant, especially with pain on palpation combined with inspiration, known as Murphy's sign due to elevated pressure within the gallbladder due to obstruction.[185] Chronic cholecystitis (or cholelithiasis) is the most common clinical presentation of symptomatic gallstones and presents as episodic biliary pain usually in the right upper abdominal quadrant or epigastric area, which can radiate to the right subscapular area, midback or right shoulder. Episodes of biliary pain generally last between 30 minutes and a few hours and episodes may occur daily or every few months. Nausea is common, but vomiting and fevers are not.

DIFFERENTIAL DIAGNOSIS

- Angina pectoris
- Appendicitis
- Bowel obstruction
- Epigastric pain from myocardial infarction
- Gastro-oesophageal reflux

- Irritable bowel syndrome
- Liver disease
- Oesophagitis
- Pancreatitis
- Peptic ulcer disease

Source: Portincasa et al. 2006[186]

Risk factors

- Age—increased biliary cholesterol secretion due to a decrease in cholesterol 7-α-hydroxylase activity[187] and decreased biliary salt excretion[188]
- Obesity—increased biliary secretion of bile from the liver with cholesterol supersaturation[186]
- Females—in pregnancy, endogenous oestrogens linked to increased hepatic cholesterol uptake and synthesis, gallbladder hypomotility and decreased cholesterol 7-α-hydroxylase activity.[181,185] The risk for women is two to three times that of males of the same age.[185,189] Women with a BMI over 32 are six times more likely to develop gallstones than women with a BMI over 22[190]
- Rapid weight loss and weight cycling and a prolonged fat-restricted diet is thought to exacerbate gallbladder stasis
- Diet—high carbohydrates in the diet[182] and high triglyceride levels in the blood[183] are linked to gallstone formation
- Dyspepsia—particularly *Helicobacter* species and slow transit time

Conventional treatment[191]

- An ultrasound is the common diagnostic tool.
- A cholescintigraphy scan is also used.
- If acute cholecystitis is suspected, refer the patient to their general practitioner or a hospital emergency department.
- Current medical treatment for cholelithiasis is surgery. Single incision laparoscopic cholecystectomy (SILC) is associated with a 90.7% success rate and a 6.1% complication rate. Critical reviews of clinical guidelines for gallstones have been articulated in the literature.[192–194]

Key treatment protocols

- Encourage beneficial dietary and lifestyle changes. (See Chapter 3 on wellness.)
- Promote optimal bile formation in the liver with choleretics such as ***Curcuma longa***,[195] ***Cynara scolymus*** and ***Peumus boldo***.
- Promote effective gallbladder motility and function with cholagogues such as ***Cynara scolymus, Peumus boldo*** and ***Taraxacum officinale***.
- As a specific for cholelithiasis use the cholerectic and cholagogue ***Peumus boldo***.
- Reduce bile and cholesterol reabsorption in the small intestine by reducing cholesterol intake, synthesis and output with niacin (B3),[196] red yeast rice,[197,198] ***Cynara scolymus***,[199] ***Taraxacum officinale***,[200] fibre and probiotics.
- Support optimal digestive function. See Chapters 4–6 on the gastrointestinal system.
- There is limited evidence of the role of Chinese herbal medicines in the treatment of cholecystitis[201] and cholelithiasis.

Pancreatitis

Pancreatitis is a progressive inflammatory disease characterised by irreversible destruction of exocrine pancreatic tissue.[202] Repeated episodes of acute pancreatitis lead to tissue remodelling and fibrosis.[202] Pancreatitis can be due to obstruction of the pancreatic duct. Obstruction leads to an overproduction of ROS in pancreatic acinar cells, affecting the mitochondria and inducing apoptosis and necrosis.[203,204] Alcohol is the most common cause of pancreatitis. Excessive alcohol consumption may cause the deposition of protein plugs in the pancreatic ducts, leading to obstruction. The presence of gallstones account for 25–40% of cases of pancreatitis; gallstone impaction at the ampulla of Vater causes hypertension in the pancreatic duct, initiating inflammation.[205] Infectious organisms account for 10% of acute pancreatitis cases, including viruses (e.g. mumps, Coxsackie B and hepatitis), bacteria (e.g. *Mycoplasma pneumoniae* and leptospirosis) and parasites (e.g. *Ascaris lumbricoides, Fasciola hepatica,* and hydatid disease).[206]

Autoimmune pancreatitis is a chronic fibroinflammatory disease of the pancreas. There are two main subtypes. Autoimmune type 1 is a multi-organ disease associated with immunoglobulin G4 (IgG4) and may include proximal bile duct strictures, retroperitoneal fibrosis, renal and salivary gland lesions and swelling of the pancreas. Autoimmune type 2 is a pancreas-specific disorder without systemic involvement.[207]

Pancreatitis usually presents with abdominal pain consistent with acute pancreatitis (acute onset of a persistent, severe, epigastric pain often radiating to the back). Serum lipase or amylase activity elevated more than three times the upper limit of normal (ULN) is a common finding. Characteristic findings of acute pancreatitis are revealed on contrast-enhanced computed tomography and magnetic resonance imaging or transabdominal ultrasonography.[208] The most common clinical presentation of chronic pancreatitis is midepigastric postprandial pain that radiates to the back that is relieved by sitting upright or leaning forwards.[209] Steatorrhoea, malabsorption, vitamin deficiencies (A, D, E, K, B12), diabetes, weight loss or obstructive jaundice may be present.[209,210]

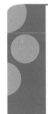

DIFFERENTIAL DIAGNOSIS

- Acute cholecystitis
- Acute pancreatitis
- Intestinal ischaemia or infarction
- Obstruction of the common bile duct
- Pancreatic cancer
- Peptic ulcers or gastritis
- Renal insufficiency

Source: Nair et al. 2007[209]

Risk factors

- Excessive alcohol consumption—leads to endoplasmic reticulum stress and abnormal unfolded protein responses in pancreas, up-regulation of autophagy and ROS[211]
- Cholelithiasis
- Abdominal trauma
- Infectious organisms: viruses, bacteria and parasites[206]
- Hyperlipidaemia
- Viral infections
- Medications (azathioprine, thiazides and oestrogens)
- Obesity and smoking increase the risk of progression to severe pancreatitis[212]
- Genetics—patients with mutations in genes linked to cationic and anionic trypsinogen, serine protease inhibitor Kazal 1, cystic fibrosis transmembrane conductance

regulator, chymotrypsinogen C and calcium-sensing receptor have been shown to be at increased risk of pancreatitis[212]
- Environmental (petrochemical fumes)[210]
- Untreated acute pancreatitis
- Possible autoimmune factor
- HIV/AIDS (comorbid factors and HAART)[213]

Conventional treatment
- Autoimmune pancreatitis: corticosteroids[207.]
- Strong opioids for acute pain
- Removal of gallstones
- Antimicrobials—broad-spectrum antibiotics
- No effective treatment for chronic pancreatitis pain
- Acute: restoration of blood volume and electrolyte balance, replace fluids and minimise pancreatic ischaemia[212]
- Enteral feeding[212] to support/avoid malnutrition and development of chronic pancreatitis
- If pancreatitis with hypertriglyceridaemia: weight loss, exercise, blood sugar control, lipid-restriction diet

Key treatment protocols
- *Encourage beneficial dietary and lifestyle changes.* Cease alcohol and tobacco use. Eat low-fat and small meals.[209] (See Chapter 3 on wellness.)
- *Reduce oxidative stress and pain.* Daily antioxidant supplementation of 600 mcg selenium, 0.54 g ascorbic acid, 9000 IU beta-carotene, 270 IU alpha-tocopherol and 2 g methionine was effective in the reduction of pain and oxidative stress of chronic pancreatitis.[210]
- *Reduce inflammation.* In experimental pancreatitis (rat model) curcumin reduced inflammation via inhibition of NF-kappa-B and activator protein-1,[214] and *Taraxacum officinale* reduced IL-6 and TNF-α levels in acute pancreatitis.[215] A TCM formulation targeting pancreatitis contained: *Bupleurum falcatum* (anti-inflammatory), *Glycyrrhiza glabra* (anti-inflammatory and secretin-stimulating), *Panax ginseng* (tonic and free radical scavenging antioxidant) and *Paeonia lactiflora* (proton pump inhibition). This herbal combination improved pancreatic ischaemia.[216]

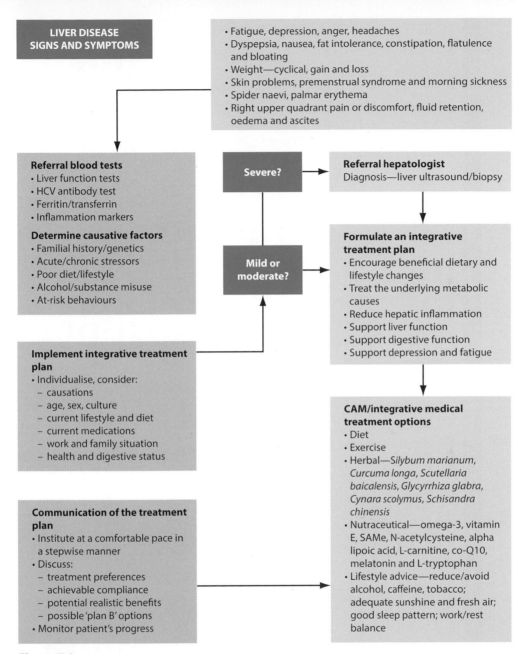

LIVER DISEASE SIGNS AND SYMPTOMS
- Fatigue, depression, anger, headaches
- Dyspepsia, nausea, fat intolerance, constipation, flatulence and bloating
- Weight—cyclical, gain and loss
- Skin problems, premenstrual syndrome and morning sickness
- Spider naevi, palmar erythema
- Right upper quadrant pain or discomfort, fluid retention, oedema and ascites

Referral blood tests
- Liver function tests
- HCV antibody test
- Ferritin/transferrin
- Inflammation markers

Determine causative factors
- Familial history/genetics
- Acute/chronic stressors
- Poor diet/lifestyle
- Alcohol/substance misuse
- At-risk behaviours

Severe?

Mild or moderate?

Referral hepatologist
Diagnosis—liver ultrasound/biopsy

Formulate an integrative treatment plan
- Encourage beneficial dietary and lifestyle changes
- Treat the underlying metabolic causes
- Reduce hepatic inflammation
- Support liver function
- Support digestive function
- Support depression and fatigue

Implement integrative treatment plan
- Individualise, consider:
  - causations
  - age, sex, culture
  - current lifestyle and diet
  - current medications
  - work and family situation
  - health and digestive status

CAM/integrative medical treatment options
- Diet
- Exercise
- Herbal—*Silybum marianum, Curcuma longa, Scutellaria baicalensis, Glycyrrhiza glabra, Cynara scolymus, Schisandra chinensis*
- Nutraceutical—omega-3, vitamin E, SAMe, N-acetylcysteine, alpha lipoic acid, L-carnitine, co-Q10, melatonin and L-tryptophan
- Lifestyle advice—reduce/avoid alcohol, caffeine, tobacco; adequate sunshine and fresh air; good sleep pattern; work/rest balance

Communication of the treatment plan
- Institute at a comfortable pace in a stepwise manner
- Discuss:
  - treatment preferences
  - achievable compliance
  - potential realistic benefits
  - possible 'plan B' options
- Monitor patient's progress

Figure 7.3
Naturopathic treatment decision tree—liver disease

Table 7.2
Review of the major evidence for liver disease

Intervention	Mechanisms of action	Literature	Summary of results	Comment
Realsil: Silybin 94 mg, phosphatidylcholine 194 mg and α-tocopherol 30 mg	Inhibits and scavenges free radicals; protects lipid membranes; regulates cell signalling pathways involved in obesity and insulin resistance; reduces cell migration, TGF-beta-induced synthesis of procollagen type I and secretion of MMP-2 phosphatidylcholine protects against oxidative stress-mediated liver damage	Loguerico et al. 2012[217]	Significant normalisation of ALT, AST and GGT over 12 months Blood glucose was 31% lower in the treated group compared with placebo	Realsil significantly reduced liver inflammation and improved dysglycaemia in NAFLD patients without increases in body weight
Silybum marianum (active isolate: silibinin) Silibinin	Antiviral, antioxidant, anti-inflammatory, hepatoprotective and antifibrotic effects	Fried et al. 2012[218] Guedj et al. 2012[219] Kim et al. 2012[220] Polyak et al. 2010[221] Salomone et al. 2017[222] Wah et al. 2017[223] Zhong et al. 2017[224]	A range of studies have revealed activities that may be beneficial in liver dysfunction and disease including reduced inflammatory cytokines activity: IL-4, IL-10, TNF-α, IFN-γ, VEGF-A, TGF-β and NF-κB activity Silibinin has prevented viral infection Silibinin inhibited TGF-β induced *de novo* synthesis of pro-collagen I Silibinin inhibits de novo lipogenesis, restores NAD⁺ levels, induces SIRT1/AMPK signaling and promotes mitochondrial β-oxidation in vivo and in vitro[222] Positive efficacy to reduce transaminases levels in NAFLD patients[224]	Intravenous use of silibinin is promising as an antiviral in HCV[175]
Scutellaria baicalensis (active isolate: baicalin)	Baicalin ameliorates ischaemia/reperfusion-induced hepatocellular damage by suppressing TLR4-mediated inflammatory responses in ALD[74] Alleviates palmitic-acid-induced cytotoxicity in AML-12 cells via suppression of ER stress and TXNIP/NLRP3 inflammasome activation[225]	Guo et al. 2009[73] Kim et al. 2012[74] Zhang et al. 2017[225]	Results have found baicalin reduces dyslipidaemia, hepatic lipid accumulation and visceral fat mass in vivo, improves hepatic steatosis[73] Reduced serum ALT, TNF-α and IL-6 in alcoholic fatty liver	The antioxidant and anti-inflammatory actions of baicalin and *Scutellaria baicalensis* make it a very useful clinical tool in NAFLD[73] and ALD[74]

Table 7.2
Review of the major evidence for liver disease (continued)

Intervention	Mechanisms of action	Literature	Summary of results	Comment
Curcuma longa	Shown in a range of studies to have antioxidant, anti-inflammatory and anti-fibrotic actions	Ak et al. 2008[226] Honda et al. 2006[54] Rahmani et al. 2016[227] Chenari et al. 2017[228]	Antioxidant, radical scavenging and metal chelating effects in animal models Prevented thioacetamide-induced cirrhosis, and hepatic fibrosis, inhibited hepatic stellate cell (HSC) activation Suppressed connective tissue growth factor expression in HSC activation	*Curcuma longa* reduces liver injury through down-regulation of inflammatory processes[229]
Cynara scolymus	Shown in a range of studies to have antioxidant, anti-inflammatory, choleretic and hepatoprotective actions, which may be of benefit for a range of liver conditions Anti-hyperglycemic, hypolipidemic	Speroni et al. 2003[88] Qiang et al. 2012[199] Ben Salem et al. 2017[230] Mocelin et al. 2016[231] Sahebkar et al. 2018[232]	Normalisation of AST and ALT Reduction of histological changes and accumulation of triglycerides[88] Lowered hamster plasma cholesterol levels by a mechanism involving the greater excretion of fecal bile acids and neutral sterols after feeding for 42 days[199]	Lowers cholesterol and triglyceride levels through stimulating bile production and flow
Glycyrrhiza glabra	Shown in a range of studies to have several beneficial actions for liver conditions including antiviral, anti-inflammatory and hepatoprotective effects Antimicrobial, antioxidative, antidiabetic, anticancer activities as well as immunomodulatory, gastro-protective, neuro-protective and cardio-protective effects	Hajiaghamohammadi et al. 2012[75] Wu et al. 2008[76] Rhee et al. 2012[77] Wang et al. 2013[233] Hosseinzadeh et al. 2017[234]	Lowered ALT and AST Prevented lipotoxicity and regulated apoptosis Reversed FFA-induced mitochondrial membrane depolarisation in HepG2 cells	Glycyrrhiza's anti-inflammatory and protective actions have significant benefits in treating NAFLD via altering gene expression pathways seen in fibrosis and reducing hepatic inflammation
Schisandra chinensis	Shown in a range of studies to have antioxidant, hepatoprotective, antiobesity and antidiabetic actions, which may benefit several liver conditions Hypolipidemic	Pan et al. 2008[89] Park et al. 2012[235] Chung et al. 2017[236]	Decreased hepatic total cholesterol and triglyceride levels (by up to 50% and 52%, respectively) in hypercholesterolaemic mice[89] Antiobesity action: reduced the accumulation of cellular triglycerides and induced inhibited differentiation and adipogenesis in 3T3-L1 cells in high-fat diet rats[229]	Hepatoprotective, especially in terms of lipid metabolism

Table 7.2
Review of the major evidence for liver disease (continued)

Intervention	Mechanisms of action	Literature	Summary of results	Comment
Alpha-lipoic acid 300–600 mg/day	Improves glucose uptake via up-regulation of GLUT4 receptors Antioxidant—scavenger and up-regulation of endogenous antioxidants via Nrf2/ARE Antifibrotic via inhibition of TGF-β and anti-inflammatory via inhibition of TNF-α induced NF-κB	Kaya-Dagistanlia et al. 2013[237] Castro et al. 2012[84] Hultberg et al. 2006[238] Min et al. 2010[239] Petersen Shay et al. 2008[240] Kim et al. 2004[241] Pilar Valdecantos et al. 2015[242]	Antidiabetic, antihyperlipidaemic, antioxidant, anti-inflammatory, antifibrotic	Decrease in fatty degeneration, inflammation and cell vacuolisation in hepatocytes
L-carnitine	Modulator of fatty acid transport and oxidation Improves beta-oxidation through protection and stimulation of mitochondrial function	Meta-analysis NAFLD Musso et al. 2010[243] Fujisawa et al. 2017[244]	Improves insulin sensitivity, modulates lipid profiles, glucose metabolism, oxidative stress and is anti-inflammatory and antifibrotic	Improves insulin sensitivity and promotes beta-oxidation
Berberine	Antimicrobial, antidiabetic, hypoglycemic, hypocholesterolemic, anti-tumoral, immunomodulatory properties, anti-inflammatory and antioxidant	Zhu et al. 2016[56] Zhao et al. 2017[57] Pirillo et al. 2015[58] Wei et al. 2017[59]	Berberine improves mitochondrial function[56] and inhibited hepatic lipogenesis[57]	Berberine is found in *Berberis vulgaris, Mahonia aquifolium, Hydrastis canadensis, Phellodendron amurense, Coptis chinensis, Eschscholzia californica*
Probiotics	Reduction of aminotransferases Immune support: inhibition of epithelial invasion, bacterial translocation, production of antimicrobial peptides Enhancement of insulin sensitivity Reduction in hepatic inflammation/steatosis, suppression of the TNFα/IKK-β signaling pathway, reduction of activity of Jun N-terminal kinase, decrease DNA binding activity of NF-κB	Doulberis et al. 2017[135]	Amelioration of hepatic steatosis and endotoxemia, prevention of NAFLD progression and tumorigenesis	Encouraging, though preliminary evidence which needs further study

KEY POINTS

- There is a cyclic relationship between metabolic syndrome and liver disease.

- Oxidative stress and inflammation drives pathology in liver disease and pancreatitis. This reduces liver and pancreatic function with systemic consequences for health.

- Effective detoxification can regulate hormones and have anti-carcinogenic effects through inhibition of phase I and induction of phase II enzymes.[94,102]

- Adjunctive naturopathic protocols, herbal medicines, nutraceuticals, probiotics, Mediterranean diet, exercise and lifestyle can attenuate disease progression by reducing inflammation and oxidative stress driven liver diseases such as NAFLD, NASH, ALD and HCV.

FURTHER READING

Buzzetti E, Pinzani M, Tsochatzis EA. The multiple-hit pathogenesis of non-alcoholic fatty liver disease (NAFLD). Metabolism 2016;65:1038–48.

Hernandez-Rodas MC, Valenzuela R, Videla LA. Relevant aspects of nutritional and dietary interventions in non-alcoholic fatty liver disease. Int J Mol Sci 2015;16:25168–98.

Katsagoni CN, Georgoulis M, Papatheodoridis GV, et al. Effects of lifestyle interventions on clinical characteristics of patients with non-alcoholic fatty liver disease: a meta-analysis. Metab Clin Exp 2017;68:119–32.

Kirpich IA, Marsano LS, McClain CJ. Gut-liver axis, nutrition, and non-alcoholic fatty liver disease. Clin Biochem 2015;48:923–30.

Reccia I, Kumar J, Akladios C, et al. Non-alcoholic fatty liver disease: a sign of systemic disease. Metab Clin Exp 2017;72:94–108.

Acknowledgments: Grateful acknowledgment goes to research assistant Hannah Boyd. This chapter contains material authored by Jon Wardle, which was previously in the *Endometriosis* chapter in the first edition.

REFERENCES

1. Mosely RH. Function of the normal liver. In: O'Grady JG, Lake JR, Howdle PD, editors. Comprehensive clinical hepatology. London: Harcourt Publishers Limited; 2000. p. 3, 1–16.

2. Finkel T, Holbrook NJ. Oxidants, oxidative stress and the biology of ageing. Nature 2000;408(6809):239–47.

3. Kung G, Konstantinidis K, Kitsis RN. Programmed necrosis, not apoptosis, in the heart. Circ Res 2011; 108(8):1017–36.

4. Medina-Santillán R, López-Velázquez JA, Chávez-Tapia N, et al. Hepatic manifestations of metabolic syndrome. Diabetes Metab Res Rev 2013;doi:10.1002/dmrr.2410.

5. Cave M, Deaciuc I, Mendez C, et al. Nonalcoholic fatty liver disease: predisposing factors and the role of nutrition. J Nutr Biochem 2007;18(3):184–95.

6. de Alwis NM, Day CP. Non-alcoholic fatty liver disease: the mist gradually clears. J Hepatol 2008;48(Suppl. 1): S104–12.

7. Younossi ZM. Review article: current management of non-alcoholic fatty liver disease and non-alcoholic steatohepatitis. Aliment Pharmacol Ther 2008;28(1): 2–12.

8. Chitturi S, Farrell GC, Hashimoto E, et al. Non-alcoholic fatty liver disease in the Asia-Pacific region: definitions and overview of proposed guidelines. J Gastroenterol Hepatol 2007;22(6):778–87.

9. Smith BW, Adams LA. Non-alcoholic fatty liver disease. Crit Rev Clin Lab Sci 2011;48(3):97–113.

10. Moore JB. Non-alcoholic fatty liver disease: the hepatic consequence of obesity and the metabolic syndrome. Proc Nutr Soc 2010;69(2):211–20.

11. Bhala N, Angulo P, van der Poorten D, et al. The natural history of nonalcoholic fatty liver disease with advanced fibrosis or cirrhosis: an international collaborative study. Hepatology 2011;54(4):1208–16.

12. Weinstein AA, Kallman Price J, Stepanova M, et al. Depression in patients with nonalcoholic fatty liver disease and chronic viral hepatitis B and C. Psychosomatics 2011;52(2):127–32.

13. Neuschwander-Tetri BA, Clark JM, Bass NM, et al. Clinical, laboratory and histological associations in adults with nonalcoholic fatty liver disease. Hepatology 2010;52(3):913–24.

14. Benhamed F, Denechaud PD, Lemoine M, et al. The lipogenic transcription factor ChREBP dissociates hepatic steatosis from insulin resistance in mice and humans. J Clin Invest 2012;122(6):2176–94.

15. Donnelly KL, Smith CI, Schwarzenberg SJ, et al. Sources of fatty acids stored in liver and secreted via lipoproteins in patients with nonalcoholic fatty liver disease. J Clin Invest 2005;115(5):1343–51.

16. Johnson NA, George J. Fitness versus fatness: moving beyond weight loss in nonalcoholic fatty liver disease. Hepatology 2010;52(1):370–81.

17. Reccia I, Kumar J, Akladios C, et al. Non-alcoholic fatty liver disease: a sign of systemic disease. Metabolism 2017;72:94–108. PubMed PMID: 28641788.

18. Brunt EM, Tiniakos DG. Histopathology of nonalcoholic fatty liver disease. World J Gastroenterol 2010;16(42):5286–96.

19. Kim D, Choi SY, Park EH, et al. Nonalcoholic fatty liver disease is associated with coronary artery calcification. Hepatology 2012;56(2):605–13.

20. Kalhan SC, Edmison J, Marczewski S, et al. Methionine and protein metabolism in non-alcoholic steatohepatitis: evidence for lower rate of transmethylation of methionine. Clin Sci 2011;121(4):179–89.

21. Vernon G, Baranova A, Younossi ZM. Systematic review: the epidemiology and natural history of non-alcoholic fatty liver disease and non-alcoholic steatohepatitis in adults. Aliment Pharmacol Ther 2011;34(3):274–85.

22. Adams LA, Lymp JF, St Sauver J, et al. The natural history of nonalcoholic fatty liver disease: a population-based cohort study. Gastroenterology 2005;129(1):113–21.

23. Zein CO, Unalp A, Colvin R, et al. Smoking and severity of hepatic fibrosis in nonalcoholic fatty liver disease. J Hepatol 2011;54(4):753–9.

24. Lombardi R, Onali S, Thorburn D, et al. Pharmacological interventions for non-alcohol related fatty liver disease (NAFLD): an attempted network meta-analysis. Cochrane Database Syst Rev 2017;(3):CD011640. PubMed PMID: 28358980.

25. Lomonaco R, Sunny NE, Bril F, et al. Nonalcoholic fatty liver disease: current issues and novel treatment approaches. Drugs 2013;73(1):1–14.

26. Mahady SE, Webster AC, Walker S, et al. The role of thiazolidinediones in non-alcoholic steatohepatitis— a systematic review and meta analysis. J Hepatol 2011;55(6):1383–90.

27. Keating SE, Hackett DA, George J, et al. Exercise and non-alcoholic fatty liver disease: a systematic review and meta-analysis. J Hepatol 2012;57(1):157–66.

28. Romero-Gomez M, Zelber-Sagi S, Trenell M. Treatment of NAFLD with diet, physical activity and exercise. J Hepatol 2017;67(4):829–46. PubMed PMID: 28545937.

29. European Association for the Study of the L, European Association for the Study of D, European Association for the Study of O. EASL-EASD-EASO Clinical Practice Guidelines for the management of non-alcoholic fatty liver disease. J Hepatol 2016;64(6):1388–402. PubMed PMID: 27062661.

30. Eslamparast T, Tandon P, Raman M. Dietary composition independent of weight loss in the management of non-alcoholic fatty liver disease. Nutrients 2017;9(8):PubMed PMID: 28933748. PubMed Central PMCID: 5579594.

31. Zelber-Sagi S, Salomone F, Mlynarsky L. The Mediterranean dietary pattern as the diet of choice for non-alcoholic fatty liver disease: evidence and plausible mechanisms. Liver Int 2017;37(7):936–49. PubMed PMID: 28371239.

32. Mayes PA. Intermediary metabolism of fructose. Am J Clin Nutr 1993;58(5 Suppl.):754S–765S.

33. Yki-Jarvinen H. Nutritional modulation of nonalcoholic fatty liver disease and insulin resistance: human data. Curr Opin Clin Nutr Metab Care 2010;13(6):709–14.

34. Kohli R, Kirby M, Xanthakos SA, et al. High-fructose, medium chain trans fat diet induces liver fibrosis and elevates plasma coenzyme Q9 in a novel murine model of obesity and nonalcoholic steatohepatitis. Hepatology 2010;52(3):934–44.

35. Song M, Schuschke DA, Zhou Z, et al. High fructose feeding induces copper deficiency in Sprague-Dawley rats: a novel mechanism for obesity related fatty liver. J Hepatol 2012;56(2):433–40.

36. Garcia-Caraballo SC, Comhair TM, Verheyen F, et al. Prevention and reversal of hepatic steatosis with a high-protein diet in mice. Biochim Biophys Acta 2013;1832(5):685–95.

37. Kirk E, Reeds DN, Finck BN, et al. Dietary fat and carbohydrates differentially alter insulin sensitivity during caloric restriction. Gastroenterology 2009;136(5):1552–60.

38. Somi MH, Rezaeifar P, Ostad Rahimi A, et al. Effects of low dose zinc supplementation on biochemical markers in non-alcoholic cirrhosis: a randomized clinical trial. Arch Iran Med 2012;15(8):472–6.

39. Lee S, Bacha F, Hannon T, et al. Effects of aerobic versus resistance exercise without caloric restriction on abdominal fat, intrahepatic lipid, and insulin sensitivity in obese adolescent boys: a randomized, controlled trial. Diabetes 2012;61(11):2787–95.

40. Hallsworth K, Fattakhova G, Hollingsworth KG, et al. Resistance exercise reduces liver fat and its mediators in non-alcoholic fatty liver disease independent of weight loss. Gut 2011;60(9):1278–83.

41. Hashida R, Kawaguchi T, Bekki M, et al. Aerobic vs. resistance exercise in non-alcoholic fatty liver disease: a systematic review. J Hepatol 2017;66(1):142–52. PubMed PMID: 27639843.

42. Rodriguez-Hernandez H, Cervantes-Huerta M, Rodriguez-Moran M, et al. Decrease of aminotransferase levels in obese women is related to body weight reduction, irrespective of type of diet. Ann Hepatol 2011;10(4):486–92.

43. Tilg H, Moschen A. Weight loss: cornerstone in the treatment of non-alcoholic fatty liver disease. Minerva Gastroenterol Dietol 2010;56(2):159–67.

44. Golabi P, Locklear CT, Austin P, et al. Effectiveness of exercise in hepatic fat mobilization in non-alcoholic fatty liver disease: systematic review. World J Gastroenterol 2016;22(27):6318–27. PubMed PMID: 27468220. PubMed Central PMCID: 4945989.

45. Sreenivasa Baba C, Alexander G, Kalyani B, et al. Effect of exercise and dietary modification on serum aminotransferase levels in patients with nonalcoholic steatohepatitis. J Gastroenterol Hepatol 2006;21(1 Pt 1):191–8.

46. Kistler KD, Brunt EM, Clark JM, et al. Physical activity recommendations, exercise intensity, and histological severity of nonalcoholic fatty liver disease. Am J Gastroenterol 2011;106(3):460–8, quiz 469.

47. Fealy CE, Haus JM, Solomon TP, et al. Short-term exercise reduces markers of hepatocyte apoptosis in nonalcoholic fatty liver disease. J Appl Physiol 2012;113(1):1–6.

48. Simpson KA, Singh MA. Effects of exercise on adiponectin: a systematic review. Obesity (Silver Spring) 2008;16(2):241–56.

49. Mann DA, Marra F. Fibrogenic signalling in hepatic stellate cells. J Hepatol 2010;52(6):949–50.

50. Coker RH, Williams RH, Yeo SE, et al. The impact of exercise training compared to caloric restriction on hepatic and peripheral insulin resistance in obesity. J Clin Endocrinol Metab 2009;94(11):4258–66.

51. Nobili V, Bedogni G, Alisi A, et al. Docosahexaenoic acid supplementation decreases liver fat content in children with non-alcoholic fatty liver disease: double-blind randomised controlled clinical trial. Arch Dis Child 2011;96(4):350–3.

52. Sanyal AJ, Chalasani N, Kowdley KV, et al. Pioglitazone, vitamin E, or placebo for nonalcoholic steatohepatitis. N Engl J Med 2010;362(18):1675–85.

53. Sato K, Gosho M, Yamamoto T, et al. Vitamin E has a beneficial effect on nonalcoholic fatty liver disease: a

meta-analysis of randomized controlled trials. Nutrition 2015;31(7–8):923–30. PubMed PMID: 26059365.

54. Honda S, Aoki F, Tanaka H, et al. Effects of ingested turmeric oleoresin on glucose and lipid metabolisms in obese diabetic mice: a DNA microarray study. J Agric Food Chem 2006;54(24):9055–62.

55. Rahmani S, Asgary S, Askari G, et al. Treatment of non-alcoholic fatty liver disease with curcumin: a randomized placebo-controlled trial. Phytother Res 2016;30(9):1540–8. PubMed PMID: 27270872.

56. Zhu X, Bian H, Gao X. The potential mechanisms of berberine in the treatment of nonalcoholic fatty liver disease. Molecules 2016;21(10):PubMed PMID: 27754444.

57. Zhao L, Cang Z, Sun H, et al. Berberine improves glucogenesis and lipid metabolism in nonalcoholic fatty liver disease. BMC Endocr Disord 2017;17(1):13. PubMed PMID: 28241817. Pubmed Central PMCID: 5329945.

58. Pirillo A, Catapano AL. Berberine, a plant alkaloid with lipid- and glucose-lowering properties: from in vitro evidence to clinical studies. Atherosclerosis 2015;243(2):449–61. PubMed PMID: 26520899.

59. Wei X, Wang C, Hao S, et al. The therapeutic effect of berberine in the treatment of nonalcoholic fatty liver disease: a meta-analysis. Evid Based Complement Alternat Med 2016;2016:3593951. PubMed PMID: 27446224. Pubmed Central PMCID: 4947506.

60. Polyak SJ, Oberlies NH, Pecheur EI, et al. Silymarin for HCV infection. Antivir Ther 2013;18(2):141–7.

61. Son TG, Camandola S, Mattson MP. Hormetic dietary phytochemicals. Neuromolecular Med 2008;10(4):236–46.

62. Ristow M, Schmeisser S. Extending life span by increasing oxidative stress. Free Radic Biol Med 2011;51(2):327–36.

63. Ristow M, Zarse K. How increased oxidative stress promotes longevity and metabolic health: the concept of mitochondrial hormesis (mitohormesis). Exp Gerontol 2010;45(6):410–18.

64. Villanueva C, Kross RD. Antioxidant-induced stress. Int J Mol Sci 2012;13(2):2091–109.

65. Surh YJ. Xenohormesis mechanisms underlying chemopreventive effects of some dietary phytochemicals. Ann N Y Acad Sci 2011;1229:1–6.

66. Kim J, Cha YN, Surh YJ. A protective role of nuclear factor-erythroid 2-related factor-2 (Nrf2) in inflammatory disorders. Mutat Res 2010;690(1–2):12–23.

67. Chlopcikova S, Psotova J, Miketova P, et al. Chemoprotective effect of plant phenolics against anthracycline-induced toxicity on rat cardiomyocytes. Part I. Silymarin and its flavonolignans. Phytother Res 2004;18(2):107–10.

68. Aghazadeh S, Amini R, Yazdanparast R, et al. Anti-apoptotic and anti-inflammatory effects of Silybum marianum in treatment of experimental steatohepatitis. Exp Toxicol Pathol 2011;63(6):569–74.

69. Polyak SJ, Morishima C, Shuhart MC, et al. Inhibition of T-cell inflammatory cytokines, hepatocyte NF-kappaB signaling, and HCV infection by standardized Silymarin. Gastroenterology 2007;132(5):1925–36.

70. Hernandez-Gea V, Friedman SL. Pathogenesis of liver fibrosis. Annu Rev Pathol 2011;6:425–56.

71. Trappoliere M, Caligiuri A, Schmid M, et al. Silybin, a component of silymarin, exerts anti-inflammatory and anti-fibrogenic effects on human hepatic stellate cells. J Hepatol 2009;50(6):1102–11.

72. Lin J, Zheng S, Chen A. Curcumin attenuates the effects of insulin on stimulating hepatic stellate cell activation by interrupting insulin signaling and attenuating oxidative stress. Lab Invest 2009;89(12):1397–409.

73. Guo HX, Liu DH, Ma Y, et al. Long-term baicalin administration ameliorates metabolic disorders and hepatic steatosis in rats given a high-fat diet. Acta Pharmacol Sin 2009;30(11):1505–12.

74. Kim SJ, Lee SM. Effect of baicalin on toll-like receptor 4-mediated ischemia/reperfusion inflammatory responses in alcoholic fatty liver condition. Toxicol Appl Pharmacol 2012;258(1):43–50.

75. Hajiaghamohammadi AA, Ziaee A, Samimi R. The efficacy of licorice root extract in decreasing transaminase activities in non-alcoholic fatty liver disease: a randomized controlled clinical trial. Phytother Res 2012;26(9):1381–4.

76. Wu X, Zhang L, Gurley E, et al. Prevention of free fatty acid-induced hepatic lipotoxicity by 18beta-glycyrrhetinic acid through lysosomal and mitochondrial pathways. Hepatology 2008;47(6):1905–15.

77. Rhee SD, Kim CH, Park JS, et al. Carbenoxolone prevents the development of fatty liver in C57BL/6-Lep ob/ ob mice via the inhibition of sterol regulatory element binding protein-1c activity and apoptosis. Eur J Pharmacol 2012;691(1–3):9–18.

78. Kar P, Laight D, Rooprai HK, et al. Effects of grape seed extract in Type 2 diabetic subjects at high cardiovascular risk: a double blind randomized placebo controlled trial examining metabolic markers, vascular tone, inflammation, oxidative stress and insulin sensitivity. Diabet Med 2009;26(5):526–31.

79. Khoshbaten M, Aliasgarzadeh A, Masnadi K, et al. Grape seed extract to improve liver function in patients with nonalcoholic fatty liver change. Saudi J Gastroenterol 2010;16(3):194–7.

80. White DL, Richardson PA, Al-Saadi M, et al. Dietary history and physical activity and risk of advanced liver disease in veterans with chronic hepatitis C infection. Dig Dis Sci 2011;56(6):1835–47.

81. Rolo AP, Teodoro JS, Palmeira CM. Role of oxidative stress in the pathogenesis of nonalcoholic steatohepatitis. Free Radic Biol Med 2012;52(1):59–69.

82. Lim CY, Jun DW, Jang SS, et al. Effects of carnitine on peripheral blood mitochondrial DNA copy number and liver function in non-alcoholic fatty liver disease. Korean J Gastroenterol 2010;55(6):384–9.

83. Jun DW, Cho WK, Jun JH, et al. Prevention of free fatty acid-induced hepatic lipotoxicity by carnitine via reversal of mitochondrial dysfunction. Liver Int 2011;31(9): 1315–24.

84. Castro MC, Massa ML, Schinella G, et al. Lipoic acid prevents liver metabolic changes induced by administration of a fructose-rich diet. Biochim Biophys Acta 2012; 1830(1):226–32.

85. Gane EJ, Weilert F, Orr DW, et al. The mitochondria-targeted anti-oxidant mitoquinone decreases liver damage in a phase II study of hepatitis C patients. Liver Int 2010;30(7):1019–26.

86. Cichoz-Lach H, Celinski K, Konturek PC, et al. The effects of L-tryptophan and melatonin on selected biochemical parameters in patients with steatohepatitis. J Physiol Pharmacol 2010;61(5):577–80.

87. Di Pierro F, Villanova N, Agostini F, et al. Pilot study on the additive effects of berberine and oral type 2 diabetes agents for patients with suboptimal glycemic control. Diabetes Metab Syndr Obes 2012;5:213–17.

88. Speroni E, Cervellati R, Govoni P, et al. Efficacy of different Cynara scolymus preparations on liver complaints. J Ethnopharmacol 2003;86(2–3):203–11.

89. Pan SY, Dong H, Zhao XY, et al. Schisandrin B from Schisandra chinensis reduces hepatic lipid contents in hypercholesterolaemic mice. J Pharm Pharmacol 2008;60(3):399–403.

90. Anstee QM, Day CP. S-adenosylmethionine (SAMe) therapy in liver disease: a review of current evidence and clinical utility. J Hepatol 2012;57(5):1097–109.

91. Khoshbaten M, Aliasgarzadeh A, Masnadi K, et al. N-acetylcysteine improves liver function in patients with non-alcoholic fatty liver disease. Hepat Mon 2010;10(1):12–16.

92. Salmond S. The hepatobiliary system. In: Hechtman L, editor. Clinical naturopathic medicine. Australia: Elsevier; 2011. p. 210–79.

93. Walter-Sack I, Klotz U. Influence of diet and nutritional status on drug metabolism. Clin Pharmacokinet 1996;31(1):47–64.

94. Moon YJ, Wang X, Morris ME. Dietary flavonoids: effects on xenobiotic and carcinogen metabolism. Toxicol In Vitro 2006;20(2):187–210.

95. Cornelis MC, El-Sohemy A, Kabagambe EK, et al. Coffee, CYP1A2 genotype, and risk of myocardial infarction. J Am Med Assoc 2006;295(10):1135–41.

96. Hornsby LB, Hester EK, Donaldson AR. Potential interaction between warfarin and high dietary protein intake. Pharmacotherapy 2008;28(4):536–9.

97. Cermak R. Effect of dietary flavonoids on pathways involved in drug metabolism. Expert Opin Drug Metab Toxicol 2008;4(1):17–35.

98. Horváthová E, Slameňová D, Navarová J. Administration of rosemary essential oil enhances resistance of rat hepatocytes against DNA-damaging oxidative agents. Food Chem 2010;123(1):151–6.

99. Di Marco MP, Edwards DJ, Wainer IW, et al. The effect of grapefruit juice and Seville orange juice on the pharmacokinetics of dextromethorphan: the role of gut CYP3A and P-glycoprotein. Life Sci 2002;71(10):1149–60.

100. Wason S, DiGiacinto JL, Davis MW. Effects of grapefruit and Seville orange juices on the pharmacokinetic properties of colchicine in healthy subjects. Clin Ther 2012;34(10):2161–73.

101. Johri RK. Cuminum cyminum and Carum carvi: an update. Pharmacogn Rev 2011;5(9):63–72.

102. Konsue N, Ioannides C. Modulation of carcinogen-metabolising cytochromes P450 in human liver by the chemopreventive phytochemical phenethyl isothiocyanate, a constituent of cruciferous vegetables. Toxicology 2010;268(3):184–90.

103. Munday R, Munday CM. Induction of phase II enzymes by aliphatic sulfides derived from garlic and onions: an overview. Methods Enzymol 2004;382:449–56.

104. Chen C, Pung D, Leong V, et al. Induction of detoxifying enzymes by garlic organosulfur compounds through transcription factor Nrf2: effect of chemical structure and stress signals. Free Radic Biol Med 2004;37(10):1578–90.

105. Iwata H, Tezuka Y, Kadota S, et al. Identification and characterization of potent CYP3A4 inhibitors in Schisandra fruit extract. Drug Metab Dispos 2004;32(12):1351–8.

106. Jeong HG, You HJ, Park SJ, et al. Hepatoprotective effects of 18beta-glycyrrhetinic acid on carbon tetrachloride-induced liver injury: inhibition of cytochrome P450 2E1 expression. Pharmacol Res 2002;46(3):221–7.

107. Subehan, Zaidi SF, Kadota S, et al. Inhibition on human liver cytochrome P450 3A4 by constituents of fennel (Foeniculum vulgare): identification and characterization of a mechanism-based inactivator. J Agric Food Chem 2007;55(25):10162–7.

108. Kiruthiga PV, Karthikeyan K, Archunan G, et al. Silymarin prevents benzo(a)pyrene-induced toxicity in Wistar rats by modulating xenobiotic-metabolizing enzymes. Toxicol Ind Health 2015;31(6):523–41. doi:10.1177/0748233713475524.

109. Balstad TR, Carlsen H, Myhrstad MC, et al. Coffee, broccoli and spices are strong inducers of electrophile response element-dependent transcription in vitro and in vivo—studies in electrophile response element transgenic mice. Mol Nutr Food Res 2011;55(2):185–97.

110. Nirmala K, Krishna PT, Polasa K. Modulation of xenobiotic metabolism in ginger (Zingiber officinale Roscoe) fed rats. Int J Nutr Metab 2010;2(3):56–62.

111. Munday R, Munday CM. Induction of phase II enzymes by 3H-1,2-dithiole-3-thione: dose-response study in rats. Carcinogenesis 2004;25(9):1721–5.

112. Lee SB, Kim CY, Lee HJ, et al. Induction of the phase II detoxification enzyme NQO1 in hepatocarcinoma cells by lignans from the fruit of Schisandra chinensis through nuclear accumulation of Nrf2. Planta Med 2009;75(12):1314–18.

113. Son TG, Camandola S, Mattson MP. Hormetic dietary phytochemicals. Neuromolecular Med 2008;10(4):236–46.

114. Dietz BM, Hagos GK, Eskra JN, et al. Differential regulation of detoxification enzymes in hepatic and mammary tissue by hops (Humulus lupulus) in vitro and in vivo. Mol Nutr Food Res 2013;57(6):1055–66.

115. Moon A, Kim SH. Effect of Glycyrrhiza glabra roots and glycyrrhizin on the glucuronidation in rats. Planta Med 1997;63(2):115–19.

116. Zegura B, Dobnik D, Niderl MH, et al. Antioxidant and antigenotoxic effects of rosemary (Rosmarinus officinalis L.) extracts in Salmonella typhimurium TA98 and HepG2 cells. Environ Toxicol Pharmacol 2011;32(2):296–305.

117. Huisman EJ, Trip EJ, Siersema PD, et al. Protein energy malnutrition predicts complications in liver cirrhosis. Eur J Gastroenterol Hepatol 2011;23(11):982–9.

118. Chadalavada R, Sappati Biyyani RS, Maxwell J, et al. Nutrition in hepatic encephalopathy. Nutr Clin Pract 2010;25(3):257–64.

119. Ambuhl PM. Protein intake in renal and hepatic disease. Int J Vitam Nutr Res 2011;81(2–3):162–72.

120. Plank LD, Gane EJ, Peng S, et al. Nocturnal nutritional supplementation improves total body protein status of patients with liver cirrhosis: a randomized 12-month trial. Hepatology 2008;48(2):557–66.

121. Mukherjee PK, Ponnusankar S, Pandit S, et al. Botanicals as medicinal food and their effects on drug metabolizing enzymes. Food Chem Toxicol 2011;49(12):3142–53.

122. Talalay P. Mechanisms of induction of enzymes that protect against chemical carcinogenesis. Adv Enzyme Regul 1989;28:237–50.

123. Enomoto N, Ikejima K, Bradford BU, et al. Role of Kupffer cells and gut-derived endotoxins in alcoholic liver injury. J Gastroenterol Hepatol 2000;15(Suppl.):D20–5.

124. Gurley BJ, Gardner SF, Hubbard MA, et al. Cytochrome P450 phenotypic ratios for predicting herb-drug interactions in humans. Clin Pharmacol Ther 2002;72(3):276–87.

125. Mullerova D, Kopecky J. White adipose tissue: storage and effector site for environmental pollutants. Physiol Res 2007;56(4):375–81.

126. Stiefelhagen P. Functional disorders call for total therapy—Kneipp's hydrotherapy instead of psychopharmaceuticals. MMW Fortschr Med 2005;147(18):4–6, 8.

127. Krop J. Chemical sensitivity after intoxication at work with solvents: response to sauna therapy. J Altern Complement Med 1998;4(1):77–86.

128. Hannuksela ML, Ellahham S. Benefits and risks of sauna bathing. Am J Med 2001;110(2):118–26.

129. Duncan K, Harris S, Ardies CM. Running exercise may reduce risk for lung and liver cancer by inducing

activity of antioxidant and phase II enzymes. Cancer Lett 1997;116(2):151–8.

130. Yiamouyiannis CA, Sanders RA, Watkins JB 3rd, et al. Chronic physical activity: hepatic hypertrophy and increased total biotransformation enzyme activity. Biochem Pharmacol 1992;44(1):121–7.

131. Cohen M. 'Detox': science or sales pitch? Aust Fam Physician 2007;36(12):1009–10.

132. Aller R, De Luis DA, Izaola O, et al. Effect of a probiotic on liver aminotransferases in nonalcoholic fatty liver disease patients: a double blind randomized clinical trial. Eur Rev Med Pharmacol Sci 2011;15(9):1090–5.

133. Malaguarnera M, Vacante M, Antic T, et al. Bifidobacterium longum with fructo-oligosaccharides in patients with non alcoholic steatohepatitis. Dig Dis Sci 2012;57(2):545–53.

134. Bashiardes S, Shapiro H, Rozin S, et al. Non-alcoholic fatty liver and the gut microbiota. Mol Metab 2016;5(9):782–94. PubMed PMID: 27617201. Pubmed Central PMCID: 5004228.

135. Doulberis M, Kotronis G, Gialamprinou D, et al. Non-alcoholic fatty liver disease: an update with special focus on the role of gut microbiota. Metab Clin Exp 2017;71:182–97. PubMed PMID: 28521872.

136. Shen F, Zheng RD, Sun XQ, et al. Gut microbiota dysbiosis in patients with non-alcoholic fatty liver disease. HBPD INT 2017;16(4):375–81. PubMed PMID: 28823367.

137. Xue L, He J, Gao N, et al. Probiotics may delay the progression of nonalcoholic fatty liver disease by restoring the gut microbiota structure and improving intestinal endotoxemia. Sci Rep 2017;7:45176. PubMed PMID: 28349964. Pubmed Central PMCID: 5368635.

138. Jiang W, Wu N, Wang X, et al. Dysbiosis gut microbiota associated with inflammation and impaired mucosal immune function in intestine of humans with non-alcoholic fatty liver disease. Sci Rep 2015;5:8096. PubMed PMID: 25644696. Pubmed Central PMCID: 4314632.

139. Eliades M, Spyrou E. Vitamin D: a new player in non-alcoholic fatty liver disease? World J Gastroenterol 2015;21(6):1718–27. PubMed PMID: 25684936. Pubmed Central PMCID: 4323447.

140. Paolella G, Mandato C, Pierri L, et al. Gut-liver axis and probiotics: their role in non-alcoholic fatty liver disease. World J Gastroenterol 2014;20(42):15518–31. PubMed PMID: 25400436. Pubmed Central PMCID: 4229517.

141. Leung C, Rivera L, Furness JB, et al. The role of the gut microbiota in NAFLD. Nat Rev Gastroenterol Hepatol 2016;13(7):412–25. PubMed PMID: 27273168.

142. Machado MV, Cortez-Pinto H. Diet, microbiota, obesity, and NAFLD: a dangerous quartet. Int J Mol Sci 2016;17(4):481. PubMed PMID: 27043550. Pubmed Central PMCID: 4848937.

143. Yasutake K, Kohjima M, Kotoh K, et al. Dietary habits and behaviors associated with nonalcoholic fatty liver disease. World J Gastroenterol 2014;20(7):1756–67. PubMed PMID: 24587653. Pubmed Central PMCID: 3930974.

144. Ashrafi M, Modabbernia A, Dalir M, et al. Predictors of mental and physical health in non-cirrhotic patients with viral hepatitis: a case control study. J Psychosom Res 2012;73(3):218–24.

145. Lee K, Otgonsuren M, Younoszai Z, et al. Association of chronic liver disease with depression: a population-based study. Psychosomatics 2013;54(1):52–9.

146. WHO. Hepatitis C. Fact sheet. WHO; 2017 (updated October 2017; cited 15 November 2017). Available from: http://www.who.int/mediacentre/factsheets/fs164/en/.

147. Dore GJ, Law M, MacDonald M, et al. Epidemiology of hepatitis C virus infection in Australia. J Clin Virol 2003;26(2):171–84.

148. Hoofnagle JH. Course and outcome of hepatitis C. Hepatology 2002;36(5 Suppl. 1):S21–9.

149. Barrett S, Goh J, Coughlan B, et al. The natural course of hepatitis C virus infection after 22 years in a unique homogenous cohort: spontaneous viral clearance and chronic HCV infection. Gut 2001;49(3):423–30.

150. Farrell GC. Chronic viral hepatitis. Med J Aust 1998;168(12):619–26.

151. Missiha SB, Ostrowski M, Heathcote EJ. Disease progression in chronic hepatitis C: modifiable and nonmodifiable factors. Gastroenterology 2008;134(6):1699–714.

152. Ioannou GN, Beste LA, Chang MF, et al. Effectiveness of sofosbuvir, ledipasvir/sofosbuvir, or paritaprevir/ritonavir/ombitasvir and dasabuvir regimens for treatment of patients with hepatitis C in the Veterans Affairs National Health Care system. Gastroenterology 2016;151(3):457–71, e5. PubMed PMID: 27267053.

153. Sarrazin C, Zeuzem S. Resistance to direct antiviral agents in patients with hepatitis C virus infection. Gastroenterology 2010;138(2):447–62. [Epub 2009/12/17]; PubMed PMID: 20006612. eng.

154. Costantino A, Spada E, Equestre M, et al. Naturally occurring mutations associated with resistance to HCV NS5B polymerase and NS3 protease inhibitors in treatment-naive patients with chronic hepatitis C. Virol J 2015;12:186. PubMed PMID: 26577836. Pubmed Central PMCID: 4650141.

155. Asselah T, Thompson AJ, Flisiak R, et al. A predictive model for selecting patients with HCV genotype 3 chronic infection with a high probability of sustained virological response to peginterferon alfa-2a/ribavirin. PLOS ONE 2016;11(3):e0150569. PubMed PMID: 26991780. Pubmed Central PMCID: 4798721.

156. Bertino G, Ardiri A, Proiti M, et al. Chronic hepatitis C: this and the new era of treatment. World J Hepatol 2016;8(2):92–106. PubMed PMID: 26807205. Pubmed Central PMCID: 4716531.

157. Banerjee D, Reddy KR. Review article: safety and tolerability of direct-acting anti-viral agents in the new era of hepatitis C therapy. Aliment Pharmacol Ther 2016;43(6):674–96. PubMed PMID: 26787287.

158. Renard S, Borentain P, Salaun E, et al. Severe pulmonary arterial hypertension in patients treated for hepatitis C with sofosbuvir. Chest 2016;149(3):e69–73. PubMed PMID: 26965976.

159. Chin-Loy K, Galaydh F, Shaikh S. Retinopathy and uveitis associated with sofosbuvir therapy for chronic hepatitis C infection. Cureus 2016;8(5):e597. PubMed PMID: 27335709. Pubmed Central PMCID: 4895080.

160. Kozbial K, Moser S, Schwarzer R, et al. Unexpected high incidence of hepatocellular carcinoma in cirrhotic patients with sustained virologic response following interferon-free direct-acting antiviral treatment. J Hepatol 2016;65(4):856–8. PubMed PMID: 27318327.

161. Reig M, Marino Z, Perello C, et al. Unexpected high rate of early tumor recurrence in patients with HCV-related HCC undergoing interferon-free therapy. J Hepatol 2016;65(4):719–26. PubMed PMID: 27084592.

162. Cheung MC, Walker AJ, Hudson BE, et al. Outcomes after successful direct-acting antiviral therapy for patients with chronic hepatitis C and decompensated cirrhosis. J Hepatol 2016;65(4):741–7. PubMed PMID: 27388925.

163. Kobayashi M, Suzuki F, Fujiyama S, et al. Sustained virologic response by direct antiviral agents reduces the incidence of hepatocellular carcinoma in patients with

HCV infection. J Med Virol 2017;89(3):476–83. PubMed PMID: 27531586.

164. ANRS collaborative study group on hepatocellular carcinoma (ANRS CO22 HEPATHER, CO12 CirVir and CO23 CUPILT cohorts). Lack of evidence of an effect of direct-acting antivirals on the recurrence of hepatocellular carcinoma: data from three ANRS cohorts. J Hepatol 2016;65(4):734–40. PubMed PMID: 27288051.

165. Stedman C. Sofosbuvir, a NS5B polymerase inhibitor in the treatment of hepatitis C: a review of its clinical potential. Therap Adv Gastroenterol 2014;7(3):131–40. PubMed PMID: 24790644.

166. Missale G, Bertoni R, Lamonaca V, et al. Different clinical behaviors of acute hepatitis C virus infection are associated with different vigor of the anti-viral cell-mediated immune response. J Clin Invest 1996;98(3):706–14.

167. Semmo N, Klenerman P. CD4+ T cell responses in hepatitis C virus infection. World J Gastroenterol 2007;13(36):4831–8.

168. Cooper S, Erickson AL, Adams EJ, et al. Analysis of a successful immune response against hepatitis C virus. Immunity 1999;10(4):439–49.

169. Lechner F, Wong DK, Dunbar PR, et al. Analysis of successful immune responses in persons infected with hepatitis C virus. J Exp Med 2000;191(9):1499–512.

170. Bowen DG, Walker CM. Adaptive immune responses in acute and chronic hepatitis C virus infection. Nature 2005;436(7053):946–52.

171. Tsai SL, Liaw YF, Chen MH, et al. Detection of type 2-like T-helper cells in hepatitis C virus infection: implications for hepatitis C virus chronicity. Hepatology 1997;25(2):449–58.

172. Yang X, Huang S, Chen J, et al. Evaluation of the adjuvant properties of Astragalus membranaceus and Scutellaria baicalensis GEORGI in the immune protection induced by UV-attenuated Toxoplasma gondii in mouse models. Vaccine 2010;28(3):737–43.

173. Kapai NA, Anisimova NY, Kiselevskii MV, et al. Selective cytokine-inducing effects of low dose Echinacea. Bull Exp Biol Med 2011;150(6):711–13.

174. Chowdhury S, Mukherjee T, Mukhopadhyay R, et al. The lignan niranthin poisons Leishmania donovani topoisomerase IB and favours a Th1 immune response in mice. EMBO Mol Med 2012;4(10):1126–43.

175. Ferenci P, Scherzer TM, Kerschner H, et al. Silibinin is a potent antiviral agent in patients with chronic hepatitis C not responding to pegylated interferon/ribavirin therapy. Gastroenterology 2008;135(5):1561–7.

176. Neumann UP, Biermer M, Eurich D, et al. Successful prevention of hepatitis C virus (HCV) liver graft reinfection by silibinin mono-therapy. J Hepatol 2010;52(6):951–2.

177. Romano M, Vacante M, Cristaldi E, et al. L-carnitine treatment reduces steatosis in patients with chronic hepatitis C treated with alpha-interferon and ribavirin. Dig Dis Sci 2008;53(4):1114–21.

178. Bitetto D, Fabris C, Fornasiere E, et al. Vitamin D supplementation improves response to antiviral treatment for recurrent hepatitis C. Transpl Int 2011;24(1):43–50.

179. Bitetto D, Fattovich G, Fabris C, et al. Complementary role of vitamin D deficiency and the interleukin-28B rs12979860 C/T polymorphism in predicting antiviral response in chronic hepatitis C. Hepatology 2011;53(4):1118–26.

180. Petta S, Camma C, Scazzone C, et al. Low vitamin D serum level is related to severe fibrosis and low responsiveness to interferon-based therapy in genotype 1 chronic hepatitis C. Hepatology 2010;51(4):1158–67.

181. Toouli J, Wright TA. Gallstones. Med J Aust 1998;169(3):166–71.

182. Cuevas A, Miquel JF, Reyes MS, et al. Diet as a risk factor for cholesterol gallstone disease. J Am Coll Nutr 2004;23(3):187–96.

183. Jonkers IJ, Smelt AH, Ledeboer M, et al. Gall bladder dysmotility: a risk factor for gall stone formation in hypertriglyceridaemia and reversal on triglyceride lowering therapy by bezafibrate and fish oil. Gut 2003;52(1):109–15.

184. Lammert F, Miquel JF. Gallstone disease: from genes to evidence-based therapy. J Hepatol 2008;48(Suppl. 1): S124–35.

185. Kalloo AN, Kantsevoy SV. Gallstones and biliary disease. Prim Care 2001;28(3):591–606, vii.

186. Portincasa P, Moschetta A, Petruzzelli M, et al. Gallstone disease: symptoms and diagnosis of gallbladder stones. Best Pract Res Clin Gastroenterol 2006;20(6):1017–29.

187. Donovan JM. Physical and metabolic factors in gallstone pathogenesis. Gastroenterol Clin North Am 1999;28(1):75–97.

188. Grunhage F, Lammert F. Gallstone disease. Pathogenesis of gallstones: a genetic perspective. Best Pract Res Clin Gastroenterol 2006;20(6):997–1015.

189. Shaffer EA. Gallstone disease: epidemiology of gallbladder stone disease. Best Pract Res Clin Gastroenterol 2006;20(6):981–96.

190. Mendez-Sanchez N, Zamora-Valdes D, Chavez-Tapia NC, et al. Role of diet in cholesterol gallstone formation. Clin Chim Acta 2007;376(1–2):1–8.

191. Kiewiet JJ, Leeuwenburgh MM, Bipat S, et al. A systematic review and meta-analysis of diagnostic performance of imaging in acute cholecystitis. Radiology 2012;264(3):708–20.

192. van Dijk AH, de Reuver PR, Besselink MG, et al. Assessment of available evidence in the management of gallbladder and bile duct stones: a systematic review of international guidelines. HPB (Oxford) 2017;19: 297–309.

193. Portincasa P, Di Ciaula A, de Bari O, et al. Management of gallstones and its related complications. Expert Rev Gastroenterol Hepatol 2016;10:93–112.

194. Internal Clinical Guidelines Team (UK). Gallstone disease: diagnosis and management of cholelithiasis, cholecystitis and choledocholithiasis. National Institute for Health and Care Excellence: Clinical Guidelines. London: National Institute for Health and Care Excellence (UK); 2014.

195. Gupta SC, Patchva S, Aggarwal BB. Therapeutic roles of curcumin: lessons learned from clinical trials. AAPS J 2013;15(1):195–218.

196. Hamoud S, Kaplan M, Meilin E, et al. Niacin administration significantly reduces oxidative stress in patients with hypercholesterolemia and low levels of high-density lipoprotein cholesterol. Am J Med Sci 2013;345(3):195–9.

197. Yang CW, Mousa SA. The effect of red yeast rice (Monascus purpureus) in dyslipidemia and other disorders. Complement Ther Med 2012;20(6):466–74.

198. Feuerstein JS, Bjerke WS. Powdered red yeast rice and plant stanols and sterols to lower cholesterol. J Diet Suppl 2012;9(2):110–15.

199. Qiang Z, Lee SO, Ye Z, et al. Artichoke extract lowered plasma cholesterol and increased fecal bile acids in Golden Syrian hamsters. Phytother Res 2012;26(7):1048–52.

200. Gonzalez-Castejon M, Visioli F, Rodriguez-Casado A. Diverse biological activities of dandelion. Nutr Rev 2012;70(9):534–47.

201. Dong ZY, Wang GL, Liu X, et al. Treatment of cholecystitis with Chinese herbal medicines: a systematic review of the literature. World J Gastroenterol 2012;18(14):1689–94.

202. Saurer L, Reber P, Schaffner T, et al. Differential expression of chemokines in normal pancreas and in chronic pancreatitis. Gastroenterology 2000;118(2):356–67.

203. Gerasimenko OV, Gerasimenko JV. Mitochondrial function and malfunction in the pathophysiology of pancreatitis. Pflugers Arch 2012;464(1):89–99.

204. Grigsby B, Rodriguez-Rilo H, Khan K. Antioxidants and chronic pancreatitis: theory of oxidative stress and trials of antioxidant therapy. Dig Dis Sci 2012;57(4):835–41.

205. Everson GT. Biliary and cholestatic diseases. In: O'Grady JG, Lake JR, Howdle PD, editors. Comprehensive clinical hepatology. London: Harcourt Publishers Limited; 2000. p. 26, 1–17.

206. Rawla P, Bandaru SS, Vellipuram AR. Review of infectious etiology of acute pancreatitis. Gastroenterology Res 2017;10:153–8.

207. Sah RP, Chari ST, Pannala R, et al. Differences in clinical profile and relapse rate of type 1 versus type 2 autoimmune pancreatitis. Gastroenterology 2010;139(1):140–8, quiz e12–13.

208. Banks PA, Bollen TL, Dervenis C, et al. Classification of acute pancreatitis–2012: revision of the Atlanta classification and definitions by international consensus. Gut 2013;62(1):102–11.

209. Nair RJ, Lawler L, Miller MR. Chronic pancreatitis. Am Fam Physician 2007;76(11):1679–88.

210. Bhardwaj P, Garg PK, Maulik SK, et al. A randomized controlled trial of antioxidant supplementation for pain relief in patients with chronic pancreatitis. Gastroenterology 2009;136(1):149–59, e2.

211. Ji C. Mechanisms of alcohol-induced endoplasmic reticulum stress and organ injuries. Biochem Res Int 2012;2012:216450. doi:10.1155/2012/216450.

212. Grant JP. Nutritional support in acute and chronic pancreatitis. Surg Clin North Am 2011;91(4):805–20, viii.

213. Dragovic G. Acute pancreatitis in HIV/AIDS patients: an issue of concern. Asian Pac J Trop Biomed 2013;3(6):422–5.

214. Gukovsky I, Reyes CN, Vaquero EC, et al. Curcumin ameliorates ethanol and nonethanol experimental pancreatitis. Am J Physiol Gastrointest Liver Physiol 2003;284(1):G85–95.

215. Seo SW, Koo HN, An HJ, et al. Taraxacum officinale protects against cholecystokinin-induced acute pancreatitis in rats. World J Gastroenterol 2005;11(4):597–9.

216. Motoo Y, Su SB, Xie MJ, et al. Effect of herbal medicine Saiko-keishi-to (TJ-10) on rat spontaneous chronic pancreatitis: comparison with other herbal medicines. Int J Pancreatol 2000;27(2):123–9.

217. Loguercio C, Andreone P, Brisc C, et al. Silybin combined with phosphatidylcholine and vitamin E in patients with nonalcoholic fatty liver disease: a randomized controlled trial. Free Radic Biol Med 2012;52(9):1658–65.

218. Fried MW, Navarro VJ, Afdhal N, et al. Effect of silymarin (milk thistle) on liver disease in patients with chronic hepatitis C unsuccessfully treated with interferon therapy: a randomized controlled trial. JAMA 2012;308(3):274–82.

219. Guedj J, Dahari H, Pohl RT, et al. Understanding silibinin's modes of action against HCV using viral kinetic modeling. J Hepatol 2012;56(5):1019–24.

220. Kim M, Yang SG, Kim JM, et al. Silymarin suppresses hepatic stellate cell activation in a dietary rat model of non-alcoholic steatohepatitis: analysis of isolated hepatic stellate cells. Int J Mol Med 2012;30(3):473–9.

221. Polyak SJ, Morishima C, Lohmann V, et al. Identification of hepatoprotective flavonolignans from silymarin. Proc Natl Acad Sci USA 2010;107(13):5995–9.

222. Salomone F, Barbagallo I, Godos J, et al. Silibinin restores NAD(+) levels and induces the SIRT1/AMPK pathway in non-alcoholic fatty liver. Nutrients 2017;9(10):PubMed PMID: 28973994. Pubmed Central PMCID: 5691703.

223. Wah Kheong C, Nik Mustapha NR, Mahadeva S. A randomized trial of silymarin for the treatment of nonalcoholic steatohepatitis. Clin Gastroenterol Hepatol 2017;15(12):1940–9, e8. PubMed PMID: 28419855.

224. Zhong S, Fan Y, Yan Q, et al. The therapeutic effect of silymarin in the treatment of nonalcoholic fatty disease: a meta-analysis (PRISMA) of randomized control trials. Medicine 2017;96(49):e9061. PubMed PMID: 29245314. Pubmed Central PMCID: 5728929.

225. Zhang J, Zhang H, Deng X, et al. Baicalin protects AML-12 cells from lipotoxicity via the suppression of ER stress and TXNIP/NLRP3 inflammasome activation. Chem Biol Interact 2017;278:189–96. PubMed PMID: 29031535.

226. Ak T, Gülçin I. Antioxidant and radical scavenging properties of curcumin. Chem Biol Interact 2008;174(1):27–37.

227. Rahmani S, Asgary S, Askari G, et al. Treatment of non-alcoholic fatty liver disease with curcumin: a randomized placebo-controlled trial. Phytother Res 2016;30(9):1540–8. PubMed PMID: 27270872.

228. Chenari S, Safari F, Moradi A. Curcumin enhances liver SIRT3 expression in the rat model of cirrhosis. Iran J Basic Med Sci 2017;20(12):1306–11. PubMed PMID: 29238464. Pubmed Central PMCID: 5722989.

229. Bruck R, Ashkenazi M, Weiss S, et al. Prevention of liver cirrhosis in rats by curcumin. Liver Int 2007;27(3):373–83.

230. Ben Salem M, Ben Abdallah Kolsi R, Dhouibi R, et al. Protective effects of Cynara scolymus leaves extract on metabolic disorders and oxidative stress in alloxan-diabetic rats. BMC Complement Altern Med 2017;17(1):328. PubMed PMID: 28629341. Pubmed Central PMCID: 5477270.

231. Mocelin R, Marcon M, Santo GD, et al. Hypolipidemic and antiatherogenic effects of Cynara scolymus in cholesterol-fed rats. Rev Bras Farmacogn 2016;26(2):233–9. https://doi.org/10.1016/j.bjp.2015.11.004.

232. Sahebkar A, Pirro M, Banach M, et al. Lipid-lowering activity of artichoke extracts: a systematic review and meta-analysis. Crit Rev Food Sci Nutr 2018;58:2549–56. PubMed PMID: 28609140.

233. Frasinariu OE, Ceccarelli S, Alisi A, et al. Gut-liver axis and fibrosis in nonalcoholic fatty liver disease: an input for novel therapies. Dig Liver Dis 2013;45(7):543–51.

234. Hosseinzadeh H, Nassiri-Asl M. Pharmacological effects of Glycyrrhiza spp. and its bioactive constituents: update and review. Phytother Res 2015;29(12):1868–86. PubMed PMID: 26462981.

235. Park HJ, Cho J-Y, Kim MK, et al. Anti-obesity effect of Schisandra chinensis in 3T3-L1 cells and high fat diet-induced obese rats. Food Chem 2012;134(1):227–34.

236. Chung MY, Shin EJ, Choi HK, et al. Schisandra chinensis berry extract protects against steatosis by inhibiting histone acetylation in oleic acid-treated HepG2 cells and in the livers of diet-induced obese mice. Nutr Res 2017;46:1–10. PubMed PMID: 29173646.

237. Kaya-Dagistanli F, Tanriverdi G, Altinok A, et al. The effects of alpha lipoic acid on liver cells damages and apoptosis induced by polyunsaturated fatty acids. Food Chem Toxicol 2013;53:84–93.

238. Hultberg M, Hultberg B. The effect of different antioxidants on glutathione turnover in human cell lines and their interaction with hydrogen peroxide. Chem Biol Interact 2006;163(3):192–8.

239. Min AK, Kim MK, Seo HY, et al. Alpha-lipoic acid inhibits hepatic PAI-1 expression and fibrosis by inhibiting the TGF-beta signaling pathway. Biochem Biophys Res Commun 2010;393(3):536–41.

240. Petersen Shay K, Moreau RF, Smith EJ, et al. Is alpha-lipoic acid a scavenger of reactive oxygen species in vivo? Evidence for its initiation of stress signaling pathways that promote endogenous antioxidant capacity. IUBMB Life 2008;60(6):362–7.

241. Kim MS, Park JY, Namkoong C, et al. Anti-obesity effects of alpha-lipoic acid mediated by suppression of hypothalamic AMP-activated protein kinase. Nat Med 2004;10(7):727–33.

242. Pilar Valdecantos M, Prieto-Hontoria PL, Pardo V, et al. Essential role of Nrf2 in the protective effect of lipoic acid against lipoapoptosis in hepatocytes. Free Radic Biol Med 2015;84:263–78. PubMed PMID: 25841776.

243. Musso G, Gambino R, Cassader M, et al. A meta-analysis of randomized trials for the treatment of nonalcoholic fatty liver disease. Hepatology 2010;52(1):79–104.

244. Fujisawa K, Takami T, Matsuzaki A, et al. Evaluation of the effects of L-carnitine on medaka (Oryzias latipes) fatty liver. Sci Rep 2017;7(1):2749. PubMed PMID: 28584294. Pubmed Central PMCID: 5459862.

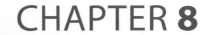

CHAPTER **8**

Respiratory infections and immune insufficiency

David Casteleijn
ND, MHSc

OVERVIEW

Respiratory tract infections (RTIs) are among the most commonly experienced illnesses, and place large economic costs on the community in terms of absences from work and school and in visits to medical professionals.[1,2] While most are self-limiting and resolve with time, they can be quite serious. Influenza kills approximately 36 000 in the United States every year,[3] with higher mortality rates in the elderly, who have weaker immune systems.[4] Many more Americans (exceeding 200 000) experience complications that require hospital admission.[3]

Respiratory infections are caused by pathogenic invasion and colonisation.[1] Upper respiratory tract infections (URTI) involve the nose, sinuses, pharynx or larynx, while lower respiratory tract infections (LRTI) involve the lungs and bronchi, and include pneumonia, lung abscess, acute bronchitis and bronchiectasis.

The term coryza (symptoms of a common cold) encompasses a number of viral URTIs with heterogeneous presentation.[1] They may in turn lead to secondary LRTI, or predispose to secondary bacterial URTI. The common cold is most frequently experienced with nasal congestion and drainage, sneezing, sore or scratchy throat, cough and general malaise.[1,2] Influenza is regarded as a separate disease entity, although the two often overlap. Manifestations of influenza commonly include fever, myalgia, fatigue, malaise, headache, pain behind the eyes, dry cough, runny nose and sore throat (Table 8.1).[3,5]

General clinical features of respiratory infections	
URTI	**LRTI**
• Nasal congestion and discharge	• Cough
• Sneezing	• Dyspnoea
• Sore or scratchy throat	• Weakness
• Cough	• High fever
• General malaise	• Fatigue
• Fever (sometimes)	
• Headache (sometimes)	
• Myalgia (sometimes)	

URTIs are more commonly experienced in the cooler months of the year, and in the rainy periods of tropical areas.[1] Children contract a greater number of infections throughout the year than adults, possibly due to their close socialisation in daycare and at school.[3,7]

Transmission occurs by one of three main methods[1–3,7]:

- hand contact with virus-containing secretions, from either the environment or an infected person
- inhalation of small-particle aerosols
- direct exposure to large-particle aerosols from an infected person (e.g. via a sneeze or cough).

Most acute respiratory illnesses are viral in origin.[8] Several viruses can cause the common cold, with rhinovirus (HRV) playing a prominent aetiological role.[1,2,9] In autumn, the peak time for colds, HRV accounts for up to 80% of URTIs.[10] Other predominant viral agents include respiratory syncytial virus (RSV), influenza virus (INF) and parainfluenza viruses (PIV).[1,3,8]

Genetics play a large role in immune function, and innate resistance to infection is principally inherited rather than acquired.[11] The set of host genes controlling this is termed the 'resistome', and this varies from person to person.[11] Defective genes in the resistome present most strikingly in congenital immunodeficiency syndromes, but variance in the genetic set may also lead to variability in the individual capacity of resistance to infections.[12,13]

Epidemiological data and the evidence from viral-challenge studies suggest that psychological stress is a risk factor for developing URTI.[14] Diet also has a key role in immune capacity. Many nutrients play a role in responding to microbial and viral challenge, with deficiencies in zinc, vitamin A, vitamin C, vitamin B6, iron, copper, selenium, protein and omega-3 fatty acids all shown to negatively affect immune capacity.[4,15–20] Malnourished children in developing countries, particularly those with vitamin A deficiency, are at far higher risk of contracting respiratory infection and also experience more severe illness.[21]

Table 8.1
The symptoms of influenza and cold

Symptom	Common cold	Influenza
Onset	Gradual: 1–3 days	Sudden: within a few hours
Site of infection	Upper respiratory tract	Entire respiratory tract
Nasal congestion	Frequent	Occasionally
Rhinorrhoea	Frequent	Occasionally
Sneezing	Frequent	Occasionally
Sore throat	Frequent	Occasionally
Cough	Less common	Can be quite severe
Chest discomfort	Mild	Pronounced
Fever	Rare	High
Myalgia	Occasional or insignificant	Severe
Fatigue/malaise	Mild	Long lasting
Headache	Rare, more mild	Prominent and severe
Exhaustion	Rare	Early and prominent

Source: Adapted from Meissner 2005[3] and Roxas & Jurenka 2007[6]

Environmental chemicals are considered to be immunotoxic and children exposed to these chemicals at an early age (pre- and postnatally) experience higher rates of respiratory infection than comparative populations with low levels of exposure.[21,22] An inverse relationship has been demonstrated between the level of physical activity and the number of URTIs experienced by adult males.[23] However, while moderate exercise enhances immune function and lowers the risk of URTI, intensive exertion produces a temporary suppressive effect on both the adaptive and the innate immune systems.[24]

The common concept of 'catching a chill' was examined in healthy subjects, who each received a 20-minute foot chill at 10°C. Approximately 29% of those receiving a foot chill were diagnosed with a cold four days after the chill experience, compared with 9% of control subjects (statistically significant).[25] In another study, a clear connection was demonstrated between the incidence of URTI and LRTI and decreases in average ambient temperature.[26]

Pathophysiology

The pathogenesis of URTI differs depending on the organism but generally involves interaction between viral replication and the host immune inflammatory response.[1] Viral infection stimulates a local inflammatory response, which causes the classic symptoms of the common cold—rhinorrhoea and nasal obstruction.[1,9] Sneezing and excess mucus production are precipitated by increased cholinergic stimulation in the area.[1] Inflammatory mediators interleukin-6 (IL-6) and IL-8 appear to be particularly involved, with some studies correlating their concentration in nasal secretions directly with the severity of cold symptoms.[27,28] Contrastingly, influenza viruses inhabit and replicate in the epithelium of the tracheobronchial area.[5] Here they generate a similar inflammatory response but also cause overt epithelial toxicity, which contributes to the severity of symptoms.[5,9]

DIFFERENTIAL DIAGNOSIS

- Viral infection (common cold)
- Influenza, or 'the flu'
- Pneumonia
- Bronchitis
- Asthma exacerbation
- Tuberculosis (in certain parts of the world) or mycobacterial infection
- Allergies—food, environmental

CONVENTIONAL TREATMENT

As the common cold is caused by a multitude of different virus types with varying pathogenic mechanisms, a universal medical treatment remains elusive, with most common over-the-counter treatments found to be ineffective.[29] Even increasing fluids has been brought into question when (particularly in children) there are no signs of dehydration.[30] A 2012 review of commonly prescribed and used treatments for the common cold found that antibiotics, antihistamines, antitussives, decongestants, codeine and bronchodilators along with vitamin C were no more effective than placebo in decreasing the symptoms or duration of a common cold,[31] although placebo was remarkably effective, particularly if the subject thought it was something they believed in.[32]

Antibiotic use is particularly contentious in treating URTI. The general consensus is that there is no benefit in treating the common cold with antibiotics and they should not be used.[33] Most studies show no difference in symptom improvement between those treated with antibiotics immediately and those with delayed prescriptions.[34] However, in patients who are more predisposed to complications, such as those with underlying lung disease, evidence does exist to support the use of antibiotics in the treatment of URTIs.[33,35]

At present, specific antiviral treatments for respiratory viruses are commercially available only for influenza viruses.[36] Although rhinoviral agents exist, they are still in the developmental stages, and often are not as clinically efficacious as in vitro studies would suggest; they must be taken early and frequently in order to have an effect, and it is often too late by the time a patient presents to their general practitioner.[2]

KEY TREATMENT PROTOCOLS

From a clinical perspective, it is important to address the acute presentation first. Amelioration of symptoms, limitation of causative pathogens and strengthening immune defences and clearance will address the patient's immediate concerns and help them feel better. Interestingly, in a study using echinacea, the importance of 'feeling one is being treated' has been highlighted where participants in a no-pill group tended to have longer and more severe illnesses than those who received pills, and for a subgroup who believed in echinacea and received pills (regardless of whether the pills contained echinacea), illnesses were substantively shorter and less severe.[32] This provides more evidence for the power of the 'placebo effect' (for further detail refer to Chapter 14 on anxiety).

The next steps are to restore the health and wellbeing of the patient, and address causes of immune dysregulation that may predispose to future infections. **Zinc sulphate**, **nasal irrigation**, **menthol rubs**, **honey**, *Pelargonium sidoides* and *Andrographis paniculata* may reduce the symptoms of the common cold.[31] **Frequent hand washing** reduced the spread of respiratory viruses, although antibacterial soaps were not significantly better.[37] **Vitamin C** and *Alium sativum*[31] have been found to be notably beneficial in prophylaxis of the common cold.

Addressing the symptoms

While it is important to take a holistic view of the disease process and underlying causes, symptomatic treatment of URTI is also essential (Table 8.2). Clearing the infection and ameliorating the symptoms can be accomplished concurrently. Overall, many symptoms are the result of an inflammatory response, and thus reducing this will address the symptom cluster as a whole.

Quercetin demonstrates a potent ability to inhibit inflammatory cytokine and chemokine production in acute and chronic inflammation, including IL-6 and IL-8, which are both implicated in the aetiology of cold symptoms.[43,44] *Echinacea* **spp.** may also be of use in this regard, as it is known to modulate levels of these two cytokines.[45] (See the section Immune modulation—humoral and cellular immune system later in this chapter.)

Naturopathic Treatment Aims

During acute infection:
- Treat symptoms (e.g. catarrh/phlegm, cough, fever).
- Address pathogens (e.g. bacteria, viruses).
- Support and modulate the immune system.

After cessation of acute infection:
- Tonify and restore vitality.
- Modulate cortisol response and HPA axis activity (if required).
- Address gastrointestinal dysregulation (if required).
  - Correct poor digestion and malabsorption.
  - Reduce intestinal permeability.
  - Rebalance intestinal microflora.

Table 8.2
Suggested actions and agents for symptomatic relief

Symptom	Action required	Herbal and nutritional remedies
Nasal congestion/ sinusitis	Mucolytic	*Foeniculum vulgare, Trigonella foenum-graecum, Armoracia rusticana, Pimpinella anisum,* N-acetylcysteine, onion, garlic, mustard seeds, papain, bromelain, amylase, sodium chloride, sodium bicarbonate
	Anticatarrhal (upper respiratory tract)	*Glycyrrhiza glabra, Euphrasia officinalis, Hydrastis canadensis, Plantago lanceolata, Sambucus nigra,* bromelain, papain
	Mucous membrane trophorestorative	*Euphrasia officinalis, Hydrastis canadensis,* vitamin A, zinc glutamine, vitamin C
Phlegm and cough	Mucolytic	*Foeniculum vulgare, Trigonella foenum-graecum, Armoracia rusticana, Pimpinella anisum,* N-acetylcysteine, onion, garlic, mustard seeds, papain, bromelain, amylase, sodium chloride, sodium bicarbonate
	Anticatarrhal (lower respiratory tract)	*Verbascum thapsus, Plantago lanceolata, Salvia officinalis,* bromelain, papain
	Expectorant	*Glycyrrhiza glabra, Verbascum thapsus, Inula helenium, Marrubium vulgare, Adhatoda vasica, Allium sativum*
	Antitussive	*Prunus serotina, Althaea officinalis, Glycyrrhiza glabra*
Fever	Diaphoretic	*Achillea millefolium, Sambucus nigra, Bupleurum falcatum, Zingiber officinale, Tilia* spp.
Sore and/or scratchy throat	Emollient	*Althaea officinalis, Glycyrrhiza glabra*
	Astringent (topical)	*Salvia officinalis, Commiphora myrrha, Euphrasia officinalis*
	Lymphatic	*Phytolacca decandra, Echinacea* spp., *Calendula officinalis, Iris versicolor*
	Respiratory antiseptic (topical)	*Salvia officinalis, Thymus vulgaris, Commiphora myrrha, Hydrastis canadensis*
	Anti-inflammatory	*Glycyrrhiza glabra, Aloe* spp., *Calendula officinalis, Commiphora myrrha, Euphrasia officinalis,* quercetin, eicosapentaenoic acid, docosahexaenoic acid
	Topical anaesthetic	*Piper methysticum, Syzygium aromaticum*

Sources: Bone 2003,[38] Fischer 1996,[39] Mills & Bone 2000,[40] Osiecki 2004,[41] and Scientific Committee of the British Herbal Medical Association 1983[42]

For the protocols for addressing symptoms such as phlegm, cough and nasal congestion, refer to Chapter 10 on congestive respiratory disorders.

Fever management

Overview

'Fever phobia' was first named in 1980[46] but continues to be widespread among care givers[47] and nurses (fuelling parent fever phobia).[48] Nurses administer antipyretic agents in an effort to prevent febrile convulsions[49] (possibly also to be seen to be doing something about an observed vital sign deviation from the norm) despite these anti-pyretic agents being ineffective in doing so[50] and despite the potential beneficial effect from fever and, potentially, adverse effects from suppressing the fever (with antipyretics) on infection outcomes.

A state of elevated core temperature is a normal part of the defence response to matter recognised as pathogenic or foreign.[51] This is part of a complex physiological reaction involving a cytokine-mediated rise in core temperature, generation of acute phase reactants and activation of numerous physiological, endocrinological and immunological systems (Figure 8.1).[51]

A positive correlation was found between maximum temperature on the day of bacteraemia and survival in a retrospective analysis of 218 patients with bacteraemia.[52] In addition, a temperature greater than 38°C was positively correlated with likelihood of survival.[53] A trend towards longer duration of rhinoviral shedding has been found in association with antipyretic therapy, with this study also showing that the use of aspirin or paracetamol is associated with suppression of the serum neutralising antibody response, and increased nasal signs and symptoms.[54] Suppressing a fever with paracetamol appeared to prolong chicken pox, with a longer time to total crusting of lesions than placebo-treated controls,[55] potentially allowing for a longer period of viral

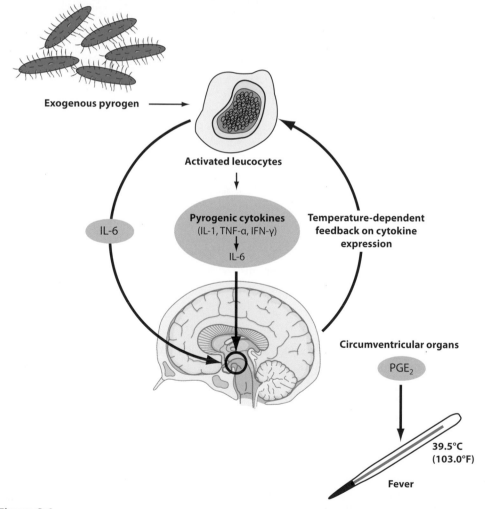

Figure 8.1
Hypothetical model for the febrile response

IL = indicates interleukin; TNF = tumour necrosis factor; IFN = interferon; PGE_2 = prostaglandin E_2 [6].

spread. A final study demonstrated that adults infected with HRV exhibit more nasal viral shedding when they receive aspirin than when administered placebo.[56] It therefore appears the current evidence does not support the practice of administering antipyretic therapies routinely to patients with fever.[50]

Naturopathic management of fever

Key pyrogenic cytokines have demonstrated immune-potentiating capabilities that may enhance resistance to infection, supporting the idea of fever as beneficial.[57] Therefore, treating moderate fever with antipyretic or direct cooling therapies may be counter-productive.[58]

According to traditional naturopathic principles, first-line treatments for fever have a 'normalising' effect, being regarded as mildly heating **diaphoretics**. Herbal examples of these include *Achillea millefolium*, *Verbena officinalis*, *Hyssopus officinalis*, *Tilia europaea*, *Sambucus nigra*, *Eupatorium perfoliatum*, *Thymus vulgaris*, *Nepeta cataria*, *Tanacetum vulgare*, *Melissa officinalis*, *Oxalis acetosella* and *Polygonum bistorta*.[59,60]

It is possible that a fever may require enhancement if it is considered that it is not adequately materialising and sufficient effort has also been made to ensure there is no underlying pathology or life-threatening infection.[59,60] Here, moderately warming/circulation-stimulating remedies such as *Cinnamomum zeylanicum*, *Allium sativum* and *Elettaria cardamomum* can be used readily. Stronger heating remedies like *Capsicum* spp., *Zingiber officinale* and *Armoracia rusticana* require additional care as they can prove more stimulating to the fever process.[59]

Just as there may be reason to enhance a fever, it is possible that it may need to be controlled. In this instance **cooling bitters** such as *Taraxacum officinale*, *Cinnamomum cassia*, *Gentiana lutea* and *Andrographis paniculata* are recommended.[59,60]

One trial found that **zinc** supplementation resolved fever 3.1 times more rapidly in two- to 24-month-old boys.[61] It is suggested that this nutrient is most beneficial in treating fever when the patient has suboptimum zinc serum levels (see Table 8.4 for a review of the evidence).

Address pathogens

For a discussion of the role of antimicrobials, antivirals and antifungal agents in respiratory illness, refer to Chapter 10 on congestive respiratory disorders.

Immune modulation—humoral and cellular immune system

Any factor that depletes immune function may predispose a person to develop an RTI, and those who suffer immune insufficiency, such as the elderly, those with co-existent disease and the immunocompromised, are particularly at risk of recurrent or severe infection.[62]

The causes of lowered innate and adaptive immune resistance are multiple and dynamic in interaction, and immune resistance varies throughout life.[63] The innate homoeostasis of individual immune response is influenced by genes, stress, diet, environmental influences, age and prior infection or inflammatory events.[63]

Adequate host defence mechanisms play a role in the symptom severity and clinical outcome of URTIs. While both specific and humoral immunity are important in host response to rhinoviral infection, it seems that the innate response is dominant early after infection, and modulates the symptomatic presentation.[9] This is also the division that is responsible for immunosurveillance of pathogens and for preventing initial entry.[64] Therefore, it is important to strengthen this general defence mechanism.

Antigen-specific humoral and cellular immune responses to URTI are elicited but are generally not detectable until after symptoms have abated.[9] Enhancement of these systems is therefore more relevant with regard to preventing re-infection.

Vitamins

Nitric oxide (NO) production by epithelial cells has a role in the body's antiviral responses,[9] reducing epithelial cell release of cytokines and chemokines induced by viral infections.[65] **Vitamin C** has demonstrated the ability in cell lines to increase NO production, and therefore may aid in viral clearance and symptom reduction via this mechanism.[66] Other studies show effects on phagocyte function, production of interferon and gene expression of monocyte adhesion molecules, thereby enhancing immune function.[15,67,68] A 2013 Cochrane review[69] examined trials exploring the effect of vitamin C on common cold duration taken both regularly each day and as a treatment (commenced once the symptoms of a cold appeared). The severity of colds was reduced by regular vitamin C, while therapeutic vitamin C gave less consistent effects. They conclude vitamin C was a low-cost and generally safe option that may be useful on an individual basis.

One of the most widely used immune modulating nutrients is **zinc**. Low levels affect almost all aspects of innate and adaptive immunity. It is crucial for the development and function of natural killer cells, phagocytes, macrophages and neutrophils and lack of zinc predisposes a person to lymphocytopenia, reduced type 1 T helper (Th1) cells and decreased thymus function.[15,70–72] Prolonged states of deficiency effectively 'reprogram' the immune system by increasing glucocorticoid secretion, which accelerates pre-T-cell and pre-B-cell apoptosis.[63] Zinc is also essential for cytokine production and secretion.[15,70–72]

A 2011 Cochrane review found the incidence of developing a cold was less in zinc-treated groups, that zinc-supplemented children were absent for fewer days from school and that an antibiotic prescription was more likely in placebo than in zinc-supplemented groups.[73]

The most bioavailable forms of zinc supplementation appear to be glycinates, gluconates and zinc-enriched yeast.[74–76] An assessment of randomised trials[77] indicated that zinc lozenges can shorten the duration of colds by 20–40%.

Quercetin may be a useful additional supplement in acute respiratory illness. It seems to exert antiviral effects via Th1:Th2 modulation, encouraging the production of Th1-derived cytokine IFN-γ, which eliminates or blocks viral replication in infected cells.[78] Quercetin did not alter exercise-induced changes in several measures of immune function, but it significantly reduced URTI incidence in cyclists during the two-week period after intensified exercise.[79] The mechanism seems to be directly antiviral rather than correction of immune dysregulation,[64] with some evidence that quercetin supplementation may decrease expression of IL-8[80] possibly reducing nasal inflammation in the common cold. In influenza, it may protect the lungs from the damaging free radicals generated in the disease process.[81]

Low levels of **vitamin A** cause a wide range of immunological defects, and may predispose a person to develop respiratory (and other) infections.[15,82] Theoretically, vitamin A should be of benefit in LRTI due to its ability to up-regulate Th1 and down-regulate Th2-mediated immune responses.[83] The nutrient also enhances innate defences by supporting healthy mucosal barriers and the function of macrophages, neutrophils and natural killer cells.[84] However, a Cochrane review in 2008 found that while supplementation could prevent LRTI in retinol-deficient children or those with a poor nutritional status or weight, it made symptoms worse in normal children.[83] One factor that may be responsible for this puzzling result is that many of these studies were mega-dose studies, and vitamin A supplementation seems more efficacious when administered via frequent low-dosing,[83,84] similar to obtaining it from a balanced diet.

The immunological activity of different herbal medicines is being increasingly documented, with labels such as 'immuno-stimulant' and 'immune-enhancer' being ascribed to herbs such as **Echinacea spp**.[85] While 'stimulation' of certain immunological systems does occur, the term 'immuno-modulation' is perhaps more apt, as the modulation of the immune system by phytoconstituents is more complex than a purely 'stimulating' effect. Various plant constituents modulate the humoral and/or the cellular components of the immune system.[86] While up-regulating the humoral immune system (increasing macrophage activity and phagocytosis) is often beneficial in cases of pathogenic challenge or in a deficient immune system, the workings of the cellular immune system are more complex. Some studies show that herbal medicines may 'up' or 'down' regulate varying aspects of the cellular immune system, and in isolation some constituents may modulate cytokines that individually are anti-inflammatory and/or inflammatory.

Herbal medicines modulate a unique combination of immune pathways, with different medicinal plants often used for similar therapeutic outcomes (e.g. acute infection). They express varying biological activities to achieve this effect. Herbal medicines may enhance the activity of immune components that are beneficial in fighting pathogens via: increased humoral activity; natural killer cell, leucocyte, selective cytokine and immunoglobulin production; modulation of Th1 and Th2 cells; and/or down-regulation of NF-κB and TNF-α[79] (Table 8.3).

It should be noted that some herbals, for example, **Hemidesmus indicus** and **Tylophora indica**, may actually 'suppress' many components of the immune system.[85] While it is advised that these plants be avoided in acute conditions,[45] they have a place in treating disease processes where an 'over-activated' cellular immune system is apparent (see Chapter 31 on autoimmunity). The clinician may find the complexities of the modulation of individual immune components by herbal medicines to be complex and confusing.

Herbal remedies

Echinacea spp. exert a strong inhibitory effect in vitro on the expression of IL-6 and IL-8 expression by bronchial cells infected with a number of common respiratory pathogens.[45,99] This helps ameliorate URTI symptoms, and is effective both prophylactically *and* symptomatically.[45] Meta-analyses and reviews of *Echinacea* spp. efficacy have shown differing results, as, in general, they have not screened studies for use of a particular plant part. One meta-analysis included a subgroup of standardised products, and found that these generated reductions in the incidence of infection by 58% and symptom duration by 1.4 days.[100] *Echinacea angustifolia/purpurea* root blend commenced 14 days prior to international jet travel (a known precursor to URT symptoms) significantly reduced the expected increase in the rate of respiratory symptoms compared with placebo[101] and *Echinacea purpurea* fresh plant extract inhibited virally confirmed colds particularly preventing enveloped virus infections, with maximal effects as a preventer of recurrent infections.[102] Both trials found echinacea to be as safe as placebo.[101,102]

Andrographis paniculata is used in Ayurvedic medicine to treat a range of illnesses including influenza, pneumonia and bronchitis.[103] *Andrographis paniculata* decreased the symptoms of viral URTI significantly better than placebo over a five-day period; only a few minor adverse effects were noted, with no significant difference in occurrence between the treated and placebo groups.[104] Previous trials indicate the effect may be dose-dependent,

Table 8.3
Key herbal medicines with immune enhancing/modulating properties

Phytomedicine	Actions[†]	Biological activity	Medicinal uses
Andrographis paniculata[87–92]	Immune enhancing Antiviral Antipyretic	Andrographolides:[‡] Inhibits NF-κB and COX-2 ↑ Phagocytosis, white blood cell count ↓ TNF-α, GM-CSF ↓ IL-2, IFN-γ production	Common cold/flu Nasopharyngeal infections/ inflammations Fever Hepatic conditions
Uncaria tomentosa[85,93]	Immune modulating Anti-inflammatory	Oxindoles:[‡] ↓ NF-κB activation ↓ TNF-α production ↑ IL-6 ↓ IL-1 Modulates lymphocytes Enhances phagocytosis	Chronic infections Inflammatory conditions Autoimmune disease Adjuvant treatment of cancer
Eleuterococcus senticosus[94–96]	Immune tonic Tonic Adaptogen	Eleutherosides:[‡] ↑ Lymphocyte and T-cell production ↑ NK activity and production ↑ Phagocytosis ↑ COX-2 inhibition ↑ IL-1, IL-6 activity	Weakened immunity Chronic infections Convalescence Fatigue
Astragalus membranaceus[85,94,97]	Immune tonic Tonic Adaptogen Cardiotonic	Astragalosides and flavonoids:[‡] ↑ Leucocyte production, phagocytosis ↑ Mononuclear, NK cells ↓ IL-6, PGE$_2$ ↑ IgG, IgM, IgE Improved T4:T8 ratios	Weakened immunity Chronic infections Convalescence
Panax ginseng[85,94]	Tonic Adaptogen Immune tonic Anti-carcinogenic	Ginsenosides:[‡] ↑ NK, IL-2 ↑ Phagocytotic activity ↑ T-cell, T helper production Modulates IFN-γ, TNF-α	Fatigue Convalescence Weakened immunity Adjuvant treatment of cancer
Ganoderma spp.[98]	Immune enhancing Anti-inflammatory Anti-tumoural	Polysaccharides:[‡] Macrophage activating ↑ NK, B lymphocytes ↑ IL-12	Chronic infections or inflammation Adjuvant treatment of cancer

†Key relevant traditional or modern-validated actions
‡Regarded as the main constituent responsible for activity

increasing in effectiveness with higher quantities of andrographolides.[105,106] There is also preliminary evidence indicating a protective effect against infection.[107] In one study, very low doses (200 mg/day) decreased the relative risk of URTI contraction by 2.1 times in the active group by the third month.[108] Adverse effects appear minimal, although the herb should be used with caution in pregnancy and bleeding disorders, and with patients taking hypoglycaemic or antiplatelet medication.[107,108] It should be noted that high doses can occasionally lead to gastric discomfort, anorexia and, in extreme cases, vomiting.[109] One way to mitigate this when prescribing high doses is to give smaller doses more frequently.

In contrast to *Andrographis paniculata*, **Astragalus membranaceus** is considered more specific for chronic or recurrent infection and in instances of immune depletion. In traditional Chinese medicine it is used for 'all diseases caused by "insufficient Qi",

---

Echinacea quality issues

Alkylamides have been found to be the most active immune-enhancing constituents in *Echinacea* spp., with a combination of *E. purpurea* and *E. angustifolia*[110–112] enhancing the bioavailability of these compounds. Combining the two extracts provides a protective effect on the alkylamides from *E. angusti-folia*, as alkyamides from *E. purpurea* protect them from liver metabolism via the P450 pathway.[111] In order to obtain the highest amounts of these active constituents, not only is the species important but also the plant part. Research has identified the following differences in the alkylamide content (mg/g) of the various parts of *E. purpurea*: flower 2.7, leaf 0.2, rhizome 5.7 and root 1.7.[113] This would suggest that the rhizome is the preferable plant part to use, though a synergy has been shown between the alkylamides from the aerial parts and the root of *E. purpurea*.[114] Therefore, a combination of root and herb tinctures may also provide enhanced immunomodulatory and anti-inflammatory effects.

Finally, the effectiveness of *Echinacea* spp. is also dose-dependent, and a thorough understanding of the therapeutic dosage range is imperative when prescribing the herb. It is important to significantly increase the dose prescribed in the presence of an acute infection. Failure to do this can contribute to echinacea not being as clinically effective as possible, even when good-quality botanical product is used.

Any one of the above may be a confounding factor in research, providing insight into why some negative trial results have emerged. However, while in vitro and in vivo studies assist in the understanding of mechanisms of action, the key clinical principle is always to prescribe in relation to traditional usage and evidence from human clinical trials.

Three main species of *Echinacea* are used medicinally: *E. palladia*, *E. purpurea* and *E. angustifolia*. There is a long history of *Echinacea* spp. use in infectious conditions, and both *E. purpurea* and *E. angustifolia* were used by the eclectics for respiratory illness such as catarrh and chronic bronchitis.[115] Given the quality issues noted here, the only relevant studies are those that use the correct plant part at reasonable doses.

---

typically those manifesting in weakness, fatigue, and vulnerability to infection'.[94,116] Clinically, *Astragalus membranaceus* improves lymphocyte function in both immune-depressed and healthy patients.[94] While no clinical studies examining the use of this botanical agent in respiratory illness could be found so far, centuries of traditional use and demonstrated immune stimulating activity suggest that it would be of benefit in treating and preventing URTI.

Sambucus nigra has strong traditional indications for respiratory tract diseases.[117] Constituents in the berries neutralise the spikes on a number of enveloped viruses, including influenza types A and B, rendering them unable to enter cells and replicate.[6,118] They also have an ability to modulate cytokine expression in vitro, and therefore potentially enhance phagocytic activity and chemotaxis for clearance of infection.[6,119] A standardised elderberry liquid extract demonstrated antimicrobial activity against both gram-positive bacteria of *Streptococcus pyogenes* and group C and G streptococci, and the gram-negative bacterium *Branhamella catarrhalis* as well as an inhibitory effect on pathogenic human influenza viruses in liquid cultures.[120] Specifically, two flavonoid compounds bound to and prevented H1N1 infection *in vitro*. This H1N1 inhibition activity compared favourably with the known anti-influenza activities of oseltamivir (Tamiflu) and amantadine. A 2009 clinical double-blind randomised controlled trial of ***Sambucus nigra*** extract demonstrated rapid and significant relief from influenza symptoms.[121] Due to concerns regarding the stability of the actives in a *Sambucus nigra* extract, a tablet form is considered preferable.[122]

For further information and other herbs with immune-stimulating activity refer to Table 8.2. Any one of these may be of use in treating RTI presentations, depending upon the patient. Their use should be guided by the indications suggested.

Pelargonium sidoides significantly reduced the severity of symptoms and shortened the duration of the common cold, proving safe and well tolerated in a study of 207 adult outpatients from eight hospitals.[123]

Preventing respiratory infections and the role of herbal 'tonics' and adaptogens

Many traditional medical systems incorporate treatments in order to maintain the vitality of the body, or keep it 'in tune'.[124] In the Malaysian and Indonesian systems, these are called *jamu*, in Ayurvedia they are *rasayanas* (for rejuvenation) and in Russia the term *toniziruyuzhie sredstva* literally translates to 'tonic substances'.[124] In the Western tradition, they are referred to as adaptogens or tonics. The general understanding of these remedies is that they are plants containing 'biologically active substances which … induce a state of … increase[d] resistance to … aversive assaults which threaten internal homeostasis'.[125]

In modern life, there are many obstacles to attaining and maintaining a state of ultimate wellness, but much can be done to move closer towards it. A healthy diet and lifestyle, with regular amounts of moderate exercise and low stress levels, contribute to a strong and healthy individual who is resistant to infection and disease.

Traditionally, **immune tonics** were used to fortify the immune system in infection or immune challenge from pathogens, or to 'tonify' and restore the immune system if deemed deficient.[59] A state of dysregulation was perceived to exist in people with recurrent infections, or presenting with symptoms such as a lingering cough or unresolved infection. In traditional Chinese medicine this is seen as Qi (vital force) deficiency, and the patient often appears with a pale face and tongue, a weak pulse, fatigue and shortness of breath.[126]

The concept of an immune tonic implies a degree of bidirectionality. While immune stimulants/modulators may, for example, encourage the up-regulation of bodily processes (such as an increase in natural killer cell function), they do not possess the ability to down-regulate this function in cases of over activity. Therefore, they are unidirectional. A true immune tonic expresses an ability to restore the immune system to balance no matter which way it departs from homoeostasis.[127] An example is *Echinacea* spp., which exhibits the ability to regulate and balance T helper cell function, with differing actions depending upon the existing state (basal or stimulated) of the immune response.[100] Therefore, an immune tonic is a 'true balancer of dysregulated immune function'. Beneficial immune tonic herbs include *Senticosus membranaceus*, *Eleutherococcus senticosus*, *Panax ginseng*, *Ganoderma* spp. and *Echinacea* spp.

There is sometimes controversy over the use of certain herbs for either 'acute' or 'chronic' conditions. A core naturopathic principle is to first use immune enhancers/modulators to help eliminate the pathogen, and follow this with a tonic to strengthen immunity. For example, the use of *Echinacea* spp. and *Andrographis paniculata* for an

---

Keep it simple

Basic elements of lifestyle and care are often the most effective in treating and preventing infection:

- adequate clean (filtered) water
- fresh air
- exposure to (safe levels of) sunshine
- regular exercise
- balanced diet
- rest—adults should be advised to get at least eight hours' sleep a night, in addition to adequate relaxation during the waking hours; this should be increased in the case of acute infection
- the 'healing relationship'—practitioner empathy significantly predicts the duration and severity of symptoms of illness[129]
- strong interpersonal relationships and social networks
- a positive attitude to life[130] and a strong sense of self-worth.

acute cold/flu would initially be employed, followed by *Astragalus membranaceus* and *Eleutherococcus senticosus* to tonify. However, it is not always so clear-cut. Evidence does not preclude the long-term use of immune modulators in chronic conditions as they may be beneficial in preventing infection and RTIs.[128] Using tonics is considered contra-indicated in most acute cases, as a strong stimulating effect can lead to more florid immune/inflammatory responses and promote a short-term worsening of the condition/symptoms. However, as an exception to the rule, these may traditionally be prescribed in cases of acute cold/flu where the person's energy is so low they struggle to fight the pathogen (presenting with marked fatigue, shortness of breath and daytime sweating).[128]

Psychoneuroimmunology, adrenal and nervine tonics

Psychoneuroimmunology is the study of the interactions between the central nervous system, the autonomic and endrocrine systems and the immune system,[131,132] demonstrating that stress, depression, anxiety, insomnia and other nervous conditions common in today's society may all have detrimental effects on immune function.[130,133,134] Epidemiological data have long shown a link between life stress and higher likelihood of infectious and inflammatory disease,[135] but it is only relatively recently that the mechanisms behind this connection have begun to be elucidated. It is likely that the effect is mediated by hormones of the hypothalamus-pituitary-adrenal (HPA) axis (see Chapter 18 on stress and fatigue).[129,136] Generally, these hormones are immune suppressing, and even the transient cortisol spike after intensive exertion may increase susceptibility to URTI.[134] Animal studies illustrate that early-life stress is likely to promote lifelong immune dysregulation.[137] Prolonged psychological stress results in chronic exposure to these hormones, and may predispose a person to lowered immunity and repeated infection.

Additionally, viral illnesses and infections are, in themselves, physiologically stressful, as they induce concomitant activation of the HPA axis, and may favour the evolution of psychological illnesses.[135] Therefore, there is a clear role for adrenal support where patients suffer from both repeated infection / poor immunity and chronic or high levels of stress.

This is an area of overlap with the previous treatment goal—boosting vitality and immune resistance. The key distinction in the decision of which actions and interventions to use depends upon the amount of stress, tension and nervous system compromise existing in a patient. If these are a core cause of immune depletion, then adrenal tonics and nervines are indicated. However, if the patient's vitality is weakened more by lifestyle considerations such as a poor diet and a lack of sleep, then adaptogens and immune tonics may be more appropriate. In many cases both will need to be used.

Useful nutrients include **vitamin C** and **zinc**. Human and animal studies suggest that vitamin C supplementation may be beneficial in reducing circulating cortisol levels both post-exercise and in situations of psychosocial stress.[133,135] It is also an important cofactor for both adrenal medulla and adrenal cortex hormone synthesis, and will be rapidly depleted in situations of over-activity and secretion.[138] Zinc deficiency, rather than impairing adrenal function, directly leads to HPA activation and chronically high circulating levels of glucocorticoids.[139] In populations at risk of low levels of zinc, this mineral may be useful to mediate HPA overactivity. Given that stress also predisposes many patients to poor digestion and absorption of nutrients, a deficiency may be present despite an adequate diet. Zinc can be toxic at high levels, and so a zinc test should be employed before supplementation.

Of the **botanical adaptogens** available, *Eleutherococcus senticosus*, *Glycyrrhiza glabra*, *Rehmannia glutinosa*, *Bupleurum falcatum*, *Rhodiola rosea*, *Panax ginseng* and *Withania* *somnifera* all demonstrate activity on the adrenal glands or hormones. The beneficial stress-protective effect of adaptogens is related to regulation of homoeostasis via several mechanisms of action associated with the HPA axis and the control of key mediators of stress response.[140] *Eleutherococcus senticosus* is native to Russia and northern Asia and has been used in traditional Chinese medicine since 190 AD and, more recently, in Russia as an adaptogen.[97,141] Clinical trials demonstrate that *Eleutherococcus senticosus* elicits a biphasic stress response from the adrenal glands, raising cortisol levels when they are too low, and reducing them in elevated states.[142] This may be due to an increased binding of the natural ligands to receptors involved in the feedback systems of stress hormones.[142] It is suggested that it inhibits catechol-O-methyl transferase, an enzyme that normally catalyses the degradation of stress hormones and, in doing so, prolongs their action in the body. This activates the negative feedback loop, lowering glucocorticoid secretion, and thus potentially diminishing the immune suppressive effects of stress.

Withania somnifera also demonstrates activity on the adrenal glands, and an ability to reduce adrenal hypertrophy and circulating levels of glucocorticoids.[146–148] In doing so, it improves the chronic stress-induced decrease of the T-lymphocyte population (CD3$^+$, CD4$^+$/CD8$^+$ T-cells).[146–148] *Rhodiola rosea* may also reduce secretion of CRF and prevent depletion of adrenal hormones in chronic stress.[149,150]

Panax ginseng has renowned adaptogenic and tonic activity, which is suspected to be due to activity on the adrenal glands.[151–153] In chronic stress the herb has demonstrated the ability to normalise adrenal gland weight and serum corticosteroid levels via restoration of regular HPA feedback cycles.[154] Restoration of regular feedback loops will decrease abnormally high levels of cortisol that may depress immune function. *Panax ginseng* also increases adrenal capacity, therefore toning the organs and promoting normal functioning.[155] Caution needs to be applied when using *Panax ginseng* as there is potential for overstimulation; concomitant use with caffeine, nicotine or other stimulants should be avoided.[156]

Glycyrrhiza glabra and *Rehmannia glutinosa* delay the breakdown of cortisol and hence, eventually, lower the levels expressed.[157,158]

Traditionally, nervine tonics such as *Avena sativa*, *Scutellaria lateriflora* and *Hypericum perforatum* are employed to nourish and strengthen the nervous system in cases of stress and nervous debility.[59] *Avena sativa* may be given green or as seed—each has slightly different actions, but both are nervine tonics.[109] The fresh green juice has demonstrated efficacy in reducing nicotine cravings and assisting in smoking cessation,[159] possibly through a stress-relieving, anxiolytic activity. *Scutellaria lateriflora* also has a history of use,[160,161] and demonstrated clinical efficacy as a nervine tonic.[162] Finally, *Hypericum perforatum*, best known for its antidepressant activity, has traditionally been suggested to be of 'value in nervous disorders'.[161] Doses between 300 and 1200 mg have shown clinical efficacy in reducing symptoms of many stress-related disorders including depression,[163] premenstrual syndrome[164] and anxiety (see Chapters 14–17 on the nervous system).

Correction of digestive function

The gastrointestinal tract plays a key role in immune function (see Chapters 4–6 on the gastrointestinal system). Not only can hypochlorhydria and malabsorption lead to key nutrient deficiencies, they can also predispose a patient to increased intestinal permeability (leaky gut), which then contributes to systemic immune dysregulation via gut-associated lymphatic tissue (GALT) dysfunction. This can then disrupt the mucosal immunity of extra-gastrointestinal tissues including the respiratory tract.[165,166]

Altered intestinal microflora may also contribute to immune deficiency, and may be a further underlying cause of recurrent URTIs. **Probiotic supplementation** with *Lactobacillus* GG, *Lactobacillus casei rhamnosus*, *Lactobacillus plantarum*, *Lactobacillus rhamnosus* and *Bifidobacterium lactis* has been shown to be useful in controlling respiratory infection.[167–169] A meta-analysis of 14 trials reported that supplementation of a number of different strains of probiotics may reduce the symptoms and duration of respiratory tract infection.[170]

INTEGRATIVE MEDICAL CONSIDERATIONS

Acupuncture

Most of the studies using acupuncture as a treatment method have been undertaken in China—and to a lesser extent Japan—and therefore many published results are unavailable in English.[171] Additionally, acupuncture trials are complicated by the difficulty of practising sham acupuncture as placebo treatment.[172] In traditional Chinese medicine, URTI may be viewed as 'pathogenic invasion of wind' (wind-cold or wind-heat) into the lung.[173] The studies available do show benefit using this treatment in respiratory infections but not as prophylaxis.[174] Acupuncture manipulation on the neck produces a significant decrease in the symptoms of the common cold, potentially via immune system activation.[145,172,174,175]

CLINICAL SUMMARY

The immediate aim of naturopathic treatment of respiratory infections should be amelioration of symptoms via strengthening immune defences and increasing inflammation clearance while limiting the causative pathogens. Once the acute stage has passed, treatment should focus on supporting vitality and addressing underlying imbalances such as gastrointestinal dysfunction, psychological and physiological stress and chronically lowered vitality. Longer term immune support may be warranted, but the power of basic lifestyle interventions—fresh air, clean water, sunshine, fresh fruit and vegetables, a balance of proteins and beneficial fats—should not be disregarded, and more interventionist treatment may not be necessary if utilised properly.

Not all naturopathic treatments are targeted at all stages of respiratory infection. Some interventions are effective for prophylaxis but not treatment. Likewise, some treatments are more appropriate in the acute stages of infection, compared with others that should be considered for chronic use. It is important to have an understanding of which interventions are best suited to each stage, rather than attempting to use a 'one-size-fits-all' approach. In this respect, when the infection is acute the primary focus is to clear the infection, while a 'tonifying' formulation can be used in the aftermath. Acute infections should resolve quickly; however, if they persist (especially in the infirm and elderly) then altering the treatment approach and prescription may be advised, in addition to appropriate medical referral.

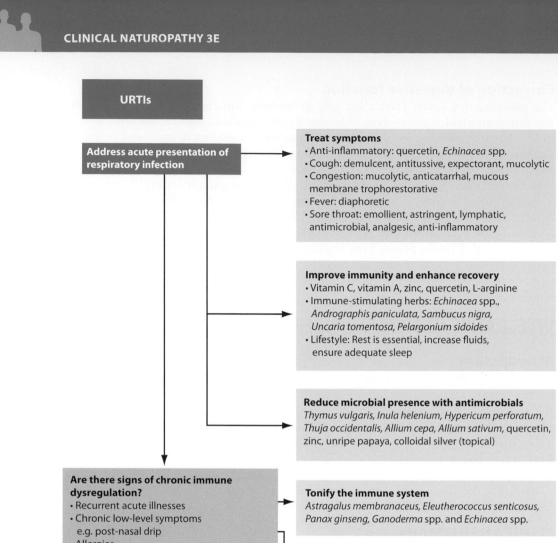

URTIs

Address acute presentation of respiratory infection

Treat symptoms
- Anti-inflammatory: quercetin, *Echinacea* spp.
- Cough: demulcent, antitussive, expectorant, mucolytic
- Congestion: mucolytic, anticatarrhal, mucous membrane trophorestorative
- Fever: diaphoretic
- Sore throat: emollient, astringent, lymphatic, antimicrobial, analgesic, anti-inflammatory

Improve immunity and enhance recovery
- Vitamin C, vitamin A, zinc, quercetin, L-arginine
- Immune-stimulating herbs: *Echinacea* spp., *Andrographis paniculata*, *Sambucus nigra*, *Uncaria tomentosa*, *Pelargonium sidoides*
- Lifestyle: Rest is essential, increase fluids, ensure adequate sleep

Reduce microbial presence with antimicrobials
Thymus vulgaris, *Inula helenium*, *Hypericum perforatum*, *Thuja occidentalis*, *Allium cepa*, *Allium sativum*, quercetin, zinc, unripe papaya, colloidal silver (topical)

Are there signs of chronic immune dysregulation?
- Recurrent acute illnesses
- Chronic low-level symptoms e.g. post-nasal drip
- Allergies

Tonify the immune system
Astragalus membranaceus, *Eleutherococcus senticosus*, *Panax ginseng*, *Ganoderma* spp. and *Echinacea* spp.

Are there signs of digestive dysfunction?
- Bloating
- Burping, flatulence
- Stool irregularity
- Abdominal pain or discomfort

Is the client under stress?

Support adrenal function
Vitamin C, zinc

Panax ginseng, *Eleutherococcus senticosus*, *Glycyrrhiza glabra*, *Rehmannia glutinosa*, *Bupleurum falcatum*, *Withania somnifera*

Lifestyle: ensure adequate rest and sleep. Relaxation techniques such as yoga, meditation

Improve digestion
- Digestive enzymes, hydrochloric acid, apple cider vinegar
- Eat more slowly and mindfully, ensure properly chewed
Reduce gut permeability
Hydrastis canadensis, *Ulmus fulva*, glutamine, vitamin A
Rebalance microflora
Probiotics including *Lactobacillus GG*, *Lactobacillus casei rhamnosus*, *Lactobacillus plantarum*, *Lactobacillus rhamnosus* and *Bifidobacterium lactis*

Figure 8.2
Naturopathic treatment decision tree—URTI

Table 8.4
Review of the major evidence

Intervention	Mechanisms of action	Key literature	Summary of results	Comment
Vitamin C	Enhances natural killer cell numbers and activity by up to 10 times[176] Enhances T- and B-cell function[176] Effects on phagocyte function and production of interferon Effects on gene expression of monocyte adhesion molecules[134,177]	Anderson et al. 1980[178] Heuser & Vojdani 1997[176] Carrillo et al. 2008[134]	Prophylactic use of at least 0.2 g/day is beneficial, with a reduction in cold duration of 8% for adults and 13.6% for children[179] Evidence does not, at this stage, show that vitamin C prophylaxis reduces common cold incidence in the general population[179] 1.5 g/day for the first day of the common cold and 1 g/day for the following four days have been shown to have a significant effect on cold symptoms[178,179]	Useful for cold prophylaxis if exposed to physical stressors but not for the general population May reduce duration of illness, possibly more efficacious in pneumonia than the common cold Effects dependent upon using therapeutic dosage
Zinc	Immune supportive Necessary for the development and function of natural killer cells, phagocytes, macrophages and neutrophils Deficiency causes reduced Th1 cells Deficiency leads to decreased thymic function[15,70–72] Prolonged deficiency increases glucocorticoid secretion, which accelerates pre-T-cell and pre-B-cell apoptosis[180] Essential for cytokine production and secretion	Marshall 2000[181] Wintergerst et al. 2006[18] Caruso et al. 2007[182] Marshall 2007[183] Mahalanabis et al. 2004[61] Hirt et al. 2007[184]	Overall, trials of zinc on the common cold report conflicting results[18,181–183] In about half of studies zinc lozenges seem to have beneficial effects on naturally acquired colds; however, many of these studies are poorly designed, so more research is needed[181–183] (Note: One later Cochrane study[183] has been withdrawn) Trials of oral supplementation (up to 30 mg) reduce pneumonia incidence in adults and children by 41% and 26% respectively[18] Zinc nasal gel reduces duration of cold symptoms when taken within 24 hours of onset[184]	Supplementation probably only of benefit in zinc-deficient individuals

183

Table 8.4
Review of the major evidence (continued)

Intervention	Mechanisms of action	Key literature	Summary of results	Comment
Echinacea spp.	Immune modulatory Suppresses/modulates expression of IL-6 and IL-8 expression by bronchial cells infected with a number of common respiratory pathogens Modifies T helper cell populations Antiviral properties in vitro Particularly enveloped viruses Antimicrobial properties in vitro Preventive effects against the development of respiratory symptoms	Sharma et al. 2009[45] Sharma et al. 2009[99] Shah et al. 2007[100] Schoop et al. 2006[185] O'Neil et al. 2008[186] Tiralongo et al. 2012[187]	In 14 unique studies, echinacea decreased the odds of developing the common cold by 58% and the duration of a cold by 1.4 days[100] The likelihood of experiencing a clinical cold was 55% higher with placebo than with echinacea[185] Over eight weeks of treatment the echinacea group experienced fewer sick days, but the result was not significant against a placebo of parsley[186] Supplementation with standardised *Echinacea* tablets, if taken before and during travel, may have preventive effects against the development of respiratory symptoms during travel involving long-haul flights	May be more beneficial as a prophylactic rather than for acute use
Andrographis paniculata	Immune supportive, especially in acute infection Inhibits NF-κB and COX-2 ↑ Phagocytosis, white blood cell count ↓ TNF-α, GM-CSF ↓ IL-2, IFN-γ production Antiviral effects in vitro	Kligler et al. 2006[108] Poolsup et al. 2004[105] Coon & Ernst 2004[107]	Systematic literature reviews collectively suggest that *Andrographis paniculata* is superior to placebo in alleviating the subjective symptoms of uncomplicated upper respiratory tract infection[107] There is also preliminary evidence of a preventative effect[107]	Potentially effective as an acute treatment of URTI
Acupuncture	Modulates a range of cytokines and immunological functions	Kawakita et al. 2008[174] Suzuki et al. 2009[171] Kawakita et al. 2004[172]	Overall, the available reviews suggest that[174]: – acupuncture is effective for treating common cold symptoms – there is lack of convincing evidence to recommend Japanese acupuncture or moxibustion for prevention of the common cold – the studies reviewed had several limitations, so further research is advisable	Most of the literature is in Chinese or Japanese, making a thorough review of the evidence difficult[171] Rigorous trial design is complicated by the difficulty of supplying a placebo equivalent[171]

KEY POINTS

- RTIs may be viral, bacterial or (rarely) fungal or (less commonly) mycobacterial.

- Remember the importance of basic lifestyle interventions—fresh air, clean water, sunshine etc.

- If a person is ill, always consider longer term immune support once the acute infection has been addressed.

- Amelioration of symptoms, limitation of causative pathogens and strengthening immune defences and clearance address a patient's immediate needs.

- Post-infection, look to support vitality and address underlying imbalances such as gastrointestinal dysfunction, psychological and physiological stress and chronically lowered vitality.

- Some interventions are effective for prophylaxis but not treatment and vice versa for others. Likewise, some treatments are more appropriate in the acute stages of infection, compared with others that should be considered for chronic use.

FURTHER READING

Barrett B, Brown R, Rakel D, et al. Placebo effects and the common cold: a randomized controlled trial. Ann Fam Med 2011;9(4):312–22.

Cunningham-Rundles S, et al. Mechanisms of nutrient modulation of the immune response. J Allergy Clin Immunol 2005;115(6):1119–28.

Karsch-Völk M, Barrett B, Kiefer D, et al. Echinacea for preventing and treating the common cold. Cochrane Database Syst Rev 2014;(2):CD000530, doi:10.1002/14651858.CD000530.pub3.

Mousa HA. Prevention and treatment of influenza, influenza-like illness, and common cold by herbal, complementary, and natural therapies. J Evid Based Complementary Altern Med 2017;22(1):166–74. [Epub 2016 Apr 6]; Review.

Spelman K, et al. Modulation of cytokine expression by traditional medicines: a review of herbal immunomodulators. Altern Med Rev 2006;11(2):128–50.

Acknowledgment: The author would like to acknowledge Tessa Finney-Brown, who authored this chapter in previous editions.

REFERENCES

1. Heikkinen T, Jarvinen A. The common cold. Lancet 2003;361(9351):51–9.

2. Mackay IM. Human rhinoviruses: the cold wars resume. J Clin Virol 2008;42(4):297–320.

3. Meissner HC. Reducing the impact of viral respiratory infections in children. Pediatr Clin North Am 2005;52(3):695–710, v.

4. Wardwell L, Chapman-Novakofski K, Herrel S, et al. Nutrient intake and immune function of elderly subjects. J Am Diet Assoc 2008;108(12):2005–12.

5. Kuiken T, Taubenberger JK. Pathology of human influenza revisited. Vaccine 2008;26(Suppl. 4):D59–66.

6. Roxas M, Jurenka J. Colds and influenza: a review of diagnosis and conventional, botanical, and nutritional considerations. Altern Med Rev 2007;12(1):25–48.

7. Hemming VG. Viral respiratory diseases in children: classification, etiology, epidemiology, and risk factors. J Pediatr 1994;124(5 Pt 2):S13–16.

8. Sloots TP, Whiley DM, Lambert SB, et al. Emerging respiratory agents: new viruses for old diseases? J Clin Virol 2008;42(3):233–43.

9. Proud D. Upper airway viral infections. Pulm Pharmacol Ther 2008;21(3):468–73.

10. Arruda E, Pitkaranta A, Witek TJ Jr, et al. Frequency and natural history of rhinovirus infections in adults during autumn. J Clin Microbiol 1997;35(11):2864–8.

11. Beutler B, Crozat K, Koziol JA, et al. Genetic dissection of innate immunity to infection: the mouse cytomegalovirus model. Curr Opin Immunol 2005;17(1):36–43.

12. Leonard WJ. Genetic effects on immunity: editorial overview. Curr Opin Immunol 2000;12(4):465–7.

13. Mouton D, Stiffel C, Biozzi G. Genetic factors of immunity against infection. Ann Inst Pasteur Immunol 1985;136D(2):131–41.

14. Cohen S. Psychological stress and susceptibility to upper respiratory infections. Am J Respir Crit Care Med 1995;152(4 Pt 2):S53–8.

15. Cunningham-Rundles S, McNeeley DF, Moon A. Mechanisms of nutrient modulation of the immune response. J Allergy Clin Immunol 2005;115(6):1119–28, quiz 1129.

16. Villamor E, Fawzi WW. Effects of vitamin A supplementation on immune responses and correlation with clinical outcomes. Clin Microbiol Rev 2005;18(3):446–64.

17. Schaible UE, Kaufmann SH. Malnutrition and infection: complex mechanisms and global impacts. PLoS Med 2007;4(5):e115.

18. Wintergerst ES, Maggini S, Hornig DH. Immune-enhancing role of vitamin C and zinc and effect on clinical conditions. Ann Nutr Metab 2006;50(2):85–94.

19. Trakatellis A, Dimitriadou A, Trakatelli M. Pyridoxine deficiency: new approaches in immunosuppression and chemotherapy. Postgrad Med J 1997;73(864):617–22.

20. Arredondo M, Nunez MT. Iron and copper metabolism. Mol Aspects Med 2005;26(4–5):313–27.

21. Cashat-Cruz M, Morales-Aguirre JJ, Mendoza-Azpiri M. Respiratory tract infections in children in developing countries. Semin Pediatr Infect Dis 2005;16(2):84–92.

22. Glynn A, Thuvander A, Aune M, et al. Immune cell counts and risks of respiratory infections among infants exposed pre- and postnatally to organochlorine compounds: a prospective study. Environ Health 2008;7:62.

23. Kostka T, Drygas W, Jegier A, et al. Physical activity and upper respiratory tract infections. Int J Sports Med 2008;29(2):158–62.

24. Neiman D. Exercise and Immunity: Clinical Studies. Psychoneuroimmunology (Fourth Edition). 2007, p. 661–73.

25. Johnson C, Eccles R. Acute cooling of the feet and the onset of common cold symptoms. Fam Pract 2005;22(6):608–13.

26. Falagas ME, Theocharis G, Spanos A, et al. Effect of meteorological variables on the incidence of respiratory tract infections. Respir Med 2008;102(5):733–7.

27. Zhu Z, Tang W, Ray A, et al. Rhinovirus stimulation of interleukin-6 in vivo and in vitro. Evidence for nuclear factor kappa B-dependent transcriptional activation. J Clin Invest 1996;97(2):421–30.

28. Turner RB, Weingand KW, Yeh CH, et al. Association between interleukin-8 concentration in nasal secretions and severity of symptoms of experimental rhinovirus colds. Clin Infect Dis 1998;26(4):840–6.

29. Smith S, Schroeder K, Fahey T. Over-the-counter medications for acute cough in children and adults in ambulatory settings. Cochrane Database Syst Rev 2008;(1):CD001831.

30. Guppy M, Mickan S, Del Mar C. 'Drink plenty of fluids': a systematic review of evidence for this recommendation in acute respiratory infections. BMJ 2004;328(7238):499–500.

31. Fashner J, Ericson K, Werner S. Treatment of the common cold in children and adults. Am Fam Physician 2012;86(2):153–9.

32. Barrett B, Brown R, Rakel D, et al. Placebo effects and the common cold: a randomized controlled trial. Ann Fam Med 2011;9(4):312–22.

33. Arroll B. Non-antibiotic treatments for upper-respiratory tract infections (common cold). Respir Med 2005;99(12):1477–84.

34. Spurling G, Del Mar C, Dooley L, et al. Delayed antibiotics for respiratory infections. Cochrane Database Syst Rev 2007;(3):CD004417.

35. Ram F, Rodriguez-Roisin R, Granados-Navarrete A, et al. Antibiotics for exacerbations of chronic obstructive pulmonary disease. Cochrane Database Syst Rev 2006;(2):CD004403.

36. Nicholson KG, Aoki FY, Osterhaus AD, et al. Efficacy and safety of oseltamivir in treatment of acute influenza: a randomised controlled trial. Neuraminidase Inhibitor Flu Treatment Investigator Group. Lancet 2000;355(9218):1845–50.

37. Jefferson T, Del Mar C, Dooley L, et al. Physical interventions to interrupt or reduce the spread of respiratory viruses: a Cochrane review. Health Technol Assess 2010;14(34):347–476.

38. Bone KM. A clinical guide to blending liquid herbs. Philadelphia: Churchill Livingstone; 2003.

39. Fischer C, Painter G. Materia medica of western herbs for the Southern Hemisphere. Victoria, BC: AbeBooks; 1996.

40. Mills S, Bone K. Principles and practice of phytotherapy. Edinburgh: Churchill Livingstone; 2000.

41. Osiecki H, editor. The nutrient bible. 6th ed. Eagle Farm: Bio Concepts Publishing; 2004.

42. Scientific Committee of the British Herbal Medical Association. British herbal pharmacopoeia. 1st ed. Bournemouth: British Herbal Medicine Association; 1983.

43. Kim BH, Lee IJ, Lee HY, et al. Quercetin 3-O-beta-(2''-galloyl)-glucopyranoside inhibits endotoxin LPS-induced IL-6 expression and NF-kappa B activation in macrophages. Cytokine 2007;39(3):207–15.

44. Liu J, Li X, Yue Y, et al. The inhibitory effect of quercetin on IL-6 production by LPS-stimulated neutrophils. Cell Mol Immunol 2005;2(6):455–60.

45. Sharma M, Schoop R, Hudson JB. Echinacea as an antiinflammatory agent: the influence of physiologically relevant parameters. Phytother Res 2009;23(6):863–7.

46. Schmitt B. Fever phobia: misconceptions of parents about fevers. Am J Dis Child 1980;134(2):176–81.

47. Betz M, Grunfeld A. 'Fever phobia' in the emergency department: a survey of children's caregivers. Eur J Emerg Med 2006;13(3):129–33.

48. Greensmith L. Nurses' knowledge of and attitudes towards fever and fever management in one Irish children's hospital. J Child Health Care 2013.

49. Poirier M, Davis P, Gonzalez-del Rey J, et al. Pediatric emergency department nurses' perspectives on fever in children. Pediatr Emerg Care 2000;16(1):9–12.

50. Carey J. Literature review: should antipyretic therapies routinely be administered to patient fever? J Clin Nurs 2010;19(17–18):2377–93.

51. Mackowiak PA. Concepts of fever. Arch Intern Med 1998;158(17):1870–81.

52. Bryant RE, Hood AF, Hood CE, et al. Factors affecting mortality of gram-negative rod bacteremia. Arch Intern Med 1971;127(1):120–8.

53. Weinstein MI, Iannini PB, Staton CW, et al. Spontaneous bacterial peritonitis: a review of 28 cases with emphasis on improved survival and factors influencing prognosis. A J Med 1978;64(4):592–8.

54. Graham NM, Burrell CJ, Douglas RM, et al. Adverse effects of aspirin, acetaminophen, and ibuprofen on immune function, viral shedding, and clinical status in rhinovirus-infected volunteers. J Infect Dis 1990;162(6):1277–82.

55. Doran T, DeAngelis C, Baumgardner RA, et al. Acetaminophen: more harm than good for chicken pox? J Pediatr 1989;114(6):1045–8.

56. Stanley E, Jackson G, Panusarn C, et al. Increased viral shedding with aspirin treatment of rhinovirus infection. JAMA 1975;231(12):1248–51.

57. Dinarello C. Endogenous pyrogens: the role of cytokines in the pathogenesis of fever. In: Mackowiak P, editor. Fever: basic mechanisms and management. New York: Raven Press; 1997. p. 23–47.

58. Laupland KB. Fever in the critically ill medical patient. Crit Care Med 2009;37(7 Suppl.):S273–8.

59. Mills S, Bone K. Principles and practice of phytotherapy. Edinburgh: Churchill Livingstone; 2000.

60. Scientific Committee of the British Herbal Medical Association. British herbal pharmacopoeia. 1st ed. Bournemouth: British Herbal Medicine Association; 1983.

61. Mahalanabis D, Lahiri M, Paul D, et al. Randomized, double-blind, placebo-controlled clinical trial of the efficacy of treatment with zinc or vitamin A in infants and young children with severe acute lower respiratory infection. Am J Clin Nutr 2004;79(3):430–6.

62. Canton R, Lode H, Graninger W, et al. Respiratory tract infections: at-risk patients, who are they? Implications for their management with levofloxacin. Int J Antimicrob Agents 2006;28(Suppl. 2):S115–27.

63. Wissinger E, Goulding J, Hussell T. Immune homeostasis in the respiratory tract and its impact on heterologous infection. Semin Immunol 2009;21(3):147–55.

64. Nieman DC. Immunonutrition support for athletes. Nutr Rev 2008;66(6):310–20.

65. Proud D. Nitric oxide and the common cold. Curr Opin Allergy Clin Immunol 2005;5(1):37–42.

66. Mizutani A, Maki H, Torii Y, et al. Ascorbate-dependent enhancement of nitric oxide formation in activated macrophages. Nitric Oxide 1998;2(4):235–41.

67. Hemila H. Vitamin C, respiratory infections and the immune system. Trends Immunol 2003;24(11):579–80.

68. Rayment SJ, Shaw J, Woollard KJ, et al. Vitamin C supplementation in normal subjects reduces constitutive ICAM-1 expression. Biochem Biophys Res Commun 2003;308(2):339–45.

69. Hemila H, Chalker E. Vitamin C for preventing and treating the common cold. Cochrane Database Syst Rev 2013;(1):CD000980.

70. Fraker PJ. Roles for cell death in zinc deficiency. J Nutr 2005;135(3):359–62.

71. Fraker PJ, King LE, Laakko T, et al. The dynamic link between the integrity of the immune system and zinc status. J Nutr 2000;130(5S Suppl.):1399S–406S.

72. Prasad AS. Clinical, immunological, anti-inflammatory and antioxidant roles of zinc. Exp Gerontol 2008;43(5):370–7.

73. Singh M, Das RR. Zinc for the common cold. Cochrane Database Syst Rev 2011;(2):CD001364.

74. Gandia P, Bour D, Maurette JM, et al. A bioavailability study comparing two oral formulations containing zinc (Zn bis-glycinate vs. Zn gluconate) after a single administration to twelve healthy female volunteers. Int J Vitam Nutr Res 2007;77(4):243–8.

75. Siepmann M, Spank S, Kluge A, et al. The pharmacokinetics of zinc from zinc gluconate: a comparison with zinc oxide in healthy men. Int J Clin Pharmacol Ther 2005;43(12):562–5.

76. Tompkins TA, Renard NE, Kiuchi A. Clinical evaluation of the bioavailability of zinc-enriched yeast and zinc gluconate in healthy volunteers. Biol Trace Elem Res 2007;120(1–3):28–35.

77. Hemila H. Zinc lozenges may shorten common cold duration. Expert Rev Respir Med 2012;6(3):253–4.

78. Nair MP, Kandaswami C, Mahajan S, et al. The flavonoid, quercetin, differentially regulates Th-1 (IFNgamma) and Th-2 (IL4) cytokine gene expression by normal peripheral blood mononuclear cells. Biochim Biophys Acta 2002;1593(1):29–36.

79. Nieman DC, Henson DA, Davis JM, et al. Quercetin's influence on exercise-induced changes in plasma cytokines and muscle and leukocyte cytokine mRNA. J Appl Physiol 2007;103(5):1728–35.

80. Nieman DC, Henson DA, Gross SJ, et al. Quercetin reduces illness but not immune perturbations after intensive exercise. Med Sci Sports Exerc 2007;39(9):1561–9.

81. Kumar P, Khanna M, Srivastava V, et al. Effect of quercetin supplementation on lung antioxidants after experimental influenza virus infection. Exp Lung Res 2005;31(5):449–59.

82. Cameron C, Dallaire F, Vezina C, et al. Neonatal vitamin A deficiency and its impact on acute respiratory infections among preschool Inuit children. Can J Public Health 2008;99(2):102–6.

83. Chen H, Zhuo Q, Yuan W, et al. Vitamin A for preventing acute lower respiratory tract infections in children up to seven years of age. Cochrane Database Syst Rev 2008;(1):CD006090.

84. Stephensen CB. Vitamin A, infection, and immune function. Annu Rev Nutr 2001;21:167–92.

85. Spelman K, Burns J, Nichols D, et al. Modulation of cytokine expression by traditional medicines: a review of herbal immunomodulators. Altern Med Rev 2006;11(2):128–50.

86. Huang CF, Lin SS, Liao PH, et al. The immunopharmaceutical effects and mechanisms of herb medicine. Cell Mol Immunol 2008;5(1):23–31.

87. Abu-Ghefreh AA, Canatan H, Ezeamuzie CI. In vitro and in vivo anti-inflammatory effects of andrographolide. Int Immunopharmacol 2009;9(3):313–18.

88. Burgos RA, Seguel K, Perez M, et al. Andrographolide inhibits IFN-gamma and IL-2 cytokine production and protects against cell apoptosis. Planta Med 2005;71(5):429–34.

89. Shen YC, Chen CF, Chiou WF. Andrographolide prevents oxygen radical production by human neutrophils: possible mechanism(s) involved in its anti-inflammatory effect. Br J Pharmacol 2002;135(2):399–406.

90. Hidalgo MA, Romero A, Figueroa J, et al. Andrographolide interferes with binding of nuclear factor-kappaB to DNA in HL-60-derived neutrophilic cells. Br J Pharmacol 2005;144(5):680–6.

91. Naik SR, Hule A. Evaluation of immunomodulatory activity of an extract of andrographolides from Andographis paniculata. Planta Med 2009;75(8):785–91.

92. Qin LH, Kong L, Shi GJ, et al. Andrographolide inhibits the production of TNF-alpha and interleukin-12 in lipopolysaccharide-stimulated macrophages: role of mitogen-activated protein kinases. Biol Pharm Bull 2006;29(2):220–4.

93. Laus G. Advances in chemistry and bioactivity of the genus Uncaria. Phytother Res 2004;18(4):259–74.

94. Block KI, Mead MN. Immune system effects of echinacea, ginseng, and astragalus: a review. Integr Cancer Ther 2003;2(3):247–67.

95. Bleakney TL. Deconstructing an adaptogen: eleutherococcus senticosus. Holist Nurs Pract 2008;22(4):220–4.

96. Drozd J, Sawicka T, Prosinska J. Estimation of humoral activity of Eleutherococcus senticosus. Acta Pol Pharm 2002;59(5):395–401.

97. Prieto JM, Recio MC, Giner RM, et al. Influence of traditional Chinese anti-inflammatory medicinal plants on leukocyte and platelet functions. J Pharm Pharmacol 2003;55(9):1275–82.

98. Zhou X, Lin J, Yin Y, et al. Ganodermataceae: natural products and their related pharmacological functions. Am J Chin Med 2007;35(4):559–74.

99. Sharma M, Anderson SA, Schoop R, et al. Induction of multiple pro-inflammatory cytokines by respiratory viruses and reversal by standardized Echinacea, a potent antiviral herbal extract. Antiviral Res 2009;83(2):165–70.

100. Shah S, Sander S, White C, et al. Evaluation of echinacea for the prevention and treatment of the common cold: a meta-analysis. Lancet Infect Dis 2007;7(7):347–8.

101. Tiralongo E, Lea RA, Wee SS, et al. Randomised, double blind, placebo-controlled trial of echinacea supplementation in air travellers. Evid Based Complement Alternat Med 2012;2012:417267. doi:10.1155/2012/417267.

102. Jawad M, Schoop R, Suter A, et al. Safety and efficacy profile of Echinacea purpurea to prevent common cold episodes: a randomized, double-blind, placebo-controlled

trial. Evid Based Complement Alternat Med 2012;2012:841315.

103. Williamson E. Major herbs of Ayurveda. London: Churchill Livingstone; 2002.

104. Saxena RC, Singh R, Kumar P, et al. A randomized double blind placebo controlled clinical evaluation of extract of Andrographis paniculata (KalmCold) in patients with uncomplicated upper respiratory tract infection. Phytomedicine 2010;17(3–4):178–85.

105. Poolsup N, Suthisisang C, Prathantararug S, et al. Andrographis paniculata in the symptomatic treatment of uncomplicated upper respiratory tract infection: systematic review of randomized controlled trials. J Clin Pharm Ther 2004;29(1):37–45.

106. Thamlikitkul V, Dechatiwongse T, Theerapong S, et al. Efficacy of Andrographis paniculata Nees for pharyngotonsillitis in adults. J Med Assoc Thai 1991;74(10):437–42.

107. Coon JT, Ernst E. Andrographis paniculata in the treatment of upper respiratory tract infections: a systematic review of safety and efficacy. Planta Med 2004;70(4):293–8.

108. Kligler B, Ulbricht C, Basch E, et al. Andrographis paniculata for the treatment of upper respiratory infection: a systematic review by the natural standard research collaboration. Explore (NY) 2006;2(1):25–9.

109. Bone KM. A clinical guide to blending liquid herbs. Philadelphia: Churchill Livingstone; 2003.

110. Matthias A, Blanchfield JT, Penman KG, et al. Permeability studies of alkylamides and caffeic acid conjugates from echinacea using a Caco-2 cell monolayer model. J Clin Pharm Ther 2004;29(1):7–13.

111. Matthias A, Addison RS, Penman KG, et al. Echinacea alkamide disposition and pharmacokinetics in humans after tablet ingestion. Life Sci 2005;77(16):2018–29.

112. Agnew LL, Guffogg SP, Matthias A, et al. Echinacea intake induces an immune response through altered expression of leucocyte hsp70, increased white cell counts and improved erythrocyte antioxidant defences. J Clin Pharm Ther 2005;30(4):363–9.

113. Perry NB, van Klink JW, Burgess EJ, et al. Alkamide levels in Echinacea purpurea: a rapid analytical method revealing differences among roots, rhizomes, stems, leaves and flowers. Planta Med 1997;63(1):58–62.

114. Chicca A, Raduner S, Pellati F, et al. Synergistic immunomopharmacological effects of N-alkylamides in Echinacea purpurea herbal extracts. Int Immunopharmacol 2009;9(7–8):850–8.

115. Felter H, Lloyd J. King's American Dispensatory, 1898. Echinacea. Online. Available: http://www.henriettesherbal.com/eclectic/kings/echinacea.html 1 Nov 2013.

116. Brush J, Mendenhall E, Guggenheim A, et al. The effect of Echinacea purpurea, Astragalus membranaceus and Glycyrrhiza glabra on CD69 expression and immune cell activation in humans. Phytother Res 2006;20(8):687–95.

117. Boericke W. Boericke's materia medica. Henriette's Herbal Homepage, 1901. Online. Available: http://www.henriettesherbal.com/eclectic/boericke/intro.html 1 Nov 2013.

118. Zakay-Rones Z, Varsano N, Zlotnik M, et al. Inhibition of several strains of influenza virus in vitro and reduction of symptoms by an elderberry extract (Sambucus nigra L.) during an outbreak of influenza B Panama. J Altern Complement Med 1995;1(4):361–9.

119. Barak V, Halperin T, Kalickman I. The effect of Sambucol, a black elderberry-based, natural product, on the production of human cytokines: I. Inflammatory cytokines. Eur Cytokine Netw 2001;12(2):290–6.

120. Krawitz C, Mraheil M, Stein M, et al. Inhibitory activity of a standardized elderberry liquid extract against clinically-relevant human respiratory bacterial pathogens and influenza A and B viruses. BMC Complement Altern Med 2011;11(16):1–6.

121. Kong F. Pilot clinical study on a proprietary elderberry extract: efficacy in addressing influenza symptoms. Online J Pharmacol and PharmacoKinet 2009;5:32–43.

122. Bone K. Personal Communication. 2013.

123. Riley DS, Lizogub VG, Zimmermann A, et al. Efficacy and tolerability of high-dose Pelargonium extract in patients with the common cold. Altern Ther Health Med 2018;24(2):16–26.

124. Davydov M, Krikorian AD. Eleutherococcus senticosus (Rupr. & Maxim.) Maxim. (Araliaceae) as an adaptogen: a closer look. J Ethnopharmacol 2000;72(3):345–93.

125. Kannur DM, Kulkarni AA, Paranjpe MP, et al. Screening of anti-stress properties of Herbal Extracts and Adaptogenic Agents. Pharmacognosy Rev 2008;2(3):95–101.

126. Mowery DB. Herbal tonic therapies. New York: Wings Books; 1993.

127. Matthias A, Banbury L, Bone KM, et al. Echinacea alkylamides modulate induced immune responses in T-cells. Fitoterapia 2008;79(1):53–8.

128. Maciocia G. The practice of Chinese medicine: the treatment of diseases with acupuncture and Chinese herbs. London: Churchill Livingstone; 1994.

129. Kemeny ME, Schedlowski M. Understanding the interaction between psychosocial stress and immune-related diseases: a stepwise progression. Brain Behav Immun 2007;21(8):1009–18.

130. Maciocia G. The foundations of Chinese medicine. Singapore: Churchill Livingstone; 1989.

131. Strausbaugh H, Irwin M. Central corticotropin-releasing hormone reduces cellular immunity. Brain Behav Immun 1992;6(1):11–17.

132. Kainuma E, Watanabe M, Tomiyama-Miyaji C, et al. Association of glucocorticoid with stress-induced modulation of body temperature, blood glucose and innate immunity. Psychoneuroendocrinology 2009;34(10):1459–68.

133. Kemeny M. Emotions and the Immune System. In: Ader R, editor. Psychoneuroimmunology. 4th ed. San Diego: Elsevier Academic Press; 2007.

134. Carrillo AE, Murphy RJ, Cheung SS. Vitamin C supplementation and salivary immune function following exercise-heat stress. Int J Sports Physiol Perform 2008;3(4):516–30.

135. Gibb J, Audet MC, Hayley S, et al. Neurochemical and behavioral responses to inflammatory immune stressors. Front Biosci (Schol Ed) 2009;1:275–95.

136. DeRijk R, Michelson D, Karp B, et al. Exercise and circadian rhythm-induced variations in plasma cortisol differentially regulate interleukin-1 beta (IL-1 beta), IL-6, and tumor necrosis factor-alpha (TNF alpha) production in humans: high sensitivity of TNF alpha and resistance of IL-6. J Clin Endocrinol Metab 1997;82(7):2182–91.

137. Avitsur R, Hunzeker J, Sheridan JF. Role of early stress in the individual differences in host response to viral infection. Brain Behav Immun 2006;20(4):339–48.

138. Satterlee DG, Aguilera-Quintana I, Munn BJ, et al. Vitamin C amelioration of the adrenal stress response in broiler chickens being prepared for slaughter. Comp Biochem Physiol A Comp Physiol 1989;94(4):569–74.

139. Roth DE, Caulfield LE, Ezzati M, et al. Acute lower respiratory infections in childhood: opportunities for reducing the global burden through nutritional interventions. Bull World Health Organ 2008;86(5):356–64.

140. Panossian A, Wikman G. Evidence-based efficacy of adaptogens in fatigue, and molecular mechanisms related to their stress-protective activity. Curr Clin Pharmacol 2009;4(3):198–219.

141. Grieve M. A modern herbal. New York: Dover Publications; 1931.

142. Gaffney BT, Hugel HM, Rich PA. Panax ginseng and Eleutherococcus senticosus may exaggerate an already existing biphasic response to stress via inhibition of enzymes which limit the binding of stress hormones to their receptors. Med Hypotheses 2001;56(5):567–72.

143. Singh A, Zelazowska EB, Petrides JS, et al. Lymphocyte subset responses to exercise and glucocorticoid suppression in healthy men. Med Sci Sports Exerc 1996;28(7): 822–8.

144. Moser M, De Smedt T, Sornasse T, et al. Glucocorticoids down-regulate dendritic cell function in vitro and in vivo. Eur J Immunol 1995;25(10):2818–24.

145. Irwin MR. Human psychoneuroimmunology: 20 years of discovery. Brain Behav Immun 2008;22(2):129–39.

146. Bhattacharya SK, Muruganandam AV. Adaptogenic activity of Withania somnifera: an experimental study using a rat model of chronic stress. Pharmacol Biochem Behav 2003;75(3):547–55.

147. Kaur P, Sharma M, Mathur S, et al. Effect of 1-oxo-5beta, 6beta-epoxy-witha-2-ene-27-ethoxy-olide isolated from the roots of Withania somnifera on stress indices in Wistar rats. J Altern Complement Med 2003;9(6):897–907.

148. Kour K, Pandey A, Suri KA, et al. Restoration of stress-induced altered T cell function and corresponding cytokines patterns by Withanolide A. Int Immunopharmacol 2009;9(10):1137–44.

149. Perfumi M, Mattioli L. Adaptogenic and central nervous system effects of single doses of 3% rosavin and 1% salidroside Rhodiola rosea L. extract in mice. Phytother Res 2007;21(1):37–43.

150. Kelly GS. Rhodiola rosea: a possible plant adaptogen. Altern Med Rev 2001;6(3):293–302.

151. Blumenthal M, Goldberg A, Brinckmann J, editors. Herbal medicine: expanded commission E monographs (English translation). Austin: Integrative Medicine Communications; 2000.

152. Tachikawa E, Kudo K. Proof of the mysterious efficacy of ginseng: basic and clinical trials: suppression of adrenal medullary function in vitro by ginseng. J Pharmacol Sci 2004;95(2):140–4.

153. Nocerino E, Amato M, Izzo AA. The aphrodisiac and adaptogenic properties of ginseng. Fitoterapia 2000;71(Suppl. 1):S1–5.

154. Rai D, Bhatia G, Sen T, et al. Anti-stress effects of Ginkgo biloba and Panax ginseng: a comparative study. J Pharmacol Sci 2003;93(4):458–64.

155. Fulder SJ. Ginseng and the hypothalamic-pituitary control of stress. Am J Chin Med 1981;9(2):112–18.

156. Braun L, Cohen M. Herbs and natural supplements: an evidence-based guide. 3rd ed. Marrickville: Elsevier; 2010.

157. Kato H, Kanaoka M, Yano S, et al. 3-Monoglucuronyl-glycyrrhetinic acid is a major metabolite that causes licorice-induced pseudoaldosteronism. J Clin Endocrinol Metab 1995;80(6):1929–33.

158. Zhang RX, Li MX, Jia ZP. Rehmannia glutinosa: review of botany, chemistry and pharmacology. J Ethnopharmacol 2008;117(2):199–214.

159. Anand CL. Effect of Avina Sativa on cigarette smoking. Nature 1971;233(5320):1.

160. Cook W. The Physiomedical Dispensatory, 1896. Online. Available: http://www.henriettesherbal.com/eclectic/cook/ 1 Nov 2013.

161. Felter H. The Eclectic Materia Medica, Pharmacology and Therapeutics, 1922. Online. Available: http://www.henriettesherbal.com/eclectic/felter/ 1 Nov 2013.

162. Wolfson P, Hoffmann D. An investigation into the efficacy of Scutellaria lateriflora in healthy volunteers. Altern Ther Health Med 2003;9(2):4.

163. Kasper S, Anghelescu I, Szegedi A, et al. Superior efficacy of St John's wort extract WS 5570 compared to placebo in patients with major depression: a randomized, double-blind, placebo-controlled, multi-center trial [ISRCTN77277298]. BMC Med 2006;4.

164. Stevinson C, Ernst E. A pilot study of hypericum perforatum for the treatment of premenstrual syndrome. BJOG 2000;107(7):870–6.

165. Fasano A. Physiological, pathological, and therapeutic implications of zonulin-mediated intestinal barrier modulation: living life on the edge of the wall. Am J Pathol 2008;173(5):1243–52.

166. Lamblin C, Saelens T, Bergoin C, et al. [The common mucosal immune system in respiratory disease]. Rev Mal Respir 2000;17(5):941–6.

167. Hatakka K, Savilahti E, Pönkä A, et al. Effect of long term consumption of probiotic milk on infections in children attending day care centres: double blind, randomised trial. BMJ 2001;322(7298):1327.

168. Lin JS, Chiu YH, Lin NT, et al. Different effects of probiotic species/strains on infections in preschool children: a double-blind, randomized, controlled study. Vaccine 2009;27(7):1073–9.

169. Pregliasco F, Anselmi G, Fonte L, et al. A new chance of preventing winter diseases by the administration of synbiotic formulations. J Clin Gastroenterol 2008;42(Suppl. 3 Pt 2):S224–33.

170. Vouloumanou EK, Makris GC, Karageorgopoulos DE, et al. Probiotics for the prevention of respiratory tract infections: a systematic review. Int J Antimicrob Agents 2009;34(3):197, e1–10.

171. Suzuki M, Yokoyama Y, Yamazaki H. Research into acupuncture for respiratory disease in Japan: a systematic review. Acupunct Med 2009;27(2):54–60.

172. Kawakita K, Shichidou T, Inoue E, et al. Preventive and curative effects of acupuncture on the common cold: a multicentre randomized controlled trial in Japan. Complement Ther Med 2004;12(4):181–8.

173. Zhou Z, Jin HD. Clinical manual of Chinese herbal medicine and acupuncture. Oxford: Churchill Livingstone; 1996.

174. Kawakita K, Shichidou T, Inoue E, et al. Do Japanese style acupuncture and moxibustion reduce symptoms of the common cold? Evid Based Complement Alternat Med 2008;5(4):481–9.

175. Sato T, Yu Y, Guo SY, et al. Acupuncture stimulation enhances splenic natural killer cell cytotoxicity in rats. Jpn J Physiol 1996;46(2):131–6.

176. Heuser G, Vojdani A. Enhancement of natural killer cell activity and T and B cell function by buffered vitamin C in patients exposed to toxic chemicals: the role of protein kinase-C. Immunopharmacol Immunotoxicol 1997;19(3):291–312.

177. Patak P, Willenberg HS, Bornstein SR. Vitamin C is an important cofactor for both adrenal cortex and adrenal medulla. Endocr Res 2004;30(4):871–5.

178. Anderson R. The Effects of increasing weekly doses of ascorbate on certain cellular and humoral immune functions in normal volunteers. Am J Clin Nutr 1980;33(1):5.

179. Douglas R, Hemilä H, Chalker E, et al. Vitamin C for preventing and treating the common cold. Cochrane Database Syst Rev 2007;(3):CD000980.

180. Fraker PJ, King LE. Reprogramming of the immune system during zinc deficiency. Annu Rev Nutr 2004;24:277–98.

181. Marshall I. Zinc for the common cold. Cochrane Database Syst Rev 2000;(2):CD001364.

182. Caruso TJ, Prober CG, Gwaltney JM Jr. Treatment of naturally acquired common colds with zinc: a structured review. Clin Infect Dis 2007;45(5):569–74.

183. Marshall I. WITHDRAWN: zinc for the common cold. Cochrane Database Syst Rev 2006;(3):CD001364.

184. Hirt M, Nobel S, Barron E. Zinc nasal gel for the treatment of common cold symptoms: a double-blind, placebo-controlled trial. Ear Nose Throat J 2000;79(10):778–80, 782.

185. Schoop R, Klein P, Suter A, et al. Echinacea in the prevention of induced rhinovirus colds: a meta-analysis. Clin Ther 2006;28(2):174–83.

186. O'Neil J, Hughes S, Lourie A, et al. Effects of echinacea on the frequency of upper respiratory tract symptoms: a randomized, double-blind, placebo-controlled trial. Ann Allergy Asthma Immunol 2008;100(4): 384–8.

187. Tiralongo E, Lea RA, Wee SS, et al. Randomised, double blind, placebo-controlled trial of echinacea supplementation in air travellers. Evid Based Complement Alternat Med 2012;2012:417267. doi:10.1155/2012/417267.

CHAPTER 9

Asthma

David Casteleijn
ND, MHSc

OVERVIEW

Asthma is a chronic inflammatory disorder of the airways and may be classed as atopic (extrinsic) or intrinsic.[1] It is an obstructive airways disease marked by recurrent attacks of paroxysmal dyspnoea with cough and wheeze, due to spasmodic contraction of the bronchi.[1,2] Key clinical features include wheeze, cough, shortness of breath, chest tightness and sputum production. The signs and symptoms of asthma may be subtle, and some children present with atypical features such as recurrent respiratory tract infections, seasonal asthma and night-time cough. Classically symptoms will present or worsen in relation to certain characteristic triggers.

The inflammation present in asthma is understood as being driven by airway hyperresponsiveness, which may lead to longer term airway remodelling and potentially a degree of permanent bronchial obstruction.[3,4] This inflammation is due to multiple mediators, particularly the recruitment and activation of mast cells and eosinophils, macrophages, dendritic cells and neutrophils, with resultant cellular infiltration and airway inflammation.[3,4] With cellular activation, preformed and generated cytokines and growth factors are released, resulting in the remodelling of the airways with amplified goblet cell production, smooth muscle hypertrophy and deposition of extracellular proteins.[5] The inflammatory mediators also seem to induce changes in the noradrenergic and parasympathetic nervous systems that may lead to bronchial hyperresponsiveness.[4]

In atopic asthma, it is thought that allergen exposure in genetically predisposed people leads to T helper type 2 (Th2) proliferation. Th2 cells stimulate B-lymphocytes

Asthma triggers	
• Inhaled allergens (animal dander or fur, dust mites, fungi, pollen)	• Changes in weather
• Inhaled irritants (tobacco smoke, air pollution)	• Exercise
	• Viral infection
• Occupational exposure to dust, chemicals, fumes or aerosols of industrial material	• Stress or high levels of emotion
	• Menstrual cycles
• Cold air	

Source: McCunney 2005[2]

to produce specific IgE antibodies, which then activate an inflammatory cascade upon subsequent exposure to the allergen (Figure 9.1).[6]

In general, infants are born with a disposition towards pro-allergic and pro-inflammatory Th2 immune responses, but early childhood exposure to infections and endotoxins shifts the body towards a predominance of Th1 responses, which suppress Th2 cells and induce tolerance.[7] The hygiene hypothesis suggests that, in developed countries, the trend towards smaller families,[8] cleaner environments[9] and early use of vaccinations and antibiotics may deprive children of these Th2-suppressing, tolerance-inducing exposures, partly explaining the continuous increase in asthma prevalence in developed countries.[7] It should be noted that, in contrast to this hypothesis, certain studies have identified a pathogenic role for viral respiratory infection in the development of asthma in atopic infants.[10] Yet others have pointed towards a strong dietary influence upon the development of asthma and allergic conditions (discussed later under Digestive and dietary factors), with some suggestion that factors such as these play more of a role than environmental cleanliness, with researchers noting that the exceptional hygiene and low rates of allergy in Japan don't fit the hygiene hypothesis model.[11]

In exercise-induced (intrinsic) asthma, mast cell activation and bronchoconstriction seems to be stimulated by moisture loss from the respiratory tract and increased airway cooling due to an increase in ventilation.[12] However, despite the lack of identifiable allergenic triggers, immune dysregulation, in the form of inappropriate IgE production and activated T-cells, still seems to be a feature.[13]

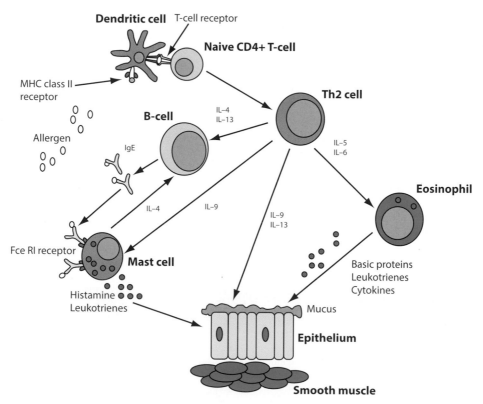

Figure 9.1
Mechanism of atopic asthma
Source: Ryanna et al 2009[6]

RISK FACTORS

Familial, genetic and environmental factors

Having first-degree relatives with a history of asthma, or a personal or family history of atopy, is a risk factor for the condition.[1] Atopic responsiveness is inherited, and genes have been identified that influence bronchial hyperresponsiveness, even in the absence of allergies.[14,15]

The environment also affects asthma development, particularly during early childhood. Breastfeeding during the neonatal period seems to prevent the development of atopy, perhaps as a desensitisation response to continual oral intake of the allergen.[16,17] However, antigen exposure later in infancy seems to promote atopic responses.[14] This may partially explain why the early introduction of formula seems to lead to an increase in child body mass index (BMI) and early asthma and atopy.[18] Childhood exposure to air pollution has been found to be associated with the development of persistent wheeze and atopy in children living in urban environments.[19] Additionally, mouldy and/or damp home environments in the first two years of life are associated with increased asthma risk.[20] Paracetamol use in infancy has also been associated with an increased risk of current wheeze in young children.[21] Some of the latest analysis of large data pools show that pet ownership in early life does not appear to increase or decrease the risk of allergic asthma in children aged 6 to 10,[22] although there is some evidence for an association between furry pet ownership in the first two years of life and reduced sensitisation to aeroallergens.[22] Higher levels of aluminium have been found in the plasma of some asthmatics, associated with altered biochemical parameters, suggesting abnormal distribution of this mineral may precipitate inflammation and oxidative stress, alter Th1–Th2 balance and contribute to the development of asthma.[23] High levels of urinary bisphenol A have been correlated with increased levels of allergic asthma in females.[24]

Digestive and dietary factors

Gastrointestinal symptoms appear to be common in children with asthma.[25] An increased prevalence of increased intestinal permeability and cytokines in patients with asthma may support naturopathic theory that leaky gut is associated with the condition.[26,27]

Gastro-oesophageal reflux has been recognised as a common trigger of asthma,[28] via oesophageal acid-induced reflex bronchoconstriction, or microaspiration of acid. A connection has also been made between hypochlorhydria and bronchial asthma.[29] This correlation may be the result of inadequate protein digestion,[30] increasing atopic allergic reactions. It may also cause poorer nutrient absorption in general,[30] affecting the development of atopy and/or bronchial hyperresponsiveness through various deficiencies.

Nutrient deficiencies, in particular of vitamins C, D and E, magnesium, potassium, and fatty acids, are associated with asthma.[31–33] Poor maternal diet has been correlated with a rise in asthma at the ages of two and five years.[32] Despite early suspicions, maternal peanut and tree nut consumption has not been associated with the development of asthma in children, and may even offer a protective effect.[34] Asthma is also known to have a number of dietary triggers such as specific 'allergenic' foods or food additives.[35,36] Hen's eggs, cow's milk, soy, wheat, tree nuts, peanuts, fish (and shellfish), monosodium glutamate (MSG), tartrazine and sulfites have all been implicated.[33]

One study has linked high fast-food intake (three or more times a week) and/or low fruit consumption (three or fewer serves per week) with a greater likelihood of severe asthma, possibly due to fatty acid balance, or increased levels of sodium, carbohydrates, sugar or preservatives.[37]

Antibiotic use in the first year of life was associated with an increased risk of wheeze in New Zealand children,[21] suggesting dysbiosis may be a risk factor. This theory is supported by evidence showing atopic infants have higher levels of i-caproic acid (a marker of *Clostridium difficile*) and lower populations of lactobacilli, bifidobacteria and *Bacteroides* than non-atopic children.[38]

Stress

Stress is a well-known asthma trigger, but it may also play a role in its pathogenesis.[2,39] Parental divorce or separation, exposure to violence and severe disease of a family member all increase the risk of developing atopic conditions.[40] Lower socioeconomic status is associated with elevated levels of stress and threat perception, as well as heightened production of IL-5 and IL-13 and higher eosinophil counts in children with asthma.[34] Children from this background are more likely to develop asthma, and exhibit poorer health outcomes.[41,42] Anxiety disorders and asthma are also common comorbidities, although the exact relationship is unclear.[43]

Metabolic syndrome

Abdominal obesity and hypertension are both components of metabolic syndrome that increase the risk of asthma-like symptoms.[44] Epidemiological studies show that, generally, people with asthma tend to be heavier than those without—a relationship that is more consistent in adults than children.[38] Additionally, the risk of asthma seems to increase as BMI rises.[45] As both obesity and asthma begin in early life, some researchers have proposed common predisposing factors including genetics, early life weight gain, low physical activity, prenatal diet and nutrition, altered intestinal microflora and adipocytokines.[38]

DIFFERENTIAL DIAGNOSIS

- Chronic obstructive pulmonary disease (wheeze, cough—usually productive)
- Bronchiectasis (cough)
- Lung cancer (cough, chest symptoms)
- Post-nasal drip (cough)
- Allergic reaction (chest tightness and wheeze)
- Gastro-oesophageal reflux (chronic cough)
- Medications (e.g. ACE inhibitor) (chronic cough)

CONVENTIONAL TREATMENT

Medical management of asthma includes four main components:[46]

- routine symptom and lung function monitoring
- patient education
- control or avoidance of environmental triggers and comorbidities that contribute to the severity of the condition
- pharmacological therapy.

Patient attitudes towards medical professionals and asthma treatment have been found to predict the degree of asthma control a patient is likely to achieve with conventional therapies.[47] In Australia the best practice asthma management standard is set by the *Asthma management handbook*.[48] Globally, standards are set by the Global Initiative for Asthma (GINA) and their published guidelines.[49] These generally propose a stepwise approach to the pharmacological management of asthma, based upon severity. Medications fall into two categories: short-acting agents designed to relieve airway obstruction in an acute exacerbation, and longer term prevention therapy.[45]

- Inhaled short-acting β_2-agonists (SABA), as a short-term reliever therapy, act to dilate the bronchioles.
- Inhaled corticosteroids (ICS) are recommended as prevention therapy. They reduce hyperresponsiveness of the airways, reduce inflammatory cell migration and block late-stage allergic responses. These drugs reduce exacerbation risk and impairment of functioning, and early treatment may help prevent the development of irreversible airflow limitation (compared with later treatment).[48]
- A leukotriene receptor antagonist (LTRA) may be considered as an alternative to ICS in some patients in order to combat the increased airway inflammation via modulation of leukotriene mediators released from mast cells, eosinophils and basophils.
- Cromolyn sodium and nedocromil sodium stabilise mast cells and interfere with chloride channel function, and may be used as additional preventive therapy if needed. They may also be used before exercise or unavoidable exposure to known allergens.
- Long-acting β_2-agonists (LABA) have a duration of bronchodilation for up to 12 hours and are useful as preventers. They improve symptom control in patients with moderate to severe asthma who experience asthma symptoms despite treatment with inhaled corticosteroids.[48]
- Sustained-release theophylline is a mild to moderate bronchodilator.

KEY TREATMENT PROTOCOLS

The main role of naturopathic treatment is to prevent acute exacerbations and ultimately address the chronic aspects of asthma. It is essential to remember (and remind the patient) that asthma attacks may be life-threatening and should always be taken seriously. Any severe acute exacerbation requires urgent medical assistance.

A **symptom diary** and **elimination diet** are useful tools to identify trigger factors (see Chapter 6 on food intolerance and allergy). Once known, these should be avoided wherever possible. As recommended by conventional medical practitioners, all efforts should be made to minimise dust mites, mould and pet dander in the home. Pillows, mattress and cushions should be covered with allergen-blocking bedding, and beds should be

> ### Naturopathic Treatment Aims
>
> - Identify allergic triggers and encourage avoidance or control.
> - Enhance patient understanding of and education about their condition and its management.
> - Modulate the immune response appropriately.
> - Reduce airway hypersensitivity and prevent/reduce longer term airway remodelling.
> - Enhance brochodilation.
> - Promote expectoration if required.
> - Correct underlying digestive dysregulation
>   - GIT dysbiosis
>   - increased intestinal permeability.
> - Support the nervous system to reduce the stress response.

raised off the ground. It is best to avoid carpets and upholstered furniture, and preference wood or tiles. Enhancing airflow through the house may assist with reducing mould growth, or a dehumidifier may be used. The house should be cleaned regularly, ideally with a vacuum cleaner that has a HEPA or ULPA filter. With time, and naturopathic treatment (including digestive repair and immune support), the patient may be well enough that certain factors cease to be problematic. As the underlying mechanism of airway obstruction is inflammation, a key priority is to manage the inflammatory response with anti-inflammatory, antiallergic and immune-modulating substances, and reduce airway hypersensitivity. On a symptomatic level, respiration will be most efficient and uncomplicated when the bronchioles are clear. Bronchodilation and expectoration are central actions to open the airways and promote symptom-free ventilation. Given the sizeable role of digestive dysfunction in the aetiogenesis of asthma, once symptoms are stabilised, better control and prevention may then be established by redressing intestinal permeability and dysbiosis.

Dampen the inflammatory cascade

Reducing airway inflammation in asthma will improve symptoms and assist in moderating disease progression. A number of herbal agents demonstrate anti-inflammatory actions specific to asthma. ***Boswellia serrata*** inhibits 5-lipoxygenase,[50] a key cytokine implicated in asthmatic inflammation. Seventy per cent of patients treated with *Boswellia serrata* showed improvement in their asthma symptoms, as opposed to 27% of controls.[51] The anti-inflammatory, antioxidant and antiviral activity of curcumin in ***Curcuma longa*** has been effective in treating airway hyperresponsiveness in allergic inflammatory diseases.[52,53] The oil of this botanical is also significantly active in removing sputum, relieving cough and preventing asthma,[54] and phytochemicals derived from *Curcuma longa* may interrupt the action of NF-κB (which induces inflammation) and diminish Th2 responses, with a concurrent reduction in asthmatic symptoms.[55] Asthmatics taking a combination extract of *Boswellia serrata, Curcuma longa* and ***Glycyrrhiza glabra*** have been shown to have significantly lower plasma levels of inflammatory cytokines when compared with patients on placebo (although this did not affect pulmonary function test results).[56] ***Zingiber officinale*** may also inhibit the release of prostaglandins,[57] suppress Th2-mediated immune responses[58] and inhibit airway contraction, possibly via blockade of plasma membrane Ca^{2+} channels.[59] ***Astragalus membranaceus*** has shown the ability to attenuate lung inflammation, airway responsiveness and other markers associated with allergen-induced asthma in mice.[60] It may also help to modulate some of the pathological processes involved in the development of chronic asthma.[61] Murine models also suggest that ***Crataegus pinnatifida*** may assist in reduction of allergic airway inflammation.[62,63] Dietary supplementation with **omega-3 fatty acids**, **zinc** and **vitamin C** significantly improved asthma control, pulmonary function tests and pulmonary inflammatory markers in children with moderately persistent bronchial asthma.[64] Benefits from essential fatty acids may be derived as far back as fetal development, with adequate maternal intake corresponding with lower rates of asthma in offspring (Figure 9.2)[65] The ingestion of 2.7 g of omega-3 polyunsaturated fatty acids for the last 10 weeks of pregnancy was shown to have a significant protective effect against the development of asthma in offspring by the age of 16 years.[66]

   Omega-3 fatty acids may also be beneficial in direct treatment, as 3.2 g EPA and 2.2 g DHA daily for 3 to 10 weeks reduces inflammatory markers, pulmonary compromise (fall in FEV_1) by nearly 80% and bronchodilator use by up to 20% in exercise-induced asthma.[67,68]

In the airways of asthmatics, inflammation is often associated with increased generation of reactive oxygen species and free radical damage.[69] Therefore the antioxidants **vitamins A**, **C** and **E** may be useful. By reducing the effect of the reactive oxygen species produced in the inflammatory process, these modulate the development of asthma and the impairment of pulmonary function. Vitamin C supplementation demonstrates a protective effect against exercise-induced airway narrowing in asthmatic subjects.[70] Serum levels of the **antioxidants** alpha- and beta-carotene have also been positively correlated to lung function and FEV_1 and FVC in epidemiological studies.[71,72]

Quercetin has the ability to inhibit inflammatory cytokine and chemokine production in acute and chronic inflammatory conditions.[73,74] High levels of this flavonoid are found in onions, apples, blueberries, curly kale, hot peppers, broccoli and green and black tea.[75,76]

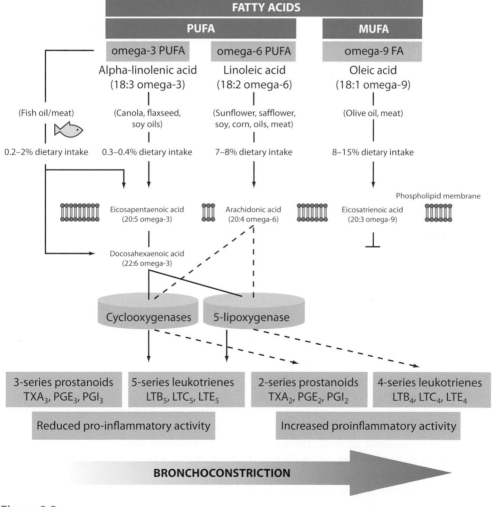

Figure 9.2
Metabolism of fatty acids and their contribution to inflammatory asthma responses

In asthma, platelet-activating factor (PAF) is released in response to exposure to allergens and induces an inflammatory airway response.[77] It is a potent bronchoconstrictor,[78] and elicits pulmonary and bronchial oedema, leading to airway obstruction and difficulty breathing.[79] While pharmaceutical PAF antagonists have not displayed absolute therapeutical efficacy alone, they may be a useful part of a combined treatment strategy.[80]

Ginkgo biloba is best known for its well-demonstrated neurological effects.[81,82] However, it has also shown activity as a PAF antagonist, exerting an anti-inflammatory action and reducing airway hyperresponsiveness and bronchospasm.[83] The most active constituents appear to be quercetin and the ginkgolides, in particular ginkgolide B.[84] Some researchers also suggest that *Ginkgo biloba* may modulate lymphocyte activation in asthma,[85] and in murine models of asthma the herb appears to impede the disease progress by alleviating all established chronic histological changes of lung except smooth muscle thickness.[86] *Pelargonium sidoides* prevented asthma attacks during viral infections of the upper respiratory tract, with less cough frequency and nasal congestion and less frequency of asthma attacks.[87] Glycyrrhizin from *Glycyrrhiza glabra* has also demonstrated ability to inhibit PAF production by human neutrophils in a dose-dependent manner.[88] *Allium cepa* exerts antiasthmatic and anti-PAF effects through its thiosulfinate content. In one study, allergen-induced asthma attacks were almost completely inhibited by an *Allium cepa* extract.[89] Therefore, garlic, onions and shallots are recommended to be included in dietary management of asthma.

Immune regulation

Immune dysregulation is a key feature of atopic asthma (and perhaps intrinsic asthma— see earlier). Strengthening immune resistance generally, rebalancing T-cell levels and restoring immune homoeostasis in the lung may decrease sensitisation to allergens and triggers.[6] In addition, viral infections are known to worsen asthma symptoms, and immune enhancement will help to prevent these.

Herbal immune modulators such as *Echinacea angustifolia* may be beneficial in supporting the body's natural resistance to infection and is particularly efficacious in prophylaxis/treatment of upper respiratory tract infections.[90,91] In addition to its significant immune-enhancing properties,[92] *Andrographis paniculata* may also be anti-inflammatory via inhibition of the NF-κB pathway.[93] *Astragalus membranaceus* has good traditional evidence as an immune-enhancing herb, and may potentially play a specific role in treating allergic asthma[94] by: reducing the expression of interleukin 4 and interleukin 5 (key initiators of allergic Th2-associated cytokines); attenuating lung inflammation, goblet cell hyperplasia and airway hyperresponsiveness; decreasing eosinophils and lymphocytes; and potentially inhibiting NF-κB expression and suppressing NF-κB translocation from the cytoplasm to the nucleus in lung tissue.[60] Also useful is *Picrorhiza kurroa*, which helps to prevent allergen- and PAF-induced bronchial obstruction.[89] **Triphala**, a Tibetan herbal mix of *Terminalia chebula*, *Emblica officinalis* and *Terminalia belerica*, has been shown to ameliorate functional and histological bronchial hyperresponsiveness (in murine models) through an increase in lung and spleen CD4 counts and its general antioxidant properties.[95] *Glycyrrhiza uralensis* flavonoids show in vitro and in vivo ability to modulate Th2 cytokines profiles in ways that may be beneficial for asthma-related inflammation.[96]

General **immune supportive nutrients** are vitamin C, vitamin A, zinc and selenium (for further immune modulators refer to Chapter 8 on infectious respiratory disease). A number of epidemiological studies have linked farming childhoods with reduced rates of allergic conditions, which some researchers suggest may be linked to early ingestion of unheated cow's milk and the resultant immunological effects.[97] The hypothesis proposes that allergenic proteins ingested in addition to milk proteins reach the infant gastrointestinal tract more intact than in adults due to more immature/milder digestion in infants. When allergenic proteins come into contact with allergen-specific IgG or IgA in raw cow's milk, it is suggested that they form immune complexes in the gastrointestinal tract, which are then taken up by Peyer's patches and induce efficient immune response in the infant. Other components of raw milk that may contribute to an immune balance favouring IgA production (over IgE and Treg production) are vitamins A and D, conjugated linoleic acid (CLA) and immunomodulary cytokines such as osteopontin, IL-10 and TGF-β_2.[97] Please note it is illegal to sell or recommend raw cow's milk for human consumption/ingestion in Australia and New Zealand. Isolated **genistein** extracts (a flavonoid in legumes, particularly soy) have been shown to alter Th1:Th2 balance in murine models of asthma.[98]

Manage allergies

Albizia lebbeck stabilises mast cell membranes in murine models, suggesting that it may inhibit histamine release in allergenic asthma,[99] appearing to deliver best results in asthma of less than two years' duration[100] **Scutellaria baicalensis** contains various flavonoids that suppress eotaxin—a chemokine associated with recruitment of eosinophils to sites of allergic inflammation—indicating a theoretical mechanism for its traditional use in asthma.[101] Skullcap flavone II has been shown to reduce airway hyperresponsiveness, airway levels of eosinophils and Th2 and TGF-β1 in bronchoalveolar lavage (BAL) fluids of treated mice.[102] It acts as a bradykinin antagonist, and had additional positive benefits in suppressive subepithelial collagen deposition and goblet cell hyperplasia, suggesting the potential to treat inflammation and modulate disease progression in allergic asthma.[102] The flavonoid baicalin was associated with significant reductions in inflammatory mediators in patients with bronchial asthma and was five to 10 times more potent than the antiallergic drug azelastine.[103] Early murine studies have shown **Panax ginseng** to have the ability to modulate various biochemical pathways involved in atopic asthma pathogenesis.[104]

In severe cases the practitioner may consider **immunosuppressive herbs**, such as *Tylophora indica* or *Hemidesmus indicus*, but caution is urged with regard to dosage, and the patient should be monitored closely. (For protocol on using these herbs, see Chapter 31 on autoimmunity.) Four small, early studies using *Tylophora indica* for short periods indicate beneficial effects (such as increased peak expiratory flow rate and ventilatory capacity).[105–107]

In addition to an anti-inflammatory role, **quercetin** is useful for its antiallergic qualities. In animal models it reduced the production of IL-4 (a Th2 cytokine) and increased the production of IFN-γ (a Th1 cytokine), potentially indicating a T-cell regulatory effect.[108] Dietary intake of **antioxidant nutrients** such as vitamins A, C, E and selenium may also help to regulate this balance. Supplementation of vitamin E and selenium are reported to promote Th1 differentiation.[109–113]

Enhance brochodilation

A key priority for the practitioner is to facilitate the ease of ventilation, and remove airway obstruction. This will reduce the symptoms of asthma caused by bronchospasm and constriction.

Adhatoda vasica is considered a specific for asthma, and is generally thought to be safe for long-term treatment.[114] The alkaloids in *Adhatoda vasica* have been compared to theophylline for their bronchodilator and antiasthmatic actions,[115] as they exhibit pronounced protection against allergen-induced bronchial obstruction.[89] ***Euphorbia*** **spp.** are also considered a reliable antiasthmatic, particularly in spasmodic forms of the condition. These promote expectoration, allay cough[116] and have antiproliferative properties.[117]

Forskolin from ***Coleus forskohlii*** has been shown to increase the levels of cAMP in cells, making it a natural bronchodilator.[118] In a model using guinea pig trachea, it showed efficacy in reducing antigen-induced constriction,[119] and in early trials it improved forced expiratory volume and decreased airway resistance in male asthmatics.[101] In vitro studies suggest that ***Zingiber officinale*** and some of its isolated constituents modulate intracellular calcium balance in airway smooth muscle and promote significant and rapid bronchodilation and therefore reduced airway hyperresponsiveness.[120] Other useful bronchospasmolytics and bronchodilators with traditional evidence are ***Grindelia camporum*** and ***Glycyrrhiza glabra***.[121,122]

Magnesium is also a renowned bronchodilator. It antagonises the movement of calcium across cell membranes, decreasing the uptake and release of the mineral in bronchial smooth muscle, and leading to relaxation and dilation of the airways.[123] In acute situations, magnesium sulfate administered intravenously or via a nebuliser appears to be effective in improving the pulmonary function of asthmatics.[124,125] In a short-term trial, 400 mg of magnesium was added to a low-magnesium diet for three weeks, producing an improvement in symptom scores.[126] In asthmatic children, 300 mg/day for two months produced reduced bronchial and skin hyperreactivity to known antigens, in addition to fewer asthma exacerbations and less medication use.[127]

Tea, **yerba maté** and **coffee**[128] are all agents that may be useful in bronchodilation. The pharmaceutical agent theophylline was derived from tea, and the caffeine that these agents contain may improve lung function for up to four hours in people with asthma.[129]

Promote expectoration if required
Refer to Chapter 10 on congestive respiratory disorders.

Consider the digestive connection
The development of asthma has been variously linked to increased digestive permeability,[27] oesophageal reflux[130] and dysbiosis,[131,132] making these the key areas to address. Inflammation may be attenuated, and the healing of the mucosal lining facilitated, by interventions including vitamin A,[133] glutamine[134,135] and *Aloe vera*.[136] Improving overall digestive capacity involves using **herbal bitters** such as *Gentiana lutea* or *Peumus boldus* and **warming digestives** such as *Zingiber officinale* or *Cinnamomum cassia* in association with enzyme therapy.[116,137–139]

With dysbiosis, the aim is to reduce overgrowth of detrimental strains of microflora and enhance beneficial strains, following a protocol known colloquially as a 'weed, seed and feed'. In various animal models, **probiotic** strains significantly reduce IgE production, airway hyperresponsiveness and/or inflammatory infiltration of the lungs.[140]

As already noted, early ingestion of raw milk is hypothesised to help reduce the likelihood of asthma and allergies. It contains antimicrobial proteins (lactoferrin and others) and non-digested sugars, which may help to promote a certain antiallergic microbial flora balance.[97] TGF-β_2 and short-chain fatty acids may also help to promote healthy gastrointestinal barrier function and epithelial health, preventing the leakage of allergens into the intestinal mucosa[97] (also noted earlier, it is illegal to sell or recommend raw cow's milk for human consumption/ingestion in Australia and New Zealand). For complete protocol and treatment suggestions, refer to Chapters 4–6 on the gastro-intestinal system.

Modification of lifestyle

Dietary advice

An elimination diet may be the most successful method of identifying allergens in asthmatic patients (see Figure 6.1 for the elimination diet protocol).[141] Egg, shellfish, tree nuts and peanuts are the foods most associated with immediate onset, while those most commonly associated with delayed onset are milk, chocolate, wheat, citrus and food colourings.[142] A diet high in sodium may be associated with more severe asthma symptoms in some patients (Figure 9.3)[143] and fast food intake is directly correlated with asthma risk.[144]

It has been suggested that oxidative stress may contribute to respiratory patholo-gies, particularly asthma.[145–147] A reduced intake of antioxidant-rich foods induces a worsening of asthma symptoms, and the levels of antioxidants are often lower in patients with asthmatic or respiratory distress.[148,149] **Antioxidant-rich diets** are associated with reduced asthma prevalence[150] and improved respiratory function.[151]

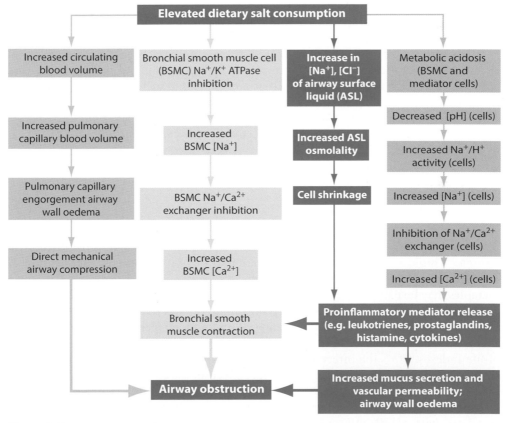

Figure 9.3
The mechanisms by which salt may contribute to airway obstruction and worsening of asthma symptoms
Source: Mickleborough 2008[128]

Antioxidant supplementation with 50 mg vitamin E and 250 mg vitamin C daily has been found to modulate the effects of pollution on children with asthma.[152] Improved beta-carotene levels are associated with a lower incidence of asthma[153] and improved FEV_1.[71] Lycopene supplementation has been linked with reduced airway neutrophil influx.[149] These relationships do not automatically imply a causal relationship and may instead be used as a marker of healthy diets more broadly. This is confirmed by epidemiological evidence that suggests that eating a **Mediterranean-style diet**, with high levels of fresh fruit, vegetables, omega-3 fatty acid and nuts, may reduce asthma risk in children by up to 80%.[154,155] Further cross-sectional studies assessing Mediterranean diet adherence in childhood generally suggest preventative benefits for asthma and wheeze.[156] Interventional and cross-sectional studies have also shown small but consistent improvements in lung function tests and quality of life, and improved asthma control in adult asthmatics consuming a Mediterranean diet.[156,157] The inclusion of **omega-3 fatty acids** should be a key priority, as there are significant correlations between low levels of omega-3 intake and asthma incidence.[128,158] An avoidance of heavy meals at night has also been proposed in order to manage asthma.[159]

Although caffeine is a known bronchodilator, studies show that the amount in a single cup of coffee (175 mL) does not provide significant bronchoprotection or bronchodilation and so should not be recommended for preventing or treating asthma attacks.[160]

Trials with multinutrient and food-based therapeutic extracts have shown benefits in allergic asthma patients, with improvements in lung function and quality of life, and reduced medication use.[160,161] Supplementation regimens in such trials typically included a mix of fish oil, **probiotics** (see Chapter 4 on probiotics – *Lactobacillus plantarum* ATCC 8014, *Lactobacillus reuteri* ATCC 23272 LGG, *Bifidobacterium animalis* sp. *Lactis* Bb 12, *Lactobacillus acidophilus* L92 and *Lactobacillus fermentum* CP34 appear to be the most useful strains in asthma),149 freeze-dried fruit and vegetable extracts, green barley powder, antioxidant complexes (coQ10, vitamins A, C, E and B6, green tea, grapeseed, citrus bioflavonoids, zinc, selenide, calcium).[160,161]

Lifestyle advice

The association between asthma symptom severity and stress is strong. It is thought that stress exacerbates the immune reactions responsible for airway inflammation in asthma,[162] indicating that relaxation therapies may be of particular use. **Meditation**,[163] **Tai Chi**[164] and **yoga**[165–168] have shown efficacy in this area. The benefits of these therapies may be partly related to their focus on breathing exercises. The yogic science of **pranayama** is designed to promote deep breathing, expand the lungs and reduce stress. These exercises may help reduce histamine response to allergens, produce decreases in FEV_1, peak expiratory flow rate, symptom score and inhaler use, and improve quality-of-life indexes.[169–172] The interventions have little or no effect on lung physiology and are presumed to have a secondary or indirect effect on the condition due in part due to their relaxation effects.

Journalling about stressful experiences not previously disclosed to others has been associated with a 13% improvement in lung function,[173] and may be a useful adjunct to treatment.

Regular **exercise** increases overall quality of life for asthmatics,[174] an approach that seems particularly relevant in children.[175–177] Swimming is often recommended as a way to improve fitness and lung function in asthmatics;[178] however, practitioners should be aware that there are concerns that exposure to chlorine may promote the development of a specific phenotype of asthmatic airways, and an increase in airway hyperresponsiveness, rhinitis and allergies.[179] Maintenance of a healthy weight is important, as asthma prevalence has a positive association with obesity;[45] weight loss in overweight patients improves asthma symptoms.[180] One study has shown a link with wheeze and asthma exacerbation and low levels of **vitamin D** in adults, but the same relationship does not seem apparent in juvenile study cohorts.[156]

INTEGRATIVE MEDICAL CONSIDERATIONS

The **Buteyko** breathing technique—which involves making breathing shallow and slow—has demonstrated an ability to reduce medication use and produce improvements in quality-of-life scores in patients with asthma.[181–184]

A Cochrane review of the English-language evidence determined that more research is needed to make a definitive conclusion as to whether **acupuncture** is useful for asthmatic patients.[185] A recent systemic review and meta-analysis suggested that pharmacopuncture (combining acupuncture and herbal therapies) may have benefits for adults with asthma.[186] Approaches in acupuncture generally address 'excessive or deficient Qi' in the respiratory system.[187] Reports suggest that it can decrease symptom severity and improve lung function (at least in the short term),[187,188] with an immediate bronchodilatory effect and improvements in FEV after even one treatment.[189]

CLINICAL SUMMARY

While naturopathic treatments have a significant role in preventing and managing asthma, patients with asthma should be strongly counselled about the importance of continuing conventional treatments for asthma in the acute phase of treatment. They should be informed that they need to continue to carry acute treatment medication with them at all times, even during naturopathic treatment, as acute asthma is a medical emergency, one that also requires immediate referral and medical intervention.

While it is pertinent to identify and remove obvious reactive triggers, a primary aim of naturopathic treatment of asthma should be to treat the underlying causes of immune hyperreactivity, and as such moderate reactions to such triggers. With time, not all triggers may need to be continually avoided. However, true allergic reactions are likely to persist.

Initially, naturopathic treatment should enhance bronchodilation and promote expectoration, and then modulate the immune response through correction of underlying factors, such as dysbiosis and increased intestinal permeability. Supporting the nervous system to reduce the stress response, which is likely to be both a contributing factor and a response to illness, should also be a significant part of naturopathic treatment in asthma. The clinical value of reassurance and the therapeutic relationship between practitioner and patient should also not be underestimated, and may help elicit improved clinical outcomes in asthma patients.

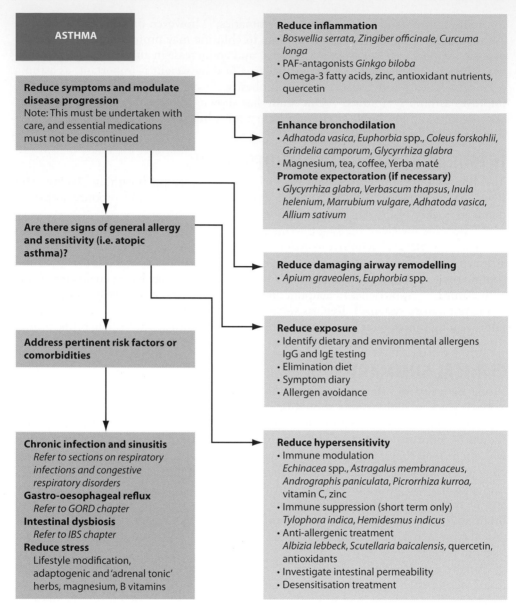

ASTHMA

Reduce symptoms and modulate disease progression
Note: This must be undertaken with care, and essential medications must not be discontinued

Are there signs of general allergy and sensitivity (i.e. atopic asthma)?

Address pertinent risk factors or comorbidities

Chronic infection and sinusitis
  Refer to sections on respiratory infections and congestive respiratory disorders
Gastro-oesophageal reflux
  Refer to GORD chapter
Intestinal dysbiosis
  Refer to IBS chapter
Reduce stress
  Lifestyle modification, adaptogenic and 'adrenal tonic' herbs, magnesium, B vitamins

Reduce inflammation
• *Boswellia serrata, Zingiber officinale, Curcuma longa*
• PAF-antagonists *Ginkgo biloba*
• Omega-3 fatty acids, zinc, antioxidant nutrients, quercetin

Enhance bronchodilation
• *Adhatoda vasica, Euphorbia* spp., *Coleus forskohlii, Grindelia camporum, Glycyrrhiza glabra*
• Magnesium, tea, coffee, Yerba maté
Promote expectoration (if necessary)
• *Glycyrrhiza glabra, Verbascum thapsus, Inula helenium, Marrubium vulgare, Adhatoda vasica, Allium sativum*

Reduce damaging airway remodelling
• *Apium graveolens, Euphorbia* spp.

Reduce exposure
• Identify dietary and environmental allergens IgG and IgE testing
• Elimination diet
• Symptom diary
• Allergen avoidance

Reduce hypersensitivity
• Immune modulation
  Echinacea spp., *Astragalus membranaceus, Andrographis paniculata, Picrorrhiza kurroa,* vitamin C, zinc
• Immune suppression (short term only)
  Tylophora indica, Hemidesmus indicus
• Anti-allergenic treatment
  Albizia lebbeck, Scutellaria baicalensis, quercetin, antioxidants
• Investigate intestinal permeability
• Desensitisation treatment

Figure 9.4
Naturopathic treatment decision tree—asthma

Table 9.1
Review of the major evidence

Intervention	Mechanisms of action	Key literature	Summary of results	Comment
Vitamin C	Antioxidant and immune modulator (enhances natural killer cell numbers and activity, and T- and B-cell function) Antihistamine effects	Kaur et al. 2009[190] Bielory et al. 1994[191] Hatch 1995[192] Monteleone & Sherman 1997[36] Romieu et al. 2002[152] Fogarty et al. 2006[193] Tecklenburg et al. 2007[70]	Meta-analysis found insufficient evidence from trials due to small numbers, varied designs and poor reporting[190] Varying trials found: • role of vitamin C was unclear due to lack of evidence • vitamin C showed efficacy in reversing or improving asthma symptoms in a majority of trials • it may have a short-term protective effect on airway responsiveness • a significant attenuation of post-exercise bronchoconstriction[70]	Vitamin C appears to be an effective adjuvant treatment; it should be used in therapeutic amounts in divided doses and titrate to bowel tolerance Consider also dietary forms
Boswellia serrata	Anti-inflammatory effects from boswellic acids Inhibits the synthesis of leukotrienes, which are responsible for the second wave of asthma-related inflammation	Ammon et al. 1991[194] Ammon et al. 1993[50] Singh & Atal 1986[195] Gupta et al. 1998[51]	In a six-week double-blind RCT, *Boswellia serrata* (300 mg three times a day) improved asthma symptoms in 70% of treated patients versus 27% in controls	Best used in a tablet form due to the active constituents being resinoids
Ginkgo biloba	Anti-inflammatory, decreases IL-5 production and modulates lymphocyte cytokine production[196] Also has anti-PAF and antiallergic effects, reducing airway hyperresponsive-ness and bronchospasm[83]	Mahmoud et al. 2000[85] Vogensen et al. 2003[197] Babayigit et al. 2009[86] Li et al. 1997[83] Tang et al. 2007[196]	Reduces PAF activity, thus modulating the allergic and inflammatory reactions in atopic asthma[197] Concentrated *Ginkgo* leaf liquor produced significant clinical improvement in FEV_1 at eight weeks[83]	Effective in modulating allergic and inflammatory reactions—better effects over longer term dosing May improve healing due to enhancement of mucosal blood flow and antioxidant properties

Table 9.1
Review of the major evidence (continued)

Intervention	Mechanisms of action	Key literature	Summary of results	Comment
Breathing exercises	Enhanced muscular strength and lung capacity	**Buteyko** Bowler et al. 1998[184] Opat et al. 2000[182] Cooper et al. 2003[181] McHugh et al. 2003[198] Cowie et al. 2008[183] **Pranayama** Nagendra & Nagarathna 1986[199] Singh et al. 1990[172] Vedanthan et al. 1998[165]	Regular use of Buteyko breathing over four weeks to six months reduces asthma symptoms and bronchodilator use and increases quality of life; in one trial patients were also able to reduce inhaled corticosteroid treatment by 50% and β_2-agonist use by 85% after six months Asthmatics practising yogic techniques, including pranayama (or pranayama solely) on a regular basis exhibit: – better exercise tolerance – a trend towards less β_2-agonist use – a trend towards improvement in FEV_1, peak expiratory flow rate, symptom score and inhaler use – reduced FEV_1 decrease in response to histamine Older studies show that up to 66% of patients may be able to stop or reduce corticosteroid treatment with regular breathing practice[199]	Easy to teach and a cheap intervention that clients can use Encourages active client engagement in the healing process
Acupuncture	In addition to immunological modulatory activity, may enhance bronchodilation	Leake & Broderick 1999[188] McCarney et al. 2004[185] Ngai & Jones 2006[187] Chu et al. 2007[189]	Cochrane review suggests that more evidence is required to reach definitive conclusion Other reviews suggest that treatment can decrease symptom severity and improve lung function, at least in the short term Trials show immediate bronchodilating effect and ability to improve quality of life and reduce bronchodilator medication	Given the method of treatment, it is difficult to find a suitable placebo, complicating trial design

KEY POINTS

- Acute asthma is a medical emergency and requires immediate referral.

- Patients should be strongly counselled about not stopping conventional treatments for asthma in the acute phase of treatment and should be informed that they need to ensure they continue to carry acute treatment medication with them at all times.

- While it is pertinent to identify and remove obvious reactive triggers, the aim of naturopathic treatment is to treat the underlying causes of hyperreactivity. With time, not all triggers may need to be avoided. True allergic reactions, however, are likely to persist.

- Acutely, enhance brochodilation and promote expectoration.

- Modulate the immune response appropriately, which may involve direct modulation and correction of underlying factors such as dysbiosis and increased intestinal permeability.

- Support the nervous system to reduce the stress response, which is likely to not only be a contributing factor but also a response to illness. Never undervalue the role of reassurance and the therapeutic relationship between practitioner and patient.

FURTHER READING

Borchers AT, et al. Probiotics and immunity. J Gastroenterol 2009;44(1):26–46.

Mali R, Dhake A. A review on herbal antiasthmatics. Orient Pharm Exp Med 2011;11:77–90.

Mickleborough TD. A nutritional approach to managing exercise-induced asthma. Exerc Sport Sci Rev 2008;36(3):135–44.

von Mutius E, et al. Exposure to endotoxin or other bacterial components might protect against the development of atopy. Clin Exp Allergy 2000;30:1230–4.

Yeh GY, Horwitz R. Integrative medicine for respiratory conditions: asthma and chronic obstructive pulmonary disease. Med Clin North Am 2017;101(5):925–41.

Acknowledgment: The author would like to acknowledge Tessa Finney-Brown, who authored this chapter in previous editions.

REFERENCES

1. Barnes P. Asthma. In: Fauci AS, editor. Harrison's principles of internal medicine. 17th ed. New York: McGraw-Hill Companies, Inc.; 2008.

2. McCunney RJ. Asthma, genes, and air pollution. J Occup Environ Med 2005;47(12):1285–91.

3. Anderson GP. Endotyping asthma: new insights into key pathogenic mechanisms in a complex, heterogeneous disease. Lancet 2008;372(9643):1107–19.

4. Linzer JFS. Review of asthma: pathophysiology and current treatment options. Clin Pediatr Emerg Med 2007;8(2):87–95.

5. Holgate ST, Davies DE, Lackie PM, et al. Epithelial-mesenchymal interactions in the pathogenesis of asthma. J Allergy Clin Immunol 2000;105(2 Pt 1):193–204.

6. Ryanna K, Stratigou V, Safinia N, et al. Regulatory T-cells in bronchial asthma. Allergy 2009;64(3):335–47.

7. Beers MH, Porter RS, Jones TV, et al Merck manual of diagnosis and therapy. 18th ed. 2006.

8. Strachan D. Hay fever, hygiene, and household size. BMJ 1989;299:1259–60.

9. Braun-Fahrländer C, Eder W, Schreuer M, et al. Exposure to farming environment during the first year of life protects against the development of asthma and allergy. Am J Respir Crit Care Med 2001;163:A157.

10. Kusel MM, de Klerk NH, Kebadze T, et al. Early-life respiratory viral infections, atopic sensitization, and risk of subsequent development of persistent asthma. J Allergy Clin Immunol 2007;119(5):1105–10.

11. Corderoy A. Asthma 'link' in eating fast food. The Age. 2013;16 Jan.

12. Carlsen KH, Carlsen KC. Exercise-induced asthma. Paediatr Respir Rev 2002;3(2):154–60.

13. Jayaratnam A, Corrigan CJ, Lee TH. The continuing enigma of non-atopic asthma. Clin Exp Allergy 2005;35(7):835–7.

14. Kay AB. Allergy and allergic diseases. First of two parts. N Engl J Med 2001;344(1):30–7.

15. Holgate ST, Yang Y, Haitchi HM, et al. The genetics of asthma: ADAM33 as an example of a susceptibility gene. Proc Am Thorac Soc 2006;3(5):440–3.

16. Friedman NJ, Zeiger RS. The role of breast-feeding in the development of allergies and asthma. J Allergy Clin Immunol 2005;115(6):1238–48.

17. Verhasselt V, Milcent V, Cazareth J, et al. Breast milk-mediated transfer of an antigen induces tolerance and protection from allergic asthma. Nat Med 2008;14(2):170–5.

18. Oddy WH, Sherriff JL. Breastfeeding, body mass index, asthma and atopy in children. Asia Pac J Public Health 2003;15(Suppl.):S15–17.

19. Salvi S. Health effects of ambient air pollution in children. Paediatr Respir Rev 2007;8(4):275–80.

20. Tischer CG, Hohmann C, Thiering E, et al. Meta-analysis of mould and dampness exposure on asthma and allergy in eight European birth cohorts: an ENRIECO initiative. Allergy 2011;66(12):1570–9.

21. Mitchell EA, Stewart AW, Clayton T, et al. Cross-sectional survey of risk factors for asthma in 6–7-year-old children in New Zealand: international Study of Asthma and Allergy in Childhood Phase Three. J Paediatr Child Health 2009;45(6):375–83.

22. Lodrup Carlsen KC, Roll S, Carlsen KH, et al. Does pet ownership in infancy lead to asthma or allergy at school age? Pooled analysis of individual participant data from 11 European birth cohorts. PLOS ONE 2012;7(8):e43214.

23. Guo CH, Chen PC, Hsia S, et al. The relationship of plasma aluminum to oxidant-antioxidant and inflammation status in asthma patients. Environ Toxicol Pharmacol 2013;35(1):30–8.

24. Vaidya SV, Kulkarni H. Association of urinary bisphenol A concentration with allergic asthma: results from the National Health and Nutrition Examination Survey 2005–2006. J Asthma 2012;49(8):800–6.

25. Caffarelli C, Deriu FM, Terzi V, et al. Gastrointestinal symptoms in patients with asthma. Arch Dis Child 2000;82(2):131–5.

26. Hijazi Z, Molla A, Al-Habashi H, et al. Intestinal permeability is increased in bronchial asthma. Arch Dis Child 2004;89(3):227–9.

27. Benard A, Desreumeaux P, Huglo D, et al. Increased intestinal permeability in bronchial asthma. J Allergy Clin Immunol 1996;97:1173–8.

28. Peterson KA, Samuelson WM, Ryujin DT, et al. The role of gastroesophageal reflux in exercise-triggered asthma: a randomized controlled trial. Dig Dis Sci 2009;54(3):564–71.

29. Gonzalez H, Ahmed T. Suppression of gastric H2-receptor mediated function in patients with bronchial asthma and ragweed allergy. Chest 1986;89(4):491–6.

30. Kelly G. Hydrochloric acid: physiological functions and clinical implications. Altern Med Rev 1997;2(2):116–27.

31. Litonjua AA, Weiss ST. Is vitamin D deficiency to blame for the asthma epidemic? J Allergy Clin Immunol 2007;120(5):1031–5.

32. Seaton A. From nurture to nature—the story of the Aberdeen asthma dietary hypothesis. QJM 2008;101(3):237–9.

33. Roberts G, Lack G. Food allergy and asthma—what is the link? Paediatr Respir Rev 2003;4(3):205–12.

34. Chen E, Hanson MD, Paterson LQ, et al. Socioeconomic status and inflammatory processes in childhood asthma: the role of psychological stress. J Allergy Clin Immunol 2006;117(5):1014–20.

35. Ozol D, Mete E. Asthma and food allergy. Curr Opin Pulm Med 2008;14(1):9–12.

36. Monteleone C, Sherman A. Nutrition and asthma. Arch Intern Med 1997;157(1):23–34.

37. Ellwood P, Innes Asher M, García-Marcos L, et al. Do fast foods cause asthma, rhinoconjunctivitis and eczema? Global findings from the International Study of Asthma and Allergies in Childhood (ISAAC) Phase Three. Thorax 2013;68:351–60.

38. Litonjua AA, Gold DR. Asthma and obesity: common early-life influences in the inception of disease. J Allergy Clin Immunol 2008;121(5):1075–84, quiz 1085–6.

39. Dupler D. Asthma. In: Krapp KL, editor. The Gale encyclopedia of alternative medicine. Farmington Hills, USA: Gale Group; 2001. p. 126–32.

40. Williams DR, Sternthal M, Wright RJ. Social determinants: taking the social context of asthma seriously. Pediatrics 2009;123(Suppl. 3):S174–84.

41. Claudio L, Tulton L, Doucette J, et al. Socioeconomic factors and asthma hospitalization rates in New York City. J Asthma 1999;36(4):343–50.

42. Ernst P, Demissie K, Joseph L, et al. Socioeconomic status and indicators of asthma in children. Am J Respir Crit Care Med 1995;152(2):570–5.

43. Goodwin RD. Asthma and anxiety disorders. Adv Psychosom Med 2003;24:51–71.

44. Lee EJ, In KH, Ha ES, et al. Asthma-like symptoms are increased in the metabolic syndrome. J Asthma 2009;46(4):339–42.

45. Beuther D, Sutherland E. Overweight, obesity, and incident asthma: a metaanalysis of prospective epidemiologic studies. Am J Respir Crit Care Med 2007;175(7):661–6.

46. Fanta C. An overview of asthma management. In: Basow DS, editor. UpToDate. Waltham, MA: UpToDate; 2013.

47. Jones CA, Bender BG, Haselkorn T, et al. Predicting asthma control using patient attitudes toward medical care: the REACT score. Ann Allergy Asthma Immunol 2009;102(5):385–92.

48. National Asthma Council Australia. Asthma management handbook 2006. Melbourne: National Asthma Council Australia; 2006.

49. Global Initiative For Asthma. Global strategy for asthma management and prevention. Bethesda: Global Initiative For Asthma; 2011.

50. Ammon H, Safayhi H, Mack T, et al. Mechanism of antiinflammatory actions of curcumine and boswellic acids. J Ethnopharmacol 1993;38(2–3):113–19.

51. Gupta I, Gupta V, Parihar A, et al. Effects of Boswellia serrata gum resin in patients with bronchial asthma: results of a double-blind, placebo-controlled, 6-week clinical study. Eur J Med Res 1998;3(11):511–14.

52. Ram A, Das M, Ghosh B. Curcumin attenuates allergen-induced airway hyperresponsiveness in sensitized guinea pigs. Biol Pharm Bull 2003;26(7):1021–4.

53. Kobayashi T, Hashimoto S, Horie T. Curcumin inhibition of Dermatophagoides farinea-induced interleukin-5 (IL-5) and granulocyte macrophage-colony stimulating factor (GM-CSF) production by lymphocytes from bronchial asthmatics. Biochem Pharmacol 1997;54(7):819–24.

54. Li C, Li L, Luo J, et al. Effect of turmeric volatile oil on the respiratory tract. Zhongguo Zhong Yao Za Zhi 1998;23(10):624–5.

55. Kurup VP, Barrios CS, Raju R, et al. Immune response modulation by curcumin in a latex allergy model. Clin Mol Allergy 2007;25(5):1.

56. Houssen ME, Ragab A, Mesbah A, et al. Natural anti-inflammatory products and leukotriene inhibitors as complementary therapy for bronchial asthma. Clin Biochem 2010;43(10–11):887–90.

57. Mascolo N, Jain R, Jain SC, et al. Ethnopharmacologic investigation of ginger (Zingiber officinale). J Ethnopharmacol 1989;27(1–2):129–40.

58. Ahui M, Champy P, Ramadan A, et al. Ginger prevents Th2-mediated immune responses in a mouse model of airway inflammation. Int Immunopharmacol 2008;8(12):1626–32.

59. Ghayur MN, Gilani AH, Janssen LJ. Ginger attenuates acetylcholine-induced contraction and Ca2+ signalling in murine airway smooth muscle cells. Can J Physiol Pharmacol 2008;86(5):264–71.

60. Yang ZC, Qu ZH, Yi MJ, et al. Astragalus extract attenuates allergic airway inflammation and inhibits nuclear factor kappaB expression in asthmatic mice. Am J Med Sci 2013;346(5):390–5.

61. Yuan X, Sun S, Wang S, et al. Effects of astragaloside IV on IFN-gamma level and prolonged airway dysfunction

in a murine model of chronic asthma. Planta Med 2011;77(4):328–33.

62. Shin IS, Lee MY, Lim HS, et al. An extract of Crataegus pinnatifida fruit attenuates airway inflammation by modulation of matrix metalloproteinase-9 in ovalbumin induced asthma. PLOS ONE 2012;7(9):e45734.

63. Lee MY, Seo CS, Lee NH, et al. Anti-asthmatic effect of schizandrin on OVA-induced airway inflammation in a murine asthma model. Int Immunopharmacol 2010;10(11):1374–9.

64. Biltagi MA, Baset AA, Bassiouny M, et al. Omega-3 fatty acids, vitamin C and Zn supplementation in asthmatic children: a randomized self-controlled study. Acta Paediatr 2009;98(4):737–42.

65. Salam M, Li Y, Langholz B, et al. Maternal fish consumption during pregnancy and risk of early childhood asthma. J Asthma 2005;42(6):513–18.

66. Olsen SF, Osterdal ML, Salvig JD, et al. Fish oil intake compared with olive oil intake in late pregnancy and asthma in the offspring: 16 y of registry-based follow-up from a randomized controlled trial. Am J Clin Nutr 2008;88(1):167–75.

67. Mickleborough TD, Murray RL, Ionescu AA, et al. Fish oil supplementation reduces severity of exercise-induced bronchoconstriction in elite athletes. Am J Respir Crit Care Med 2003;168(10):1181–9.

68. Arm J, Horton C, Mencia-Huerta J, et al. Effect of dietary supplementation with fish oil lipids on mild asthma. Thorax 1998;43(2):84–91.

69. Riccioni G, Barbara M, Bucciarelli T, et al. Antioxidant vitamin supplementation in asthma. Ann Clin Lab Sci 2007;37(1):96–101.

70. Tecklenburg S, Mickleborough T, Fly A, et al. Ascorbic acid supplementation attenuates exercise-induced bronchoconstriction in patients with asthma. Respir Med 2007;101(8):1770–8.

71. Grievink L, de Waart F, Schouten E, et al. Serum carotenoids, alpha-tocopherol, and lung function among Dutch elderly. Am J Respir Crit Care Med 2000;161(3):790–5.

72. Hu G, Cassano PA. Antioxidant nutrients and pulmonary function: the Third National Health and Nutrition Examination Survey (NHANES III). Am J Epidemiol 2000;151(10):975–81.

73. Geraets L, Moonen HJ, Brauers K, et al. Dietary flavones and flavonoles are inhibitors of poly(ADP-ribose) polymerase-1 in pulmonary epithelial cells. J Nutr 2007;137(10):2190–5.

74. Lim M, Citardi MJ, Leong JL. Topical antimicrobials in the management of chronic rhinosinusitis: a systematic review. Am J Rhinol 2008;22(4):381–9.

75. Erdman JW Jr, Balentine D, Arab L, et al. Flavonoids and heart health: proceedings of the ILSI North America flavonoids workshop, May 31–June 1, 2005, Washington, DC. J Nutr 2007;137(3 Suppl. 1):718S–37S.

76. Manach C, Williamson G, Morand C, et al. Bioavailability and bioefficacy of polyphenols in humans. I. Review of 97 bioavailability studies. Am J Clin Nutr 2005; 81(1 Suppl.):230S–42S.

77. Kaplan M, Mutlu EA, Benson M, et al. Use of herbal preparations in the treatment of oxidant-mediated inflammatory disorders. Complement Ther Med 2007;15(3):207–16.

78. Hsieh KH. Effects of PAF antagonist, BN52021, on the PAF-, methacholine-, and allergen-induced bronchoconstriction in asthmatic children. Chest 1991;99:877–82.

79. Page CP. The role of platelet-activating factor in asthma. J Allergy Clin Immunol 1988;81(1):144–52.

80. Kasperska-Zajac A, Brzoza Z, Rogala B. Platelet-activating factor (PAF): a review of its role in asthma and clinical efficacy of PAF antagonists in the disease therapy. Recent Pat Inflamm Allergy Drug Discov 2008;2(1):72–6.

81. Mix JA, Crews WD. A double-blind, placebo-controlled, randomized trial of Ginkgo biloba extract EGb 761* in a sample of cognitively intact older adults: neuropsychological findings. Hum Psychopharmacol 2002;17:267–77.

82. Kennedy DO, Scholey AB, Wesnes KA. The dose-dependent cognitive effects of acute administration of Ginkgo biloba to healthy young volunteers. Psychopharmacology (Berl) 2000;151:416–23.

83. Li M, Zhang H, Yang B. Effects of ginkgo leaf concentrated oral liquor in treating asthma. Zhongguo Zhong Xi Yi Jie He Za Zhi 1997;17:216–18.

84. Shi C, Zhao L, Zhu B, et al. Protective effects of Ginkgo biloba extract (EGb761) and its constituents quercetin and ginkgolide B against beta-amyloid peptide-induced toxicity in SH-SY5Y cells. Chem Biol Interact 2009;181(1):115–23.

85. Mahmoud F, Abul H, Onadeko B, et al. In vitro effects of Ginkgolide B on lymphocyte activation in atopic asthma: comparison with cyclosporin A. Jpn J Pharmacol 2000;83(3):241–5.

86. Babayigit A, Olmez D, Karaman O, et al. Effects of Ginkgo biloba on airway histology in a mouse model of chronic asthma. Allergy Asthma Proc 2009;30(2):186–91.

87. Tahan F, Yaman M. Can the Pelargonium sidoides root extract EPs(R) 7630 prevent asthma attacks during viral infections of the upper respiratory tract in children? Phytomedicine 2013;20(2):148–50. doi:10.1016/j.phymed.2012.09.022.

88. Nakamura T, Kuriyama M, Kosuge E, et al. Effects of saiboku-to (TJ-96) on the production of platelet-activating factor in human neutrophils. Ann N Y Acad Sci 1993;685:572–9.

89. Dorsch W, Wagner H. New antiasthmatic drugs from traditional medicine? Int Arch Allergy Appl Immunol 1991;94(1–4):262–5.

90. Barrett B. Medicinal properties of Echinacea: a critical review. Phytomedicine 2003;10(1):66–86.

91. Tiralongo E, Lea RA, Wee SS, et al. Randomised, double blind, placebo-controlled trial of echinacea supplementation in air travellers. Evid Based Complement Alternat Med 2012;2012:417267.

92. Poolsup N, Suthisisang C, Prathanturarug S, et al. Andrographis paniculata in the symptomatic treatment of uncomplicated upper respiratory tract infection: systematic review of randomized controlled trials. J Clin Pharm Ther 2004;29(1):37–45.

93. Bao ZGS, Cheng C, Wu S, et al. A novel antiinflammatory role for andrographolide in asthma via inhibition of the nuclear factor-kappaB pathway. Am J Respir Crit Care Med 2009;179(8):657–65.

94. Shen HH, Wang K, Li W, et al. Astragalus membranaceus prevents airway hyperreactivity in mice related to Th2 response inhibition. J Ethnopharmacol 2008;116(2):363–9.

95. Horani A, Shoseyov D, Ginsburg I, et al. Triphala (PADMA) extract alleviates bronchial hyperreactivity in a mouse model through liver and spleen immune modulation and increased anti-oxidative effects. Ther Adv Respir Dis 2012;6(4):199–210.

96. Yang N, Patil S, Zhuge J, et al. Glycyrrhiza uralensis Flavonoids Present in Anti-Asthma Formula, ASHMI™, inhibit memory Th2 responses in vitro and in vivo. Phytother Res 2013;27(9):1381–91.

97. van Neerven RJ, Knol EF, Heck JM, et al. Which factors in raw cow's milk contribute to protection against allergies? J Allergy Clin Immunol 2012;130(4):853–8.

98. Gao F, Wei D, Bian T, et al. Genistein attenuated allergic airway inflammation by modulating the transcription factors T-bet, GATA-3 and STAT-6 in a murine model of asthma. Pharmacology 2012;89(3–4):229–36.

99. Johri RK, Zutshi U, Kameshwaran L, et al. Effect of quercetin and Albizia saponins on rat mast cell. Indian J Physiol Pharmacol 1985;29(1):43–6.

100. Bone KM. A clinical guide to blending liquid herbs. Philadelphia: Churchill Livingstone; 2003.

101. Nakajima T, Imanishi M, Yamamoto K, et al. Inhibitory effect of baicalein, a flavonoid in Scutellaria Root, on eotaxin production by human dermal fibroblasts. Planta Med 2001;67(2):132–5.

102. Jang HY, Ahn KS, Park MJ, et al. Skullcapflavone II inhibits ovalbumin-induced airway inflammation in a mouse model of asthma. Int Immunopharmacol 2012;12(4):666–74.

103. Niitsuma T, Morita S, Hayashi T, et al. Effects of absorbed components of saiboku-to on the release of leukotrienes from polymorphonuclear leukocytes of patients with bronchial asthma. Methods Find Exp Clin Pharmacol 2001;23(2):99–104.

104. Kim DY, Yang WM. Panax ginseng ameliorates airway inflammation in an ovalbumin-sensitized mouse allergic asthma model. J Ethnopharmacol 2011;136(1):230–5.

105. Shivpuri DN, Menon MP, Prakash D. A crossover double-blind study on Tylophora indica in the treatment of asthma and allergic rhinitis. J Allergy 1969;43(3):145–50.

106. Shivpuri DN, Singhal SC, Parkash D. Treatment of asthma with an alcoholic extract of Tylophora indica: a cross-over, double-blind study. Ann Allergy 1972;30(7):407–12.

107. Thiruvengadam KV, Haranath K, Sudarsan S, et al. Tylophora indica in bronchial asthma (a controlled comparison with a standard anti-asthmatic drug). J Indian Med Assoc 1978;71(7):172–6.

108. Park HJ, Lee CM, Jung ID, et al. Quercetin regulates Th1/Th2 balance in a murine model of asthma. Int Immunopharmacol 2009;9(3):261–7.

109. Broome CS, McArdle F, Kyle JA, et al. An increase in selenium intake improves immune function and poliovirus handling in adults with marginal selenium status. Am J Clin Nutr 2004;80(1):154–62.

110. Zheng K, Adjei AA, Shinjo M, et al. Effect of dietary vitamin E supplementation on murine nasal allergy. Am J Med Sci 1999;318(1):49–54.

111. Han SN, Wu D, Ha WK, et al. Vitamin E supplementation increases T helper 1 cytokine production in old mice infected with influenza virus. Immunology 2000;100(4):487–93.

112. Malmberg KJ, Lenkei R, Petersson M, et al. A short-term dietary supplementation of high doses of vitamin E increases T helper 1 cytokine production in patients with advanced colorectal cancer. Clin Cancer Res 2002;8(6):1772–8.

113. Jeong DW, Yoo MH, Kim TS, et al. Protection of mice from allergen-induced asthma by selenite: prevention of eosinophil infiltration by inhibition of NF-kappa B activation. J Biol Chem 2002;277(20):17871–6.

114. Claeson U, Malmfors T, Wikman G, et al. Adhatoda vasica: a critical review of ethnopharmacological and toxicological data. J Ethnopharmacol 2000;72(1–2):1–20.

115. Williamson E. Major herbs of ayurveda. London: Churchill Livingstone; 2002.

116. Felter H, Lloyd J. King's American Dispensatory [Online at Henriette's Herbal Homepage]; 1898. Available

from: http://www.henriettesherbal.com/eclectic/kings/echinacea.html. 1 Nov 2013.

117. Chaabi M, Freund-Michel V, Frossard N, et al. Anti-proliferative effect of Euphorbia stenoclada in human airway smooth muscle cells in culture. J Ethnopharmacol 2007;109(1):134–9.

118. Laurenza A, Sutkowski EM, Seamon KB. Forskolin: a specific stimulator of adenylyl cyclase or a diterpene with multiple sites of action? Trends Pharmacol Sci 1989;10(11):442–7.

119. Burka JF. Inhibition of antigen and calcium ionophore A23187 induced contractions of guinea pig airways by isoprenaline and forskolin. Can J Physiol Pharmacol 1983;61(6):581–9.

120. Townsend EA, Siviski ME, Zhang Y, et al. Effects of ginger and its constituents on airway smooth muscle relaxation and calcium regulation. Am J Respir Cell Mol Biol 2013;48(2):157–63.

121. Scientific Committee of the British Herbal Medical Association. British herbal pharmacopoeia. 1st ed. Bournemouth: British Herbal Medicine Association; 1983.

122. Liu B, Yang J, Wen Q, et al. Isoliquiritigenin, a flavonoid from licorice, relaxes guinea-pig tracheal smooth muscle in vitro and in vivo: role of cGMP/PKG pathway. Eur J Pharmacol 2008;587(1–3):257–66.

123. Jaber R. Respiratory and allergic diseases: from upper respiratory tract infections to asthma. Prim Care 2002;29(2):231–61.

124. Rowe B, Bretzlaff J, Bourdon C, et al. Magnesium sulfate is effective for severe acute asthma treated in the emergency department. West J Med 2000;172(2):96.

125. Blitz M, Blitz S, Beasely R, et al. Inhaled magnesium sulfate in the treatment of acute asthma. Cochrane Database Syst Rev 2005;(4):CD003898.

126. Hill J, Micklewright A, Lewis S, et al. Investigation of the effect of short-term change in dietary magnesium intake in asthma. Eur Respir J 1997;10(10):2225–9.

127. Gontijo-Amaral C, Ribeiro MA, Gontijo LS, et al. Oral magnesium supplementation in asthmatic children: a double-blind randomized placebo-controlled trial. Eur J Clin Nutr 2007;61(1):54–60.

128. Mickleborough TD. A nutritional approach to managing exercise-induced asthma. Exerc Sport Sci Rev 2008;36(3):135–44.

129. Bara AI, Barley EA. Caffeine for asthma. Cochrane Database Syst Rev 2001;(4):CD001112.

130. Harding SM. Gastroesophageal reflux and asthma: insight into the association. J Allergy Clin Immunol 1999;104(2 Pt 1):251–9.

131. Fukuda S, Ishikawa H, Koga Y, et al. Allergic symptoms and microflora in schoolchildren. J Adolesc Health 2004;35(2):156–8.

132. Noverr MC, Huffnagle GB. The 'microflora hypothesis' of allergic diseases. Clin Exp Allergy 2005;35(12):1511–20.

133. McCullough FS, Northrop-Clewes CA, Thurnham DI. The effect of vitamin A on epithelial integrity. Proc Nutr Soc 1999;58(2):289–93.

134. Scheppach W, Loges C, Bartram P, et al. Effect of free glutamine and alanyl-glutamine dipeptide on mucosal proliferation of the human ileum and colon. Gastroenterology 1994;107(2):429–34.

135. Ban K, Kozar RA. Enteral glutamine: a novel mediator of PPARgamma in the postischemic gut. J Leukoc Biol 2008;84(3):595–9.

136. Hamman JH. Composition and applications of Aloe vera leaf gel. Molecules 2008;13(8):1599–616.

137. Speisky H, Cassels BK. Boldo and boldine: an emerging case of natural drug development. Pharmacol Res 1994;29(1):1–12.

138. Ali B, Blunden G, Tanira M, et al. Some phytochemical, pharmacological and toxicological properties of ginger (Zingiber officinale Roscoe): a review of recent research. Food Chem Toxicol 2008;46(2):409–20.

139. Low Dog T. A reason to season: the therapeutic benefits of spices and culinary herbs. Explore (NY) 2006;2(5):446–9.

140. Borchers AT, Selmi C, Meyers FJ, et al. Probiotics and immunity. J Gastroenterol 2009;44(1):26–46.

141. Ogle K, Bullocks J. Children with allergic rhinitis and/or bronchial asthma treated with elimination diet: a five year follow-up. Ann Allergy 1980;44:273–8.

142. Carey O, Locke C, Cookson J. Effect of alterations of dietary sodium on the severity of asthma in men. Thorax 1993;48(7):714–18.

143. Wickens K, Barry D, Friezema A, et al. Fast foods—are they a risk factor for asthma? Allergy 2005;60(12):1537–41.

144. Rahman I, Biswas S, Kode A. Oxidant and antioxidant balance in the airways and airway diseases. Eur J Pharmacol 2006;533(1–3):222–39.

145. Wood L, Fitzgerald D, Gibson P, et al. Lipid peroxidation as determined by plasma isoprostanes is related to disease severity in mild asthma. Lipids 2000;35(9):967–74.

146. Wood L, Gibson P, Garg M. Biomarkers of lipid peroxidation, airway inflammation and asthma. Eur Respir J 2003;21(1):177–86.

147. Misso N, Brooks-Wildhaber J, Ray S, et al. Plasma concentrations of dietary and nondietary antioxidants are low in severe asthma. Eur Respir J 2005;26:257–64.

148. Wood L, Garg M, Powell H, et al. Lycopene-rich treatments modify noneosinophilic airway inflammation in asthma: proof of concept. Free Radic Res 2008;42(1):94–102.

149. Patel B, Welch A, Bingham S, et al. Dietary antioxidants and asthma in adults. Thorax 2006;61:388–93.

150. Hodge L, Tan K, Loblay R. Assessment of food chemical intolerance in adult asthmatic patients. Thorax 1996;51:805–9.

151. Schünemann H, Grant B, Freudenheim J, et al. The relation of serum levels of antioxidant vitamins C and E, retinol and carotenoids with pulmonary function in the general population. Am J Respir Crit Care Med 2001;163(5):1246–55.

152. Romieu I, Sienra-Monge J, Ramírez-Aguilar M, et al. Antioxidant supplementation and lung functions among children with asthma exposed to high levels of air pollutants. Am J Respir Crit Care Med 2002;166(5):703–9.

153. Rubin R, Navon L, Cassano P. Relationship of serum antioxidants to asthma prevalence in youth. Am J Respir Crit Care Med 2004;169(3):393–8.

154. Chatzi L, Apostolaki G, Bibakis I, et al. Protective effect of fruits, vegetables and the Mediterranean diet on asthma and allergies among children in Crete. Thorax 2007;62(8):677–83.

155. Castro-Rodriguez JA, Garcia-Marcos L, Alfonseda Rojas JD, et al. Mediterranean diet as a protective factor for wheezing in preschool children. J Pediatr 2008;152(6):823–8, 8 e1–2.

156. Varraso R. Nutrition and asthma. Curr Allergy Asthma Rep 2012;12(3):201–10.

157. Sexton P, Black P, Metcalf P, et al. Influence of Mediterranean diet on asthma symptoms, lung function, and systemic inflammation: a randomized controlled trial. J Asthma 2013;50(1):75–81.

158. Li J, Xun P, Zamora D, et al. Intakes of long-chain omega-3 (n-3) PUFAs and fish in relation to incidence of asthma among American young adults: the CARDIA study. Am J Clin Nutr 2013;97(1):173–8.

159. Singh V, Sinha H, Gupta R. Barriers in the management of asthma and attitudes towards complementary medicine. Respir Med 2002;96(10):835–40.

160. Yurach MT, Davis BE, Cockcroft DW. The effect of caffeinated coffee on airway response to methacholine and exhaled nitric oxide. Respir Med 2011;105(11):1606–10.

161. Guo CH, Liu PJ, Lin KP, et al. Nutritional supplement therapy improves oxidative stress, immune response, pulmonary function, and quality of life in allergic asthma patients: an open-label pilot study. Altern Med Rev 2012;17(1):42–56.

162. Chen E, Miller G. Stress and inflammation in exacerbations of asthma. Brain Behav Immun 2007;21(8):993–9.

163. Wilson A, Honsberger R, Chiu J, et al. Transcendental meditation and asthma. Respiration 1975;32(1):74–80.

164. Chang Y, Yang Y, Chen C, et al. Tai Chi Chuan training improves the pulmonary function of asthmatic children. J Microbiol Immunol Infect 2008;41(1):88–95.

165. Vedanthan P, Kesavalu L, Murthy K, et al. Clinical study of yoga techniques in university students with asthma: a controlled study. Allergy Asthma Proc 1998;19(1):3–9.

166. Manocha R, Marks G, Kenchington P, et al. Sahaja yoga in the management of moderate to severe asthma: a randomised controlled trial. Thorax 2002;57(2):110–15.

167. Nagarathna R, Nagendra H. Yoga for bronchial asthma: a controlled study. Br Med J 1985;291(6502):1077–9.

168. Galantino M, Galbavy R, Quinn L. Therapeutic effects of yoga for children: a systematic review of the literature. Pediatr Phys Ther 2008;20(1):66–80.

169. Thomas M, McKinley R, Mellor S, et al. Breathing exercises for asthma: a randomised controlled trial. Thorax 2009;64(1):55–61.

170. Holloway E, West R. Integrated breathing and relaxation training (the Papworth method) for adults with asthma in primary care: a randomised controlled trial. Thorax 2007;62(12):1039–42.

171. von Steinaecker K, Welke J, Bühring M, et al. [Pilot study of breathing therapy in groups for patients with bronchial asthma]. Forsch Komplementmed 2007;14(2):86–91, [in German].

172. Singh V, Wisniewski A, Britton J, et al. Effect of yoga breathing exercises (pranayama) on airway reactivity in subjects with asthma. Lancet 1990;335(8702):1381–3.

173. Smyth J, Stone A, Hurewitz A, et al. Effects of writing about stressful experiences on symptom reduction in patients with asthma or rheumatoid arthritis: a randomized trial. JAMA 1999;281(14):1304–9.

174. Lucas SR, Platts-Mills TA. Physical activity and exercise in asthma: relevance to etiology and treatment. J Allergy Clin Immunol 2005;115(5):928–34.

175. Bonsignore M, La Grutta S, Cibella F, et al. Effects of exercise training and montelukast in children with mild asthma. Med Sci Sports Exerc 2008;40(3):405–12.

176. Fanelli A, Barros Cabral A, Neder J, et al. Exercise training on disease control and quality of life in asthmatic children. Med Sci Sport Exerc 2007;39(9):1474–80.

177. Welsh L, Kemp J, Roberts R. Effects of physical conditioning on children and adolescents with asthma. Sport Med 2005;35(2):127–41.

178. Swimming improves fitness in children with asthma. BMJ 2013;346:f2714.

179. Bougault V, Boulet LP. Airways disorders and the swimming pool. Immunol Allergy Clin North Am 2013;33(3):395–408.

180. Eneli I, Skybo T, Camargo C. Weight loss and asthma: a systematic review. Thorax 2008;63(8):671–8.

181. Cooper S, Oborne J, Newton S, et al. Effect of two breathing exercises (Buteyko and pranayama) in asthma: a randomised controlled trial. Thorax 2003;58(8): 674–9.

182. Opat A, Cohen M, Bailey M, et al. A clinical trial of the Buteyko Breathing Technique in asthma as taught by a video. J Asthma 2000;37(7):557–64.

183. Cowie R, Conley D, Underwood M, et al. A randomised controlled trial of the Buteyko method as an adjunct to conventional management of asthma. Respir Med 2008;102(5):726–32.

184. Bowler S, Green A, Mitchell C. Buteyko breathing techniques in asthma: a blinded randomised controlled trial. Med J Aust 1998;169(11–12):575–8.

185. McCarney RW, Brinkhaus B, Lasserson TJ, et al. Acupuncture for chronic asthma. Cochrane Database Syst Rev 2004;(1):CD000008.

186. Shen FY, Lee MS, Jung SK. Effectiveness of pharmacopuncture for asthma: a systematic review and meta-analysis. Evid Based Complement Alternat Med 2011;doi:10.1155/2011/678176.

187. Ngai SP, Hui-Chan CW, Jones A. A short review of acupuncture and bronchial asthma—western and traditional Chinese medicine concepts. Hong Kong Physiother J 2006;24:28–38.

188. Leake R, Broderick J. Treatment efficacy of acupuncture: a review of the research literature. Integr Med 1999;1(3):107–15.

189. Chu KA, Wu YC, Ting YM, et al. Acupuncture therapy results in immediate bronchodilating effect in asthma patients. J Chin Med Assoc 2007;70(7):265–8.

190. Kaur B, Rowe BH, Arnold E. Vitamin C supplementation for asthma. Cochrane Database Syst Rev 2009;(1):CD000993.

191. Bielory L, Gandhi R. Asthma and vitamin C. Ann Allergy 1994;73(2):89–96, quiz–100.

192. Hatch GE. Asthma, inhaled oxidants, and dietary antioxidants. Am J Clin Nutr 1995;61(3 Suppl.): 625S–30S.

193. Fogarty A, Lewis SA, Scrivener SL, et al. Corticosteroid sparing effects of vitamin C and magnesium in asthma: a randomised trial. Respir Med 2006;100(1):174–9.

194. Ammon H, Mack T, Singh G, et al. Inhibition of leukotriene B4 formation in rat peritoneal neutrophils by an ethanolic extract of the gum resin exudate of Boswellia serrata. Planta Med 1991;57(3):203–7.

195. Singh GB, Atal CK. Pharmacology of an extract of salai guggal ex-Boswellia serrata, a new non-steroidal anti-inflammatory agent. Agents Actions 1986;18(3–4):407–12.

196. Tang Y, Xu Y, Xiong S, et al. The effect of Ginkgo Biloba extract on the expression of PKCalpha in the inflammatory cells and the level of IL-5 in induced sputum of asthmatic patients. J Huazhong Univ Sci Technol Med Sci 2007;27(4):375–80.

197. Vogensen SB, Stromgaard K, Shindou H, et al. Preparation of 7-substituted ginkgolide derivatives: potent platelet activating factor (PAF) receptor antagonists. J Med Chem 2003;46(4):601–8.

198. McHugh P, Aitcheson F, Duncan B, et al. Buteyko Breathing technique for asthma: an effective intervention. N Z Med J 2003;116(1187):U710.

199. Nagendra HR, Nagarathna R. An integrated approach of yoga therapy for bronchial asthma: a 3–54-month prospective study. J Asthma 1986;23(3):123–37.

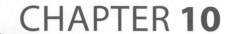

CHAPTER **10**

Congestive respiratory disorders

David Casteleijn
ND, MHSc

OVERVIEW

Congestive respiratory disorders are conditions that present with mucus build-up in the upper and/or lower respiratory tract. Rhinitis and sinusitis are the most common upper respiratory expressions of congestion. Sinusitis is an inflammatory condition of one or more of the four (paired) paranasal sinuses.[1] The condition may be classified by symptom duration (acute if less than four weeks, chronic if more than 12 weeks) or by aetiology (viral, bacterial, fungal or non-infectious).[1,2] Chronic sinusitis is one of the most common chronic illnesses worldwide, estimated to affect 2–16% of people in the United States and 7–27% in Europe (estimates vary depending upon differences in diagnostic criteria).[3] Acute sinusitis is also common, affecting on average one in seven people in the United States every year.

Sinusitis presents with clinical features including:[1–3]

- mucopurulent nasal drainage (it may be difficult to distinguish bacterial sinusitis from preceding viral upper respiratory tract infection (URTI), since both can be associated with thick, purulent or discoloured nasal discharge)
- nasal congestion, blockage or obstruction
- facial pain or pressure that is worse when bending over or supine
- tenderness over affected sinus (particularly with maxillary infection)
- reduction or loss of smell
- other symptoms of acute rhinosinusitis including headache, fever, cough, fatigue, halitosis and ear pressure or fullness.

Sinusitis is usually bacterial in origin, although this may be difficult to assess on clinical presentation alone.[3] Common organisms include *Streptococcus pneumoniae, Haemophilus influenzae, Streptococcus pyogenes,* other streptococci and *Neisseria* spp.[1,4] Cases of chronic sinusitis may be associated with high levels of fungal colonisation.[5]

Lower respiratory congestion, presenting as a productive cough, is usually associated with an acute infection (see Chapter 8) or chronic obstructive process, either reversible (such as asthma) or non-reversible (such as chronic obstructive pulmonary disease [COPD], previously known as chronic obstructive airways disease).[6]

RISK FACTORS

Key factors in the development of sinusitis are sinus obstruction and/or impaired ciliary clearance of secretions (e.g. due to anatomical abnormalities or other conditions). Other disorders that may exacerbate or contribute to developing chronic rhinosinusitis include allergic rhinitis, chronic exposure to environmental irritants (e.g. tobacco smoke), immunodeficiency states, recurrent URTI or systemic diseases (e.g. granulomatosis with polyangiitis).[3] Inflammatory polyps were found to be a cause of chronic frontal sinusitis (requiring frontal sinus surgery) in 53% of sinus surgery cases.[4,7] Other local conditions that predispose children to rhinosinusitis include swimming and diving, enlarged and infected adenoids, vasomotor disturbance leading to obstruction of drainage and deflection of the nasal septum.[8]

Chronic sinusitis is often a concomitant presentation with other forms of respiratory atopy, such as allergic rhinitis[9] or asthma.[3] Suppressive treatment of hayfever is thought to lead to the development of chronic sinus inflammation. A recent study out of Korea strongly linked chronic sinusitis to persistent allergic rhinitis, and showed a significant association with heavy stress.[10]

Dietary factors are often suggested to contribute to excess mucus production. Dairy, wheat and corn have been proposed to promote a more globular mucus, disable sinus drainage and promote antigen exposure.[11] While certain individuals may be predisposed to inflammatory responses with certain foods, the concept that some foods are universally mucus-promoting is an oversimplification of this process.[12] In people who believe this, however, the consumption of such products does dispose them to greater subjective respiratory symptoms,[12] demonstrating a potential psychosomatic component. (For risk factors for lower respiratory tract [LRT] congestion, see Chapter 8 on respiratory infections and immune insufficiency and Chapter 9 on asthma.)

DIFFERENTIAL DIAGNOSIS

- Infection—viral, bacterial, fungal
- Allergic rhinitis
- Vasomotor rhinitis
- Food allergy/intolerance symptoms
- Nasal polyp
- Nasal tumour

CONVENTIONAL TREATMENT

The predominant conventional treatment of sinusitis centres around antibiotics to control infection and medications such as topical (in acute cases) or oral (in chronic cases) corticosteroids to reduce acute inflammation.[11,13] Adjunctive treatments include topical and oral decongestants, analgesics and antihistamines to reduce mucosal blood flow, decrease tissue oedema and perhaps enhance drainage of secretions from the sinus ostia.[3,11,13] In chronic or unresponsive cases, nasal endoscopic surgery may assist in clearance of the sinuses and restoration of mucociliary activity.[14]

While antibiotics are frequently prescribed, a Cochrane review of 49 studies concluded that they produced insignificant cure rates, with only a small treatment effect on patients in a primary care setting.[15] (For conventional treatment of LRT congestion see Chapter 8 on respiratory infections and immune insufficiency and Chapter 9 on asthma.)

KEY TREATMENT PROTOCOLS

As congestive respiratory disorders differ significantly from one another (e.g. COPD and allergic rhinitis), general treatment protocols will require adaptation to suit the presentation. However, for all of these conditions, an overwhelming priority will be the reduction of congestion and easing of airway blockage by using mucolytic and anticatarrhal herbs and nutrients. Obstruction may also be eased by reducing inflammation and, in LRT disorders, enhancing bronchodilation. If there is a cough, this may be relieved and/or used to assist mucociliary airway clearance.

Acute immune support and reduction of pathogens will also be necessary in acute infection. If congestion is chronic or

> ### Naturopathic Treatment Aims
>
> * Reduce congestion (clear the paranasal sinuses or bronchioles).
> * Reduce bacterial or viral load.
> * Support immune response.
> * Support the integrity of the mucous membranes.
> * If chronic, support elimination via the lymphatic system.
> * Use tonifying protocols to boost immunity and vitality after acute infection is cleared.

repeated, then longer term immune tonics and adaptogens should be used in order to strengthen the resistance of the individual. In forms of congestion linked to atopy, anti-allergic substances and those that modulate hypersensitivity are indicated.

In chronic conditions there are often underlying factors to be addressed. Digestive disturbance or lymphatic stagnation may play a role in exacerbating and/or perpetuating the complaint.

Whenever there is an overproduction of catarrh, the respiratory mucous membrane health is likely to be compromised. Trophorestoratives and nutritive support are necessary to nourish these back to health. Their integrity is vital as they are one of the few body surfaces exposed continually to the external environment, and play a large role in first-line innate immune defence.

Reduce congestion in the sinuses and airways

Blocked sinuses: steam inhalations, heat therapy and nasal irrigation

With sinusitis it is important to liquefy the congested secretions in an effort to clear the sinus passages. **Herbal mucolytics** act to thin out mucosal secretions and make them easier to expel.[16] *Trigonella foenum-graecum*[17] is useful, especially as a hot infusion, with the heat and steam being an integral part of the process. It is important to warn your patient that they should expect a nasal discharge to result, so they can plan the best time for the intervention. If they know, they are also less likely to take antihistamines, which would suppress the desired effect. Other mucolytic herbs to consider are *Foeniculum vulgare*, *Allium cepa*, *Armoracia rusticana* and *Allium sativum*.[18,19] Extracts of **Myrtol** (an essential oil blend derived from *Pinus* spp., *Citrus aurantifolia* and *Eucalyptus globulus*) standardised to contain the secretolytic and secretomotor essential oils limonene 75 mg, cineole 75 mg and alpha-pinene 20 mg may be used to improve nasal mucociliary clearance and nasal patency in cases of chronic rhinitis.[20,21]

An additional category of herbs applied in sinus congestion are upper respiratory tract (URT) **anticatarrhals**, such as *Euphrasia* spp.*, Plantago lanceolata*, *Sambucus nigra* and *Hydrastis canadensis*.[19] Anticatarrhals differ from mucolytics in that their action involves reducing mucus production, rather than clearance.[22] Few well-designed clinical trials were found to substantiate the effectiveness of these interventions, but they have a history of traditional use.[19,23] *Hydrastis canadensis* is traditionally contraindicated in acute inflammatory conditions of the mucous membranes and may also be used in subacute or chronic conditions.[19] A combination of *Gentiana lutea*, *Primula veris*, *Rumex* spp., *Sambucus nigra* and *Verbena officinalis* is approved by Commission E to treat sinusitis and seems to exert mucolytic or anticatarrhal, antiviral and anti-inflammatory effects in a number of trials.[24,25] It may not offer additional benefits for olfactory dysfunction if utilised following administration of oral corticosteroids.[26]

Nutritional mucolytics may also be included in a supplement regimen. **N-acetylcysteine** (NAC) is the most researched and broadly used mucolytic.[27,28] The sulfhydryl group works to cleave disulphide bonds in mucous glycoproteins, making nasal secretions easier to expel.[29] NAC has demonstrated the ability to increase the mucociliary clearance rate by 35%, in comparison with no effect by placebo.[30] In vitro studies in human mucosal tissue also suggest that vitamin C has the ability to increase cilia beat frequency and therefore improve mucociliary clearance.[31]

Proteolytic enzymes, including bromelain, show an ability to break down the naked peptide region of mucous glycoproteins when applied topically.[29] There have been questions surrounding the bioavailability of these agents upon oral ingestion, but these have been answered by studies showing that ingestion of the compounds leads to appreciable increases in their serum concentration.[32–34] In a number of trials conducted on patients with chronic sinusitis or allergic rhinitis, the administration of bromelain (in addition to individualised conventional treatment) produced significant improvements in parameters including nasal mucosal inflammation, overall symptoms, breathing difficulties and nasal discomfort.[34–36]

Possible fenugreek allergy

One study has found that fenugreek seed powder may contain a number of potential allergenic proteins. In most cases, this reactivity seems to be due to cross-reactivity with peanut sensitisation.[2,22] While true fenugreek allergy is unlikely to be a concern, practitioners should be aware of the potential for cross-reactivity when using this mucolytic agent in patients with peanut allergies.

A longstanding traditional remedy for blocked sinuses and nasal congestion is the inhalation of steam. Often this is with an additive (see below). Studies are mixed on the use of hot, moist air alone, with some positive trials[37,38] and others showing no effect greater than room-temperature air.[39–41] As an extension of this principle, local application of heat more generally has also been shown to alleviate the symptoms of allergic rhinitis.[42,43]

The 'old wives' cure of **chicken soup** may not be such a myth. The inhalation of hot air (from hot water) is known to help clear nasal congestion,[39,40] and research has shown that hot chicken soup is more effective than hot water.[44] The addition of aromatic spices and culinary herbs will also help to open up the nasal passages and clear secretions.[45] As an additional benefit, eating the soup inhibits neutrophil migration, possibly helping to reduce symptoms in infection.[45]

The use of botanicals may improve therapeutic effectiveness of steam inhalation. Commission E supports inhaling *Matricaria recutita* for inflammation and irritation of the respiratory tract.[24] The **essential oils** of *Cinnamomum zeylanicum*, *Thymus vulgaris*, *Mentha piperita*, *Perilla frutescens*, *Cymbopogon* spp. and *Eucalyptus* spp. have demonstrated antibacterial activity against common respiratory pathogens through vapour contact, and therefore may also be of use.[46–48] One of the most common inhalants is *Eucalyptus* spp. oil; when administered via inhalation or as a chest rub, it has demonstrated ability to reduce nasal congestion and improve breathing function in those with respiratory infection.[47,49] Myrtol, a German inhalant product combining cineol, limonene and alpha-pinene, also has great efficacy in treating purulent mucosinusitis.[50] These phytochemicals are constituents of many essential oils including *Mentha* *piperita*, citrus oils, *Anethum graveolens*, *Pinus* spp., *Piper nigrum*, *Eucalyptus* spp. and *Melaleuca cajuputi*.[51] Other suggested inhalations include *Mentha piperita*, *Lavandula* spp., *Pinus sylvestris, Melaleuca alternifolia* and *Rosmarinus officinalis*.[52] Essential oil inhalations should be avoided in infants due to the danger of laryngeo- or bronchospasm (Kratschmer reflex).

Nasal irrigation is another method of clearing sinus congestion. The origins of this technique lie in yogic and homeopathic traditions.[53,54] **Jala neti** is a hatha yoga technique of pouring water in through one nostril using a neti pot so that it pours out the other. The method is believed to be an essential part of health maintenance, and is recommended three or four times a week.[55,56] A number of trials evince the positive benefits of nasal irrigation among people with allergic rhinitis or chronic sinusitis.[57] A Cochrane review in 2007 reported that nasal irrigation could improve the symptoms of chronic rhinosinusitis in the majority of patients, with few adverse effects.[53] Benefits are derived not solely from the initial mechanical clearance of the airways but also due to the physiological benefits of topical **saline** (sodium chloride), which has been proposed to: improve mucus clearance; enhance ciliary beat activity; remove antigens, biofilm or inflammatory mediators; and be protective of the mucous membranes.[53] **Sodium bicarbonate** is also mucolytic in nature and may be useful in nasal irrigation.[57]

One method of nasal irrigation is suggested in Figure 10.1, but there are many slight variations, and it is recommended that the practitioner become comfortable with their chosen technique themselves first before recommending it to others. It should also be

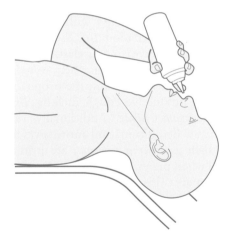

Figure 10.1
Nasal irrigation

How to perform nasal irrigation

1. Lie on a bed with the head extended off the end of the bed or over a bathtub or sink.
2. Direct saline solution into the right nostril.
3. Slowly release the saline solution to comfortably fill the nasal and sinus cavities.
4. Repeat in the left nostril directing the nozzle towards the left ear.
5. Remain in this position for two minutes.
6. Turn the head to the side and allow the saline solution to drain.
7. Return to an upright position.
8. If necessary, gently blow the nose when finished.

noted that bulb syringe irrigators have been found to be a potential source of contamination in rhinosinusitis,[58] so attempts should be made to ensure the cleanliness of the equipment and procedure.

Address phlegm and cough

There are a number of different treatment strategies to address respiratory congestion and cough. Dry (non-productive) or particularly severe coughs can benefit from suppression with an antitussive agent. Otherwise, although it may be annoying, it is best not to suppress the productive cough reflex, as it helps to clear infectious organisms and cellular debris from the airways.[59]

Expectorants may enhance a productive cough, allowing greater clearance of abnormal and thick phlegm and mucus. This will help remove pathogens, speeding recovery and decreasing the fatiguing effort required to cough. The majority of expectorants fall into one of two categories:

- stimulating expectorants, which provoke cough by reflex irritation of the upper digestive tract membranes[60]
- warming expectorants, which increase blood flow to the respiratory mucosa, provide reflex stimulation of the upper digestive lining and alter the mucopolysaccharide constituents of mucus, making it runnier and easier to expel.[61]

Mucolytics and anticatarrhals may also be useful where there is a great deal of phlegm, mucus and/or congestion present. These agents will help to reduce catarrhal congestion of the upper or lower respiratory system. As with mucolytic pharmaceuticals, their mechanism of action is not fully understood, but they may act by altering the mucopolysaccharide structure of mucus, decreasing its elasticity or viscosity.[28]

Herbal medicines with demulcent action may help to reduce a cough if it is a reflex response to hyperactive or irritated receptors in the oropharynx.[59] Treatments used in Western herbal traditions for productive cough include *Thymus vulgaris*, *Glycyrrhiza glabra*, *Lobelia inflata* and *Polygala senega*.[24] Additionally, *Verbascum thapsus*, *Tussilago farfara* and *Althaea officinalis* are demulcents and antitussives indicated for dry or unproductive coughs.[24] Herbs, such as *Prunus serotina*, are primary antitussives; however, caution needs to be applied when prescribing these as they can suppress a cough despite there being mucus to expectorate. This may exacerbate an acute respiratory infection.

Glycyrrhiza glabra is approved by Commission E to treat upper respiratory catarrh and cough.[24] In addition to its expectorant and antitussive actions, *Glycyrrhiza glabra* has anti-inflammatory, immune-enhancing and mucoprotective effects, the traditional reason behind its use in respiratory tract infections. The herb has demonstrated antitussive effects in animal studies, most likely due to the component liquiritin and its metabolite, liquiritigenin.[62] *Thymus vulgaris* has been used successfully in a large trial for the treatment of bronchial cough.[63] It demonstrates an ability to improve mucociliary clearance in vivo, although the mechanism remains to be elucidated.[64] In conjunction with *Sambucus nigra*, *Primula veris*, *Rumex acetosa*, *Verbena officinalis* and *Thymus vulgaris*, *Gentiana lutea* (the extract) has a demonstrated ability to reduce the frequency of symptomatic coughing fits.[65,66] It is also traditionally recommended for use in respiratory tract infections as an extract or gargle due to its antimicrobial and antitussive qualities.[24,61,67]

In the case of productive cough, *Inula helenium* is another key herb to use due to its combined effects as a stimulating expectorant and antibacterial agent.[68] Given that it contains a high level of mucilage, it also contributes to soothing the mucous membranes, therefore covering a wide range of the required therapeutic actions. It is also a respiratory spasmolytic that is well tolerated in long-term therapy.[63] Traditional eclectic texts purport *Althaea officinalis* to be useful in the case of catarrh or irritated mucous membranes.[18,69] The polysaccharide constituent has demonstrated inhibition of coughs caused by laryngopharangeal and tracheobronchial irritation.[69] New research indicates a relatively pronounced antibacterial effect (stronger than that of *Thymus vulgaris*) on various strains of *Escherichia coli*, exerted via inhibition of microbial metabolism.[70] *Althaea officinalis* is more indicated for an irritating than a congestive cough.[24]

Chronic obstructive pulmonary disease

Overview

Chronic obstructive pulmonary disease (COPD), includes emphysema and chronic bronchitis. Unlike asthma, the airflow obstruction is only partially, or not, reversible and the disease process is progressive.[71] Airflow obstruction is usually associated with abnormal inflammation and remodelling of the airways, parenchyma and pulmonary vasculature in response to chronic inhalation of noxious particles or gases.[4,71,72]

COPD is diagnosed when a patient has spirometry readings of:

- $FEV_1/FVC*$ of less than or equal to 70%
- FEV_1 of less than or equal to 80% after administration of a bronchodilator[71] and symptoms that may include cough, dyspnoea, wheezing and sputum or mucus production.[73]

Risk factor includes[71,74]

- smoking (the major environmental factor)
- heavy exposure to occupational dusts and chemicals (vapours, irritants and fumes)
- indoor/outdoor air pollution
- genetic factors
- repeated/severe respiratory infections.

Treatment protocols

- Support smoking cessation.[75]
- Reduce/remove exposure to irritants.
- Reduce mucus congestion.
- Reduce airway inflammation and constriction.
- Support the mucous membranes.
- Improve immunity and address any acute infection.
- Support special needs nutritionally—adequate caloric intake and protein intake,[76] possibly a high-fat, low-carbohydrate diet.[77–79]

Nutraceutical interventions

- Mucolytics and anticatarrhals: *Trigonella foenum-graecum*, *Plantago lanceolata*, *Hydrastis canadensis*, *Foeniculum vulgare*, *Allium cepa*, *Armoracia rusticana*, *Allium sativum*, N-acetylcysteine,[27,80,81] bromelain, trypsin, papain and aromatic inhalants[82]
- Anti-inflammatory: *Boswellia serrata*, *Curcuma longa*, *Zingiber officinale*, omega-3 fatty acids, quercetin, fish, antioxidant foods (fruit and vegetables)[83–86] and possibly antioxidant nutrients,[7,87,88] *Camellia sinensis*[85]
- Bronchodilating: *Adhatoda vasica*, *Euphorbia* spp., *Coleus forskohlii*, *Grindelia camporum*, *Glycyrrhiza glabra*, magnesium[89] (dietary and supplemental)
- Acute immune enhancement (in the case of infection): vitamin C, vitamin A, zinc, quercetin, *Echinacea* spp., *Andrographis paniculata*, *Picrorhiza kurroa*, *Uncaria tomentosa*
- Immune tonics (during chronic stages where there is no acute infection): *Astragalus membranaceus*, *Eleutherococcus senticosus*, *Withania somnifera* and *Echinacea* spp. may be used throughout both periods of remission and exacerbation
- Mucous membrane trophorestoratives: *Hydrastis canadensis*, vitamins A and C, zinc, selenium, adequate protein intake[90]

Adhatoda vasica is mentioned in the Vedas for treatment of a number of respiratory illnesses, and is also listed in the *Pharmacopoeia of India*.[91] Extracts of the aerial parts administered orally exhibit the ability to inhibit both mechanical and chemically induced coughs.[91] When this treatment was combined with *Echinacea* spp. and *Eleutherococcus senticosus* extracts in clinical trials, it produced additive benefits in treating URTI.[92] Patients showed greater improvement in many of the parameters tested, including severity of coughing, frequency of coughing, efficacy of mucus discharge in the respiratory tract, nasal congestion and general feeling of sickness.[92]

Inhaled preparations containing menthol, such as *Eucalyptus* spp. oil, have shown the ability to significantly increase tracheobronchial clearance of mucus from the lungs[93] and help to reduce cough.[94] Add-on therapy with **Pelargonium sidoides** led to an improvement in health-related quality of life and other patient-reported outcomes in adult patients with chronic obstructive pulmonary disease compared to placebo, while showing good long-term tolerability.[95] As discussed earlier, **nutritional mucolytic agents** such as N-acetylcysteine, vitamin C and proteolytic enzymes may be useful in LRT congestion. Dietary treatment should also be employed. **Allium spp.** are antimicrobial, expectorant, mucolytic and anti-inflammatory.[61] The respiratory system is one of the main systems to benefit from the antimicrobial action of this volatile oil, as it is excreted from the lungs. **Culinary herbs** such as *Pimpinella anisum*, *Foeniculum vulgare*, *Trigonella foenum-graecum* and *Zingiber officinale* are warming expectorants and can be incorporated into treatment, either in food or as hot beverages.[61]

Reduce microbial load

Herbal antimicrobials (encompassing antivirals, antibacterials and antifungals) differ from some pharmaceutical products in that they usually exert a bacteriostatic effect on the pathogen rather than being directly biocidal. Biocidal agents act via a number of mechanisms, at a number of different target sites in the cell. The combined overall activity seems to result in the bactericidal death of the microbe.[96] According to Maillard, when used at lower doses, biocides exert a bacteriostatic effect, inhibiting the growth and colonisation of a pathogen.[96] Although more research is needed in the area, it seems that herbal agents (given at the right doses) exert a bacteriostatic, rather than a cytotoxic or even biocidal, effect.

While there are many individual constituents that have been identified as antimicrobial, whole plant extracts seem to be more efficacious at clearing pathogens due to synergism between components.[97] For further information on plant compounds and their antimicrobial efficacy, see Table 10.1.

In the case of respiratory infections, antimicrobials are useful to address the primary infection, inhibiting further replication of the causative organism and additionally to prevent secondary infection. However, they are unlikely to 'cure' an infection when used alone. Rather, they are most effective when combined with other botanicals, such as those with immune-modulating activity.

Antimicrobial herbs traditionally recommended for the respiratory system are *Allium sativum*, *Inula helenium*, *Hydrastis canadensis* and *Thymus vulgaris*. The essential oil of *Thymus vulgaris* exhibits some of the most pronounced antimicrobial effects of herb that have been scientifically evaluated. It contains a multitude of compounds with activity against microorganisms, including thymol, carvacrol, luteolin and linalool.[97,119] The combined effect of these is more potent than the individual constituents alone, illustrating the importance of using whole plant extracts for the most rapid antimicrobial effects.[97] When tested against a number of the most common bacterial respiratory

Table 10.1
Plant constituents and their antimicrobial effects

Constituent class	Subclass	Antimicrobial effects	Examples
Phenolics	Simple phenols	Substrate deprivation Membrane disruption[98,99]	*Picrorhiza kurroa*
	Phenolic acids	Cell membrane interaction as protonophores?[100]	*Amphipterygium adstringens* *Arctostaphylos uva-ursi* *Anacardium pulsatilla* *Matricaria recutita*[100,101]
	Quinones	Bind to adhesions Complex with cell wall Weaken cell membrane Inactivate enzymes[101,102]	*Salvia miltiorrhiza*
	Flavonoids	Bind to adhesins[103,104]	*Camellia sinensis*[101]
	Flavones	Complex with cell wall Inactivate enzymes Inhibit HIV reverse transcriptase[105–108]	*Zingiber officinale* *Piper solmsianum*[75,106]
	Flavonols[109]	Action on the cytoplasmic membrane causing bacterial aggregation[110]	Quercetin (e.g. from *Allium Cepa*)[52]
	Tannins	Bind to proteins Bind to adhesins Enzyme inhibition Substrate deprivation Complex with cell wall Membrane disruption Metal ion complexation[101,111,112]	*Potentilla* spp. *Arctium lappa* *Rhamnus purshiana* *Eucalyptus globulus* *Melissa officinalis* *Thymus vulgaris*[101,112]
	Coumarins	Interaction with eucaryotic DNA (antiviral activity)[101]	*Carum carvi*[101]
Terpenoids, essential oils		Membrane disruption[113]	*Capsicum* spp. *Melaleuca* spp. *Berberis vulgaris* *Syzygium aromaticum* *Armoracia rusticana* *Mentha piperita* *Rosmarinus officinalis* *Thymus vulgaris* *Curcuma longa*[101]
Alkaloids		Intercalate into cell wall and/or DNA[101,114–116]	*Piper nigrum* *Hydrastis canadensis* *Mahonia aquifolium*[101]
Lectins and polypeptides		Block viral fusion or adsorption Form disulfide bridges[101,117,118]	*Phytolacca decandra* *Viscum album* *Urtica dioica* *Juglans nigra*

Adapted from Cowan 1999[101]

pathogens, *Thymus vulgaris* oil exhibited marked inhibitory effects on bacterial cell growth.[120] The two other oils with marked significant action against these pathogens were *Cinnamomum zeylanicum* and *Syzygium aromaticum*.[120] It is interesting to note that these effects were just as strong in antibiotic multiresistant strains of bacteria, suggesting a role for increasing use of botanical agents in clearing respiratory infection.[120] When combined with either primrose herb or ivy leaf extract, *Thymus vulgaris* shows marked efficacy in treating the symptoms and shortening the duration of acute bronchitis, an effect that is likely to be due in part to its antimicrobial action.[66,67,121]

Inula helenium also exhibits antimicrobial activity in vitro, but clinical trials of the herb are lacking.[18] Among its constituents, *Inula helenium* contains thymol derivatives, and therefore, at least in theory, some of the results of research with thyme oil may be applicable.[122] Among the most potent **antivirals** in the herbal repertory are *Hypericum perforatum* and *Thuja occidentalis*. The hypericin component of *Hypericum perforatum* is especially active against enveloped viruses, such as HIV and herpes simplex, while *Thuja occidentalis* has a broader spectrum of viricidal targets.[123] When *Thuja occidentalis* is given in combination with *Baptisia tinctoria* radix, *Echinacea purpurea* radix and *Echinacea pallida* radix, the mixture exhibits the ability to inhibit influenza A virus pathology in animals.[124] *Verbascum thapsus* is a herb traditionally used in both Western and other medical traditions as an expectorant and trophorestorative. At present, scientific information about its properties is limited to in vitro and in vivo animal studies, but results suggest that it may have some anthelmintic, antispasmosdic,[125] antiviral[126] and antimicrobial[127] activity.

One widely available antimicrobial is *Allium sativum*.[128] It has demonstrated activity against a number of bacteria, fungi and viruses implicated in respiratory infection, with some of its most potent constituents being allicin and allitridin.[129–132] In a recent trial, intranasal garlic powder was shown to decrease the likelihood of contracting an airborne infection while travelling.[133]

Increasing food intake of shallots (*Allium ascalonicum*), garlic and onions (*Allium cepa*) will also provide the active **organosulfur compounds** and exert an antimicrobial effect, and be beneficial in treating respiratory infection.[128,134,135] These foods will be at their most potent fresh or as close to fresh as possible.[135] Other nutrients and foods that exhibit bacteriostatic qualities are **zinc** and **unripe papaya**.[136,137]

If considering a topical throat spray or gargle, suspended nanoparticles of **colloidal zinc** and **silver** may be useful, as they demonstrate antimicrobial (bacteriostatic and bactericidal) efficacy against a range of organisms including *Enterococcus faecalis*, *Staphylococcus* spp., *Streptococcus pyogenes*, *Pseudomonas aeruginosa* and *Escherichia coli*.[137,138]

Support immune response

In congestive respiratory disorders, it is important to identify the cause, as this will affect what type of immune modulation is necessary. In cases of infection or an altered immune response the practitioner should boost general immunity and, if allergies are present or contributing, then give antiallergic agents. In asthma, immune modulation may be necessary. Chronic diseases are very likely to benefit from immune tonics.

Pelargonium sidoides has been found to be significantly superior to placebo in treating acute rhinosinusitis,[139] with decreased debilitating symptoms and faster recovery. The activity of this herb is likely to be due to moderate antimicrobial activity and marked immune modulating activity, including an ability to alter the release of tumour-necrosis factor (TNF-α) and nitric oxide.[140]

Vitamin C has proven efficacious in the treatment of chronic sinusitis and allergic rhinitis. As a nutrient, it enhances both innate and adaptive components of the immune system, including natural killer cells, T-cells and B-cells.[141] It is also antiallergic, in that it stabilises mast cells and inhibits histamine release.[142] Levels of ascorbic acid, vitamin E, copper and zinc were found to be lower in children with chronic rhinosinusitis than in controls without the condition.[143] Treatment of allergic rhinitis with an ascorbic acid solution intranasally three times daily has been shown to reduce symptoms in up to 74% of treated subjects. They experienced a decrease in nasal secretions, blockage and oedema.[144]

Allergic concerns may also be treated with ***Urtica dioica***, which may inhibit inflammation through its histamine content, which inhibits leukotriene formation.[145] The herb has demonstrated success in treating allergic rhinitis, with all treated patients in a randomised controlled trial reporting improved global assessments.[146] ***Nigella sativa*** may also have antiallergic and anti-inflammatory benefits, with the ability to reduce congestion, nasal itching, rhinorrhoea, sneezing and other symptoms of allergic rhinitis within two weeks of administration.[147] Other antiallergic agents include quercetin and the herbs ***Albizia lebbeck*** and ***Scutellaria baicalensis***.

Reducing inflammation in mucosal tissue (as with conventional corticosteroid application) may also help to relieve congestion, and in this sense, anti-inflammatory botanicals may be utilised. A combination of ***Scutellaria baicalensis*** and ***Eleuthrococcus senticosus*** has been shown to significantly block early- and late-phase inflammatory mediators such as PGE_2, histamine and IL-5 in ex vivo human mucosal tissue.[31] The combination also inhibited bacterial stimulation of pro-inflammatory cytokines from T-cells to a similar or greater extent than fluticasone propionate.[31] Small pilot interventional studies have also demonstrated a role for silymarin (an extract of ***Silybum marianum***) as an adjunct to conventional treatment for allergic rhinitis, acting as an antioxidant and anti-inflammatory. Oral administration of the extract produced significant improvements in clinical symptoms (above that of the control group).[148]

Support the integrity of the mucous membranes

Continual goblet cell activation and mucus production may compromise the mucosal linings of the airways. This necessitates support of the mucous membranes themselves through herbal **mucous membrane trophorestoratives** and nutritionally with *collagen supportive nutrients*. *Hydrastis canadensis* and *Euphrasia* spp. are traditionally indicated for supporting mucosal surfaces in the body, especially in the URT.[19,68] At present, no pharmacological research or clinical trials have been found to substantiate these effects.

Nutrients that are important in the healing of wounds and help to support the integrity of collagen, epithelium and mucous membranes are vitamins A and C, lysine, proline and zinc. In addition to its antioxidant role, **vitamin C** is required for converting proline and lysine to hydroxyproline and hydroxylysine so that they may be incorporated into collagen structures.[111] **Zinc** is a cofactor for RNA and DNA polymerase, meaning that it is essential for DNA replication, repair and cell proliferation.[149] It also stimulates reepithelialisation, fibroblast proliferation and is involved with collagen synthesis,[149,150] and therefore is essential for healing of the airways. **Copper** is also essential for collagen and elastin cross-linking.[149] **Vitamin A** is essential for the strength and health of the mucous membranes and epithelial integrity.[151,152] It assists 'normal endodermal differentiation as well as maintaining balanced cell proliferation, differentiation and apoptosis'.[153] Studies have repeatedly demonstrated the beneficial effects of vitamin A supplementation on gastrointestinal mucosa,[154] and the benefits may be extrapolated to also apply to the respiratory mucosa.

Support elimination via the lymphatic system

The idea of lymphatic cleansing is a traditional naturopathic approach to many chronic congestive conditions, including respiratory, musculoskeletal and skin disorders. The beneficial herbal actions are **lymphatic** and **alterative**, and herbs such as *Phytolacca decandra*, *Echinacea* spp., *Urtica* spp., *Galium aparine* and *Calendula officinalis* are viable options.[23]

INTEGRATIVE MEDICAL CONSIDERATIONS

Yoga

Participation in yoga programs may be of benefit in congestive disorders. After participating in a specially adapted program, elderly COPD sufferers were able to tolerate more activity without dyspnoea-related distress and improved functional performance.[155] One session of yogic breathing techniques alone may produce favourable respiratory changes in sufferers.[156]

Acupuncture and traditional chinese medicine

A review[157] examined seven high-quality randomised controlled trials and concluded that there was sufficient evidence to recommend acupuncture for improving symptoms of perennial rhinitis. Chinese medicine acupoint herbal patching also seems to improve general health and quality of life in patients with allergic rhinitis.[158] Vasomotor rhinitis has also been shown to respond favourably to acupuncture. Patients in a recent trial showed significant improvement in nasal sickness score both over baseline and in comparison to controls given sham acupuncture.[157] A meta-analysis performed in 2012 concluded that Chinese herbal medicine interventions appear to have beneficial effects in persistent allergic rhinitis, but the published efficacy studies are too small to draw firm conclusions.[159]

In COPD, acupuncture may be useful due to its ability to reduce disease-related dyspnoea.[160,161] Acu-TENS also produces increased FEV and decreased dyspnoea in patients compared with controls, even after a single 45-minute session.[162]

Reflexology, massage and aromatherapy

An early trial examining reflexology treatment of COPD shows some moderate improvements, perhaps relating to the increased relaxation felt by patients.[163] In a small trial of five patients treated with 24 weekly treatments of neuromuscular release massage therapy, four of these experienced increases in thoracic gas volume, peak flow and FVC.[164] Aromatherapy is most useful in these conditions when used as an inhaled preparation. Most of the beneficial essential oils have been covered earlier. As well as antimicrobial actions, some constituents depolarise thermoreceptors in the nasal mucosa by inhibiting cellular calcium influx and therefore lead to subjective improvements in airflow, although nasal resistance is not decreased.[41]

CLINICAL SUMMARY

While congestive respiratory disorders present in a variety of forms, all require naturopathic treatment focused on immune modulation, subject to the stage of treatment. In many chronic instances this will focus on stimulation; however, stimulating the immune system in the acute stage is contraindicated as this can exacerbate inflammation and even worsen acute illness. Acute inflammation instead requires down-regulation of the immune system, and thick secretions need to be liquefied (along with bronchodilation to facilitate removal) and mucous membrane integrity enhanced.

During naturopathic treatment of congestive respiratory disorders, underlying causes such as psychological stress, immune dysregulation, food intolerance and/or altered intestinal permeability need to be addressed. Once the initial symptoms have been controlled tonifying the immune system should be considered to prevent reoccurence.

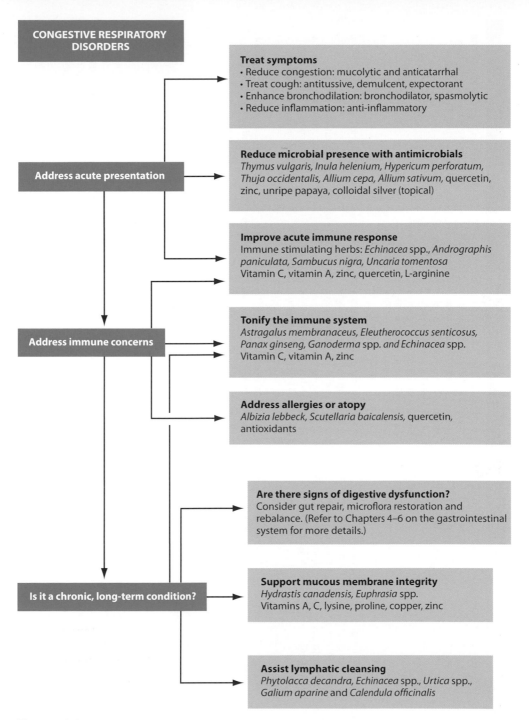

CONGESTIVE RESPIRATORY DISORDERS

Treat symptoms
• Reduce congestion: mucolytic and anticatarrhal
• Treat cough: antitussive, demulcent, expectorant
• Enhance bronchodilation: bronchodilator, spasmolytic
• Reduce inflammation: anti-inflammatory

Address acute presentation

Reduce microbial presence with antimicrobials
Thymus vulgaris, Inula helenium, Hypericum perforatum, Thuja occidentalis, Allium cepa, Allium sativum, quercetin, zinc, unripe papaya, colloidal silver (topical)

Improve acute immune response
Immune stimulating herbs: *Echinacea* spp., *Andrographis paniculata, Sambucus nigra, Uncaria tomentosa*
Vitamin C, vitamin A, zinc, quercetin, L-arginine

Address immune concerns

Tonify the immune system
Astragalus membranaceus, Eleutherococcus senticosus, Panax ginseng, Ganoderma spp. *and Echinacea* spp.
Vitamin C, vitamin A, zinc

Address allergies or atopy
Albizia lebbeck, Scutellaria baicalensis, quercetin, antioxidants

Are there signs of digestive dysfunction?
Consider gut repair, microflora restoration and rebalance. (Refer to Chapters 4–6 on the gastrointestinal system for more details.)

Is it a chronic, long-term condition?

Support mucous membrane integrity
Hydrastis canadensis, Euphrasia spp.
Vitamins A, C, lysine, proline, copper, zinc

Assist lymphatic cleansing
Phytolacca decandra, Echinacea spp., *Urtica* spp., *Galium aparine* and *Calendula officinalis*

Figure 10.2
Naturopathic treatment decision tree—congestive respiratory disorders

Table 10.2
Review of the major evidence

Intervention	Mechanisms of action	Key literature	Summary of results	Comment
N-acetylcysteine (NAC)	Mucolytic and increases the mucociliary clearance rate[30]	Todisco et al. 1985[30] Grandjean et al. 2000[27] Stey et al. 2000[81] Sadowska et al. 2007[165]	Prolonged NAC administration results in fewer acute exacerbations of bronchopulmonary disease[27] Reduces the risk of exacerbations and improves symptoms in patients with chronic bronchitis when given orally for 12–24 weeks[81] At dosages used in COPD treatment, it reduces exacerbation rate and limits the number of hospitalisation days but has little or no influence on lung function parameters[165]	Useful in chronic conditions and for preventing exacerbations May take time to be effective
Thymus vulgaris	Antimicrobial, mucolytic, anti-catarrhal and expectorant properties	Fabio et al. 2007[120] Wienkötter et al. 2007[64] Büechi et al. 2005[166] Kemmerich et al. 2007[66] Marzian 2007[121]	Demonstrated antimicrobial activity against a number of common respiratory pathogens[120] In animal studies, improves mucociliary clearance by an unknown mechanism[64] Clinical trials have all used the herb as part of a combination formula, whereby it reduces the frequency of symptomatic cough[66,121,166]	Consider in both acute URTI and LRTI Efficacy often shown in combination with other herbs, so may be due to synergistic effects of the formulation
Proteolytic enzymes	Separates the peptide bond of naked mucous glycoprotein when applied topically[25]	Majima 2002[29] Seltzer 1967[34] Ryan 1967[35] Taub 1967[36]	Older clinical trials are quite old but demonstrate that bromelain may decrease nasal inflammation and breathing difficulties while mitigating nasal discomfort in allergic rhinitis and sinusitis[34–36]	More efficacious as supplements, but food sources may have synergistic ingredients (e.g. vitamin C)
Nasal irrigation	Physical cleansing of the nasal passages	Harvey et al. 2007[54] Rabago et al. 2002[56] Rabago et al. 2006[167] Raza et al. 2008[168]	Nasal lavage with saline or additional sodium hypochlorite is well tolerated, with only minor side effects[54] It improves a range of nasal and respiratory symptoms[56,167–169]	A traditional safe method that has supportive evidence
Inhalation of essential oils	Many essential oils (especially from the lamiaceae family) have antimicrobial, anticatarrhal, mucolytic and expectorant properties	Cowan 1999[101] Inouye et al. 2001[46] Fabio et al. 2007[120] Lim et al. 2008[170] Federspil et al. 1997[50] Meister 1999[82] Matthys et al. 2000[82] Hasani et al. 2003[93]	Many plant constituents, especially essential oils, show marked antimicrobial activity[46,101,120] A systemic review shows that topical antimicrobial agents appear effective in treating chronic rhinosinusitis[170] Trials using essential oils have shown: – improvement of mucociliary clearance from the lungs of patients with chronic bronchitis[93] – decreased symptoms of mucopurulent sinusitis[50] – more rapid regression of acute bronchitis[82]	Effective, with multiple benefits; however, be aware that some oils should not be used for children, and many are not recommended in pregnancy

KEY POINTS

- Congestive disorders present in a variety of clinical forms.
- They may be infectious or non-infectious and generally all require some form of immune support or modulation.
- Liquefy and remove the secretions that can be a reservoir for infection.
- Support of mucous membrane integrity via herbal, nutritional or dietary measures is necessary.
- Once the initial symptoms have been controlled, address the underlying causes such as immune dysregulation, food intolerance and/or altered intestinal permeability and psychological stress.
- Consider a tonifying protocol once acute exacerbations have ceased.

FURTHER READING

Anushiravani M, Bakhshaee M, Taghipour A, et al. A systematic review of randomized controlled trials with herbal medicine on chronic rhinosinusitis. Phytother Res 2018;32(3):395–401. doi:10.1002/ptr.5968. Epub 2017 Nov 12.

Lim M, Citardi MJ, Leong JL. Topical antimicrobials in the management of chronic rhinosinusitis: a systematic review. Am J Rhinol 2008;22(4):381–9.

Sadowska AM, Manuel YKB, De Backer WA. Antioxidant and anti-inflammatory efficacy of NAC in the treatment of COPD: discordant in vitro and in vivo dose-effects: a review. Pulm Pharmacol Ther 2007;20(1):9–22.

Acknowledgment: The author would like to acknowledge Tessa Finney-Brown, who authored this chapter in previous editions.

REFERENCES

1. Rubin M, Gonzales R, Sande M. Infections of the upper respiratory tract. In: Kasper D, Fauci A, Longo D, et al, editors. Harrison's principles of internal medicine. 16th ed. New York: McGraw-Hill Companies Inc.; 2005.
2. Piccirillo JF. Clinical practice. Acute bacterial sinusitis. N Engl J Med 2004;351(9):902–10.
3. Hamilos D. Clinical manifestations, pathophysiology, and diagnosis of chronic rhinosinusitis. In: UpTodate [internet]. Waltham MA: UpToDate; 2013.
4. Rabe KF, Hurd S, Anzueto A, et al. Global strategy for the diagnosis, management, and prevention of chronic obstructive pulmonary disease: GOLD executive summary. Am J Respir Crit Care Med 2007;176(6):532–55.
5. Murr AH, Goldberg AN, Pletcher SD, et al. Some chronic rhinosinusitis patients have elevated populations of fungi in their sinuses. Laryngoscope 2012;122(7):1438–45.
6. Health NIo. National Asthma Education and Prevention Program: Guidelines for the diagnosis and management of asthma. National Asthma Education and Prevention Program Expert Panel Report 3. Washington; 2007.
7. Han JK, Ghanem T, Lee B, et al. Various causes for frontal sinus obstruction. Am J Otolaryngol 2009;30(2):80–2.
8. Benjamin B. Sinusitis in children—general considerations. Int J Pediatr Otorhinolaryngol 1983;5(3):281–4.
9. Spector SL. The role of allergy in sinusitis in adults. J Allergy Clin Immunol 1992;90(3 Pt 2):518–20.
10. Kim YS, Kim NH, Seong SY, et al. Prevalence and risk factors of chronic rhinosinusitis in Korea. Am J Rhinol Allergy 2011;25(3):117–21.
11. Helms S, Miller A. Natural treatment of chronic rhinosinusitis. Altern Med Rev 2006;11(3):196–207.
12. Wuthrich B, Schmid A, Walther B, et al. Milk consumption does not lead to mucus production or occurrence of asthma. J Am Coll Nutr 2005;24(6 Suppl.): 547S–55S.
13. Slavin RG, Spector SL, Bernstein IL, et al. The diagnosis and management of sinusitis: a practice parameter update. J Allergy Clin Immunol 2005;116(6 Suppl.):S13–47.
14. Lanza DC, Kennedy DW. Current concepts in the surgical management of chronic and recurrent acute sinusitis. J Allergy Clin Immunol 1992;90(3 Pt 2):505–10, discussion 511.
15. Ahovuo-Saloranta A, Borisenko OV, Kovanen N, et al. Antibiotics for acute maxillary sinusitis. Cochrane Database Syst Rev 2008;(2):CD000243.
16. Rogers DF. Mucoactive agents for airway mucus hypersecretory diseases. Respir Care 2007;52(9):1176–93, discussion 1193–7.
17. Wichtl M, editor. Herbal drugs and phytopharmaceuticals: a handbook for practice on a scientific basis. 3rd ed. Stuttgart: Medpharm GmbH Scientific Publishers; 2004.
18. Felter H, Lloyd J King's American Dispensatory; 1898. Online. Available: http://www.henriettesherbal.com/ eclectic/kings/echinacea.html 1 Nov 2013.
19. Agency EM. Community monograph on Foeniculum vulgare [monograph]. London: EMEA Committee on Herbal Medicinal Products; 2007.
20. Han D, Wang N, Zhang L. The effect of myrtol standardized on human nasal ciliary beat frequency and mucociliary transport time. Am J Rhinol Allergy 2009;23(6):610–14.
21. Behrbohm H, Kaschke O, Sydow K. [Effect of the phytogenic secretolytic drug Gelomyrtol forte on mucociliary clearance of the maxillary sinus]. Laryngorhinootologie 1995;74(12):733–7.
22. Bone KM. A clinical guide to blending liquid herbs. Philadelphia: Churchill Livingstone; 2003.

23. Mittman P. Ask the experts. Severe recurring sinusitis. Explore (NY) 2005;1(6):496. 495.

24. Blumenthal M, Goldberg A, Brinckmann J, editors. Herbal medicine: expanded commission E monographs (English translation). Austin: Integrative Medicine Communications; 2000.

25. Guo R, Canter PH, Ernst E. Herbal medicines for the treatment of rhinosinusitis: a systematic review. Otolaryngol Head Neck Surg 2006;135(4):496–506.

26. Reden J, El-Hifnawi D, Zahnert T, et al. The effect of a herbal combination of primrose, gentian root, vervain, elder flowers, and sorrel on olfactory function in patients with a sinonasal olfactory dysfunction. Rhinology 2011;49(3):342–6.

27. Grandjean E, Berthet P, Ruffmann R, et al. Efficacy of oral long-term N-acetylcysteine in chronic bronchopulmonary disease: a meta-analysis of published double-blind, placebo-controlled clinical trials. Clin Ther 2000;22(2):209–21.

28. Henke MO, Ratjen F. Mucolytics in cystic fibrosis. Paediatr Respir Rev 2007;8(1):24–9.

29. Majima Y. Mucoactive medications and airway disease. Paediatr Respir Rev 2002;3(2):104–9.

30. Todisco T, Polidori R, Rossi F, et al. Effect of N-acetylcysteine in subjects with slow pulmonary mucociliary clearance. Eur J Respir Dis Suppl 1985;139:136–41.

31. Zhang N, Van Crombruggen K, Holtappels G, et al. A herbal composition of Scutellaria baicalensis and Eleutherococcus senticosus shows potent anti-inflammatory effects in an ex vivo human mucosal tissue model. Evid Based Complement Alternat Med 2012;2012:673145.

32. Maurer HR. Bromelain: biochemistry, pharmacology and medical use. Cell Mol Life Sci 2001;58(9):1234–45.

33. Castell JV, Friedrich G, Kuhn CS, et al. Intestinal absorption of undegraded proteins in men: presence of bromelain in plasma after oral intake. Am J Physiol 1997;273(1 Pt 1):G139–46.

34. Seltzer AP. Adjunctive use of bromelains in sinusitis: a controlled study. Eye Ear Nose Throat Mon 1967;46(10):1281–8.

35. Ryan RE. A double-blind clinical evaluation of bromelains in the treatment of acute sinusitis. Headache 1967;7(1):13–17.

36. Taub SJ. The use of bromelains in sinusitis: a double-blind clinical evaluation. Eye Ear Nose Throat Mon 1967;46(3):361–2, passim.

37. Ophir D, Elad Y. Effects of steam inhalation on nasal patency and nasal symptoms in patients with the common cold. Am J Otolaryngol 1987;8(3):149–53.

38. Tyrrell D, Barrow I, Author J. Local hyperthermia benefits natural and experimental common colds. BMJ 1989;298:1280–3.

39. Forstall G, Macknin L, Yen-Lieberman B, et al. Effect of inhaling heated vapor on symptoms of the common cold. JAMA 1994;271(14):1109–11.

40. Macknin M, Mathew S, Medendorp S. Effect of inhaling heated vapor on symptoms of the common cold. JAMA 1990;264:989–91.

41. Ciuman RR. Phytotherapeutic and naturopathic adjuvant therapies in otorhinolaryngology. Eur Arch Otorhinolaryngol 2012;269(2):389–97.

42. Yerushalmi A, Karman S, Lwoff A. Treatment of perennial allergic rhinitis by local hyperthermia. Proc Natl Acad Sci 1982;79(15):4766–9.

43. Elad Y, Fink A, Fishler E, et al. Effects of elevated intranasal temperature on subjective and objective findings in perennial rhinitis. Ann Otol Rhinol Laryngol 1988;97(3):259–63.

44. Saketkhoo K, Januszkiewicz A, Sackner MA. Effects of drinking hot water, cold water, and chicken soup on nasal mucus velocity and nasal airflow resistance. Chest 1978;74(4):408–10.

45. Rennard BO, Ertl RF, Gossman GL, et al. Chicken soup inhibits neutrophil chemotaxis in vitro. Chest 2000;118(4):1150–7.

46. Inouye S, Yamaguchi H, Takizawa T. Screening of the antibacterial effects of a variety of essential oils on respiratory tract pathogens, using a modified dilution assay method. J Infect Chemother 2001;7(4):251–4.

47. Burrows A. The effects of camphor, eucalyptus and menthol vapour on nasal resistance to airflow and nasal sensation. Acta Otolaryngol 1983;96:157–63.

48. Shubina L, Siurin S, Savchenko V. [Inhalations of essential oils in the combined treatment of patients with chronic bronchitis]. Vrach Delo 1990;5:66–7.

49. Food and Drug Administration. Over the counter drugs: monograph for OTC nasal decongestent drug products. Fed Reg 1994;41:38408–9.

50. Federspil P, Wulkow R, Zimmermann T. [Effects of standardized Myrtol in therapy of acute sinusitis–results of a double-blind, randomized multicenter study compared with placebo]. Laryngorhinootologie 1997;76(1):23–7.

51. Pengelly A. The constituents of medicinal plants. 2nd ed. Crows Nest, NSW: Allen & Unwin; 2004.

52. Purchon N. Nerys Purchon's handbook of aromatherapy. 2nd ed. Sydney: Hodder Headline Australia; 1999.

53. Burton MJ, Eisenberg LD, Rosenfeld RM. Extracts from The Cochrane Library: nasal saline irrigations for the symptoms of chronic rhinosinusitis. Otolaryngol Head Neck Surg 2007;137(4):532–4.

54. Harvey R, Hannan SA, Badia L, et al. Nasal saline irrigations for the symptoms of chronic rhinosinusitis. Cochrane Database Syst Rev 2007;(3):CD006394.

55. Jefferson W. The neti pot for better health. Summertown: Healthy Living Publications; 2005.

56. Rabago D, Zgierska A, Mundt M, et al. Efficacy of daily hypertonic saline nasal irrigation among patients with sinusitis: a randomized controlled trial. J Fam Pract 2002;51(12):1049–55.

57. Rhee C, Majima Y, Cho J, et al. Effects of mucokinetic drugs on rheological properties of reconstituted human nasal mucus. Arch Otolaryngol Head Neck Surg 1999;125:101–5.

58. Williams GB, Ross LL, Chandra RK. Are bulb syringe irrigators a potential source of bacterial contamination in chronic rhinosinusitis? Am J Rhinol 2008;22(4):399–401.

59. Ziment I. Herbal antitussives. Pulm Pharmacol Ther 2002;15(3):327–33.

60. Gunn J. The action of expectorants. BMJ 1927;2:972–5.

61. Mills S, Bone K. Principles and practice of phytotherapy. Edinburgh: Churchill Livingstone; 2000.

62. Kamei J, Saitoh A, Asano T, et al. Pharmacokinetic and pharmacodynamic profiles of the antitussive principles of Glycyrrhizae radix (licorice), a main component of the Kampo preparation Bakumondo-to (Mai-men-dong-tang). Eur J Pharmacol 2005;507(1–3):163–8.

63. Ernst E, März R, Sieder C. [Acute bronchitis: effectiveness of Sinupret. Comparative study with common expectorants in 3,187 patients]. Fortschr Med 1997;115(11):52–3.

64. Wienkotter N, Begrow F, Kinzinger U, et al. The effect of thyme extract on beta2-receptors and mucociliary clearance. Planta Med 2007;73(7):629–35.

65. Kemmerich B. Evaluation of efficacy and tolerability of a fixed combination of dry extracts of thyme herb and primrose root in adults suffering from acute bronchitis with productive cough. A prospective,

double-blind, placebo-controlled multicentre clinical trial. Arzneimittelforschung 2007;57(9):607–15.

66. Kemmerich B, Eberhardt R, Stammer H. Efficacy and tolerability of a fluid extract combination of thyme herb and ivy leaves and matched placebo in adults suffering from acute bronchitis with productive cough. A prospective, double-blind, placebo-controlled clinical trial. Arzneimittelforschung 2006;56(9):652–60.

67. Scientific Committee of the British Herbal Medical Association. British herbal pharmacopoeia. 1st ed. Bournemouth: British Herbal Medicine Association; 1983.

68. Deriu A, Zanetti S, Sechi LA, et al. Antimicrobial activity of Inula helenium L. essential oil against gram-positive and gram-negative bacteria and Candida spp. Int J Antimicrob Agents 2008;31(6):588–90.

69. Nosal'ova G, Strapkova A, Kardosova A, et al. [Antitussive action of extracts and polysaccharides of marsh mallow (Althea officinalis L., var. robusta)]. Pharmazie 1992;47(3):224–6.

70. Watt K, Christofi N, Young R. The detection of antibacterial actions of whole herb tinctures using luminescent Escherichia coli. Phytother Res 2007;21(12):1193–9.

71. Pauwels RA, Buist AS, Ma P, et al. Global strategy for the diagnosis, management, and prevention of chronic obstructive pulmonary disease: national Heart, Lung, and Blood Institute and World Health Organization Global Initiative for Chronic Obstructive Lung Disease (GOLD): executive summary. Respir Care 2001;46(8):798–825.

72. Barnes PJ. Mechanisms in COPD: differences from asthma. Chest 2000;117(2 Suppl.):10S–4S.

73. Celli BR, MacNee W. Standards for the diagnosis and treatment of patients with COPD: a summary of the ATS/ERS position paper. Eur Respir J 2004;23(6):932–46.

74. Radin A, Cote C. Primary care of the patient with chronic obstructive pulmonary disease-part 1: frontline prevention and early diagnosis. Am J Med 2008;121(7 Suppl.):S3–12.

75. White P. COPD: challenges and opportunities for primary care. Respiratory Medicine: COPD Update 2005;1:43–52.

76. Brug J, Schols A, Mesters I. Dietary change, nutrition education and chronic obstructive pulmonary disease. Patient Educ Couns 2004;52(3):249–57.

77. Frankfort JD, Fischer CE, Stansbury DW, et al. Effects of high- and low-carbohydrate meals on maximum exercise performance in chronic airflow obstruction. Chest 1991;100(3):792–5.

78. Angelillo VA, Bedi S, Durfee D, et al. Effects of low and high carbohydrate feedings in ambulatory patients with chronic obstructive pulmonary disease and chronic hypercapnia. Ann Intern Med 1985;103(6 Pt 1):883–5.

79. Efthimiou J, Mounsey PJ, Benson DN, et al. Effect of carbohydrate rich versus fat rich loads on gas exchange and walking performance in patients with chronic obstructive lung disease. Thorax 1992;47(6):451–6.

80. Sadowska AM, Verbraecken J, Darquennes K, et al. Role of N-acetylcysteine in the management of COPD. Int J Chron Obstruct Pulmon Dis 2006;1(4):425–34.

81. Stey C, Steurer J, Bachmann S, et al. The effect of oral N-acetylcysteine in chronic bronchitis: a quantitative systematic review. Eur Respir J 2000;16(2):253–62.

82. Meister R, Wittig T, Beuscher N, et al. Efficacy and tolerability of myrtol standardized in long-term treatment of chronic bronchitis. A double-blind, placebo-controlled study. Study Group Investigators. Arzneimittelforschung 1999;49(4):351–8.

83. Smit HA, Grievink L, Tabak C. Dietary influences on chronic obstructive lung disease and asthma: a review of the epidemiological evidence. Proc Nutr Soc 1999;58(2):309–19.

84. Britton JR, Pavord ID, Richards KA, et al. Dietary antioxidant vitamin intake and lung function in the general population. Am J Respir Crit Care Med 1995;151(5):1383–7.

85. Celik F, Topcu F. Nutritional risk factors for the development of chronic obstructive pulmonary disease (COPD) in male smokers. Clin Nutr 2006;25(6):955–61.

86. Rautalahti M, Virtamo J, Haukka J, et al. The effect of alpha-tocopherol and beta-carotene supplementation on COPD symptoms. Am J Respir Crit Care Med 1997;156(5):1447–52.

87. Hu G, Cassano PA. Antioxidant nutrients and pulmonary function: the Third National Health and Nutrition Examination Survey (NHANES III). Am J Epidemiol 2000;151(10):975–81.

88. Fujimoto S, Kurihara N, Hirata K, et al. Effects of coenzyme Q10 administration on pulmonary function and exercise performance in patients with chronic lung diseases. Clin Investig 1993;71(8 Suppl.):S162–6.

89. Bhatt SP, Khandelwal P, Nanda S, et al. Serum magnesium is an independent predictor of frequent readmissions due to acute exacerbation of chronic obstructive pulmonary disease. Respir Med 2008;102(7):999–1003.

90. Faeste CK, Namork E, Lindvik H. Allergenicity and antigenicity of fenugreek (Trigonella foenum-graecum) proteins in foods. J Allergy Clin Immunol 2009;123(1):187–94.

91. Dhuley JN. Antitussive effect of Adhatoda vasica extract on mechanical or chemical stimulation-induced coughing in animals. J Ethnopharmacol 1999;67(3):361–5.

92. Narimanian M, Badalyan M, Panosyan V, et al. Randomized trial of a fixed combination (KanJang) of herbal extracts containing Adhatoda vasica, Echinacea purpurea and Eleutherococcus senticosus in patients with upper respiratory tract infections. Phytomedicine 2005;12(8):539–47.

93. Hasani A, Pavia D, Toms N, et al. Effect of aromatics on lung mucociliary clearance in patients with chronic airways obstruction. J Altern Complement Med 2003;9(2):243–9.

94. Morice AH, Marshall AE, Higgins KS, et al. Effect of inhaled menthol on citric acid induced cough in normal subjects. Thorax 1994;49(10):1024–6.

95. Matthys H, Funk P. Pelargonium sidoides preparation EPs 7630 in COPD: health-related quality-of-life and other patient-reported outcomes in adults receiving add-on therapy. Curr Med Res Opin 2018;1–7:doi:10.1080/03007995.2017.1416344.

96. Maillard JY. Bacterial target sites for biocide action. Symp Ser Soc Appl Microbiol 2002;31:16S–27S.

97. Iten F, Saller R, Abel G, et al. Additive antimicrobial effects of the active components of the essential oil of Thymus vulgaris—Chemotype Carvacrol. Planta Med 2009;75(11):1231–6.

98. Peres MT, Delle Monache F, Cruz AB, et al. Chemical composition and antimicrobial activity of Croton urucurana Baillon (Euphorbiaceae). J Ethnopharmacol 1997;56(3):223–6.

99. Toda M, Okubo S, Ikigai H, et al. The protective activity of tea catechins against experimental infection by Vibrio cholerae O1. Microbiol Immunol 1992;36(9):999–1001.

100. Castillo-Juarez I, Rivero-Cruz F, Celis H, et al. Anti-Helicobacter pylori activity of anacardic acids from Amphipterygium adstringens. J Ethnopharmacol 2007;114(1):72–7.

101. Cowan MM. Plant products as antimicrobial agents. Clin Microbiol Rev 1999;12(4):564–82.

102. Alves DS, Perez-Fons L, Estepa A, et al. Membrane-related effects underlying the biological activity of the

anthraquinones emodin and barbaloin. Biochem Pharmacol 2004;68(3):549–61.

103. Perrett S, Whitfield PJ, Sanderson L, et al. The plant molluscicide Millettia thonningii (Leguminosae) as a topical antischistosomal agent. J Ethnopharmacol 1995;47(1):49–54.

104. Rojas A, Hernandez L, Pereda-Miranda R, et al. Screening for antimicrobial activity of crude drug extracts and pure natural products from Mexican medicinal plants. J Ethnopharmacol 1992;35(3):275–83.

105. Brinkworth RI, Stoermer MJ, Fairlie DP. Flavones are inhibitors of HIV-1 proteinase. Biochem Biophys Res Commun 1992;188(2):631–7.

106. Sookkongwaree K, Geitmann M, Roengsumran S, et al. Inhibition of viral proteases by Zingiberaceae extracts and flavones isolated from Kaempferia parviflora. Pharmazie 2006;61(8):717–21.

107. Ono K, Nakane H, Fukushima M, et al. Inhibition of reverse transcriptase activity by a flavonoid compound, 5,6,7-trihydroxyflavone. Biochem Biophys Res Commun 1989;160(3):982–7.

108. Taniguchi M, Kubo I. Ethnobotanical drug discovery based on medicine men's trials in the African savanna: screening of east African plants for antimicrobial activity II. J Nat Prod 1993;56(9):1539–46.

109. Li M, Xu Z. Quercetin in a lotus leaves extract may be responsible for antibacterial activity. Arch Pharm Res 2008;31(5):640–4.

110. Cushnie TP, Hamilton VE, Chapman DG, et al. Aggregation of Staphylococcus aureus following treatment with the antibacterial flavonol galangin. J Appl Microbiol 2007;103(5):1562–7.

111. Haslam E. Natural polyphenols (vegetable tannins) as drugs: possible modes of action. J Nat Prod 1996;59(2):205–15.

112. Tomczyk M, Latte KP. Potentilla—a review of its phytochemical and pharmacological profile. J Ethnopharmacol 2009;122(2):184–204.

113. Cichewicz RH, Thorpe PA. The antimicrobial properties of chile peppers (Capsicum species) and their uses in Mayan medicine. J Ethnopharmacol 1996;52(2):61–70.

114. Atta ur R, Choudhary MI. Diterpenoid and steroidal alkaloids. Nat Prod Rep 1995;12(4):361–79.

115. Freiburghaus F, Kaminsky R, Nkunya MH, et al. Evaluation of African medicinal plants for their in vitro trypanocidal activity. J Ethnopharmacol 1996;55(1):1–11.

116. Houghton PJ, Woldemariam TZ, Khan AI, et al. Antiviral activity of natural and semi-synthetic chromone alkaloids. Antiviral Res 1994;25(3–4):235–44.

117. Meyer JJ, Afolayan AJ, Taylor MB, et al. Antiviral activity of galangin isolated from the aerial parts of Helichrysum aureonitens. J Ethnopharmacol 1997;56(2):165–9.

118. Kokoska L, Janovska D. Chemistry and pharmacology of Rhaponticum carthamoides: a review. Phytochemistry 2009;70(7):842–55.

119. Lopez-Lazaro M. Distribution and biological activities of the flavonoid luteolin. Mini Rev Med Chem 2009;9(1):31–59.

120. Fabio A, Cermelli C, Fabio G, et al. Screening of the antibacterial effects of a variety of essential oils on microorganisms responsible for respiratory infections. Phytother Res 2007;21(4):374–7.

121. Marzian O. [Treatment of acute bronchitis in children and adolescents. Non-interventional postmarketing surveillance study confirms the benefit and safety of a syrup made of extracts from thyme and ivy leaves]. MMW Fortschr Med 2007;149(11):69–74.

122. Stojakowska A, Malarz J, Kisiel W. Thymol derivatives from a root culture of Inula helenium. Z Naturforsch [C] 2004;59(7–8):606–8.

123. Miskovsky P. Hypericin—a new antiviral and antitumor photosensitizer: mechanism of action and interaction with biological macromolecules. Curr Drug Targets 2002;3(1):55–84.

124. Bodinet C, Mentel R, Wegner U, et al. Effect of oral application of an immunomodulating plant extract on Influenza virus type A infection in mice. Planta Med 2002;68(10):896–900.

125. Ali N, Ali Shah SW, Shah I, et al. Anthelmintic and relaxant activities of Verbascum thapsus Mullein. BMC Complement Altern Med 2012;12:29.

126. Rajbhandari M, Mentel R, Jha PK, et al. Antiviral activity of some plants used in Nepalese traditional medicine. Evid Based Complement Alternat Med 2009;6(4):517–22.

127. Turker AU, Gurel E. Common mullein (Verbascum thapsus L.): recent advances in research. Phytother Res 2005;19(9):733–9.

128. Low Dog T. A reason to season: the therapeutic benefits of spices and culinary herbs. Explore (NY) 2006;2(5):446–9.

129. Zhen H, Fang F, Ye DY, et al. Experimental study on the action of allitridin against human cytomegalovirus in vitro: inhibitory effects on immediate-early genes. Antiviral Res 2006;72(1):68–74.

130. Adeleye IA, Opiah L. Antimicrobial activity of extracts of local cough mixtures on upper respiratory tract bacterial pathogens. West Indian Med J 2003;52(3):188–90.

131. Luo DQ, Guo JH, Wang FJ, et al. Anti-fungal efficacy of polybutylcyanoacrylate nanoparticles of allicin and comparison with pure allicin. J Biomater Sci Polym Edn 2009;20(1):21–31.

132. Liu ZF, Fang F, Dong YS, et al. Experimental study on the prevention and treatment of murine cytomegalovirus hepatitis by using allitridin. Antiviral Res 2004;61(2):125–8.

133. Hiltunen R, Josling PD, James MH. Preventing airborne infection with an intranasal cellulose powder formulation (Nasaleze travel). Adv Ther 2007;24(5):1146–53.

134. Amin M, Kapadnis BP. Heat stable antimicrobial activity of Allium ascalonicum against bacteria and fungi. Indian J Exp Biol 2005;43(8):751–4.

135. Al-Waili NS, Saloom KY, Akmal M, et al. Effects of heating, storage, and ultraviolet exposure on antimicrobial activity of garlic juice. J Med Food 2007;10(1):208–12.

136. Osato JA, Santiago LA, Remo GM, et al. Antimicrobial and antioxidant activities of unripe papaya. Life Sci 1993;53(17):1383–9.

137. Jones N, Ray B, Ranjit KT, et al. Antibacterial activity of ZnO nanoparticle suspensions on a broad spectrum of microorganisms. FEMS Microbiol Lett 2008;279(1):71–6.

138. Djokic S. Synthesis and antimicrobial activity of silver citrate complexes. Bioinorg Chem Appl 2008;436–58.

139. Bachert C, Schapowal A, Funk P, et al. Treatment of acute rhinosinusitis with the preparation from Pelargonium sidoides EPs 7630: a randomized, double-blind, placebo-controlled trial. Rhinology 2009;47(1):51–8.

140. Lizogub VG, Riley DS, Heger M. Efficacy of a Pelargonium sidoides preparation in patients with the common cold: a randomized, double blind, placebo-controlled clinical trial. Explore (NY) 2007;3(6):573–84.

141. Heuser G, Vojdani A. Enhancement of natural killer cell activity and T and B cell function by buffered vitamin C in patients exposed to toxic chemicals: the role of protein kinase-C. Immunopharmacol Immunotoxicol 1997;19(3):291–312.

142. Murray MT. A comprehensive review of Vitamin C. Am J Nat Med 1996;3:8–21.

143. Unal M, Tamer L, Pata YS, et al. Serum levels of antioxidant vitamins, copper, zinc and magnesium in children with chronic rhinosinusitis. J Trace Elem Med Biol 2004;18(2):189–92.

144. Podoshin L, Gertner R, Fradis M. Treatment of perennial allergic rhinitis with ascorbic acid solution. Ear Nose Throat J 1991;70(1):54–5.

145. Flamand N, Plante H, Picard S, et al. Histamine-induced inhibition of leukotriene biosynthesis in human neutrophils: involvement of the H2 receptor and cAMP. Br J Pharmacol 2004;141(4):552–61.

146. Mittman P. Randomized, double-blind study of freeze-dried Urtica dioica in the treatment of allergic rhinitis. Planta Med 1990;56(1):44–7.

147. Nikakhlagh S, Rahim F, Aryani FH, et al. Herbal treatment of allergic rhinitis: the use of Nigella sativa. Am J Otolaryngol 2011;32(5):402–7.

148. Bakhshaee M, Jabbari F, Hoseini S, et al. Effect of silymarin in the treatment of allergic rhinitis. Otolaryngol Head Neck Surg 2011;145(6):904–9.

149. Demling RH. Nutrition, anabolism, and the wound healing process: an overview. Eplasty 2009;9:e9.

150. Barbul A, Purtill WA. Nutrition in wound healing. Clin Dermatol 1994;12(1):133–40.

151. Ross AC, Ternus ME. Vitamin A as a hormone: recent advances in understanding the actions of retinol, retinoic acid, and beta carotene. J Am Diet Assoc 1993;93(11):1285–90, quiz 1291–2.

152. Osiecki H. The nutrient bible. 6th ed. Eagle Farm: Bio concepts Publishing; 2004.

153. Kohlmeier M. Nutrient metabolism. Oxford: Elsevier; 2003.

154. McCullough FS, Northrop-Clewes CA, Thurnham DI. The effect of vitamin A on epithelial integrity. Proc Nutr Soc 1999;58(2):289–93.

155. Donesky-Cuenco D, Nguyen HQ, Paul S, et al. Yoga therapy decreases dyspnea-related distress and improves functional performance in people with chronic obstructive pulmonary disease: a pilot study. J Altern Complement Med 2009;15(3):225–34.

156. Pomidori L, Campigotto F, Amatya TM, et al. Efficacy and tolerability of yoga breathing in patients with chronic obstructive pulmonary disease: a pilot study. J Cardiopulm Rehabil Prev 2009;29(2):133–7.

157. Fleckenstein J, Raab C, Gleditsch J, et al. Impact of acupuncture on vasomotor rhinitis: a randomized placebo-controlled pilot study. J Altern Complement Med 2009;15(4):391–8.

158. Hsu WH, Ho TJ, Huang CY, et al. Chinese medicine acupoint herbal patching for allergic rhinitis: a randomized controlled clinical trial. Am J Chin Med 2010;38(4):661–73.

159. Wang S, Tang Q, Qian W, et al. Meta-analysis of clinical trials on traditional Chinese herbal medicine for treatment of persistent allergic rhinitis. Allergy 2012;67(5):583–92.

160. Suzuki M, Namura K, Ohno Y, et al. The effect of acupuncture in the treatment of chronic obstructive pulmonary disease. J Altern Complement Med 2008;14(9):1097–105.

161. Jobst K, Chen JH, McPherson K, et al. Controlled trial of acupuncture for disabling breathlessness. Lancet 1986;2(8521–22):1416–19.

162. Lau KS, Jones AY. A single session of Acu-TENS increases FEV1 and reduces dyspnoea in patients with chronic obstructive pulmonary disease: a randomised, placebo-controlled trial. Aust J Physiother 2008;54(3):179–84.

163. Wilkinson IS, Prigmore S, Rayner CF. A randomised-controlled trail examining the effects of reflexology of patients with chronic obstructive pulmonary disease (COPD). Complement Ther Clin Pract 2006;12(2):141–7.

164. Beeken JE, Parks D, Cory J, et al. The effectiveness of neuromuscular release massage therapy in five individuals with chronic obstructive lung disease. Clin Nurs Res 1998;7(3):309–25.

165. Sadowska AM, Manuel YKB, De Backer WA. Antioxidant and anti-inflammatory efficacy of NAC in the treatment of COPD: discordant in vitro and in vivo dose-effects: a review. Pulm Pharmacol Ther 2007;20(1):9–22.

166. Buechi S, Vogelin R, von Eiff MM, et al. Open trial to assess aspects of safety and efficacy of a combined herbal cough syrup with ivy and thyme. Forsch Komplementarmed Klass Naturheilkd 2005;12(6):328–32.

167. Rabago D, Barrett B, Marchand L, et al. Qualitative aspects of nasal irrigation use by patients with chronic sinus disease in a multimethod study. Ann Fam Med 2006;4(4):295–301.

168. Raza T, Elsherif HS, Zulianello L, et al. Nasal lavage with sodium hypochlorite solution in Staphylococcus aureus persistent rhinosinusitis. Rhinology 2008;46(1):15–22.

169. Rabago D, Pasic T, Zgierska A, et al. The efficacy of hypertonic saline nasal irrigation for chronic sinonasal symptoms. Otolaryngol Head Neck Surg 2005;133(1):3–8.

170. Lim M, Citardi MJ, Leong JL. Topical antimicrobials in the management of chronic rhinosinusitis: a systematic review. Am J Rhinol 2008;22(4):381–9.

CHAPTER 11

Atherosclerosis and dyslipidaemia

Matthew Leach
ND, PhD

OVERVIEW

The association between elevated serum cholesterol and coronary heart disease (CHD) was first reported in the 1930s, with subsequent large epidemiological studies confirming the strong relationship between serum cholesterol and CHD.[1–3] Current predictions estimate that by the year 2020 cardiovascular diseases, notably atherosclerosis, will become the leading global cause of total disease burden.[4] Lipoprotein disorders or dyslipidaemias are common and are an important risk factor for coronary artery disease and all types of atherosclerotic vascular disease.[5] Cardiovascular risk has been shown to be positively associated with low-density lipoprotein cholesterol (LDL-C) levels and inversely with high-density lipoprotein cholesterol (HDL-C) levels.[6] The relationship between fasting serum triglyceride (TG) and cardiovascular risk has been confounded by the inverse association between TG and HDL-C, as well as by the association of TG with other risk factors such as diabetes mellitus and body mass.[6] TGs alone are now considered an important independent predictor of cardiovascular risk.[1]

Atherosclerosis affects various regions of the circulation and will present with unique clinical symptoms depending on the particular vascular bed affected. In coronary arteries, atherosclerosis contributes to myocardial infarction and angina, whereas stroke and transient cerebral ischaemia can occur when atherosclerosis is present in the arteries of the central nervous system.[2,7] In the peripheral circulation, atherosclerosis can result in intermittent claudication and gangrene, which can jeopardise limb viability.[4]

Atherogenesis or the pathogenesis of atherosclerosis usually occurs over decades in a discontinuous fashion, with relative periods of quiescence punctuated with periods of rapid evolution.[3] The eventual clinical manifestation may be chronic, as is the case in angina, or acute, such as a heart attack, stroke or sudden death. In some cases, individuals may experience no symptoms at all.

The 'fatty streak' represents the initial lesion of atherosclerosis, usually due to focal increases in the density of lipoproteins within the intima of a blood vessel, hence the reason for vigilance in maintaining low levels of these particles in the bloodstream.[8] The lipoproteins often associate with glycosaminoglycans in the arterial extracellular matrix and become more 'fixed' in the vasculature. These lipoprotein macromolecules undergo oxidative modifications, giving rise to hydroperoxides, lysophospholipids, oxysterols and aldehydic breakdown products.[4] Constituents of oxidatively modified LDL-C can augment expression of leucocyte adhesion molecules, recruiting leucocytes and macrophages into the area, which initiate inflammation.[9]

Areas of inflammation produce altered laminar flow in the arteries affected, and reduce the production of nitric oxide, which is vasodilatory and anti-inflammatory. The inflammatory process eventually penetrates or tears the endothelial layer with the products of lipoprotein oxidation, inducing the release of cytokines and tumour necrosis factor alpha (TNF-α) from the vascular cell walls.[4] Once inside the walls of the artery, mononuclear phagocytes mature into macrophages and become foam cells.

The cytokines and TNF-α produce growth factors that induce the smooth muscle to produce local growth factors such as platelet-derived growth factor and fibroblast growth factors.[9] This fibro-fatty material recruits more smooth muscle cells into the intima from the tunica media layer of the vessel. At this point, transforming growth factor beta (TGF-β), among other mediators, stimulates collagen production by the smooth muscle cells, transforming the fatty streak into a more fibrous smooth muscle cell and extracellular-rich lesion.[4] In addition to this process, products of blood coagulation and thrombosis contribute to atheroma evolution, which explains the alternative term for the process, 'atherothrombosis' (Figure 11.1).

Unfortunately, the prevalence of traditional risk factors is almost as high in those without cardiovascular disease as in subsequently affected people.[1] Several novel key biomarkers have been implicated in the pathology of atherosclerosis, but those receiving the most attention are C-reactive protein (CRP), homocysteine (Hcy) and indicators of oxidative stress.[5,8–10]

C-reactive protein

C-reactive protein (CRP) is a calcium-binding pentameric protein consisting of five identical, non-covalently linked 23-kDa subunits.[1] It is present in trace amounts in humans and appears to have been highly conserved over hundreds of millions of years. It is synthesised primarily by hepatocytes in response to activation of several cytokines, such as interleukins 1 and 6, and TNF-α.[1] In healthy people, and in the absence of

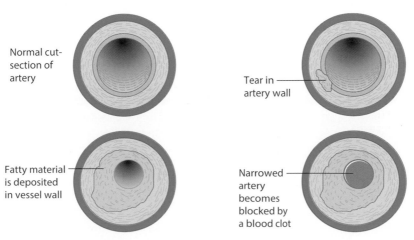

Figure 11.1
Progression of atherosclerosis

active inflammatory states, CRP levels are usually below 1 mg/L. CRP is expressed in atherosclerotic plaques and may enhance expression of local adhesion molecules, increase expression of endothelial plasminogen activation inhibitor 1, reduce endothelial nitric oxide bioactivity and alter LDL-C by macrophages.[10]

Homocysteine

The homocysteine (Hcy) theory of arteriosclerosis attributes one of the underlying causes of vascular disease to elevation of blood Hcy concentrations as the result of dietary, genetic, metabolic, hormonal and/or toxic factors.[11] Dietary deficiency of vitamin B6 and folic acid and absorptive deficiency of vitamin B12, which result from traditional food processing or abnormal absorption of B vitamins, are important factors contributing to elevations in blood Hcy.[10,11] It is believed that homocysteinylation of lipoproteins increases their atherogenicity and hence their cytotoxic effects on endothelial tissue.[12] It is also thought that oxidative stress and methylative modification is the mechanism by which Hcy is proatherosclerotic.[13]

Oxidative stress

Endothelial dysfunction is the initial step in the pathogenesis of atherosclerosis.[14,15] Nitric oxide (NO) plays an important role in the regulation of vascular tone and the suppression of smooth muscle cell proliferation. An increase in oxidative stress inactivates NO, impairing endothelium-dependent vasodilation and creating endothelial dysfunction.[16] Dyslipidaemia may be primary or secondary. The secondary causes are shown in Table 11.1. If secondary causes have been excluded, primary dyslipidaemia due to genetic and environmental (particularly dietary) factors is diagnosed.[17]

RISK FACTORS

The general risk factors applicable to atherosclerosis relate to lifestyle choices and genetics. Overall estimates of the heritability of myocardial infarction, one of the major clinical outcomes of atherosclerosis, have varied widely, ranging from 50 to 60%.[20,21] It is important to note that heritability varies from population to population. In populations where the environment is relatively homogeneous (e.g. Iceland), genetics will tend to predominate, whereas in populations exhibiting large environmental differences

Table 11.1
Common secondary causes of dyslipidaemia

Cause	Effect on lipid profile
Hypothyroidism Nephrotic syndrome Cholestasis Anorexia nervosa	Increased LDL-C
Type 2 diabetes Obesity Renal impairment Smoking	Increased TG and/or decreased HDL-C
Alcohol use Oestrogen use	Increased TG, HDL-C may increase rather than decrease; cardiovascular risk may not be increased

Source: Therapeutic Guidelines (Cardiovascular)[17]

DIFFERENTIAL DIAGNOSIS

- Primary/familial dyslipidaemia
- Diabetes mellitus
- Alcohol overuse
- Chronic kidney disease
- Hypothyroidism
- HIV infection
- Inflammatory disease (e.g. psoriasis, rheumatoid arthritis)
- Overweight/obesity
- Polycystic ovary syndrome
- Primary biliary cirrhosis
- Medication adverse effects (e.g. thiazide diuretics, beta-blockers, retinoids)

Sources: National Heart, Lung and Blood Institute 2013[18] and Merck & Co, Inc.[19]

(e.g. Los Angeles) genetics are relatively less important.[1] The known risk factors for atherosclerosis generally exhibit significant heritability estimates as well (Figure 11.2). Smoking and alcohol consumption as well as a diet rich in refined sugars, sodium and trans fats will adversely influence the condition.[22] Hypertension, diabetes and obesity have a pronounced negative influence on the disease.[1] Exercise is also a significant factor.[3] In women, the protective effects of oestrogen are greatly diminished in menopause.[1] There are several medical conditions that drastically increase the risk of developing this condition, and all of these may cause altered blood fat profiles secondary to their

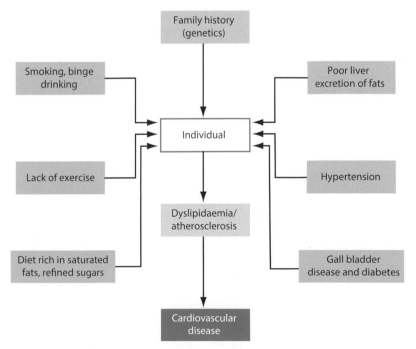

Figure 11.2
Aetiology of cardiovascular disease

primary condition. The influence of environmental factors on lipoprotein metabolism and cardiovascular disease has been revealed through comparisons of different populations.[3] Studies have shown that intrauterine under-nutrition is associated with obesity and other detrimental metabolic characteristics in adulthood.[1] In particular, under-nutrition is shown to be associated with a premature onset of neonatal leptin surge, which appears to be involved in the formation of the energy-regulation circuits in the hypothalamus that affect metabolism in adults.[1]

Genetic and environmental risk factors for cardiovascular disease

Risk factors with a significant genetic component

- Total cholesterol (TC) (40–60%)
- HDL-C (45–75%)
- Total TGs (40–80%)
- Body mass index (BMI) (25–60%)
- Systolic blood pressure (30–70%)
- Diastolic blood pressure (30–65%)
- Lipoprotein(a) levels (90%)
- Hcy levels (45%)
- Type 2 diabetes (40–80%)
- Fibrinogen (20–50%)
- CRP (~40%)
- Myeloperoxidase
- Carotid intima-media thickness (~40%)
- Gender (100%)

Environmental risk factors

- Smoking
- Diet
- Exercise
- Infection
- Fetal environment
- Air pollution (particulates)

Source: Topol 2007[1]

CONVENTIONAL TREATMENT

The assessment of dyslipidaemia involves measuring fasting TC, HDL-C, LDL-C and TG.[17] Fasting usually takes place from midnight prior to the blood test.

Determining when to initiate pharmacological treatment for dyslipidaemia is generally based on the presence of:

- LDL-C elevation and/or clinical indicators for the initiation of pharmacological treatment for mild to moderate hypertriglyceridaemia (see box on next page), particularly if associated with reduced HDL-C (which increases the risk of cardiovascular disease)
- TG exceeding 10 mmol/L (which increases the risk of pancreatitis).

Of course, the thresholds for initiating pharmacological treatment vary depending on the level of patient risk, as outlined in Table 11.2. Treatment aims to reduce the progression of atherosclerosis and improve survival rates. It also aims to prevent myocardial infarction (heart attack) and stroke in patients with established cardiovascular disease. A reduction in TG levels should also prevent the occurrence of pancreatitis in susceptible people. Current targets for lipid management are outlined in the box on the next page. Common pharmacological interventions for dyslipidaemia are listed in Table 11.2.

Table 11.2
Pharmacological treatment of dyslipidaemia

Drug	Benefit	Disadvantage
Statin	Reduces LDL-C by 25–55%, TGs by 10–20% Best tolerated	Reduces coenzyme Q10
Bile-acid binding resin	Reduces LDL-C by 15–30%, TGs by 25–30%	Poorly tolerated, may worsen hypertriglyceridaemia
Nicotinic acid	Reduces LDL-C by 15–30%, TGs by 25–40% Increases HDL-C by 20–35%	Causes severe flushing, which limits use
Ezetimibe	Reduces LDL-C by 15–25%. Well tolerated	Generally not used alone
Fibrate	Reduces LDL-C by 5–15%, TGs by 40–80% Increases HDL-C by 10–30%	Can increase LDL-C in some instances

Source: Australian Medicines Handbook 2009[23].

The most frequently prescribed treatment for hypercholesterolaemia is the statin group of medications, which includes simvastatin, atorvastatin, rosuvastatin and others. A commonly occurring side effect of this class of drugs is muscular problems. The presence of these muscle-related adverse effects (including myalgia, myasthenia and muscle fatigue) is a leading reason why patients discontinue statin therapy. These side effects may be effectively managed with the supplementation of coenzyme Q10 (daily doses ranging between 100 and 600 mg).[24]

Target lipid levels

LDL-C < 2.0 mmol/L (< 1.8 mmol/L for high-risk patients with existing cardiovascular disease)

TC < 4.0 mmol/L

HDL-C > 1.0 mmol/L, non-HDL-C <2.5 mmol/L

TGs < 2.0 mmol/L

These target levels are adapted from the National Heart Foundation of Australia and the Cardiac Society of Australia and New Zealand. Guidelines on reducing risk in heart disease. 2012.

Source: Therapeutic Guidelines (Cardiovascular)[17]

Patients in the 'very high risk' category*

- Patients with symptomatic coronary heart, cerebrovascular or peripheral vascular disease
- Patients with diabetes mellitus who:
  - are aged 60 years or older, or
  - are Aboriginal or Torres Strait Islander, or
  - have microalbuminuria (urinary albumin excretion rate of > 20 mg/minute, or urinary albumin to creatinine ratio of > 2.5 [males], > 3.5 [females])
- Patients who have a family history of premature coronary heart disease (one or more first-degree relatives symptomatic before the age of 45 years, or two or more first-degree relatives symptomatic before the age of 55 years).

*Regardless of their fasting lipid levels

Source: Therapeutic Guidelines (Cardiovascular)[17]

KEY TREATMENT PROTOCOLS

The aim of dyslipidaemia treatment is to restore blood chemistry to acceptable levels within a specified range and reduce the production of potentially harmful metabolites. The cardioprotective effects of HDLs have been well documented and omega fats are useful in raising their levels. Oxidised lipids can be prevented through the use of herbs and the excretion of harmful fats can be encouraged. This can be achieved through dietary modification, exercise and nutrients (dietary or supplemental).

> **Naturopathic Treatment Aims**
>
> - Reduce excess Hcy levels where appropriate.
> - Reduce levels of CRP.
> - Treat oxidative stress.
> - Alter the lipid profile via diet (reduced saturated/*trans* fats).
> - Encourage beneficial lifestyle changes.
> - Encourage exercise.

Lower homocysteine

Plasma Hcy has been associated with cardiovascular risk in multiple large-scale observational studies, and is considered an independent risk factor for atherosclerosis.[25] Evidence indicates that although mild hyper-Hcy may be regarded as a minor risk factor for CHD in low-risk patients, it can play a role in triggering new events in patients with known CHD by interacting with 'classical' cardiovascular risk factors.[25] In spite of this association between elevated Hcy and risk of atherosclerosis, there is still much uncertainty about the clinical implications of treating hyper-Hcy. The findings of a recent Cochrane review of 15 RCTs (involving 71 422 participants) concluded that vitamin B6, B9 or B12 supplementation (administered alone or in combination), at any dosage, was no more effective than placebo, or standard care, in preventing myocardial infarction or reducing all-cause mortality in patients at risk of, or living with, cardiovascular disease.[26,27]

Lower C-reactive protein

CRP is an inflammatory protein that may play a role in the pathogenesis of atherosclerosis. Evidence now suggests that a single nucleotide polymorphism that results in the CRP-757C allele may be responsible for an increase in the intima thickness in the carotid arteries of patients with cardiovascular disease.[28] In terms of modifiable factors, a loss of body fat has been shown to be positively correlated with lower CRP levels. In an RCT of 450 overweight/obese subjects, loss of body fat was found to be significantly associated with reductions in high-sensitivity CRP within 18 months.[29] In epidemiological studies, high fibre intakes have consistently been associated with a reduction in cardiovascular disease risk and CRP levels. A meta-analysis of 14 RCTs reported small but statistically significantly lower CRP concentrations among overweight/obese adults consuming dietary fibre or fibre-rich foods (at dosages above 8 g/day) when compared with controls, with dosages ranging between 3.3 and 7.8 g/MJ.[30]

Inflammatory reactions in coronary plaques play an important role in the pathogenesis of acute atherothrombotic events. A meta-analysis of 160 309 records of patients without vascular disease found CRP concentration had a continuous association with the risk of ischaemic stroke, coronary heart disease and vascular mortality.[31] Antioxidants may play a role in reducing levels of CRP. **Vitamin C** supplementation at 515 mg daily reduced CRP levels by 24% in an RCT involving 160 active and passive smokers.[32] **Alpha-tocopherol** (vitamin E) supplementation (especially at higher doses) in human subjects and animal models has been shown to be both antioxidant and anti-inflammatory, decreasing CRP and the release of pro-inflammatory cytokines such as chemokines IL-8 and PAI-1.[33]

Attenuate oxidative stress

Oxidative stress plays a pivotal role in atherogenesis, and some antioxidants, such as **lipoic acid**, can have an effect on attenuating dyslipidaemia. Supplementation with lipoic acid induced decreases in lipid peroxidation, plasma cholesterol, triacylglycerols and LDL-C, and an increase in HDL in mice fed a high-fat diet.[34] Similarly, rabbits on a high-cholesterol diet had significantly lower levels of LDL-C and TC when given 4.2 mg/kg of lipoic acid daily.[35] It is posited that lipoic acid reduces oxidative stress by increasing free radical scavenger enzyme expression in the cell.[34] In mice, **vitamin E** has a modest effect at best on experimental atherosclerosis, and only in situations of severe vitamin E deficiency.[36] However, the benefits of vitamin E may be due to its effects on smooth muscle proliferation. Cell culture studies have shown that alpha–tocopherol inhibits smooth muscle cell proliferation, possibly via inhibition of protein kinase C activity. In a review of human trials, nutritional supplementation (particularly with omega-3 fatty acids, niacin, resveratrol or red yeast extract) showed promise in reducing LDL and TG levels, LDL particle size, oxidised LDL and inflammation.[37]

CoQ10 may also play a role in reducing oxidative stress in dyslipidaemia by improving antioxidant capacity (i.e. recycling oxidised tocopherol and ascorbate), reducing oxidative stress (i.e. reducing free radicals) and improving endothelial function (i.e. upregulating endothelial NO synthase).[38] In a case-controlled study, 51 patients with at least 50% stenosis of one major coronary artery were found to have significantly lower plasma CoQ10, catalase and glutathione peroxidase levels compared with 102 healthy controls. The authors concluded that there was a significant association between high plasma CoQ10 levels and lower risk of coronary artery disease.[38,39]

A number of plant extracts have been shown to reduce lipid peroxidation and improve lipid profiles in animal models, including *Curcuma longa* (turmeric), *Trigonella foenum-graecum* (fenugreek) and *Zingiber officinale* (ginger). However, there is limited clinical evidence demonstrating such activity in human subjects.[40] **Cocoa** is rich in plant-derived flavonoids, which has been shown to exhibit both antioxidant and anti-inflammatory effects. In an RCT involving 100 patients with type 2 diabetes, those randomised to cocoa treatment (10 g, twice daily for six weeks) demonstrated a significant reduction in lipid peroxidation and markers of inflammation (i.e. interleukin-6, tissue necrosis factor-alpha and high-sensitivity CRP), relative to those receiving a similar dosage of milk powder.[41]

Modify lipid profile with natural products

Nicotinic acid, or niacin, has established efficacy for treating dyslipidaemia, but the clinical use of niacin has been limited by cutaneous flushing—a well-recognised associated adverse effect. Flushing has been cited as the main reason for discontinuing niacin therapy, estimated at rates as high as 25–40%.[42] A meta-analysis of 13 RCTs involving 35 206 participants has found niacin therapy (dosage range not reported) for 6–74 months to be effective in improving HDL-C levels when compared with controls. However, changes in TC and LDL-C levels failed to reach statistical significance.[43] The Australian *Therapeutic Guidelines*[17] recommend daily dosing of niacin of 500 mg, with slow titration to 3 g daily.

Policosanol is a mixture of higher primary aliphatic alcohols purified from sugarcane wax with cholesterol-lowering effects proven in patients with type II hypercholesterolaemia and dyslipidaemia due to type 2 diabetes mellitus.[44] In a meta-analysis of 22 RCTs (comprising a pool of 1886 participants with dyslipidaemia), sugarcane policosanol, at a dose of 5–10 mg/day for 1–52 weeks, was found to be significantly more effective than placebo at increasing HDL-C levels, and reducing TC and LDL-C levels, but not TG.[45]

Allium sativum (garlic) studies have suggested a multitude of physiological effects, including inhibition of platelet activity and increased levels of antioxidant enzymes.[46] Garlic has been shown to inhibit the enzymes involved in lipid synthesis, decrease platelet aggregation, prevent lipid peroxidation of oxidised erythrocytes and LDL, increase antioxidant status and inhibit angiotensin-converting enzyme.[47] A meta-analysis of 39 RCTs (*n* = 2298 participants) found garlic (in various forms and dosages), for 2–8 weeks, significantly improved TC, LDL-C and HDL-C, but not TG, when compared with controls. Effects were shown to be more pronounced with longer term treatment.[48] Concerns have been raised about the use of garlic in patients on blood-thinning medication. Notwithstanding, a 2008 study by Abdul and Jiang failed to show any pharmacodynamic interaction.[49] This opinion reiterates a 2006 study on the use of aged garlic in patients on oral anticoagulant therapy that concluded that aged garlic extract (AGE) was relatively safe and posed no serious haemorrhagic risk.[49]

The principal **essential fatty acids** in fish oil are eicosapentaenoic acid (EPA) and docosahexaenoic acid (DHA).[50] Fish oil has been reported to have anti-inflammatory and immunosuppressive effects, and EPA competitively inhibits synthesis of thromboxane A_2. Both EPA and DHA interfere with prostaglandin synthesis in platelets and blood vessels, resulting in decreased platelet activity.[50] The beneficial effect of dietary fish oil on plasma TGs is thought to be related to the high quantities of omega-3 polyunsaturated fatty acids found in many types of fish.[17] In an attempt to further explain the mechanism of action of fish oil, a study of a fish oil-rich diet administered to apolipoprotein E-deficient mice resulted in reduced adhesion molecule expression in atherosclerotic lesions.[51] Because these molecules are involved in lesion progression, the effect of fish oil may explain the observed decrease in atherogenesis. Evidence from a Cochrane review of 23–28 RCTs (*n* = 35 035–37 281 participants) has shown high omega-3 fatty acid intake (from supplementation, diet or dietary advice) to have a significant effect on serum TG levels when compared with low omega-3 fatty acid intake. The effect of omega-3 fatty acid intake on LDL-C, TC and HDL-C levels was negligible.

Cocoa butter, a fat derived from cocoa plants and found predominantly in dark chocolate, contains an average of 33% monounsaturated oleic acid and 33% stearic acid.[41] In a meta-analysis of 21 RCTs involving 986 patients, daily consumption of cocoa or chocolate was found to have a marginally significant effect on HDL (−0.07 mmol/L) and LDL (0.03 mmol/L) cholesterol levels.[41,52]

A number of plant extracts have been shown to exhibit hypolipidaemic activity in vivo. Those demonstrating beneficial effects on multiple lipid parameters (i.e. LDL-C, TG, TC, HDL-C) include *Ocimum basilicum* (basil), *Vaccinium myrtillus* (blueberry), *Apium graveolens* (celery), *Taraxacum officinale* (dandelion), *Eugenia jambolana* (eugenol), *Trigonella foenum-graecum* (fenugreek), *Zingiber officinale* (ginger), *Panax ginseng* (ginseng), grape seed procyanidin extract, *Camellia sinensis* (green tea) and *Nigella sativa* (black caraway). Those demonstrating evidence of efficacy under clinical trial conditions are summarised on the next page.[53]

- ***Zingiber officinale*** (ginger): A meta-analysis of six RCTs ($n = 328$ participants) found ginger to be significantly more effective than placebo in reducing LDL-C, TC and TG, and improving HDL-C.[54]

- ***Trigonella foenum-graecum*** (fenugreek): A double-blind RCT of 56 patients with borderline hyperlipidaemia found fenugreek seed powder (8 g/day) to be significantly more effective than placebo at reducing LDL-C, TC and TG, but not HDL-C at eight weeks.[55]

- ***Cinnamomum spp.*** (cinnamon): The effectiveness of cinnamon (in various forms and dosages) for dyslipidaemia in patients with and without type 2 diabetes was examined in a systematic review of 15 RCTs, comprising a total of 1127 patients. The body of evidence was found to be inconclusive.[56]

- ***Crocus sativus*** (saffron): Two double-blind RCTs (involving 48 patients with metabolic syndrome and 54 patients with type 2 diabetes) have examined the effectiveness of saffron (i.e. 15 mg hydroalcoholic extract twice daily for eight weeks, or 100 mg Crocin daily for six weeks) on lipid profile. Both trials found saffron/crocin to be no more effective than placebo at improving serum lipid levels.[57,58]

- ***Curcuma longa*** (turmeric): A meta-analysis of seven RCTs, involving a total of 649 patients with cardiovascular risk factors, found turmeric and curcumin to be significantly more effective than controls in improving LDL-C and TG levels, but not HDL-C or TC levels.[59]

- **Anthocyanin**: In a meta-analysis of six RCTs ($n = 586$ patients with dyslipidaemia), anthocyanin supplementation (90–320 mg daily for 4–24 weeks) was found to be significantly more effective than placebo at reducing TC, TG and LDL-C levels, and improving HDL-C levels.[60]

- **Grape seed extract**: A meta-analysis of nine RCTs, involving 390 participants, found grape seed extract (150–2000 mg daily for 2–24 weeks) had no significant effect on LDL-C, HDL-C, TC or TG when compared with controls.[61]

- ***Nigella sativa*** (black caraway): Authors of a meta-analysis of 17 RCTs ($n = 1185$) reported significant improvements in TC, LDL-C and TG levels following *Nigella sativa* supplementation (in various forms and dosages) when compared with controls. Improvements in HDL-C were only observed with *Nigella sativa* powder.[62]

Promote liver choleresis

Bile acids and their salts are essential in managing cholesterol levels, and are synthesised from cholesterol in the liver. There are three groups of bile salts: primary (cholic and chenodeoxycholic acids and their salts); secondary, made from the action of bacteria on primary bile salts (deoxycholate and lithocholate); and tertiary, the result of modifications of secondary bile salts (sulfate ester of lithocholate, ursodeoxycholate and 7-β-epimer of chenodeoxycholate).[63] Saponins interfere with the absorption of cholesterol, bile acids and fats and have shown potential in reducing blood cholesterol levels.[64] Their cholesterol-lowering effect may also be linked to their binding of bile salts and increasing their faecal excretion (see Chapter 7 on liver disease for more detail).

Choleretics stimulate bile production by hepatocytes and most have effective cholagogue properties as well.[64] One such compound is ***Cynara scolymus***. Evidence from a meta-analysis of nine RCTs ($n = 702$ subjects) showed artichoke extract to be significantly more effective than controls at reducing TC, LDL-C and TG; however, the effect on HDL-C was not statistically significant.[65] An in vitro study demonstrated that artichoke leaf extract may increase the activity of an endothelial nitric oxide synthase (eNOS) promoter.[66] The compounds thought responsible were the flavonoids luteolin and cynaroside, with the activity suspected to occur through an increase in eNOS gene transcription.[66] Apart from this choleretic activity, *Cynara scolymus* has long been known for its antioxidant ability. The antioxidant activity of the herbal medicine was confirmed by its in vitro inhibition of LDL oxidation in rats. It also raised levels of glutathione peroxidase activity.[67] A methanolic extract of *Cynara scolymus* was found to suppress serum TG elevation in olive-loaded mice, with the components responsible identified as sesquiterpenes (cynaropicrin, aguerin B and grosheimin) together with new sesquiterpene glycosides (cynarascolosides A, B and C).[68]

Silymarin marianum (milk thistle) is another herb with choleretic and antioxidant properties. Silymarin, a mixture of flavonolignans from milk thistle, has demonstrated hypolipidaemic activity in several clinical trials, including improvements in LDL-C, TG and TC when compared with placebo. The effects of silymarin on HDL-C levels, however, have been inconsistent.[69,70]

INTEGRATIVE MEDICAL CONSIDERATIONS

Lifestyle modification

As a minimum, all patients should be given **dietary advice as first-line therapy for dyslipidaemia**, irrespective of whether the patient is in a high-risk category. This includes enriching the diet with a good source of fibre, both soluble and insoluble, between 10 and 60 g daily.[71,72] This is because increasing dietary fibre intake may have a beneficial effect on lipid profiles. The findings of a Cochrane review (23 RCTs, 1513 participants) support this position, revealing that increased fibre was associated with lower TC levels, and to a lesser extent, elevated HDL-C levels; however, increased dietary fibre intake was found to have no effect on LDL-C levels.[73] Subjects taking 70 g of oats (3 g soluble fibre) twice daily for four weeks demonstrated significant reductions in both TC and LDL-C when compared to control in an RCT of 80 adults with mild hypercholesterolaemia.[71]

The National Cholesterol Education Program Adult Treatment Panel III (ATP III)[74] recommends a low saturated fat diet with nutritional supplementation (fish oil, oat bran or plant sterol). These diets have generally lowered TC (7–18%) and LDL-C (7–15%) concentrations respectively.[74] A comparative trial in 2008 examined the impact of this low-fat diet versus a very low carbohydrate diet in 40 overweight men and women. Each diet provided around 1500 kcal daily and around 20–30 g protein. The diets differed in the amount of carbohydrate, being 12% for the low-carbohydrate diet and 56% for the low-fat diet. The low-carbohydrate diet was higher in fats, particularly omega-6 fatty acids. The very low carbohydrate diet resulted in profound alterations in fatty acid composition and reduced inflammation compared with a low-fat diet, as well as reducing atherosclerosis.[75]

Smoking cessation is also recommended in the management of dyslipidaemia.[32,74] Free radicals in cigarette smoke cause oxidative damage to proteins, DNA and lipids, contributing to the pathobiology of atherosclerosis, heart disease and cancer. Active and passive smoking also raise plasma levels of CRP,[32] which causes oxidative damage to vascular endothelium via raised plasma fats. In a meta-analysis of 530 905 participants of the CHANCES consortium (a large study examining age-related chronic conditions), cessation of smoking was found to be associated with a substantial reduction in risk of cardiovascular mortality, with risk reducing by 10% within 5 years of smoking cessation, 16% within 5–9 years, 22% within 10–19 years and 39% after 20 years of smoking cessation.[69,76]

Alcohol intake should also be reduced to a moderate level (one to two glasses of wine daily).[77] Light to moderate alcohol intake has been shown in a meta-analysis of 31 studies (*n* = 1267 patients) to have cardioprotective properties; in particular, it was found to be associated with small but significant improvements in LDL-C and HDL-C concentration, but not TC or TG concentration.[77] An analysis of Atherosclerosis Risk in Communities (ARIC) study data failed to show any differential benefit on lipid profile with the type of alcoholic beverage consumed.[77,78]

Exercise is well known to have positive effects on lipid levels. An RCT of 111 sedentary, overweight adults with mild-to-moderate dyslipidaemia showed that a level of exercise equivalent to jogging 32.0 km per week at 65–80% of peak oxygen consumption resulted in greater improvements in lipid levels relative to lower amounts of exercise, which were the equivalent of jogging 19.2 km a week at 65–80% of peak oxygen consumption and the equivalent of walking 19.2 km per week at 40–55% of peak oxygen consumption. All three interventions were superior to the control condition in all 11 lipid variables.[79] In a review of the National Cholesterol Education Program mentioned above, exercise intervention increased HDL-C levels (5–14%) and lowered TG levels (4–18%) respectively.[80] By contrast, a meta-analysis of 79 RCTs involving a total of 15 618 participants found that the effects of physical activity interventions on lipid levels, versus usual care, was inconclusive. However, when exercise was combined with dietary interventions, participants demonstrated significant improvements in TC, LDL-C, HDL-C and TG; these improvements were far greater than that observed with dietary intervention alone.[81]

CLINICAL SUMMARY

Cardiovascular disease is very common and usually a patient will seek advice after being diagnosed by their doctor from a routine fasting blood test. In most instances, there will be a window of opportunity to make lifestyle changes before prescriptive medicine is employed. As detailed in the decision tree (Figure 11.3), cases are complicated by hypertension, diabetes and other conditions that may require referral. Most patients will be motivated to make changes, but the aim of a successful relationship is to create a healthy result that is sustainable in the long term. It is important to consider that not all patients will want to use natural therapies exclusively and combinations of orthodox and complementary medicine may work well.

Most people know the basics of a good diet, but very few actually know how much they should eat and the finer details of an appropriate tailored diet; thus, dietary education is crucial for all patients with cardiovascular disease. Losing body fat is only achievable through appropriate food consumption, and exercise is an important additive to good basic nutrition and lifestyle education. Fish or krill oil can be the cornerstone of any nutraceutical prescription, as they have benefits that far outweigh their role in modifying blood fats (particularly triglycerides). Supplements like garlic, anthocyanin, black caraway, and policosanol all assist the foundations of a healthy diet and lifestyle, with encouraging evidence also emerging for a number of other plant extracts and constituents.

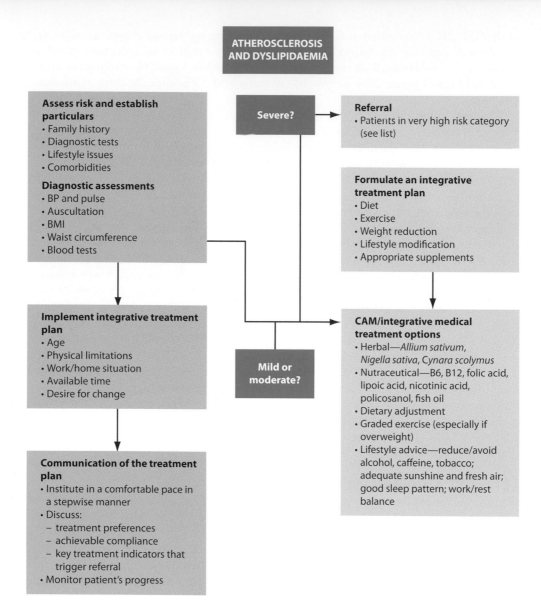

Figure 11.3
Naturopathic treatment decision tree—atherosclerosis and dyslipidaemia

Table 11.3
Review of the major evidence

Intervention	Mechanisms of action	Key literature	Summary of results	Comment
Omega-3 fish oil	Reduction in oxidative damage and markers of inflammation[82,83] Reduction in plasma Hcy[84]	Meta-analysis of 23–28 RCTs with a total of 35 035–37 281 participants (depending on lipid parameter assessed) examining omega-3 fatty acid intake from supplementation, diet or dietary advice[82] Meta-analysis of 38 clinical trials and observational studies (n = 2270 participants) examining omega-3 fatty acid intake from supplementation or dietary intervention[83] Nineteen randomised, placebo-controlled trials were included in this meta-analysis of omega-3 fatty acids and homocysteine[84]	Omega-3 fatty acids significantly reduced serum TG when compared with controls (mean difference −0.24 mmol/L, 95% CI −0.31 to −0.16). Omega-3 fatty acids had little to no effect on TC, HDL-C and LDL-C levels[82] Omega-3 fatty acid intake from marine or EPA/DHA-enriched food sources (≥ 4 g/day) lowered TG by 9–26%. Omega-3 fatty acid intake from EPA/DHA supplementation (1–5 g/day) lowered TG by 4–51%[83]	Fish oil supplementation produces a clinically significant dose-dependent reduction of fasting blood TG[82,83] Another meta-analysis suggested that omega-3 PUFA supplementation can decrease plasma Hcy levels The implications of these findings remain to be elucidated[84]
Krill oil (*Euphausia superba*)	Krill oil—antioxidant effect on blood fats Astaxanthin component found to have a reduction of CRP	Meta-analysis of seven RCTs (n = 662 participants) examining the effectiveness of krill oil supplementation[85] Ahn et al. 2018[86]	Krill oil supplementation, at a daily dose of 0.5–4.0 g for 4–12 weeks, is significantly more effective than controls at reducing LDL-C (WMD, −15.52 mg/dL; 95%CI, −28.43 to −2.61) and TG (WMD, −14.03 mg/dL; 95%CI, −21.38 to −6.67), and increasing HDL-C (WMD, 6.65 mg/dL; 95%CI, 2.30 to 10.99)[85]	Krill oil is effective for managing hyperlipidaemia High content of free EPA and DHA in krill oil increases bioavailability in blood, brain and lipids[86]

Table 11.3
Review of the major evidence (continued)

Intervention	Mechanisms of action	Key literature	Summary of results	Comment
Cynara scolymus	Beneficial effects for dyslipidaemia from choleretic, antioxidant and anticholesterol properties[87]	Meta-analysis of nine RCTs (*n* = 702 participants) examining the effectiveness of artichoke extract.[65]	Artichoke extract is significantly more effective than controls in reducing plasma TC (WMD: −17.6 mg/dL, 95%CI: −22.0 to −13.3), LDL-C (WMD: −14.9 mg/dL, 95%CI: −20.4 to −9.5) and TG (WMD: −9.2 mg/dL, 95%CI: −16.2 to −2.1).[65] Anti-hyperlipidaemic effect due to suppression of inhibition of cholesterol biosynthesis, lipid peroxidation, and intestinal reuptake of bile salts[87]	Artichoke extract may be an effective and well-tolerated treatment for dyslipidaemia[65,87]
Lipoic acid	Increases free radical scavenger enzyme to reduce oxidative stress and lipid peroxidation[88] Modulates lipid metabolism by increasing beta-oxidation of and decreasing synthesis of cholesterol	Meta-analysis of 11 clinical trials (*n* = 452 participants) examining the effectiveness of alpha-lipoic acid supplementation[34]	Alpha-lipoic acid (ALA) supplementation significantly reduced serum TG (WMD, −29.185 mg/dL; 95% CI: −51.454 to −6.916), TC (WMD, −10.683 mg/dL; 95% CI: −19.816 to −1.550) and LDL-C (WMD, −12.906 mg/dL; 95% CI: −22.133 to −3.679) when compared with placebo[89]	Patients with overweight/ obesity and receiving daily doses of ALA > 600 mg demonstrate greater improvements in serum lipids[89]
Alium sativum	A range of actions that are beneficial in cardiovascular disease including: choleretic, hypo-lipidaemic, hypotensive, antioxidant, hypo-glycaemic and antiplatelet properties	Meta-analysis of six RCTs examining the effectiveness of garlic supplementation[90] Meta-analysis of 39 RCTs (*n* = 2298 participants) examining the effectiveness of garlic in various forms and dosages[48]	Garlic supplementation did not significantly reduce lipoprotein(a) concentration when compared with controls[90] Garlic (administered in various forms and dosages for 2–8 weeks) was significantly more effective than controls at improving TC (MD, −15.25 mg/dL; 95%CI: −20.72 to −9.78), LDL-C (MD, −6.41; 95%CI: −11.77 to −1.05) and HDL-C (MD, 1.49; 95%CI: 0.19 to 2.79)[48]	Garlic may be an effective treatment for dyslipidaemia[48] Effects of garlic supplementation may be more pronounced with longer term treatment[48]

Table 11.3
Review of the major evidence (continued)

Intervention	Mechanisms of action	Key literature	Summary of results	Comment
Cocoa-polyphenols	Multiple cardioprotective effects including antiatherogenic, antioxidant, antiinflammatory, antihypertensive and antiplatelet activity[91]	Meta-analysis of 21 RCTs (n = 986 participants) examining the effectiveness of cocoa, chocolate and flavan-3-ols[92] Review of the mechanisms of action of cocoa polyphenols on the cardiovascular system[91]	Cocoa/chocolate/flav-3-ols were significantly more effective than controls in improving LDL-C ((MD −0.07 mmol/L; 95% CI: −0.14 to −0.00) and HDL-C concentration (MD 0.03 mmol/L; 95% CI: 0.00 to 0.06)[92] Cocoa polyphenols reduce lipid peroxidation, intestinal cholesterol absorption and hepatic biosynthesis of cholesterol, and improve flow-mediated dilatation[91]	Cocoa polyphenols show promise as a cardioprotective agent[91] The effect of cocoa polyphenols on lipid profile is small and may not be clinically significant[92]
Aerobic activity (e.g. walking, swimming, resistance training)	Beneficial effects on improving strength of cardiac muscle, reduces blood pressure and stress levels, and alters lipid profile	Meta-analysis and reviews: Systematic review and meta-analysis of RCTs: Seventy-nine RCTs involving a total of 15 618 participants[81] Sixty-five RCTs/comparative trials (total number of participants not reported)[93]	Physical activity interventions alone had no significant effect on TC, LDL-C, HDL-C or TG when compared with usual care[81] High-intensity interval training had no significant effect on TC, LDL-C, HDL-C or TG in normal weight or overweight/obese individuals[93]	The evidence of the effectiveness of exercise in improving lipid levels is inconclusive[93]

TC = total cholesterol; TG = triglycerides

KEY POINTS

- Recommend reduction of smoking and consumption of alcohol.
- Educate the patient on a healthy diet.
- Reduce body fat (keep BMI below 25).
- Advise adequate exercise.
- Use omega-3 fats to beneficially modify blood fat profile.
- Increase excretion of fats through the use of choleretics.
- Reduce Hcy to reduce arterial stiffness.
- Prevent production of oxidised products and CRP.

FURTHER READING

Anand SS, et al. Food consumption and its impact on cardiovascular disease: importance of solutions focused on the globalized food system: a report from the workshop convened by the World Heart Federation. J Am Coll Cardiol 2015;66(14):1590–614.

Fioranelli M, editor. Integrative cardiology: a new therapeutic vision. Switzerland: Springer; 2017.

Martí-Carvajal AJ, Solà I, Lathyris D. Homocysteine-lowering interventions for preventing cardiovascular events. Cochrane Database Syst Rev 2015;(1):CD006612.

Santini A, Novellino E. Nutraceuticals in hypercholesterolaemia: an overview. Brit J Pharmacol 2017;174(11):1450–63.

Therapeutic guidelines, cardiovascular (version 7). Online. Therapeutic Guidelines Limited; 2018.

REFERENCES

1. Topol EJ, editor. Textbook of cardiovascular medicine. 3rd ed. Philadelphia: Lippincott Williams & Wilkins; 2007.
2. Peck MD, Ai AL. Cardiac conditions. J Gerontol Soc Work 2008;50(Suppl. 1):13–44.
3. Vanuzzo D, et al. Cardiovascular risk and cardiometabolic risk: an epidemiological evaluation. G Ital Cardiol (Rome) 2008;9(4 Suppl. 1):6S–17S.
4. Libby P. The pathogenesis, prevention, and treatment of atherosclerosis. In: Harrison's principles of internal medicine. 19th ed. New York: McGraw-Hill; 2015. p. np.
5. Yu E, et al. Diet, lifestyle, biomarkers, genetic factors, and risk of cardiovascular disease in the nurses' health studies. Am J Public Health 2016;106(9):1616–23.
6. Rizzo M, et al. Atherogenic dyslipidemia and oxidative stress: a new look. Transl Res 2009;153(5):217–23.
7. Easton JD, et al. Definition and evaluation of transient ischemic attack: a scientific statement for healthcare professionals from the American Heart Association/American Stroke Association Stroke Council; Council on Cardiovascular Surgery and Anesthesia; Council on Cardiovascular Radiology and Intervention; Council on Cardiovascular Nursing; and the Interdisciplinary Council on Peripheral Vascular Disease. The American Academy of Neurology affirms the value of this statement as an educational tool for neurologists. Stroke 2009;40(6):2276–93.
8. Sobenin IA, et al. Reduction of cardiovascular risk in primary prophylaxy of coronary heart disease. Klin Med (Mosk) 2005;83(4):52–5.
9. Wong BW, Meredith A, Lin D, et al. The biological role of inflammation in atherosclerosis. Can J Cardiol 2012;28(6):631–41.
10. Adukauskienė D, et al. Clinical relevance of high sensitivity C-reactive protein in cardiology. Medicina (Kaunas) 2016;52(1):1–10.
11. Cybulska B, Klosiewicz-Latoszek L. Homocysteine—is it still an important risk factor for cardiovascular disease? Kardiol Pol 2015;73:1092–6.
12. Ferretti G, et al. Homocysteinylation of low-density lipoproteins (LDL) from subjects with Type 1 diabetes: effect on oxidative damage of human endothelial cells. Diabet Med 2006;23(7):808–13.
13. Su J, et al. A comparative study on pathogenic effects of homocysteine and cysteine on atherosclerosis. Wei Sheng Yan Jiu 2009;38(1):43–6.
14. Harrison DG, Gongora MC. Oxidative stress and hypertension. Med Clin North Am 2009;93(3):621–35.
15. Roberts CK, Sindhu KK. Oxidative stress and metabolic syndrome. Life Sci 2009;84(21–22):705–12.
16. Kelly FJ, Fussell JC. Role of oxidative stress in cardiovascular disease outcomes following exposure to ambient air pollution. Free Rad Biol Med 2017;110:345–67.
17. Therapeutic guidelines, cardiovascular (version 7). Online. Therapeutic Guidelines Limited; 2018.
18. National Heart, Lung and Blood Institute. High blood cholesterol. Online. Available: https://www.nhlbi.nih.gov/health-topics/high-blood-cholesterol. [Accessed 30 November 2018].
19. Merck & Co, Inc. MSD Manual: professional version. Kenilworth, USA: Merck & Co; 2019.
20. Dai X, Wiernek S, Evans JP, et al. Genetics of coronary artery disease and myocardial infarction. World J Cardiol 2016;8(1):1–23.
21. Khera AV, et al. Genetic risk, adherence to a healthy lifestyle, and coronary disease. N Engl J Med 2016;375:2349–58.
22. Silvennoinen R, et al. Attitudes and actions: a survey to assess statin use among Finnish patients with increased risk for cardiovascular events. J Clin Lipidol 2017;11(2):485–94.
23. Australian Medicines Handbook Pty Ltd. Australian medicines handbook, Adelaide; 2018.
24. Qu H, et al. Effects of coenzyme Q10 on statin-induced myopathy: an updated meta-analysis of randomized controlled trials. J Am Heart Assoc 2018;7(19):e009835.
25. McCully KS. Homocysteine and the pathogenesis of atherosclerosis. Expert Rev Clin Pharmacol 2015;8:211–19.
26. Martí-Carvajal AJ, Solà I, Lathyris D, et al. Homocysteine-lowering interventions (B-complex vitamin therapy) for preventing cardiovascular events. Cochrane Database Syst Rev 2009;7(4):CD006612.
27. Debrecini B, Debreceni L. The role of homocysteine-lowering B-vitamins in the primary prevention of cardiovascular disease. Cardiovasc Ther 2014;32(3):130–8.
28. Ben-Assayag E, et al. Association of the –757T>C polymorphism in the CRP gene with circulating C-reactive protein levels and carotid atherosclerosis. Thromb Res 2009;24(4):458–62.
29. Beavers KM, et al. Effects of total and regional fat loss on plasma CRP and IL-6 in overweight and obese, older adults with knee osteoarthritis. Osteoarthritis Cartilage 2015;23(2):249–56.
30. Jiao J, et al. Effect of dietary fiber on circulating C-reactive protein in overweight and obese adults: a meta-analysis of randomized controlled trials. Int J Food Sci Nutr 2015;66:114–19.
31. Emerging Risk Factors Collaboration, et al. C-reactive protein concentration and risk of coronary heart disease, stroke, and mortality: an individual participant meta-analysis. Lancet 2010;375(9709):132–40.
32. Block G, et al. Plasma C-reactive protein concentrations in active and passive smokers: influence of antioxidant supplementation. J Am Coll Nutr 2004;23(2):141–7.
33. Singh U, Devaraj S. Vitamin E: inflammation and atherosclerosis. Vitam Horm 2007;76:519–49.

34. Yang RL, et al. Lipoic acid prevents high-fat diet-induced dyslipidemia and oxidative stress: a microarray analysis. Nutrition 2008;24(6):582–8.

35. Amom Z, et al. Lipid lowering effect of antioxidant alpha-lipoic acid in experimental atherosclerosis. J Clin Biochem Nutr 2008;43(2):88–94.

36. Suarna C, et al. Protective effect of vitamin E supplements on experimental atherosclerosis is modest and depends on preexisting vitamin E deficiency. Free Radic Biol Med 2006;41(5):722–30.

37. Houston M. The role of nutrition and nutritional supplements in the treatment of dyslipidemia. Clin Lipidol 2014;9(3):333–54.

38. Tousoulis D, et al. Oxidative stress and early atherosclerosis: novel antioxidant treatment. Cardiovasc Drugs Ther 2015;29(1):75–88.

39. Lee BJ, et al. The relationship between coenzyme Q10, oxidative stress, and antioxidant enzymes activities and coronary artery disease. Sci World J 2012;2012:Article ID 792756.

40. Nammour MA, et al. Selected edible plant-derived therapies for controlling dyslipidemia. J Food Nutr Disord 2016;5(5):np.

41. Parsaeyan N, Mozaffari-Khosravi H, Absalan A, et al. Beneficial effects of cocoa on lipid peroxidation and inflammatory markers in type 2 diabetic patients and investigation of probable interactions of cocoa active ingredients with prostaglandin synthase-2 (PTGS-2/COX-2) using virtual analysis. J Diabetes Metab Disord 2014;13(1):30.

42. Davidson M. Niacin use and cutaneous flushing: mechanisms and strategies for prevention. Am J Cardiol 2008;101(8 Suppl. 1):S14–19.

43. Gary A, et al. Role of niacin in current clinical practice: a systematic review. Am J Med 2017;130(2):173–87.

44. Castano G, et al. A randomized, double-blind, placebo-controlled study of the efficacy and tolerability of policosanol in adolescents with type II hypercholesterolemia. Curr Ther Res Clin Exp 2002;63(4):286–303.

45. Gong J, et al. Efficacy and safety of sugarcane policosanol on dyslipidemia: a meta-analysis of randomized controlled trials. Mol Nutr Food Res 2018;62(1):ePub.

46. Mansoor GA. Herbs and alternative therapies in the hypertension clinic. Am J Hypertens 2001;14:971–5.

47. Rahman K, Lowe GM. Garlic and cardiovascular disease: a critical review. J Nutr 2006;136(3 Suppl.):736S–740S.

48. Reid K, Toben C, Fakler P. Effect of garlic on serum lipids: an updated meta-analysis. Nutr Rev 2013;71(5):282–99.

49. Mohammed Abdul MI, Jiang X, et al. Pharmacodynamic interaction of warfarin with cranberry but not with garlic in healthy subjects. Br J Pharmacol 2008;154(8):1691–700.

50. Tassoni D, et al. The role of eicosanoids in the brain. Asia Pac J Clin Nutr 2008;17(Suppl. 1):220–8.

51. Casos K, et al. Atherosclerosis prevention by a fish oil-rich diet in apoE(–/–) mice is associated with a reduction of endothelial adhesion molecules. Atherosclerosis 2008;201(2):306–17.

52. Hooper L, et al. Effects of chocolate, cocoa, and flavan-3-ols on cardiovascular health: a systematic review and meta-analysis of randomized trials. Am J Clin Nutr 2012;95(3):740–51.

53. Rouhi-Boroujeni H, et al. Herbs with anti-lipid effects and their interactions with statins as a chemical anti-hyperlipidemia group drugs: a systematic review. ATYA Atheroscler 2015;11(4):244–51.

54. Zhu J, Chen H, Song Z, et al. Effects of ginger (Zingiber officinale Roscoe) on type 2 diabetes mellitus and components of the metabolic syndrome: a systematic review and meta-analysis of randomized controlled trials. Evid Based Complement Altern Med 2018;2018:Article ID 5692962.

55. Yousefi E, et al. Fenugreek: a therapeutic complement for patients with borderline hyperlipidemia: a randomised, double-blind, placebo-controlled, clinical trial. Adv Integr Med 2017;4(1):31–5.

56. Santos HO, Silva GAR. To what extent does cinnamon administration improve the glycemic and lipid profiles? Clin Nutr ESPEN 2018;27:1–9.

57. Kermani T, et al. The efficacy of crocin of saffron (Crocus sativus L.) on the components of metabolic syndrome: a randomized controlled clinical trial. J Res Pharm Pract 2017;6(4):228–32.

58. Milajerdi A, et al. The effect of saffron (Crocus sativus L.) hydroalcoholic extract on metabolic control in type 2 diabetes mellitus: a triple-blinded randomized clinical trial. J Res Med Sci 2018;23:16.

59. Qin S, et al. Efficacy and safety of turmeric and curcumin in lowering blood lipid levels in patients with cardiovascular risk factors: a meta-analysis of randomized controlled trials. Nutr J 2017;16:68.

60. Liu C, Sun J, Lu Y, et al. Effects of anthocyanin on serum lipids in dyslipidemia patients: a systematic review and meta-analysis. PLoS ONE 2016;11(9):e0162089.

61. Feringa HH, Laskey DA, Dickson JE, et al. The effect of grape seed extract on cardiovascular risk markers: a meta-analysis of randomized controlled trials. J Am Diet Assoc 2011;111(8):1173–81.

62. Sahebkar A, et al. Nigella sativa (black seed) effects on plasma lipid concentrations in humans: a systematic review and meta-analysis of randomized controlled trials. Pharmacol Res 2016;106:37–50.

63. Francini-Pesenti F, et al. Sugar cane policosanol failed to lower plasma cholesterol in primitive, diet-resistant hypercholesterolemia: a double blind, controlled study. Complement Ther Med 2008;16(2):61–5.

64. Mills S, Bone K. Principles and practice of phytotherapy. 2nd ed. St Louis: Churchill Livingstone; 2013.

65. Sahebkar A, et al. Lipid-lowering activity of artichoke extracts: a systematic review and meta-analysis. Crit Rev Food Sci Nutr 2017;Epub ahead of print.

66. Li H, et al. Flavonoids from artichoke (Cynara scolymus L.) up-regulate endothelial-type nitric-oxide synthase gene expression in human endothelial cells. J Pharmacol Exp Ther 2004;310(3):926–32.

67. Jimenez-Escrig A, et al. In vitro antioxidant activities of edible artichoke (Cynara scolymus L.) and effect on biomarkers of antioxidants in rats. J Agric Food Chem 2003;51(18):5540–5.

68. Shimoda H, et al. Anti-hyperlipidemic sesquiterpenes and new sesquiterpene glycosides from the leaves of artichoke (Cynara scolymus L.): structure requirement and mode of action. Bioorg Med Chem Lett 2003;13(2):223–8.

69. Ebrahimpour-koujan S, et al. Lower glycemic indices and lipid profile among type 2 diabetes mellitus patients who received novel dose of Silybum marianum (L.) Gaertn. (silymarin) extract supplement: a triple-blinded randomized controlled clinical trial. Phytomedicine 2018;44:39–44.

70. Huseini HF, et al. The efficacy of Silybum marianum (L.) Gaertn. (silymarin) in the treatment of type II diabetes: a randomized, double-blind, placebo-controlled, clinical trial. Phytother Res 2006;20(12):1036–9.

71. Gulati S, Misra A, Pandey RM. Effects of 3 g of soluble fiber from oats on lipid levels of Asian Indians—a randomized controlled, parallel arm study. Lipids Health Dis 2017; 16:71.

72. Mia MA, et al. Dietary fibre and coronary heart disease. Mymensingh Med J 2002;11(2):133–5.

73. Hartley L, et al. Dietary fibre for the primary prevention of cardiovascular disease. Cochrane Database Syst Rev 2016;(1):CD011472.

74. Critchley JA, Capewell S. Smoking cessation for the secondary prevention of coronary heart disease. Cochrane Database Syst Rev 2012;(2):CD003041.

75. Forsythe CE, et al. Comparison of low fat and low carbohydrate diets on circulating fatty acid composition and markers of inflammation. Lipids 2008;1:65–77.

76. Mons U, et al. Impact of smoking and smoking cessation on cardiovascular events and mortality among older adults: meta-analysis of individual participant data from prospective cohort studies of the CHANCES consortium. BMJ 2015;350:1551.

77. Huang Y, et al. Moderate alcohol consumption and atherosclerosis: meta-analysis of effects on lipids and inflammation. Wien Klin Wochenschr 2017;129(21–22):835–43.

78. Volcik KA, et al. Relationship of alcohol consumption and type of alcoholic beverage consumed with plasma lipid levels: differences between whites and African Americans of the ARIC Study. Ann Epidemiol 2008;18(2):101–7.

79. Kraus WE, et al. Effects of the amount and intensity of exercise on plasma lipoproteins. N Engl J Med 2002;347(19):1483–92.

80. Varady KA, Jones PJ. Combination diet and exercise interventions for the treatment of dyslipidemia: an effective preliminary strategy to lower cholesterol levels? J Nutr 2005;135(8):1829–35.

81. Zhang X, et al. Effect of lifestyle interventions on cardiovascular risk factors among adults without impaired glucose tolerance or diabetes: a systematic review and meta-analysis. PLOS ONE 2017;12(5):e0176436.

82. Abdelhamid AS, et al. Omega-3 fatty acids for the primary and secondary prevention of cardiovascular disease. Cochrane Database Syst Rev 2018;(11):CD003177.

83. Leslie MA, et al. A review of the effect of omega-3 polyunsaturated fatty acids on blood triacylglycerol levels in normolipidemic and borderline hyperlipidemic individuals. Lipids Health Dis 2015;14:53.

84. Dawson SL, Bowe SJ, Crowe TC. A combination of omega-3 fatty acids, folic acid and B-group vitamins is superior at lowering homocysteine than omega-3 alone: a meta-analysis. Nutr Res 2016;36(6):499–508.

85. Ursoniu S, et al. Lipid-modifying effects of krill oil in humans: systematic review and meta-analysis of randomized controlled trials. Nutr Rev 2017;75(5):361–73.

86. Ahn SH, et al. Absorption rate of krill oil and fish oil in blood and brain of rats. Lipids Health Dis 2018;17:162.

87. Shimoda H, et al. Anti-hyperlipidemic sesquiterpenes and new sesquiterpene glycosides from the leaves of artichoke (Cynara scolymus L.): structure requirement and mode of action. Bioorg Med Chem Lett 2003;13(2):223–8.

88. Serhiyenko V, Serhiyenko L, Suslik G, et al. Alpha-lipoic acid: mechanisms of action and beneficial effects in the prevention and treatment of diabetic complications. MOJ Public Health 2018;7(4):174–8.

89. Mousavi SM, et al. Effect of alpha-lipoic acid supplementation on lipid profile: a systematic review and meta-analysis of controlled clinical trials. Nutrition 2019;5:121–30.

90. Sahebkar A, et al. Effect of garlic on plasma lipoprotein(a) concentrations: a systematic review and meta-analysis of randomized controlled clinical trials. Nutrition 2016;32(1):33–40.

91. Aprotosoaie AC, et al. The cardiovascular effects of cocoa polyphenols—an overview. Diseases 2016;4:39.

92. Hooper L, et al. Effects of chocolate, cocoa, and flavan-3-ols on cardiovascular health: a systematic review and meta-analysis of randomized trials. Am J Clin Nutr 2012;95(3):740–51.

93. Batacan RB, et al. Effects of high-intensity interval training on cardiometabolic health: a systematic review and meta-analysis of intervention studies. Br J Sports Med 2017;51:494–503.

CHAPTER 12

Hypertension and stroke

Matthew Leach
ND, PhD

OVERVIEW

Hypertension or high blood pressure (BP) is a *sustained* rise in *resting* BP—specifically, a persistent systolic BP ≥ 140 mmHg and diastolic BP ≥ 90 mmHg.[1] Diagnosis is by sphygmomanometry, usually over at least two consecutive visits to a doctor.[1] The readings can be confounded by some clinically pertinent conditions, namely 'masked' and 'white coat' hypertension. The phenomenon of masked hypertension (MH) is defined as a clinical condition in which a patient's office BP level is less than 140/90 mmHg but ambulatory or home BP readings are in the hypertensive range. The prevalence of MH has been estimated at 7.5% and 29.3% among people with optimal BP and prehypertension in-office, respectively.[2] White coat hypertension (WCHT) occurs in patients who have a rise in BP in the clinic yet record normotensive readings at home, possibly related to anxiety experienced by patients during the clinical encounter. WCHT has a population prevalence of approximately 13% and is associated with non-smoking, age > 50 years and slightly elevated clinic BP. Compared with normotensives, subjects with WCHT are at increased cardiovascular risk due to a higher prevalence of glucose dysregulation, increased left ventricular mass index and increased risk of future diabetes and hypertension.[3]

Hypertension is a common condition, affecting approximately one-third of the population. It is an important risk factor in coronary heart disease and in cerebrovascular accident or 'stroke', and may also lead to kidney failure and left ventricular failure or 'heart failure'.[4-6]

Left ventricular hypertrophy usually develops in response to some factor, such as high BP, that requires the left ventricle to work harder. As ventricular workload increases, the walls of the chamber grow thicker, lose elasticity and eventually may fail to pump with as much force as a healthy heart.[7] Left ventricular hypertrophy presents with increased risk of heart disease, including heart attack, heart failure, irregular heartbeat (arrhythmia) and sudden cardiac arrest.[8]

The term 'stroke' encompasses a heterogeneous group of cerebrovascular disorders. Ischaemic stroke or cerebral infarction accounts for 80–85% of all strokes and typically presents as a sudden, painless, focal neurological deficit with preserved consciousness.[4,9] Haemorrhagic stroke accounts for 15–20% of all strokes, and presents as an acute focal neurological deficit but continues to worsen as the haematoma expands, with headache and altered consciousness resulting.[9] Haemorrhagic stroke involves bleeding within or around the brain, which may be secondary to uncontrolled hypertension, arteriovenous malformation or aneurysms. Ischaemic strokes usually occur at night or in the early morning and are caused by a thrombus (blood clot) forming in an artery inside or leading to the brain, chiefly as a result of atherosclerosis.[10]

The pathophysiology of hypertension is complex but may be classified as:

- primary or essential (no known cause), which is the most common classification (90%)
- secondary (identifiable cause), with kidney disease the most common cause; other causes may include coarctation of the aorta, endocrine disease and pregnancy.[9]

DIFFERENTIAL DIAGNOSIS*

- Renal artery or vascular disease or aortic coarctation
- Unexplained hypokalaemia
- Phaeochromocytoma
- Abdominal/lumbar trauma
- Kidney disease—chronic glomerulonephritis, pyelonephritis, obstructive nephropathy
- Medication-induced hypertension (e.g. birth control pills)
- Endocrine diseases—Cushing's disease, hyperaldosteronism, hyper-/hypothyroidism
- Psychiatric disorders (anxiety/stress disorders)
- Medication/drug adverse effects—prednisolone, licorice, cocaine, antidepressants

*Primary/secondary hypertension
Source: Charles et al. 2017[11]

RISK FACTORS

Hypertension[12,13]
- Obesity (BMI above 25 kg/m^2)
- Occupational stress
- Poor-quality diet, high salt intake, high alcohol intake
- High homocysteine (Hcy)
- Physical inactivity
- Social isolation
- Poor sleep hygiene
- Housing instability
- Depression or exposure to traumatic events

Stroke[14]
- Smoking
- Abdominal obesity
- Hypertension
- Diabetes
- Hypercholesterolaemia
- Physical inactivity
- High alcohol intake
- Poor-quality diet
- Cardiac pathology

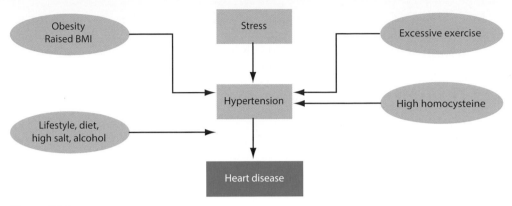

Figure 12.1
Risk factors for hypertension

Figure 12.1 illustrates the risk factors for hypertension. The risk of high BP increases with age, and is more prevalent in middle-aged men and postmenopausal women.[15] It develops at an earlier age in black ethnicity than it does in Caucasians and is influenced by family history. Although the long-term effect of stress on BP is not well understood, chronic stress (particularly occupational stress) has been shown to be associated with higher rates of hypertension.[13] Dietary factors that may affect hypertension include high levels of salt, reduced levels of potassium and heavy drinking. Other social behaviours such as smoking and physical inactivity can have long-term detrimental effects on BP.[16]

CONVENTIONAL TREATMENT

The initial medical approach for managing non-life-threatening hypertension centres around weight loss and dietary change.[17] Patients are encouraged to increase the level of fruits and vegetables in their diet while reducing salt and alcohol intake. These interventions, combined with regular aerobic exercise, can reduce systolic BP by 7–13 mmHg.[1]

If the hypertension is high (> 140/90 mmHg) on several occasions or unresponsive to lifestyle modification, then drug therapy is instigated.[9] Generally, confirmed hypertension treated with a single drug at the lowest recommended dose will provide satisfactory reduction of BP in about 25–50% of people.[18] For uncomplicated hypertension, unless there is a contraindication or a specific indication for another drug, the order of consideration is:

- angiotensin-converting enzyme (ACE) inhibitor (or sartan), or
- a dihydropyridine calcium channel blocker, or
- thiazide diuretic (low dose) if 65 years or older.[18]

For all patients, treatment aims to reduce BP to under 130/80 mmHg. Elderly and frail can tolerate a diastolic BP as low as 60–65 mmHg without an increase in cardiovascular events.[9]

> **Naturopathic Treatment Aims**
>
> - Reduce stress and advise relaxation techniques.
> - Focus on attaining a healthy weight.
> - Give dietary advice.
> - Encourage graded exercise.
> - Modify Hcy levels.
> - Reduce arterial stiffening.
> - Support key organs of assistance (e.g. kidneys).

In the event of an acute ischaemic stroke, alteplase (rt-PA) is recommended for eligible patients within 4.5 hours of symptom onset. The rationale for this treatment is to prevent stroke-related disability. Aspirin given within 48 hours is also effective but its effect is more modest than that of alteplase.[18]

KEY TREATMENT PROTOCOLS

Unlike orthodox medicine that categorises most cases of hypertension as primary (or idiopathic), a naturopathic approach assumes the presence of an underlying cause, even in primary (idiopathic) hypertension. Differing hypertension prevalence among certain population and age groups is partially due to differences in the intake of certain nutrients. Sustained raised BP is positively associated with higher sodium, alcohol and protein intakes, and is inversely associated with potassium, calcium and magnesium intake.[19] Due to this, dietary and lifestyle measures are a primary focus in the naturopathic management of hypertension.

Reduce stress

The stress response increases sympathetic nervous activity, which can adversely affect the cardiovascular system (see Chapter 18 on stress and fatigue). Cardiovascular disease (particularly hypertension) is due in part to stress-induced mechanisms mediated primarily through increased adrenergic stimulation.[7] These stress-induced mechanisms may be physiological (e.g. elevations in serum lipids, alterations in blood coagulation, atherogenesis, endothelial dysfunction), social (e.g. discrimination, socioeconomic status), psychological (e.g. anxiety, depression) or occupational (e.g. job insecurity, job strain).[13,17]

There are causal relationships between stress and pathophysiological behaviours that, in turn, have detrimental effects on health including hypertension. A landmark study conducted over a period of seven years and involving 6576 subjects clearly indicated that stress leads to increased consumption of alcohol, smoking and a reduction in physical activity.[20] One therapy that has undergone extensive investigation because of its positive effects on stress and parasympathetic activity is yoga. A systematic review of 120 RCTs, non-randomised controlled trials, cohort studies and case reports, involving 6693 normotensive and hypertensive participants, found yoga to be generally effective in reducing blood pressure and lowering antihypertensive medication use. However, it is important to note that the methodological quality of included studies was generally low and the level of methodological heterogeneity was high.[21] Another mind-body therapy with demonstrable antihypertensive activity is transcendental meditation (TM). An umbrella review of eight systematic reviews and analyses concluded that TM may be effective in lowering BP, yielding potential reductions in systolic BP of −4 mmHg and diastolic BP of −2 mmHg.[22]

Several interventions for managing coronary heart disease-prone behaviour patterns have demonstrated some success. A large evaluation study of a community-based program was found to support the effect of multiple therapeutic lifestyle changes on hypertension (see Table 12.2 at the end of the chapter for a review of the evidence).[16] A number of herbs also show some promise. *Valeriana officinalis* has a long history of use as an anxiolytic, and has been shown in a double-blind RCT to be more effective than oxazepam and placebo at reducing total and state anxiety in 61 hospitalised patients with coronary artery disease.[23] As well as reducing 'psychological stress', animal studies indicate that *Valeriana officinalis* has cardioprotective activity, including vasodilatory, hypotensive and negative chronotropic effects.[24] However, these effects have yet to be confirmed in clinical trials.

Findings from earlier clinical studies also indicate a possible benefit of *Passiflora* spp. for anxiety;[25] more recent evidence suggests that this plant may also help improve cardiovascular function. In a double-blind RCT of 90 university students with any somatic or mental health disorder, *P. incarnata* extract (500 mg/day for six days) was found to be more effective than placebo at reducing systolic BP following exposure to experimental anxiety. However, no significant effect on diastolic BP or heart rate was observed.[26] Similarly, in a double-blind RCT of 41 subjects with type 2 diabetes, purple passion fruit peel extract (*P. edulis*, 220 mg/day for 16 weeks) was shown to significantly reduce systolic BP, but not diastolic BP or blood lipids, over time.[27] (see Chapters 14–17 on the nervous system and Chapters 18–20 on the endocrine system).

Modify body mass index

Obesity and hypertension are highly correlated[28]; however, the concept of ideal body weight may raise more questions than it answers. The body mass index (BMI) attempts to create a standardised framework that can be used as a clinical tool to assess 'normal, healthy' human weight. The National Institutes of Health has based its classification of body weight on the concept of BMI, which is derived by dividing body weight by the square of height. A classification based on a measurement such as this inevitably is somewhat arbitrary and is designed simply to provide an approximate guide for identifying people at differing levels of risk for cardiovascular events. A normal or acceptable BMI is lower than 25 kg/m^2, overweight is between 25 and 29.9 kg/m^2 and obesity is 30 kg/m^2 or higher. Some critics have argued that these definitions are too generous, particularly as an optimal cardiovascular prognosis appears to be associated with a BMI equal to or less than 21 kg/m^2.[29] While the method may provide an understanding of ideal weight for people of varying heights, it does not take into account muscle mass and body frame.

The BMI is a ratio:

$$\frac{\text{Weight of person (in kilograms)}}{\text{Height of person (in metres}^2)}$$

The results of the BMI can be interpreted using Table 12.1.

Table 12.1
BMI chart

BMI (kg/m^2)	Weight category	BMI (kg/m^2)	Weight category
Less than 18.5	Underweight	25–29.9	Pre-obesity
18.5–24.9	Normal weight	30 or higher	Obesity

Source: WHO 2018[30]

The impact of BMI on cardiovascular risk has been well documented. The Korean Health Insurance Service Study—one of the largest population-based longitudinal studies to date (i.e. 2.61 million young adults first assessed in 2002/03 and followed up to 2015)—found increasing BMI to be associated with increasing risk of coronary heart disease. Importantly, obese subjects that demonstrated weight loss to normal levels over the follow-up period were shown to have a reduced risk of coronary heart disease.[31] A BMI over 30 plus any two of triglycerides ≥ 1.7 mmol/L, high-density lipoprotein < 1.03, BP ≥ 130/85 mmHg and fasting glucose ≥ 5.6 mmol/L is considered to be metabolic syndrome[32] (discussed further in Chapter 19 on diabetes). As there is a continuous linear relationship between excess body fat, BP and the prevalence of hypertension,[33] weight loss to achieve normal BMI should always be attempted.

Modify diet

The Dietary Approaches to Stop Hypertension (DASH) diet is a healthy eating plan specifically developed to facilitate the lowering of blood pressure. The diet emphasises a reduction in sodium, saturated fat and total fat intake, and the increased consumption of dietary potassium, calcium and magnesium (through fruits, vegetables, wholegrains and low-fat dairy).[34] A meta-analysis of 17 RCTs, involving 2561 adult participants with and without hypertension, found the DASH diet (for 2–26 weeks) significantly reduced systolic BP by 6.74 mmHg (95% CI: −8.25 to −5.23) and diastolic BP by 3.54 mmHg (95% CI: −4.29 to −2.79) when compared with control diets.[34] In terms of the role of sodium in the DASH diet, it is assumed that salt plays an important role in the inactivation of nitric oxide (NO) synthase in endothelial cells of arteries, causing a reduction in elasticity and an increase in pressure.[35] Females of an older age are most sensitive to the hypertensive effects of dietary sodium, so sodium consumption should be monitored in this population.[36] There is a belief that sea salt is more beneficial and less harmful than table salt. Sea salt is obtained directly through the evaporation of seawater. It is usually not processed, or undergoes minimal processing, and therefore retains trace levels of minerals like magnesium, potassium, calcium and other nutrients. Table salt, on the other hand, is mined from salt deposits and then processed to give it a fine texture so it's easier to mix and use in recipes. Processing strips table salt of any trace minerals it may have contained, and additives are also usually incorporated to prevent clumping or caking. Other than the trace levels of minerals in sea salt, both forms contain around 40% sodium.[37] As for the role of caffeine in hypertension management, there is currently insufficient evidence to indicate that caffeine-containing beverages should be omitted from the diets of people living with hypertension.[38]

Ensure adequate exercise

Evidence from a meta-analysis of 93 randomised controlled trials (involving 5223 participants) supports the positive effects of exercise (including endurance, dynamic resistance and isometric resistance training) on systolic and diastolic BP. The review reported reductions in systolic BP ranging between 1.8 mmHg and 10.9 mmHg (depending on exercise type), and reductions in diastolic BP ranging between 2.2 mmHg and 6.2 mmHg. The largest reductions in BP were observed with isometric exercise.[39] Aerobic exercise that uses large muscle groups for 20–60 minutes a day for a minimum of three days a week is advisable.[9] It is interesting to note, however, that exercise over 758 minutes a week (108 minutes per day) increases methionine metabolism, which also increases its amino acid metabolic intermediate Hcy, known to increase cardiovascular risk.[40] It is important to remember that optimal exercise activity should be implemented in a graded fashion, under the direction of an exercise physiologist and/or medical practitioner (see Chapter 3 on wellness and Chapter 26 on fibromyalgia).

Lower homocysteine

As mentioned previously, excessive exercise as well as deficiency of folic acid, vitamin B6 and/or vitamin B12 can result in elevated total plasma Hcy concentrations, which is considered a risk factor for vascular disease.[41] As discussed in Chapter 11 on atherosclerosis, a considerable body of evidence suggests that Hcy plays a significant role in the pathology of cardiovascular disease. In fact, recent evidence indicates that elevated levels of Hcy may be an independent risk factor of blood pressure variability—a predictor of hypertension-associated end-organ damage.[41] Some antihypertensive medications, such as candesartan and amlodipine, are effective in reducing cellular oxidative stress, but this effectiveness can be reduced in the presence of raised Hcy levels.[42] Experimentally increasing plasma Hcy concentrations by methionine loading rapidly impairs both conduit and resistance vessel endothelial function in healthy humans. Endothelial dysfunction in conduit and resistance vessels may underlie the reported associations between Hcy, atherosclerosis and hypertension. Increased oxidant stress appears to play a pathophysiological role in the deleterious endothelial effects of Hcy.[43]

Despite the strong association between elevated homocysteine and risk of hypertension, there is still some uncertainty about the clinical implications of treating hyperhomocystinaemia. The findings of a recent Cochrane review of 15 RCTs, involving 71 422 participants, indicated that vitamin B6, B9 or B12 supplementation (administered alone or in combination), at any dosage, was no more effective than placebo, or standard care, in preventing myocardial infarction, or reducing all-cause mortality, in patients at risk of or living with cardiovascular disease.[44]

Enhance arterial elasticity and integrity

Age-related changes in the arterial system begin from the age of 20 years and accelerate through midlife.[45] Increased collagen deposition and weakened vascular elastin result in altered elasticity, distensibility and dilation.[45] Stiffening of the central arteries results in higher wave velocities and augmentation of systolic arterial pressure.[45] Lifestyle modification is one way by which arterial stiffness can be improved. In a small comparative study of 45 overweight and obese men, a well-balanced diet (containing 1680 kcal/day) was found to be as effective as regular exercise (walking 40–60 minutes daily, three times a week) in improving carotid arterial compliance, as well as body mass and waist circumference (all independent risk factors for cardiovascular disease).[46] The role of **omega-3 fatty acids** on arterial elasticity is currently uncertain. While the findings of a meta-analysis of 23 RCTs (1385 participants) indicated that fish oil supplementation may be more effective than controls at improving flow-mediated dilatation (WMD 1.49; 95% CI: 0.48 to 2.50), when the review was limited to higher quality studies (Jadad scores > 2) fish oil was found to have no significant effect on endothelial function.[47]

Antioxidants, such as vitamins C and E, may play a role in improving vascular integrity and elasticity by reducing oxidative stress and atherogenesis.[48] Evidence from a meta-analysis of 46 RCTs (1817 participants) supports this earlier work, revealing that vitamin C (500–2000 mg/day; SMD: 0.25; 95% CI: 0.02 to 0.49) and vitamin E supplementation alone (300–1800 IU/day; SMD: 0.48; 95% CI: 0.23 to 0.72), but not together, were significantly more effective than controls in improving endothelial function.[49]

Pycnogenol, an extract of the bark from *Pinus pinaster*, consists of a concentrate of water-soluble polyphenols, the bioflavonoids catechin and taxifolin, as well as phenolcarbonic acids. Pycnogenol augments endothelium-dependent vasodilation by increasing NO production in the vascular wall.[50] Findings from a meta-analysis of nine RCTs, involving 549 subjects suggest pycnogenol (150–200 mg/day for 2–25 weeks) may be significantly more effective than controls at reducing systolic BP (WMD −3.22 mmHg; 95% CI: −6.20 to −0.24) and diastolic BP (WMD −3.11 mmHg; 95% CI: −4.60 to −1.62). However, when the review was limited to high-quality studies (Jadad scores > 2), pycnogenol was found to have no significant effect on systolic BP.[51]

Dietary flavonoids, such as quercetin and epicatechin, can augment NO status and reduce endothelin-1 concentrations, and may thereby improve endothelial function.[52] **Cocoa** is rich in plant-derived flavonoids, and has been the subject of much research on hypertension. A Cochrane review of 35 RCTs, involving 1804 generally healthy participants, found flavanol-rich cocoa products (mean 670 mg flavanol in 1.4–105 grams cocoa product daily, for 2–18 weeks) had a small but statistically significant effect on systolic BP (MD –1.76 mmHg; 95% CI: –3.09 to –0.43) and diastolic BP (MD –1.76 mmHg; 95% CI: –2.57 to –0.94) relative to low-flavanol-containing cocoa products (mean 55 mg flavanols). Much larger improvements in systolic BP (up to 4 mmHg) were observed among hypertensive populations relative to prehypertensive or normotensive populations.[53] A range of potential mechanisms through which flavonols and cocoa might exert their benefits on cardiovascular health include activation of NO (hypotensive effect), scavenging of free radicals (antioxidant effect), inhibition of thromboxane A2 (antiplatelet effect), inhibition of LDL oxidation (anti-atherogenic effect) and inhibition of inflammatory cytokine production (anti-inflammatory effect).[54]

Magnesium plays a role in a number of chronic disease-related conditions, including hypertension. Magnesium acts as a calcium channel antagonist, stimulates production of vasodilator prostacyclins and NO and alters vascular responses to vasoactive agonists.[55] Accordingly, it has been studied in more than 34 RCTs involving 2028 normotensive and hypertensive adults. Findings from a meta-analysis of these studies revealed magnesium supplementation (administered at a median daily dose of 368 mg over a median period of three months) was significantly more effective than placebo at reducing systolic BP (MD –2.00 mmHg; 95% CI: –0.43 to –3.58) and diastolic BP (MD –1.78 mmHg; 95% CI: –0.73 to –2.82). Higher quality trials were associated with larger reductions in BP.[56]

Most of the herbal treatments for hypertension probably act as peripheral vasodilators.[9] One herb that has gained increasing attention as a hypotensive agent is *Allium sativum* (garlic). **Garlic** may facilitate reductions in blood pressure through various mechanisms, including reduced oxidative stress, enhanced NO generation, partial angiotensin-converting enzyme inhibition, and increased urinary sodium excretion.[57] These hypotensive effects have been demonstrated clinically, with a meta-analysis of 17 RCTs (*n* = 578 normotensive and hypertensive subjects) finding garlic supplementation (primarily garlic powder, 300–2400 mg daily for 2–24 weeks) to be significantly more effective than control in reducing systolic BP (MD –3.75 mmHg; 95% CI: –5.04 to –2.45) and diastolic BP (MD –3.39 mmHg; 95% CI: –4.14 to –2.65). When the analysis was limited to high-quality trials, the effect of garlic on systolic BP was larger, whereas the effect on diastolic BP was smaller.[58]

Consider vasopressin and diuresis

Diuretics have long been used to treat hypertension in general practice. Technically, a 'diuretic' is an agent that increases urine volume, while a 'natriuretic' causes an increase in renal sodium excretion. Because natriuretics almost always increase water excretion, they are usually called diuretics.[33] Generally, diuretics should be initiated at the lowest effective dose of the class chosen. Problems that may occur with both short- and long-term use of diuretics include hyponatraemia, hypokalaemia, metabolic alkalosis and increased uric acid levels. Carbohydrate metabolism is frequently disturbed, with resultant hyperglycaemia and insulin resistance.[59]

Many herbs are reported to have diuretic effects (e.g. *Agropyron repens* [couch grass] *Apium graveolens* [celery], *Zea mays* [cornsilk]); however, few have demonstrated diuretic activity in human subjects, with the exception of *Taraxacum officinale* (dandelion) and *Equisetum arvense* (horsetail), both of which contain trace amounts of potassium which may assist in averting a common adverse effect of many diuretics—hypokalaemia.

A small pilot study of 17 healthy women found the hydroethanolic extract of *T. officinale* fresh leaf (8 mL three times for one day) significantly increased urinary frequency and volume when compared with control day values.[60] Similarly, in a double-blind crossover trial of 36 healthy men, treatment with standardised dried extract of *E. arvense* (900 mg daily for four days) resulted in a significantly greater level of diuresis when compared with negative control, and an effect that was equivalent to that of hydrochlorothiazide.[61] Whether these results translate into clinical improvements in hypertensive populations is yet to be determined.

Prevention and adjunctive treatment of stroke

Ginkgo biloba

- The use of *Ginkgo biloba* extract leads to a significant increase in cerebral blood flow and glucose uptake into brain tissue.[62]
- Ginkgo extract, EGb 761, administered orally to wild mice produced 50.9% less neurological dysfunction and 48.2% smaller infarct volumes than non-treated mice after cerebral infarct (stroke).[62]
- A 2005 Cochrane review of 10 trials (792 patients) found no convincing evidence to support the routine use of *Ginkgo biloba* to promote recovery between 14 and 35 days after stroke.[62]
- More recent evidence from an RCT of 348 patients with acute ischaemic stroke suggests the administration of *Ginkgo biloba* extract (450 mg daily, plus 100 mg aspirin daily, for six months) within seven days of an acute stroke, may be significantly more effective than aspirin alone in improving Montreal Cognitive Assessment scores, National Institutes of Health Stroke Scale scores, modified Rankin Scale scores for independent rate, Barthel Index scores and Mini-Mental State Examination scores at 30, 90 and 180 days.[63]

Acupuncture

- A meta-analysis of 25 RCTs involving 2224 subjects with ischaemic stroke found acupuncture (when administered daily for 2–4 weeks) to be significantly more effective than controls at improving stroke recovery, functional deficit, disability with activities of daily living, and neurologic deficit.[64]
- Evidence from a meta-analysis of 72 predominantly low-quality studies (6134 patients with stroke) suggests acupuncture may be significantly more effective than controls at improving stroke-related dysphagia.[65]
- Findings from a meta-analysis of five RCTs (involving 291 patients post-stroke) indicate acupuncture (8–30 sessions over an undisclosed period of time) may significantly reduce post-stroke spasticity of the wrists, knees and elbows when compared with controls.[66]

INTEGRATIVE MEDICAL CONSIDERATIONS

The influence of stress in cardiovascular disease should not be underestimated. In fact exposure to long-term stress can be a contributing factor in the pathogenesis of hypertension.[13] **Massage** therapy may play a role in the management of hypertension by eliciting the relaxation response, which in turn may help in lowering BP and hypertension. Findings from two open-label RCTs involving a total of 140 patients with pre-hypertension/hypertension) found Swedish massage (administered for 10–15 minutes, 2–3 times a week, for 3.5–6 weeks) significantly reduced systolic and diastolic BP when compared with controls.[67,68] If the person's stress stems from environmental factors (such as work, home life and financial problems), then referral to a counsellor or psychologist may be a consideration.

Practitioners may also consider referral to an acupuncturist. There is some evidence to suggest that **acupuncture** may play a role in the management of hypertension by inhibiting neural activity in the rostral ventrolateral medulla (rVLM), thereby reducing sympathetic nerve activity and blood pressure.[69] However, the effectiveness of acupuncture in hypertensive human subjects is unclear. While a meta-analysis of 30 RCTs (2107 patients) found acupuncture plus antihypertensive medication to be significantly more effective than antihypertensive medication alone in reducing systolic and diastolic BP, the overall quality of included trials was low.[70] Other therapies known to elicit the relaxation response include yoga, Tai Chi and meditation. Indeed, meta-analyses/reviews of RCTs measuring the effectiveness of these three therapies have reported positive results, with yoga (120 RCTs),[21] Tai Chi (20 RCTs)[71] and transcendental meditation (eight systematic reviews/meta-analyses)[72] all shown to be more effective than controls in reducing systolic and diastolic BP.

Acute myocardial infarct: is there a case for natural medicines?

Intravenous magnesium supplementation

- During the first hour of administration for myocardial infarct (MI), IV magnesium may produce antiarrhythmic effects and calcium channel-blocking effects, improve NO release from coronary endothelium and prevent serum coagulation. While the hypotensive and antiarrhythmic effects of intravenous magnesium are supported to some extent in meta-analyses of RCTs, the effect of magnesium on mortality post MI is still inconclusive.[73]

Salvia miltiorrhiza

- *Salvia miltiorrhiza* exhibits a number of effects that may support recovery from acute myocardial infarction, including sedative, antioxidant and antiplatelet effects, as well as improving coronary micro-circulation.
- Danshen is widely used in China for the prevention and treatment of angina pectoris and MI.
- A meta-analysis of six RCTs (2368 participants) found insufficient evidence to support an effect of *S. miltiorrhiza* on total mortality in patients with acute MI.[74]

Ginkgo biloba

- *Ginkgo biloba* leaf extract exhibits a number of actions that may mitigate the destruction of myocardial tissue post MI, including antioxidant and anti-inflammatory effects, and the inhibition of myocardial remodelling.[75]
- *Ginkgo biloba* extract has been shown to be effective in reducing infarct size in acute MI mouse models.[75] The translation of these effects into human subjects, however, is not yet certain.

Allium sativum

- *Allium sativum* demonstrates a range of cardioprotective effects that may mitigate myocardial damage following MI, including antioxidant, anti-arrhythmic, fibrinolytic and vasorelaxant activity.[76]
- Various constituents of *Allium sativum* have been shown to prevent MI, prevent myocardial necrosis and reduce myocardial ischaemia-reperfusion injury in animal models.[77] The clinical effectiveness of garlic for the management of acute MI is still unclear.

CLINICAL SUMMARY

Fortunately hypertension is clinically 'clear-cut' if clinicians adopt the accepted medical classification of the condition. Determination of a primary or secondary cause is useful for guiding treatment. In primary hypertension, a full history (diet, weight, age, sex, stress, smoking, alcohol, sedentary lifestyle, illicit drug use) will provide the information required to inform an appropriate treatment plan. A patient who displays symptoms but has less obvious causes may require blood work to elicit the root of the problem. This may include investigating blood components such as Hcy and C-reactive protein (CRP). Secondary hypertension can involve disease states that require referral. If the condition is mild to moderate, then there is usually a window of opportunity of three to six months to make significant changes to health before medical intervention is required.

Treatment should include as a minimum, the modification of both dietary and lifestyle factors that impact health. Therapeutic supplements might include: *Passiflora* spp. (to help lower BP and anxiety), *Taraxacum officinalis* and *Equisetum arvense* (to faciliate diuresis); magnesium; omega-3 fats and cocoa flavanols (to improve endothelial function); and magnesium and *Allium sativum* (to promote vasodilation) (see Figure 12.2). These treatments should be considered alongside other therapies, such as acupuncture, transcendental meditation, yoga and Tai Chi. Lastly, it is important to note that hypertension may be a lifetime condition, and any treatment has to be sustainable and capable of being maintained over a lifetime.

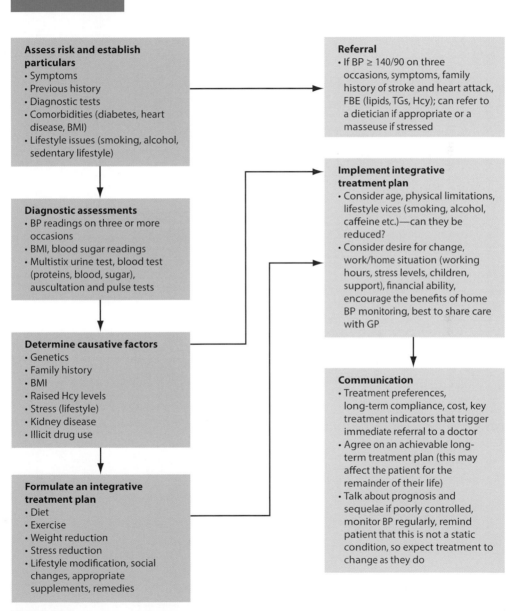

Figure 12.2
Naturopathic treatment decision tree—hypertension and stroke

Table 12.2
Review of the major evidence

Intervention	Mechanisms of action	Key literature	Summary of results	Comment
Allium sativum	Reduces oxidative stress, enhances NO generation, partially inhibits angiotension converting enzyme activity, increases urinary sodium excretion[57]	Meta-analysis (17 RCTs, 578 patients); garlic versus control. Wang et al. 2015[58]	Garlic supplementation (primarily garlic powder, 300–2400 mg daily for 2–24 weeks) was significantly more effective than control in reducing systolic BP (MD –3.75 mmHg; 95% CI: –5.04 to –2.45) and diastolic BP (MD –3.39 mmHg; 95% CI: –4.14 to –2.65). When the analysis was limited to high-quality trials, the effect of garlic on systolic BP was larger, whereas the effect on diastolic BP was smaller[58]	Garlic exhibits a range of cardioprotective effects, which may make it a suitable adjunct for the management of hypertension and other cardiovascular diseases
Magnesium	Calcium channel antagonist, stimulates production of vasodilator prostacyclins and NO, and alters vascular responses to vasoactive agonists[55]	Meta-analysis (34 RCTs, 2028 adults); magnesium versus placebo Zhang et al. 2016[56]	Magnesium supplementation significantly reduced systolic BP (MD –2.00 mmHg; 95% CI: –0.43 to –3.58) and diastolic BP (MD –1.78 mmHg; 95% CI: –0.73 to –2.82) when compared with placebo. Higher quality trials were associated with larger reductions in BP[56]	The 34 trials included in this review reported the use of seven different magnesium supplement formulations. The comparative effectiveness of these different formulations in lowering BP is not yet clear[56]
Cocoa flavanols	Activates NO, scavenges free radicals, inhibits thromboxane A2, inhibits LDL oxidation and inhibits inflammatory cytokine production[54]	Meta-analysis (35 RCTs, 1804 participants): High-flavanol cocoa products versus low-flavanol cocoa products Ried et al. 2017[53]	High-flavanol cocoa products produced a small but statistically significant effect on systolic BP (MD –1.76 mmHg; 95% CI: –3.09 to –0.43) and diastolic BP (MD –1.76 mmHg; 95% CI: –2.57 to –0.94) compared with low-flavanol cocoa products. Much larger improvements in systolic BP (up to 4 mmHg) were observed among hypertensive populations relative to prehypertensive or normotensive populations[53]	Some patients may find it difficult to consume 670 mg cocoa flavanols daily (i.e the median dose reported in this review) through diet alone. For these patients, supplementation may be an alternative option[56]
Therapeutic lifestyle changes (TLCs)	Reducing salt intake reduces the inactivation of NO synthase and increases arterial elasticity. Exercise may reduce BP by decreasing oxidative stress, psychosocial stress, inflammation, arterial stiffness and sympathetic activity[78]	Baseline and six-month evaluation after participation in community TLCs (exercise training, weight and stress management and smoking cessation): Bavikati et al. 2008[16] Meta-analysis (93 RCTs, 5223 participants): endurance versus dynamic resistance versus isometric resistance versus combined training: Cornelissen et al. 2013[39] Meta-analysis (17 RCTs, 2561 adults): DASH diet versus control diet[34]; Saneei et al. 2014[34]	Baseline systolic and diastolic BP reduced subjects with BMI < 30 kg/m² had greater reduction than those with BMI > 30 kg/m².[16] Significant reduction in systolic BP (ranging between 1.8 mmHg and 10.9 mmHg) and diastolic BP (ranging between 2.2 mmHg and 6.2 mmHg) following 4–52 weeks of any exercise category. Larger reductions in BP were observed with isometric exercise[39] The DASH diet (which focuses on reducing sodium, saturated fat and total fat intake, and increasing consumption of dietary potassium, calcium and magnesium through fruits, vegetables, wholegrains and low-fat dairy), when consumed for 2–26 weeks, was effective at reducing systolic BP (–6.74 mmHg; 95% CI: –8.25 to –5.23) and diastolic BP (–3.54 mmHg; 95% CI: –4.29 to –2.79) when compared with control diets[34]	Effectiveness of TLC on cardiovascular parameters supported in real-world setting Recommendations can be extended for a range of lifestyle interventions to lower BP

KEY POINTS

- Establish the correct diagnosis of hypertension.
- Determine the primary or secondary cause.
- Consider referral if < 35-year-old female; history of abdominal or lumbar trauma; chronic cystitis; kidney disease; kidney stones; pregnancy; secondary causes.
- Facilitate dietary and lifestyle changes.
- Consider treatments to support a normotensive state.
- Make treatment decisions based on long-term maintenance of the condition.

FURTHER READING

Fioranelli M, editor. Integrative cardiology: a new therapeutic vision. Switzerland: Springer; 2017.

Sacre JW, Jennings GLR, Kingwell BA. Exercise and dietary influences on arterial stiffness in cardiometabolic disease. Hypertension 2014;63:888–93.

Shatnawi A, et al. Complementary and alternative medicine use in hypertension: the good, the bad, and the ugly: hypertension treatment from nature—myth or fact? In: Emerging applications, perspectives, and discoveries in cardiovascular research. Hershey, USA: IGI Global; 2017. p. 255–87.

Therapeutic Guidelines Limited. Therapeutic guidelines, cardiovascular (version 7). 2018.

REFERENCES

1. National Heart Foundation of Australia. Guideline for the diagnosis and management of hypertension in adults—2016. Melbourne: National Heart Foundation of Australia; 2016.
2. Franklin SS, O'Brien E, Staessen JA. Masked hypertension: understanding its complexity. Eur Heart J 2016;38(15):1112–18.
3. Cobos B, Haskard-Zolnierek K, Howard K. White coat hypertension: improving the patient–health care practitioner relationship. Psychol Res Behav Manag 2015;8:133–41.
4. Easton JD, et al. Definition and evaluation of transient ischemic attack: a scientific statement for healthcare professionals from the American Heart Association/ American Stroke Association Stroke Council; Council on Cardiovascular Surgery and Anesthesia; Council on Cardiovascular Radiology and Intervention; Council on Cardiovascular Nursing; and the Interdisciplinary Council on Peripheral Vascular Disease. The American Academy of Neurology affirms the value of this statement as an educational tool for neurologists. Stroke 2009;40(6):2276–93.
5. Grossman E, Messerli F. Drug-induced hypertension: an unappreciated cause of secondary hypertension. Am J Med 2012;125(1):14–22.
6. Vardaxis NJ. Pathology for the health sciences. South Melbourne: Macmillan Education Australia; 1996. p. 106.
7. Lazzeroni D, Rimoldi O, Camici PG. From left ventricular hypertrophy to dysfunction and failure. Circ J 2016;80(3):555–64.
8. Griffin BP, editor. Manual of cardiovascular medicine. 4th ed. Philadelphia: Lippincott Williams & Wilkins; 2012.
9. Merck, Sharp & Dohme. MSD Manual: professional version. Kenilworth: Merck & Co; 2018.
10. Hisham NF, Bayraktutan U. Epidemiology, pathophysiology and treatment of hypertension in ischaemic stroke patients. J Stroke Cerebrovasc Dis 2013;22(7):e4–14.
11. Charles L, Trsicott J, Dobbs B. Secondary hypertension: discovering the underlying cause. Am Fam Physician 2017;96(7):453–61.
12. Australian Institute of Health & Welfare (AIHW). Risk factors to health. Canberra, Australia: AIHW; 2017.
13. Cuffee Y, et al. Psychosocial risk factors for hypertension: an update of the literature. Curr Hypertens Rep 2014;16:483.
14. O'Donnell MJ, et al. Global and regional effects of potentially modifiable risk factors associated with acute stroke in 32 countries (INTERSTROKE): a case-control study. Lancet 2016;388(10046):761–75.
15. The Mayo clinic. High blood pressure (hypertension). Online. Available: https://www.mayoclinic.org/ diseases-conditions/high-blood-pressure/symptoms-causes/ syc-20373410. Accessed 2 November 2018.
16. Bavikati VV, et al. Effect of comprehensive therapeutic lifestyle changes on prehypertension. Am J Cardiol 2008;102(12):1677–80.
17. Cuevas AG, Williams DR, Albert MA. Psychosocial factors and hypertension: a review of the literature. Cardiol Clin 2017;35(2):223–30.
18. Australian Medicines Handbook 2018. Online. Available: https://amh.net.au/ Accessed 2 November 2018.
19. Suter P, et al. Nutritional factors in the control of blood pressure and hypertension. Nutr Clin Care 2002;5(1):9–19.
20. Hamer M, et al. Psychological distress as a risk factor for cardiovascular events: pathophysiological and behavioural mechanisms. J Am Coll Cardiol 2008;52(25):2163–5.
21. Tyagi A, Cohen M. Yoga and hypertension: a systematic review. Altern Ther Health Med 2014;20(2):32–59.
22. Ooi SL, Giovino M, Pak SC. Transcendental meditation for lowering blood pressure: an overview of systematic reviews and meta-analyses. Complement Ther Med 2017;34:26–34.
23. Rafiee M, et al. The effects of lavender, valerian, and oxazepam on anxiety among hospitalized patients with

coronary artery disease. Mod Care J 2018;ePub ahead of print.

24. Chen H-W, et al. Chemical components and cardiovascular activities of Valeriana spp. Evid Based Complement Alternat Med 2015;2015:Article ID 947619.

25. Circosta C, et al. Biological and analytical characterization of two extracts from Valeriana officinalis. J Ethnopharmacol 2007;112(2):361–7.

26. da Silva JA, et al. Effects of the single supplementation and multiple doses of Passiflora incarnata L. on human anxiety: a clinical trial, double-blind, placebo-controlled, randomized. Int Arch Med 2017;10(6):1–9.

27. Raju IN, Reddy KK, Kumari CK. Efficacy of purple passion fruit peel extract in lowering cardiovascular risk factors in type 2 diabetic subjects. J Evid Based Integr Med 2013;18(3):183–90.

28. Bowman TS, et al. Eight-year change in body mass index and subsequent risk of cardiovascular disease among healthy non-smoking men. Prev Med 2007;45(6):436–41.

29. Fontana L, Hu FB. Optimal body weight for health and longevity: bridging basic, clinical, and population research. Aging Cell 2014;13(3):391–400.

30. World Health Organisation. Body mass index—BMI. Online. Available: http://www.euro.who.int/en/health-topics/disease-prevention/nutrition/a-healthy-lifestyle/body-mass-index-bmi Accessed 4 December 2018.

31. Choi S, Kim K, Kim SM. Association of obesity or weight change with coronary heart disease among young adults in South Korea. JAMA Intern Med 2018;178(8):1060–8.

32. Longmore JM, et al. Oxford handbook of clinical medicine. 7th ed. Oxford: Oxford University Press; 2014. p. 199.

33. Katzung BG. Basic and clinical pharmacology. 14th ed. USA: McGraw-Hill; 2018.

34. Saneei P, et al. Influence of Dietary Approaches to Stop Hypertension (DASH) diet on blood pressure: a systematic review and meta-analysis on randomized controlled trials. Nutr Metab Cardiovasc Dis 2014;24(12):1253–61.

35. Li J, et al. Salt inactivates endothelial nitric oxide synthase in endothelial cells. J Nutr 2009;139(3):447–51.

36. He J, et al. Gender difference in blood pressure responses to dietary sodium intervention in the GenSalt study. J Hypertens 2009;27(1):48–54.

37. American Heart Association. Sea Salt vs Table Salt. Available: http://www.heart.org/en/healthy-living/healthy-eating/eat-smart/sodium/sea-salt-vs-table-salt Accessed 5 Dec 2018.

38. Guessous I, Eap CB, Bochud M. Blood pressure in relation to coffee and caffeine consumption. Curr Hypertens Rep 2014;16:468.

39. Cornelissen VA, Smart NA. Exercise training for blood pressure: a systematic review and meta-analysis. J Am Heart Assoc 2013;2(1):e004473.

40. Joubert LM, Manore MM. The role of physical activity level and B-vitamin status on blood homocysteine levels. Med Sci Sports Exerc 2008;40(11):1923–31.

41. Gu G, et al. Correlation between homocysteine levels and 24-h ambulatory blood pressure variability in Chinese hypertensive patients. Int J Clin Exp Med 2016;9(6):11715–22.

42. Muda P, et al. Effect of antihypertensive treatment with candesartan or amlodipine on glutathione and its redox status, homocysteine and vitamin concentrations in patients with essential hypertension. J Hypertens 2005;23(1):105–12.

43. Kanani PM, et al. Role of oxidant stress in endothelial dysfunction produced by experimental hyperhomocyst(e)inemia in humans. Circulation 1999;100(11):1161–8.

44. Martí-Carvajal AJ, Solà I, Lathyris D, et al. Homocysteine-lowering interventions (B-complex vitamin therapy) for preventing cardiovascular events. Cochrane Database Syst Rev 2009;(4):CD006612.

45. Fleg JL, Strait J. Age-associated changes in cardiovascular structure and function: a fertile milieu for future disease. Heart Fail Rev 2012;17(0):545–54.

46. Maeda S, et al. Lifestyle modification decreases arterial stiffness in overweight and obese men: dietary modification vs. exercise training. Hum Kinetics J 2015;25(1):69–77.

47. Xin W, Wei W, Li X. Effect of fish oil supplementation on fasting vascular endothelial function in humans: a meta-analysis of randomized controlled trials. PLoS ONE 2012;7(9):e46028.

48. Rodriguez JA, et al. Vitamins C and E prevent endothelial VEGF and VEGFR-2 overexpression induced by porcine hypercholesterolemic LDL. Cardiovasc Res 2005;65:665–73.

49. Ashor A, et al. Effect of vitamin C and vitamin E supplementation on endothelial function: a systematic review and meta-analysis of randomised controlled trials. Br J Nutr 2015;113(8):1182–94.

50. Nishioka K, et al. Pycnogenol, French maritime pine bark extract, augments endothelium-dependent vasodilation in humans. Hypertens Res 2007;30(9):775–80.

51. Zhang Z, et al. Effect of pycnogenol supplementation on blood pressure: a systematic review and meta-analysis. Iran J Public Health 2018;47(6):779–87.

52. Loke WM, et al. Pure dietary flavonoids quercetin and (–)-epicatechin augment nitric oxide products and reduce endothelin-1 acutely in healthy men. Am J Clin Nutr 2008;88(4):1018–25.

53. Ried K, Fakler P, Stocks NP. Effect of cocoa on blood pressure. Cochrane Database Syst Rev 2017;(4):CD008893.

54. Aprotosoaie AC, et al. The cardiovascular effects of cocoa polyphenols—an overview. Diseases 2016;4(4):39.

55. Sontia B, Touyz RM. Magnesium transport in hypertension. Pathophysiology 2007;14(3–4):205–11.

56. Zhang X, et al. Effects of magnesium supplementation on blood pressure: a meta-analysis of randomized double-blind placebo-controlled trials. Hypertension 2016;68(2):324–33.

57. Shouk R, et al. Mechanisms underlying the antihypertensive effects of garlic bioactives. Nutr Res 2014;34(2):106–15.

58. Wang HP, et al. Effect of garlic on blood pressure: a meta-analysis. J Clin Hypertens 2015;17(3):223–31.

59. Roush GC, Siza DA. Diuretics for hypertension: a review and update. Am J Hypertens 2016;29(10):1130–7.

60. Clare BA, Conroy RS, Spelman K. The diuretic effect in human subjects of an extract of Taraxacum officinale folium over a single day. J Altern Complement Med 2009;15(8):929–34.

61. Carneiro DM, et al. Randomized, double-blind clinical trial to assess the acute diuretic effect of Equisetum arvense (field horsetail) in healthy volunteers. Evid Based Complement Alternat Med 2014;2014:760683.

62. Zeng X, et al. Ginkgo biloba for acute ischaemic stroke. Cochrane Database Syst Rev 2005;(4):CD003691, doi:10.1002/14651858.CD003691.pub2.

63. Li S, et al. Ginkgo biloba extract improved cognitive and neurological functions of acute ischaemic stroke: a randomised controlled trial. Stroke Vasc Neurol 2017;2:189–97.

64. Li L, Meng SQ, Qian HZ. An updated meta-analysis of the efficacy and safety of acupuncture treatment for cerebral infarction. PLoS ONE 2014;9(12):e114057.

65. Long YB, Wu XP. A meta-analysis of the efficacy of acupuncture in treating dysphagia in patients with a stroke. Acupunct Med 2012;30:291–7.

66. Lim SM, et al. Acupuncture for spasticity after stroke: a systematic review and meta-analysis of randomized controlled trials. Evid Based Complement Alternat Med 2015;2015:870398.

67. Mohebbi Z, et al. The effect of back massage on blood pressure in the patients with primary hypertension in 2012-2013: a randomized clinical trial. Int J Community Based Nurs Midwifery 2014;2(4):251–8.

68. Givi M. Durability of effect of massage therapy on blood pressure. Int J Prev Med 2013;4(5):511–16.

69. Zhou W, Longhurst JC. Neuroendocrine mechanisms of acupuncture in the treatment of hypertension. Evid Based Complement Alternat Med 2012;2012:878673.

70. Chen H, et al. Efficacy and safety of acupuncture for essential hypertension: a meta-analysis. Med Sci Monit 2018;24:2946–69.

71. Lian Z, et al. Effects of Tai chi on adults with essential hypertension in China: a systematic review and meta-analysis. Eur J Integr Med 2017;12:153–62.

72. Ooi SL, Giovino M, Pak SC. Transcendental meditation for lowering blood pressure: an overview of systematic reviews and meta-analyses. Complement Ther Med 2017;34:26–34.

73. Li J, Zhang Q, Zhang M, et al. Intravenous magnesium for acute myocardial infarction. Cochrane Database Syst Rev 2007;(2):CD002755.

74. Wu T, Ni J, Wei J. Danshen (Chinese medicinal herb) preparations for acute myocardial infarction. Cochrane Database Syst Rev 2008;(2):CD004465.

75. Li Y, et al. Ginkgo biloba extract prevents acute myocardial infarction and suppresses the inflammation- and apoptosis-regulating p38 mitogen-activated protein kinases, nuclear factor-κB and B-cell lymphoma 2 signaling pathways. Mol Med Rep 2017;16(3):3657–63.

76. Khatua TN, Adela R, Banerjee SK. Garlic and cardioprotection: insights into the molecular mechanisms. Can J Physiol Pharmacol 2013;91:448–58.

77. Banerjee SK, Dinda AK, et al. Chronic garlic administration protects rat heart against oxidative stress induced by ischemic reperfusion injury. BMC Pharmacol 2002;2:16.

78. Diaz KM, Shimbo D. Physical activity and the prevention of hypertension. Curr Hypertens Rep 2013;15(6):659–68.

CHAPTER **13**

Chronic venous insufficiency

Matthew Leach
ND, PhD

OVERVIEW

Chronic venous insufficiency (CVI) is a pathological disorder of the venous system characterised by impaired venous blood flow in the lower limbs. The condition is manifested by pathological changes to the skin, subcutaneous tissue and vascular tissue.[1] These manifestations, which can range from mild to severe, can be grouped into symptomatic complaints, such as leg heaviness, discomfort and pruritus, or advanced physical signs, including leg oedema, ochre pigmentation and lipodermatosclerosis. The condition, which is a precursor to varicose veins and venous leg ulceration, is not uncommon, affecting 0.1–17% of men and 0.2–20% of women.[1] The global prevalence of CVI is approximately 32%, according to data collected from 99 359 subjects across 23 countries.[2]

This chronic and sometimes disabling disorder (which is associated with increasing difficulty in performing activities of daily living)[3] is believed to originate from an inherent weakness in the venous architecture (primary CVI) or an episode of macrovascular injury (secondary CVI), which may be attributed to lower limb surgery, trauma, deep vein thrombosis (DVT) or pregnancy.[3] This insult to the venous system, which may or may not lead to thrombus formation, can result in valvular incompetence, venous reflux (or retrograde blood flow), ambulatory venous hypertension, venous wall dilation and a subsequent rise in capillary filtration. As well as contributing to the formation of interstitial oedema, increased capillary filtration may also lead to localised hypoxia, malnutrition and eventual tissue destruction (Figure 13.1). The extravasation of fibrinogen and the subsequent formation of pericapillary cuffs, and the intraluminal trapping of leucocytes and subsequent release of toxic metabolites, proteolytic enzymes and tissue necrosis factor alpha (TNF-α),[5] are some of the mechanisms linking elevated capillary filtration pressure to changes in tissue perfusion and local architecture, although there is a paucity of clinical evidence to support these theories. The extravasation of fibrinogen and leucocyte products into pericapillary tissue may also mediate inflammation, suggesting that CVI may be a disease of chronic inflammation.[3]

RISK FACTORS

Many risk factors, both modifiable and non-modifiable, reportedly contribute to the pathogenesis of venous insufficiency. Occupations requiring periods of prolonged

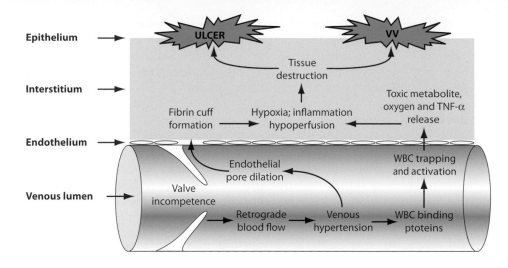

VV = varicose vein

Figure 13.1
The pathophysiology of chronic venous insufficiency
Source: Leach 2006[4]

standing (such as nurses, flight attendants and factory workers) have been observed across a number of studies to have a higher prevalence and severity of CVI and varicose veins.[1] This could be attributed in part to excessive lower limb venous congestion secondary to reduced calf-muscle pump activity. However, evidence linking other modifiable risk factors to CVI, such as obesity, smoking, constipation, hormone therapy and hypertension, has been inconsistent.[1,3]

In terms of non-modifiable risk factors, both family history and increasing age appear to be associated with an increased risk of CVI.[1] Advancing age is also correlated with an increased prevalence of varicose veins[1] and venous leg ulceration.[6] While female gender has also been associated with an increased risk of varicose veins[1] and venous leg ulceration,[7] there is conflicting evidence regarding the link between sex and CVI risk.

DIFFERENTIAL DIAGNOSIS

- Cellulitis
- Congestive heart failure
- DVT
- Hepatic disease

- Hypothyroidism
- Idiopathic oedema
- Lymphoedema
- Renal disease

Adapted from Beebe-Dimmer et al. 2005,[1] Raju & Neglen[8]

CONVENTIONAL TREATMENT

There are a number of different approaches to managing CVI. Two approaches often recommended in conventional practice are compression therapy and surgery. Compression therapy is advocated in conventional practice because it helps to reduce leg oedema, venous reflux, venous hypertension and lipodermatosclerosis, while improving deep vein blood flow velocity, capillary clearance, calf-muscle pump function, venous refilling time and venous ejection volume.[8] Compression therapy targets a number of processes associated with the pathogenesis of venous insufficiency, with a meta-analysis of 11 randomised controlled trials (RCTs) ($n = 1453$) finding compression therapy (10–15 mmHg) to be significantly more effective than low-grade compression, placebo stockings and no treatment at reducing the symptoms of CVI, including lower limb oedema and discomfort.[9] These results need to be interpreted with caution, however, given the heterogeneous populations and diverse assessment techniques used in these studies. It is also possible that the reported effectiveness of compression therapy may not reflect that observed in clinical practice due to the poor level of compliance observed with this treatment. Some of the reasons for the poor adherence to compression therapy may relate to the long duration of therapy, the visible appearance of the stockings, associated discomfort, skin reactions and the cost and maintenance of the therapy.[10]

The surgical restoration or removal of diseased vessels also may be advised in the overall management of CVI. The array of surgical techniques that may be recommended include sclerotherapy, venous ligation and stripping, endovenous laser treatment, phlebectomy and valvuloplasty. Evidence from a meta-analysis of four RCTs suggests that venous ligation and valvuloplasty may be more effective than ligation alone in improving ambulatory venous pressure and quality of life, although these outcomes were only reported in one trial.[11] Another meta-analysis of three RCTs found subfascial endoscopic perforator vein surgery to be significantly more effective than conventional surgery at reducing venous ulcer recurrence, wound infection and length of hospital stay in patients with CVI.[12] It is not clear from either of these reviews, however, whether the benefits of these techniques outweigh the risks and costs of surgery, and whether these approaches are relatively more effective (both economically and clinically) than the conservative management of CVI.

KEY TREATMENT PROTOCOLS

One of the core principles of naturo-pathic practice is to identify the underlying aetiology of the presenting condition. While some measures may be put in place to prevent macrovascular injury (such as adequate hydration and mobilisation), prevention of venous insufficiency may not always be possible, given that many individuals only present to their practitioner after CVI is well established. The naturopath can, however, target a number of mechanisms to prevent further progression of venous insufficiency, including chronic inflammation, enzymatic degradation and oxidative damage.

> **Naturopathic Treatment Aims**
>
> - Identify the underlying cause of the venous insufficiency.
> - Improve venous vessel tone and integrity.
> - Improve venous haemodynamics.
> - Alleviate unpleasant symptoms of venous insufficiency.
> - Prevent further progression of venous insufficiency.
> - Educate the patient about appropriate lifestyle choices.

Enhance venous integrity

Enzymatic degradation

The abnormal venous tone observed in CVI may be linked to an increase in lysosomal enzyme activity, as evidenced by the elevated levels of these enzymes in patients with CVI[13] and in the exudate and wound bed of recalcitrant venous ulcers.[14,15] The lysosomal enzymes hyaluronidase and elastase are believed to be responsible for this extravascular and extracellular matrix degradation[16] and the subsequent increase in capillary permeability and oedema formation. It is therefore thought that a reduction in lysosomal enzyme activity could decrease the symptoms of CVI by restoring venous elasticity and contractility through improvements in collagen biosynthesis[12] and proteoglycan recovery.[16]

The saponins and sapogenins of **Hedera helix** and **Aesculus hippocastanum**[16] and the aerial parts of **Lythrum salicaria**[17] have been shown to inhibit hyaluronidase activity in vitro, whereas **Ruscus aculeatus** saponins,[16] rutin,[18] **grapeseed** procyanidins,[19] the lyophilised juice of **Cucumis sativus**[20] and the bark of *Aesculus hippocastanum*[17] have been found to inhibit elastase activity in vitro. By attenuating overactive lysosomal enzyme activity, these compounds may shift the equilibrium between proteoglycan synthesis and degradation, towards net synthesis. This reduction in enzyme activity against capillary wall mucopolysaccharides may improve vessel wall integrity and subsequently reduce oedema formation.[21–23] Although the saponins appear to be responsible for the anti-exudative and vascular-tightening effect of several of these plant extracts, the effect of other constituents (such as flavonoids and tannins) cannot be dismissed.

Oxidative damage

Another process implicated in the pathogenesis of CVI is oxidative injury. This process involves the peroxidation of venous lipids, production of oxygen free radicals[24,25] and consequent destruction of lipids, proteins, collagen, proteoglycan and hyaluronic acid.[26] Agents that exhibit significant antioxidant activity may interrupt this cascade of events and, as a result, preserve venous tissue and improve venous integrity.

Many phlebotonic agents exhibit good antioxidant activity in experimental models, particularly free radical scavenging activity, including **Aesculus hippocastanum** (**horse chestnut seed extract: HCSE**),[24] **Centella asiatica** flavonoids,[27] **Vaccinium myrtillus** extract,[28] grapeseed extract, pine bark extract,[29] quercetin, rutin[18,30] and **Vitis vinifera** leaf extracts.[31] When the active-oxygen scavenging activity of 65 plant extracts were compared in vitro, HCSE and **Hamamelis virginiana** demonstrated the greatest antioxidant activity. Both extracts were found to be more potent than ascorbic acid and α-tocopherol in scavenging superoxide anions, but less effective than ascorbic acid in scavenging hydroxyl radicals and inhibiting singlet-oxygen generation.[25] As an indicator of cell protection, Masaki et al.[25] explored the effect of plant extracts on fibroblast survival. HCSE, *Hamamelis virginiana* and **Quercus robur** were the most protective, increasing fibroblast survival at least threefold. As fibroblasts are a key source of collagen, elastin, proteoglycans and matrix metalloproteinases,[14] increasing fibroblast survival is likely to improve venous integrity.

There is a large body of evidence to support the use of HCSE in managing mild to moderate CVI. A Cochrane review of 17 RCTs found orally administered HCSE (standardised to 50–150 mg aescin daily and administered for 20 days to 16 weeks [mean = six weeks]) to be more effective than placebo and as effective as other phlebotonic agents at reducing leg pain, oedema, pruritus, leg volume and ankle and calf circumference in patients with mild to moderate CVI.[32] As for severe or advanced cases of CVI, it appears that HCSE may not be as effective.[33]

Reduce inflammation

Chronic inflammation is another contributing factor in developing CVI. It is thought that the manifestation of venous hypertension leads to widened capillary pore diameter, causing intravascular components such as fibrinogen, erythrocytes and α_2-macroglobulin to be leached into the interstitium.[4] These potent chemoattractants up-regulate the expression of intracellular adhesion molecule 1 (ICAM-1) and, together with increased platelet reactivity,[34] increase the expression of platelet-derived growth factor (PDGF) and vascular endothelial growth factor (VEGF). These growth factors trigger leucocyte migration. Once recruited, the white blood cells secrete or activate transforming growth factor-β_1 (TGF-β_1). Since TGF-β_1 has been located in pericapillary cuffs, it is believed that this growth factor may be responsible for tissue remodelling and fibrosis, as well as capillary angiogenesis, increased capillary tortuosity and density.[5] This factor may therefore contribute to some of the defining features of CVI, including varicose veins and lipodermatosclerosis. The increased expression of ICAM-1,[35-37] TGF-β_1,[38] PDGF and VEGF[39] in the dermis of patients with CVI lends some support to this sequelae of events.

Venotonic agents exhibiting anti-inflammatory activity may attenuate the progression of CVI through a number of different pathways. Aescin (from HCSE)[40] and *Ruscus aculeatus* extract,[41] for instance, both inhibit histamine-induced vascular permeability in vivo, an important step in the pathogenesis of CVI. Aescin,[40] grapeseed extract,[42] *Vaccinium myrtillus* anthocyanosides,[43] *Vaccinium corymbosum* extract[44] and *Centella asiatica* extract[45] have also been shown to inhibit carrageenan-induced paw oedema, another measure of acute anti-inflammatory activity. French maritime pine bark extract (**Pycnogenol**), on the other hand, exhibits anti-inflammatory activity by inhibiting nuclear factor kappa B (NFκB) and the pro-inflammatory cytokine interleukin-1 (IL-1),[46] whereas rutin and quercetin reduce inflammation by inhibiting the secretion of TNF-α, IL-1, IL-6, IL-8 and immunoglobulin E-induced histamine release.[47] **Other plant extracts** shown to markedly reduce macrophage-secreted TNF-α, IL-1 and IL-10 in vitro include *Malus domestica Borkh.*, *Laurus nobilis*, *Piper nigrum*, *Carum carvi*, *Cinnamomum cassia*, *Glycyrrhiza glabra*, *Myristica fragrans* and *Salvia officinalis*.[48] Apart from grapeseed extract,[49] few of these agents have yet been found to inhibit the key chemical mediators of CVI pathogenesis, including PDGF, VEGF, ICAM-1 and TGF-β_1.

The body of mechanistic data that supports many of these aforementioned treatments is supported by a growing body of clinical evidence. Many of these studies have, however, used complex formulations. This is problematic because it is almost impossible to extrapolate the effect of an individual agent from the effect of a complex formulation. Therefore, when reviewing the best available evidence for these treatments, only those studies using monopreparations were included (Table 13.1). In brief, evidence from RCTs indicates that: *Ruscus aculeatus* extract is statistically significantly superior to placebo in reducing leg volume, ankle and leg girth and leg heaviness, fatigue, paresthesia, feeling of swelling and tension[59]; *Centella asiatica* extract is significantly more effective than placebo at reducing ankle swelling,[60] leg pain,[61] heaviness and oedema[62]; Pycnogenol is significantly more effective than placebo or compression stockings alone at reducing leg heaviness and subcutaneous oedema[51-54]; and *Vitis vinifera* leaf extract is statistically significantly superior to placebo at reducing calf circumference[56,57] and lower limb volume and pain.[58]

INTEGRATIVE MEDICAL CONSIDERATIONS

The naturopathic management of CVI can be complemented by a range of conventional treatments including compression therapy and surgery. Both of these approaches have already been described in detail under 'conventional treatment'. In more advanced cases of venous insufficiency (such as venous leg ulceration), other health professionals will need to be involved in the patient's care, including a nurse (for wound management) and vascular surgeon (for clinical review, surgical intervention and/or monitoring of vascular function). Other interventions that may be integrated into the patient's management plan are massage and reflexology. While **massage** may help to alleviate venous congestion, and therefore may be theoretically justified as a treatment for CVI, there is still uncertainty about the safety and clinical effectiveness of massage in CVI. Other modalities for which clinical evidence of effectiveness is either lacking or insufficient include acupuncture, aromatherapy, chiropractic, homeopathy and osteopathy.

Reflexology

Reflexology is a tactile therapy that manipulates specific points in the hands, feet and/or ears to initiate a reflex or physiological response in distant organs and tissues. A single-blind RCT tested whether this treatment may be effective in CVI by randomly assigning 55 healthy pregnant women with foot oedema to one of three groups: relaxation foot reflexology, lymphatic foot reflexology and rest.[63] Up to four 15-minute treatments were provided, though the mean number of visits in each group was not clear. The study found no statistically significant difference between groups in mean ankle and foot circumference measurements over time. While all groups demonstrated a significant reduction in pain, discomfort and tiredness, it is not clear if these symptoms related to the pregnancy or to CVI specifically. Therefore, at this point in time, it is uncertain whether reflexology would be useful in alleviating the symptoms of venous insufficiency.

Dietary and lifestyle advice

Many lifestyle changes may be recommended for the management of CVI. However, much of this advice is based on theoretical or pathophysiological rationale. In fact, many lifestyle factors (smoking, obesity, constipation, physical inactivity) have not been shown conclusively to increase the risk of CVI. There is also insufficient evidence linking the modification of these risk factors to clinical improvements in venous insufficiency. There is weak evidence, however, to suggest that lower limb elevation, prescribed exercise and hydrotherapy may be helpful in CVI.[64]

Leg elevation is often recommended to people with CVI to help reduce lower limb venous pressure, leg discomfort and oedema. Although lower limb elevation (to 30 cm above heart level) has been shown to enhance microcirculatory flow velocity in liposclerotic skin of patients with CVI,[65] it is uncertain whether leg elevation offers any significant clinical benefit to patients with CVI. Given that many patients experience some relief of symptoms following lower limb elevation, there is no reason why this practice should not be recommended at this point in time.

A **structured exercise** program also may be recommended to individuals with CVI in order to facilitate calf-muscle pump function and reduce venous congestion. Findings from a small RCT ($n = 31$) have demonstrated that a supervised calf-muscle strength exercise program, together with compression hosiery, significantly improves mean venous ejection fraction at six months when compared with control. Between-group differences in venous reflux, venous severity scores and quality of life, however, were not statistically significant.[66] Nevertheless, given that long periods of standing may contribute to the pathogenesis of CVI, it is probable that a structured exercise program may still be useful in preventing the onset and/or progression of the disease.

Haemorrhoids

Overview

- Internal haemorrhoids are a complex of dilated blood vessels, including branches of the superior haemorrhoidal artery and veins of the internal haemorrhoidal venous plexus.
- The underlying causes of haemorrhoidal disease are similar to that of varicose veins.
- As the portal venous system contains no valves, factors that increase venous congestion in the region—including intraabdominal pressure from causes such as strained defecation, pregnancy, cirrhosis of the liver or standing or sitting for prolonged periods of time can hasten haemorrhoid formation.[67-69]
- Haemorrhoids are common and tend to develop between the ages of 20 and 50 years—in the Western world, they are extremely common and half of all people are likely to experience them by the time they reach 50 years of age.[69]
- Bleeding is the first and often only symptom of haemorrhoids. Other symptoms may include itching and irritation, prolapse, mucoid discharge, incomplete bowel evacuation and pain.

Conventional treatment

- *Surgery*. Treatment to remove haemorrhoids revolves around a number of surgical options, including rubber band ligation, cryotherapy, infrared coagulation, radiofrequency ablation and haemorrhoidectomy.[67-69] Notwithstanding, conventional management of haemorrhoids is becoming increasingly focused on prevention.
- *Diet*. One factor contributing to the exacerbation of haemorrhoids is constipation due to lack of fibre. Accordingly, conventional treatment centres around the promotion of a soft, bulky stool through dietary modification and/or supplementation.[68]
- *Pharmaceutical agents*. Topical treatment for pruritus ani or pain may be recommended, most often in the form of steroid or anaesthetic medication.[69]

CAM interventions

- *Fibre*. With overwhelming evidence to support increased fibre in the diet, appropriate dietary adjustments should be suggested. However, supplementation with bulking agents such as *Ulmus fulva* or *Plantago ovata* husks may also be beneficial. Not only is supplementation with *Plantago ovata* husks approved by Commission E for relieving constipation in haemorrhoids,[21] a meta-analysis of seven RCTs has found fibre (including *Plantago ovata*, sterculia and unprocessed bran) to be more effective than non-fibre controls at reducing overall haemorrhoidal symptoms and bleeding.[70]
- *Hydrotherapy*. A warm sitz bath may be an effective, non-invasive treatment for haemorrhoids, most likely due to mechanisms involving relaxation of the internal anal sphincter[71,72]; although, the evidence of effectiveness in support of this practice is not convincing.[73]
- *Herbal medicine (oral)*. The internal use of herbs for varicose veins and venous insufficiency as suggested earlier in the chapter are equally well indicated in restoring venous integrity in haemorrhoid treatment. Herbal medicines may be useful both internally and topically. Nonetheless, few trials of herbal or nutritional supplementation for haemorrhoids exist. In one double-blind, placebo-controlled trial, oral *Aesculus hippocastanum* (equivalent to 40 mg aescin three times daily) for six days or more was found to relieve symptoms (82% compared with 32% with placebo) and reduce swelling (87% versus 38% with placebo) in 72 patients with acute symptomatic haemorrhoids.[23] Similarly, an RCT of 84 subjects with acute haemorrhoidal episodes found oral Pycnogenol (300 mg daily for four days, then 150 mg daily for three days) to be significantly more effective than placebo at reducing overall haemorrhoidal symptom scores; this effect was further improved when oral Pycnogenol was administered concomitantly with topical (0.5%) Pycnogenol.[74] Findings from a registry study ($n = 49$) suggest pycnogenol may also be of benefit for women with postpartum symptomatic haemorrhoids; the study found the use of pycnogenol (150 mg/day for six months) in conjunction with best practice care to be more effective than best practice alone in reducing the signs and symptoms of haemorrhoids.[75]
- *Herbal medicine (topical)*. Topical therapy in most instances provides only temporary relief of symptoms. Astringent therapy may be beneficial in restoring venous tone and has been traditionally used for this purpose.[21,76] Astringent ointments containing *Hamamelis virginiana*, for instance, have been shown in clinical studies to be beneficial in alleviating the symptoms of haemorrhoids, demonstrating similar efficacy to conventional topical applications.[77,78] Other topical herbs that have traditionally been used include *Matricaria recutita* and *Calendula officinalis*.

Hydrotherapy shows some promise as a treatment for CVI. Evidence from two earlier RCTs indicates that the daily application of alternating hot and cold water to the bilateral lower limbs for a period of 24 days may significantly improve lower limb haemodynamics and the symptoms of varicose veins when compared with no-treatment controls.[79,80] However, these findings should be interpreted with caution as these trials were conducted by the same research team more than 20 years ago and the results have yet to be independently replicated. In another RCT, exposure to 18 days of 50-minute balneohydrotherapy (comprising Kneipp therapy, walking in a pool, underwater massage and bathing in a tub) plus 20 minutes rest was shown to be significantly more effective than usual care at improving CVI severity and quality of life in persons with moderate CVI.[81] However, given the complexity and duration of this therapy, and the need for specialised equipment, this therapy may have limited application in most naturopathic practices.

Dietary modification is a central feature of the naturopathic prescription. Even though there is a paucity of clinical evidence to justify dietary modification in CVI management, the potential benefit of this approach should not be overlooked. It is possible that many of the pathological processes of CVI, such as inflammation and oxidation, may be attenuated by reducing the dietary intake of saturated, omega-6 and *trans*-fatty acids, and by increasing the consumption of foods high in omega-3 fatty acids (such as salmon), flavonoids (such as onion) and procyanidins (such as berries).

CLINICAL SUMMARY

For a person presenting with CVI, it is unlikely that this chronic condition will ever be cured. The naturopathic treatment approach (Figure 13.2) may, however, prevent further progression of the disease by attenuating the pathogenesis of CVI and, in turn, prevent the development of more serious pathologies, including varicose veins and venous leg ulceration.

Once the underlying causes of the CVI have been identified, and measures introduced to address the causes (where possible), the naturopath should focus their attention on the pathological processes of the disease. Agents with venotonic activity, as well as anti-oxidant, anti-inflammatory, antienzymatic and antioedema effects, are most desirable in this case. Interventions that exhibit more than one of these actions and, more importantly, have demonstrable clinical efficacy in patients with CVI should be afforded the highest priority in the naturopathic management of venous insufficiency. Examples of interventions that fulfil these criteria include HCSE, *Ruscus aculeatus*, *Vaccinium myrtillus*, *Centella asiatica*, French maritime pine bark extract, red vine leaf extract and grapeseed extract. Other herbs with purported venotonic effects for which clinical evidence is currently insufficient include *Ginkgo biloba* and *Melilotus officinalis*. Data from mechanistic[30,47] and in vivo studies[64] also suggest a possible role for mixed bioflavonoid supplementation in the management of CVI; though this is based on theoretical evidentiary support only, with clinical evidence currently lacking.

In summary, if the patient adheres to the naturopathic treatment plan (herbal and nutritional prescriptions, and dietary and lifestyle advice), a clinically significant reduction in CVI manifestations (such as leg heaviness, discomfort and oedema) should be evident within four weeks. If no clinical improvement is observed after 12 weeks, the patient should be referred to a vascular surgeon for review.

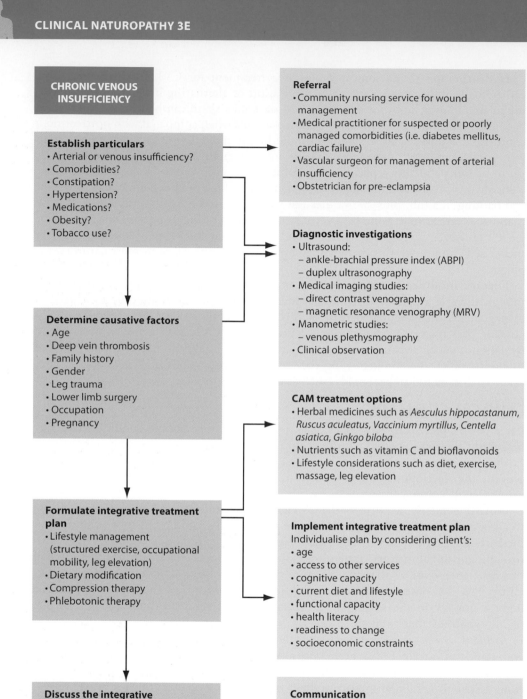

CHRONIC VENOUS INSUFFICIENCY

Establish particulars
- Arterial or venous insufficiency?
- Comorbidities?
- Constipation?
- Hypertension?
- Medications?
- Obesity?
- Tobacco use?

Determine causative factors
- Age
- Deep vein thrombosis
- Family history
- Gender
- Leg trauma
- Lower limb surgery
- Occupation
- Pregnancy

Formulate integrative treatment plan
- Lifestyle management (structured exercise, occupational mobility, leg elevation)
- Dietary modification
- Compression therapy
- Phlebotonic therapy

Discuss the integrative treatment plan
- Communicate with client clearly and honestly
- Engage with client in a participative manner
- Communicate with pertinent members of the healthcare team

Referral
- Community nursing service for wound management
- Medical practitioner for suspected or poorly managed comorbidities (i.e. diabetes mellitus, cardiac failure)
- Vascular surgeon for management of arterial insufficiency
- Obstetrician for pre-eclampsia

Diagnostic investigations
- Ultrasound:
  - ankle-brachial pressure index (ABPI)
  - duplex ultrasonography
- Medical imaging studies:
  - direct contrast venography
  - magnetic resonance venography (MRV)
- Manometric studies:
  - venous plethysmography
- Clinical observation

CAM treatment options
- Herbal medicines such as *Aesculus hippocastanum*, *Ruscus aculeatus*, *Vaccinium myrtillus*, *Centella asiatica*, *Ginkgo biloba*
- Nutrients such as vitamin C and bioflavonoids
- Lifestyle considerations such as diet, exercise, massage, leg elevation

Implement integrative treatment plan
Individualise plan by considering client's:
- age
- access to other services
- cognitive capacity
- current diet and lifestyle
- functional capacity
- health literacy
- readiness to change
- socioeconomic constraints

Communication
Discuss:
- treatment options
- client expectations
- client preferences
- safety of treatment
- efficacy of treatment
- rationale for treatment plan
- implications of untreated CVI

Figure 13.2
Naturopathic treatment decision tree—chronic venous insufficiency

Table 13.1
Review of the major evidence

Intervention	Mechanisms of action	Key literature	Summary of results	Comment
Centella asiatica	*Centella asiatica* has a range of activities that may be beneficial in CVI, including: antioxidant[22] and anti-inflammatory[45] properties	Systematic review: Chong & Aziz 2013[50]	Extracts of *Centella asiatica* (60–180 mg/day for 4–8 weeks) were more effective than placebo at reducing ankle swelling and lower leg pain, heaviness and oedema	It is not yet clear if the long-term use of high-dose *Centella asiatica* is safe or effective in CVI
Pycnogenol	Has a range of activities that may be beneficial in CVI including antioxidant,[29] inhibition of pro-oxidative enzymes[51] and anti-inflammatory[46] effects	Clinical trials: Arcangeli 2000[52] Cesarone et al. 2010[53] Petrassi et al. 2000[54] Schoonees et al. 2012[51]	Pycnogenol (300 mg/day) was more effective than placebo/compression stockings alone at reducing leg heaviness and subcutaneous oedema at eight weeks	Changes in venous haemodynamics were not consistent between the two studies Overall, findings are inconclusive due to the small sample sizes and wide confidence intervals
Aeculus hippocastanum	Inhibits hyaluronidase activity[13] and has antioxidant[24] and antiinflammatory[40] properties	Cochrane review: Pittler & Ernst 2006[32]	*Aesculus hippocastanum* (standardised to 50–150 mg aescin daily and administered for 20 days to 16 weeks) was more effective than placebo, and as effective as other phlebotonic agents, at reducing leg pain, oedema, pruritus, leg volume and ankle and calf circumference in patients with mild to moderate CVI	The saponins in *Aesculus hippocastanum* may cause gastric irritation and/or nausea in some individuals Enteric-coated *Aesculus hippocastanum* formulations may reduce the risk of these adverse events
Vitis vinifera leaf extract	Antioxidant[31] and vasoprotective properties; also facilitates endothelial repair[55]	Clinical trials: Kalus et al. 2004[56] Kiesewetter et al. 2000[57] Rabe et al. 2011[58]	Red vine leaf extract (360–720 mg/day) was more effective than placebo at reducing calf circumference/volume at 6–12 weeks	Changes in ankle circumference were reported in two studies,[56,57] but findings were not consistent
Ruscus aculeatus	Inhibits elastase activity[16] and has antiinflammatory[41] properties	Systematic review: Kakkos & Allaert 2017[59]	*Ruscus aculeatus* extract (varied dosages, for 2–14 weeks) was more effective than placebo at reducing leg volume, ankle and leg girth and leg heaviness, fatigue, paresthesia and tension at 12 weeks	Dosage and type of extract were not clearly reported in all studies, making translation to practice difficult

KEY POINTS

- CVI is a chronic and often disabling disorder of the lower limbs.
- The treatment of CVI should focus primarily on addressing and resolving the underlying cause and pathological processes of the condition.
- The naturopathic management of CVI should give preference to agents with venotonic, anti-inflammatory, antioxidant, antienzymatic and antioedema activity, particularly those with demonstrable clinical efficacy in patients with CVI.
- Patients with advanced CVI should be referred for compression therapy, surgery, wound management and/or further assessment where applicable.

FURTHER READING

Pittler MH, Ernst E. Horse chestnut seed extract for chronic venous insufficiency. Cochrane Database Syst Rev 2012;(11):CD003230.

Santler B, Goerge T. Chronic venous insufficiency—a review of pathophysiology, diagnosis, and treatment. J Dtsch Dermatol Ges 2017;15(5):538–56.

Shammas NW. Management of chronic venous insufficiency. In: Bhatt DL, editor. Cardiovascular intervention: a companion to Braunwald's heart disease. Philadelphia: Elsevier; 2016.

REFERENCES

1. Beebe-Dimmer JL, et al. The epidemiology of chronic venous insufficiency and varicose veins. Ann Epidemiol 2005;15:175–84.
2. Vuylsteke ME, Colman R, Thomis S, et al. An epidemiological survey of venous disease among general practitioner attendees in different geographical regions on the globe: the final results of the Vein Consult Program. Angiology 2018;[Epub ahead of print].
3. Chiesa R, Marone EM, Limoni C, et al. Effect of chronic venous insufficiency on activities of daily living and quality of life: correlation of demographic factors with duplex ultrasonography findings. Angiology 2007;58(4):440–9.
4. Leach MJ. Making sense of the venous leg ulcer debate: a literature review. J Wound Care 2004;13(2):52–7.
5. Deoranie N, et al. Pathogenesis of varicose veins and cellular pathophysiology of chronic venous insufficiency. In: Gloviczki P, editor. Handbook of venous and lymphatic disorders: guidelines of the American Venous Forum. 4th ed. Boca Raton, Florida: Taylor & Francis; 2017.
6. Margolis DJ, Bilker W, Santanna J, et al. Venous leg ulcer: incidence and prevalence in the elderly. J Am Acad Dermatol 2002;46(3):381–6.
7. Callam M, et al. Chronic ulcer of the leg: clinical history. BMJ 1987;294(6584):1389–91.
8. Raju S, Neglen P. Chronic venous insufficiency and varicose veins. N Engl J Med 2009;360(22):2319–27.
9. Amsler F, Blattler W. Compression therapy for occupational leg symptoms and chronic venous disorders—a meta-analysis of randomised controlled trials. Eur J Vasc Endovasc Surg 2008;35(3):366–72.
10. Raju S, et al. Use of compression stockings in chronic venous disease: patient compliance and efficacy. Ann Vasc Surg 2008;21(6):790–5.
11. Goel RR, Abidia A, Hardy SC. Surgery for deep venous incompetence. Cochrane Database Syst Rev 2015;(2):CD001097.
12. Luebke T, Brunkwall J. Meta-analysis of subfascial endoscopic perforator vein surgery (SEPS) for chronic venous insufficiency. Phlebology 2009;24(1):8–16.
13. Kreysel H, et al. A possible role of lysosomal enzymes in the pathogenesis of varicosis and the reduction in their serum activity by Venostasin. VASA 1983;12(4):377–82.
14. Schultz G, Mast B. Molecular analysis of the environment of healing and chronic wounds: cytokines, proteases, and growth factors. Wounds 1998;10(Suppl.F):1F–9F.
15. Moor AN, Vachon DJ, Gould LJ. Proteolytic activity in wound fluids and tissues derived from chronic venous leg ulcers. Wound Repair Regen 2009;17(6):832–9.
16. Facino R, et al. Anti-elastase and anti-hyaluronidase activities of saponins and sapogenins from Hedera helix, Aesculus hippocastanum, and Ruscus aculeatus: factors contributing to their efficacy in the treatment of venous insufficiency. Arch Pharm 1995;328(10):720–4.
17. Piwowarski JP, Kiss AK, Kozłowska-Wojciechowska M. Anti-hyaluronidase and anti-elastase activity screening of tannin-rich plant materials used in traditional Polish medicine for external treatment of diseases with inflammatory background. J Ethnopharmacol 2011;137(1):937–41.
18. Makarenko O, Levitsky A. Biochemical mechanisms of therapeutic and prophylactic effects of bioflavonoids. J Pharm Pharmacol 2016;4:451–6.
19. Carini M, et al. Procyanidins from Vitis vinifera seeds inhibit the respiratory burst of activated human neutrophils and lysosomal enzyme release. Planta Med 2001;67(8):714–17.
20. Nema NK, Maity N, Sarkar B, et al. Cucumis sativus fruit—potential antioxidant, anti-hyaluronidase, and anti-elastase agent. Arch Dermatol Res 2011;303(4):247–52.
21. Blumenthal M, editor. The complete German Commission E monographs: therapeutic guide to herbal medicines. Austin: American Botanical Council; 1998.
22. Thomson Healthcare. PDR for herbal medicines. 4th ed. Montvale: Thomson Reuters; 2007.
23. Sirtori C. Aescin: pharmacology, pharmacokinetics and therapeutic profile. Pharmacol Res 2001;44(3):183–93.
24. Guillaume M, Padioleau F. Veinotonic effect, vascular protection, antiinflammatory and free radical scavenging

properties of horse chestnut extract. Arzneimittelforschung 1994;44(1):25–35.

25. Masaki H, et al. Active-oxygen scavenging activity of plant extracts. Biol Pharm Bull 1995;18(1):162–6.

26. Yeoh S. The influence of iron and free radicals on chronic leg ulceration. Prim Inten 2000;8(2):47–55.

27. Zheng CJ, Qin LP. Chemical components of Centella asiatica and their bioactivities. Chin J Integr Med 2007;5(3):348–51.

28. Faria A, et al. Antioxidant properties of prepared blueberry (Vaccinium myrtillus) extracts. J Agric Food Chem 2005;53(17):6896–902.

29. Busserolles J, et al. In vivo antioxidant activity of procyanidin-rich extracts from grape seed and pine (Pinus maritima) bark in rats. Int J Vitam Nutr Res 2006;76(1):22–7.

30. Zhang J, et al. Free radical scavenging and cytoprotective activities of phenolic antioxidants. Mol Nutr Food Res 2006;50(11):996–1005.

31. Katalinic V, Mozina SS, Generalic I, et al. Phenolic profile, antioxidant capacity, and antimicrobial activity of leaf extracts from six vitis vinifera L. Varieties. Int J Food Properties 2013;16(1):45–60.

32. Pittler MH, Ernst E. Horse chestnut seed extract for chronic venous insufficiency. Cochrane Database Syst Rev 2013;(11):CD003230.

33. Leach MJ, et al. Clinical efficacy of horsechestnut seed extract in the treatment of venous ulceration. J Wound Care 2006;15(4):159–67.

34. Lu X, Chen Y, Huang Y, et al. Venous hypertension induces increased platelet reactivity and accumulation in patients with chronic venous insufficiency. Angiology 2006;57(3):321–9.

35. Ciuffetti G, et al. Circulating leucocyte adhesion molecules in chronic venous insufficiency. VASA 1999;28(3):156–9.

36. Peschen M, et al. Expression of the adhesion molecules ICAM-1, VCAM-1, LFA-1 and VLA-4 in the skin is modulated in progressing stages of chronic venous insufficiency. Acta Derm Venereol 1999;79(1):27–32.

37. Wilkinson LS, et al. Leukocytes: their role in the etiopathogenesis of skin damage in venous disease. J Vasc Surg 1993;17:669–75.

38. Pappas PJ, et al. Dermal tissue fibrosis in patients with chronic venous insufficiency is associated with increased transforming growth factor-β1 gene expression and protein production. J Vasc Surg 1999;30(6):1129–45.

39. Peschen M, et al. Increased expression of platelet-derived growth factor receptor alpha and beta and vascular endothelial growth factor in the skin of patients with chronic venous insufficiency. Arch Dermatol Res 1998;290(6):291–7.

40. Matsuda H, et al. Effects of escins Ia, Ib, IIa, and IIB from Horse chestnut, the seeds of Aesculus hippocastanum L., on acute inflammation in animals. Biol Pharm Bull 1997;20(10):1092–5.

41. Bouskela E, et al. Possible mechanisms for the inhibitory effect of Ruscus extract on increased microvascular permeability induced by histamine in hamster cheek pouch. J Cardiovasc Pharmacol 1994;24(2):281–5.

42. Greenspan P, et al. Antiinflammatory properties of the muscadine grape (Vitis rotundifolia). J Agric Food Chem 2005;53(22):8481–8.

43. Lietti A, et al. Studies on Vaccinium myrtillus anthocyanosides. I. Vasoprotective and antiinflammatory activity. Arzneimittelforschung 1976;26(5):829–32.

44. Torri E, Lemos M, Caliari V, et al. Anti-inflammatory and antinociceptive properties of blueberry extract (Vaccinium corymbosum). J Pharm Pharmacol 2007;59(4):591–6.

45. George M, Joseph L, Ramaswamy. Anti-allergic, anti-pruritic, and anti-inflammatory activities of centella asiatica extracts. Afr J Tradit Complement Altern Med 2009;6(4):554–9.

46. Cho KJ, et al. Effect of bioflavonoids extracted from the bark of Pinus maritima on proinflammatory cytokine interleukin-1 production in lipopolysaccharide-stimulated RAW 264.7. Toxicol Appl Pharmacol 2000;168(1):64–71.

47. Park HH, et al. Flavonoids inhibit histamine release and expression of pro-inflammatory cytokines in mast cells. Arch Pharm Res 2008;31(10):1303–11.

48. Mueller M, Hobiger S, Jungbauer A. Anti-inflammatory activity of extracts from fruits, herbs and spices. Food Chem 2010;122(4):987–96.

49. Wen W, et al. Grape seed extract inhibits angiogenesis via suppression of the vascular endothelial growth factor receptor signalling pathway. Cancer Prev Res (Phila) 2008;1(7):554–61.

50. Chong NJ, Aziz Z. A systematic review of the efficacy of Centella asiatica for improvement of the signs and symptoms of chronic venous insufficiency. Evid Based Complement Alternat Med 2013;2013:627182.

51. Schoonees A, Visser J, Musekiwa A, et al. Pycnogenol (extract of French maritime pine bark) for the treatment of chronic disorders. Cochrane Database Syst Rev 2012;(4):CD008294.

52. Arcangeli P. Pycnogenol in chronic venous insufficiency. Fitoterapia 2000;71(3):236–44.

53. Cesarone MR, et al. Improvement of signs and symptoms of chronic venous insufficiency and microangiopathy with Pycnogenol: a prospective, controlled study. Phytomedicine 2010;17(11):835–9.

54. Petrassi C, et al. Pycnogenol in chronic venous insufficiency. Phytomedicine 2000;7(5):383–8.

55. Nees S, et al. Protective effects of flavonoids contained in the red vine leaf on venular endothelium against the attack of activated blood components in vitro. Arzneimittelforschung 2003;53(5):330–41.

56. Kalus U, et al. Improvement of cutaneous microcirculation and oxygen supply in patients with chronic venous insufficiency by orally administered extract of red vine leaves AS 195: a randomised, double-blind, placebo-controlled, crossover study. Drugs R D 2004;5(2):63–71.

57. Kiesewetter H, et al. Efficacy of orally administered extract of red vine leaf AS 195 (folia vitis viniferae) in chronic venous insufficiency (stages I-II). A randomized, double-blind, placebo-controlled trial. Arzneimittelforschung 2000;50(2):109–17.

58. Rabe E, Stücker M, Esperester A, et al. Efficacy and tolerability of a red-vine-leaf extract in patients suffering from chronic venous insufficiency—results of a double-blind placebo-controlled study. Eur J Vasc Endovasc Surg 2011;41(4):540–7.

59. Kakkos SK, Allaert FA. Efficacy of Ruscus extract, HMC and vitamin C, constituents of Cyclo 3 fort, on improving individual venous symptoms and edema: a systematic review and meta-analysis of randomized double-blind placebo-controlled trials. Int Angiol 2017;36(2):93–106.

60. De Sanctis MT, et al. Treatment of edema and increased capillary filtration in venous hypertension with total triterpenic fraction of Centella asiatica: a clinical, prospective, placebo-controlled, randomized, dose-ranging trial. Angiology 2001;52(Suppl. 2):S55–9.

61. Cesarone MR, et al. Microcirculatory effects of total triterpenic fraction of Centella asiatica in chronic venous hypertension: measurement by laser Doppler, TcPO2–CO2, and leg volumetry. Angiology 2001;52(Suppl. 2):S45–8.

62. Pointel JP, et al. Titrated extract of Centella asiatica (TECA) in the treatment of venous insufficiency of the lower limbs. Angiology 1987;38(1 Pt 1):46–50.

63. Mollart L. Single-blind trial addressing the differential effects of two reflexology techniques versus rest, on ankle and foot oedema in late pregnancy. Complement Ther Nurs Midwifery 2003;9(4):203–8.

64. Ivanov IS, et al. Antioxidant composition causes antiexsudorific effect in the model of chronic venous insufficiency. Bull Exp Biol Med 2011;152(1):25–7.

65. Abu-Own A, et al. Effect of leg elevation on the skin microcirculation in chronic venous insufficiency. J Vasc Surg 1994;20(5):705–10.

66. Padberg FT, et al. Structured exercise improves calf muscle pump function in chronic venous insufficiency: a randomized trial. J Vasc Surg 2004;39(1):79–87.

67. Lohsiriwat V. Hemorrhoids: from basic pathophysiology to clinical management. World J Gastroenterol 2012;18(17):2009–17.

68. Acheson AG, Scholefield JH. Management of haemorrhoids. BMJ 2008;336(7640):380–3.

69. Murtagh J. General practice. 6th ed. Sydney: McGraw-Hill; 2015.

70. Alonso-Coello P, et al. Laxatives for the treatment of haemorrhoids. Cochrane Database Syst Rev 2005;(4):CD004649.

71. Shafik A. Role of warm-water bath in anorectal conditions. The 'thermosphincteric reflex'. J Clin Gastroenterol 1993;16(4):304–8.

72. Shirah BH, Shirah HA. Fallata AH, et al. Hemorrhoids during pregnancy: sitz bath vs. ano-rectal cream: a comparative prospective study of two conservative treatment protocols. Women Birth 2017;[Epub ahead of print].

73. Ping DL, Chi TP, Li GM, et al. The effectiveness of sitz bath in managing adult patients with anorectal disorders: a systematic review. JBI Reports 2010;8(11):447–69.

74. Belcaro G, et al. Pycnogenol treatment of acute hemorrhoidal episodes. Phytother Res 2010;24(3):438–44.

75. Belcaro G, et al. Pycnogenol in postpartum symptomatic haemorrhoids. Minerva Ginecol 2014;66(1):77–84.

76. Scientific Committee of the British Herbal Medical Association: British herbal pharmacopoeia, 1983, Bournemouth: British Herbal Medicine Association.

77. Drug therapy of hemorrhoids: proven results of therapy with a hamamelis containing hemorrhoid ointment. Results of a meeting of experts. Fortschr Med 1991;116(Suppl.):1–11.

78. Knoch HG, et al. Ointment treatment of 1st degree hemorrhoids: comparison of the effectiveness of a phytogenic preparation with two new ointments containing synthetic drugs. Fortschr Med 1992;110(8):135–8.

79. Ernst E, Saradeth T, Resch KL. A single blind randomized, controlled trial of hydrotherapy for varicose veins. VASA 1991;20(2):147–52.

80. Ernst E, Saradeth T, Resch KL. Hydrotherapy for varicose veins: a randomized, controlled trial. Phlebology 1992;7(4):154–7.

81. Forestier RJ, Briancon G, Francon A, et al. Balneohydrotherapy in the treatment of chronic venous insufficiency. VASA. 2014;43:365–71.

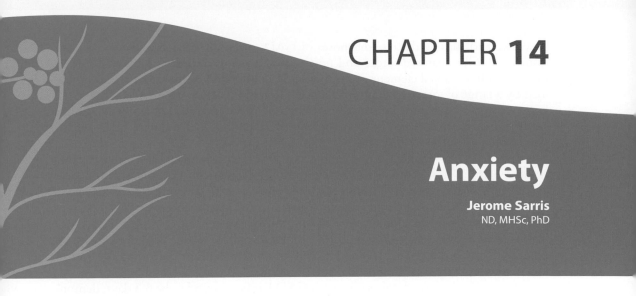

CHAPTER **14**

Anxiety

Jerome Sarris
ND, MHSc, PhD

OVERVIEW

Generalised anxiety disorder (GAD) is diagnosed in people with excessive worry and anxiety, which the person finds difficult to control. Somatic complaints and sleeping problems often accompany the anxiety. According to the *Diagnostic and Statistical Manual of Mental Disorders* (DSM-5) diagnostic criteria, in addition to uncontrollable worrying, there must also be at least three of six somatic symptoms (restlessness, fatigue, concentration problems, irritability, tension or sleep disturbance) occurring for a period of at least six months.[1] For a diagnosis of GAD to be reached, significant distress or impaired functioning from the condition must be present. As in major depressive disorder (MDD), a number of exclusion criteria must also be ruled out (e.g. symptoms must not be confined to features of another mental disorder or due to substance use or general medical conditions).

Occasional worry and situational anxiety is a normal human experience; true chronic generalised anxiety is a disorder whereby the worrying becomes self-perpetuating and uncontrollable, has a number of distressing somatic features and causes marked impairment of work or social functioning. It should be noted that the diagnosis of GAD is fairly restrictive in terms of the requirement of a long duration and multiple somatic symptoms. As the condition commonly waxes and wanes, the DSM-5 diagnosis may be excessively restrictive in clinical practice.[2] A utilitarian diagnosis may involve a period of anxiety or worry that is bothersome to the patient and has occurred for longer than two weeks. It is also worth considering that in some people GAD may reflect 'trait anxiety'— that is, a person whose personality archetype is that of a chronic worrier.

Anxiety disorders are second only to MDD as the most commonly diagnosed psychiatric conditions in primary care.[3] As a whole diagnostic entity, anxiety disorders are prevalent and affect marked societal suffering and economic cost.[4,5] In 2007 the Australian Bureau of Statistics National Survey of Mental Health and Wellbeing[6] approximated that around one in seven Australians suffer from an anxiety disorder at any one time, with women being almost twice as likely as men to experience a disorder, being most prevalent between the ages of 16 and 54 years.[6] Anxiety disorders are ubiquitous and persistent, usually have an early onset and are highly comorbid with affective disorders and substance misuse.[7] Anxiety disorders as a collective entity are pervasive and include discrete diagnoses of GAD, social phobia, obsessive-compulsive disorder (OCD), panic disorder and post-traumatic stress disorder.[1] Anxiety disorders present with a marked element of psychological tension and distress, and are accompanied by a range of somatic symptoms such as palpitations, shortness of breath, dizziness, hyperthermia and digestive disturbance.[1] Lifetime prevalence rates of anxiety disorders are approximately 3–6% for GAD, 4–6% for social phobia, 1–3% for OCD, 1–2% for post-traumatic stress disorder and 1–3% for panic disorder.[8,9]

In respect to GAD, the data reveal high or very high psychological distress is experienced by 53.2% of people with the condition.[10] People with GAD may also not be able to fully participate in the labour force and this has individual impacts on a person's income, in addition to wider economic impacts and negative effects on social participation and self-esteem. One recent estimate found that 55.1% of people with GAD had used services for their mental health problems in the previous 12 months, with an estimated cost in Australia at more than $20 billion per annum (including the cost of loss of productivity and labour force participation).[10] The average number of days per month out of role or work for people with GAD has been found to be 6.3 days, demonstrating that this condition needs to be assertively treated.[10]

Anxiety symptoms are endemic in depression, and true comorbidity of depressive and anxious conditions commonly occurs.[11] Studies have revealed that approximately 60–80% of patients with GAD will suffer from a mood disorder within their lifetime.[12] Comorbidity of GAD with other anxiety disorders is the rule, not the exception. Other psychiatric disorders such as depression (unipolar and bipolar), social phobia, panic disorder, OCD, post-traumatic stress disorder and attention deficit hyperactivity disorder (ADHD) commonly co-exist.[13,14]

Mental disorders co-occurring with GAD

Unipolar depression: Persistent low mood or lack of pleasure in combination with changes in sleep patterns, appetite, self-esteem, sexual drive, motivation and possible suicidal ideation.

Bipolar (hypo)mania: Hypomania—a distinct period of elevated, expansive or irritable mood lasting fewer than four days in addition to an increase in signs such as self-esteem/goal-oriented, activity/grandiosity/pleasurable activities, and reduced need for sleep. Mania—the previous signs plus possible hospitalisation, psychotic features, marked social impairment.

Social phobia: Significant anxiety provoked by exposure to social or performance situations, leading to avoidance of social situations.

Panic disorder: Regular experience of panic attacks (acute anxiety and fear with signs and symptoms such as tachycardia, sweating, rapid breathing, fear of 'losing control' and persistent worry about another panic attack occurring). This causes distress and interferes with social and work functioning.

OCD: Persistent chronic compulsive or obsessive thoughts or activities. Compulsions cause anxiety and are allayed by repetitive actions. It must cause distress and social or work impairment, be noticeable by others and be time consuming.

ADHD: Several signs of inattention, hyperactivity and/or impulsiveness such as poor focus, poor self-control, difficulty sitting still and difficulty controlling speech. Must first occur before the age of seven years.

Source: Abstracted from DSM-5 diagnostic criteria[1]

DIFFERENTIAL DIAGNOSIS

- Anxiety symptoms from medications
- Other psychiatric disorders
- Alcoholism or substance misuse
- Hyperthyroidism

RISK FACTORS

Several risk factors and protective factors exist for GAD (Figure 14.1). The primary risk factor for developing GAD appears to be genetic.[15] Significant familial aggregation also exists, with a strong correlation between the sufferer and a first-order relative with the disorder.[16] An anxiogenic familial environment appears also to contribute to the development of the pathology, although the data suggest that genetics are the dominant factor.[17] Women are twice more likely to experience GAD than men, and a diagnosis of GAD is uncommon in children and adolescents with the incidence of GAD greatly increasing later in life (onset is usually after 25 years of age).[16] As discussed above, comorbidity with depression is common, so it is salient to do a screening for GAD when depressive symptomatology is present. The diagnosis of GAD may be seen as a risk factor for developing these other psychiatric disorders and also of alcohol and substance abuse disorders.[18] People with alcohol or substance use disorders are more likely to develop an anxiety disorder,[19] and there appears to be a bidirectional relationship in that people with clinical anxiety may increase alcohol misuse or abuse.

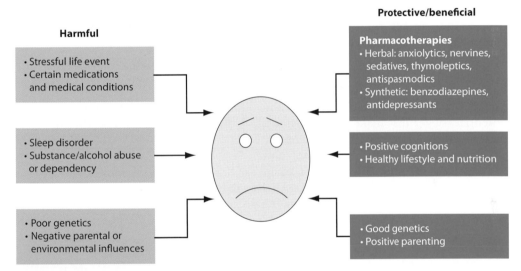

Figure 14.1
Anxiety: harmful and beneficial factors

Adapted from Kessler et al. 2010[13] and Tyrer & Baldwin 2006[17]

CONVENTIONAL TREATMENT

Medical treatment of anxiety disorders primarily focuses on pharmaceutical and psychological interventions. Pharmacotherapies include synthetic anxiolytics (e.g. benzodiazepines, pregabalin, beta-blockers and buspirone) and antidepressants (e.g. tricyclics, monoamine oxidase inhibitors [MAOIs] and selective serotonin reuptake inhibitors [SSRIs] or serotonin–noradrenaline reuptake inhibitors [SNRIs]).[20] Current evidence supports the use of both antidepressants and benzodiazepines, with some studies indicating that paroxetine and venlafaxine are the preferable choices. Several issues are present with respect to treating anxiety disorders with benzodiazepines. Common side effects include sedation, motor disturbance and cognitive interference (due to GABA-$\alpha_{1,2}$ agonism), while long-term treatment (more than two weeks) may cause dependence and withdrawal issues.[21] Abrupt cessation of benzodiazepines may cause rebound symptoms such as insomnia, agitation and digestive disturbance, and the patient's anxiety may return to an even higher level than before treatment. There are currently various effective psychological therapies and pharmacological treatments available for anxiety disorders. The recommended first-line treatment strategies for most anxiety disorders include antidepressants and/or cognitive behaviour therapy (CBT).[22] Combination approaches using psychological and pharmacotherapy treatments are commonly recommended; also, evidentiary support does not currently endorse this approach over using each as a monotherapy.[22] The combination does, however, seem to make sense, as pharmacotherapies such as benzodiazepines (or natural alternatives such as *Piper methysticum*) may elicit an immediate benefit while psychology techniques have been shown to lessen the chance of relapse over the long term.[17,22]

KEY TREATMENT PROTOCOLS

As outlined in the box on the right, anxiety disorders need to be treated both symptom-atically and systemically (as in the case of depression). Initially, thorough case taking is necessary to determine the causes, onset and duration of the episode, the level of impairment, comorbidities and their individual presentation. With respect to causes, practitioners should ask about any potential trigger that makes them anxious, their cognitive state and any potentially anxiogenic factors—caffeine, alcohol and illicit drugs, pharmaceuticals, poor sleep pattern or excessive work-to-rest ratio. Anxiety-reducing herbal pharmacotherapies may be useful as an initial treatment to ameliorate anxiety. See Table 14.1 for an evidence summary on integrative treatments for anxiety.

> ### Naturopathic Treatment Aims
>
> - Reduce anxiety, worrying, and somatic symptoms.
> - Support and normalise adrenal function.
> - Regulate hypothalamic–pituitary–adrenal (HPA) axis activity.
> - Teach 'worry management' techniques.
> - Encourage stress management via lifestyle changes.
> - Improve diet and reduce stimulants.
> - Prevent or lessen chance of relapsing anxiety.

Placebo response

Placebo response is endemic in sufferers of anxiety, with approximately 25% receiving marked benefit from a placebo (dummy) intervention!

Psychological intervention might also be beneficial by working on interpersonal and behavioural skills and eliminating anxiogenic self-talk. It is also worth noting that a depressive phase often occurs after an episode of GAD,[47] so patient education and prevention strategies are vital. The final main protocol in treating GAD is to educate the patient about self-help interventions they can use to better manage their stress. The use of bibliotherapy, massage, aromatherapy and exercise, and the adoption of calming euthymic activities or hobbies, may also be beneficial (these are reviewed on the following pages). While individually each of the aforementioned interventions may possess limited evidence, or have a small clinical effect, the use of many of these self-help techniques in the context of an overall lifestyle pattern may provide a sustained beneficial effect.

Although the goal is to use evidence-based treatments, it is encouraging to know that any therapeutic interface will commonly promote an anxiolytic effect. Evidence reveals that sufferers of GAD commonly experience other presentations of anxiety such as panic attacks and social phobias.[18] Because of this, thorough case taking needs to be employed to assess for any comorbidities. Panic attacks are a severe manifestation of anxiety and their co-occurrence with GAD or MDD indicates a more severe condition, resulting in a potentially poorer prognosis and more demanding treatment protocol. In the case of comorbid social phobia, behavioural and interpersonal issues need to be explored via an appropriate psychological intervention. As detailed below, several theories and models exist.

GABA pathway modulation

The key biological pathway involved in presenting and modulating anxiety disorders involves gamma aminobutyric acid (GABA).[17] GABAergic neurons and receptors are involved in the main mode of inhibitory transmission in the central nervous system, and these innervations densely occupy parts of the anxiety/fear-modulating corticolimbic system such as the hippocampus and amygdala.[48] GABA-α receptors are the principal target of benzodiazepines, exerting affects such as anxiolysis, sedation and anticonvulsant effects.[49] Stimulation of GABAergic pathways also modulates the release of several key neurochemicals (e.g. noradrenaline, serotonin and dopamine), although the exact effects are still disputed. A range of herbal medicines may exert GABA-modulating activity. Reviews of **herbal medicines with anxiolytic GABAergic activity** included *Scutellaria lateriflora, Ziziphus jujuba, Valeriana officinalis, Damiana diffusa, Magnolia* spp., *Euphorbia hirta, Eschscholzia californica, Crocus sativus, Citrus aurantium, Matricaria recutita, Melissa officinalis, Passiflora incarnata, Piper methysticum* and *Withania somnifera*.[50–52] Valerenic acid from *Valeriana officinalis* has demonstrated GABA-A receptor (β_3 subunit) agonism; this mechanism has been identified as an important pharmacodynamic action responsible for the plant's anxiolytic and hypnotic action.[53]

The phytotherapy that has received the greatest attention regarding GABAergic activity is ***Piper methysticum*** (kava). Current evidence indicates that kavalactones (the resinoid lipid-soluble constituents found primarily in the root and stem) modulate GABA activity via altering lipid membrane structures and sodium channel, rather than by significant GABA-$\alpha_{1,2}$ agonism.[23] Importantly, this activity in animal models was found to occur in the anxiety/fear-modulating hippocampus and amygdala. Other neuromodulatory activity effecting anxiolysis are considered to involve a down-regulation of beta-adrenergic activity and MAO-B inhibition.[23] Interestingly, inhibition of the reuptake of noradrenaline in the prefrontal cortex has been demonstrated in animal models.[54] This facilitates kava's unique effect of enhancing mental acuity while relaxing the body and calming the mind. This effect is of a distinct advantage compared with alcohol and benzodiazepines, which cause deleterious cognitive effects.[55] Another advantage of using kava in anxiety disorders is that kavalactones have also demonstrated relaxation of muscular contractibility via modulation of sodium and calcium channels.[56] Somatic tension is a common occurrence in anxiety disorders.[17]

Strong evidence supports the use of kava in treating anxiety disorders. A Cochrane review of 12 double-blind randomised controlled trials (RCTs) of rigorous methodology using kava mono-preparations (60 mg to 280 mg of kavalactones) in anxious conditions revealed positive results in favour of the phytomedicine.[24] Medicinal use of kava is currently restricted in the European Union and Canada over hepatotoxicity. The World Health Organization (WHO) has recommended research into 'aqueous' extracts of the plant to establish its safety and efficacy in treating anxiety disorders.[57] This is in preference to previous acetonic or ethanolic extracts, which may be implicated in hepatotoxic reactions. Hepatotoxicity caused by European kava products may in part be due to a commercial cost-motivated preference for the aerial parts and root or stem peelings, which contain the alkaloid pipermethystine, and due to the use of non-traditional solvents (ethanol and acetone).[58] The use of a water-soluble extract of the peeled rootstock of a 'noble' cultivar of kava may be the solution.[59] Prescriptive advice is to use kava away from alcohol and drugs, and within therapeutic dosage range. An occasional liver function test is also advised if regularly consuming the plant. Short-term, intermittent courses with occasional liver function tests being conducted to monitor for the rare occurrence of liver dysfunction are indicated.

Other herbal medicines that may affect anxiolysis via limbic system interaction (with evidence from human studies) include *Passiflora incarnata*, *Scutellaria lateriflora*, *Melissa officinalis*, *Ginkgo biloba and Galphimia glauca*.[51] **Passiflora incarnata** has traditional usage in the treatment of anxiety and neurosis.[51] As detailed in the evidence table, clinical trials support the use of the plant for general anxiety and for amelioration of preoperative anxiety. The fragrant herbal medicine **Melissa officinalis** has traditional usage as a mild sedative and an antispasmodic.[51] Studies using the plant for the acute reduction of anxiety and perceived stress have revealed beneficial effects (also seen when combined with *Valeriana officinalis*). **Scutellaria lateriflora** is a traditional anxiolytic herbal medicine that has been used to treat a variety of nervous system disorders in Native American and eclectic medicine.[51] In preclinical models, the herb has displayed anxiolytic effects, with the compounds baicalin and baicalein purported to be involved in this activity via GABA-α binding.[60] Aside from a poorly designed and reported study, there has not been a study of sufficient methodological strength to test the plant for clinical anxiety.

Matricaria recutita is consumed in many countries in tea form, being imbibed for a perceived calming effect.[61] Preclinical research has revealed a range of GABAergic effects from constituents such as apigenin.[62,63] An eight-week double-blind RCT ($n = 57$) using a standardised extract (220–1100 mg depending on response; 1.2% apigenin) for adults diagnosed with GAD found a statistically significant reduction in anxiety symptoms on the Hamilton Anxiety Scale (HAMA) compared with placebo.[61] Two further clinical trials by the authors reported both short and long term (i.e. 8 and 38 weeks) effects of anxiety treatment using 1500 mg of chamomile (500 mg capsule three times daily) in 179 patients with GAD. At week eight, 58% of the sample met the criteria for clinical response in the Chamomile group, with significant reductions in mean anxiety across the entire sample.[64] However, in the long-term study, clinical responders randomly assigned to continued active or placebo treatment for a further 26 weeks found no difference in relapse rates between the groups.[65]

Eschscholzia californica, *Ziziphus jujuba*, *Magnolia* spp. and *Damiana diffusa* are other plant medicines with encouraging preclinical activity supported by traditional knowledge[50]; however, to date no human clinical studies have been conducted using these as monotherapies to treat anxiety disorders. **Eschscholzia californica** has preclinical research revealing an anxiolytic and sedative effect via a binding affinity to GABA receptors, with flumazenil (a benzodiazepine receptor antagonist) suppressing these sedative and anxiolytic effects.[66] *Eschscholzia californica* is non-narcotic and only acts as a milder sedative, due to a chemical composition of alkaloids, than opium poppies.[67,68] Animal models have revealed that the jujubosides in **Ziziphus jujuba** inhibit glutamate-mediated pathways (excitory pathway) in the hippocampus.[69] Other studies using Suanzaoren (a traditional Chinese medicine formula containing *Ziziphus jujuba* as the principal herbal medicine) in animal models have demonstrated modulation of central monoamines and limbic system interaction and effects in humans.[70,71]

The bark of **Magnolia spp.** is used in traditional Asian medicine for anxiety and mood disorders, being a major ingredient of certain Kampo and traditional Chinese medicine formulas.[50] In vitro assays have revealed that whole *Magnolia* spp. extract has an affinity with GABA and adenosine pathways (and is also a 5-HT_6 receptor antagonist).[72] Anxiolytic effects have also been revealed in animal models, with active anxiolytic constituents considered to date to be honokiol,[73] 4-O-methylhonokiol,[74] magnolol[75] and obovatol.[76] **Tilia spp.** aerial parts (in particular the flowers) have been used in traditional South and Central American medicine for anxiety and insomnia.[50] While no human studies have been conducted exploring this use, the anxiolytic and sedative effects have been revealed in several preclinical models (tiliroside, quercetin, quercitrin and kaempherol considered to contribute to activity).

Magnesium has an important role in neurological activity, and deficiency of the nutrient may cause neuropathologies.[77] Magnesium ions regulate calcium ion flow in neuronal calcium channels, helping to regulate neuronal nitric oxide production.[78] The deficit of neuronal magnesium ions may be induced by stress hormones, excessive dietary calcium and dietary deficiencies of magnesium.[78] Studies using animal models have demonstrated that magnesium deficiency can cause depression and anxiety-like behaviour. After magnesium was administered to deficient animals, anxiolytic activity was demonstrated in mice during elevated plus-maze and forced swim tests.[79] Magnesium appears to exert its anxiolytic effect by the involvement of the N-methyl-D-aspartic (NMDA)/glutamate pathway, and this activity may involve the glycine B sites.[80] Interaction between magnesium and benzodiazepine/GABA-α receptors may also be involved in producing anxiolytic-like activity.[81] While no study has explored the use of magnesium monotherapy in humans to ameliorate anxiety, a preliminary controlled study for relieving mild premenstrual symptoms using combinations of magnesium, vitamin B6, magnesium and vitamin B6 (and placebo) for one menstrual cycle in women ($n = 44$) showed no overall difference between individual treatments.[82] Further specific subanalysis, however, showed a significant effect on reducing anxiety-related premenstrual symptoms (nervous tension, mood swings, irritability or anxiety).

The Kava-Anxiety Lowering Medication (KALM) Study

- A six-week placebo-controlled, double-blind trial involving 75 adult participants with diagnosed GAD and no comorbid mood disorder.
- Participants were prescribed either kava tablets (equivalent of 120/240 mg of kavalactones per day, depending on response) or matching placebo.
- The aqueous extract of kava was found to significantly reduce participants' HAMA anxiety score over placebo with a moderate clinical effect size.
- Within the kava group, GABA transporter genetic polymorphisms rs2601126 and rs2697153 were associated with HAMA reduction, indicating that these polymorphisms appear to potentially modify the anxiolytic response to kava.
- Interestingly, kava significantly increased sexual drive in females compared with placebo on a sub-domain of the Arizona Sexual Experience Scale (ASEX), with no negative effects seen in males. A highly significant correlation was also found between ASEX reduction (improved sexual function and performance) and anxiety reduction in the whole sample.
- The extract was found to be safe, with no serious adverse effects and no clinical hepatotoxicity.

Sources: Sarris et al. 2013[83,84]

Monoamine pathway modulation

Aside from the monoamine system being involved in the underpinning of depression, dysregulation of this pathway is linked to anxiety disorders.[16] Several herbal medicines have monoamine modulatory effects that may be useful for anxiety disorders (primarily via the serotonergic system). While *Ginkgo biloba* is primarily studied for neuromodulatory activity for the treatment of cognitive conditions, studies have documented mood modulation in cognitively impaired subjects. A 2006 RCT involving 82 subjects with GAD using *Ginkgo biloba* EGb 761 extract (480 mg or 240 mg per day) or placebo for four weeks revealed a significant dose-dependent reduction of HAMA over placebo in the 480 mg/day and the 240 mg/day *Ginkgo biloba* groups.[85] The leaves and stem from *Galphimia glauca* is used in traditional Mexican and Central American cultures for a range of conditions, including nervous disorders.[51] The nor-seco-triterpene 'galphimine B' is regarded as an active constituent, which has been shown to interact with serotonergic transmission in the dorsal hippocampus in an animal model. Two RCTs have shown that *Galphimia glauca* is equal to and potentially more effective than the benzodiazepine lorazepam in reducing anxiety in adults with GAD. Tolerability of *Galphimia glauca* was good, with a side-effects analysis also demonstrating no difference between treatments.

Centella asiatica has been used in traditional Ayurvedic and Chinese medicine for centuries to treat a range of conditions (including anxiety) and to provide relaxation. The anxiolytic action of gotu kola has been supported by preclinical research that found the triterpene asiaticoside to be the main active constituent responsible for the anxiolytic activity.[86,87] While an animal model linked triterpenes in gotu kola to increased brain levels of 5-HT, NE and DA together with reduced serum corticosterone levels,[87] a recent eight-week open-label study used *Centella asiatica* hydroethanolic extract of the leaves (500 mg twice daily) in 33 adults with GAD.[88] Results revealed a significantly reduced anxiety by 26% at study endpoint in addition to a reduction in stress and depression ratings. While no studies have been conducted using the amino acid **L-tryptophan** or **5-HTP** for anxiety disorders, it has a theoretical place as a precursor of serotonin for use in anxiety disorders with comorbid insomnia.[89]

Hypericum perforatum for anxiety disorders

Hypericum perforatum (St John's wort: SJW) has been used throughout Europe and studied extensively in depression; however, despite anecdotal clinical use for anxiety, no study has been conducted on the efficacy of SJW in 'generalised anxiety' or GAD to date. SJW has, however, been studied in OCD and in social phobia in 12-week RCTs, and results revealed no significant effect beyond placebo. While it may be effective for reducing anxiety that may co-occur with depression, no evidence supports it currently as a treatment for any anxiety disorder.

Endocrinological factors

Although not entirely understood yet, the endocrine system has a distinct role in stress and anxiety, with HPA-axis hyperactivation being regarded as a prime component in chronic anxiogenesis.[83] Complementary and alternative medicine (CAM) interventions that modulate the HPA axis may have a role in treating stress and anxiety (see Chapters 18–20 on the endocrine system). Among CAM interventions that may provide HPA-axis modulation are herbal 'adaptogens' and 'tonics', including *Panax ginseng*, *Withania somnifera* and *Rhodiola rosea*. **Withania somnifera** is classified in Ayurvedic medicine as a 'rasayana', being considered to enhance physical and mental performance.[19] *Withania* *somnifera* has been shown in preclinical models to exert an anxiolytic effect via GABA-mimetic activity.[90] One six-week double-blind RCT using 500 mg of a root extract in 39 patients with a range of ICD-10 diagnosed anxiety disorders, revealed a 2.4 point difference on HAMA in favour of *Withania somnifera*; however, this effect was not statistically significant.[91]

Rhodiola rosea may also have a place in treating generalised anxiety, especially if presenting with fatigue and cardiovascular problems. A small pilot trial used a standardised *Rhodiola rosea* (Rhodax) formulation in 10 participants with diagnosed GAD. Participants received 340 mg of Rhodax in two divided doses for a period of 10 weeks.[87] Results demonstrated a significant drop on the HAMA. While this study yielded a positive outcome, the uncontrolled design and small sample temper confidence in the results. A more recent larger study concerning a two-week clinical trial involving 80 mildly anxious patients given either two lots of 200 mg per day of roseroot (Vitano) or a non-placebo control condition (no treatment),[92] revealed that *R. rosea* demonstrated a significant reduction in self-reported anxiety, stress, anger, confusion and depression and improvements in total mood. Once again, caution needs to be extended to this result due to the lack of a credible control. A caveat that should be observed by clinicians using *Rhodiola rosea* root for anxious presentations is that the herb has (dose-dependently) been found to cause anxiety, irritability and insomnia in some people.

Panax ginseng has traditional Asiatic use as a 'tonic' due to its adaptogenic properties.[93] While clinical studies have shown cognitive enhancing[94] and adaptogenic effects,[95] preclinical models have also revealed anxiolytic activities. To date, however, it has not been studied in humans for any anxiety disorder, and due to its stimulatory effects would not be advised in treating acute anxiety, having more of an application in chronic anxiety presenting in the 'exhaustion' phase (see Chapter 18 on stress and fatigue).

Traditional approaches for reducing anxiety

While the modern application of naturopathy often focuses on the prescriptive use of nutraceuticals, it is important to consider lifestyle factors that may assist in reducing anxiety and stress. As advocated by Hippocrates, this may include having ample exposure to nature and fresh air, while going on retreats or attending 'sanatoriums' may also be of benefit. One example of a traditional therapy that may be useful in reducing anxiety is the use of 'balneotherapy' (BT), which involves bathing in mineral-rich spas in addition to potentially experiencing a massage from bubbling water currents. An eight-week study of four spa resorts was conducted to assess the efficacy of BT compared with paroxetine in DSM-IV-diagnosed GAD.[96] A total of 237 outpatients were recruited, with 117 being assigned randomly to BT and 120 to paroxetine. The mean change in HAMA scores revealed an improvement in both groups, with a significant advantage of BT compared with paroxetine. Remission and sustained response rates were also significantly higher in the BT group.

Somatic treatment

Anxiety disorders commonly present with the somatic manifestations of perceived muscular tension or pain.[1] The therapeutic technique of **progressive muscle relaxation**, developed by Jacobson in 1938, reduces anxiety and stress by first tensing a muscle and then releasing that tension.[36] By releasing physical tension the sympathetic nervous system-activated 'fight or flight' response may be reduced. This technique may be of value in GAD, which commonly presents with somatic tension. Aside from the physiological relaxation that ensues from progressive muscle relaxation, the technique may have additional anxiolytic benefits by focusing the person's mind away from worries and allowing them to develop a sense of self-mastery over their anxiety. Evidence supports the use of muscular relaxation therapy techniques to reduce anxiety and tension. A review of 60 studies concluded that these techniques are as effective as pharmacological and cognitive techniques.[97] A review of the effect sizes from five controlled studies revealed a moderate pooled effect size.

Acupuncture may be effective in reducing acute anxiety (not withstanding people's fear of needles) via modification of the opioid and monoamine systems.[34,98] A meta-analysis of the efficacy of acupuncture in treating anxiety and anxiety disorders included 12 controlled trials of sufficient methodological standard.[35] All trials reported positive findings, but the reports lacked many basic methodological details. Evidence of studies involving perioperative anxiety was generally supportive of acupuncture. Acupuncture, and in particular auricular (ear) acupuncture, was found to be more effective than acupuncture at sham points. The authors note, however, that most results were based on subjective measures and blinding could not be guaranteed.

Massage therapy has been used extensively by many cultures for millennia for a variety of curative purposes. Theories of massage therapy's mechanism of action involve the 'gate control theory of pain reduction' (whereby manual pressure creates a stimulus that interferes with the pain signal), promotion of parasympathetic nervous system activity, stimulation of serotonergic and endorphin activity, reduction of somatic tension and via interpersonal attention.[99] One 12-week study assessed the effectiveness of therapeutic massage for treating GAD in 68 patients.[100] Compared with thermotherapy or relaxation-room therapy for a total of 10 sessions all treatments showed similar effects with no difference between groups. **Aromatherapy** may be used for anxiety reduction via inhalation, topical application or in massage oils. A standardised *Lavendula spp.* formula (Silexan) has revealed notable anxiolytic effects. A 10-week RCT involving 221 adults suffering from a range of anxiety disorders found that the oral preparation had a clinically meaningful anxiolytic effect and also assisted in reducing disturbed sleep.[101] The volatile constituents responsible for purported anxiolytic activity include linalool, linalyl acetate and geraniol, which may have interaction with the limbic system. Plants rich in these constituents include lavender, lemon balm, neroli, rose and ylang ylang.[41]

The biological and psychosomatic role of the 'heart'

Crataegus oxyacantha has traditional use as a phytomedicine to treat cardiovascular complaints and is considered to have cardiovascular modifying properties.[102] *Crataegus* spp. is usually prescribed in phytomedicine for cardiovascular complaints, an arena in which it possesses robust evidence of efficacy.[103]

Emerging data indicate a use in anxiety, especially where somatic cardiovascular symptoms present (e.g. palpitations or tachycardia). In a double-blind RCT involving participants presenting with mild to moderate GAD (assessed via DSM-III-R), 264 adults were prescribed two tablets containing fixed quantities of a fixed combination of *Crataegus oxyacantha* (300 mg), *Eschscholzia californica* (80 mg) and magnesium (300 mg elemental) twice daily for three months.[104] Total and somatic HAMA scores, subjective patient-rated anxiety and doctor's Clinical Global Impressions Scale were used as outcome measures. The results demonstrated that the formula markedly ameliorated anxiety in comparison to placebo as determined by HAMA and subjectively assessed anxiety.

The heart and anxiety

- The connection between cardiovascular conditions and anxiety has evidence.
- Cardiovascular disease may cause anxiety or vice versa.
- A somatic effect of anxiety is heart palpitations and tachycardia.
- This reflects traditional medicine knowledge of the heart–emotion/mental connection.

Sources: Tyrer & Baldwin 2006,[17] Culpeper 1652,[102] Peck & Ai 2008[105] and Maciocia 1989[106]

INTEGRATIVE MEDICAL CONSIDERATIONS

As in all psychiatric disorders, an integrative approach is advised in managing GAD. Aside from judicious prescription of complementary or synthetic pharmacotherapies and the recommendation of psychological interventions, options such as massage, acupuncture and an exercise and relaxation program may be of additional benefit. A key integrative management technique of chronic anxiety is to screen, or refer for assessment, alcohol or substance abuse or dependency issues and other comorbid medical and psychiatric disorders.

N-acetylcysteine for obsessive-compulsive disorder

Aside from use in paracetamol overdose and as a mucolytic, N-acetylcysteine (NAC) has been used as a novel treatment of OCD due to an inhibitory effect on synaptic glutamate release, as well as an ability to reduce oxidative stress and attenuate inflammatory pathways. Emerging research has found that in OCD and trichotillomania (compulsive repetitive hair pulling), two small pilot double-blind RCTs have revealed beneficial effects; however, a more recent RCT only found effects on the compulsive symptomatology of OCD.[107] The recommended dose for OCD is between 2 g and 3 g per day, while it should be noted that beneficial effects may take 10 or more weeks before occurring in some patients.

Sources: Camfield et al. 2011,[108] Dean et al. 2012,[109] Afshar et al. 2012[110] and Grant et al. 2009[111]

Psychological intervention

As documented in Chapter 15 on depression, various psychological techniques including cognitive and/or behavioural therapy and interpersonal techniques may be of benefit in treating GAD.[17] Some people may be 'wired to worry' via genetic and/or familial upbringing. Although the understanding of people with trait anxiety is limited, it is possible that CAM and pharmaceutical interventions may be only of supportive value in people who are prone to worry. Techniques that modify anxiogenic behaviours, such as hyperventilation, and assist patients to understand how their thoughts may affect their anxiety and how to alter these cognitive patterns may reduce the intensity and frequency of the anxiety. While practitioners are encouraged to refer to clinical psychologists or a qualified counsellor, they can still employ a 'person-centred' approach (empathy, active listening and genuineness) to the therapeutic encounter. A Cochrane meta-analysis was conducted involving 22 controlled studies (1060 participants) using psychological interventions to treat GAD.[112] Results based on a subsection of 13 studies using CBT found the technique to be more effective than 'treatment as usual' or 'waitlist' control in achieving a reduction of anxiety. However, six studies comparing CBT against basic supportive therapy revealed no significant difference in clinical response at post-treatment. Psychological therapies based on CBT or interpersonal supportive principles are effective treatments in reducing anxiety.

Naturopathic medicine for treating anxiety

While therapeutic components of typical naturopathic treatment have been studied only two studies have been performed exploring the whole practice of the modality in the area of anxiety disorders.[113]

A double-blind 12-week RCT involving 87 adults with chronic anxiety by Cooley et al.[114] compared a structured naturopathic therapy protocol (including *Withania somnifera*—300 mg twice daily, dietary counselling, breathing relaxation techniques and a standard multivitamin) to control. The control group received a standardised psychotherapy intervention, matched deep breathing relaxation techniques and placebo pill supplement over 12 weeks. Results revealed that Beck anxiety inventory scores decreased significantly by 56.5% in the naturopathy group compared with 30.5% in the control group.

Another more recent study involved an analysis of naturopathic consultations of adults with self-reported anxiety or depression.[115] Outcomes from consultations (from two or three visits over approximately four to six weeks) were assessed via a mixed methods approach. From the 11 naturopaths who provided data for analysis (consisting of 31 consultations from 15 patients), eight participants had follow-up data across time from baseline to their final follow-up consultation. A significant reduction occurred for anxiety, depression and stress on a range of psychiatric scales. An evaluation of clinicians' prescriptions found nutrient supplementation was prescribed by 67% of practitioners, with 84% prescribing a herbal medicine. Dietary or exercise advice was recommended in 52% and 32% of consultations, respectively. Meditation/relaxation techniques were taught in 35% of consultations. Sleep hygiene advice was provided in 32% of cases and counselling was offered 38% of the time. While preliminary evidence in this uncontrolled study revealed that naturopathic medicine may be beneficial in improving mood and reducing anxiety the small study sample and the uncontrolled unblinded design restrict the strength of this conclusion.

Homeopathy and Bach flowers

The clinical practice of **homeopathy** has its beginnings in the 1800s in Germany.[43] A systematic review by Pilkington et al.[45] identified eight RCTs using homeopathy to treat anxiety, with results revealing that no determination of efficacy was possible based on the available evidence. This was due to the identified studies all exhibiting significant methodological issues (e.g. small samples, lack of control group). Another stricter systematic review by Davidson et al.[44] of homeopathy in psychiatry revealed that in four out of five studies located for anxiety (two on GAD), homeopathy was not superior to placebo. A review of three **Bach flower** RCTs for use in anxiety disorders also found no significant effect beyond placebo.[46] In summary, on the basis of the current literature it is not possible to provide support for the use of homeopathy for treatment of anxiety-based disorders.

Dietary and lifestyle advice

Dietary programs designed to treat depression have to date not been rigorously evaluated. Although evidence supporting specific dietary advice is currently absent, a basic balanced diet (see Chapter 3 on wellness) with foods rich in individual nutrients such as folate, omega-3, tryptophan, B and C vitamins, zinc and magnesium can be recommended. These foods include whole grains, lean meat, deep-sea fish, green leafy vegetables, coloured berries and nuts (walnuts and almonds). A low glycaemic index diet may be beneficial in stabilising blood sugar levels, which may in turn reduce the 'fight or flight' response of low blood sugar levels (see Chapters 18–20 on the endocrine system).

General lifestyle advice should focus on encouraging a balance between meaningful work, adequate rest, judicious exercise, positive social interaction and pleasurable hobbies. Behavioural therapy techniques have shown positive effects in reducing anxiety by training the person to reduce or better manage stressful situations, and to increase pleasurable activities. These may enhance self-esteem and self-mastery and increase physical and mental wellbeing. With respect to sleep, insomnia is common in anxiety sufferers (see Chapter 16 on insomnia) and treating this is of primary importance as poor sleep may in turn deleteriously affect neuroendocrine balance and subsequently exacerbate the anxiety. Removing caffeine from the person's diet is a vital component to reduce anxiety and improve sleep.[116] Caffeine causes arousal, hypervigilance and possible anxiogenesis in certain individuals via stimulation of beta-adrenergic receptors and up-regulation of noradrenaline and dopamine; additionally, adenosine receptor antagonism interferes with sleep.[116] 'Decaffeinated' coffee and tea products still provide for the experience to be had without the sweaty palms and heart palpitations.

Exercise or physical activity

Physical activity is anecdotally regarded as having a positive effect on reducing stress and anxiety, with people often participating in activities such as walking, swimming, cycling, doing yoga or going to the gym in order to improve their wellbeing. A recent meta-analysis conducted to examine the effects of exercise on anxiety included 49 studies and showed an overall moderate effect size, indicating larger reductions in anxiety among exercise groups than no-treatment control groups.[33] A non-significant trend towards a dose-dependent effect for moderate exercise occurred, while both lower and higher intensity exercise appears less effective. Exercise was found to have a stronger effect than stress management and education, while it was shown as having similar effects to CBT and slightly less efficacy than pharmacotherapies. Caution should be adopted with anxious people who present with respiratory or cardiovascular symptoms, as these symptoms may be exacerbated with exercise and this in turn may increase anxiety. In some cases respiratory distress may also provoke a panic attack. Graded exercise programs that may be appropriate for anxiety may involve either aerobic or anabolic exercise for a minimum of 20 minutes three to five times per week.

Meditation techniques

Meditative techniques have been documented to reduce the arousal state and may also ameliorate anxiety symptoms and improve mood.[117] The concept of meditation is varied, with a key attribute of the practice involving 'mindfulness', commonly defined as the awareness that arises through 'paying attention in a particular way: on purpose, in the present moment, and non-judgmentally'.[118] A Cochrane review conducted included two RCTs of sufficient methodological rigour.[39] Both studies were of moderate quality and used active control comparisons (another type of meditation, relaxation, biofeedback or anxiolytic drugs). The small numbers of studies included in this review, however, do not permit any conclusions to be drawn on the effectiveness of meditation therapy for anxiety disorders. One particular formalised mindfulness technique with evidence is '**mindfulness-based stress reduction**' (MBSR).[38] MBSR is an 8–10-week structured program that involves: training in mindfulness meditation practice; mindful awareness such as during yoga postures; and mindfulness during stressful everyday situations and social interaction. There is evidence to suggest that among the general population the MBSR technique may bring about a reduction in trait and state anxiety and symptoms.[119,120]

Yoga and breathing techniques

Yoga incorporates a range of meditative, postural and breathing techniques that may be beneficial for reducing anxiety. Kirkwood et al.[121] reviewed eight studies of yoga for anxiety disorders but methodological limitations preclude firm conclusions. Since then, however, nine additional RCTs have shown significant benefits for patients with varying anxiety and stress-related disorders.[122] **Traditional breathing techniques** have been used for centuries in various spiritual traditions. 'Voluntarily regulated breathing practices' include traditional yoga breathing, paced breathing and technology-assisted breathing interventions.[122] Slow yoga breathing can begin with focusing attention on the rate and depth of breath while increasing awareness (or mindfulness) of the breath technique. Slow rhythmic deep breathing should produce calming effects, with a breathing rate of four to six breaths per minute (with equal inhalation and exhalation) having an effect to balance sympatho vagal tone (Figure 14.2).

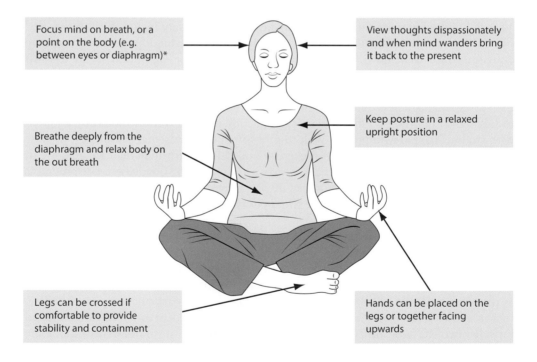

Focus mind on breath, or a point on the body (e.g. between eyes or diaphragm)*

View thoughts dispassionately and when mind wanders bring it back to the present

Keep posture in a relaxed upright position

Breathe deeply from the diaphragm and relax body on the out breath

Legs can be crossed if comfortable to provide stability and containment

Hands can be placed on the legs or together facing upwards

*After 5–15 minutes of 'focused attention', mindfulness awareness can optionally be alternatively extended to external environment (present location and sounds) or 'open monitoring' of internal thoughts (dispassionate observation).

Figure 14.2
Mindfulness meditation

CLINICAL SUMMARY

As in the case of major depressive disorder, GAD sufferers with comorbid mental disorders have increased psychological and social impairment, require more treatment and present with a poorer prognosis.[18] While specific diagnosis is previously the domain of psychiatrists and psychologists, it is important that practitioners take a methodical case study to determine more detail beyond the presentation of 'anxiety'. As illustrated an initial presentation of 'stress' or 'anxiety' may be confused with other disorders—for example, a depressive disorder, bipolar (hypo)mania, ADHD, OCD or social phobia—or may co-present with other disorders such as panic disorder. If the patient presents with an obvious bipolar disorder, delusions or self-harm/suicidality, referral to a medical practitioner or to psychiatric assessment is advised. In the case of co-occurring social phobia, OCD or ADHD, CAM interventions currently do not have firm evidentiary support (although they may have a beneficial adjuvant role). Psychological support to assist in behavioural and cognitive modification may be helpful as part of an integrative solution. When advising alcohol withdrawal in cases of comorbid alcohol dependence, acute anxiety may occur via an increased level of stimulatory glutamate and a desensitisation of GABA pathways,[123] thus appropriate medical care is needed. Furthermore, long-term alcohol use may reduce levels of critical nutrients required for neurological function, such as B vitamins.[124] GAD often presents with a current recurring course. Due to this a therapeutic position of chronic condition management is potentially needed. See Figure 14.3 for a clinical decision tree on the integrative treatment of anxiety.

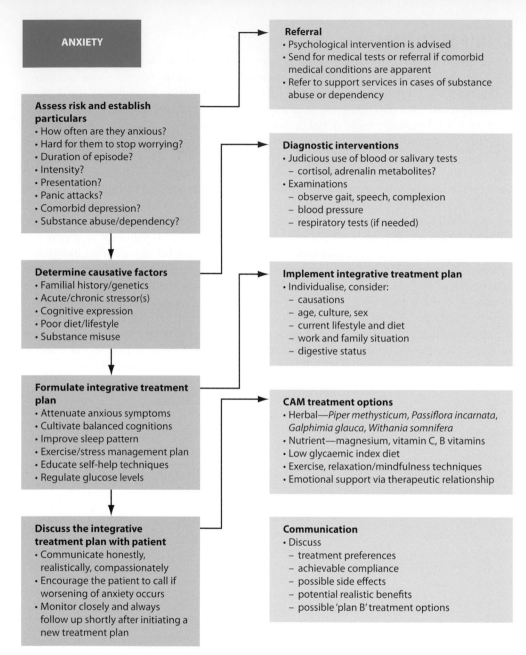

Figure 14.3
Naturopathic treatment decision tree—anxiety

Table 14.1
Review of the major evidence

Intervention	Mechanims of action	Key literature	Summary of results	Comment
Piper methysticum	GABA membrane modulation and weak GABA binding Blockage of voltage-gated channels Noradrenaline reuptake inhibition Beta-adrenergic downregulation MAO-B inhibition[23]	Meta-analysis, review: Pittler et al. 2003[24] Sarris et al. 2011[23]	$n = 345$ HAMA 5.0 point reduction over placebo (95% CI: 1.1–8.8)	Significant anxiolysis occurred with *Piper methysticum* over placebo Occasional liver tests advised in chronic use
Passiflora incarnata	GABA pathway modulation[25]	RCTs: Two acute RCTs ($n = 60$[26] and $n = 60$)[27] using *Passiflora incarnata* for preoperative anxiety; a four-week RCT *Passiflora incarnata* versus oxazepam ($n = 36$)[28]	All studies revealed positive anxiety reduction: greater than placebo or equivalent to oxazepam	Solid evidence as an anxiolytic, needs a larger RCT for anxiety disorders to confirm efficacy
Galphimia glauca	Anxiolysis occurs via serotonergic system modulation[29]	RCTs: Two GAD studies (four-week $n = 153$,[30] 15-week $n = 191$)[31]; *Galphimia glauca* versus lorazepam	Four-week study found equivocal efficacy, 16-week study *Galphimia glauca* was superior to lorazepam	Encouraging data supports the use of the plant for anxiety Not available yet in some countries
Exercise	Increase in circulating endorphins, anandamide and various neurotransmitters Increases tryptophan hydroxylase Modulates the HPA axis[32]	Meta-analysis Wipfli et al. 2008[33]: 49 RCTs	Moderate effect size (0.48) Small–moderate effect size	Exercise groups showed a greater reduction than other forms of exercise Adults with higher stress baseline may have greater benefit
Acupuncture	Opioid pathway modulation Increased release of serotonin and noradrenaline Cortisol modulation[34]	Systematic review: Pilkington et al. 2007[35]: 12 controlled trials, six on GAD	Positive results in all studies; however, bias may be present	Overall most studies included had poor methodology No studies included assessing other anxiety disorders such as OCD or panic disorder

Table 14.1
Review of the major evidence (continued)

Intervention	Mechanims of action	Key literature	Summary of results	Comment
Relaxation therapy	A range of neurosomatic effects; however, perceived anxiolysis may not be a result of physical effects[3b]	Systematic review: Jorm et al. 2004[37]: 60 RCTs	Effect sizes from five controlled studies revealed a moderate pooled effect size of $d = 0.49$ (glass effect size technique)	Good evidence but needs to be conducted by a person trained in relaxation techniques
Meditation	Increases release of neurotransmitters May increase brain tissue thickness Increased oxygenation of brain tissue[38]	Systematic reviews: Krisanaprakornkit et al. 2008[39] Cochrane review: two RCTs	Insufficient controlled studies to make any firm conclusion	More studies are required to assess different types of meditation
Massage	Somatic relaxation with potential effects on the opioid and neuroendocrine system[40]	Systematic review/ meta-analysis Moyer et al. 2004[40]: 37 RCTs	A moderate effect size; state anxiety $g = 0.37$ moderate–strong effect size for trait anxiety $g = 0.75$	Practitioner training level varied markedly, as well as the length of the treatment, body parts massaged and environment and gender factors
Aromatherapy	Inhalation has effects on multiple neurotransmitters GABAergic activity[41]	Systematic review: Lee et al. 2011[42]: 16 clinical trials	Positive effect for reducing anxiety found in most studies	A safe and low-cost intervention with potentially a mild clinical effect for anxiety Not supported for clinical anxiety disorders
Homeopathy and Bach flowers	Considered to work on the principle of 'vibrational medicine'[43]	Systematic reviews: Davidson et al. 2011[44]: homeopathy Pilkington et al. 2007[45]: Bach flowers[46]	Data does not provide supportive evidence of homeopathy or Bach flowers for any anxiety disorder	Homeopathy and Bach flowers appear to only have an effect equal to placebo for treating anxiety

KEY POINTS

- 'Stress' in patients should be further screened for anxiety disorders.
- Chronic worry needs to not be dismissed as a personality trait—it could be GAD.
- The first responsibility is to reduce acute suffering, especially in panic disorder.
- Check for co-occurring substance/alcohol abuse or dependence, depression and insomnia.

FURTHER READING

Craske MG, Stein MB. Anxiety. Lancet 2016;388(10063):3048–59. doi:10.1016/S0140-6736(16)30381-6.

Firth J, Torous J, Nicholas J, et al. Can smartphone mental health interventions reduce symptoms of anxiety? A meta-analysis of randomized controlled trials. J Affect Disord 2017;218:15–22.

Hoge EA, Ivkovic A, Fricchione GL. Generalized anxiety disorder: diagnosis and treatment. BMJ 2012;345:e7500. doi:10.1136/bmj.e7500.

Sarris J, Moylan S, Camfield DA, et al. Complementary medicine, exercise, meditation, diet, and lifestyle modification for anxiety disorders: a review of current evidence. Evid Based Complement Alternat Med 2012;2012:809653.

Sarris J, Gadsden S, Schweitzer I. Naturopathic medicine for treating self-reported depression and anxiety: an observational pilot study of naturalistic practice. Adv Integr Med 2014;1(2):87–92.

Sarris J. Herbal medicines in the treatment of psychiatric disorders: 10-year updated review. Phytother Res 2018;32(7):1147–62.

Savage K, Firth J, Stough C, et al. GABA-modulating phytomedicines for anxiety: a systematic review of preclinical and clinical evidence. Phytother Res 2018;32(1):3–18.

REFERENCES

1. American Psychiatric Association. Diagnostic and statistical manual of mental disorders. 5th ed. Arlington: American Psychiatric Association; 2013.
2. Shearer SL. Recent advances in the understanding and treatment of anxiety disorders. Prim Care 2007;34(3):475–504, v–vi.
3. Antai-Otong D. Current treatment of generalized anxiety disorder. J Psychosoc Nurs Ment Health Serv 2003;41(12):20–9.
4. Baxter AJ, Scott KM, Vos T, et al. Global prevalence of anxiety disorders: a systematic review and meta-regression. Psychol Med 2013;43(5):897–910.
5. Wittchen HU, Jacobi F, Rehm J, et al. The size and burden of mental disorders and other disorders of the brain in Europe 2010. Eur Neuropsychopharmacol 2011;21(9):655–79.
6. Australian Bureau of Statistics. National Survey of Mental Health and Wellbeing. Canberra: ABS; 2007.
7. McEvoy PM, Grove R, Slade T. Epidemiology of anxiety disorders in the Australian general population: findings of the 2007 Australian National Survey of Mental Health and Wellbeing. Aust N Z J Psychiatry 2011;45(11):957–67.
8. Alonso J, Angermeyer MC, Bernert S, et al. Prevalence of mental disorders in Europe: results from the European Study of the Epidemiology of Mental Disorders (ESEMeD) project. Acta Psychiatr Scand Suppl 2004;420(420):21–7.
9. Kessler RC, Chiu WT, Demler O, et al. Prevalence, severity, and comorbidity of 12-month DSM-IV disorders in the National Comorbidity Survey Replication. Arch Gen Psychiatry 2005;62(6):617–27.
10. Department of Health and Ageing. The mental health of Australians: anxiety disorders in Australia. Canberra: Australian Government; 2012.
11. Hunt C, Slade T, Andrews G. Generalized anxiety disorder and major depressive disorder comorbidity in the National Survey of Mental Health and Well-Being. Depress Anxiety 2004;20(1):23–31.
12. Gorwood P. Generalized anxiety disorder and major depressive disorder comorbidity: an example of genetic pleiotropy? Eur Psychiatry 2004;19(1):27–33.
13. Kessler RC, Ruscio AM, Shear K, et al. Epidemiology of anxiety disorders. Curr Top Behav Neurosci 2010;2: 21–35.
14. Gadermann AM, Alonso J, Vilagut G, et al. Comorbidity and disease burden in the National Comorbidity Survey replication (NCS-R). Depress Anxiety 2012;29(9):797–806.
15. Hettema JM, Neale MC, Kendler KS. A review and meta-analysis of the genetic epidemiology of anxiety disorders. Am J Psychiatry 2001;158(10):1568–78.
16. Nutt DJ, Ballenger JC, Sheehan D, et al. Generalized anxiety disorder: comorbidity, comparative biology and treatment. Int J Neuropsychopharmacol 2002;5(4):315–25.
17. Tyrer P, Baldwin D. Generalised anxiety disorder. Lancet 2006;368(9553):2156–66.
18. Nutt D, Argyropoulos S, Hood S, et al. Generalized anxiety disorder: a comorbid disease. Eur Neuropsychopharmacol 2006;16(Suppl. 2):S109–18.
19. Kushner MG, Abrams K, Borchardt C. The relationship between anxiety disorders and alcohol use disorders: a review of major perspectives and findings. Clin Psychol Rev 2000;20(2):149–71.
20. Huh J, Goebert D, Takeshita J, et al. Treatment of generalized anxiety disorder: a comprehensive review of the literature for psychopharmacologic alternatives to newer antidepressants and benzodiazepines. Prim Care Companion CNS Disord 2011;13(2).
21. Hoffman EJ, Mathew SJ. Anxiety disorders: a comprehensive review of pharmacotherapies. Mt Sinai J Med 2008;75(3):248–62.
22. Bandelow B, Seidler-Brandler U, Becker A, et al. Meta-analysis of randomized controlled comparisons of psychopharmacological and psychological treatments for anxiety disorders. World J Biol Psychiatry 2007;8(3):175–87.
23. Sarris J, LaPorte E, Schweitzer I. Kava: a comprehensive review of efficacy, safety, and psychopharmacology. Aust N Z J Psychiatry 2011;45(1):27–35.
24. Pittler MH, Ernst E. Kava extract for treating anxiety. Cochrane Database Syst Rev 2003;(1):CD003383.
25. Appel K, Rose T, Fiebich B, et al. Modulation of the gamma-aminobutyric acid (GABA) system by Passiflora incarnata L. Phytother Res 2011;25(6):838–43.
26. Aslanargun P, Cuvas O, Dikmen B, et al. Passiflora incarnata Linneaus as an anxiolytic before spinal anesthesia. J Anesth 2012;26(1):39–44.
27. Movafegh A, Alizadeh R, Hajimohamadi F, et al. Preoperative oral Passiflora incarnata reduces anxiety in ambulatory surgery patients: a

double-blind, placebo-controlled study. Anesth Analg 2008;106(6):1728–32.

28. Akhondzadeh S, Naghavi HR, Vazirian M, et al. Passionflower in the treatment of generalized anxiety: a pilot double-blind randomized controlled trial with oxazepam. J Clin Pharm Ther 2001;26(5): 363–7.

29. Jimenez-Ferrer E, Herrera-Ruiz M, Ramirez-Garcia R, et al. Interaction of the natural anxiolytic Galphimine-B with serotonergic drugs on dorsal hippocampus in rats. J Ethnopharmacol 2011;137(1):724–9.

30. Herrera-Arellano A, Jimenez-Ferrer E, Zamilpa A, et al. Efficacy and tolerability of a standardized herbal product from Galphimia glauca on generalized anxiety disorder. A randomized, double-blind clinical trial controlled with lorazepam. Planta Med 2007;73(8):713–17.

31. Herrera-Arellano A, Jimenez-Ferrer JE, Zamilpa A, et al. Therapeutic effectiveness of galphimia glauca vs. lorazepam in generalized anxiety disorder. A controlled 15-week clinical trial. Planta Med 2012;78(14):1529–35.

32. Sarris J, Kavanagh D, Newton R. Depression and exercise. J Complement Med 2008;May/June(3):48–50, 61.

33. Wipfli BM, Rethorst CD, Landers DM. The anxiolytic effects of exercise: a meta-analysis of randomized trials and dose-response analysis. J Sport Exerc Psychol 2008;30(4):392–410.

34. Samuels N, Gropp C, Singer SR, et al. Acupuncture for psychiatric illness: a literature review. Behav Med 2008;34(2):55–64.

35. Pilkington K, Kirkwood G, Rampes H, et al. Acupuncture for anxiety and anxiety disorders—a systematic literature review. Acupunct Med 2007;25(1–2):1–10.

36. Conrad A, Roth W. Muscle relaxation therapy for anxiety disorders: it works but how? J Anxiety Disord 2007;21:243–64.

37. Jorm AF, Christensen H, Griffiths KM, et al. Effectiveness of complementary and self-help treatments for anxiety disorders. Med J Aust 2004;181(7 Suppl.):S29–46.

38. Sarris J, Moylan S, Camfield DA, et al. Complementary medicine, exercise, meditation, diet, and lifestyle modification for anxiety disorders: a review of current evidence. Evid Based Complement Alternat Med 2012;2012:809653.

39. Krisanaprakornkit T, Krisanaprakornkit W, Piyavhatkul N, et al. Meditation therapy for anxiety disorders. Cochrane Database Syst Rev 2006;(1):CD004998.

40. Moyer C, Rounds J, Hannum J. A meta-analysis of massage therapy research. Psychol Bull 2004;130(1):3–18.

41. Perry N, Perry E. Aromatherapy in the management of psychiatric disorders. CNS Drugs 2006;20(4):257–80.

42. Lee YL, Wu Y, Tsang HW, et al. A systematic review on the anxiolytic effects of aromatherapy in people with anxiety symptoms. J Altern Complement Med 2011;17(2):101–8.

43. Di Stefano V. Holism and complementary medicine: origins and principles. Sydney: Allen & Unwin Academic; 2006.

44. Davidson JR, Crawford C, Ives JA, et al. Homeopathic treatments in psychiatry: a systematic review of randomized placebo-controlled studies. J Clin Psychiatry 2011;72(6):795–805.

45. Pilkington K, Kirkwood G, Rampes H, et al. Homeopathy for anxiety and anxiety disorders: a systematic review of the research. Homeopathy 2006;95(3):151–62.

46. Thaler K, Kaminski A, Chapman A, et al. Bach Flower Remedies for psychological problems and pain: a systematic review. BMC Complement Altern Med 2009;9:16.

47. Kessler RC, Gruber M, Hettema JM, et al. Co-morbid major depression and generalized anxiety disorders in the National Comorbidity Survey follow-up. Psychol Med 2008;38(3):365–74.

48. Millan M. The neurobiology and control of anxious states. Prog Neurobiol 2003;70:83–244.

49. Baldwin DS, Ajel KI, Garner M. Pharmacological treatment of generalized anxiety disorder. Curr Top Behav Neurosci 2010;2:453–67.

50. Sarris J, McIntyre E, Camfield D. Plant-based medicines for anxiety disorders part 1: a systematic review of preclinical studies. CNS Drugs 2013;27(8):675.

51. Sarris J, McIntyre E, Camfield D. Plant-based medicines for anxiety disorders part 2: a systematic review of clinical studies with supportive preclinical evidence. CNS Drugs 2013;27(4):301–19.

52. Savage K, Stough C, Firth J, et al. GABA-modulating phytomedicines for anxiety: a systematic review of preclinical and clinical evidence. Phytother Res 2018;32(1):3–18.

53. Benke D, Barberis A, Kopp S, et al. GABA(A) receptors as in vivo substrate for the anxiolytic action of valerenic acid, a major constituent of valerian root extracts. Neuropharmacology 2009;56(1):174–81.

54. Seitz U, Schule A, Gleitz J. [3H]-monoamine uptake inhibition properties of kava pyrones. Planta Med 1997;63(6):548–9.

55. LaPorte E, Sarris J, Stough C, et al. Neurocognitive effects of kava (Piper methysticum): a systematic review. Hum Psychopharmacol 2011;26(2):102–11.

56. Martin HB, McCallum M, Stofer WD, et al. Kavain attenuates vascular contractility through inhibition of calcium channels. Planta Med 2002;68(9):784–9.

57. Coulter D. Assessment of the risk of hepatotoxicity with kava products. Geneva: WHO appointed committee, World Health Organization; 2007.

58. Teschke R, Sarris J, Glass X, et al. Kava, the anxiolytic herb: back to basics to prevent liver injury? Br J Clin Pharmacol 2011;71(3):445–8.

59. Teschke R, Sarris J, Lebot V. Kava hepatotoxicity solution: a six-point plan for new kava standardization. Phytomedicine 2011;18(2–3):96–103.

60. Awad R, Arnason JT, Trudeau V, et al. Phytochemical and biological analysis of skullcap (Scutellaria lateriflora L.): a medicinal plant with anxiolytic properties. Phytomedicine 2003;10(8):640–9.

61. Amsterdam JD, Li Y, Soeller I, et al. A randomized, double-blind, placebo-controlled trial of oral Matricaria recutita (chamomile) extract therapy for generalized anxiety disorder. J Clin Psychopharmacol 2009;29(4):378–82. doi:10.1097/JCP.0b013e3181ac935c.

62. Avallone R, Zanoli P, Puia G, et al. Pharmacological profile of apigenin, a flavonoid isolated from Matricaria chamomilla. Biochem Pharmacol 2000;59(11):1387–94.

63. Awad R, Levac D, Cybulska P, et al. Effects of traditionally used anxiolytic botanicals on enzymes of the γ-aminobutyric acid (GABA) system. Can J Physiol Pharmacol 2007;85(9):933–42.

64. Keefe JR, Mao JJ, Soeller I, et al. Short-term open-label chamomile (Matricaria chamomilla L.) therapy of moderate to severe generalized anxiety disorder. Phytomedicine 2016;23:1699–705.

65. Mao JJ, Xie SX, Keefe JR, et al. Long-term chamomile (Matricaria chamomilla L.) treatment for generalized anxiety disorder: a randomized clinical trial. Phytomedicine 2016;23:1735–42.

66. Rolland A, Fleurentin J, Lanhers MC, et al. Neurophysiological effects of an extract of Eschscholzia californica Cham. (Papaveraceae). Phytother Res 2001;15(5):377–81.

67. Klvana M, Chen J, Lépine F, et al. Analysis of secondary metabolites from Eschscholzia californica by high-performance liquid chromatography. Phytochem Anal 2006;17(4):236–42.

68. Abascal K, Yarnell E. Nervine herbs for treating anxiety. Altern Complement Ther 2004;10(6):309–15.

69. Zhang M, Ning G, Shou C, et al. Inhibitory effect of jujuboside A on glutamate-mediated excitatory signal pathway in hippocampus. Planta Med 2003;69(8):692–5.

70. Hsieh MT, Chen HC, Hsu PH, et al. Effects of Suanzaorentang on behavior changes and central monoamines. Proc Natl Sci Counc Repub China B 1986;10(1):43–8.

71. Chen HC, Hsieh MT, Shibuya TK. Suanzaorentang versus diazepam: a controlled double-blind study in anxiety. Int J Clin Pharmacol Ther Toxicol 1986;24(12):646–50.

72. Koetter U, Barrett M, Lacher S, et al. Interactions of Magnolia and Ziziphus extracts with selected central nervous system receptors. J Ethnopharmacol 2009;124(3):421–5.

73. Kuribara H, Kishi E, Hattori N, et al. The anxiolytic effect of two oriental herbal drugs in Japan attributed to honokiol from magnolia bark. J Pharm Pharmacol 2000;52(11):1425–9.

74. Han H, Jung JK, Han SB, et al. Anxiolytic-like effects of 4-O-methylhonokiol isolated from Magnolia officinalis through enhancement of GABAergic transmission and chloride influx. J Med Food 2011; 14(7–8):724–31.

75. Alexeev M, Grosenbaugh DK, Mott DD, et al. The natural products magnolol and honokiol are positive allosteric modulators of both synaptic and extra-synaptic GABA(A) receptors. Neuropharmacology 2012;62(8):2507–14.

76. Seo JJ, Lee SH, Lee YS, et al. Anxiolytic-like effects of obovatol isolated from Magnolia obovata: involvement of GABA/benzodiazepine receptors complex. Prog Neuropsychopharmacol Biol Psychiatry 2007;31(7):1363–9.

77. Jacka FN, Maes M, Pasco JA, et al. Nutrient intakes and the common mental disorders in women. J Affect Disord 2012;141(1):79–85.

78. Eby GA, Eby KL. Rapid recovery from major depression using magnesium treatment. Med Hypotheses 2006;67(2):362–70.

79. Spasov AA, Iezhitsa IN, Kharitonova MV, et al. Depression-like and anxiety-related behaviour of rats fed with magnesium-deficient diet. Zh Vyssh Nerv Deiat Im I P Pavlova 2008;58(4):476–85.

80. Poleszak E, Wlaz P, Wrobel A, et al. NMDA/glutamate mechanism of magnesium-induced anxiolytic-like behavior in mice. Pharmacol Rep 2008;60(5):655–63.

81. Poleszak E. Benzodiazepine/GABA(A) receptors are involved in magnesium-induced anxiolytic-like behavior in mice. Pharmacol Rep 2008;60(4):483–9.

82. De Souza MC, Walker AF, Robinson PA, et al. A synergistic effect of a daily supplement for 1 month of 200 mg magnesium plus 50 mg vitamin B6 for the relief of anxiety-related premenstrual symptoms: a randomized, double-blind, crossover study. J Womens Health Gend Based Med 2000;9(2):131–9.

83. Sarris J, Stough C, Bousman C, et al. Kava in the Treatment of Generalized Anxiety Disorder: a double-blind, randomized, placebo-controlled study. J Clin Psychopharmacol 2013;33(5):643–8.

84. Sarris J, Stough C, Teschke R, et al. Kava for the Treatment of Generalized Anxiety Disorder RCT: analysis of adverse reactions, liver function, addiction, and sexual effects. Phytother Res 2013;27(11):1723–8.

85. Woelk H, Arnoldt K, Kieser M, et al. Ginkgo biloba special extract EGb 761 in generalized anxiety disorder and adjustment disorder with anxious mood: a randomized, double-blind, placebo-controlled trial. J Psychiatr Res 2007;41(6):472–80.

86. Wijeweera P, Arnason JT, Koszycki D, et al. Evaluation of anxiolytic properties of Gotukola, Äì (Centella asiatica) extracts and asiaticoside in rat behavioral models. Phytomedicine 2006;13(9, 10):668–76.

87. Chen Y, Han T, Rui Y, et al. Effects of total triterpenes of Centella asiatica on the corticosterone levels in serum and contents of monoamine in depression rat brain. Zhong Yao Cai 2005;28(6):492–6.

88. Jana U, Sur TK, Maity LN, et al. A clinical study on the management of generalized anxiety disorder with Centella asiatica. Nepal Med Coll J 2010;12(1):8–11.

89. Sarris J, Kavanagh DJ, Byrne G. Adjuvant use of nutritional and herbal medicines with antidepressants, mood stabilizers and benzodiazepines. J Psychiatr Res 2010;44(1):32–41.

90. Mehta AK, Binkley P, Gandhi SS, et al. Pharmacological effects of Withania somnifera root extract on GABAA receptor complex. Indian J Med Res 1991;94: 312–15.

91. Andrade C, Aswath A, Chaturvedi SK, et al. A double-blind, placebo-controlled evaluation of the anxiolytic efficacy of an ethanolic extract of withania somnifera. Indian J Psychiatry 2000;42(3):295–301.

92. Cropley M, et al. The effects of Rhodiola rosea L. extract on anxiety, stress, cognition and other mood symptoms. Phytother Res 2015;29(12):1934–9.

93. Panossian A, Wikman G. Evidence-based efficacy of adaptogens in fatigue, and molecular mechanisms related to their stress-protective activity. Curr Clin Pharmacol 2009;4(3):198–219.

94. Geng J, Dong J, Ni H, et al. Ginseng for cognition. Cochrane Database Syst Rev 2010;(12):CD007769.

95. Panossian A. Stimulating effect of adaptogens: an overview with particular reference to their efficacy following single dose administration. Phytother Res 2005;19:819–38.

96. Dubois O, Salamon R, Germain C, et al. Balneotherapy versus paroxetine in the treatment of generalized anxiety disorder. Complement Ther Med 2010;18(1):1–7.

97. Jorm AF, Morgan AJ, Hetrick SE. Relaxation for depression. Cochrane Database Syst Rev 2008;(4):CD007142.

98. Cabyoglu MT, Ergene N, Tan U. The mechanism of acupuncture and clinical applications. Int J Neurosci 2006;116(2):115–25.

99. Bender TS, Nagy GR, Barna IN, et al. The effect of physical therapy on beta-endorphin levels. Eur J Appl Physiol 2007;100(4):371–82.

100. Sherman KJ, Cherkin DC, Hawkes RJ, et al. Randomized trial of therapeutic massage for chronic neck pain. Clin J Pain 2009;25(3):233–8.

101. Kasper S, et al. Silexan, an orally administered Lavandula oil preparation, is effective in the treatment of 'subsyndromal' anxiety disorder: a randomized, double-blind, placebo controlled trial. Int Clin Psychopharmacol 2010;25(5):277–87.

102. Culpeper N. Culpeper's complete herbal. Hertfordshire: Wordsworth Editions Ltd.; 1652.

103. Pittler MH, Schmidt K, Ernst E. Hawthorn extract for treating chronic heart failure: meta-analysis of randomized trials. Am J Med 2003;114(8):665–74.

104. Hanus M, Lafon J, Mathieu M. Double-blind, randomised, placebo-controlled study to evaluate the efficacy and safety of a fixed combination containing two plant extracts

(Crataegus oxyacantha and Eschscholzia californica) and magnesium in mild-to-moderate anxiety disorders. Curr Med Res Opin 2004;20(1):63–71.

105. Peck MD, Ai AL. Cardiac conditions. J Gerontol Soc Work 2008;50(Suppl. 1):13–44.

106. Maciocia G. The foundations of Chinese medicine. Singapore: Churchill Livingstone; 1989.

107. Sarris J, et al. N-acetyl cysteine (NAC) in the treatment of obsessive-compulsive disorder: a 16-week, double-blind, randomised, placebo-controlled study. CNS Drugs 2015;29(9):801–9.

108. Camfield DA, Sarris J, Berk M. Nutraceuticals in the treatment of obsessive compulsive disorder (OCD): a review of mechanistic and clinical evidence. Prog Neuropsychopharmacol Biol Psychiatry 2011;35(4):887–95.

109. Dean OM, Bush A, Berk M. Translating the Rosetta stone of N-acetyl cysteine. Biol Psychiatry 2012;71(11):935–6.

110. Afshar H, Roohafza H, Mohammad-Beigi H, et al. N-acetylcysteine add-on treatment in refractory obsessive-compulsive disorder: a randomized, double-blind, placebo-controlled trial. J Clin Psychopharmacol 2012;32(6):797–803.

111. Grant JE, Odlaug BL, Kim SW. N-acetylcysteine, a glutamate modulator, in the treatment of trichotillomania: a double-blind, placebo-controlled study. Arch Gen Psychiatry 2009;66(7):756–63.

112. Hunot V, Churchill R, Silva de Lima M, et al. Psychological therapies for generalised anxiety disorder. Cochrane Database Syst Rev 2007;(1):CD001848.

113. Sarris J. Whole system research of naturopathy and medical herbalism for improving mood and reducing anxiety. Aust J Med Herbal 2011;23(3):116–19.

114. Cooley K, Szczurko O, Perri D, et al. Naturopathic care for anxiety: a randomized controlled trial ISRCTN78958974. PLOS ONE 2009;4(8):e6628.

115. Sarris J, Gadsden S, Schweitzer I. Naturopathic medicine for treating self-reported depression and anxiety: an observational pilot study of naturalistic practice. Adv Integr Med 2014;In Press.

116. Lara DR. Caffeine, mental health, and psychiatric disorders. J Alzheimers Dis 2010;20(Suppl. 1):S239–48.

117. Manocha R, Black D, Sarris J, et al. A randomized, controlled trial of meditation for work stress, anxiety and depressed mood in full time workers. Evid Based Complement Alternat Med 2011;2011:960583.

118. Kabat-Zinn J. Wherever you go, there you are: mindfulness meditation in everyday life. New York: Hyperion; 1994.

119. Anderson ND, Lau MA, Segal ZV, et al. Mindfulness-based stress reduction and attentional control. Clin Psychol Psychother 2007;14(6):449–63.

120. Shapiro SL, Schwartz GE, Bonner G. Effects of mindfulness-based stress reduction on medical and premedical students. J Behav Med 1998;21(6):581–99.

121. Kirkwood G, Rampes H, Tuffrey V, et al. Yoga for anxiety: a systematic review of the research evidence. Br J Sports Med 2005;39(12):884–91, discussion 891.

122. Brown RP, Gerbarg PL, Muench F. Breathing practices for treatment of psychiatric and stress-related medical conditions. Psychiatr Clin North Am 2013;36(1):121–40.

123. Olive MF. Metabotropic glutamate receptor ligands as potential therapeutics for addiction. Curr Drug Abuse Rev 2009;2(1):83–98.

124. Ryle PR, Thomson AD. Nutrition and vitamins in alcoholism. Contemp Issues Clin Biochem 1984;1:188–224.

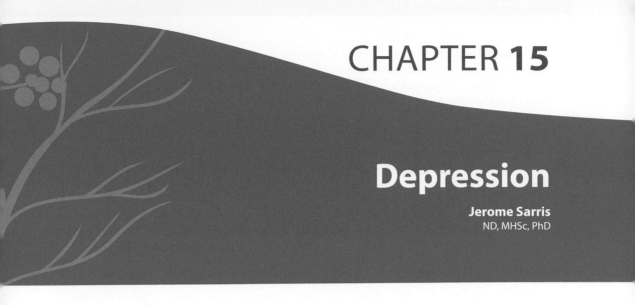

CHAPTER 15

Depression

Jerome Sarris
ND, MHSc, PhD

OVERVIEW

Depression is associated with normal emotions of sadness and loss, and can be seen as part of the natural adaptive response to life's stressors. True 'clinical depression', however, is a disproportionate ongoing state of sadness or absence of pleasure that persists after the exogenous stressors have abated. Clinical depression is commonly characterised by either a low mood or a loss of pleasure in combination with changes in, for example, appetite, sleep and energy, and is often accompanied by feelings of guilt or worthlessness or suicidal thoughts.[1] The *Diagnostic and Statistical Manual of Mental Disorders* (DSM-5) classifies 'major depressive disorder' (MDD) as a clinical depressive episode that lasts longer than two weeks and is uncomplicated by recent grief, substance abuse or a medical condition.[1] MDD diagnostic guidelines according to the new DSM-5 allows for clinical depression to potentially be diagnosed during the initial stage of bereavement (assuming low mood and/ or loss of pleasure is the predominant feature, not grief). Depression presents a significant socioeconomic burden, with the condition being projected by the year 2020 to effect the second greatest increase in morbidity after cardiovascular disease.[2] The lifetime prevalence of depressive disorders varies depending on the country, age, sex and socioeconomic group, and approximates about one in six people.[3] The 12-month prevalence of MDD is approximately 5–8%, with women approximately twice as likely as men to experience an episode.[4]

Pathophysiology of depression

- Dysfunction in monoamine expression and receptor activity, or a lowering of monoamine production
- Secondary messenger system malfunction; for example, G proteins or cyclic adenosine monophosphate (AMP)
- Neuroendocrinological abnormality concerning hyperactivity of the hypothalamic–pituitary–adrenal (HPA) axis, which increases serum cortisol and thereby subsequently reduces brain-derived neurotrophic factor (BDNF) and neurogenesis
- Impaired endogenous opioid function
- Changes in GABAergic and/or glutamatergic transmission, and cytokine or steroidal alterations
- Abnormal circadian rhythm

Adapted from Raison et al. 2006,[5] Belmaker & Agam 2008[6] and Chopra et al. 2011[7]

Several biological and psychological models theorising the causes of depression have been proposed. The predominant biological model of depression in the past 60 years is the monoamine hypothesis.[8] Other key biological theories involve the homocysteine hypothesis[9] and the inflammatory cytokine depression theory.[5] An emerging hypothesis concerns mitochondrial dysfunction, with an association between energy metabolism and depression being documented. A 'mitochondrial psychiatry' model is proposed in which oxidative damage, impaired mitochondrial energy metabolism and dysregulation of multiple mitochondrial genes may provoke neuronal damage and subsequent depression.[10]

Psychologically, cognitive and behavioural causes (or manifestations) of MDD are also commonly present in variations of negative or erroneous thought patterns or schemas, impaired self-mastery, challenged social roles and depressogenic behaviours or lifestyle choices.[11–13] A prominent psychological model is the stress-diathesis model, which promulgates the theory that a combination of vulnerabilities (genetic, parenting, health status and cognitions) are exploited by a life stressor—for example, relationship break-up, job loss or family death.[13,14] These stressful events may trigger a depressive disorder. Some scholars have advanced the theory of a biopsychosocial model, which aims to understand depression in terms of a dynamic interrelationship between the biological, psychological and social causes (discussed later).[12]

DIFFERENTIAL DIAGNOSIS

- Depressive symptoms from medications
- Other psychiatric disorders
- Hypothyroidism
- Chronic pain
- Chronic fatigue syndrome
- Cancer

Adapted from American Psychiatric Association 2013[1] and Raison et al. 2006[15]

RISK FACTORS

Various factors that increase the risk of MDD exist, and such an episode may in turn cause certain health disorders/issues. Genetic vulnerability may play an important part in developing MDD. Genetic studies have revealed that polymorphisms relevant to monoaminergic neurotransmission exist in some people who experience MDD.[16] Some hypotheses suggest that genes related to neuroprotective/toxic/trophic processes and to the overactivation of the hypothalamic–pituitary axis may be involved in the pathogenesis of MDD.[16] Early life events or proximal stressful events increase the risk of an episode.[17] Twin studies provide evidence of the effect of environmental stressors on depression and many studies have revealed that a range of stressful events are involved, affecting remission and relapse of the disorder. Recurrence of depressive episodes and early age at onset present with the greatest familial risk.[18] Current evidence suggests that the primary risk factors involved in MDD are a complex interplay of genetics and exposure to depressogenic life events (see Figure 15.1).

A consistent theme revealed by epidemiological data is that females have higher rates of MDD than males, approximating two times higher in some community samples.[20] This is associated with a higher risk of first onset, and not due to differential persistence

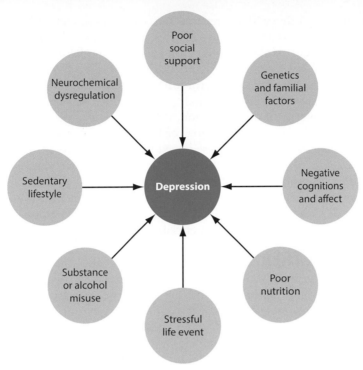

Figure 15.1
Aetiological factors and depression

Depression: at-risk groups
• Females
• Separated or unmarried people (especially for men)
• Unemployed or under financial pressure
• People with disabilities
• Possibly those living in large urban areas
• Major health conditions (especially cardiovascular disease)
• Obesity/metabolic disorders
• Chronic insomnia
• Alcohol/drug abuse or dependency
Adapted from Bromet et al. 2011,[3] McIntyre et al. 2012[19] and Kessler et al. 2003[20]

or recurrence. It appears that hormonal factors are not responsible (e.g. oestrogen levels, pregnancy or the use of oral contraceptives). Biological vulnerabilities and environmental psychosocial factors appear to be responsible for the increased incidence of depression among women.[20]

Practitioners should be aware of the existence of conditions that commonly co-occur with MDD. People who are clinically depressed have a far greater risk of having co-occurring generalised anxiety, sleep disorders and substance abuse or dependency.[21] It should be noted that these conditions may cause MDD and may also result from MDD. Depression is also often misdiagnosed as 'unipolar' when in fact it is the presentation of the depressive phase of 'bipolar' depression.[22] Appropriate screening needs to occur in patients presenting with depression. Initial questioning should assess the length and frequency of previous and current episodes, the severity, what triggers an episode and whether the patient thinks about death regularly or has felt so low lately that they have considered suicide. Assessment should also include a drug and alcohol screen. As chronic insomnia is a prominent risk factor for MDD, it is critical to review the patient's sleep pattern (see Chapter 16 on insomnia).

To assess any bipolarity of the depression, it is important to determine whether they have ever experienced several days or more of feeling very happy or 'high' in addition to behavioural changes such as a decreased need for sleep, rapidity of cognition or ideas and any increases in planning, spending money or sexual drive[1] (see Chapter 36 on bipolar disorder). Appropriate referral in the case of suspected alcohol/substance abuse or dependency or bipolar disorder is recommended, as complementary or alternative medicine (CAM) currently lacks evidence as a primary intervention in these areas (although CAM may be adjunctively beneficial).

CONVENTIONAL TREATMENT

Current medical treatment strategies for MDD primarily involves synthetic antidepressants[6] (e.g. tricyclics, monoamine oxidase inhibitors or selective serotonin reuptake inhibitors [SSRIs]) and psychological interventions (e.g. cognitive behaviour therapy [CBT], interpersonal therapy [IPT] and behavioural therapy).[23] Antidepressant response in Caucasians tends to be modified by several neurochemical polymorphisms. A systematic review and meta-analysis found that genetic differences of 5-HTTLPR, STin2, HTR1A, HTR2A, TPH1 and BDNF neurochemicals modified people's response to SSRIs (although heterogeneity was present across studies).[24] Genetic tests can be given to patients assessing which polymorphisms they have and their likely response to specific medications (see Chapter 2 on diagnostics).

Medical treatment guidelines usually involve options such as providing counselling, CBT or IPT for mild depression, antidepressants and/or CBT for moderate depression and antidepressants and electroconvulsive therapy (ECT) (and hospitalisation if required) for severe depression.[25,26] As only 30–40% of people achieve a satisfactory response to first-line antidepressant prescription and approximately 40% do not achieve remission after several antidepressant prescriptions, further pharmacotherapeutic developments are required.[27] Future novel antidepressant mechanisms of action may involve modulating cytokines, mitochondrial function, secondary messengers and glucocorticoid, or opioid, dopaminergic or melatoninergic pathways.[10,28]

KEY TREATMENT PROTOCOLS

From a clinical perspective, the goal of treating depression is to as safely and quickly as possible reduce depressive symptoms and improve mood. An integrative approach is advised, targeting the multiple pathophysiological underpinnings of the disorder. Suicide is a great concern, and is a devastating potential consequence of depression. If suicidal ideation is significant, or if self-harm is a distinct possibility at any stage, referral to a medical practitioner or to a hospital emergency department for immediate psychiatric assessment is crucial.

> **Naturopathic Treatment Aims**
>
> - Reduce depression and enhance mood.
> - Improve energy level if required.
> - Promote positive balanced cognition.
> - Encourage beneficial lifestyle changes.
> - Educate about depressogenic factors and create a plan to combat them.

The socioeconomic cost of untreated depression is massive, and treated depression reduces the burden on healthcare systems.[29] Evidence advocates early intervention to effectively treat depression and to enhance remission, thereby decreasing human suffering and socioeconomic burden.[30]

Although medical research has not currently advanced to the state of tailoring pharmacotherapy prescriptions to individual neurochemical or genetic profiles, 'whole-system' naturopathic diagnosis and treatment has an advantage in being able to prescribe in an individualised manner, with an uncontrolled pilot study revealing naturopathic medicine to significantly improve self-reported depression.[31] First, in order to treat depression effectively, it helps to understand the psychological and biological factors that are involved. Causes of depression are multifaceted, and individual presentations vary markedly. Because of this, tailoring the prescription for the individual may assist in compliance and recovery. Causative factors can be classified into pre-existing 'vulner-abilities' to depression, which may be 'triggered' by a stressor (commonly a series of stressors or one key event), then 'maintaining' factors may exacerbate or prolong the episode.

Herbal medicines used to treat mental health disorders have central nervous system modulating activity, and most are particularly adept at affecting neuroreceptor binding and activity to achieve an antidepressant effect. Common actions can involve monoamine activity modulation, stimulation or sedation of central nervous system activity[32] and regulation or support of healthy hypothalamic pituitary adrenal axis function (see Table 15.1).

Biopsychosocial model of depression

The most suitable model consistent with the holistic paradigm is a biopsychosocial model. The essence of the model is that the cause of depression is multifactorial, with many interrelated influences involved in its growth. Genetics and biochemistry (biological), cognitions and personality traits (psychological), environmental factors (environmental) and social interactions (sociological) all affect the level of a person's 'vulnerability' to a depressive disorder, which is commonly triggered by chronic or acute stressors. Protective factors are considered to be good genetics, balanced positive cognitions, spirituality and healthy interpersonal relations and social support.[11,33]

Table 15.1
Nervous system herbal medicine actions

Traditional herbal action	Proposed mechanisms	Applications
Nervines (tonics, stimulants)	HPA-modulation, beta-adrenergic activity	Depression, fatigue, convalescence
Adaptogens, thymoleptics, antidepressants	Monoamine interactions HPA-modulation	Depression, fatigue, convalescence
Anxiolytics, hypnotics, sedatives	GABA or adenosine-receptor binding or modulation	Anxiety disorders, insomnia
Antispasmodics, analgesics	Calcium/sodium channel modulation Substance P or enkephalin effects	Muscular tension (dysmenorrhoea, irritable bowel syndrome, headaches), visceral spasm, pain
Cognitive enhancers	Cholinergic activity Acetylcholine esterase inhibition	Cognitive decline, dementia

Source: Sarris et al. 2011[32]

A balanced and integrative naturopathic treatment plan needs to address all aspects concerning the biopsychosocial model.[34] Nutraceutical and dietary prescription can modulate the biological component of depression; psychological therapies and counselling support is advised to reconfigure negative cognitions, resolve underlying issues and build resilience; social concerns (e.g. healthy work, lifestyle, exercise, rest balance and sufficient family/friend/community interaction) should also be addressed. Depression may provide a context for developing meaning from the experience, thereby promoting spiritual growth. Displayed below is a model developed by the author for treating depression: the ALPS model (Figure 15.2). This treatment model is based on the biopsychosocial model, outlining specific strategies for treating depression holistically. The model advocates: a combined approach of antidepressant agents (natural or synthetic); lifestyle adjustments such as dietary improvement and reduction/elimination of alcohol, cigarettes and illicit substances and increased relaxation and exercise; psychological interventions; and improved social functioning and integration.

Monoamine hypothesis

The monoamine hypothesis concerns the theory that depression is primarily caused by dysregulation of serotonin, dopamine and noradrenaline pathways (receptor activity and density, neurotransmitter production and neurochemical transport and transmission).[7,35] Herbal and nutritional/dietary modulation may be helpful in modulating monoaminergic transmission. To date, the phytotherapy with the most evidence of monoamine modulation is *Hypericum perforatum* (**St John's wort [SJW]**). During the past two decades, more than 40 clinical trials of varying methodological quality have been conducted assessing the efficacy of SJW in treating depressed mood. Several meta-analyses have been conducted, including a Cochrane review (Table 15.2). The Cochrane meta-analyses have revealed that *Hypericum perforatum* provides a significant antidepressant effect compared with placebo and an equivalent efficacy compared with synthetic antidepressants. SJW has demonstrated several beneficial effects on

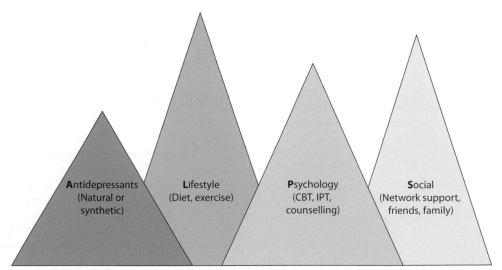

Figure 15.2
The ALPS model

modulating monoamine transmission. The herb contains a range of constituents, including the naphthodianthrones hypericin and pseudohypericin, the phloroglucinol hyperforin and a range of flavonoids, volatile oils and tannins.[36] Preclinical studies suggest that a range of neurochemical activity is involved with the antidepressant effect of SJW. In vitro and in vivo research has revealed nonselective inhibition of the neuronal re-uptake of serotonin, dopamine and noradrenaline, and weak monoamine oxidase A and B inhibition (see Table 15.2 for other mechanisms of action). However, it should be noted that the neurochemical effects revealed in preclinical studies have used exceedingly high doses of SJW or its isolated constituents (far above normal clinical doses). Further, the poor bioavailability of many constituents and the lack of penetration across the blood–brain barrier (e.g. hypericin) suggest that caution needs to be applied when extrapolating from preclinical studies to human clinical activity.[64]

Aside from **SJW**, *Rhodiola rosea* and *Crocus sativus* currently possess the most evidence as monoamine and neuroendocrine modulators, and have provided preliminary human clinical evidence of efficacy in treating MDD.[32] *Rhodiola rosea* is a stimulating adaptogen, which possesses antidepressant, antifatigue and tonic activity.[65] The phytochemicals salidroside, rosvarin and tyrosol are considered to be some of the active constituents.[65] In animal models, *Rhodiola rosea* has been documented to increase noradrenaline, dopamine and serotonin in the brainstem and hypothalamus, and to increase the blood–brain permeability to neurotransmitter precursors.[65] In an earlier small-scale study using the herb for depression,[66] the effect size was small, with a low response in comparison with a very low placebo response (usually there is a 20–50% reduction of depression in a placebo group). A more recent study of a standardised *R. rosea* extract in MDD ($n = 57$) sought to determine whether it was more effective than sertraline and placebo, in a 12-week double-blind RCT.[67] Results revealed a nonsignificant difference between treatments for depression and anxiety outcomes. However, side effects were far less pronounced in the *R. rosea* group compared to the sertraline. *Crocus sativus* is developing clinical evidence as an effective antidepressant, with several RCTs showing it to be effective in reducing depression. A meta-analysis of published RCTs examining the effects of saffron supplementation on symptoms of depression in MDD revealed a significant result with a large effect size in favour of saffron treatment versus placebo control.[68] Longer studies with larger samples, in more diverse jurisdictions, are now advised. Crocin and safranal are currently regarded as the constituents responsible for *Crocus sativus*'s antidepressant action.[69]

Other herbal medicines that have been documented to exert monoamine modulation include *Bacopa monnieri*, *Ginkgo biloba* and *Panax ginseng*; however, aside from a small isolated positive study for MDD in females,[70] to date insufficient clinical trials have confirmed antidepressant effects in humans.

HPA axis modulation

In the past two decades, cortisol has achieved increased attention in the study of the pathogenesis of depression. Substantial evidence exists for the role of cortisol and the HPA axis in depression.[5] Postmortem studies and cerebral spinal fluid sampling have found that corticotrophin-releasing hormone (or factor) (CRF) can be elevated in samples from depressed patients.[71] A combination of vulnerability factors (genetic, age and early life events) and precipitating factors (psychological, physiological stressors, substance misuse and comorbid disease) may provoke an increase in CRF.[11] This stimulates the secretion of adrenocorticotrophic hormone (ACTH), and subsequent cortisol release from the adrenal glands (see Chapters 18–20 on the endocrine system). In vitro and animal models have demonstrated that HPA-axis dysfunction and increased cortisol attenuate the production of BDNF in the brain.[5,35] BDNF is an important growth factor that nourishes nerve cells, and lower BDNF is correlated with depressive states.[6,16] Synthetic antidepressants and electroconvulsive therapy appear to regulate the HPA axis and increase the production of BDNF.[72] In animal models, hypericin and the flavonoid derivatives have demonstrated to down-regulate plasma ACTH and corticosterone levels.[64] In particular, an animal model demonstrated that eight weeks of SJW or hypericin administration decreased the expression of genes involved in the regulation of the HPA axis; however, human studies have found that SJW increases salivary and serum cortisol levels.[73,74] An interesting cross-sectional investigation was conducted of the serum BDNF levels in 962 depressed patients, 700 fully remitted persons (≥ six months) and 382 healthy controls.[75] Results revealed that SJW use was associated with higher serum BDNF in depressed patients compared with non-medicated controls.

It should be noted that while evidence does suggest that HPA modulation does occur with SJW administration, the complex pharmacodynamics of the effect has not been fully elucidated to date, with variables such as differing human or animal models, stress study methodology and types of SJW extracts obfuscating the conclusion. Clinicians should be mindful of potential drug interactions if using products with higher (> 1 mg) hyperforin and in co-administration with other psychotrophic medications. SJW should not be prescribed at significantly higher doses, while caution is advised for use in those with bipolar disorder who are not receiving a mood stabiliser.

Herbal adaptogens and tonics may play a beneficial role in modulating ACTH (refer further to Chapters 18–20 on the endocrine system). Stimulating adaptogens such as *Eleutherococcus senticosus*, *Schisandra chinensis* and *Rhodiola rosea* have demonstrated significant adaptogenic effects, posited as occurring from HPTA modulation.[76] Although *Eleutherococcus senticosus*, *Schisandra chinensis* and other adaptogens such as *Panax ginseng* and *Withania somnifera* have not demonstrated specific antidepressant activity, they may provide a supportive role in depressive presentations with HPA-axis dysregulation.

Antidepressant response of St John's wort

An analysis was conducted on two pooled eight-week RCTs (*n* = 483) to determine the response pattern of participants with MDD to SJW compared with two antidepressants and placebo. Of the participants who were taking SJW and were 'responders' at the week 8 study endpoint (> 50% reduction of depressive symptoms), they showed an early response rate (25–50%) depression reduction of 44% by week 1, 79% by week 2 and 85% by week 4. Of participants with no clinical response at any time-point by week 8, the majority had no early improvement compared with those who had an early partial response. The clinical conclusion indicates that participants who ultimately respond to SJW respond early. Therefore if no signs of an antidepressant effect from SJW occur within two weeks, switching to other treatments or medical referral is advised.

Source: Sarris et al. 2013[77]

Homocysteine hypothesis

The homocysteine hypothesis centres on the theory that genetic and environmental factors elevate levels of homocysteine, which in turn provokes changes in neuronal architecture and neurotransmission, resulting in depression.[9] The sulfur compound homocysteine (formed from methionine) has been demonstrated to be directly toxic to neurons and can induce DNA strand breakage. Higher serum levels of homocysteine have been noted in depressive populations compared with healthy controls[78]; however a recent cross-sectional study only found this association in older adults.[79] Metabolism of homocysteine to *S*-adenosyl methionine (SAMe) or back to methionine requires folate, B6 and B12.[9] An adjunctive RCT on responsiveness to SSRIs found response (Hamilton Depression Rating Scale: HAMD ≥ 50% reduction) and remission rates were significantly higher for patients treated with adjunctive SAMe (36.1% and 25.8%, respectively) than adjunctive placebo (17.6% versus 11.7%, respectively).[46]

Folate is involved with the methylation pathways in the 'one-carbon' cycle, and is responsible for metabolising and synthesising various monoamines.[78] Folate is also most notably involved with the synthesis of SAMe, an endogenous antidepressant formed from homocysteine. Folate deficiency is implicated in causing increased homocysteine levels, and has been consistently demonstrated in depressive populations and in poor responders to antidepressants.[80] Folate deficiency has been reported in approximately one-third of people suffering from depressive disorders.[80] Mixed evidence has been found for a correlation between the methylenetetrahydrofolate (MTHF) reductase C677T gene (a folate-metabolising enzyme) polymorphism and depression.[50,81]

Several studies exist assessing the antidepressant effect of **folic acid** in humans with concomitant antidepressant use.[49] All of these studies yielded positive results with regard to enhancing antidepressant response rates or increasing the onset of response. The study demonstrated a statistically significant reduction after 10 weeks on the HAMD for women. This effect was not, however, replicated in the male sample. A two-year prospective Australian community-based RCT[82] involving a sub-sample of 209 antidepressant users examined the effects of folic acid supplementation (400 mcg/day plus vitamin B12 100 mcg/day) in older adults (aged 60–74) with depressive symptoms. Results revealed no significant interaction between the supplement group and antidepressant use. Along with a good dietary intake of folate-rich leafy vegetables or folic acid supplementation, a multivitamin high in B vitamins (especially B6 and B12) may assist in reducing homocysteine and maintaining adequate levels of SAMe. This will also assist in maintaining of energy production and adrenal function and creating neurotransmitters. The folinic acid or 5-MTHF (L-methylfolate) active forms are advised as they do not require the MTHF reductase enzyme to convert into the active form.

Inflammatory factors causing depression

A cytokine-mediated pro-inflammatory event has been considered as a factor involved with the pathophysiology of MDD.[83] Studies have demonstrated that otherwise healthy patients with depression have presented with activated inflammatory pathways.[83] It has been posited that pro-inflammatory cytokines produced from inflammation may influence neuroendocrine function via entry through the 'leaky regions' of the brain (e.g. the circumventricular organs) and subsequent modulation of cytokine-specific transport molecules or cytokine stimulation of vagal afferent fibres.[5] Modulation of both cortisol and neurotransmitters is known to be effected by cytokines. The main pro-inflammatory cytokines implicated in depressogenesis centres on IFN-α producing IL-1β, IL-6 and TNF-α cytokines (see Chapter 31 on autoimmunity). In laboratory studies, animals exposed to a variety of stressors have demonstrated an increase in these pro-inflammatory cytokines. Synthetic antidepressants have been shown to inhibit the production of various inflammatory cytokines and to stimulate the production of anti-inflammatory cytokines.[10]

Attenuation of pro-inflammatory cytokines may be of benefit in individuals who present with either a preceding or a comorbid inflammatory condition, or a chronic latent infection. Appropriate screening to determine any infections (or inflammatory process) with reference to the chronology of the onset of depression is advised. If an association is plausible, herbal medicines and nutrients that dampen the inflammatory cascade and attenuate the production of pro-inflammatory cytokines may be advised (see Chapters 8–10 on the respiratory system and Chapter 4–6 on the gastrointestinal system).

A link between bowel microflora and depression?

Raised in a seminal publication by Raison is the potential link between bowel microfloral imbalance and increased GIT inflammation and permeability causing systemic immune dysregulation and depression. Significant data suggest that a loss of exposure to a variety of beneficial microorganisms may promote depression by increasing systemic levels of inflammatory cytokines.

Source: Raison et al. 2010[84]

In brief, herbal and nutritional medicines that may potentially benefit the treatment of pro-inflammatory-evoked MDD include ***Albizia* spp.**, ***Echinacea* spp.**, **vitamin C** and **bioflavonoids** (see Chapters 8–10 on the respiratory system). Aside from its culinary use, *Curcuma longa* has been used in traditional Ayurvedic and Chinese medicine, possessing anti-inflammatory, antioxidant, neuroprotective and monoaminergic modulatory activities.[85] A meta-analysis in 2017 by Ng and colleagues included six clinical trials (four to eight weeks in duration) involving 377 participants with depression, and compared either turmeric or curcumin (the active constituent) to placebo.[86] Results revealed a significant effect in favour of curcumin in reducing depressive symptoms. **Zinc** is another compound that dampens inflammation via inhibition of TNF-alpha and IL-1β[87] and is critical to neurobiological function. The mineral is one of the most prevalent trace elements in the amygdala, hippocampus and neocortex brain regions. Zinc is involved with hippocampal neurogenesis via upregulation of BDNF, while also modifying N-methyl-D-aspartate (NMDA) and glutamate activity.[88] Zinc also modulates the HPA axis and has been shown to be neuroprotective in animal models.[89] Low zinc serum level is associated with depression risk and correlated with an increase in the activation immune system biomarkers, suggesting that this effect may result in part from a depression-related alteration in the immune-inflammatory system.[88]

A cross-sectional study examined the relationship between dietary intake of zinc and depression in 402 postgraduate students.[90] Results revealed an inverse relationship between dietary intake of zinc and depression. The results persisted even after being controlled for several potential confounding variables related to depressive symptoms, such as sex, years of education and smoking status. Currently there is emerging evidence for zinc in improving depressed mood. A recent review by Lai et al.[48] aimed to synthesise results from all published RCTs on the efficacy of zinc supplementation for reducing or preventing depressive symptoms. The review revealed two adjunctive RCTs showing significant effects beyond placebo in reducing depression.

Albizia spp. (in particular *Albizia lebbeck*) have been documented to exert anti-inflammatory and antiallergic activity.[91] In addition to this activity, anxiolytic and antidepressant effects have been demonstrated in ***Albizia julibrissin***, the plant curiously is known as 'happy bark' in traditional Chinese medicine.[92] Aside from the previously mentioned herbal and nutritional medicines, **omega-3 fatty acids** also have a role in reducing inflammation-based MDD. Epidemiological studies have demonstrated that a rise in depressive symptoms may be correlated with lower dietary omega-3 fish oil (eicosapentaenoic acid [EPA] and docosahexaenoic acid [DHA]).[93,94] Studies have also revealed that people with depression have a tendency towards a higher ratio of serum arachidonic acid to essential fatty acids, and an overall lower serum level of omega-3 compared with healthy controls.[95] Urbanised Western cultures tend to have a far higher ratio of dietary omega-6 oils compared with omega-3 oils, and this has been regarded as a possible factor in the rise of depression over the past several decades.[96] The pathophysiology occurring from a pro-omega-6 diet may involve an increased promotion of inflammatory eicosanoids, a lessening of BDNF and a decrease in neuronal cell membrane fluidity and communication.[97]

Evidence currently suggests that omega-3 fatty acids exert antidepressant activity via beneficial effects on neurotransmission including modulation of neurotransmitter (noradrenaline, dopamine and serotonin) reuptake, degradation, synthesis and receptor binding, anti-inflammation and BDNF increase.[42] Several human clinical trials have been conducted assessing the efficacy of EPA, DHA or a combination of both of these essential fatty acids, with current evidence strongly supporting EPA over DHA as being responsible for the antidepressant effect.[43]

Suicide
• Screen for presence of a clearly articulated plan to suicide, any preparations being made and any past serious attempts.
• If a patient is suicidal, immediately refer them to an emergency department for psychiatric assessment.
• Extreme caution should be observed for patients who, in light of a recent suicidal disposition, suddenly appear happy with no clear reason (they may be at peace with their decision to suicide).
• Initial antidepressant use may increase the risk of suicide. Be especially aware of antidepressant use in adolescents.

INTEGRATIVE MEDICAL CONSIDERATIONS

As detailed, an evidence-based integrative prescriptive plan should be provided to comprehensively treat depression. Other treatments include acupuncture and psychological interventions. If the patient is unresponsive to CAM treatment (after two to four weeks of treatment), the prescription should be altered or additional interventions

Lifestyle medicine for depression
There is now compelling evidence that a range of lifestyle factors are involved in the pathogenesis of depression. The term 'lifestyle medicine' has been coined for a treatment approach of prescribing physical activity or exercise, dietary modification, adequate relaxation/sleep and social interaction, the reduction of recreational substances such as nicotine, drugs and alcohol, in addition to consideration of environmental issues (e.g. urbanisation and exposure to air, water, noise and chemical pollution) and the increasing human interface with technology. Source: Sarris et al. 2014[98]

provided. Antidepressants may be required if the depressive episode worsens and suicidal ideation is present, or if symptoms persist after several prescription modifications to non-response. Aside from the interventions discussed above, current evidence supports various psychological techniques, exercise, dietary improvement (longitudinal and cross-sectional relationship) and acupuncture (although study designs are often poor) to improve mood. Evidence does not currently support other interventions such as chiropractics or homeopathy.

Acupuncture and massage

The use of acupuncture to treat depressive disorders has been documented in traditional Chinese medicine texts.[99] In traditional Chinese medicine the two main organs (energetically) involved in depression are the liver and the heart, and the two primary patterns of depression are diagnosed in traditional Chinese medicine: 'stagnation of liver Qi' (excess pattern) and 'deficiency of Qi, blood, or kidney Jing' (deficient pattern).[99] Results of a recent Cochrane review (Smith et al.) found low-quality evidence revealing mainly positive effects on reducing depression versus non-specific or sham acupuncture and waitlist.[100] It should, however, be noted that many studies had poor methodological design.

Massage may also be of benefit in improving mood and reducing depression. Studies of varying methodological rigour have shown that massage increases relaxation, decreases stress and elevates the mood.[101] A rigorous review of massage techniques in treating clinical depression commented that, while positive studies exist, a lack of evidence from RCTs does not support this intervention.[101] While evidence currently does not support massage as a primary monotherapy in treating depression, use of massage adjunctively can be advised, especially in cases of co-occurring muscular tension.

Psychological intervention

As outlined under the ALPS model, psychological intervention is an important component in treating MDD. Guidelines support the use of psychological interventions such as CBT and IPT in mild depression rather than synthetic medication.[26] CBT and IPT are accepted psychological interventions, both having equal evidence of efficacy in treating MDD.[23] CBT involves learning cognitive skills to 'reprogram' erroneous or negative thought patterns with positive balanced cognitions, and to institute positive behavioural modifications. The theory is based on the concept that a person's negative, critical, erroneous thought patterns provoke deleterious emotional and physiological responses. By intervening before this cascade occurs, and establishing a positive balanced inner dialogue, this spiral can be avoided. IPT focuses on identifying problematic social situations that are depressogenic and developing interpersonal techniques (such as social skills) to manage interpersonal relationships. By increasing confidence and competency in managing social interactions, a robust self-esteem may develop. The use of psychoeducation to explain to the patient what depression is and a variety of ways to manage the condition is also of benefit, as found in a 2009 meta-analysis.[102] Psychoeducational interventions can be easily implemented and are not expensive.

Other techniques, such as teaching problem-solving skills to identify and deal with depressogenic triggers, may be of assistance. Finally, it is important to assist the patient to identify external triggers that may cause an episode (e.g. the anniversary of a death or a change in weather) and help them to formulate a 'pro-euthymic' plan to combat this. Naturopaths may learn basic skills in teaching CBT and IPT, and a caring humanistic

---

Adjunctive use of nutraceuticals with antidepressants

If the patient is taking antidepressant medication without adequate response, adjunctive options are a potential option to enhance the thymoleptic effect or reduce side effects (see Sarris et al.[103] for review). Consideration of serotonin syndrome or switching to bipolar (hypo)mania should be considered.

- Evidence exists for combining SAMe, L-tryptophan, zinc, folic acid or EPA with antidepressants to increase response or speed the onset of action.[42]
- Novel adjuvant prescription includes the use of aromatic or bitter herbs such as *Zingiber officinale*[104] or *Cynara scolymus*[105] to reduce nausea and relieve dyspepsia, or to address some common digestive symptoms manifesting from depression.
- Co-occurring fatigue could potentially be reduced via co-administration of adaptogens such as *Rhodiola rosea*[65] or *Panax ginseng*.[44]
- Insomnia and irritability can be treated via herbal anxiolytics such as *Passiflora incarnata*[106] or *Piper methysticum*.[107]
- Sexual dysfunction may be alleviated in some patients by using *Leidium meyenii* (maca root)[108] or *Ginkgo biloba*,[109] although not all studies show positive results.
- The occurrence of hepatotoxicity could be potentially reduced by using antioxidant hepatics such as *Silybum marianum* or *Schisandra chinensis*.[110]

---

approach should always be present. However, for skilled psychological intervention, referral to a clinical psychologist or highly trained counsellor is advised.

Dietary modification

Major changes in dietary patterns have occurred globally in the past century, with a shift in Western societies towards a typical high-calorific diet rich in saturated fats and refined sugar.[111] Cross-sectional[59] and longitudinal data[58] show that poor diets are associated with an increase in depressive symptoms. Diet modulates several key biological processes that underscore mood disorders, including oxidative processes and inflammation, brain plasticity and function, the endocrine system and mitochondrial function.[56,57]

To date, one well-designed RCT ($n = 67$) examining dietary modification for MDD exists. Results revealed that the dietary support group showed a significantly greater reduction in depression symptoms compared to the social support control.[53] Although evidence supporting specific dietary advice is currently insufficient (aside from a Mediterranean diet approach), a basic balanced diet (see Chapter 3 on wellness) including foods rich in a spectrum of nutrients can be recommended. Foods rich in folate, omega-3, tryptophan, B and C vitamins, zinc and magnesium are necessary for the production of neurotransmitters and neuronal communication.[112] These include whole grains, lean meat, deep-sea fish, green leafy vegetables, coloured berries and nuts (e.g. walnuts, almonds and Brazil nuts).[96] See Chapter 3 for more comprehensive dietary advice.

Exercise and physical activity

Increasing physical activity is advised in cases of underactivity. Modernity has similarly reduced the amount of physical activity and formalised exercise undertaken by the average person. Our lifestyles are increasingly sedentary, with the resultant side effect of obesity being currently recognised as a major health problem worldwide.[113,114] Epidemiological studies have shown that adequate physical activity is associated with fewer depressive symptoms, while insufficient physical activity may be a risk factor for developing depressive symptoms.[115–118] Evidence provides some support for the use of exercise. A recent Cochrane review (updated from 2009) included 32 studies ($n = 1858$) involving exercise for treating researcher-defined depression.[62] From these studies, 28 RCTs ($n = 1101$) were included in a meta-analysis revealing a moderate to large effect in favour of exercise over standard treatment or control. However, only four trials with adequate allocation concealment, blinding and intention-to-treat analysis were located, resulting in a more modest effect size in favour of exercise. Pooled data from seven trials ($n = 373$) with long-term follow-up data also found a small clinical effect in favour of exercise. Research strongly suggests that anabolic **exercise of high intensity** is more effective than that of low intensity.[119] The biological antidepressant effects of exercise include a beneficial modulation of the HPA axis, increased expression of 5-HT and increased levels of circulating testosterone (which may have a protective effect against depression).[120,121]

Evidence also exists for the use of **yoga** to reduce depression and improve mood. A review documented five RCTs using various types of yoga to treat MDD.[63] While the studies reviewed all concluded positive results, the methodologies were poorly reported and thereby no firm conclusion can be reached. It is worthwhile highlighting that certain types of yoga may actually have greater antidepressant effect. 'Mindfulness' in exercise techniques such as yoga may potentially have greater efficacy than low-intensity, low-focus yoga, although evidence does not currently confirm this theory.[122]

Evidence for the type and amount of exercise for managing MDD currently favours anabolic over aerobic activity to gain the greatest benefits, and the intensity needs to be moderate to high and performed two or three times per week.[61] Caveats exist regarding exercise prescription for MDD. Depression may be worsened if the person is unable to meet expectations, potentially promoting a sense of failure and guilt. This may be more likely to occur in severe MDD, especially where psychomotor retardation, hypersomnia, somnolence, marked fatigue or anhedonia are present. Exercise plans should be instituted after a medical assessment and initially commenced at a low intensity to allow for physical and psychological adaptation to occur to the new stimulus.

CLINICAL SUMMARY

The initial case-taking process is important to assess the causations of the depressive pattern (within a biopsychosocial framework), when the first episode occurred, the number of discrete episodes, the severity, what may trigger an episode (e.g. anniversary of a death, change in the weather), maintaining factors that may exacerbate or prolong the episode (e.g. ill health, chronic stress, unemployment) and what alleviates the depression (Figure 15.3). It is important also to screen for hypothyroidism symptoms and, if present, to refer for a blood test to determine thyroid-stimulating hormone (TSH) levels. After thorough case taking, an individual tailoring of the prescription is vital to address the specific underlying causes of the depression, therefore assisting in compliance and recovery. It is important to address in the prescription a range of common symptoms that often present with depression, such as changes in sleep pattern, energy levels and digestive function. After initial case taking and prescription, a follow-up appointment (approximately one week later) is especially important not only to monitor for any lowering of mood but also to ensure compliance, to check for adverse reactions and to provide a supportive therapeutic role.

Any lifestyle modifications in the prescription should consider that any changes need to be incorporated to form a normal ongoing lifestyle adjustment. Motivational issues, time restrictions, financial limitations, the perspective about the source of their difficulties and their treatment priorities may influence a patient's ability to make those changes. Adherence and engagement is increased by having ownership of the treatment plan and a sense of shared partnership in its development and planning. Due to this, all treatment strategies should be developed considering the above factors, and the treatment package should be individually tailored and offered in a stepwise manner. General lifestyle advice should focus on encouraging a balance between meaningful work, adequate rest and sleep, judicious exercise, positive social interaction and pleasurable hobbies. Behavioural therapy techniques have shown positive effects on reducing depression by training the person to reduce or better manage stressful situations and to increase pleasurable activities that enhance self-esteem and self-mastery. If substance or alcohol dependence or misuse is apparent, supportive advice on curtailing this, or appropriate referral, should be communicated.

In addition to evidence-based prescriptions, lifestyle medicine can always be offered, focusing on encouraging a balance between meaningful work, adequate rest, judicious exercise, positive social interaction and pleasurable hobbies.

A final clinical consideration is to encourage exploration of fun activities in the patient's life. Pleasurable euthymic activities (especially involving social contact) offer a powerful antidote to life's stressors.

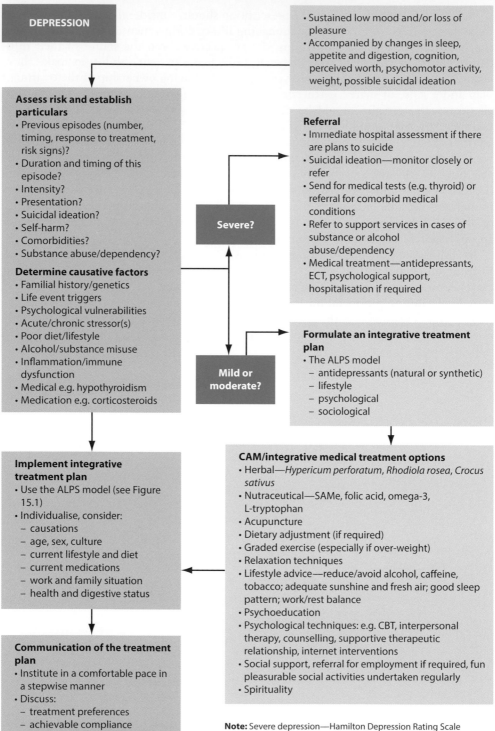

DEPRESSION

- Sustained low mood and/or loss of pleasure
- Accompanied by changes in sleep, appetite and digestion, cognition, perceived worth, psychomotor activity, weight, possible suicidal ideation

Assess risk and establish particulars
- Previous episodes (number, timing, response to treatment, risk signs)?
- Duration and timing of this episode?
- Intensity?
- Presentation?
- Suicidal ideation?
- Self-harm?
- Comorbidities?
- Substance abuse/dependency?

Determine causative factors
- Familial history/genetics
- Life event triggers
- Psychological vulnerabilities
- Acute/chronic stressor(s)
- Poor diet/lifestyle
- Alcohol/substance misuse
- Inflammation/immune dysfunction
- Medical e.g. hypothyroidism
- Medication e.g. corticosteroids

Severe?

Mild or moderate?

Referral
- Immediate hospital assessment if there are plans to suicide
- Suicidal ideation—monitor closely or refer
- Send for medical tests (e.g. thyroid) or referral for comorbid medical conditions
- Refer to support services in cases of substance or alcohol abuse/dependency
- Medical treatment—antidepressants, ECT, psychological support, hospitalisation if required

Formulate an integrative treatment plan
- The ALPS model
  - antidepressants (natural or synthetic)
  - lifestyle
  - psychological
  - sociological

Implement integrative treatment plan
- Use the ALPS model (see Figure 15.1)
- Individualise, consider:
  - causations
  - age, sex, culture
  - current lifestyle and diet
  - current medications
  - work and family situation
  - health and digestive status

CAM/integrative medical treatment options
- Herbal—*Hypericum perforatum, Rhodiola rosea, Crocus sativus*
- Nutraceutical—SAMe, folic acid, omega-3, L-tryptophan
- Acupuncture
- Dietary adjustment (if required)
- Graded exercise (especially if over-weight)
- Relaxation techniques
- Lifestyle advice—reduce/avoid alcohol, caffeine, tobacco; adequate sunshine and fresh air; good sleep pattern; work/rest balance
- Psychoeducation
- Psychological techniques: e.g. CBT, interpersonal therapy, counselling, supportive therapeutic relationship, internet interventions
- Social support, referral for employment if required, fun pleasurable social activities undertaken regularly
- Spirituality

Communication of the treatment plan
- Institute in a comfortable pace in a stepwise manner
- Discuss:
  - treatment preferences
  - achievable compliance
  - potential realistic benefits
  - possible 'plan B' options
- Monitor patient's progress

Note: Severe depression—Hamilton Depression Rating Scale (HAMD) > 24, suicidal thoughts, psychotic symptoms, mood very low e.g. ≤ 2/10, may have non-responded to previous medication; Moderate depression—HAMD 17–24, low mood e.g. 3–4; Mild depression—HAMD 7–16, average–low mood 5–6/10

Figure 15.3
Naturopathic treatment decision tree—depression

Table 15.2
Review of the major evidence

Intervention	Mechanisms of action	Key literature	Summary of results	Comment
Hypericum perforatum (St John's wort [SJW])	Nonselective reuptake inhibition of monamines Weak monoamine oxidase A and B inhibition Decreased degradation of neurochemicals Increased dopaminergic activity in the prefrontal cortex Neuroendocrine modulation[36]	Meta-analysis: Linde 2008[37]	SJW versus placebo on HAMD: Relative risk (RR) of 1.48 (1.23, 1.77) from 18 combined studies for response versus placebo (significant effect) SJW versus synthetics on HAMD: Equivocal effect with SSRIs. RR of 1.00 (0.90, 1.15)	SJW consistently demonstrates greater efficacy than placebo in treating MDD Efficacy is equal to synthetic antidepressants Lower hyperforin extracts are advised to minimise drug interactions
Crocus sativus	Reuptake inhibition of dopamine, noradrenaline and serotonin NMDA receptor antagonism GABA-α agonism, opioid receptor modulation[32]	RCTs: Akhondzadeh et al. 2005, 2007 Noorbala et al. 2005, Moshiri et al 2006[38–41]	Four RCTs: more effective than placebo; equivalent efficacy to synthetic antidepressants	Effective, but expensive Potential adverse reactions include nausea, diarrhoea, tachycardia, dyspepsia and appetite changes[32]
Omega-3 fatty acids	Modulation and increase of several neurotransmitters Benefits neurotransmission via ↑ cell fluidity Reduces inflammation[42]	Meta-analysis: Sublette et al. 2011[43]	High EPA supplements (≥ 60%) versus placebo on HAMD: Significant effect size = 0.532 (0.277, 0.733) High DHA supplements (≥ 60%) versus placebo on HAMD: non-significant effect size = 0.026 (−0.200, 0.148)	Evidence supports EPA and not DHA Most positive studies included were 'adjunctive' trials Recommend in deficient states, or in comorbid inflammatory conditions or CVD or adjunctively with antidepressants
L-tryptophan	Required for conversion into serotonin via intermediary step to active form 5-HTP[44]	Systematic review and meta-analysis: Shaw et al. 2002[45] Positive augmentation studies[44]	Tryptophan augmentation with MAOIs, SSRIs and some TCAs is effective in increasing the antidepressant response No difference occurred compared with placebo with other tricyclics	May be of use in subjects taking antidepressants, in tryptophan deficiency or in depression caused by serotonergic pathway dysregulation High dosage may cause adverse reactions such as GIT complaints, nausea or serotonin syndrome

Table 15.2
Review of the major evidence (continued)

Intervention	Mechanisms of action	Key literature	Summary of results	Comment
S-adenosyl methionine (SAMe)	Enhanced methylation of catecholamines Increased serotonin turnover, reuptake inhibition of noradrenaline Enhanced dopaminergic activity Decreased prolactin secretion Increased phosphatidylcholine conversion[46]	Systematic review: Williams et al. 2005[47] Key adjunctive study: Papakostas et al. 2010[46]	Intramuscular and oral augmentation of SAMe with antidepressants has demonstrated ↑ response and remission rates May enhance response in antidepressant non-responders	Stability and cost an issue Parenteral administration may be more efficacious than oral administration Caution in bipolar patients to avoid switching to mania
Zinc	Increases hippocampal neurogenesis via upregulation of BDNF Modifies N-methyl-D-aspartate (NMDA) and glutamate activity Modulates the HPA axis Neuroprotective in animal models[48]	Systematic review: Lai et al. 2012[48] RCTs: Two key 12-week RCTs that examined the effects of zinc (25 mg/d) monotherapy supplementation as an adjunct with antidepressants	Zinc significantly lowered depressive symptom scores of depressed patients (pooled standard mean difference over placebo on HAMD of −2.84 points)	This evidence suggests potential benefits of zinc as a stand-alone intervention or as an adjunct to conventional antidepressant drug therapy for depression Picolinate or glycinate the best forms
Folic acid	Involved in the one carbon cycle in addition to B12 and SAMe[49]	RCTs: Several adjunctive studies using antidepressants and folic acid (see Taylor et al. 2004 for a review[50])	Several studies have assessed the antidepressant effect of folic acid with concomitant antidepressant use,[49] with most yielding positive results in either enhancing antidepressant response rates or increasing the onset of response	In cases of folate deficiency supplementation can be cautiously recommended with antidepressants to potentially ↑ response and efficacy Caution should be observed in pernicious anaemia (addition of B12 required) Currently no study confirming folic acid as a monotherapy for depression Folinic acid or 5-MTHF active forms best

Table 15.2
Review of the major evidence (continued)

Intervention	Mechanisms of action	Key literature	Summary of results	Comment
Acupuncture	Opioid pathway modulation Increased release of serotonin and noradrenaline Cortisol modulation[51]	Meta-analyses and reviews: Smith et al. 2010[52] Jacka et al. 2017[53] Wang et al. 2008[54] Leo & Ligot 2007[55]	A review of eight small RCTs suggested that acupuncture significantly reduces the severity of depression; however, a Cochrane review found most studies were of poor design and therefore no firm conclusion could be reached	Study design issues are common, restricting confidence of results Skills and technique differences may occur between clinicians Electro-acupuncture may be more potent than normal acupuncture
Diet	Modulates brain plasticity and function, the stress response system, mitochondria, inflammation and oxidative processes[56,57]	Cross-sectional and longitudinal studies: Sanchez-Villegas et al. 2009[58] Jacka et al. 2010[59] O'Neil et al. 2013[60]	A traditional or Mediterranean dietary pattern is protective against depressive symptoms compared with Western processed dietary pattern	Evidence currently links a poor diet with increased depressive symptoms One RCT shows benefit of dietary modification as a treatment Can still advise a high-quality diet in the management of depression
Exercise	Increase in circulating— endorphins, anandamide and various neurotransmitters Increases tryptophan hydroxylase Modulates the HPA axis[61]	Meta-analysis: exercise[62] Systematic review: Yoga: Pilkington 2000[63]	Cochrane meta-analysis (28 studies $n = 1101$) found a moderate to large effect size (standard mean difference) of -0.67 (-0.90 to -0.43) in favour of exercise over standard treatment or control Yoga more effective in reducing depression versus no treatment or waitlist control	All modes of physical activity have antidepressant effects Higher intensity exercise and weights appear to have the greatest antidepressant effect

KEY POINTS

- Depression is a condition that should be treated early and assertively.
- An integrated individualised treatment approach such as ALPS is recommended.
- Carefully monitor the prescription's effect and any change in suicidal ideation.
- If depression persists or worsens, adjust prescription and/or refer appropriately.

FURTHER READING

Jacka FN, et al. A randomised controlled trial of dietary improvement for adults with major depression (the 'SMILES' trial). BMC Med 2017;15(1):23.

Murphy J, Sarris J, Byrne G. A review of the conceptualisation and risk factors associated with treatment resistant depression. Depress Res Treat 2017;4176825.

Ng QX, et al. Clinical use of curcumin in depression: a meta-analysis. J Am Med Dir Assoc 2017;18(6):503–8.

Sarris J, et al. Lifestyle medicine for depression. BMC Psychiatry 2014;10(14):107.

Sarris J, et al Nutritional medicine as mainstream in psychiatry. Lancet Psychiatry. 2015;2(3):271–4.

Sarris J, et al. Adjunctive nutrient nutraceuticals for depression: a systematic review and meta-analyses. Am J Psychiatry 2016;173(6):575–87.

Firth J, et al. The efficacy of smartphone-based mental health interventions for depressive symptoms: a meta-analysis of randomized controlled trials. World Psychiatry 2017;16(3):287–98.

REFERENCES

1. American Psychiatric Association. Diagnostic and statistical manual of mental disorders. 5th ed. Arlington: American Psychiatric Association; 2013.
2. World Health Organization. Mental and neurological disorders: depression. Online. Available: http://www.who.int/mental_health/management/depression/definition/en/. [Accessed 1 November 2013].
3. Bromet E, Andrade LH, Hwang I, et al. Cross-national epidemiology of DSM-IV major depressive episode. BMC Med 2011;9:90.
4. Wittchen HU, Jacobi F, Rehm J, et al. The size and burden of mental disorders and other disorders of the brain in Europe 2010. Eur Neuropsychopharmacol 2011;21(9):655–79.
5. Raison CL, Capuron L, Miller AH. Cytokines sing the blues: inflammation and the pathogenesis of depression. Trends Immunol 2006;27(1):24–31.
6. Belmaker RH, Agam G. Major depressive disorder. N Engl J Med 2008;358(1):55–68.
7. Chopra K, Kumar B, Kuhad A. Pathobiological targets of depression. Expert Opin Ther Targets 2011.
8. Berton O, Nestler EJ. New approaches to antidepressant drug discovery: beyond monoamines. Nat Rev Neurosci 2006;7(2):137–51.
9. Folstein M, Liu T, Peter I, et al. The homocysteine hypothesis of depression. Am J Psychiatry 2007;164(6):861–7.
10. Maes M, Fisar Z, Medina M, et al. New drug targets in depression: inflammatory, cell-mediated immune, oxidative and nitrosative stress, mitochondrial, antioxidant, and neuroprogressive pathways. And new drug candidates-Nrf2 activators and GSK-3 inhibitors. Inflammopharmacology 2012.
11. Southwick SM, Vythilingam M, Charney DS. The psychobiology of depression and resilience to stress: implications for prevention and treatment. Annu Rev Clin Psychol 2005;1:255–91.
12. Molina J. Understanding the biopsychosocial model. Int'l J Psychiatry in Medicine 1983;13(1):29–36.
13. Haeffel GJ, Grigorenko EL. Cognitive vulnerability to depression: exploring risk and resilience. Child Adolesc Psychiatr Clin N Am 2007;16(2):435–48, x.
14. Kessler RC. The effects of stressful life events on depression. Annu Rev Psychol 1997;48:191–214.
15. Kumar P, Clark M, editors. Clinical medicine. 5th ed. London: W. B. Saunders; 2002.
16. Levinson DF. The genetics of depression: a review. Biol Psychiatry 2006;60(2):84–92.
17. Tennant C. Life events, stress and depression: a review of recent findings. Aust N Z J Psychiatry 2002;36(2):173–82.
18. Paykel E. Life events and affective disorders. Acta Psychiatr Scand Suppl 2003;418:61–6.
19. McIntyre RS, Alsuwaidan M, Goldstein BI, et al. The Canadian Network for Mood and Anxiety Treatments (CANMAT) task force recommendations for the management of patients with mood disorders and comorbid metabolic disorders. Ann Clin Psychiatry 2012;24(1):69–81.
20. Kessler RC, Berglund P, Demler O, et al. The epidemiology of major depressive disorder: results from the National Comorbidity Survey Replication (NCS-R). JAMA 2003;289(23):3095–105.
21. Kessler RC, Chiu WT, Demler O, et al. Prevalence, severity, and comorbidity of 12-month DSM-IV disorders in the National Comorbidity Survey Replication. Arch Gen Psychiatry 2005;62(6):617–27.
22. Miklowitz DJ, Johnson SL. The psychopathology and treatment of bipolar disorder. Annu Rev Clin Psychol 2006;2:199–235.
23. Parker G, Fletcher K. Treating depression with the evidence-based psychotherapies: a critique of the evidence. Acta Psychiatr Scand 2007;115(5):352–9.

24. Kato M, Serretti A. Review and meta-analysis of antidepressant pharmacogenetic findings in major depressive disorder. Mol Psychiatry 2010;15(5):473–500.

25. Ellen S, Selzer R, Norman T, et al. Depression and anxiety: pharmacological treatment in general practice. Aust Fam Physician 2007;36(4):222–8.

26. Ellis P. Australian and New Zealand clinical practice guidelines for the treatment of depression. Aust N Z J Psychiatry 2004;38(6):389–407.

27. Warden D, Rush AJ, Trivedi MH, et al. The STAR*D Project results: a comprehensive review of findings. Curr Psychiatry Rep 2007;9(6):449–59.

28. Rizvi SJ, Kennedy SH. The keys to improving depression outcomes. Eur Neuropsychopharmacol 2011;21(Suppl. 4):S694–702.

29. Kessler RC. The costs of depression. Psychiatr Clin North Am 2012;35(1):1–14.

30. Donohue J, Pincus H. Reducing the societal burden of depression: a review of economic costs, quality of care and effects of treatment. Pharmacoeconomics 2007;25(1): 7–24.

31. Sarris J, Gadsden S, Schweitzer I. Naturopathic medicine for treating self-reported depression and anxiety: an observational pilot study of naturopathic practice. Adv Integr Med 2013;In Press.

32. Sarris J, Panossian A, Schweitzer I, et al. Herbal medicine for depression, anxiety and insomnia: a review of psychopharmacology and clinical evidence. Eur Neuropsychopharmacol 2011;21(12):841–60.

33. Schotte CK, Van Den Bossche B, De Doncker D, et al. A biopsychosocial model as a guide for psychoeducation and treatment of depression. Depress Anxiety 2006;23(5):312–24.

34. Sarris J. Clinical depression: an evidence-based integrative complementary medicine treatment model. Alter Ther Health Med 2011;17:4.

35. Hindmarch I. Expanding the horizons of depression: beyond the monoamine hypothesis. Hum Psychopharmacol 2001;16(3):203–18.

36. Sarris J. St John's Wort for the Treatment of Psychiatric Disorders. Psychiatr Clin North Am 2013;36(1):65–72.

37. Linde K, Berner M, Kriston L. St John's wort for major depression. Cochrane Database Syst Rev 2008;(4):CD000448.

38. Akhondzadeh B, Moshiri E, Noorbala A, et al. Comparison of petal of Crocus sativus L. and fluoxetine in the treatment of depressed outpatients: a pilot double-blind randomized trial. Prog Neuropsychopharmacol Biol Psychiatry 2007;30(2):439–42.

39. Moshiri E, Basti AA, Noorbala AA, et al. Crocus sativus L. (petal) in the treatment of mild-to-moderate depression: a double-blind, randomized and placebo-controlled trial. Phytomedicine 2006;13(9–10):607–11.

40. Akhondzadeh S, Tahmacebi-Pour N, Noorbala AA, et al. Crocus sativus L. in the treatment of mild to moderate depression: a double-blind, randomized and placebo-controlled trial. Phytother Res 2005;19(2):148–51.

41. Noorbala AA, Akhondzadeh S, Tahmacebi-Pour N, et al. Hydro-alcoholic extract of Crocus sativus L. versus fluoxetine in the treatment of mild to moderate depression: a double-blind, randomized pilot trial. J Ethnopharmacol 2005;97(2):281–4.

42. Sarris J, Schoendorfer N, Kavanagh DJ. Major depressive disorder and nutritional medicine: a review of monotherapies and adjuvant treatments. Nutr Rev 2009;67(3):125–31.

43. Sublette M, Ellis S, Geant A, et al. Meta-analysis of the effects of eicosapentaenoic acid (EPA) in clinical trials in depression. J Clin Psychiatry 2011;72(12):1577–84.

44. Sarris J, Kavanagh DJ, Byrne G. Adjuvant use of nutritional and herbal medicines with antidepressants, mood stabilizers and benzodiazepines. J Psychiatr Res 2010;44(1):32–41.

45. Shaw K, Turner J, Del Mar C. Are tryptophan and 5-hydroxytryptophan effective treatments for depression? A meta-analysis. Aust N Z J Psychiatry 2002;36(4):488–91.

46. Papakostas GI, Mischoulon D, Shyu I, et al. S-adenosyl methionine (SAMe) augmentation of serotonin reuptake inhibitors for antidepressant nonresponders with major depressive disorder: a double-blind, randomized clinical trial. Am J Psychiatry 2010;167(8):942–8.

47. Williams AL, Girard C, Jui D, et al. S-adenosylmethionine (SAMe) as treatment for depression: a systematic review. Clin Invest Med 2005;28(3):132–9.

48. Lai J, Moxey A, Nowak G, et al. The efficacy of zinc supplementation in depression: systematic review of randomised controlled trials. J Affect Disord 2012;136(1–2):e31–9.

49. Fava M, Mischoulon D. Folate in depression: efficacy, safety, differences in formulations, and clinical issues. J Clin Psychiatry 2009;70(Suppl. 5):12–17.

50. Lizer MH, Bogdan RL, Kidd RS. Comparison of the frequency of the methylenetetrahydrofolate reductase (MTHFR) C677T polymorphism in depressed versus nondepressed patients. J Psychiatr Pract 2011;17(6):404–9.

51. Samuels N, Gropp C, Singer SR, et al. Acupuncture for psychiatric illness: a literature review. Behav Med 2008;34(2):55–64.

52. Smith CA, Hay PP, Macpherson H. Acupuncture for depression. Cochrane Database Syst Rev 2010;(1): CD004046.

53. Jacka FN, O'Neil A, Opie R, et al. A randomised controlled trial of dietary improvement for adults with major depression (the 'SMILES' trial). BMC Med 2017;15(1):23. doi:10.1186/s12916-017-0791-y.

54. Wang H, Qi H, Wang B, et al. Is acupuncture beneficial in depression: a meta-analysis of 8 randomized controlled trials? J Affect Disord 2008;111(2–3):125–34.

55. Leo R, Ligot JJ. A systematic review of randomized controlled trials of acupuncture in the treatment of depression. J Affect Disord 2007;97(1–3):13–22.

56. Berk M, Kapczinski F, Andreazza AC, et al. Pathways underlying neuroprogression in bipolar disorder: focus on inflammation, oxidative stress and neurotrophic factors. Neurosci Biobehav Rev 2010;35(3):804–17.

57. Berk M, Jacka F. Preventive strategies in depression: gathering evidence for risk factors and potential interventions. Br J Psychiatry 2012;201:339–41.

58. Sanchez-Villegas A, Delgado-Rodriguez M, Alonso A, et al. Association of the Mediterranean dietary pattern with the incidence of depression: the Seguimiento Universidad de Navarra/University of Navarra follow-up (SUN) cohort. Arch Gen Psychiatry 2009;66(10):1090–8.

59. Jacka FN, Pasco JA, Mykletun A, et al. Association of Western and traditional diets with depression and anxiety in women. Am J Psychiatry 2010;167(3):305–11.

60. O'Neil A, Berk M, Itsiopoulos C, et al. A randomised, controlled trial of a dietary intervention for adults with major depression (the 'SMILES' trial): study protocol. BMC Psychiatry 2013;13:114.

61. Sarris J, Kavanagh D, Newton R. Depression and exercise. J Complement Med 2008;(3):48–50, 61.

62. Rimer J, Dwan K, Lawlor DA, et al. Exercise for depression. Cochrane Database Syst Rev 2012;(7):CD004366.

63. Pilkington K, Kirkwood G, Rampes H, et al. Yoga for depression: the research evidence. J Affect Disord 2005;89(1–3):13–24.

64. Butterweck V, Schmidt M. St. John's wort: role of active compounds for its mechanism of action and efficacy. Wien Med Wochenschr 2007;157(13–14):356–61.

65. Panossian A, Wikman G, Sarris J. Rosenroot (Rhodiola rosea): traditional use, chemical composition, pharmacology and clinical efficacy. Phytomedicine 2010;17(7):481–93.

66. Darbinyan V, Aslanyan G, Amroyan E, et al. Clinical trial of Rhodiola rosea L. extract SHR-5 in the treatment of mild to moderate depression. Nord J Psychiatry 2007;61(5): 343–8.

67. Mao JJ, et al. Rhodiola rosea versus sertraline for major depressive disorder: a randomized placebo-controlled trial. Phytomedicine 2015;22(3):394–9.

68. Hausenblas HA, Saha D, Dubyak PJ, et al. Saffron (Crocus sativus L.) and major depressive disorder: a meta-analysis of randomized clinical trials. J Integr Med 2013;11:377–83.

69. Schmidt M, Betti G, Hensel A. Saffron in phytotherapy: pharmacology and clinical uses. Wien Med Wochenschr 2007;157(13–14):315–19.

70. Jeong HG, Ko YH, Oh SY, et al. Effect of Korean Red Ginseng as an adjuvant treatment for women with residual symptoms of major depression. Asia Pac Psychiatry 2015;7:330–6.

71. Mitchell AJ. The role of corticotropin releasing factor in depressive illness: a critical review. Neurosci Biobehav Rev 1998;22(5):635–51.

72. Pariante CM, Thomas SA, Lovestone S, et al. Do antidepressants regulate how cortisol affects the brain? Psychoneuroendocrinology 2004;29(4):423–47.

73. Schule C, Baghai T, Ferrera A, et al. Neuroendocrine effects of Hypericum extract WS 5570 in 12 healthy male volunteers. Pharmacopsychiatry 2001;34(Suppl. 1): S127–33.

74. Franklin M, Hafizi S, Reed A, et al. Effect of sub-chronic treatment with Jarsin (extract of St John's wort, Hypericum perforatum) at two dose levels on evening salivary melatonin and cortisol concentrations in healthy male volunteers. Pharmacopsychiatry 2006;39(1): 13–15.

75. Molendijk ML, Bus BA, Spinhoven P, et al. Serum levels of brain-derived neurotrophic factor in major depressive disorder: state-trait issues, clinical features and pharmacological treatment. Mol Psychiatry 2011;16(11):1088–95.

76. Panossian A, Wikman G. Evidence-based efficacy of adaptogens in fatigue, and molecular mechanisms related to their stress-protective activity. Curr Clin Pharmacol 2009;4(3):198–219.

77. Sarris J, Nierenberg A, Schweitzer I, et al. Conditional Probability of Response or Non-Response of Placebo Compared to Antidepressants or St John's wort in Major Depressive Disorder. J Clin Psychopharmacol 2013;33(6):827–30.

78. Bottiglieri T, Laundy M, Crellin R, et al. Homocysteine, folate, methylation, and monoamine metabolism in depression. J Neurol Neurosurg Psychiatry 2000;69(2):228–32.

79. Beydoun MA, Shroff MR, Beydoun HA, et al. Serum folate, vitamin B-12, and homocysteine and their association with depressive symptoms among U.S. adults. Psychosom Med 2010;72(9):862–73.

80. Taylor MJ, Carney SM, Goodwin GM, et al. Folate for depressive disorders: systematic review and meta-analysis of randomized controlled trials. J Psychopharmacol 2004;18(2):251–6.

81. Bjelland I, Tell GS, Vollset SE, et al. Folate, vitamin B12, homocysteine, and the MTHFR 677C->T polymorphism in anxiety and depression: the Hordaland Homocysteine Study. Arch Gen Psychiatry 2003;60(6):618–26.

82. Christensen H, Aiken A, Batterham PJ, et al. No clear potentiation of antidepressant medication effects by folic acid+vitamin B12 in a large community sample. J Affect Disord 2011;130(1–2):37–45.

83. Raison CL, Miller AH. Is depression an inflammatory disorder? Curr Psychiatry Rep 2011;13(6):467–75.

84. Raison CL, Lowry CA, Rook GA. Inflammation, sanitation, and consternation: loss of contact with coevolved, tolerogenic microorganisms and the pathophysiology and treatment of major depression. Arch Gen Psychiatry 2010;67(12):1211–24, E.

85. Kunnumakkara AB, Bordoloi D, Padmavathi G, et al. Curcumin, the golden nutraceutical: multitargeting for multiple chronic diseases. Br J Pharmacol 2017;174(11):1325–48.

86. Ng QX, Koh SSH, Chan HW, et al. Clinical use of curcumin in depression: a meta-analysis. J Am Med Dir Assoc 2017;18:503–8.

87. Prasad AS. Zinc: role in immunity, oxidative stress and chronic inflammation. Curr Opin Clin Nutr Metab Care 2009;12(6):646–52.

88. Szewczyk B, Kubera M, Nowak G. The role of zinc in neurodegenerative inflammatory pathways in depression. Prog Neuropsychopharmacol Biol Psychiatry 2011;35(3):693–701.

89. Takeda A. Zinc signaling in the hippocampus and its relation to pathogenesis of depression. Mol Neurobiol 2011;44(2):166–74.

90. Yary T, Aazami S. Dietary Intake of Zinc was Inversely Associated with Depression. Biol Trace Elem Res 2011.

91. Johri RK, Zutshi U, Kameshwaran L, et al. Effect of quercetin and Albizia saponins on rat mast cell. Indian J Physiol Pharmacol 1985;29(1):43–6.

92. Kim WK, Jung JW, Ahn NY, et al. Anxiolytic-like effects of extracts from Albizia julibrissin bark in the elevated plus-maze in rats. Life Sci 2004;75(23):2787–95.

93. Sanchez-Villegas A, Henriquez P, Figueiras A, et al. Long chain omega-3 fatty acids intake, fish consumption and mental disorders in the SUN cohort study. Eur J Nutr 2007;46(6):337–46.

94. Hibbeln JR. Fish consumption and major depression. Lancet 1998;351(9110):1213.

95. Parker G, Gibson N, Heruc G, et al. Omega-3 fatty acids and mood disorders. Am J Psychiatry 2006;163: 969–78.

96. Sanchez-Villegas A, Henriquez P, Bes-Rastrollo M, et al. Mediterranean diet and depression. Public Health Nutr 2006;9(8A):1104–9.

97. Tassoni D, Kaur G, Weisinger RS, et al. The role of eicosanoids in the brain. Asia Pac J Clin Nutr 2008;17(Suppl. 1):220–8.

98. Sarris J, O'Neil A, Cousan C, et al. Lifestyle medicine for depression. BMC Psychiatry 2014.

99. Maciocia G. The foundations of Chinese medicine. Singapore: Churchill Livingstone; 1989.

100. Smith CA, Armour M, Lee MS, et al. Acupuncture for depression. Cochrane Database Syst Rev 2018;(3):CD004046, doi:10.1002/14651858.CD004046.pub4.

101. Coelho HF, Boddy K, Ernst E. Massage therapy for the treatment of depression: a systematic review. Int J Clin Pract 2008;62(2):325–33.

102. Donker T, Griffiths KM, Cuijpers P, et al. Psychoeducation for depression, anxiety and psychological distress: a meta-analysis. BMC Med 2009;7:79.

103. Sarris J, et al. Adjunctive nutrient nutraceuticals for depression: a systematic review and meta-analyses. Am J Psychiatry 2016;173(6):575–87.

104. Chrubasik S, Pittler MH, Roufogalis BD. Zingiberis rhizoma: a comprehensive review on the ginger effect and efficacy profiles. Phytomedicine 2005;12(9):684–701.

105. Sarris J. Cynara scolymus (monograph). In: Mills S, Bone K, editors. Principles and Practice of Phytotherapy. Edinburgh: Churchill and Livingstone; 2013.

106. Sarris J, McIntyre E, Camfield D. Plant-based medicines for anxiety disorders part 2: a systematic review of clinical studies with supportive preclinical evidence. CNS Drugs 2013;27(4):301–19.

107. Sarris J, LaPorte E, Schweitzer I. Kava: a comprehensive review of efficacy, safety, and psychopharmacology. Aust N Z J Psychiatry 2011;45(1):27–35.

108. Dording CM, Schettler PJ, Dalton ED, et al. A double-blind placebo-controlled trial of maca root as treatment for antidepressant-induced sexual dysfunction in women. Evid Based Complement Alternat Med 2015;2015:949036. doi:10.1155/2015/949036. [Epub 2015 Apr 14].

109. Sarris J. Ginkgo biloba (monograph). In: Mills S, Bone K, editors. Principles and Practice of Phytotherapy. Edinburgh: Churchill and Livingstone; 2013.

110. Stickel F, Schuppan D. Herbal medicine in the treatment of liver diseases. Dig Liver Dis 2007;39(4):293–304.

111. Nielsen SJ, Siega-Riz AM, Popkin BM. Trends in energy intake in U.S. between 1977 and 1996: similar shifts seen across age groups. Obes Res 2002;10(5):370–8.

112. Kaplan B, Crawford S, Field C, et al. Vitamins, minerals, and mood. Psychol Bull 2007;133(5):747–60.

113. World Health Organization. Diet, nutrition, and the prevention of chronic diseases. Report of a WHO Study Group. Geneva: World Health Organization; 2003.

114. Yarborough BJ, Janoff SL, Stevens VJ, et al. Delivering a lifestyle and weight loss intervention to individuals in real-world mental health settings: lessons and opportunities. Transl Behav Med 2011;1(3):406–15.

115. Lucas M, Mekary R, Pan A, et al. Relation between clinical depression risk and physical activity and time spent watching television in older women: a 10-year prospective follow-up study. Am J Epidemiol 2011;174(9):1017–27.

116. Galper DI, Trivedi MH, Barlow CE, et al. Inverse association between physical inactivity and mental health in men and women. Med Sci Sports Exerc 2006;38(1):173–8.

117. Farmer M, Locke B, Moscicki E, et al. Physical activity and depressive symptoms: the NHANES I Epidemiologic Follow-up Study. Am J Epidemiol 1988;128(6):1340–51.

118. Brown WJ, Ford JH, Burton NW, et al. Prospective study of physical activity and depressive symptoms in middle-aged women. Am J Prev Med 2005;29(4):265–72.

119. Dunn AL, Trivedi MH, Kampert JB, et al. Exercise treatment for depression: efficacy and dose response. Am J Prev Med 2005;28(1):1–8.

120. Erickson KI, Miller DL, Roecklein KA. The aging hippocampus: interactions between exercise, depression, and BDNF. Neuroscientist 2012;18(1):82–97.

121. Deslandes A, Moraes H, Ferreira C, et al. Exercise and mental health: many reasons to move. Neuropsychobiology 2009;59(4):191–8.

122. Tsang HW, Chan EP, Cheung WM. Effects of mindful and non-mindful exercises on people with depression: a systematic review. Br J Clin Psychol 2008;47(Pt 3):303–22.

CHAPTER 16

Insomnia

Jerome Sarris
ND, MHSc, PhD

OVERVIEW

Periods of sleep disturbance due to acute stress or environmental change are common human experiences. The *Diagnostic and Statistical Manual of Mental Disorders* (DSM-5) classification of insomnia disorder is differentiated from an acute occurrence of sleep disturbance, requiring the disorder to be a major health complaint, presenting with more than three months of persistent problems (more than three nights per week) in initiating or maintaining sleep, or early morning wakening.[1] Furthermore, for this diagnosis to be met the sleep disturbance must: cause significant distress or impairment in social or occupational functioning; be exclusive of other disorders (e.g. other sleep or psychiatric disorders); and not be due to medications, drugs, alcoholism or a general medical condition. Insomnia may be secondary—that is, caused by: another medical condition; medicines, recreational drugs or alcohol consumption; or environmental factors such as altitude, jet lag, poor bedding, excess light or noise. Due to this, a thorough assessment is required to establish particulars of the causation. It is estimated that 25% of chronic insomnia can be classified as 'primary', with approximately 75% due to other aforementioned causations.[2] Interestingly, people who experience 'transient' insomnia (less than one month), usually from an environmental change, acute social stressors or the loss of a loved one, usually experience daytime sleepiness during this period. A person with chronic insomnia usually does not feel sleepy but instead may feel 'hyperstimulated', even after only four to six hours' sleep.[2]

Parameters measuring sleep outcomes involve evaluating total sleep time, sleep latency (how long it takes to get to sleep) and wake time after sleep onset.[3] Previously, prevalence of general sleep disturbance experienced by people for more than a year was estimated at approximately 85%, while the estimate of diagnosed chronic insomnia was estimated at around 10%.[2] Recent European data estimates that each year 7% of the European Union population suffers from insomnia.[4]

Prolonged poor 'sleep hygiene' may cause behavioural conditioning towards 'expecting' to have bad sleep.[5] This is reflected in the fact that population surveys indicate that of the 50% of people who have sleep difficulties, 20–36% report the duration is greater than a year.[6] Sleep hygiene is a term used to describe lifestyle interventions that help prepare for sleep. Aspects of good sleep hygiene focus on replacing stimulating activities with restful and quiescent activities (or non-activities) to establish a regulated circadian rhythm (this will be discussed further later in this chapter). Beyond the socioeconomic cost, the subjective effect of chronic sleep disturbance often involves the person experiencing a low mood or anxiety (may not meet diagnostic threshold), fatigue or daytime somnolence, poor concentration or memory, tension headaches or digestive disturbances.[7]

Pathophysiology of insomnia

- Hyperarousal of the neuroendocrine system (hypothalamic–pituitary–adrenal (HPA) axis/cortisol hyperactivation)
- Abnormalities in circadian rhythm (involving clock genes, melatonin secretion and adenosine receptors)
- Gamma-aminobutyric acid (GABA) pathway dysregulation
- Excitory pathways involving glutamate, aspartate

Sources: Roth et al. 2007,[8] Piggins 2002,[9] Lancel 1999[10] and Strecker et al. 2006[11]

RISK FACTORS

The elderly, females, shift workers, chronic pain sufferers, people with co-occurring medical conditions or psychiatric disorders (especially depression and anxiety) are at greater risk of developing chronic insomnia (Figure 16.3).[8] A sedentary life and reduced exposure to sunlight may also contribute to sleep disorders. Elderly populations frequently report that they perceive a poorer quality of sleep, commonly that they have interrupted sleep, wake early or feel inadequately rested.[12] Interestingly, studies show that statistically the elderly sleep similar hours to younger counterparts, and that the reduction of qualitative sleep experience is actually due to comorbid health issues or medications, not to do with 'being old'.[12] Chronic experience of pain increases the risk of insomnia, with a study revealing that 44% of people with chronic pain reporting that they had co-existing insomnia.[12] Furthermore, the more severe the level of pain was, the greater percentage experienced insomnia. Aside from poor sleep affecting pain, data from the Behavioral Risk Factor Surveillance System of 138,201 people found that sleep disturbance is a significant risk factor for obesity, diabetes, coronary artery disease, myocardial infarction and stroke.[13]

Adequate restful sleep is critical for mental health, and mood and anxiety disorders are associated with major disturbance in circadian rhythm.[14,15] Sleep disturbance is a frequent symptom of depression, and a strong causal link exists between insomnia and depression.[2] This effect is most likely bidirectional: insomnia can increase depression risk and vice versa. Research has shown that people with chronic insomnia have an increased risk of a depression. A review of 21 prospective studies with follow-up data by Baglioni[16] revealed that insomnia predicted a twofold increased risk for a depressive episode. Further, epidemiological data have shown that approximately 40% of chronic insomniacs suffer from a comorbid psychiatric disorder.[17]

Economic impact of insomnia

The cost that sleep disorders cause is immense, with substantial workplace costs. An American sample of 7428 employed health-plan subscribers revealed that the estimated prevalence of insomnia was 23.2%,[18] with sleep disorders being significantly associated with lost work performance due to 'presenteeism' (reduced productivity). Based on the estimates of these data, this is the equivalent to an annualised American population-level

Conditions causing chronic sleep disturbance
Medical conditions
Cancer, congestive heart failure, HIV/AIDS, stroke, benign prostatic hypertrophy, hyperthyroidism, renal disease, gastro-oesophageal reflux, psychiatric disorders
Other abnormal events
Restless leg syndrome, respiratory distress, headaches, panic attacks, pain
Source: Ramakrishnan & Scheid 2007[19]

cost of $63.2 billion. While prescriptive drug use is prevalent in insomniacs for their treatment, medications for other conditions may also cause insomnia.[12,19]

It should be noted that while the previously mentioned risk factors may cause sleep disorders, chronic sleep disturbances may also in turn cause a variety of physical and mental conditions.[6,20] The most concerning link with chronic insomnia is evidence that indicates that people with poor sleep or less than six hours per night have a significantly greater risk of: developing cardiovascular disorders (e.g. hypertension, hypercholesterolaemia); metabolic disorders (increase in weight gain, BSL, insulin resistance, increased cortisol level and decreased human growth hormone); higher incidence than healthy sleepers of experiencing more accidents, higher work absenteeism and lower productivity; and higher healthcare costs.[3,7]

Shift work sleep disorder
Shift workers are especially at risk of developing a sleep disorder. The experience of clinically significant excessive sleepiness or insomnia associated with work (during normal nocturnal sleep time) has important safety implications and socioeconomic, medical and quality-of-life consequences. Treatment protocols may involve using stimulant therapy and letting bright light in upon waking, and hypnotic agents upon retiring. To date no complementary and alternative medicine (CAM) interventions have been rigorously assessed in real life situations to manage shift work sleep disorders. The best treatment is to avoid shift work if possible!
Sources: Schwartz & Roth 2006[21] and Hein 2004[22]

DIFFERENTIAL DIAGNOSIS
- Other psychiatric disorder (e.g. mood, anxiety or adjustment disorder)
- Medication side effects or substance effects (e.g. from caffeine)
- Sleep apnoea
- Cardiovascular/respiratory disorder

CONVENTIONAL TREATMENT

Erudite advice when treating transient insomnia should be to establish the underlying cause(s), initiate good sleep hygiene changes, commence (or refer) an appropriate psychological intervention and offer lifestyle and prescriptive advice.[19] From the conventional therapeutic options available, benzodiazepine-receptor agonists and cognitive behaviour therapy (CBT) are supported by the strongest data.[23] The medical 'quick fix' is usually the use of pharmaceutical hypnotics as the primary first-line pharmacotherapy to treat chronic insomnia.[24] The use of benzodiazepines such as diazepam (or its metabolites) or non-benzodiazepine hypnotics such as zolpidem or zopiclone are preferred currently over older barbiturates, which can cause death in cases of overdose.[24] In respect to benzodiazepines, although a relatively safe medication, concerns exist over dependency and currently most guidelines endorse only short-term use.[25] Prescription of sedating antidepressants such as mirtazapine or fluvoxamine may also be prescribed, especially in cases of comorbid depression.[24] In some cases sedating antipsychotic or tricyclics medication may also be employed. Opiates also have soporific effects, and may be indicated in cases of chronic pain with insomnia. Melatonin (an endogenous hormone secreted by the pineal gland) is also prescribed in some countries, especially to treat sleep disturbance, particularly if caused by jet lag.[26] A novel melatoninergic agent called agomelatine, a melatonin 1, 2 receptor agonist and serotonin $5HT_{2c}$ receptor agonist, may also be of value in cases of comorbid depression.[27] Referral for psychological interventions such as cognitive modification or behavioural adjustments may also be recommended in primary care. CBT is an effective alternative for chronic insomnia. Although more time consuming for patients than drug therapy, CBT may produce sustained sleep improvement over time.[28]

Drugs that may cause insomnia

Alcohol, stimulants (nicotine, caffeine, amphetamines), stimulating antidepressants, attention deficit, hyperactivity disorder (ADHD), psycho-stimulants, corticosteroids, thyroxin, calcium channel blockers, bronchodilators, beta-blockers, decongestants, anticholinergic agents, oral contraceptive pill

Sources: Benca et al. 2004[12] and Ramakrishnan & Scheid 2007[19]

KEY TREATMENT PROTOCOLS

Circadian rhythm modulation

The primary circadian 'clock' in humans is found in the suprachiasmatic nuclei, located in the hypothalamus; these cells govern the daily biological rhythm over a cycle lasting approximately 24 hours and 11 minutes.[9] The sleep–wake cycle is influenced externally by light and dark, with exposure to light increasing the secretion of serotonin, while darkness increases the secretion of melatonin. The circadian rhythm governs internal temperature changes, sleep and eating patterns. Human clock genes have been identified as being involved with various sleep disorders.[9] Future gene therapy may target the expression of these clock genes to effectively re-set the circadian rhythm. In the meantime, the use of interventions that modulate the circadian rhythm and the use of sleep hygiene techniques such as 'sleep restriction' and 'light therapy' may assist in re-adjusting the circadian rhythm.

Another neurological factor involved in sleep is the endogenous compound adenosine. This inhibitory compound and the adenosine receptor binding sites are a homoeostatic sleep factor responsible for mediating the REM cycle (Figure 16.3).[29] **Adenosine** can potently inhibit cholinergic neurons that are involved with cortical

Naturopathic Treatment Aims

- Assess the cause(s) of the sleep disorder.
- Educate on good sleep hygiene practices.
- Regulate circadian rhythm, HPA function and enhance GABAergic activity.
- Regulate and support the nervous system.
- Encourage beneficial lifestyle changes.
- Appropriately address external stressors (e.g. relationship/job factors).

arousal. During periods of prolonged wakefulness adenosine accumulates in certain parts of the brain and promotes the transition from a wake state to a sleep state.[11] This is considered to be one of the factors involved in the theory of 'sleep debt', in which sleep deprivation over days accrues a chronological sleep debt (a build-up of adenosine) that then prompts a period of increased sleep to make up for the loss. Caffeine antagonises adenosine receptors, thereby increasing wakefulness.[30] The compound adenosine would appear to be a potential hypnotic substance; as discussed earlier endogenous adenosine is responsible for modulating the sleep–wake cycle via binding to adenosine (A1) and (A2) receptors. A literature search reviewing clinical evidence of this product, however, reveals no clinical evidence; this remains an area of potential exploration.

Humulus lupulus is used extensively in Europe in sleep formulations to promote sleep. The bitter herb is regarded by the eclectics as a useful remedy for imparting sedative and hypnotic actions.[31] While animal and in vitro models do not currently support sedative or anxiolytic activity, hypnotic effects involving melatoninergic and GABAergic modulation have been documented.[32] *Humulus lupulus* combines well with *Valeriana* spp. root, demonstrated by a fixed combination of the two herbs (Ze 91019) found to reduce sleep latency and waking time compared with placebo in 30 subjects after two weeks of treatment.[33] Another randomised controlled trial (RCT) comparing the combination with placebo and diphenhydramine revealed less conclusive results.[34] The four-week study involving 184 adults with mild insomnia showed no or only minor improvements of subjective sleep parameters compared with placebo, with most outcomes being similar between all groups. It is possible that the inclusion of 'mild' insomniacs diluted the response from the herbal combination. In vitro studies indicate that hops-valerian preparations invoke hypnotic activity via agonising adenosine, melatonin and serotonin receptors.[35–37]

Valeriana officinalis has a rich folkloric tradition of use in conditions of restlessness, hysteria, nervous headache and mental depression,[31,38] with Pliny regarding the powder of the root as effective in cases of spasms causing pain.[39] 'Energetically' *Valeriana* spp. root was regarded by Dioscorides as possessing warming properties[39]; this is reflected in the pungent aroma of the essential oils (valerenal, iso/valerianic acid) and terpenes (valerenic acid).[40]

The use of *Valeriana* spp. in prescriptions needs to be monitored due to its 'heating' effect, which can evoke stimulation and restlessness (the eclectics classify valerian as a 'cerebral stimulant').[31,41] *Valeriana* spp. hypnotic effect is posited as involving an increase in REM stage and delta sleep,[42,43] mediated by GABA-A receptor (β3 subunit) agonism[44] and adenosine,[1] benzodiazepine and serotonin 5-HT$_{1a}$ receptor agonism.[35,37,45]

Commission E (2000) and the World Health Organization (1999) support the use of *Valeriana* spp. for restlessness and sleep disorders[46]; however, as detailed in the review of evidence table (Table 16.1), current evidence does not provide strong evidence supporting valerian for insomnia. A further systematic review and meta-analysis by Bent et al. (2006) based on 16 eligible RCTs ($n = 1093$) found that 9 out of 16 studies did not have positive outcomes regarding improvement of sleep quality.[40] It should be noted that many studies included in the review involved combinations of valerian with other herbal medicines such as *Piper methysticum* or *Humulus lupulus*, as well as differing outcome scales, dosages and participant populations; eight trials had small sample sizes. A 2011 review by Sarris et al. also mirrored this conclusion.[47] Due to this, current evidence does not firmly support the use of *Valeriana* spp. as a stand-alone hypnotic.

Vitex agnus-castus, although used commonly for hormonal and menstrual irregularities,[56] may exert a novel melatoninergic activity. While to date no human clinical trials exist testing *Vitex agnus-castus* in insomnia, a study of 20 healthy human males demonstrated a significant dose-dependent increase of melatonin secretion using 120 mg, 240 mg and 480 mg of the extract per day compared with placebo for 14 days.[57]

Neuroendocrine and monoamine system dysregulation

Chronic primary insomnia has been characterised by a state of biopsychological arousal, which is counter to a lowering of body temperature, blood pressure and cortisol (Figure 16.1).[8] Elevations of circulating catecholamines, adrenocorticotrophic hormone and cortisol production, raised metabolic rate and core body temperature and overactive beta electroencephalogram (EEG) frequency has been documented in this hyperstimulated state responsible for chronic insomnia.[8] Interestingly, this mirrors various presentations of melancholic depression (anxiety, psychosocial unresponsiveness, early morning waking), the common link (an overactive HPA axis) possibly explaining the correlation between depression and insomnia (see Chapter 15 on depression and Chapters 18–20 on the endocrinesystem).[17,58] Herbal medicines that regulate HPA-axis activity and exercise may have a role in treating insomnia. ***Withania somnifera*** is regarded as an anxiolytic, adaptogen and nervine trophorestorative, used to assist in reducing mental tension and revitalise body/mind.[59] *Withania somnifera* is classed as a 'Rasayana' in Ayurvedic medicine, and is used to promote physical and mental health.[60] Animal studies have confirmed its efficacy in treating chronic stress and anxiety,[60,61] with the glycowithanolides regarded as the active constituents, exerting a GABA-mimetic activity. To date no RCTs exist examining the herb for use in insomnia, so caution should be adopted when extrapolating from the minor in vitro and in vivo evidence. Other herbal medicines that may exert a HPA-axis modulating effect include ***Rhodiola rosea*** and ***Panax ginseng*** (caution use in the evening due to stimulatory properties) and ***Eleutherococcus senticosus***.[41,62]

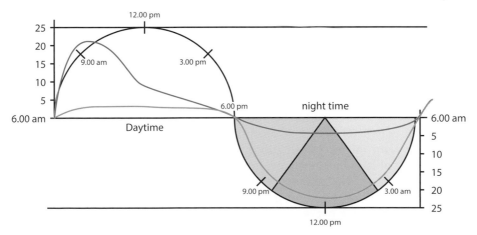

Figure 16.1
Cortisol and melatonin levels and the circadian rhythm

Cortisol (blue line) spikes in the morning and reduces throughout the day. Melatonin (grey line) starts to spike around bedtime, evoking sleepiness. Too much stress throughout the day elevates cortisol levels, which can remain elevated into the night causing insomnia or poor-quality sleep.

Exercise and physical activity is advised to assist in balancing the function of the HPA axis. Regular graded physical exercise may promote relaxation and raise core body temperature, this activity potentially benefitting the sleep pattern.[63] Exercise also addresses weight gain and obesity, which are also factors that increase the occurrence of sleep disorders. A Cochrane review found, in one trial involving a sample of 43 elderly participants with insomnia, that exercise improved sleep onset latency, total sleep and quality of sleep.[64]

The monoamine system may also be dysregulated, with serotonergic pathways also being implicated in insomnia.[8] **L-tryptophan** is used by the body to convert into serotonin. This neurochemical plays a role in non-REM deep sleep and its depletion has been shown in depression and insomnia.[51] Reviews by Hartmann[51] and Bowman[50] detail that the weight of evidence (animal and human studies) indicates that L-tryptophan produces an increase in sleepiness and a decrease in sleep latency. The authors comment that the best results seem to occur in cases of mild insomnia with long sleep latency, and in the absence of comorbid medical or psychiatric disturbance. The prescriptive use of the amino acid may be restricted in some countries (such as Australia); however, safe and reliable sources of L-tryptophan or 5-HT taken within recommended dosage should not present with any high level of risk (see a health professional for exact prescriptive advice) (see Chapter 15 on depression for more detail on interventions that modulate this system).

GABAergic system modulation

As discussed in Chapter 14 on anxiety, GABA has a role in the inhibitory effect on neurological activity by attenuating hyperarousal in both mood and sleep disturbance. GABA-α receptors play a crucial role in initiating and maintaining non-REM sleep (deep sleep).[10] Furthermore, in cases of comorbid anxiety, interventions that modulate GABA activity may have a role in reducing anxiety, which in turn may ameliorate insomnia. The use of GABA-modulating phytotherapies such as *Scutellaria lateriflora*, *Passiflora incarnata* and *Piper methysticum* (kava) may be of benefit in treating insomnia. *Scutellaria lateriflora* is regarded by eclectic doctors and physiomedicalists as a 'truly valuable medicine' used to treat nervous excitability, restlessness or wakefulness (see Chapter 14 on anxiety for evidence).[31,38] *Passiflora incarnata* has a history of use by Europeans and Native Americans, being utilised for its hypnotic and anxiolytic action (see Chapter 14 on anxiety for evidence).[31] It should be noted that while both *Scutellaria lateriflora* and *Passiflora incarnata* have documented anxiolytic activity, it does not necessarily confer a hypnotic effect, with no clinical trials having been conducted assessing this application.

Kava is a well-documented GABA-modulator that has solid evidence as an effective anxiolytic.[65] It may be of benefit in anxious insomnia and, to date, one specific study examined the plant in this presentation. A four-week RCT using 200 mg of a standardised extract of kava in 61 patients explored the effect on anxious participants with comorbid insomnia.[66] The results revealed that, compared with placebo, the extract improved the quality of sleep and the recuperative effect after sleep via a sleep questionnaire. Interestingly, a five-week RCT has also been conducted to explore the use of kava on benzodiazepine withdrawal. A standardised kava extract was used on 40 participants with chronic anxiety and a long history of benzodiazepine use.[67] Participants were tapered off their benzodiazepines over the first two weeks, while the kava was titrated from 50 mg up to 300 mg by the end of week 1. Kava produced a statistically significant reduction in anxiety, with only five subjects in the kava group displaying adverse symptoms from benzodiazepine withdrawal compared with 10 in the placebo group. During follow-up, 9 out of 14 subjects who were switched from kava to placebo experienced re-occurrence of anxiety. A qualitative study exploring the experiences of people taking kava in a clinical trial revealed that, in addition to the plant improving participants' mood and anxiety levels, some participants detailed beneficial effects on sleep outcomes.[68]

Sleep apnoea and snoring

Sleep apnoea is caused by abnormalities in the anatomy and physiology of the pharynx and upper airway muscle dilator in addition to the stability of ventilatory control, which cause pharyngeal collapse during sleep. Obstructive sleep apnoea can be diagnosed from a history of snoring and daytime sleepiness and via a physical examination and overnight polysomno-graphy. People with sleep apnoea are rarely aware of having difficulty breathing, even upon awakening.

Snoring is a common presentation of obstructive sleep apnoea and is the result of vibration of respiratory structures (uvula and soft palate), causing a sound due to obstructed air movement. Aside from structural issues, the causes of snoring may also involve obesity, smoking and use of alcohol and central nervous system depressant medications.

Treatment usually involves lifestyle changes such as avoiding alcohol or muscle relaxants, losing weight and quitting smoking. Sleeping at a 30-degree elevation of the upper body may also be of benefit. 'Breathing machines' (e.g. continuous positive airway pressure) can be used in severe cases that are unresponsive to lifestyle interventions. Surgical procedures may also assist. To date no CAM products have strong evidentiary support in treating apnoea or snoring.

A novel study assessed the use of didgeridoo playing on daytime sleepiness and other outcomes in 25 patients with moderate obstructive sleep apnoea syndrome and snoring.[69] Participants undertook didgeridoo lessons and daily practice at home with standardised instruments for four months. In the didgeridoo group, daytime sleepiness improved significantly and partners reported less sleep disturbance compared with the control group.

Source: Malhotra & White 2002[70]

INTEGRATIVE MEDICAL CONSIDERATIONS

Various integrative options exist for treating insomnia. Referral for appropriate psychological interventions and for an exercise program or relaxation techniques (and possibly acupuncture) may be of assistance. Sleep clinics are usually available in major cities. These clinics may perform EEG tests observing the person's sleep latency and arousal level during sleep, as well as other nocturnal factors such as sleep apnoea. Sleep hygiene techniques may also be taught at these clinics.

Psychological intervention

A review of the psychological and behavioural treatments of insomnia by Morin et al.[28] of 37 controlled studies involving 2246 subjects concluded that these techniques produced reliable changes in several sleep parameters, and that these improvements were well sustained over time. Five main evidence-based psychological and behavioural treatments exist in managing insomnia.

- *Stimulus control therapy.* Involving going to bed only when sleepy, getting out of bed when not sleepy, using the bed only for sleeping and arising the same time from bed.
- *Sleep restriction therapy.* Curtail time in bed to the average time the person sleeps; for example, if they only sleep six out of eight hours in bed, then reduce to six hours and work up to eight hours.

- *Relaxation training.* Techniques to reduce somatic and psychological stress via muscular relaxation, imagery or meditation.
- *Sleep hygiene education.* Instruction on health practices to enhance sleep such as exercise, diet, substance use, environmental factors (light, noise, temperature, bed quality, removal of beside clocks).
- *Cognitive therapy.* Challenging and changing erroneous beliefs about sleep. Cognitive therapy may assist some sleep sufferers who form erroneous beliefs about their sleep pattern. They may catastrophise by thinking thoughts such as 'I can never get to sleep' or 'I need a sleeping pill to sleep'. They may also present with a trait of being a chronic worrier, and may be kept up by an overactive internal dialogue (if so screen for generalised anxiety disorder). While evidence supports these interventions, more studies are required to evaluate the effect on morbidity outcomes such as daytime fatigue and cognitive functioning.

Acupuncture and chinese herbal medicine

A Cochrane review and meta-analysis of acupuncture and acupressure in treating insomnia has been conducted reviewing 33 clinical trials involving 2293 participants.[55] While the meta-analysis supported the efficacy of acupuncture for insomnia, on subgroup analysis, only needle acupuncture but not electroacupuncture showed benefits. Although promising, the small numbers of heterogenous and methodologically poor RCTs do not currently support the use of any form of acupuncture for treating insomnia. Publication bias was likely present and the effect sizes were generally small with wide confidence intervals. Further, all trials had a high risk of bias and were heterogeneous in the classification of insomnia, participant characteristics, treatment regimen and acupoints used.

Dozens of Chinese herbal medicine (CHM) formulas exist, with several being commonly used for sleep disorders. In one review, Gui Pi Tang, Xue Fu Zhu Yu Tang, Dan Zhi Xiao Yao San and Suan Zao Ren Tang were four of the most commonly studied formulas.[71] The main herbal medicine in Suan Zao Ren Tang is *Ziziphus jujuba*, being the component that was most frequently used in 190 (87.6%) of the 217 studies reviewed. While many clinical trials have been conducted using CHM for insomnia (mainly in China), a critical issue is the deficit of methodological quality.[72] In the Yeung et al.[71] review, 72% of the 217 studies located showed that CHM for insomnia was effective on sleep outcome measures; 96.3% of the studies were rated as low-quality RCTs (Jadad score ≤ 2).

Sleep, hygiene, dietary and lifestyle advice

General lifestyle advice should focus on good sleep hygiene techniques (Figure 16.2).[5] The key techniques revealed by sleep researchers focus primarily on limiting exposure to the bed (sleep restriction) such as having only a limited time to sleep and getting up at a set time in the morning regardless of quality or quantity of sleep.[5] This should in time regulate the circadian rhythm. Patients should also be advised not to 'force' sleep. If sleep does not occur within 20 minutes, then they should get up and focus the mind on an activity until they feel tired (still minimise light and mental activity). The other mainstay is to reduce exposure to light prior to sleep and increase exposure to morning sunlight upon waking. It is also best to avoid excessive daytime naps as this may disturb the circadian rhythm.

Further sleep hygiene advice includes stimulus control–avoidance of stimulating activity and stimulants close to sleep such as smoking, caffeine and external stimuli

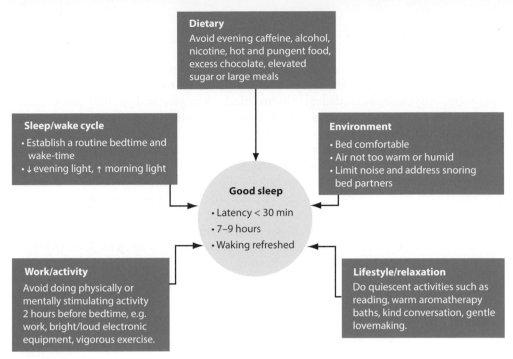

Figure 16.2
Good sleep hygiene

(stimulating TV or books)[73]—and adequate sleep preparation such as aromatherapy baths, relaxing reading material, quiescent lovemaking and calm cognition. Avoidance of excess energetically 'heating' foods such as alcohol, garlic, chillies and curries may also be of assistance,[74] while the diet (or supplementation) may provide nutrients required to create and regulate adrenal hormones and psychoactive neurotransmitters (B vitamins, magnesium, calcium and vitamin C). These will help support a healthy functioning nervous system.[75] Although evening meal portions should not be excessive (may cause rebound hypoglycaemia), sufficient calorific intake is required to avoid waking up due to hunger. Some people find a warm milk drink helpful in initiating sleep; this may be due to the effect of calcium.[76] Finally, moderating a busy work schedule is desirable to allow for regular exercise and relaxation to reduce stress levels.

The most obvious advice is to cut down or eliminate caffeine consumption. Caffeine is antagonistic to adenosine receptors and will interfere with circadian rhythm.[30] The half-life of caffeine is approximately four to six hours and in women on the oral conceptive pill it may be greatly increased (see Chapter 14 on anxiety for more detail).[30] Pharmacokinetically, the caffeine from a strong cup of coffee consumed at 1 pm may be still in the system by sleep time at 11 pm, so avoidance of caffeine after lunch may be prudent advice. Patients may also be advised to keep a sleep diary over two weeks to record their sleep pattern. This may provide more diagnostic detail and allow for a more thorough critique of their sleep hygiene. A worry diary can also be an added component, with patients writing down anything on their mind before they sleep. This technique may help the person 'let go' of these concerns, leaving them on paper to be addressed the following day.

CLINICAL SUMMARY

Insomnia is expected to be ameliorated with treatment within the week, although chronic insomniacs have a poorer prognosis and this is complicated by comorbid mental disorders and substance abuse.[77] An integrative approach involving sleep hygiene education, psychological, dietary/nutraceutical, lifestyle and herbal intervention should offer a sustained benefit if compliance is maintained (see clinical decision tree, Figure 16.3). If after two weeks of the prescription minimal benefit has occurred, the herbal prescription can be modified to include other hypnotics and anxiolytics.[31,78] The use of melatonin or L-tryptophan may also be used if the patient is non-responsive to the initial prescription. Additional psychological interventions may also be of assistance (i.e. behavioural or social-based models) to examine and aid in managing the external triggers of the anxiety. The key is to advise the person to be patient and not to 'force' the sleep process—to be disciplined if following sleep restriction techniques (i.e. no daytime napping and sticking to a regular waking time), maintain good sleep hygiene and try to address any psychosocial social factors affecting sleep.

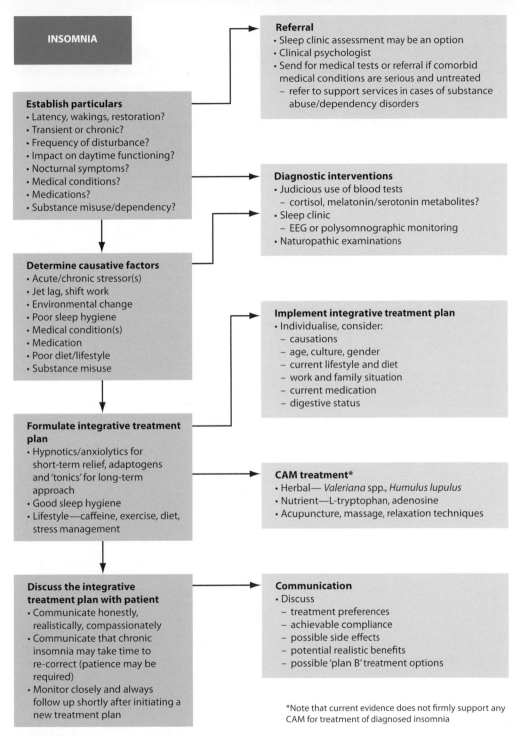

Figure 16.3
Naturopathic treatment decision tree—insomnia

Table 16.1
Review of the major evidence

Intervention	Mechanisms of action	Key literature	Summary of results	Comment
Valeriana spp. (valerian)	Adenosine (A$_1$ receptor) interactions GABA modulation (increased reuptake and decreased degradation of GABA) Valerenic acid from valerian has demonstrated GABA-A receptor (β3 subunit) agonism 5-HT$_{5a}$ partial agonism	Systematic review and meta-analysis: Fernandez-San-Martin 2010[48] A meta-analysis of 18 RCTs: Valerian versus placebo or active control	Inconclusive evidence Valerian reduced sleep latency over placebo by only 0.70 min (95% CI −3.44, 4.83), with the standardised mean differences between the groups measured being statistically equivocal −0.02 (95% CI −0.35, 0.31) Some studies found subjective improvement in quality of sleep	Caution with valerian in people with 'heat' signs, and with hops in people with depression The combination of valerian and hops may be synergistically more effective
Humulus lupulus	Melatonin receptor modulation (binding affinity to M$_1$ and M$_2$ receptors) Hypothermic activity[32]	Review: Zanoli & Zavatti 2008[32]	Inconclusive evidence for use individually in the treatment of insomnia	Caution in people with depression
L-tryptophan and 5-HTP	Required for conversion into serotonin via intermediary step to active form 5-HTP[49]	Reviews: Boman 1988[50] Hartmann 1982[51]	Good supportive evidence for use in insomnia May be better for milder types of sleep disturbance or for long sleep latency	Caution in cases of co-prescription with antidepressants Stay within prescriptive guidelines and only use reputable products
Melatonin	An endogenous hormone involved in synchronising circadian rhythm and induces sleep[52]	Meta-analysis: Buscemi et al. 2005[53]	Positive evidence supporting the use of melatonin in reducing sleep latency Lacks evidence in treating other sleep markers such as duration and quality	Product quality can be a significant issue In some countries the sale of melatonin may be restricted
Acupuncture and acupressure	Opioid pathway modulation Increased release of serotonin and noradrenaline Cortisol modulation[54]	Meta-analysis: Cheuk 2012[55]	Tentatively supportive evidence; may improve subjective quality of sleep No support in specific sleep domains such as latency and nocturnal awakenings	Only use qualified acupuncturists Caution in cases of needle phobia, which may increase distress in some people

KEY POINTS

- Determine the cause(s) of the insomnia and current sleep hygiene status.
- Assess, monitor and if required refer any substance use issues, medical or psychiatric conditions.
- Enact a comprehensive program involving sleep hygiene education, psychological techniques, natural hypnotic interventions (and judicious use of pharmaceutical hypnotics in times of critical need).
- Advise the insomniac to be patient and to be compliant with sleep hygiene techniques.

FURTHER READING

Buysse DJ. Insomnia. JAMA 2013;309(7):706–16. doi:10.1001/jama.2013.193.

Leach MJ, Page AT. Herbal medicine for insomnia: a systematic review and meta-analysis. Sleep Med Rev 2015;24:1–12. doi:10.1016/j.smrv.2014.12.003.

Sarris J, Byrne GJ. A systematic review of insomnia and complementary medicine. Sleep Med Rev 2011;15(2):99–106.

Zhou ES, Gardiner P, Bertisch SM. Integrative medicine for insomnia. Med Clin North Am 2017;101(5):865–79. doi:10.1016/j.mcna.2017.04.005.

REFERENCES

1. American Psychiatric Association. Diagnostic and statistical manual of mental disorders. 5th ed. Arlington: American Psychiatric Association; 2013.
2. Roth T, Roehrs T. Insomnia: epidemiology, characteristics, and consequences. Clin Cornerstone 2003;5(3):5–15.
3. Krystal AD, Roth T. Definitions, measurements, and management in insomnia. J Clin Psychiatry 2004;65:5–7.
4. Wittchen HU, Jacobi F, Rehm J, et al. The size and burden of mental disorders and other disorders of the brain in Europe 2010. Eur Neuropsychopharmacol 2011;21(9):655–79.
5. Stepanski EJ, Wyatt JK. Use of sleep hygiene in the treatment of insomnia. Sleep Med Rev 2003;7(3):215–25.
6. Krystal AD. The changing perspective on chronic insomnia management. J Clin Psychiatry 2004;65:20–5.
7. Roth T. Measuring treatment efficacy in insomnia. J Clin Psychiatry 2004;65:8–12.
8. Roth T, Roehrs T, Pies R. Insomnia: pathophysiology and implications for treatment. Sleep Med Rev 2007;11(1):71–9.
9. Piggins HD. Human clock genes. Ann Med 2002;34(5):394–400.
10. Lancel M. Role of GABA(A) receptors in the regulation of sleep: initial sleep responses to peripherally administered modulators and agonists. Sleep 1999;22(1):33–42.
11. Strecker RE, Basheer R, McKenna JT, et al. Another chapter in the adenosine story. Sleep 2006;29(4):426–8.
12. Benca RM, Ancoli-Israel S, Moldofsky H. Special considerations in insomnia diagnosis and management: depressed, elderly, and chronic pain populations. J Clin Psychiatry 2004;65:26–35.
13. Grandner MA, Jackson NJ, Pak VM, et al. Sleep disturbance is associated with cardiovascular and metabolic disorders. J Sleep Res 2012;21(4):427–33.
14. McClung CA. Circadian rhythms and mood regulation: insights from pre-clinical models. Eur Neuropsychopharmacol 2011;21(Suppl. 4):S683–93.
15. Monteleone P, Martiadis V, Maj M. Circadian rhythms and treatment implications in depression. Prog Neuropsychopharmacol Biol Psychiatry 2011;35(7):1569–74.
16. Baglioni C, Battagliese G, Feige B, et al. Insomnia as a predictor of depression: a meta-analytic evaluation of longitudinal epidemiological studies. J Affect Disord 2011;135(1–3):10–19.
17. Roth T. Insomnia as a risk factor for depression. Int J Neuropsychopharmacol 2004;7:S34–5.
18. Kessler RC, Berglund PA, Coulouvrat C, et al. Insomnia and the performance of US workers: results from the America insomnia survey. Sleep 2011;34(9):1161–71.
19. Ramakrishnan K, Scheid DC. Treatment options for insomnia. Am Fam Physician 2007;76(4):517–26.
20. Sateia MJ, Nowell PD. Insomnia. Lancet 2004;364(9449):1959–73.
21. Schwartz JR, Roth T. Shift work sleep disorder: burden of illness and approaches to management. Drugs 2006;66(18):2357–70.
22. Hein H. The sleep apnoea syndromes: alternative therapies. Pneumologie 2004;58(5):325–9. Epub 2004/05/27. Schlafapnoe-Syndrome: Alternative Therapieverfahren.
23. Morin CM, Benca R. Chronic insomnia. Lancet 2012;379(9821):1129–41.
24. Tariq SH. Pulisetty S. Pharmacotherapy for insomnia. Clin Geriatr Med 2008;24(1):93–105.
25. Rickels K, Rynn M. Pharmacotherapy of generalized anxiety disorder. J Clin Psychiatry 2002;63(Suppl. 14):9–16.
26. Cajochen C, Krauchi K, Wirz-Justice A. Role of melatonin in the regulation of human circadian rhythms and sleep. J Neuroendocrinol 2003;15(4):432–7.
27. Lemoine P, Guilleminault C, Alvarez E. Improvement in subjective sleep in major depressive disorder with a novel antidepressant, agomelatine: randomized, double-blind comparison with venlafaxine. J Clin Psychiatry 2007;68(11):1723–32.
28. Morin CM, Bootzin RR, Buysse DJ, et al. Psychological and behavioral treatment of insomnia: update of the recent evidence (1998–2004). Sleep 2006;29(11):1398–414.
29. Basheer R, Strecker R, Thakkar M, et al. Adenosine and sleep-wake regulation. Prog Neurobiol 2004;73:379–96.
30. Nehlig A, Daval JL, Debry G. Caffeine and the central nervous system: mechanisms of action, biochemical,

metabolic and psychostimulant effects. Brain Res Brain Res Rev 1992;17(2):139–70.

31. Felter HW, Lloyd JU. King's American Dispensatory, 1898. Online. Available: http://www.henriettesherbal.com/eclectic/kings/extracta 1 Nov 2013.

32. Zanoli P, Zavatti M. Pharmacognostic and pharmacological profile of Humulus lupulus L. J Ethnopharmacol 2008;116:383–96.

33. Fussel A, Wolf A, Brattstrom A. Effect of a fixed valerian-Hop extract combination (Ze 91019) on sleep polygraphy in patients with non-organic insomnia: a pilot study. Eur J Med Res 2000;5(9):385–90.

34. Morin C, Koetter U, Bastien C, et al. Valerian-hops combination and diphenhydramine for treating insomnia: a randomized placebo-controlled clinical trial. Sleep 2005;28(11):1465–71.

35. Abourashed EA, Koetter U, Brattstrom A. In vitro binding experiments with a Valerian, hops and their fixed combination extract (Ze91019) to selected central nervous system receptors. Phytomedicine 2004;11(7–8):633–8.

36. Muller CE, Schumacher B, Brattstrom A, et al. Interactions of valerian extracts and a fixed valerian-hop extract combination with adenosine receptors. Life Sci 2002;71(16):1939–49.

37. Schellenberg R, Sauer S, Abourashed EA, et al. The fixed combination of valerian and hops (Ze91019) acts via a central adenosine mechanism. Planta Med 2004;70(7):594–7.

38. Cook W. The Physiomedical Dispensatory, 1869. Online. Available: http://www.ibiblio.org/herbmed/eclectic/cook/main.htm 10 Oct 2005.

39. Culpeper N. Culpeper's complete herbal. Hertfordshire: Wordsworth Editions Ltd.; 1652.

40. Bent S, Padula A, Moore D, et al. Valerian for sleep: a systematic review and meta-analysis. Am J Med 2006;119:1005–12.

41. Mills S, Bone K. Principles and practice of phytotherapy. London: Churchill Livingstone; 2000.

42. Donath F, Quispe S, Diefenbach K, et al. Critical evaluation of the effect of valerian extract on sleep structure and sleep quality. Pharmacopsychiatry 2000;33(2):47–53.

43. Herrera-Arellano A, Luna-Villegas G, Cuevas-Uriostegui ML, et al. Polysomnographic evaluation of the hypnotic effect of Valeriana edulis standardized extract in patients suffering from insomnia. Planta Med 2001;67(8):695–9.

44. Benke D, Barberis A, Kopp S, et al. GABA(A) receptors as in vivo substrate for the anxiolytic action of valerenic acid, a major constituent of valerian root extracts. Neuropharmacology 2009;56(1):174–81.

45. Schumacher B, Scholle S, Holzl J, et al. Lignans isolated from valerian: identification and characterization of a new olivil derivative with partial agonistic activity at A(1) adenosine receptors. J Nat Prod 2002;65(10):1479–85.

46. Blumenthal M, Brinckmannm J, Wollschlaeger Be. The ABC clinical guide to herbs. Austin: American Botanical Council; 2004.

47. Sarris J, Byrne GJ. A systematic review of insomnia and complementary medicine. Sleep Med Rev 2011;15(2):99–106.

48. Fernandez-San-Martin MI, Masa-Font R, Palacios-Soler L, et al. Effectiveness of valerian on insomnia: a meta-analysis of randomized placebo-controlled trials. Sleep Med 2010;11(6):505–11. [Epub 2010/03/30].

49. Sarris J, Kavanagh DJ, Byrne G. Adjuvant use of nutritional and herbal medicines with antidepressants, mood stabilizers and benzodiazepines. J Psychiatr Res 2010;44(1):32–41. [Epub 2009/07/21].

50. Boman B. L-tryptophan: a rational anti-depressant and a natural hypnotic? Aust N Z J Psychiatry 1988;22(1):83–97.

51. Hartmann E. Effects of L-tryptophan on sleepiness and on sleep. J Psychiatr Res 1982;17(2):107–13.

52. Coogan AN, Thome J. Chronotherapeutics and psychiatry: setting the clock to relieve the symptoms. World J Biol Psychiatry 2011;12(Suppl. 1):40–3. [Epub 2011/09/16].

53. Buscemi N, Vandermeer B, Hooton N, et al. The efficacy and safety of exogenous melatonin for primary sleep disorders. A meta-analysis. J Gen Intern Med 2005;20(12):1151–8.

54. Samuels N, Gropp C, Singer SR, et al. Acupuncture for psychiatric illness: a literature review. Behav Med 2008;34(2):55–64.

55. Cheuk DK, Yeung WF, Chung KF, et al. Acupuncture for insomnia. Cochrane Database Syst Rev 2012;(9):CD005472.

56. Wuttke W, Jarry H, Christoffel V, et al. Chaste tree (Vitex agnus-castus)—pharmacology and clinical indications. Phytomedicine 2003;10(4):348–57.

57. Dericks-Tan JS, Schwinn P, Hildt C. Dose-dependent stimulation of melatonin secretion after administration of Agnus castus. Exp Clin Endocrinol Diabetes 2003;111(1):44–6.

58. Ayuso-Gutierrez JL. Depressive subtypes and efficacy of antidepressive pharmacotherapy. World J Biol Psychiatry 2005;6(Suppl. 2):31–7.

59. Mishra LC, Singh BB, Dagenais S. Scientific basis for the therapeutic use of Withania somnifera (ashwagandha): a review. Altern Med Rev 2000;5(4):334–46.

60. Bhattacharya SK, Bhattacharya A, Sairam K, et al. Anxiolytic-antidepressant activity of Withania somnifera glycowithanolides: an experimental study. Phytomedicine 2000;7(6):463–9.

61. Bhattacharya SK, Muruganandam AV. Adaptogenic activity of Withania somnifera: an experimental study using a rat model of chronic stress. Pharmacol Biochem Behav 2003;75(3):547–55.

62. Kelly GS. Rhodiola rosea: a possible plant adaptogen. Altern Med Rev 2001;6(3):293–302.

63. Atkinson G, Davenne D. Relationships between sleep, physical activity and human health. Physiol Behav 2007;90(2–3):229–35.

64. Montgomery P, Dennis J. Physical exercise for sleep problems in adults aged 60. Cochrane Database Syst Rev 2002;(4):CD003404.

65. Sarris J, LaPorte E, Schweitzer I. Kava: a comprehensive review of efficacy, safety, and psychopharmacology. Aust N Z J Psychiatry 2011;45(1):27–35.

66. Lehrl S. Clinical efficacy of kava WS 1490 in sleep disturbances associated with anxiety disorders. Results of a multicenter, randomized, placebo-controlled, double-blind clinical trial. J Affect Disord 2004;78:101–10.

67. Malsch U, Kieser M. Efficacy of kava-kava in the treatment of non-psychotic anxiety, following pretreatment with benzodiazepines. Psychopharmacology (Berl) 2001;157:277–83.

68. Sarris J, Adams J, Kavanagh D. An explorative qualitative analysis of participants' experience of using kava versus placebo in an RCT. Aust J Med Med Herbalism 2010;22(1):12–16.

69. Puhan MA, Suarez A, Lo Cascio C, et al. Didgeridoo playing as alternative treatment for obstructive sleep apnoea syndrome: randomised controlled trial. BMJ 2006;332(7536):266–70.

70. Malhotra A, White DP. Obstructive sleep apnoea. Lancet 2002;360(9328):237–45.

71. Yeung WF, Chung KF, Man-Ki Poon M, et al. Chinese herbal medicine for insomnia: a systematic review of randomized controlled trials. Sleep Med Rev 2012;16(6):497–507.

72. Sarris J. Chinese herbal medicine for sleep disorders: poor methodology restricts any clear conclusion. Sleep Med Rev 2012;16(6):493–5.

73. Jefferson CD, Drake CL, Scofield HM, et al. Sleep hygiene practices in a population-based sample of insomniacs. Sleep 2005;28(5):611–15.

74. Maciocia G. The foundations of Chinese medicine. Singapore: Churchill Livingstone; 1989.

75. Haas EM. Staying healthy with nutrition. Berkeley: Celestial Arts; 1992.

76. Werbach M. Nutritional influences on illness. Tarzana. California: Third Line Press; 1996.

77. Nutt D, Argyropoulos S, Hood S, et al. Generalized anxiety disorder: a comorbid disease. Eur Neuropsychopharmacol 2006;16(Suppl. 2):S109–18.

78. Bone K. A clinical guide to blending liquid herbs: herbal formulations for the individual patient. China: Churchill & Livingstone; 2003.

CHAPTER 17

Headache and migraine

Phillip Cottingham
ND

OVERVIEW

The complex set of conditions classified as headache are broadly defined as 'pain located above the orbitomeatal line'.[1] The number of classifications found in the International Classification of Headaches Disorders (ICHD)[1] illustrates the fact that headache, while classified as a condition, is primarily the result of other conditions. The types focused upon will be those that are potentially treatable in a naturopathic clinical situation. There are 14 major headache classifications (Table 17.1).[2] The naturopathic approach is to consider headaches as symptoms, rather than discrete conditions, but the ICHD codes classify primary headaches as disorders, with secondary headaches as arising from other disorders. It is useful to consider identifying primary causes and triggers when clinically investigating headaches. This will help develop a treatment plan that is effective long term as well as palliative short term.

Definition of headache compared with the definition of migraine

Headache is defined as pain in the cranial region, an isolated benign occurrence or manifestation of variety of disorders.[4] Migraine is defined as a disabling, primary headache characterised by unilateral pulsating pain.[5] Headache is more generalised pain; migraine is unilateral and generally produces several concomitant symptoms. Although the detailed definition of headache disorders is evolving, and somewhat controversial,[6] the basics of differentiation between headache and migraine remain reasonably constant. Migraine is also defined as being with or without aura (premonition of the pain and other symptoms).[7] See Tables 17.1 and 17.2a–b and Figures 17.1a–d for classifications and differential diagnostic information.

Pathophysiology of headache and migraine

The classification of headache and migraine into 13 major groups indicates considerable complexity in its biological and psychological basis. This overview will address the most significant and common causes and manifestations, particularly those that are commonly encountered in naturopathic clinical practice. Aetiological and trigger factors are often indistinguishable because of low neurochemical thresholds to triggers producing pain.[21]

Table 17.1
Major classifications of headache disorders

Primary or secondary	Primary headaches				Secondary headaches		
ICHD II code	**1.**	**2.**	**3.**	**4.**	**5.**	**6.**	**7.**
Classification	Migraine	Tension type	Cluster headaches and other trigeminal neuralgias	Other primary headaches	Attributed to head and/or neck trauma	Attributed to cranial or cervical vascular disorder	Attributed to non-vascular intracranial disorder
	Migraine with or without aura	Infrequent and frequent episodic and chronic	Episodic and chronic cluster headaches	Stabbing, cough, exertional, associated with sexual activity, hypnic, primary thunderclap, hemicranias continual, new/daily persistent headaches	Acute and chronic post-traumatic headache	Associated with: ischaemic stroke, transient ischaemic attacks (TIAs), intracranial haemorrhage (non-traumatic); sub-arachnoid haemorrhage	Attributed to high cerebrospinal fluid (CSF) pressure; intracranial hypertension; non-infectious inflammatory disease

	Secondary headaches						
ICHD II code	**8.**	**9.**	**10.**	**11.**	**12.**	**13.**	**14.**
Classification	Attributed to substance or its withdrawal	Attributed to infection	Attributed to disorder of homoeostasis	Attributed to disorder of cranium, neck, eyes, ears, nose, sinuses, teeth, mouth or other facial or cranial structures	Attributed to psychiatric disorder	Cranial neuralgias and central causes of facial pain	Other headache, cranial neuralgia or primary facial pain
Examples	Substances such as: carbon monoxide; nitric oxide; alcohol; food components or additives; MSG; cocaine; cannabis; histamine; or medication overuse	Infections such as: bacterial meningitis; lymphocytic meningitis; encephalitis; brain abcess; and systemic infections	Conditions such as: hypoxia; hypercapnia; high altitude; sleep apnoea; arterial hypertension; hypothyroidism; fasting	Cranial bone disorders; cervicogenic headaches; acute glaucoma; rhinosinusitis; TMJ disorders.	Somatisation or psychotic disorders	Trigeminal neuralgias; supraorbital neuralgia; cold stimulus headache; associated with herpes zoster	Unclassified headaches

Source: International Headache Society 2013[3]

Table 17.2a
Diagnosis of headache according to headache types

Primary headaches

	Type of headache (HA)			
Signs and symptoms	**Migraine (without aura)[8]**	**Migraine with aura[8]**	**Tension-type headache[9]**	**Cluster HA[10]**

	A. At least 5 attacks fulfilling criteria B–D
	B. Headache attacks lasting 4–72 hours (untreated or unsuccessfully treated)
	C. Headache has at least 2 of the following characteristics:
	  • unilateral location
	  • pulsating quality
	  • moderate to severe pain
	  • aggravation by or causing avoidance of routine physical activity (e.g. walking or climbing stairs)
	D. During headache at least 1 of the following:
	  • nausea and/or vomiting
	  • photophobia and phonophobia
	E. Not attributed to another disorder
		Auras include focal neurological symptoms (visual, sensory or speech disturbances) lasting 5–60 minutes, either prior or concurrent with the headache
		Otherwise the symptoms are similar to migraine without aura
			A. At least 10 previous headache episodes fulfilling criteria B–D; number of days with such headaches: less than 180 per year or 15 per month
			B. Headaches lasting from 30 minutes to 7 days
			C. At least two of the following pain characteristics:
			  • pressing or tightening (non-pulsating) quality
			  • mild to moderate intensity (nonprohibitive)
			  • bilateral location
			  • no aggravation from walking stairs or similar routine activities
			D. Both of the following:
			  • no nausea or vomiting
			  • photophobia and phonophobia absent, or only one is present
			NB. Chronic tension-type headache Same as tension-type headache, except number of days with such headaches: at least 15 days per month, for at least six months
			Chronic dailyheadache
			Features of tension-type headache
			Occurs at least 6 days per week
				A. At least 5 attacks fulfilling B–D
				B. Severe unilateral orbital, supraorbital and/or temporal pain lasting 15–180 mins. Untreated
				C. HA is associated with at least one of the following signs:
				  • conjunctival injection
				  • lachrymation
				  • nasal congestion
				  • rhinorrhoea
				  • forehead or facial swelling
				  • miosis (pupil constriction)
				  • ptosis (eyelid droop)
				  • eyelid oedema
				D. Frequency from 1 every other day to 8/day
				E. At least one of the following:
				  • history and physical exam rule out other forms of HA
				  • other forms of HA ruled out after investigation
				  • other forms of HA present but CH occurs for first time as not temporally related to the other HA

Source: Cephalalgia 1988[8-10]

Table 17.2b

Diagnosis of headache according to headache types

Secondary headaches

	Type of headache (HA)					
	Cranial neuralgia and nerve trunk pain[11]	HA associated with metabolic disorder (MD)[12]	HA related to cranial or facial disorder or cervicogenic HA[13]	HA related to head trauma (HT)[14]	HA related to vascular disorders (VDO)[15]	HA associated with non-vascular intracranial disorder (NVICD)[16]
Related disorders		1. Hypoxia (altitude sickness) 2. Hypercapnia 3. Hypoglycaemia 4. Dialysis 5. Other metabolic abnormality (possible but not yet validated) such as anaemia, ischaemic HA, fasting (without hypoglycaemia)			1. Transient ischaemic attacks 2. Thromboembolic stroke 3. Intracranial haematoma 4. Subarachnoid haemorrhage 5. Unruptured vascular formation 6. Arteritis 7. Carotid or vertebral artery pain (caused by dissection or carotidynia) 8. Venous thrombosis 9. Arterial hypertension 10. Other VDO	1. High cerebrospinal fluid (CSF) pressure 2. Low CSF pressure 3. Intracranial infection such as meningitis, encephalitis, brain abscess, subdural empyrea 4. Intracranial sarcoidosis 5. Associated with intrathecal injection 6. Intracranial neoplasm 7. Other intracranial disorder
Signs and symptoms	A. Pain in the distribution of one or more cranial nerve and or cervical roots 2 and 3 without projection into neighbouring area B. Demonstration of relevant lesion C. Onset of pain temporally related to cranial nerve lesion D. Treatment of lesion remits the pain	E. Confirmation by lab investigation F. Frequency of HA related to frequency and time of MD G. Normalisation of MD relieves HA	A. Clinical or Lab evidence of disorder B. HA located in affected structure and/or radiating to surrounding areas (Pain may refer to more distant areas) C. HA disappears with a month of successful treatment of disorder	A. Significance of HT documented by at least one of the following: • loss of consciousness • posttraumatic amnesia > 10 mins • at least two of the following examinations reveals relevant abnormality: clinical neurological exam, x-ray of skull, neuroimaging, evoked potentials, spinal fluid exam, vestibular function test, neuropsychological tests • HA occurs < 14 days after regaining consciousness or occurrence of head trauma • HA disappears within 8 weeks of regaining consciousness or occurrence of trauma	A. Signs of symptoms of VDO B. Investigations indicate VDO C. HA as a new symptom occurs in close temporal association with onset of VDO	A. Symptoms and/or signs of NVICD B. Confirmation of disorder by appropriate investigations C. HA as a new symptom or a new type temporally related to NVICD

Source: Cephalalgia 1988[11-16]

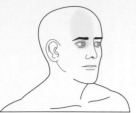
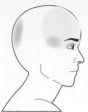

Figure 17.1a
Distribution of pain in migraine

Source: Kunkel 2001[17]

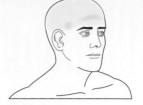
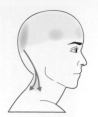

Figure 17.1b
Distribution of pain in tension-type headache

Source: Diamond 1999[18]

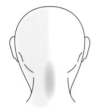
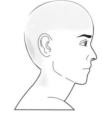

Figure 17.1c
Distribution of pain in cervicogenic headache

Source: Haldeman & Dagenais 2001[19]

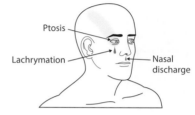

Figure 17.1d
Distribution of pain in cluster headache

Source: Lipton et al 1999[20]

Historical view of headaches and migraines

Historically, headaches have been treated with extreme methods, such as trepanning (cutting holes in the skull) and with live electric fish from the Nile.[22] Descriptions of headache are found in Mesopotamian and Egyptian artifacts, and Hippocrates exhibited extensive understanding of headaches, their causation and treatment.[23] The Byzantine era (4th–7th century) produced several texts that classified headaches into cluster headaches, migraines and traumatic headaches.[24] A wide variety of herbal treatments have been used in headaches, especially by medieval European and Arabic doctors,[22] with the famous Persian physician Ibn Sinna (Avicenna) (980–1037) classifying according to location, such as frontal or generalised.[24] Tulp (1593–1674) has left behind many case studies of headache[25] utilising cupping, bloodletting and herbal remedies.

The dawn of the 17th and 18th centuries saw a shift in perception of headache towards a more 'scientific view'.[22] In the 19th century there is one of the early references to a link with the vascular system and headaches, made by Erasmus Darwin.[24] Liveing (1832–1919) produced the first scientific exploration of migraine, followed by Gowers who, in his *Manual of diseases of the nervous system*, discusses trigger events such as cold, dietetic error, visual stimulus, fatigue and peculiar odours.[22] The 20th century saw the introduction of pharmaceutical treatments, including barbiturates and analgesics (salicylates, codeines, etc.).[26]

Vascular theory

The vascular origin of migraines is a strongly held theory that has been postulated as far back as 1664 when Thomas Willis identified the dilation of blood vessels as being the main contributor to the pain felt by sufferers.[27] While vascular conditions are held to be significant, the question arises as to why the blood vessels should alter their nature to produce migraines. Goadsby[28] considers the issue to be a trigeminovascular one, as

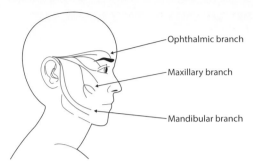

Ophthalmic branch

Maxillary branch

Mandibular branch

Figure 17.2
Trigeminal nerve pathways

the major vascular pathways surrounding the brain are innervated by branches of the trigeminal nerve. He dismisses the vascular theory in favour of a *neurovascular theory*. This could have implications for the way in which migraine and headache are approached in naturopathic practice.

Neurogenic (sensitisation) theory
Migraine and cluster headache have all been said to be caused by neurovascular or neurogenic mechanisms. The neurogenic mechanism postulates a central sensitisation of neural function,[29] with restriction of nerves, spinal cord and meninges, affecting both functional (physiological) and structural (space for movement) and blood flow around neural tissue.[30] This has implications for the use of body therapies in migraine and cluster headache.

Musculoskeletal origins
Tension-type headache has been shown to be associated with both cervical tension and temperomandibular joint (TMJ) disorders and bruxism (teeth grinding).[31,32] Cervicogenic headaches are also (as the name suggests) associated with tension in the cervical region (see Figure 17.2). A comorbidity with depression has been identified.[33] This has clinical implications and needs to considered in treatment plans.

CONVENTIONAL TREATMENT

Migraine
Acute treatment for migraine is primarily focused on pharmaceutical medication. The principles of pharmaceutical administration include: early intervention for stress (pain is still mild); adequate dosage; appropriate administration routes (for rapidity and effectiveness of medication); co-administration of other drugs for vegetative symptoms, such as nausea and to facilitate absorption; and guard against overdose and prolonged use, which can bring about chronicity and/or medication overuse headache.[34]

The goals of acute treatment include: rapid and consistent treatment; restoration of function; minimisation of use of back-up medication; optimisation of self-care; cost-effectiveness of management; and reduction of adverse effects.[37]

Risk factors—migraine

Modifiable
- Attack frequency
- Obesity
- Medication overuse
- Stressful life events
- Caffeine overuse
- Snoring (sleep apnoea)

Non-modifiable
- Age
- Low socioeconomic status
- Head injury

Source: Bigal & Lipton 2006[35]

DIFFERENTIAL DIAGNOSIS*

Types of headache: tension, trigeminal, migrainous
- Referred pain from trauma, muscular tension, inflammation
- Spinal misalignment
- Upper respiratory tract infection or nasal congestion/obstruction
- Dehydration, food allergy/intolerance
- Acute or chronic stress or anxiety disorder
- Sleep deprivation
- Cancer or brain tumour
- Reaction to biological substance (e.g. medication, caffeine)

*Sensation of a headache occurring due to range of underlying conditions
Sources: Kernick et al. 2008,[36] and Lipton et al. 1999[20]

Medications commonly used fall into three main categories[34]:

- non-specific anti-migraine drugs including: analgesics (aspirin, metoclopramide, tolfenamic acid, ibuprofen, naproxen sodium, diclofenac, ketoprofen) and non-steroidal anti-inflammatory drugs (NSAIDs)
- specific anti-migraine drugs including:
  - ergotamine and derivatives (dihydroergotamine), which have an anti-5-HT action
  - triptans (sumatriptan, zolmitriptan, eletriptan, almotriptan, rizatriptan, naratriptan, frovatriptan), either in nasal spray or tablet form—also act on 5-HT receptors
  - newer drugs, such as CGRP receptor agonists and antiepileptic drugs such as divalprox sodium and sodium valproate, which are utilised because of their effect on GABA
  - OnabotulinumtoxinA, the use of which for migraine has increased in recent times.[38]

Preventive treatment is also focused around the use of pharmaceuticals. Main classes of drugs used are[39]:

- beta-blockers (atenolol, bisoprolol, metoprolol, nadolol, propranolol, timolol)
- antidepressants (amitriptyline, doxepin, nortriptyline, protriptyline)
- selective serotonin reuptake inhibitors (SSRIs) (venlafaxine).

These drugs are primarily used to inhibit the adrenergic and serotoninergic pathways.

Calcium channel antagonists are found to be effective in migraine prevention, but the mechanisms are poorly understood. It is thought that they may inhibit '5-HT release, neurovascular inflammation or the initiation and propagation of neurocortical spreading'.[39]

Anticonvulsants have been shown to have effectiveness in migraine prophylaxis, as have ACE inhibitors and botulinum toxin type A (Botox).[39]

KEY TREATMENT PROTOCOLS

Considering the wide range of manifestation and the neurophysiological complexity of headache and migraine (Table 17.1) it is important for any treatment plans to be developed for the particular patient and adapted to their unique circumstances. A comprehensive and exhaustive case history (with referral for diagnosis when required) is essential to ensure the causative and trigger factors are identified (in particular 'red flag' signs), so that treatment addresses the pathological underpinnings of the condition. Aside from treating the underlying causations, the primary treatment focus needs to be on ameliorating acute pain and suffering.

While the pathophysiological approach targets specific systems and mechanisms, the holistic approach has a much wider perspective, addressing lifestyle issues and psychosocial make-up. It is as important to understand the person with the headache or migraine as the factors that have direct biological involvement in their development.[40] Headache has been shown to be closely linked with psychological issues and linked to such disorders as depression[41] and, as such, requires a greater analysis and understanding of the patient. Poor sleep quality has been associated with migraine, and sleep hygiene may be a factor to consider in naturopathic treatment.[42,43]

> **Naturopathic Treatment Aims**
>
> - Establish the type of headache and its underlying cause.
> - Check for risk factors and triggers.
> - Reduce pain and inflammation.
> - Ensure optimal nutrition and hydration.
> - Check for food sensitivities and allergic responses to environmental agents.
> - Consider detoxification programs to manage medication overuse headache syndrome.[44-46]
> - Manage sleep quality.
> - Assess body mechanics and spinal alignment (especially cervical region).
> - Consider cranial osteopathy, craniosacral therapy or chiropractic referral.

Addressing the neurovascular underpinnings of headache

There is a hypothesis that brainstem (the nuclei involved in nociception) dysfunction may be involved in the pathogenesis of migraines.[27] Another factor may involve brain plasticity, with a decrease of grey matter in several regions in migraine patients.[47,48]

Genetic factors may be involved in susceptibility to migraine (without aura) but not migraine with aura.[49] However, this may explain the role of hormonal factors in migraine. Hormonal factors are implicated in migraine, with oestrogens modulating neurobiological processes that initiate migraines (neuronal excitability, release of nitric oxide and neuropeptides).[50,51] A recent systematic review confirms this hypothesis, with evidence from epidemiological, pathophysiological and clinical studies linking oestrogen to migraine.[52] This is a clinically significant factor for naturopathic practitioners.

Treatment protocols for this will involve modulating the neurovascular response and reducing neural sensitisation. This will include herbal treatments and nutritional approaches. Stress management, body therapy approaches and lifestyle modifications support these protocols (Figure 17.3 and Table 17.3).

As identified, the neurovascular migraine and headache mechanisms involve a number of targets for monoamine neurotransmitters.[64] The serotonergic pathway has been specifically identified in using *Tanacetum parthenium* (TP). This inhibits phospholipase

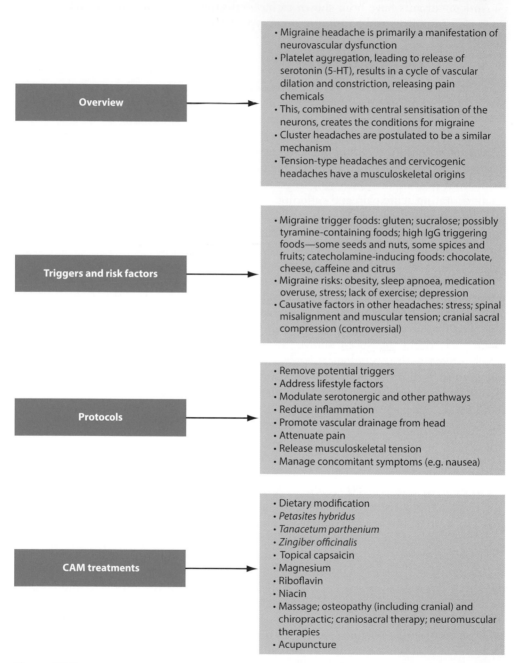

Overview
- Migraine headache is primarily a manifestation of neurovascular dysfunction
- Platelet aggregation, leading to release of serotonin (5-HT), results in a cycle of vascular dilation and constriction, releasing pain chemicals
- This, combined with central sensitisation of the neurons, creates the conditions for migraine
- Cluster headaches are postulated to be a similar mechanism
- Tension-type headaches and cervicogenic headaches have a musculoskeletal origins

Triggers and risk factors
- Migraine trigger foods: gluten; sucralose; possibly tyramine-containing foods; high IgG triggering foods—some seeds and nuts, some spices and fruits; catecholamine-inducing foods: chocolate, cheese, caffeine and citrus
- Migraine risks: obesity, sleep apnoea, medication overuse, stress; lack of exercise; depression
- Causative factors in other headaches: stress; spinal misalignment and muscular tension; cranial sacral compression (controversial)

Protocols
- Remove potential triggers
- Address lifestyle factors
- Modulate serotonergic and other pathways
- Reduce inflammation
- Promote vascular drainage from head
- Attenuate pain
- Release musculoskeletal tension
- Manage concomitant symptoms (e.g. nausea)

CAM treatments
- Dietary modification
- *Petasites hybridus*
- *Tanacetum parthenium*
- *Zingiber officinalis*
- Topical capsaicin
- Magnesium
- Riboflavin
- Niacin
- Massage; osteopathy (including cranial) and chiropractic; craniosacral therapy; neuromuscular therapies
- Acupuncture

Figure 17.3
Migraine and headache

and therefore prevents the release of 5-HT from platelets and polymorphonuclear leucocytes,[55] which may explain the perceived effectiveness of TP for headache and, in particular, migraine prophylaxis. Another pathway has also been suggested (albeit only in in-vitro studies), and that is inhibiting nitric oxide release by TP.[65] Nitric oxide is considered to sensitise migraineurs to pain[66] as well as activate vasodilation pathways, which have been suggested as possible migraine triggers,[67] although this is still uncertain.[68] An older study also suggests TP may play a role in inhibiting prostaglandin synthesis.[69]

Perhaps the most comprehensive and statistically significant study (along with a high clinical significance) is the study where a CO_2 extract of TP was given over four months, with the effect measured over a number of clinically significant parameters.[53] However, whether this finding could be extrapolated to ingestion of the raw leaf (a common administration method) or other preparations remains to be investigated.

A study that attempted to identify a possible mechanism for TP, which was performed on rats,[57] showed that it may be possible that parthenolide (a sesquiterpene lactone present in feverfew) interferes with activation of the nucleus trigeminalis caudalis (a trigeminal nerve nuclei)—a factor in migraines.[70] Lack of consistency of trial data has resulted in inconclusiveness about the efficacy of TP in migraine prophylaxis[54]; however, it has shown potential for migraine prophylaxis (probably acting on neurovascular mechanisms) and is established as relatively safe.[55]

A 1990 case study has indicated the possibility of ***Zingiber officinalis*** having effectiveness in migraines (based on Ayurvedic and Unani Tibb medicinal information).[55] Since this case study, two more recent studies[58,71] using proprietary compounds of TP and *Zingiber officinalis* showed efficacy in migraine treatment. However, neither of these studies has postulated a mechanism or a constituent that may act upon the receptors for migraine. However, it could be its antioxidant properties that may contribute to this.[72]

Similar pathways have been proposed for generalised antioxidant therapy. In a small pilot study (non-controlled) 12 patients with long-term history of migraine, resistant to standard medication, were given a standardised formulation containing extract of ***Pinus maritima*** (120 mg), vitamin C (60 mg) and vitamin E (30 IU) (Enzogenol) 10 capsules daily for three months. The Migraine Disability Assessment (MIDAS) questionnaire was used as a measurement of severity. A significant reduction in the mean measures (five domains) was seen.[73] While this study was small and non-controlled it indicates that antioxidant therapy in migraine is worth further investigation. Neutralising nitric oxide-activated vasodilation is postulated as the mechanism in this case.

Petasites hybridus has been used for migraines in Germany for more than 30 years.[74] A large study[56] ($n = 202$) has demonstrated efficacy in migraine (75 mg extract b.i.d.) over placebo. This is supported by a smaller study that also showed efficacy in reducing migraine frequency and number of migraine days. Efficacy in reducing the intensity and duration of attacks was achieved only after eight weeks (suggesting long-term treatment is important).[75] Possible mechanisms are identified as anti-inflammatory, through an anti-leukotriene activity or an effect on calcium channels. Leukotrienes and other inflammatory mediators have been implicated in migraines.[76] In other studies it has been shown to block calcium channels in hypertension, causing vascular smooth muscle relaxation.[77] A note of caution, however: it contains pyrrolizidine alkaloids. Use processed preparations that have reduced these alkaloids.[56]

Inhibition of platelet aggregation, resulting in less release of serotonin, is an important factor in migraine (and some types of headache) therapy. A number of medicinal plants have been shown to inhibit platelet aggregation. In a study of **Australian native medicinal plants** used traditionally for headache, Rogers et al.[78] found that *Crataegus monogyna, Ipomoea pes-caprae, Eremophila freelingii, Eremophila longifolia* and *Asteromyrtus symphyocarpa* all exhibited platelet aggregation inhibition in vitro.

The effect of *Mentha X piperita* in headache has undergone some investigation. In one study[59] varying dependent parameters of headaches (such as neurophysiological, psychological and experimental algesimetric) were measured using four different preparations of peppermint and *Eucalyptus* spp. (species not identified) essential oils in combinations (controls contained traces only). The main domains that were found to be significant included pain sensitivity and performance-related activity. While this study is useful, an effectiveness study looking at these parameters would further understanding. Mechanisms are not discussed in this paper; however, Atta and Alkofahi[79] have confirmed antinociceptive properties with *Mentha piperita* and Galeotti et al.[80] have confirmed a local anaesthetic activity. In a review of its efficacy in a number of conditions, McKay and Blumberg[81] have indicated a use in pericranial muscular tension (a possible application in headaches in particular).

Caffeine has been shown to reduce headache pain (albeit in an older study).[82] Plants containing caffeine (e.g. **Coffea spp.**, **Paullinia cupana**, **Cola acuminata** and **Passiflora nitida**) may prove useful, but studies using whole plant extracts are needed. Paradoxically, given its possible therapeutic effects, caffeine has been implicated in migraines, with many migraineurs reporting effects of consumption or withdrawal.[83] This may be related to cerebral blood flows and velocities.[84] A case-controlled population study showed that caffeine (in the form of coffee) is a modest risk factor across several types of headache.[85] Sucralose (a popular sweetener marketed as Splenda) has also been implicated in migraines, although not conclusively.[86,87]

Ginkgo biloba has shown some promise in migraine with aura, with gingkolide B having efficacy in a multicentric, open, preliminary trial.[88]

A small study has utilised **topical capsaicin** to address arterial pain that occurs in migraine. However, more research is required to understand possible mechanisms and to establish definite efficacy.[89]

Nutritional approaches have been primarily focused around **diet and food triggers**, but there is some evidence of supplement effectiveness in migraine and migraine prophylaxis. Specific food and drink constituents have been shown to be migraine triggers. Red wine is popularly thought to be a migraine trigger. Panconesi,[90] in a review of alcohol consumption and migraine, concludes it is more than the alcohol content that acts to induce migraines and attributes the action of the red wine to phenolic flavonoids, rather than the popular tyramine theory. One study concluded that red wine did not induce the release of 5-HT from platelets,[91] suggesting that this pathway is not the mechanism, if indeed red wine is a culprit. However, this finding is not supported by another review, concluding that it is a possibility that red wine may induce 5-HT release from platelets.[92] Tyramine is not just found in red wine. Studies of tyramine found in other foods (such as cheese, broad beans and sauerkraut) linked to migraines may still implicate it as a trigger factor.[93] There is a recent theory that SULT1A enzymes (protective against the adverse effects of catecholamines) may be inhibited by red wine, chocolate, citrus, cheese and coffee.[94]

Gluten may play a role as a migraine trigger. In a study of people with coeliac disease, four of the participants were found to have migraine, which improved on a gluten-free diet.[95] While not conclusive, it is a promising indication and may indicate excluding gluten in non-coeliac, gluten-sensitive migraineurs.

Various food antigens have been implicated in IgG-modulated migraine. A randomised, double-blind crossover study conducted with 21 migraineurs utilised a range of foods with a known low IgG antibody response, compared with those with a known high response. There was a significant difference in the number of attacks (and those requiring acute medication), as well as number of headache days. The duration and severity of the attacks was not significantly affected. Unfortunately specificity about the IgG positive or negative diets is not given, but grains with gluten, seeds and nuts, spices and fruits are listed as high IgG triggers, while salads, mushrooms, moss, sugar products and meat are low.[96] This suggests that elimination diets (with challenges) could be a useful approach to ensure that only those foods that are migraine-triggering are eliminated totally.

While not a trigger, obesity has been implicated as a causative factor in migraine[97] and any nutritional approach will need to consider weight loss as a significant part of the approach in those migraine patients who are overweight. Nutrients, particularly phyto-nutrients, have been suggested for migraine prophylaxis.[98] This would imply a diet high in vegetables and fruits, with the proviso that IgG-positive foods (test and challenge) are not included.

A mitochondrial dysfunction has been suggested in migraine, resulting in impaired oxygen metabolism (possibly in platelets, resulting in platelet aggregation and release of 5-HT).[99] **Riboflavin (B2)** (400 mg single dose) has been shown to have a significant beneficial effect in migraine over placebo (being a precursor to flavin mononucleotide and flavin adenine dinucleotide within mitochondria).[100] One study suggests that these results may not translate to paediatric migraine, but this may be dose related (50 mg/day)[101] or due to absorption rates.[102] This has been associated with different haplogroups of mitochondrial DNA.[60]

Magnesium (Mg^{++}) is another nutrient that has shown promise in migraine. An older study demonstrated that red blood cells in migraine sufferers was lower than the normal range.[103] This study has been supported by recent studies showing serum Mg^{++} reduced in migraineurs.[61,104] Possible mechanisms postulated are: increased neuroexcitability with low Mg^{++}[105] and mitochondrial dysfunction.[63] Not surprisingly both Mg^{++} oral supplementation (for prophylaxis),[62,106] along with intravenous Mg^{++} (in acute attacks),[107] show effectiveness in a number of studies.

Niacin also shows promise in several studies for the treatment of migraine.[108] A review of nine studies[109] shows significant beneficial effects of niacin in migraine. The mechanism may also relate to mitochondrial function. This same mechanism has been postulated for the demonstrated efficacy of coenzyme Q10 in reducing frequency, migraine days and severity of migraines.[110]

Nutritional protocols in migraine need to be built around removal of **dietary triggers** and inclusion of more vegetables, non-allergenic fruits, whole grains, legumes, non-allergenic nuts/seeds (vitamins B2 and B3, Mg^{++}) and cruciferous vegetables, especially grown organically (higher Mg^{++}).[111] Supplementation should be considered where there are identified deficiencies.[112]

Application of, or referral for, body therapy is an important consideration in naturopathic treatment plans in migraine. There is considerable evidence of effectiveness of a number of body therapies. Irregular exercise and alcohol consumption have been associated with migraine and tension-type headache incidence.[113] **Biofeedback** has been shown to have effectiveness in migraine,[114,115] suggesting that **stress management** is important in assisting patients in managing the condition. Medication overuse is a risk factor[3] in migraine, particularly with migraine medication[65] and often a naturopathic consultation may uncover this. Referral back to the doctor for management of this is important, but detoxification strategies may be of help to assist patients in managing this. Depression (particularly in conjunction with anxiety) is a common underlying condition for migraine and tension-type headache[116] that needs to be managed. Sleep problems (including sleep apnoea) have also been associated with headache[3] and are well managed through naturopathic and herbal strategies.

Hydrotherapy (and its sister science balneotherapy) have had some traditional usage in treating headache[117] and are widely used in naturopathic medicine worldwide.[118] Researched evidence for hydrotherapy in headache is scant, but there is some evidence from its use in musculoskeletal conditions that indicate usefulness, particularly in promoting blood flow,[119] which, as has been shown, is a critical factor in migraines and some headaches. Some positive results have been achieved using hydrotherapy with other manual therapies in fibromyalgia,[120] which may be significant given that TMJ dysfunction (a feature of many fibromyalgia patients) is a known contributor to headache.

The neurogenic theory

The neurodynamic approach to migraine focuses on the effects of neural impairment on head and neck pain (including migraine) from a central sensitisation of the nervous system.[121] Puentedura et al.[30] postulate a neural sensitisation that affects the upper dura mater as a potential headache generator. This could be because of the connection of the ligamentum nuchae and rectus capitis minor muscle to the dura.[122,123] The dura mater is directly acted upon by cranial osteopathy and craniosacral therapy,[124] which indicates a possible treatment path, particularly when the creation of greater flexibility and tissue space around the neural vessels and outputs may reduce sensitivity.[30] Gard[125] has presented a hypothesis of intracranial regulation resulting in oscillations of the CSF, in relation to vascular drainage of the skull, that may explain the clinical reports of effectiveness in the treatment of migraines.

Tension-type and cluster headaches

Protocols for these types of headache are similar to those of migraine, with some specific applications of therapy to these types. Plasma serotonin has been shown to increase in tension-type headache,[64] which points to herbal treatment as a possibly effective therapy, particularly ***Tanacetum parthenium***[55] and possibly ***Petasites hybridus***.[56] Some evidence also points to the usefulness of Ca^{++} antagonists in cluster headaches,[126] which could also indicate that *Petasites hybridus* is useful.[77]

The nasal application of capsaician (a constituent of ***Capsicum annuum***) has been shown to be effective in cluster headache, in at least three studies.[127–129] All of these studies are dated, but all show similar methodology and statistical significance.

Osteopathic treatment effectiveness in tension-type headache was shown in a single-blinded randomised trial involving 26 volunteers.[130] Significant results occurred in headache-free days, degree of improvement and frequency and intensity. Treatment included a wide range of osteopathic methods, such as cranial osteopathy, fascial unwinding and strain-counterstrain techniques, as well as joint articulation. The usefulness of this study is that it was conducted in the clinical setting, indicating that osteopathy has a significant part to play in the treatment of tension-type headaches.

Treating musculoskeletal origins

Protocols for headaches of musculoskeletal origin are centred on body therapies but can be supported by lifestyle considerations and stress management (for further detail see Chapters 25 and 26 on musculoskeletal considerations and Chapter 40 on pain management).

The ICHD II code 11 headaches are those caused by disorders of the cranium or cervicogenic headaches (CGHA).[2] The efficacy of a number of body therapy treatments has been studied. The few reviews that have been conducted have shown some promise, but the trial numbers have been small, limiting the emergent evidence to possibility, rather than probability.[131]

A systematic review of CAM for CGHA[132] found that overall CAM shows promise for CGHA, with some CAM therapies being of greater benefit. The following summary details the findings: Acupuncture was found to be no more efficacious than physio-therapy (66% rating on high quality studies); spinal manipulation shows some promise (68%); electrotherapy (TENS) was inconclusive (50%); physiotherapy (non-CAM but included in the study) came out lower than 50%; massage, homeopathy and other therapies had too few trials to be able to determine any benefit.

INTEGRATIVE MEDICAL CONSIDERATIONS

The management of acute migraine and other headache types often requires effective pain management (see Chapter 40 on pain management) or nausea management, which may often involve pharmaceutical medication,[34] compared with the more prophylactic approach. CAM therapies in acute pain management may not be as effective as modern analgesic pharmaceuticals.

Physical therapies

Body therapy is a potential therapeutic approach, given that the origin of the headache is located in the cervical spine, and most investigations have centred on various types of body therapies. Other therapies that have shown promise are: articular mobilisa-tion, stretches for increasing range of motion, traction of the cervical region, soft tissue massage, myofascial techniques for release, strengthening muscle function and postural/body mechanics adjustment.[133]

Cranial osteopathy and **craniosacral therapy** have shown some promise in the treatment of migraine. The motion of the cranial bones is controversial,[114] but a number of sutural mobilisations have been postulated to assist in migraine treatment through reducing compressive forces on the neural outflow of the cranial nerves by sutural compressive forces (among other mechanisms).[134] A randomised, waitlisted study of craniosacral therapy (the control group was waitlisted and received only eight weeks treatment, while the treatment group received 16 weeks) showed a significant difference in treatment effects (using the HIT-6 questionnaire, which uses the domains of pain, social participation, general activity, vitality, intellectual activity and biological suffering).[135] Craniosacral therapy and cranial osteopathy studies face considerable challenges in terms of devising acceptable placebo controls (similar to many CAM therapies), an issue that has required innovative measures such as magnets.[136,137]

Osteopathic and **chiropractic manipulation** have been studied in migraine and neurovascular headache with some useful outcomes. A study of osteopathic manipulative treatment (using non-treatment as a control) showed a decrease in pain intensity, reduction of migraine days and reduction of lifestyle effects (such as work days lost).[138] In general, spinal manipulation appears to have some evidence for efficacy; however, studies appear to be quite heterogeneous, which impacts on the strength of evidence.[139]

Massage has been found in one study to be effective in the treatment of tension-type headache,[140] but a systematic review of six studies found no evidence above placebo that manual therapies were effective in tension-type headache.[141] What is evident from this review is that the effectiveness (pragmatic) trial methodology would be more suited to studying manual therapy and headache because of the difficulty of designing a placebo control that cannot be distinguished from the treatment itself.

While **acupuncture** trials report good results, both in treatment[142] and in prophylaxis,[143] the reporting standards of many acupuncture trials in migraine has been questioned.[144] However, a Cochrane review of trials of acupuncture in migraine concluded that it is 'at least as effective as, and possibly more effective than, prophylactic drug treatment, with fewer side effects'.[145] It is certainly useful for naturopaths to consider incorporating acupuncture into the integrative treatment of migraine and neurovascular headache.

Where there are red flag signs and symptoms there is a need to refer to other medical providers. Severe headaches and migraines will often require conventional pain relief and it is important that the naturopathic practitioner works with patients to ensure their condition is managed effectively.

CLINICAL SUMMARY

The first consideration is to determine the causation of the headache and if concerning red flag signs and symptoms are present. Appropriate use of diagnostic techniques is needed in addition to referral when required. Taking an integrative approach, the choice of therapies (nutritional/herbal or structural, or a combination of both) can be tailored to the individual according to type of headache, patient preferences and costs (Figure 17.4). The primary initial goal is always to ameliorate pain and suffering, and while some CAM interventions may be effective, in many instances the use of pharmaceutical analgesics is advised. Regardless, chronic use of these is not recommended, and thus it is a goal of naturopathic medicine to reduce the amount of analgesic medication used by the patient while reducing the occurrence and severity of the headaches.

From the evidence that has been accumulated so far, there is some promise for CAM in headache and migraine. However, this evidence is only just emerging, and it is also important for naturopaths to understand conventional approaches detailed in the biomedical literature and apply this knowledge to naturopathic clinical practice. The potential of CAM in headache and migraine lies in an integrated approach to treatment, targeting both biochemical and structural causation and triggers. While the herbal and nutritional approaches have the potential to beneficially affect vascular and neurotransmitter pathways, there is still need to further investigate the nature of these pathways and investigate the role of individual nutritional factors, as well as nutritional regimens and herbal remedies (individually and in combination) in affecting these pathways.

In summary, naturopathic medicine provides potential in integrated treatment of headache and migraine; however, an integrative approach that utilises appropriate referral, conventional diagnostic techniques and pharmacotherapies to manage pain when needed is highly advised.

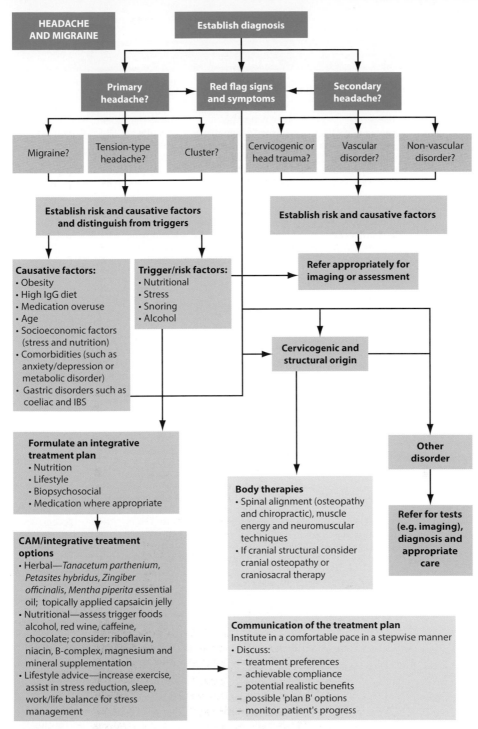

Figure 17.4
Naturopathic treatment decision tree—headache/migraine

Table 17.3
Review of the major evidence

Intervention	Mechanisms of action	Key literature	Summary of results	Comment
Tanacetum parthenium	Inhibits platelet aggregation reducing the release of serotonin (5-HT), which dilates the blood vessels, causing migraines	Pfaffenrath et al. 2002[53]: double-blind RCT	Frequency migraines reduced in a dose- dependent manner (*p* = 0.001)Adverse events similar treatment and placebo[50]	Available evidence suggests that *Tanacetum parthenium* may be effective in migraine prophylaxis; however, better quality trials are still needed
	Nitric oxide and prostaglandin pathway modulation	Some patients were on medication that may have influenced the results (not excluded for practical reasons)	After 60 days with *Tanacetum parthenium* treatment, the average pain intensity declined (*p* < 0.001)	
	Possible effect on central neural sensitisation	Palevitch et al. 1997[6]: double-blind placebo controlled study	Significant reduction in symptoms such as vomiting, nausea, photophobia and noise sensivity[55]	
		Pittler & Ernst 2009[54] meta-analysis and review	A Cochrane review concluded that no conclusive evidence of efficacy could be established; however, there were no safety concerns[54]	
Petasites hybridus	Anti-inflammatory properties through an anti-leukotriene activity or an effect on calcium channels	Lipton et al. 2004[56]: a three-arm, double-blind RCT comparing *Petasites hybridus* extract 75 mg b.i.d. (twice daily) *Petasites hybridus* extract 50 mg b.i.d. or placebo b.i.d. in 245 patients with migraine	Migraine attack frequency reduced by 48% for petasites extract 75 mg bid (*p* = 0.0012 vs placebo)[53]	Care needs to be taken with preparation and dosage due to pyrrolizidine alkaloids; preparations that removed these potentially useful
		Grossman et al. 2005[57]: double-blind study RCT, utilising a CO_2 extract of *Petasites hybridus* with pyrrolizidine alkaloids removed	Frequency reduced 60% (*p* < 0.05); intensity reduced from 4.3 to 2.8 (*p* < 0.05); duration reduced (*p* < 0.05)[57]	No adverse events reported (possibly due to the removal of pyrrolizidine alkaloids)

Table 17.3
Review of the major evidence (continued)

Intervention	Mechanisms of action	Key literature	Summary of results	Comment
Mentha piperita (essential oil)	Antinociceptive effects, with reduction in pericranial muscular tension	Gobel et al. 1994[58]: the effects of peppermint oil and *Eucalyptus* spp. oil preparations on neurophysiological, psychological and experimental algesimetric parameters investigated in 32 healthy subjects in a double-blind RCT (crossover design)	Significant reduction in EMG surface activity of the temporal muscle (by 30.6% ($p < 0.0011$) Reduction pain sensitivity 40.3% ($p < 0.001$)[59]	Topical application of *Mentha piperita* essential oil in acute treatment of headache may be effective; it can, however, aggravate some headaches
Riboflavin (vitamin B2)	Krebs cycle interaction altering mitochondrial enzymes, which affects platelet aggregation[60,61]	Schoenen et al. 1998[60]: a three-month, randomised, placebo-controlled trial, using 400 mg ribflavin daily. Lorenzo et al. 2009[61]: a four-month open trial with riboflavin (400 mg once daily) and 64 migraineurs genotyped blindly for mtDNA haplogroups (tested riboflavin association with different haplogroups)	Riboflavin was superior to placebo in reducing attack frequency ($p = 0.005$) and headache days ($p = 0.012$)[60] Mean frequency of headaches was reduced significantly from baseline to four months from riboflavin treatment ($p < 0.001$)[61]	Riboflavin (along with B vitamin combination) may provide a cheap adjunctive treatment option Dosage may be critical
Magnesium	Reduces neuroexcitability[62] and mitochondrial dysfunction[63]	Mazzotta, et al. 1999[62] utilised electromyographical tests to determine Mg^{++} levels in blood cells in migraineurs, tension-type headaches and healthy controls Samaie et al.[63] tested the relationship between blood levels of Mg^{++} in 50 migraineurs using a case-control comparison to non-migraineurs	EMG ischaemic test positive in 71% of migraineurs compared with 9.5% in tension-type headache[62] Serum total Mg^{++} level was notably lower in the group with these attacks compared with the control group (1.86 ± 0.41 mg/dL versus 2.10 ± 0.23 mg/dL, $p < 0.001$)[63]	Magnesium (along with a mineral complex) has potential usefulness in a migraine treatment regimen

KEY POINTS

- Herbal therapy provides emergent evidence for migraine and headache management.
- Nutritional management of migraine and headache provides common ground between naturopathic treatment strategies and conventional understanding, especially for trigger factors in migraine.
- Migraines and headaches that arise from structural issues respond well to body therapies.

FURTHER READING

Fernandez-de-las-Penas C, Chaitow L, Scoenen J, editors. Multidisciplinary management of migraine. Burlington: Jones and Bartlett Learning; 2013.

Millstine D, Chen CY, Bauer B. Complementary and integrative medicine in the management of headache. BMJ 2017;357:j1805.

Rizzoli P, Mullally WJ. Headache. Am J Med 2018;131(1):17–24.

REFERENCES

1. International Headache Society. IHS Classification ICHD-II: 2013. Online. Available: http://ihs-classification.org/en/02_klassifikation/06_glossar/?letter=h. 15 Jan 2013.
2. Olesen J, Bousser M-G, Diener H-C, et al. The international classification of headache disorders (abbreviated pocket version). Int Headache Soc 2004.
3. NA. IHS Classification ICHD-II. International Headache Society; 2013.
4. Headache MeSH term [Internet]. National Center for Biotechnology Information. 2006 [retrieved 15th February 2013]. Available from: http://www.ncbi.nlm.nih.gov/mesh/68006261.
5. Migraine MeSH term [Internet]. National Center for Biotechnology Information. 2006 [retrieved 15th February 2013]. Available from: http://www.ncbi.nlm.nih.gov/mesh/68008881.
6. Manzoni G, Bonavita V, Bussone G, et al. Chronic migraine classification: current knowledge and future perspectives. J Headache Pain 2011;12(6):585–92.
7. Silberstein SD. Migraine with Aura. In: Michael JA, Robert BD, editors. Encyclopedia of the neurological sciences. New York: Academic Press; 2003. p. 174–9. Editors-in-Chief.
8. Migraine. Cephalalgia 1988;8(7 Suppl.):19–28.
9. Tension-type headache. Cephalalgia 1988;8(7 Suppl.):29–34.
10. Cluster headache and chronic paroxysmal hemicrania. Cephalalgia 1988;8(7 Suppl.):35–8.
11. Cranial neuralgias, nerve trunk pain and deafferentation pain. Cephalalgia 1988;8(7 Suppl.):65–72.
12. Headache associated with metabolic disorder. Cephalalgia 1988;8(7 Suppl.):59–60.
13. Headache or facial pain associated with disorder of cranium, neck, eyes, ears, nose, sinuses, teeth, mouth or other facial or cranial structures. Cephalalgia 1988;8(7 Suppl.):61–4.
14. Headache associated with head trauma. Cephalalgia 1988;8(7 Suppl.):44–5.
15. Headache associated with vascular disorders. Cephalalgia 1988;8(7 Suppl.):46–50.
16. Headache associated with non-vascular intercranial disorder. Cephalalgia 1988;8(7 Suppl.):51–3.
17. Kunkel RS. Clinical manifestations of migraine. Clin Cornerstone 2001;4(3):18–25.
18. Diamond S. Tension-type headache. Clin Cornerstone 1999;1(6):33–44.
19. Haldeman S, Dagenais S. Cervicogenic headaches: a critical review. Spine J 2001;1(1):31–46.
20. Lipton RB, Goadsby P, Silberstein SD. Classification and epidemiology of headache. Clin Cornerstone 1999;1(6):1–10.
21. Adelman JU, Adelman RD. Current options for the prevention and treatment of migraine. Clin Ther 2001;23(6):772–88.
22. Sabatowski R, Schäfer D, Kasper SM, et al. Pain treatment: a historical overview. Curr Pharm Des 2004;10(7):701–16.
23. Trompoukis C, Vadikolias K. The 'Byzantine Classification' of headache disorders. Headache 2007;47(7):1063–8.
24. Magiorkinis E, Diamantis A, Mitsikostas D-D, et al. Headaches in antiquity and during the early scientific era. J Neurol 2009;256(8):1215–20.
25. Koehler P. Prevalence of headache in Tulp's Observationes Medicae (1641) with a Description of Cluster Headache. Cephalalgia 1993;13(5):318–20.
26. López-Muñoz F, Ucha-Udabe R, Alamo1 C. The history of barbiturates a century after their clinical introduction. Neuropsychiatr Dis Treat 2005;1(4):329–43.
27. Gatenbein A, Sandor P, Riederer F, et al. A comprehensive view of migraine pathophysiology. In: Fernandez-de-las-Penas C, Chatow L, Scoenen J, editors. Multidisciplinary management of migraine. Burlington: Jones and Bartlett Learning; 2013. p. 67–79.
28. Goadsby PJ. 6.16—Migraine. In: John BT, David JT, editors. Comprehensive medicinal chemistry II. Oxford: Elsevier; 2007. p. 369–79.
29. Chaitow L. Neuromuscular therapies in treatment of migraine. In: Fernandez-de-las-Penas C, Chaitow L, Scoenen J, editors. Multidisciplinary management of migraine. Burlington: Jones and Bartlett Learning; 2013. p. 205–23.
30. Puentedura E, Louw A, Mintken P, et al. Neurodynamic approach for migraines. In: Fernandez-de-las-Penas C, Chaitow L, Scoenen J, editors. Multidisciplinary management of migraine. Burlington: Jones and Bartlett Learning; 2013. p. 241–54.

31. Evans RW, Bassiur JP, Schwartz AH. Bruxism, temporomandibular dysfunction, tension-type headache, and migraine. Headache 2011;51(7):1169–72.

32. Klinger R, Matter N, Kothe R, et al. Unconditioned and conditioned muscular responses in patients with chronic back pain and chronic tension-type headaches and in healthy controls. Pain 2010;150(1):66–74.

33. Breslau N, Lipton RB, Stewart WF, et al. Comorbidity of migraine and depression: investigating potential etiology and prognosis. Neurology 2008;60(8):1308–12.

34. Antonaci F, Allena M. Acute anti-migraine drugs. In: Fe rnandez-de-las-Penas C, Chaitow L, Scoenen J, editors. Multidisciplinary management of migraine. Burlington: Jones and Bartlett Learning; 2013. p. 83–9.

35. Bigal ME, Lipton RB. Modifiable risk factors for migraine progression. Headache 2006;46(9):1334–43.

36. Kernick D, Stapley S, Hamilton W. GPs' classification of headache: is primary headache underdiagnosed? Br J Gen Pract 2008;58(547):102–4.

37. Matchar DB, Young WB, Rosenberg JH, et al. Evidence-based guidelines for migraine headache in the primary care setting: pharmacological management of acute attacks. Am Acad Neurol 2000;1–58.

38. Bendtsen L, Sacco S, Ashina M, et al. Guideline on the use of onabotulinumtoxinA in chronic migraine: a consensus statement from the European Headache Federation. J Headache Pain 2018;19(1):110. Available from: http://dx.doi.org/10.1186/s10194-018-0921-8.

39. Silberstein S, Latsko M, Schoenen J. Preventive anti-migraine drugs. In: Fernandez-de-las-Penas C, Chaitow L, Scoenen J, editors. Multidisciplinary management of migraine. Burlington: Jones and Bartlett Learning; 2013. p. 91–105.

40. Nicholson RA, Houle TT, Rhudy JL, et al. Psychological risk factors in headache. Headache 2007;47(3):413–26. PubMed PMID: 24350255.

41. Porter-Moffitt S, Gatchel RJ, Robinson RC, et al. Biopsychosocial profiles of different pain diagnostic groups. J Pain 2006;7(5):308–18.

42. Tae-Jin S, Soo-Jin C, Won-Joo K, et al. Poor sleep quality in migraine and probable migraine: a population study. J Headache Pain 2018;19(1):1–8. Available at: http://dx.doi.org/10.1186/s10194-018-0887-6.

43. Walters AB, Hamer JD, Smitherman TA. Sleep disturbance and affective comorbidity among episodic migraineurs. Headache 2014;54(1):116–24. doi:10.1111/head.12168.

44. Boes C, Capobianco D. Chronic migraine and medication-overuse headache through the ages. Cephalalgia 2005;25(5):378–90.

45. Krymchantowski AV, Moreira PF. Out-patient detoxification in chronic migraine: comparison of strategies. Cephalalgia 2003;23(10):982–93. PubMed PMID: 11858999.

46. Rossi P, Lorenzo CD, Faroni J, et al. Advice alone vs. structured detoxification programmes for medication overuse headache: a prospective, randomized, open-label trial in transformed migraine patients with low medical needs. Cephalalgia 2006;26(9):1097–105.

47. Kim J, Suh S-I, Seol H, et al. Regional grey matter changes in patients with migraine: a voxel-based morphometry study. Cephalalgia 2008;28(6):598–604.

48. Schmidt-Wilcke T, Gänßbauer S, Neuner T, et al. Subtle grey matter changes between migraine patients and healthy controls. Cephalalgia 2008;28(1):1–4.

49. Russell MB, Olesen J. Increased familial risk and evidence of genetic factor in migraine. BMJ 1995;311(7004):541–4.

50. Parduz A, Multon S, Malgrange B, et al. Effect of systemic nitroglycerin on CGRP and 5-HT afferents to rat caudal

51. spinal trigeminal nucleus and its modulation by estrogen. Eur J Neurosci 2002;15(11):1803–9.

51. Gupta S, Mehrotra S, Villalón CM, et al. Potential role of female sex hormones in the pathophysiology of migraine. Pharmacol Ther 2007;113(2):321–40.

52. Brandes J. The influence of estrogen on migraine: a systematic review. JAMA 2006;295(15):1824–30.

53. Diener H, Pfaffenrath V, Schnitker J, et al. Efficacy and safety of 6.25 mg t.i.d. feverfew CO2-extract (MIG-99) in migraine prevention—a randomized, double-blind, multicentre, placebo-controlled study. Cephalalgia 2005;25(11):1031–41.

54. Pittler MH, Ernst E. Feverfew for preventing migraine. Cochrane Database Syst Rev 2004;(1):CD002286, 2009 20th February 2013.

55. Palevitch D, Earon G, Carasso R. Feverfew (Tanacetum parthenium) as a prophylactic treatment for migraine: a double-blind placebo-controlled study. Phytother Res 1997;11(7):508–11.

56. Lipton RB, Göbel H, Einhäupl KM, et al. Petasites hybridus root (butterbur) is an effective preventive treatment for migraine. Neurology 2004;63(12):2240–4.

57. Tassorelli C, Greco R, Morazzoni P, et al. Parthenolide is the component of Tanacetum parthenium that inhibits nitroglycerin-induced Fos activation: studies in an animal model of migraine. Cephalalgia 2005;25(8):612–21.

58. Cady RK, Schreiber CP, Beach ME, et al. Gelstat Migraine (sublingually administered feverfew and ginger compound) for acute treatment of migraine when administered during the mild pain phase. Med Sci Monit 2005;11(9).

59. Göbel H, Schmidt G, Soyka D. Effect of peppermint and eucalyptus oil preparations on neurophysiological and experimental algesimetric headache parameters. Cephalalgia 1994;14(3):228–34.

60. Lorenzo CD, Pierelli F, Coppola G, et al. Mitochondrial DNA haplogroups influence the therapeutic response to riboflavin in migraineurs. Neurology 2009;72(18):1588–94.

61. Talebi M, Savadi-Oskouei D, Farhoudi M, et al. Relation between serum magnesium level and migraine attacks. Neurosciences 2011;16(4):320–3.

62. Mauskop A, Varughese J. Why all migraine patients should be treated with magnesium. J Neural Transm 2012;119(5):575–9.

63. Welch KMA, Ramadan NM. Mitochondria, magnesium and migraine. J Neurol Sci 1995;134(1–2):9–14.

64. Jensen R, Hindberg I. Plasma serotonin increase during episodes of tension-type headache. Cephalalgia 1994;14(3):219–22.

65. Aviram A, Tsoukias NM, Melnick SJ, et al. Inhibition of nitric oxide synthesis in mouse macrophage cells by feverfew supercritical extract. Phytother Res 2012;26(4):541–5.

66. Tommaso Md, Capuano A, Valeriani M. Peripheral and central sensitization mechanisms in migraine. In: Fern andez-de-las-Penas C, Chaitow L, Scoenen J, editors. Multidisciplinary management of migraine. Burlington: Jones and Bartlett Learning; 2013. p. 47–56.

67. Myers DE. Potential neurogenic and vascular roles of nitric oxide in migraine headache and aura. Headache 1999;39(2):118–24.

68. Charles A. The evolution of a migraine attack—a review of recent evidence. Headache 2013;53(2):413–19.

69. Collier HOJ, Butt NM, McDonald-Gibson WJ, et al. Extract of feverfew inhibits prostaglandin biosynthesis. Lancet 1980;316(8200):922–3.

70. Caudle RM, King C, Nolan TA, et al. Central sensitization in the trigeminal nucleus caudalis produced by a conjugate

of substance P and the A subunit of cholera toxin. J Pain 2010;11(9):838–46.

71. Cady RK, Goldstein J, Nett R, et al. A double-blind placebo-controlled pilot study of sublingual feverfew and ginger (LipiGesicTMM) in the treatment of migraine. Headache 2011;51(7):1078–86. PubMed PMID: 62960666.

72. Bode AM, Dong Z. The amazing and mighty ginger. In: Benzie I, Wachtel GS, editors. Herbal medicine: biomolecular and clinical aspects. 2nd ed. Boca Raton: CRC Press; 2011. p. 131–56.

73. Chayasirisobhon S. Use of a pine bark extract and antioxidant vitamin combination product as therapy for migraine in patients refractory to pharmacologic medication. Headache 2006;46(5):788–93.

74. Snyder R. Find migraine relief with butterbur. Nat Health 2003;33(1):32. PubMed PMID: 9006099.

75. Grossmann W, Schmidramsl H. An extract of Petasites hybridus is effective in the prophylaxis of migraine. Altern Med Rev 2001;6(3):303.

76. Brandes JL, Visser WH, Farmer MV, et al. Montelukast for migraine prophylaxis: a randomized, double-blind, placebo-controlled study. Headache 2004;44(6):581–6.

77. Wang G-J, Shum AY-C, Lin Y-L, et al. Calcium channel blockade in vascular smooth muscle cells: major hypotensive mechanism of S-Petasin, a hypotensive sesquiterpene from Petasites formosanus. J Pharmacol Exp Ther 2001;297(1):240–6.

78. Rogers KL, Grice ID, Griffiths LR. Inhibition of platelet aggregation and 5-HT release by extracts of Australian plants used traditionally as headache treatments. Eur J Pharm Sci 2000;9(4):355–63.

79. Atta AH, Alkofahi A. Anti-nociceptive and anti-inflammatory effects of some Jordanian medicinal plant extracts. J Ethnopharmacol 1998;60(2):117–24.

80. Galeotti N, Ghelardini C, Di Cesare Mannelli L, et al. Local anaesthetic activity of (+)-and (-)-menthol. Planta Med 2001;67(2):174–6.

81. McKay DL, Blumberg JB. A review of the bioactivity and potential health benefits of peppermint tea (Mentha piperita L.). Phytother Res 2006;20(8):619–33.

82. Ward N, Whitney C, Avery D, et al. The analgesic effects of caffeine in headache. Pain 1991;44(2):151–5.

83. Downing D. Dietary approaches. In: Fernandez-de-las-Pe nas C, Chaitow L, Scoenen J, editors. Multidisciplinary management of migraine. Burlington: Jones and Bartlett Learning; 2013. p. 413–17.

84. Couturier E, Laman D, van Duijn M, et al. Influence of caffeine and caffeine withdrawal on headache and cerebral blood flow velocities. Cephalalgia 1997;17(3):188–90.

85. Scher AI, Stewart WF, Lipton RB. Caffeine as a risk factor for chronic daily headache: a population-based study. Neurology 2004;63(11):2022–7.

86. Patel RM, Sarma R, Grimsley E. Popular sweetner Sucralose as a migraine trigger. Headache 2006;46(8):1303–4.

87. Bigal ME, Krymchantowski AV. Migraine triggered by sucralose—a case report. Headache 2006;46(3):515–17.

88. D'Andrea G, Bussone G, Allais G, et al. Efficacy of Ginkgolide B in the prophylaxis of migraine with aura. Neurol Sci 2009;30(1):121–4. doi:10.1007/s10072-009-0074-2.

89. Cianchetti C. Capsaicin jelly against migraine pain. Int J Clin Pract 2010;64(4):457–9. doi:10.1111/j.1742-1241.2009.02294.x.

90. Panconesi A. Alcohol and migraine: trigger factor, consumption, mechanisms. A review. J Headache Pain 2008;9(1):19–27.

91. Jarman J, Pattichis K, Peatfield R, et al. Red wine-induced release of [14C]5-hydroxytryptamine from platelets of migraine patients and controls. Cephalalgia 1996;16(1):41–3. PubMed PMID: 6408631.

92. Sandler M, Li N-Y, Jarrett N, et al. Dietary migraine: recent progress in the red (and white) wine story. Cephalalgia 1995;15(2):101–3.

93. Millichap JG, Yee MM. The diet factor in pediatric and adolescent migraine. Pediatr Neurol 2003;28(1):9–15.

94. Eagle K. Toxicological effects of red wine, orange juice, and other dietary SULT1A inhibitors via excess catecholamines. Food Chem Toxicol 2012;50(6):2243–9.

95. Gabrielli M, Cremonini F, Fiore G, et al. Association between migraine and celiac disease: results from a preliminary case-control and therapeutic study. Am J Gastroenterol 2003;98(3):625–9.

96. Aydinlar EI, Dikmen PY, Tiftikci A, et al. IgG-based elimination diet in migraine plus irritable bowel syndrome. Headache 2013;53(3):514–25.

97. Peterlin BL, Rosso AL, Rapoport AM, et al. Obesity and migraine: the effect of age, gender and adipose tissue distribution. Headache 2010;50(1):52–62.

98. Bengmark S. Nutritional modulation of acute- and 'chronic'-phase responses. Nutrition 2001;17(6):489–95.

99. Sangiorgi S, Mochi M, Riva R, et al. Abnormal platelet mitochondrial function in patients affected by migraine with and without aura. Cephalalgia 1994;14(1):21–3.

100. Schoenen J, Jacquy J, Lenaerts M. Effectiveness of high-dose riboflavin in migraine prophylaxis: a randomized controlled trial. Neurology 1998;50(2):466–70.

101. Bruijn J, Duivenvoorden H, Passchier J, et al. Medium-dose riboflavin as a prophylactic agent in children with migraine: a preliminary placebo-controlled, randomised, double-blind, cross-over trial. Cephalalgia 2010;30(12):1426–34.

102. O'Brien HL, Hershey AD. Vitamins and paediatric migraine: riboflavin as a preventative medication. Cephalalgia 2010;30(12):1417–18.

103. Gallai V, Sarchielli P, Morucci P, et al. Red blood cell magnesium levels in migraine patients. Cephalalgia 1993;13(2):94–8.

104. Samaie A, Asghari N, Ghorbani R, et al. Blood magnesium levels in migraineurs within and between the headache attacks: a case control study. Pan Afr Med J 2012;11:46.

105. Mazzotta G, Sarchielli P, Alberti A, et al. Intracellular Mg++ concentration and electromyographical ischemic test in juvenile headache. Cephalalgia 1999;19(9):802–9.

106. Mauskop A, Sun-Edelstein C. Role of magnesium in the pathogenesis and treatment of migraine. Expert Rev Neurother 2009;9(3):369–79.

107. Bigal M, Bordini C, Tepper S, et al. Intravenous magnesium sulphate in the acute treatment of migraine without aura and migraine with aura. A randomized, double-blind, placebo-controlled study. Cephalalgia 2002;22(5):345–53.

108. Velling DA, Dodick DW, Muir JJ. Sustained-release niacin for prevention of migraine headache. Mayo Clin Proc 2003;78(6):770–1.

109. Prousky J, Millman CG, Kirkland JB. Pharmacologic use of niacin. J Evid Based Complementary Altern Med 2011;16(2):91–101.

110. Sándor PS, Clemente LD, Coppola G, et al. Efficacy of coenzyme Q10 in migraine prophylaxis: a randomized controlled trial. Neurology 2005;64(4):713–15.

111. Kapusta-Duch J, Leszczyńska T, Florkiewicz A, et al. Comparison of calcium and magnesium contents in cruciferous vegetables grown in areas around steelworks, on

organic farms, and those available in retail. Ecol Food Nutr 2011;50(2):155–67.

112. Office of Dietary Supplements—National Institutes of Health. Dietary Supplement Fact Sheets Bethesda; 2013 [10th March 2013]. Available from: http://ods.od.nih.gov/.

113. Milde-Busch A, Blaschek A, Borggräfe I, et al. Associations of diet and lifestyle with headache in high-school students: results from a cross-sectional study. Headache 2010;50(7):1104–14.

114. Andrasik F. Behavioral management of migraine. Biomed Pharmacother 1996;50(2):52–7.

115. Bussone G, Grazzi L, D'Amico D, et al. Biofeedback-assisted relaxation training for young adolescents with tension-type headache: a controlled study. Cephalalgia 1998;18(7):463–7. PubMed PMID: 4997357.

116. Boardman HF, Thomas E, Millson DS, et al. Psychological, sleep, lifestyle, and comorbid associations with headache. Headache 2005;45(6):657–69.

117. Koehler PJ, Boes CJ. A history of non-drug treatment in headache, particularly migraine. Brain 2010;133(8):2489–500.

118. Wardle J. Hydrotherapy: a forgotten Australian therapeutic modality. Aust J Herbal Med 2013;25(1):12.

119. Ulbricht C. Peripheral vascular disease: an integrative approach: a natural standard monograph. Altern Complement Ther 2012;18(1):44–50.

120. Jerabek J, Bordon A, Pineda RM. Complex balneo-physiatric treatment in fibromyalgia: a pilot study. Int J Aesthet Antiaging Med 2008;1(1):2. PubMed PMID: 44413550.

121. Goadsby PJ. Migraine pathophysiology. Headache 2005;45:S14–24.

122. Bogduk N. The neck and headaches. Neurol Clin 2004;22(1):151–71.

123. Alix ME, Bates DK. A proposed etiology of cervicogenic headache: the neurophysiologic basis and anatomic relationship between the dura mater and the rectus posterior capitis minor muscle. J Manipulative Physiol Ther 1999;22(8):534–9.

124. Ferguson AJ, Upledger JE, McPartland JM, et al. Cranial osteopathy and craniosacral therapy: current opinions. J Bodyw Mov Ther 1998;2(1):28–37.

125. Gard G. An investigation into the regulation of intra-cranial pressure and its influence upon the surrounding cranial bones. J Bodyw Mov Ther 2009;13(3):246–54.

126. Meyer JS, Nance M, Walker M, et al. Migraine and cluster headache treatment with calcium antagonists supports a vascular pathogenesis. Headache 1985;25(7):358–67.

127. Sicuteri F, Fusco BM, Marabini S, et al. Beneficial effect of capsaicin application to the nasal mucosa in cluster headache. Clin J Pain 1989;5(1):49–54.

128. Marks DR, Rapoport A, Padla D, et al. A double-blind placebo-controlled trial of intranasal capsaicin for cluster headache. Cephalalgia 1993;13(2):114–16.

129. Fusco BM, Marabini S, Maggi CA, et al. Preventative effect of repeated nasal applications of capsaicin in cluster headache. Pain 1994;59(3):321–5.

130. Anderson RE, Seniscal C. A comparison of selected osteopathic treatment and relaxation for tension-type

headaches. Headache 2006;46(8):1273–80. PubMed PMID: 22019388.

131. Haldeman S, Dagenais S. Choosing a treatment for cervicogenic headache: when? what? how much? Spine J 2010;10(2):169–71.

132. McDermaid CS, Hagino C, Vernon H. Systematic review of randomized clinical trials of complementary/alternative therapies in the treatment of tension-type and cervicogenic headache. Complement Ther Med 1999;7(3):142–55.

133. Rana MV. Managing and treating headache of cervicogenic origin. Med Clin North Am 2013;97(2):267–80.

134. Fernandez-de-las-Penas C, Gonzalez-Iglesias J, Piekartz HV, et al. Manual therapy in the cranial region. In: Fernandez-de-las-Penas C, Chaitow L, Scoenen J, editors. Multidisciplinary management of migraine. Burlington: Jones and Bartlett Learning; 2013. p. 255–75.

135. Arnadottir TS, Sigurdardottir AK. Is craniosacral therapy effective for migraine? Tested with HIT-6 Questionnaire. Complement Ther Clin Pract 2013;19(1):11–14.

136. Curtis P, Gaylord SA, Park J, et al. Credibility of low-strength static magnet therapy as an attention control intervention for a randomized controlled study of craniosacral therapy for migraine headaches. J Altern Complement Med 2011;17(8):711–21. PubMed PMID: 63168718.

137. Mann J, Faurot K, Wilkinson L, et al. Craniosacral therapy for migraine: protocol development for an exploratory controlled clinical trial. BMC Complement Altern Med 2008;8(1):28. doi:10.1186/1472-6882-8-28. PubMed PMID.

138. Voigt K, Liebnitzky J, Burmeister U, et al. Efficacy of osteopathic manipulative treatment of female patients with migraine: results of a randomized controlled trial. J Altern Complement Med 2011;17(3):225–30.

139. Bronfort G, Assendelft WJJ, Evans R, et al. Efficacy of spinal manipulation for chronic headache: a systematic review. J Manipulative Physiol Ther 2001;24(7):457–66.

140. Tsao JCI. Effectiveness of massage therapy for chronic, non-malignant pain: a review. Evid Based Complement Alternat Med 2007;4(2):165–79.

141. Fernández-de-las-Peñas C, Alonso-Blanco C, Cuadrado ML, et al. Manual therapies in the management of tension-type headache. Headache 2005;45(2):169–71.

142. Yang C-P, Chang M-H, Liu P-E, et al. Acupuncture versus topiramate in chronic migraine prophylaxis: a randomized clinical trial. Cephalalgia 2011;31(15):1510–21.

143. Wallasch T-M, Weinschuetz T, Mueller B, et al. Cerebrovascular response in migraineurs during prophylactic treatment with acupuncture: a randomized controlled trial. J Altern Complement Med 2012;18(8):777–83.

144. Claraco AE, Hanna SE, Fargas-Babjak A. Reporting of clinical details in randomized controlled trials of acupuncture for the treatment of migraine/headaches and nausea/vomiting. J Altern Complement Med 2003;9(1):151–9.

145. Acupuncture for migraine prophylaxis [Internet]. John Wiley & Sons, Ltd. 2009 [retrieved 20th February 2013]. Available from: http://onlinelibrary.wiley.com/doi/10.1002/14651858.CD001218.pub2/abstract.

CHAPTER 18

Stress and fatigue

Tini Gruner
ND, MSc, PhD

Jerome Sarris
ND, MHSc, PhD

OVERVIEW

Stress

The nexus between stress and fatigue often occurs along a continuum, with neuroendocrine dysregulation being an underlying element. Hans Selye, in 1935, was the first to develop a theory of stress. When he imposed different types of physical stressors on rats he discovered that, regardless of the kind of stressor, the same physiological response was the result: hypertrophied adrenal glands, atrophied lymphatic organs (lymph nodes, spleen and thymus) and bleeding gastric ulcers. These symptoms developed over time. He called this the 'general adaptation syndrome' (GAS), stating 'stress is the nonspecific response of the body to any demand made upon it'.[1] This requires adjustment or adaptation to a new situation.

From his observations he hypothesised three stages: alarm, resistance and exhaustion. The alarm stage was characterised by hormonal changes such as increased sympathetic nervous system (SNS) activity, with its typical fight or flight response and noradrenaline secretions, and up-regulated cortisol. In the resistance stage the body had adapted to the stressor, the above symptoms had disappeared and body metabolism had returned to normal. In the exhaustion stage the stress triad of hypertrophied adrenals, atrophied lymph organs and gastric ulcers were noticed, together with an initial increase in cortisol, which later declined to below normal. Only in this stage, with severe stress over prolonged periods of time, did the body lose its ability to cope and eventually death ensued. However, in general the physiological changes mentioned above were thought of as being protective to ensure the animal's survival.[1,2] Therefore, stress is actually a positive occurrence needed for protection (readiness for action when in danger, increased immune particles when injured). It becomes pathological only if it is protracted or uncontrolled.[3–5]

Physiologically, a stressor causes disruptions in homoeostasis, leading to neural and endocrine changes known as the 'stress response' or 'stress cascade' (Figure 18.1).[6,7] Mental and emotional stressors stimulate the hypothalamus via the limbic system (the hippocampus and amygdala),[6–8] whereas physical and physiological processes, such as injury or hypoglycaemia, can stimulate the hypothalamus directly.

The first (and immediate) reaction to a stressor is caused by imbalances in the central nervous system (CNS) through overstimulation of the SNS and suppression of the parasympathetic nervous system (PNS). The SNS stimulates the adrenal medulla to secrete

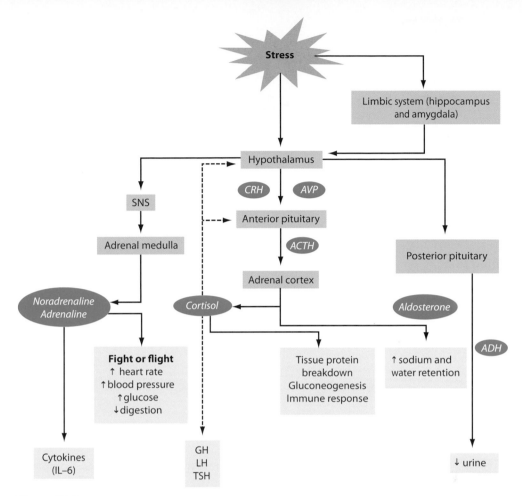

Figure 18.1
The stress cascade

Solid arrows indicate stimulation and dotted arrows indicate inhibition.
ACTH = adrenocorticotrophic system; ADH = antidiuretic hormone; AVP = arginine vasopression; CRH = corticotrophin-releasing hormone; SNS = sympathetic nervous system

the catecholamines noradrenaline and adrenaline. They are produced from phenylalanine and hence tyrosine (Figure 18.2). These hormones lead to heightened alertness to quickly judge a situation regarding its potential danger. Blood pressure, breathing and heart rate are accelerated for fight or flight, for which glycogenolysis (release of glycogen from the liver) provides the extra fuel. Endorphins are released to dampen pain from a potential injury. Digestion, relaxation and sleep are suppressed, and the body is prepared for swift action needed for survival.[3,6,9,10]

Stimulation of the anterior pituitary gland is achieved through secreting corticotrophin-releasing hormone (CRH), and to a lesser extent arginine vasopressin (AVP), which leads to the release of adrenocorticotrophic hormone (ACTH). ACTH triggers the release of vast amounts of cortisol glucocorticoid and moderate amounts of aldosterone, a mineralocorticoid, from the adrenal cortex. Both these hormones are made (a mineralocorticoid) from cholesterol (Figure 18.3).

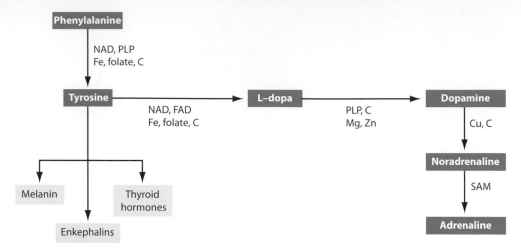

Figure 18.2
Catecholamine production

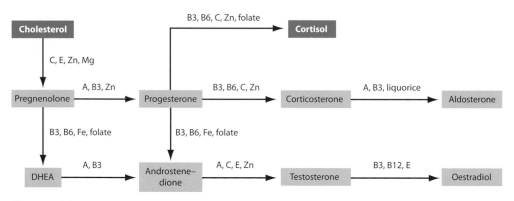

Figure 18.3
Steroid hormone production with nutrient cofactors

Under normal circumstances cortisol levels are highest in the morning and lowest in the evening. Its physiological actions control carbohydrate, protein and fat metabolism, and it inhibits prostaglandin synthesis and contributes to emotional stability. In stress, however, cortisol levels in blood are elevated, triggering an increase in protein breakdown and mobilisation of fatty acids (gluconeogenesis) in order to provide glucose for the fight or flight response. This results in a hyperglycaemic state in the liver with peripheral hypoglycaemia, temporarily leading to moderate insulin resistance. High cortisol also decreases lymphocyte and eosinophil counts, effectively dampening any inflammation or immune response.[2,6,7] Moreover, elevated glucocorticoids influence reproduction, growth and thyroid functions by inhibiting gonadotrophin-releasing hormone (GnRH) and luteinising hormone (LH), growth hormone (GH) and thyroid-stimulating hormone (TSH), respectively.[6] As a result, these functions are suppressed because the body deems them to be of minor importance in the face of an acute stressor.[6,11–14]

Cortisol, adrenaline and glucagon all have the ability to raise blood glucose levels. Due to their hyperglycaemic action they have a catabolic effect on the body. Cortisol is involved in replenishing depleted energy stores, and it converts food into glycogen and fat, and initiates hunger. Adrenaline increases mental alertness, blood pressure, breathing and heart rate, muscle tone, glycogenolysis and the release of endorphins. Simultaneously, it down-regulates appetite, digestion, elimination, relaxation and sleep.[3] Glucagon opposes insulin by mediating the release of glucose from storage.

The second hormone released by the adrenal cortex—aldosterone—retains sodium and water in the body. In addition, stimulation of the posterior pituitary gland by the hypothalamus results in antidiuretic hormone (ADH) secretion. The combined result of these actions is fluid retention and increased blood volume, which can lead to increased blood pressure.[2]

The secretion and interplay of the stress hormones will vary, depending on the type, intensity and duration of the stressor as well as its hormonal regulation.[15,16] High amounts of circulating cortisol will, via negative feedback loops, shut off the release of hormones from the hypothalamus and anterior pituitary glands. Therefore, once the acute stressor has subsided, the stress cascade abates and the physiology of the organism returns to normal. The individual becomes more resilient as a result of successful adaptation to a new situation in which wear and tear are minimised.[17] This memory is stored in the hippocampus and readily accessible when a similar stressful situation arises, so the learning from the first event can guide the (re)actions when it recurs. The role of the amygdala is to retain the emotional impact of the stressor and, together with the hippocampus, will ensure a better memory of an emotionally charged event. Both cortisol and adrenaline are needed for this memory to happen.[3] Thus mind and body can both be strengthened from a stressful experience, becoming more resilient to future stressors.

Distress

If, however, stress is chronic or intense and exceeds the person's mental and physical resources, it becomes 'distress'. Prolonged stress can cause generalised fatigue (referred to sometimes as 'adrenal exhaustion' in naturopathy), which corresponds to the final stage of Selye's GAS. The circulating hormones will not return to their normal levels and initially stay in a state of hyperarousal.[6,8] As a result, CRH, AVP and ACTH are no longer inhibited via negative feedback (leading to dysregulation of the hypothalamus–pituitary–adrenal (HPA) axis), target organs become overstimulated, receptors possibly become desensitised and tissue damage ensues.[4] This 'wear and tear' or 'cost' of adaptation or allostasis has been termed 'allostatic load'. It is implicated in numerous disease processes[4,18–20] and has been associated with an energy-deficiency state of the body.[14] It is mediated by adrenaline and cortisol. Both hormones actually serve to imprint the stressful event into long-term memory, but prolonged action will cause damage to the part of the brain that should shut them off. This in turn leads to higher levels of these hormones circulating in the blood ('cortisol resistance'), which can do more damage to the brain, especially the hippocampus. High levels of cortisol have been linked to the conditions outlined in Table 18.1. Agitation and anxiety can also be caused by glutamatergic activation. Note that the precursor for both the inhibitory and the excitatory pathways is the same amino acid: glutamine (Figure 18.4). If zinc or vitamin B6 are in short supply then adequate amounts of gamma-aminobutyric acid (GABA), the inhibitory neurotransmitter, cannot be formed. Instead, glutamate, the excitatory neurotransmitter, accumulates, leading to the above-mentioned symptoms.[21]

Fatigue

After prolonged exposure to stress there is a blunted response before cortisol levels will decline or the diurnal rhythm will flatten.[20] With lowered cortisol levels, endogenous

Table 18.1
Chronic diseases caused by high cortisol[3]

Hormonal dysregulation	Disorder
General effects	Addictions, alcoholism and obsessive-compulsive disorders[22–24] Anorexia nervosa[25] Cushing's syndrome[7]
Lowered serotonin levels	Anxiety, panic disorder and melancholic depression[5,6,26–28]
High cytokines leading to oxidative stress	Neurological diseases[28–30] Overtraining syndrome in athletes[31]
Suppression of immune function	Infections[32,33]
↑ bone demineralisation	Reduction in bone mass and osteoporosis[6,28]
↑ storage of fat around abdomen → ↑ gluconeogenesis from protein (loss of muscle mass) to meet energy demands → ↑ insulin → ↑ cortisol → ↑ eating energy-dense foods → ↑ storage of fat	Visceral adiposity, insulin resistance and loss of glycaemic control[6,8,28,34,35] Metabolic syndrome[36,37]
Shrivelling of dendrites → destruction of neurons → ↓ neurogenesis → cerebral ischaemia → ↓ hippocampus size	Depression, impaired memory and loss of cognitive function, acceleration of ageing[29]
Impaired conversion of thyroxine (T_4) to triiodothyronine (T_3)	Thyroid dysfunction[6]
Dysregulation of reproductive hormones[38]	Hormonal disturbances[6,13]

Urban environment and stress

Evidence has revealed that people who grow up or spend more time in industrialised environments such as cities have higher levels of perceived stress than their country-dwelling counterparts. A key neuroimaging study showed that hyper-reactivity of the amygdala (region of the brain responsible for the fight-or-flight reaction and storing stressful memories) is correlated to the degree of urbanisation in stress-provoked individuals.

Source: Lederbogen et al. 2011[43]

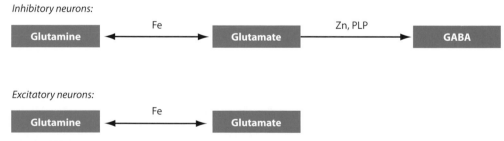

Inhibitory neurons:

Glutamine ⟷ (Fe) Glutamate → (Zn, PLP) GABA

Excitatory neurons:

Glutamine ⟷ (Fe) Glutamate

Figure 18.4
Production of GABA

glucose production is compromised, and sugar and stimulant cravings are likely as a consequence of the resultant hypoglycaemia. If untreated, this can lead to 'adrenal burnout' and subsequent chronic fatigue.[35] The results of low cortisol are shown in Table 18.2.

Table 18.2
Chronic diseases caused by low cortisol (insufficient HPA response to stress)[3]

Hormonal dysregulation	Disorder
General	Addison's disease[7] Hypopituitarism[39] Hypothyroidism[6]
Unresponsive HPA, low (exhausted) cortisol levels and blunted response to exercise, disturbances in serotonergic neurotransmission and AVP	Chronic fatigue syndrome, fibromyalgia[27,35,40] Atypical (flat) depression[27] Inflammatory conditions[41]
Burnout → loss of regulation in limbic system → brain damage and atrophy	Poor mental performance[20,42] Non-melancholic depression[3]
Depleted adrenaline/hypoarousal of the HPA	Non-melancholic depression[3]

The flow-on effect of these disturbances in neurotransmitters and stress hormones can also lead to exhausted serotonin levels, potentially resulting in anxiety and sleep disturbances. The precursor of serotonin is tryptophan (Figure 18.5). The established link between carbohydrate cravings and depression is thought to be due to its tryptophan-increasing properties,[44,45] with mood-elevating results.[46]

Testing for adrenal hormone abnormalities

Chronic stress and may cause significant demands on the neuroendocrine system and this may in turn cause fatigue. It is therefore important to assess for potential HPA axis dysregulation before treatment is instigated.[47] The tests in Table 18.3 have been shown to be useful in diagnosing HPA axis dysregulation. The information revealed in these tests will indicate not only the level of cortisol excess or depletion (and potentially which GAS phase the patient is in) but also any concomitant health conditions that may have developed as a result of stress, such as insulin resistance, hypopituitarism and inflammation.

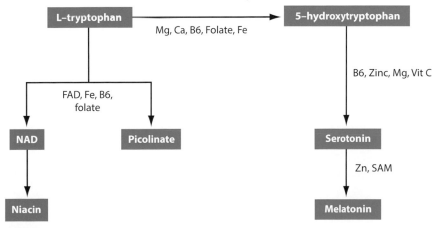

Figure 18.5
Production of serotonin

NAD = nicotanimide adenine dinucleotide; Fe = Iron; Ca = Calcium; Mg = Magnesium; Zn = Zinc; FAD = Flavin adenine dinucleotide; SAM = S-adenosyl methionine

Table 18.3
Pathology tests for evaluating stress markers

Test	Tissue	Comments
Cortisol	Serum	Cortisol is diurnal—it is highest in the morning at 6–8 am and drops throughout the day, with lowest levels occurring around midnight Therefore, tests should be performed at around 8 am, at 4 pm and then again later in the evening prior to bedtime with the morning readings close to the maximum and the afternoon values closer to the lower end of the reference range
	Urine	24-hour readings indicate whether adequate amounts of cortisol have been produced overall
	Saliva	Several readings can be taken throughout the day to determine the diurnal variation
ACTH	Serum	ACTH needs to be present to stimulate cortisol release and is therefore following the same diurnal variation as cortisol If both cortisol and ACTH are low, an ACTH stimulation test should be performed to determine whether cortisol is low because of lack of ACTH
ACTH stimulation	Serum	A synthetic form of ACTH (cosyntropin) is injected after taking a blood sample for baseline cortisol measurements Blood samples are taken in half-hourly intervals for the following one to two hours If cortisol is still low, adrenal exhaustion or Addison's disease (primary hypoadrenalism) is the likely cause If cortisol levels are within the normal range, then the problem lies with inadequate ACTH secretion (hypopituitarism or secondary hypoadrenalism)
GTT (glucose tolerance test)	Serum	A three-hour glucose tolerance test can be performed, with half-hourly measurements of glucose, insulin and cortisol If hypoglycaemia is present, then cortisol levels should increase to activate glucose release from glycogen stores Both the hypoglycaemia and low cortisol in response are indicative of adrenal exhaustion
ITT (insulin tolerance test)	Serum	This test is usually used for identifying patients with GH deficiency, but it has also been used to determine HPA status[48] Hypoglycaemia is induced by the intravenous infusion of insulin and/or arginine Blood samples for growth hormone, glucose and cortisol are taken at regular intervals for 90 minutes However, this test is contraindicated in cases of low basal plasma cortisol
Inflammatory markers	Serum	Erythrocyte sedimentation rate (ESR), C-reactive protein (CRP), homocysteine and antibodies should all be tested, as low cortisol reduces the ability of the body to control inflammatory processes
Electrolytes	Serum	Altered aldosterone levels due to mineralocorticoid insufficiency (as part of glucocorticoid insufficiency) can lead to imbalances in electrolytes, notably sodium
Aldosterone	Blood and urine	Aldosterone can be altered due to adrenal pathology However, this test is mainly used to diagnose hyperaldosteronism and may not be relevant in this scenario
Lipid studies	Serum	Cortisol is made in the body from cholesterol Further, in an insulin-resistant state it is likely that triglycerides and possibly low-density lipoprotein (LDL) are elevated, with insufficient amounts of high-density lipoprotein (HDL)
Viruses	Serum	To rule out any viral causes of fatigue

Source: Pagana & Pagana 2006[49]

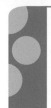

DIFFERENTIAL DIAGNOSIS*

- A general symptom from many medical conditions
- Addison's disease
- Cushing's syndrome
- Psychiatric disorders

- Chronic fatigue syndrome
- Insomnia
- Cancer
- Medication side effects

*From the clinical presentation of stress or fatigue

Source: Crowley 2004[50]

RISK FACTORS

As discussed earlier, chronic stress may manifest fatigue and the consequences of both may have a range of health consequences. An increase in stress (and resultant fatigue) may occur due to a range of external and internal factors, with obvious stressors being tensions from a person's relationships, employment, financial state, health status and their environment. The use of stimulants such as coffee increases the stress response and adrenal output, as shown by elevated catecholamines, notably adrenaline, in urine.[51,52] If coffee is used as a 'pick-me-up' without having an effect, leading to increasingly greater consumption, adrenaline production may potentially be exhausted. This kind of stimulation may therefore hasten the decline in adrenal function, thus being a stressor in its own right. Perceived unmanageable stress can be the result of multiple stressors, each of them not being enough to cause HPA dysfunction; however, the additive effects (if not addressed) can weaken the system to such an extent that other health problems could arise, such as chronic fatigue, clinical depression, hypothyroidism, hormonal disturbances and inflammatory and autoimmune conditions (outlined in Table 18.2).

CONVENTIONAL TREATMENT

'Stress' or 'fatigue' is not considered to be a diagnosis per se in conventional medicine, and are considered to be symptoms of a specific medical condition, or a transitory state due to factors such as a lack of sleep or food, or a stress-provoking event. Primary hypoadrenalism (Addison's disease) is rare. If it is part of an autoimmune endocrine disease,[53] where adrenal function has been maintained through endogenous up-regulation of corticotrophic hormone stimulation, treatment may not be required. If secondary hypoadrenalism has been diagnosed, glucocorticoids are the drugs of choice,[54,55] with mineralocorticoids if needed.[56] Didehydroepiandrosterone (DHEA) has been trialled, with mixed results.[56,57] Apart from the removal of the adrenals (as may occur in Cushing's syndrome), hypoadrenalism is mainly recognised in the medical literature as being the result of brain injury,[58] tumours, endocrine disorders or critical illness.[59,60] Conventionally, to reduce stress/anxiety, medications such as antidepressants,[61–63] beta-blockers[64,65] and anti-glutamatergic agents may be prescribed.[62] Other novel treatments include glucocorticoid receptor antagonists and atrial natriuretic peptide receptor agonists.[64] Psychostimulants such as dexamphetamine or modafinil may be prescribed in cases of chronic fatigue.[66]

KEY TREATMENT PROTOCOLS

When a patient has the clinical presentation of stress and/or fatigue (not occurring from a diagnosed medical condition), the primary protocol is to establish which GAS phase the patient is in (alarm, adaptation, exhaustion). For patients with acute stress, then adrenaline and/or cortisol is usually high. They may complain of anxiety, sleep issues and a range of somatic symptoms reflective of SNS up-regulation. In cases of chronic stress leading to fatigue, hormones such as cortisol and adrenaline are generally low, resulting in a blunted stress response and physical and mental exhaustion. There is energy depletion on a cellular level, coupled with lack of neuro-transmitter precursors and/or cofactors.

The general aim of treatment is to assist in enhancing the functioning of the neuro-endocrine system, thus increasing the energy and wellbeing in the patient. Since the HPA axis is stimulated by mental and emotional as well as physical events, giving the patient resources requires not only support with nutrients, but also teaching better coping strategies.[47] Aside from addressing nutrient deficiencies and prescribing nutraceuticals that modulate the neuroendocrine system (covered below), it is vital to consider an integrative approach to addressing stress. See

> ### Naturopathic Treatment Aims
>
> - Address external factors contributing to stress
>   - consider social stressors and stress management/psychosocial techniques.
> - Modify lifestyle
>   - work, rest, sleep, play balance.
> - Enhance physical and emotional stamina and perceived wellbeing
>   - graded exercise, nutrition, psychological techniques, relaxation/meditative techniques.
> - Resource the body and mind to be able to deal with stressors
>   - low glycaemic load diet
>   - modify stimulant use
>   - nutritional supplements to replenish metabolic pathways (cortisol and neurotransmitter synthesis)
>   - plant-based adaptogens.

the anxiety, depression and insomnia chapters for further discussion on: lifestyle considerations such as meditation, yoga and breathing techniques; sleep hygiene; exposure to fresh air and 'greenspace'; and use of traditional techniques such as balneotherapy. See Table 18.4 for an evidence summary on integrative intervention for general stress and fatigue.

Regulation of the HPA axis to reduce stress and fatigue

The HPA axis activates and is inactivated by cortisol (Figure 18.1).[74] In the case of low cortisol, the negative feedback is impaired, leading to dysregulation of other stress hormones. Diet, lifestyle and thought patterns have a key influence on the HPA axis. Adjusting these aspects are the primary concerns as they will need to be the first line of defence for future stressors. Certain herbal medicines have been used traditionally to modulate the nervous system and the stress response. They may have potential roles in the three phases of the stress-fatigue nexus (see Figure 18.6 herbal interventions in GAS scale). One of the most important herbal medicines modulating cortisol is **_Glycyrrhiza glabra_**. The constituents from _Glycyrrhiza glabra_, specifically its active constituent glycyrrhetinic acid, is a potent inhibitor of 11 beta-hydroxysteroid dehydrogenase (which converts active cortisol to inactive cortisone),[75,76] thus increasing the amount of circulating cortisol.[77–79] It is therefore ideally suited to cases of low cortisol, such as in the 'exhaustion' phase, although contraindicated in the 'alarm' or 'adaptation' phases. Care needs to be taken as _Glycyrrhiza glabra_ can lead to pseudoaldosteronism by binding to mineralocorticoid receptors, therefore promoting sodium and fluid retention as well as potassium loss, potentially leading to hypertension.[80] It is therefore not recommended in liver and kidney disease. A diet high in potassium and low in sodium is recommended if _Glycyrrhiza glabra_ is used long term.[81]

Further, herbs with anxiolytic, sedative, adaptogenic and memory-enhancing properties[82–84] may be indicated in HPA axis dysregulation. In order to treat specific diseases arising from allostatic load, other phytomedicines (such as anti-inflammatory and immune-modulating herbs) are available, and need to be carefully selected to match the condition of the patient.

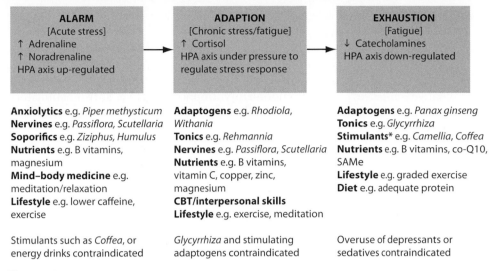

ALARM [Acute stress] ↑ Adrenaline ↑ Noradrenaline HPA axis up-regulated	**ADAPTION** [Chronic stress/fatigue] ↑ Cortisol HPA axis under pressure to regulate stress response	**EXHAUSTION** [Fatigue] ↓ Catecholamines HPA axis down-regulated
Anxiolytics e.g. *Piper methysticum* **Nervines** e.g. *Passiflora, Scutellaria* **Soporifics** e.g. *Ziziphus, Humulus* **Nutrients** e.g. B vitamins, magnesium **Mind–body medicine** e.g. meditation/relaxation **Lifestyle** e.g. lower caffeine, exercise	**Adaptogens** e.g. *Rhodiola, Withania* **Tonics** e.g. *Rehmannia* **Nervines** e.g. *Passiflora, Scutellaria* **Nutrients** e.g. B vitamins, vitamin C, copper, zinc, magnesium **CBT/interpersonal skills** **Lifestyle** e.g. exercise, meditation	**Adaptogens** e.g. *Panax ginseng* **Tonics** e.g. *Glycyrrhiza* **Stimulants*** e.g. *Camellia, Coffea* **Nutrients** e.g. B vitamins, co-Q10, SAMe **Lifestyle** e.g. graded exercise **Diet** e.g. adequate protein
Stimulants such as *Coffea*, or energy drinks contraindicated	*Glycyrrhiza* and stimulating adaptogens contraindicated	Overuse of depressants or sedatives contraindicated

Figure 18.6
General adaptation scale and therapeutics approaches
* Still use stimulants sparingly, ideally before 3 pm.
(Note: This diagram was typeset incorrectly in the previous edition of this book and has now been corrected.)

Adaptogens

Adaptogenic substances are innocuous agents, nonspecifically increasing resistance to a range of stressors by normalising body functions and strengthening systems that are compromised by stress.

Herbal adaptogens have been used to 'enhance endurance during fatigue and to reduce or prevent stress-induced impairments of neuroendocrine or immune function'.[85] Adaptogenic activity may occur from regulating the stress response via the HPA axis, from antioxidant action, and from modulation of the CNS.[11] Several herbal medicines, as shown below, have increased physical and mental stamina.[11,86] This class of herbs is therefore ideally suited to treat chronic stress and/or fatigue.

One of the phytomedicines with pronounced adaptogenic activity is ***Panax ginseng***, having a long tradition as a tonic in China, Japan, Korea and Russia. In the West, it is used to combat mental or physical fatigue and stress, and to enhance energy, wellbeing and performance.[79,87–89] It is used as an 'adrenal tonic', antidepressant, adaptogen and immunomodulator. It should be used with caution in diabetes as it may potentiate the actions of oral hypoglycaemic drugs and insulin and long-term use or high amounts may cause overstimulation. Russians have investigated ***Eleutherococcus senticosus*** and found it to be the most important substitute for *Panax ginseng*.[90] *Eleutherococcus senticosus* has shown nonspecific body resistance to stress and fatigue.[91] It has similar properties to *Panax ginseng*, in that it is an adaptogenic, a tonic and an immune modulator, and has anabolic qualities.[92] It has been suggested that a threshold exists: when stress hormones are high *Eleutherococcus senticosus* will have a lowering effect; if stress hormones are low they will be enhanced.[12]

Another adaptogen from the ginseng family is ***Panax quinquefolium***. It has tonic, immune-modulating and anti-inflammatory properties, combats stress and enhances the nervous and immune systems.[93] Both *Panax quinquefolium* and *Panax ginseng* can potentially elevate cortisol levels due to its effect on the HPA axis.[94] Research in mice has resulted in normalising dopamine, noradrenaline and 5-hydroxytryptophan after chronic unpredictable stress when *Panax quinquefolium* was given at an oral dose of 200 mg/kg, but not at 100 mg/kg.[95]

Another adaptogen with less stimulating qualities is **Withania somnifera**. Its many qualities include a regulatory effect on the HPA axis by exerting a positive influence on the endocrine, nervous and cardiovascular systems. Main actions are adaptogenic, mildly sedative, anti-stress, immunomodulatory, trophorestorative, anti-inflammatory, antioxidant and rejuvenating.[11,84,87,96,97] Application includes convalescing after illness, fatigue and weakness.[79]

Rhodiola rosea has been used traditionally to alleviate symptoms of anxiety, insomnia and depression.[70] Clinical trials have corroborated these findings.[98–101] *Rhodiola rosea* has been found to relieve fatigue,[102] increase work and exercise performance,[86,103] increase physical fitness and decrease mental fatigue in stressful situations.[104] It has therefore been used in asthenic conditions (conditions of weakness and debility, decline in function)[99] and chronic stress.[105]

Other phytomedicines with neuroendocrine modulatory activity and stress control include **Rehmannia glutinosa**,[81] **Ocimum sanctum**,[84,106] **Ginkgo biloba**[107] and **Bacopa monnieri**.[108] The latter two may also have a role in enhancing some domains of cognitive function.[81]

Address underlying nutrient deficiencies

To support nutritional status and provide the building blocks critical for the proper functioning of the neuroendocrine system, nutrients such as **B vitamins** and **vitamin C** are essential. B vitamins and **coenzyme Q10** (co-Q10) are cofactors in the Krebs cycle and oxidative phosphorylation (electron transport chain), respectively, which can be compromised (as is seen particularly in chronic fatigue syndrome).[21] These nutrients may therefore be needed to increase energy production. **Magnesium** is a cofactor in energy production and needed for glucose regulation. It is best given with an organic ligand such as citrate for optimal bioavailability.[109,110]

Phenylalanine and tyrosine are precursors for dopamine, noradrenaline and adrenaline synthesis. Reduced dopamine levels have been implicated in impaired reward/punishment processing.[111,112] Precursors for serotonin and melatonin synthesis are tryptophan or 5-hydroxytryptophan (5-HTP).[113] **Glutamine** is needed for GABA production.[21] Vitamins B2, B3 and B6 (ideally in the form of pyridoxal 5-phosphate—PLP), folate, vitamins B12 and C and minerals **iron**, **copper**, **calcium** and **zinc** are needed as cofactors for neurotransmitter synthesis (Figures 18.2, 18.4 and 18.5). In depression, it may well be the synergy of these neurotransmitters and their cofactors that is unbalanced.[111] Ensuring their optimal supply in cellular metabolism is ideal for resilience to stress.

Vitamin C has been shown to reduce adrenaline, cortisol and anti-inflammatory peptides in stress,[114] thus showing a lowered stress response and allostatic load. Most animals (except primates, guinea pigs, fruit bats and some birds) produce their own vitamin C from glucose in response to a stressor, indicating that this vitamin is indeed essential for mounting an effective stress response.[21] With high SNS and low PNS activity, digestion can be compromised due to suppression of digestive enzymes. When symptoms indicative of indigestion are reported by the patient, hydrochloric acid, pepsin and pancreatic enzymes with every meal may be indicated. These measures are taken in order to optimise digestive capacity.

With low digestive capacity, **vitamin B12** absorption will also be affected due to insufficient or absent intrinsic factor.[115] It can be administered either as sublingual troches or by intramuscular injection by a qualified health-care provider. Vitamin B12 plays an essential role in lowering homocysteine and providing methyl groups for neurotransmitter functioning.[116] Lack of vitamin B12 and folate have been linked to depression,[117] with vitamin B12 termed the 'master key' as it influences so many different systems. It may be needed even when serum levels appear normal.[118] Both nutrients are involved in **S-adenosylmethionine (SAMe)** production and are therefore crucial for methyl transfer. SAMe has been used successfully for depression and may have a role if low mood is a comorbidity of the patient's fatigue (see Chapter 15 on depression).[119] SAMe is the universal methyl donor and is needed for a range of metabolic reactions, including neurotransmitter production (Figures 18.2 and 18.4, last step). Endogenously, it is made from homocysteine and requires vitamin B12, folate and adenosine as cofactors. If homocysteine is low, methionine or SAMe can be given as a substrate for methyl groups.

Omega-3 fatty acids have been indicated for use in depression[120] and are needed to support a healthy nervous system and brain function (see Chapter 15 on depression for further comment). Due to their anti-inflammatory properties they also dampen stress-induced cytokine activation.[121] Further, antioxidants such as vitamins A, C and E, the minerals selenium and zinc, as well as bioflavonoids, **co-Q10** and glutathione are required in higher amounts to combat free-radical damage and oxidative stress.[122–124]

Co-Q10 tends to be low when cortisol is low.[125] (Abnormal thyroid function can have an influence on co-Q10 levels and should be ruled out.) The amino acids L-lysine and L-arginine have been shown to enhance ACTH, cortisol, adrenaline and noradrenaline levels in response to psychosocial stress and anxiety.[126] For more detailed discussion on allaying fatigue and enhancing energy levels, see Chapter 38 on chronic fatigue.

Reducing symptoms of stress

For psychological and physiological manifestations of stress a range of herbal anxiolytics may be appropriate[127] (see Chapter 14 on anxiety for more discussion). *Matricaria recutita* and *Melissa officinalis* are safe options as a mild nervine and antispasmodic and both herbs are suitable for children. If a stronger sedative action is desirable and insomnia is also present, *Valeriana* **spp.** can be considered. *Valeriana officinalis* and *Valeriana edulis* are both used, with the former having higher levels of terpenes and the latter higher levels of valepotriates.[81] These interventions may improve sleep quality without morning drowsiness or impairment of concentration or reaction time and are therefore preferable to drug treatment.[128] While some studies have shown hypnotic effects from *Valeriana* spp., it should be noted that current evidence does not currently strongly support its use as a soporific.[129,130] *Valeriana* spp. have nervine and soporific actions, and combine well with *Humulus lupulus*, *Matricaria recutita* and *Melissa officinalis* for sleep disorders with anxiety and restlessness.[128] These herbs are safe, but long-term use of *Valeriana* spp. can lead to insomnia. On rare occasions, this phytomedicine can have a stimulating effect in some people and should therefore be avoided in such cases. *Passiflora incarnata* and *Scutellaria lateriflora* has been used for any kind of nervous system disorders, from headaches, irritability and restlessness to insomnia.[128] Additionally, *Lavandula angustifolia* could be prescribed due to its nervine properties, antidepressant and mood-enhancing qualities, having a potentially addictive effect with some antidepressants.[131]

Piper methysticum has anxiolytic, antispasmodic and soporific qualities[127] (see Chapter 14 on anxiety for more discussion), and may have a role in the alarm and adaptation GAS phases. In the Chinese tradition *Ziziphus jujuba* var. *spinosa* has been used for nervous disorders and insomnia.[127,132] Apart from its hypnotic and sedative qualities it can be prescribed for irritability and to prevent sweating, especially at night.[127,132] In addition, it can reduce heart palpitations and hypertension.[128]

Modify lifestyle

Balance of work, relaxation/sleep, socialising, physical activities and daily chores is difficult to achieve in modern life. However, it is important to be aware of a person's commitments and how these influence their life. Chronic stress has been linked to premature death,[133] and social support networks are related to positive states of health and reduced disease burden.[134] The importance of **physical activity** cannot be under-estimated. Since the body is geared up for action when under stress ('fight or flight'), exercise is a potent tool to modulate the neuroendocrine system, reducing stress and building stamina.[135] Regular physical activity has been shown to help in reducing stress, depression and anxiety.[119] Exercising in nature (**'green exercise'**) may also have mood elevating, de-stressing effect beyond that of indoor exercise. Exercising in the presence of nature may also enhance self-esteem.[136]

Reduction or avoidance of stimulants such as tea and coffee, so commonly used to keep up alertness and functioning in times of increased work demand and fatigue, may also be of benefit as excess caffeine can over-stimulate the HPA axis. Further, caffeine within eight hours of sleep may cause insomnia which will further exacerbate stress and fatigue (see Chapter 16 on insomnia). These beverages can be replaced with decaffeinated coffee or tea, coffee-replacements such as 'dandelion coffee' and herbal teas. The change is best done slowly to reduce the risk of caffeine withdrawal symptoms such as headache and further fatigue.[52]

Stress is often accompanied by carbohydrate cravings, which can lead to blood sugar imbalances, especially if they are high in sugar and refined starches. Fruit is best limited to two pieces a day as it may increase glycaemic load. **Whole grains** are preferable due to their fibre content, thus slowing down the release of sugar,[137] and their B vitamin content. B vitamins are essential in the Krebs cycle for energy production.[21] Carbohy-drates are commonly craved during stress due to their tryptophan-serotonin enhancing qualities.[44,45] This partially explains the weight gain experienced by some people when under stress.[45] High cortisol is also known to lead to weight increases and potentially to metabolic syndrome,[116,118] although in chronic generalised fatigue cortisol is usually low (depleted). **High-protein foods** and snacks for amino acids, especially fish as the latter also contributes to a favourable EFA balance, may decrease carbohydrate cravings while at the same time providing the necessary amino acids as precursors for neurotransmitter synthesis. Protein powders can be used in smoothies to provide additional amino acids for neurotransmitter production and to help reduce hypoglycaemic episodes.

INTEGRATIVE MEDICAL CONSIDERATIONS

Mind–body medicine and psychology

Patients may respond well to talking about their problems if stress is due to known life circumstances. Sharing with friends or family members may help putting stress factors into perspective. **Mindfulness meditation** or forms which foster 'mental silence'[68,138,139] attempt to foster greater awareness of thought processes in the 'here and now' in order to increase coping ability.[140] A meta-analysis has found that mindfulness-based stress reduction is indeed able to assist patients in dealing with both mental and physical stressors.[141] Other forms of 'movement meditation' such as **yoga** and **Tai Chi** can be beneficial in reducing anxiety, stress, fatigue and pain (see Chapter 14 on anxiety for mindfulness meditation guidelines).[142] Other means to help with problem solving include imagery and creative visualisation.[135] **Art** and **music therapy**[143] have been shown to reduce stress, anxiety and pain. Spiritual or pastoral **counselling** may be needed if the stress is manifesting on an existential level.[144]

Cognitive behaviour therapy has been investigated and found to be a beneficial technique in stress-related health problems such as anxiety, depression, phobias and panic, anorexia and distress, and can be combined with mindfulness (mindfulness-based cognitive therapy).[145]

Physical therapies

Acupuncture and **massage** (with or without aromatherapy) may be beneficial techniques for the somatic and psychological manifestation of stress. An eight-week pilot randomised waitlist-controlled study using electroacupuncture in stressed medical students revealed the treatment provided a significant reduction of stress-related symptoms, with improvement in energy and mood also occurring.[146] **Touch** is one of the most ancient ways of healing and has shown beneficial effects for anxiety and depression.[147] A review of 25 studies that evaluated the effects of massage in reducing stress revealed that reductions in salivary cortisol, heart rate and blood pressure were common physiological effects.[148] There was, however, insufficient data to make definitive conclusion regarding the multiple treatment effect of massage therapy on urinary cortisol or catecholamine levels. **Progressive muscular relaxation**, where sequential muscle groups are first tensed and then relaxed, can also be used to invoke a relaxation response.[7]

CLINICAL SUMMARY

The initial therapeutic aim is to determine what the external stressors are and what stage of the GAS scale the patient is in. If in the alarm phase, this can be corrected reasonably quickly; however, with prolonged stress leading to exhaustion, a more patient road to recovery is needed. Many biological, lifestyle and psychosocial elements can be initiated by the clinician (detailed in the decision tree at Figure 18.7), and there is always scope for changing the treatment should the current prescription fail to produce the desired results (improved mood, energy and coping ability). Both the physical and the mental/emotional symptoms that present need to be taken into consideration in the design of a treatment plan. The connection between psychological, neurological and endocrine symptoms is now well established in disciplines such as psychoneuroendocrinology.[149] A healthy diet, coupled with a balanced lifestyle and regular exercise, will help to settle imbalances in the stress cascade. To replenish depleted adrenals and neurotransmitters and nourish compromised physiology, select nutritional supplements may be indicated. In longer standing problems (as is the case in chronic fatigue), cellular metabolism is further compromised with potential oxidative damage to the brain, as well as the development of a range of chronic diseases.[5,17] Treatment in that case would be more comprehensive and extended over a longer time span.

Allostatic load can be modified and even reversed. People who can ward off allostatic load best tend to have the following attributes: a positive mental attitude; acceptance of themselves and others; fulfilling relationships yet are able to retain their own autonomy; beliefs and principles that they defend; the ability to create and shape their own environment conducive to their needs for health and happiness; a purpose in life; and a sense of personal growth.[3] Having a good nutritional status and a balanced lifestyle is also a goal of any prescriptive treatment. While long-term management of stress and energy levels is something that all humans must address in an age of increased pressure and competition, the key is to 'put back in what we take out'.

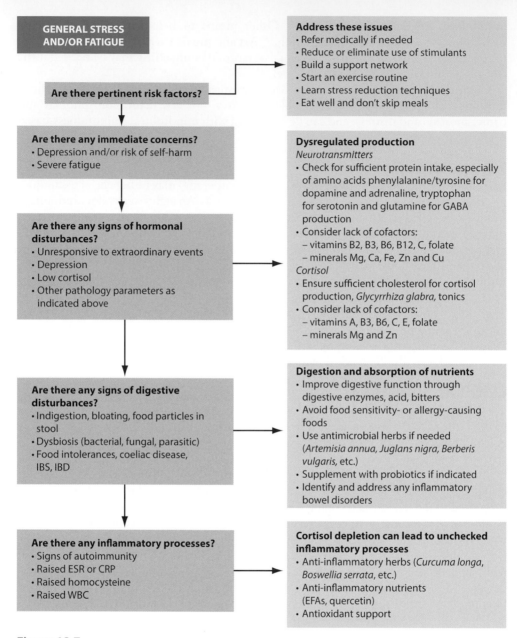

GENERAL STRESS AND/OR FATIGUE

Are there pertinent risk factors?

Address these issues
- Refer medically if needed
- Reduce or eliminate use of stimulants
- Build a support network
- Start an exercise routine
- Learn stress reduction techniques
- Eat well and don't skip meals

Are there any immediate concerns?
- Depression and/or risk of self-harm
- Severe fatigue

Dysregulated production
Neurotransmitters
- Check for sufficient protein intake, especially of amino acids phenylalanine/tyrosine for dopamine and adrenaline, tryptophan for serotonin and glutamine for GABA production
- Consider lack of cofactors:
  – vitamins B2, B3, B6, B12, C, folate
  – minerals Mg, Ca, Fe, Zn and Cu
Cortisol
- Ensure sufficient cholesterol for cortisol production, *Glycyrrhiza glabra,* tonics
- Consider lack of cofactors:
  – vitamins A, B3, B6, C, E, folate
  – minerals Mg and Zn

Are there any signs of hormonal disturbances?
- Unresponsive to extraordinary events
- Depression
- Low cortisol
- Other pathology parameters as indicated above

Are there any signs of digestive disturbances?
- Indigestion, bloating, food particles in stool
- Dysbiosis (bacterial, fungal, parasitic)
- Food intolerances, coeliac disease, IBS, IBD

Digestion and absorption of nutrients
- Improve digestive function through digestive enzymes, acid, bitters
- Avoid food sensitivity- or allergy-causing foods
- Use antimicrobial herbs if needed (*Artemisia annua, Juglans nigra, Berberis vulgaris,* etc.)
- Supplement with probiotics if indicated
- Identify and address any inflammatory bowel disorders

Are there any inflammatory processes?
- Signs of autoimmunity
- Raised ESR or CRP
- Raised homocysteine
- Raised WBC

Cortisol depletion can lead to unchecked inflammatory processes
- Anti-inflammatory herbs (*Curcuma longa, Boswellia serrata,* etc.)
- Anti-inflammatory nutrients (EFAs, quercetin)
- Antioxidant support

Figure 18.7
Naturopathic treatment decision tree—stress and fatigue

Table 18.4
Review of the major evidence*

Intervention	Mechanisms of action	Key literature	Result	Comment
Diet	Proteins, fats and certain nutrients are critical to assist in the manufacture of neurochemicals and hormones[41]	Case Control Study: Brunner et al. 2002[67] Comparative study 22 high stress (HS) prone versus 23 of low stress (LS) prone subjects submitted to stressful situations and high carbohydrate (CHO)/low protein or low CHO/high-protein diets	Only in uncontrollable stress in HS subjects, the high CHO/low protein diet reduced stress parameters	The results were attributed to the CHO-rich diet being high in tryptophan However, the long-term effects of a CHO-rich diet could be dysglycaemia, potentially leading to insulin resistance and metabolic syndrome (which is a known flow-on effect of stress) (Note: Most studies have focused on impact of stress on diet, rather than diet on individual stress parameters. Most work in this area is theoretical, and more trials are needed.)
Meditation	Long-term meditation may alter brain structure and modify neurochemistry	RCT: Manocha et al. 2011[68] 178 adult workers eight-week, three-arm RCT Meitation versus relaxation versus waitlist	Significant improvement for the meditation group compared with both the relaxation control and the waitlist groups on perceived stress while improving mood ($p = 0.026$)	Meditation is a safe and effective strategy for dealing with work stress and low mood
Multivitamins	Critical cofactors of neurochemical production and function (in particular B vitamins, vitamin C, zinc, magnesium)	Review and meta-analysis: Long & Benton 2013[69]: Eight RCTs using multivitamins > 28 days	Supplementation reduced the levels of perceived stress (standard mean difference [SMD] = 0.35; 95% confidence interval [CI] = 0.47–0.22; ($p = 0.001$), fatigue (SMD = 0.27; 95% CI = 0.40–0.146; ($p < 0.001$)	Multivitamins have a beneficial effect on perceived stress and mild psychiatric symptoms High-dose B vitamins formulations potentially more effective

Table 18.4
Review of the major evidence* (continued)

Intervention	Mechanisms of action	Key literature	Result	Comment
Rhodiola rosea	Neuroendocrine modulation (reduces cortisol and stress-induced protein kinases) Monoamine oxidase A inhibition Monoamine modulation	Review: (Panossian et al. 2010)[70] Several RCTs reviewed (n = 40–161) using *Rhodiola rosea* acutely or repeated to reduce fatigue and improve cognitive or physical performance	The weight of evidence reveals that *Rhodiola rosea* is an effective adaptogen, improving physical and mental performance while reducing fatigue	May be stimulating in some people Use an extract standardised for rosvarin and salidroside
Panax ginseng	HPA axis modulation Monoamine modulation (dopamine, serotonin) Anti-inflammatory and antioxidant effects Nitric oxide synthase inhibition	RCT (Dorling et al. 1980)[71] Twelve weeks (n = 60, aged 22–80) 200 mg extract (≈ 1 g root)	Significant improvements in visual and auditory reaction times and recovery from physical exercie	Several trials have shown no benefit over placebo regarding performance; this could be due to their shorter duration However, most trials done on athletes have shown improvements in stamina[72]
Eleutherococcus senticosus	HPA axis and monoamine modulation Immunological modulatory effects	RCT (Cicero et al. 2004)[73] Eight weeks, two-arm (n = 20, aged ≥ 65 years, hypertensive) – 300 mg/day dry extract Short form—36 health survey at baseline, weeks 4 and 8	Significant differences in social functioning between treatment and placebo groups at four weeks but not at eight weeks No difference in blood pressure	Long-term use seems to attenuate the benefits

*See anxiety and depression chapters for review of other potential interventions.

KEY POINTS

- Stress activates the HPA axis and triggers the release of a cascade of hormones and neurotransmitters, notably adrenaline and cortisol.
- With prolonged stress, nutrient status can become exhausted, leading to a gradual decline of adrenal function and neurotransmitters, and finally to a state of endocrine imbalance and subsequent fatigue.
- Practitioners need to discern between the alarm, adaptation and exhaustion phases of the GAS scale, and test for the presence of either high or low cortisol levels.
- Treatment needs to focus on both the physical *and* the mental/emotional aspects of stress.

FURTHER READING

Finsterer J, Mahjoub SZ. Fatigue in healthy and diseased individuals. Am J Hosp Palliat Care 2014;31(5):562–75. doi:10.1177/1049909113494748. [Epub 2013 Jul 26].

Hulme K, Safari R, Thomas S, et al. Fatigue interventions in long term, physical health conditions: a scoping review of systematic reviews. PLoS ONE 2018;13(10):e0203367. doi:10.1371/journal. pone.0203367. eCollection 2018.

Panossian AG. Adaptogens in mental and behavioral disorders. Psychiatr Clin North Am 2013;36(1):49–64. doi:10.1016/j.psc.2012.12.005. Review.

REFERENCES

1. Selye H. Stress without distress. London: Hodder and Stoughton; 1974. p. 27.
2. Thibodeau G, Patton K. Anatomy and physiology. 5th ed. St Louis: Mosby; 2003. [Chapter 22].
3. McEwen BS. The end of stress as we know it. Washington: The Dana Press (Joseph Henry Press); 2002.
4. McEwen BS. Interacting mediators of allostasis and allostatic load: towards an understanding of resilience in aging. Metabolism 2003;52(10 Suppl. 2):10–16.
5. McEwen BS. Protection and damage from acute and chronic stress: allostasis and allostatic overload and relevance to the pathophysiology of psychiatric disorders. Ann N Y Acad Sci 2004;1032:1–7.
6. Tsigos C, Chrousos GP. Hypothalamic-pituitary-adrenal axis, neuroendocrine factors and stress. J Psychosom Res 2002;53(4):865–71.
7. Miller DB, O'Callaghan JP. Neuroendocrine aspects of the response to stress. Metabolism 2002;51(6 Suppl. 1):5–10.
8. Vanitallie TB. Stress: a risk factor for serious illness. Metabolism 2002;51(6 Suppl. 1):40–5.
9. Haddad JJ, et al. Cytokines and neuro-immune-endocrine interactions: a role for the hypothalamic-pituitary-adrenal revolving axis. J Neuroimmunol 2002;133(1–2):1–19.
10. Eskandari F, Sternberg EM. Neural-immune interactions in health and disease. Ann N Y Acad Sci 2002;966:20–7.
11. Wilson L. Review of adaptogenic mechanisms: Eleutherococcus senticosus, Panax ginseng, Rhodiola rosea, Schisandra chinensis and Withania somnifera. AJMH 2007;19(3):126–38.
12. Gaffney BT, et al. The effects of Eleutherococcus senticosus and Panax ginseng on steroidal hormone indices of stress and lymphocyte subset numbers in endurance athletes. Life Sci 2001;70(4):431–42.
13. Cutolo M, et al. Hypothalamic-pituitary-adrenocortical and gonadal functions in rheumatoid arthritis. Ann N Y Acad Sci 2003;992:107–17.
14. Loucks AB, Redman LM. The effect of stress on menstrual function. Trends Endocrinol Metab 2004;15(10):466–71.
15. Gilad GM, Gilad VH. Overview of the brain polyamine-stress-response: regulation, development, and modulation by lithium and role in cell survival. Cell Mol Neurobiol 2003;23(4–5):637–49.
16. Goldstein DS, McEwen B. Allostasis, homeostasis, and the nature of stress. Stress 2002;5(1):55–8.
17. McEwen BS. Sex, stress and the hippocampus: allostasis, allostatic load and the aging process. Neurobiol Aging 2002;23(5):921–39.
18. McEwen BS. Stressed or stressed out: what is the difference? J Psychiatry Neurosci 2005;30(5):315–18.
19. McEwen B, Lasley EN. Allostatic load: when protection gives way to damage. Adv Mind Body Med 2003;19(1):28–33.
20. Abercrombie HC, et al. Flattened cortisol rhythms in metastatic breast cancer patients. Psychoneuroendocrinology 2004;29(8):1082–92.
21. Gropper S, et al. Advanced nutrition and human metabolism. 5th ed. Australia: Wadsworth: Cengage Learning; 2009.
22. King A, et al. Attenuated cortisol response to alcohol in heavy social drinkers. Int J Psychophysiol 2006;59(3):203–9.
23. Meyer G, et al. Casino gambling increases heart rate and salivary cortisol in regular gamblers. Biol Psychiatry 2000;48(9):948–53.
24. Lovallo WR. Cortisol secretion patterns in addiction and addiction risk. Int J Psychophysiol 2006;59(3):195–202.
25. Hellhammer J, et al. Allostatic load, perceived stress, and health: a prospective study in two age groups. Ann N Y Acad Sci 2004;1032:8–13.
26. McEwen BS. Early life influences on life-long patterns of behavior and health. Ment Retard Dev Disabil Res Rev 2003;9(3):149–54.
27. Korte SM, et al. The Darwinian concept of stress: benefits of allostasis and costs of allostatic load and the trade-offs in health and disease. Neurosci Biobehav Rev 2005;29(1):3–38.
28. McEwen BS. Mood disorders and allostatic load. Biol Psychiatry 2003;54(3):200–7.
29. Carroll BJ. Ageing, stress and the brain. Novartis Found Symp 2002;242:26–36, discussion 45.
30. Weaver JD, et al. Interleukin-6 and risk of cognitive decline: MacArthur studies of successful aging. Neurology 2002;59(3):371–8.
31. Angeli A, et al. The overtraining syndrome in athletes: a stress-related disorder. J Endocrinol Invest 2004;27(6):603–12.
32. Jefferies WM. Cortisol and immunity. Med Hypotheses 1991;34(3):198–208.
33. Butcher SK, et al. Raised cortisol:DHEAS ratios in the elderly after injury: potential impact upon neutrophil function and immunity. Aging Cell 2005;4(6):319–24.
34. Mechanick JI. Metabolic mechanisms of stress hyperglycemia. JPEN J Parenter Enteral Nutr 2006;30(2):157–63.
35. Maloney EM, et al. Chronic fatigue syndrome and high allostatic load. Pharmacogenomics 2006;7(3):467–73.
36. Björntorp P, Rosmond R. The metabolic syndrome—a neuroendocrine disorder? Br J Nutr 2000;83(Suppl. 1):S49–57.
37. Nieuwenhuizen AG, Rutters F. The hypothalamic-pituitary-adrenal-axis in the regulation of energy balance. Physiol Behav 2008;94(2):169–77.
38. Kalantaridou SN, et al. Stress and the female reproductive system. J Reprod Immunol 2004;62(1–2):61–8.
39. Anderson KN, editor. Mosby's medical, nursing and allied health dictionary. 6th ed. St Louis. London: CV Mosby; 2002.
40. Demitrack MA, Crofford LJ. Evidence for and pathophysiologic implications of hypothalamic-pituitary-

adrenal axis dysregulation in fibromyalgia and chronic fatigue syndrome. Ann N Y Acad Sci 1998;840: 684–97.

41. Harbuz M. Neuroendocrine function and chronic inflammatory stress. Exp Physiol 2002;87(5):519–25.

42. Berridge KC. Motivation concepts in behavioral neuroscience. Physiol Behav 2004;81(2):179–209.

43. Lederbogen F, Kirsch P, Haddad L, et al. City living and urban upbringing affect neural social stress processing in humans. Nature 2011;474(7352):498–501. doi:10.1038/nature10.

44. Markus R, et al. Effects of food on cortisol and mood in vulnerable subjects under controllable and uncontrollable stress. Physiol Behav 2000;70(3–4):333–42.

45. Takeda E, et al. Stress control and human nutrition. J Med Invest 2004;51(3–4):139–45.

46. Christensen L, Brooks A. Changing food preference as a function of mood. J Psychol 2006;140(4):293–306.

47. Anderson DC. Assessment and nutraceutical management of stress-induced adrenal dysfunction. Integrat Med: A Clinic J 2008;7(5):18–25.

48. Giordano R, et al. Hypothalamus-pituitary-adrenal axis evaluation in patients with hypothalamo-pituitary disorders: comparison of different provocative tests. Clin Endocrinol 2008;68(6):935–41.

49. Pagana KD, Pagana TJ. Mosby's manual of diagnostic and laboratory tests. 3rd ed. USA: CV Mosby; 2006.

50. Crowley LV. An introduction to human disease: pathology and pathophysiology correlations. 6th ed. Sudbury: Jones and Bartlett Publishers; 2004.

51. Papadelis C, et al. Effects of mental workload and caffeine on catecholamines and blood pressure compared to performance variations. Brain Cogn 2003;51(1):143–54.

52. Lane JD, et al. Caffeine affects cardiovascular and neuroendocrine activation at work and home. Psychosom Med 2002;64(4):595–603.

53. Giordano R, et al. Corticotrope hypersecretion coupled with cortisol hypo-responsiveness to stimuli is present in patients with autoimmune endocrine diseases: evidence for subclinical primary hypoadrenalism? Eur J Endocrinol 2006;155(3):421–8.

54. Debono M, Ross RJ. Doses and steroids to be used in primary and central hypoadrenalism. Ann Endocrinol (Paris) 2007;68(4):265–7.

55. Barbetta L, et al. Comparison of different regimens of glucocorticoid replacement therapy in patients with hypoadrenalism. J Endocrinol Invest 2005;28(7):632–7.

56. Libè R, et al. Effects of dehydroepiandrosterone (DHEA) supplementation on hormonal, metabolic and behavioral status in patients with hypoadrenalism. J Endocrinol Invest 2004;27(8):736–41.

57. Bhagra S, et al. Dehydroepiandrosterone in adrenal insufficiency and ageing. Curr Opin Endocrinol Diabetes Obes 2008;15(3):239–43.

58. Giordano G, et al. Variations of pituitary function over time after brain injuries: the lesson from a prospective study. Pituitary 2005;8(3–4):227–31.

59. Beishuizen A, Thijs LG. The immunoneuroendocrine axis in critical illness: beneficial adaptation or neuroendocrine exhaustion? Curr Opin Crit Care 2004;10(6):461–7.

60. Marik PE. Adrenal-exhaustion syndrome in patients with liver disease. Intensive Care Med 2006;32(2):275–80.

61. Ströhle A. The neuroendocrinology of stress and the pathophysiology and therapy of depression and anxiety. Nervenarzt 2003;74(3):279–91, quiz 292.

62. Cortese BM, Phan KL. The role of glutamate in anxiety and related disorders. CNS Spectr 2005;10(10):820–30.

63. Ströhle A, Holsboer F. Stress responsive neurohormones in depression and anxiety. Pharmacopsychiatry 2003;36(Suppl. 3):S207–14.

64. Chierichetti SM, et al. Beta-blockers and psychic stress: a double-blind, placebo-controlled study of bopindolol vs lorazepam and butalbital in surgical patients. Int J Clin Pharmacol Ther Toxicol 1985;23(9):510–14.

65. Schweizer R, et al. Effect of two beta-blockers on stress during mental arithmetic. Psychopharmacology (Berl) 1991;105(4):573–7.

66. Breitbart W, Alici Y. Psychostimulants for cancer-related fatigue. J Natl Compr Canc Netw 2010;8(8):933–42.

67. Brunner EJ, et al. Adrenocortical, autonomic, and inflammatory causes of the metabolic syndrome: nested case-control study. Circulation 2002;106(21):2659–65.

68. Manocha R, Black D, Sarris J, et al. A randomized, controlled trial of meditation for work stress, anxiety and depressed mood in full-time workers. Evid Based Complement Alternat Med 2011;2011:960583.

69. Long SJ, Benton D. Effects of vitamin and mineral supplementation on stress, mild psychiatric symptoms, and mood in nonclinical samples: a meta-analysis. Psychosom Med 2013;75(2):144–53.

70. Panossian A, Wikman G, Sarris J. Rosenroot (Rhodiola rosea): traditional use, chemical composition, pharmacology and clinical efficacy. Phytomedicine 2010;17(7):481–93.

71. Dorling E, et al. Do ginsenosides influence the performance? Notabene Med 1980;10(5):241–6.

72. Bone K. Ginseng—the regal herb part 2. Mediherb Prof Rev 1998;63:1–5.

73. Cicero AF, et al. Effects of Siberian ginseng (Eleutherococcus senticosus Maxim.) on elderly quality of life: a randomized clinical trial. Arch Gerontol Geriatr Suppl 2004;9:69–73.

74. De Kloet ER, Derijk R. Signaling pathways in brain involved in predisposition and pathogenesis of stress-related disease: genetic and kinetic factors affecting the MR/GR balance. Ann N Y Acad Sci 2004;1032:14–34.

75. Duax WL, et al. Steroid dehydrogenase structures, mechanism of action, and disease. Vitam Horm 2000;58:121–48.

76. Kohlmeier M. Nutrient metabolism. Amsterdam: Academic Press; 2003.

77. Braun L, Cohen M. Herbs and natural supplements. 2nd ed. Sydney: Churchill Livingstone; 2007.

78. Kato H, et al. 3-monoglucuronyl-glycyrrhetinic acid is a major metabolite that causes licorice-induced pseudoaldosteronism. J Clin Endocrinol Metab 1995;80(6):1929–33.

79. Morgan M, Bone K. Herbs with tonic, adaptogenic, adrenal tonic and nervine activity. Phytotherapist Perspectiv 2005;58.

80. Armanini D, et al. History of the endocrine effects of licorice. Exp Clin Endocrinol Diabetes 2002;110(6):257–61.

81. Bone K. A clinical guide to blending liquid herbs. USA: Elsevier; 2003.

82. Blumenthal M. The ABC clinical guide to herbs. Austin: American Botanical Council; 2003.

83. Mills S, Bone K. Principles and practice of phytotherapy. Sydney: Churchill Livingstone; 2000.

84. Rege NN, et al. Adaptogenic properties of six rasayana herbs used in Ayurvedic medicine. Phytother Res 1999;13(4):275–91.

85. Bone K. Rhodiola. Clin Monit 2008;23:1–2.

86. Panossian A, Wagner H. Stimulating effect of adaptogens: an overview with particular reference to their efficacy

following single dose administration. Phytother Res 2005;19(10):819–38.

87. Morgan M. Withania, ginseng: gentle tonic and adaptogenic. Phytotherapist Perspective 2005;59.

88. Beyer I, Rimpler M. Ginseng: Adaptogenitat zur Umstimmungstherapie—Teil 2. Biol Med 1996; 25(4):151.

89. Beyer I, Rimpler M. Ginseng: Adaptogenitat zur Umstimmungstherapie—Teil 1. Biol Med 1996;25(3):98.

90. Baranov AI. Medicinal uses of ginseng and related plants in the Soviet Union: recent trends in the Soviet literature. J Ethnopharmacol 1982;6(3):339–53.

91. Kimura Y, Sumiyoshi M. Effects of various Eleutherococcus senticosus cortex on swimming time, natural killer activity and corticosterone level in forced swimming stressed mice. J Ethnopharmacol 2004;95(2–3):447–53.

92. Bone K, Mills S. Principles and practice of phytotherapy. 2nd ed. London: Churchill Livingstone; 2013.

93. Kitts D, Hu C. Efficacy and safety of ginseng. Public Health Nutr 2000;3(4A):473–85.

94. Nocerino E, et al. The aphrodisiac and adaptogenic properties of ginseng. Fitoterapia 2000;71(Suppl. 1):S1–5.

95. Rasheed N, et al. Involvement of monoamines and proinflammatory cytokines in mediating the anti-stress effects of Panax quinquefolium. J Ethnopharmacol 2008;117(2):257–62.

96. Lindner S. Withania somnifera: winter cherry, Indian ginseng, ashwagandha. AJMH 1996;8(3):78.

97. Mishra LC, et al. Scientific basis for the therapeutic use of Withania somnifera (ashwagandha): a review. Altern Med Rev 2000;5(4):334–46.

98. Bystritsky A, et al. A pilot study of Rhodiola rosea (Rhodax) for generalized anxiety disorder (GAD). J Altern Complement Med 2008;14(2):175–80.

99. Kelly GS. Rhodiola rosea: a possible plant adaptogen. Altern Med Rev 2001;6(3):293–302.

100. Sarris J. Herbal medicines in the treatment of psychiatric disorders: a systematic review. Phytother Res 2007;21(8):703–16.

101. Darbinyan V, et al. Clinical trial of Rhodiola rosea L. extract SHR-5 in the treatment of mild to moderate depression. Nord J Psychiatry 2007;61(5):343–8.

102. Shevtsov VA, et al. A randomized trial of two different doses of a SHR-5 Rhodiola rosea extract versus placebo and control of capacity for mental work. Phytomedicine 2003;10(2–3):95–105.

103. De Bock K, et al. Acute Rhodiola rosea intake can improve endurance exercise performance. Int J Sport Nutr Exerc Metab 2004;14(3):298–307.

104. Spasov AA, et al. A double-blind, placebo-controlled pilot study of the stimulating and adaptogenic effect of Rhodiola rosea SHR-5 extract on the fatigue of students caused by stress during an examination period with a repeated low-dose regimen. Phytomedicine 2000;7(2):85–9.

105. Rhodiola rosea, monograph. Altern Med Rev 2002;7(5):421–3.

106. Morgan M. Holy basil. Phytotherapist Perspective 2001;19:1–3.

107. Shirai M, et al. Approach to novel functional foods for stress control 5. Antioxidant activity profiles of antidepressant herbs and their active components. J Med Invest 2005;52(Suppl.):249–51.

108. Rai D, et al. Adaptogenic effect of Bacopa monniera (brahmi). Pharmacol Biochem Behav 2003;75(4):823–30.

109. Lindberg JS, et al. Magnesium bioavailability from magnesium citrate and magnesium oxide. J Am Coll Nutr 1990;9(1):48–55.

110. Walker AF, et al. Mg citrate found more bioavailable than other Mg preparations in a randomised, double-blind study. Magnes Res 2003;16(3):183–91.

111. Roiser JP, et al. The subjective and cognitive effects of acute phenylalanine and tyrosine depletion in patients recovered from depression. Neuropsychopharmacology 2005;30(4):775–85.

112. McLean A, et al. The effects of tyrosine depletion in normal healthy volunteers: implications for unipolar depression. Psychopharmacology (Berl) 2004;171(3):286–97.

113. Freeman MP, et al. Selected integrative medicine treatments for depression: considerations for women. J Am Med Womens Assoc (1972) 2004;59(3):216–24.

114. Peters EM, et al. Vitamin C supplementation attenuates the increases in circulating cortisol, adrenaline and anti-inflammatory polypeptides following ultramarathon running. Int J Sports Med 2001;22(7):537–43.

115. Rufenacht P, et al. Vitamin B12 deficiency: a challenging diagnosis and treatment. Rev Med Suisse 2008;4(175):2212.

116. Golub MS. The adrenal and the metabolic syndrome. Curr Hypertens Rep 2001;3(2):117–20.

117. Coppen A, Bolander-Gouaille C. Treatment of depression: time to consider folic acid and vitamin B12. J Psychopharmacol 2005;19(1):59–65.

118. Epel E, et al. Are stress eaters at risk for the metabolic syndrome? Ann N Y Acad Sci 2004;1032:208–10.

119. Stear S. Health and fitness series—1. The importance of physical activity for health. J Fam Health Care 2013;13(1):10–13.

120. Appleton KM, Rogers PJ, Ness AR. Updated systematic review and meta-analysis of the effects of n-3 long-chain polyunsaturated fatty acids on depressed mood. Am J Clin Nutr 2010;91(3):757–70.

121. Kidd P. Th1/Th2 balance: the hypothesis, its limitations, and implications for health and disease. Altern Med Rev 2003;8(3):223–46.

122. Urso ML, Clarkson PM. Oxidative stress, exercise, and antioxidant supplementation. Toxicology 2003;189(1–2):41–54.

123. Mayne ST. Antioxidant nutrients and chronic disease: use of biomarkers of exposure and oxidative stress status in epidemiologic research. J Nutr 2003;133(Suppl. 3): 933S–40S.

124. Dhanasekaran M, Ren J. The emerging role of cocnzyme Q-10 in aging, neurodegeneration, cardiovascular disease, cancer and diabetes mellitus. Curr Neurovasc Res 2005;2(5):447–59.

125. Mancini A, et al. Coenzyme Q10 evaluation in pituitary-adrenal axis disease: preliminary data. Biofactors 2005;25(1–4):197–9.

126. Jezova D, et al. Subchronic treatment with amino acid mixture of L-lysine and L-arginine modifies neuroendocrine activation during psychosocial stress in subjects with high trait anxiety. Nutr Neurosci 2005;8(3):155–60.

127. Sarris J, McIntyre E, Camfield D. Plant-based medicines for anxiety disorders part 2: a systematic review of clinical studies with supportive preclinical evidence. CNS Drugs 2013;27(4):301–19.

128. Burgoyne B. Herbal treatment of insomnia. Mod Phytotherapist 2002;7(1):12–21.

129. Sarris J, Byrne GJ. A systematic review of insomnia and complementary medicine. Sleep Med Rev 2011;15(2):99–106.

130. Herrera-Arellano A, et al. Polysomnographic evaluation of the hypnotic effect of Valeriana edulis standardized extract in patients suffering from insomnia. Planta Med 2001;67(8):695–9.

131. Sarris J, Kavanagh D, Byrne G. Adjuvant use of nutritional and herbal medicines with antidepressants, mood stabilizers and benzodiazepines. J Psychiatr Res 2010;44:32–41.

132. Bone K. Clinical applications of Ayurvedic and Chinese herbs. Warwick: Phytotherapy Press; 1996.

133. Kopp MS, Rethelyi J. Where psychology meets physiology: chronic stress and premature mortality—the Central-Eastern European health paradox. Brain Res Bull 2004;62(5):351–67.

134. Singer B, et al. Protective environments and health status: cross-talk between human and animal studies. Neurobiol Aging 2005;26(Suppl. 1):113–18.

135. Fliopoulus C. Invitation to holistic health. Boston: Jones and Bartlett Publishers; 2004.

136. Barton J, Pretty J. What is the best dose of nature and green exercise for improving mental health? A multi-study analysis. Environ Sci Technol 2010;44(10):3947–55.

137. Mukherjee A. Fight stress with food. McClatchy-Tribune Business News. 2008.

138. Adelman EM. Mind-body intelligence: a new perspective integrating eastern and western healing traditions. Holist Nurs Pract 2006;20(3):147–51.

139. Shigaki CL, et al. Mindfulness-based stress reduction in medical settings. J Clin Psychol Med Settings 2006;13(3):209–16.

140. Sarris J, Moylan S, Camfield DA, et al. Complementary medicine, exercise, meditation, diet, and lifestyle modification for anxiety disorders: a review of current evidence. Evid Based Complement Alternat Med 2012;2012:809653.

141. Grossman P, et al. Mindfulness-based stress reduction and health benefits—a meta-analysis. J Psychosom Res 2004;57(1):35–43.

142. Oman D, et al. Passage meditation reduces perceived stress in health professionals: a randomized, controlled trial. J Consult Clin Psychol 2006;74(4):714–19.

143. Pratt RR. Art, dance, and music therapy. Phys Med Rehabil Clin N Am 2004;15(4):827–41.

144. Pronk K. Role of the doctor in relieving spiritual distress at the end of life. Am J Hosp Palliat Care 2005;22(6):419–25.

145. Barnhofer T, Crane C, Hargus E, et al. Mindfulness-based cognitive therapy as a treatment for chronic depression: a preliminary study. Behav Res Ther 2009;47(5):366–73.

146. Dias M, Pagnin D, de Queiroz Pagnin V, et al. Effects of electroacupuncture on stress-related symptoms in medical students: a randomised controlled pilot study. Acupunct Med 2012;30(2):89–95.

147. Robson T. An introduction to complementary medicine. Sydney: Allen & Unwin; 2003.

148. Moraska A, Pollini RA, Boulanger K, et al. Physiological adjustments to stress measures following massage therapy: a review of the literature. Evid Based Complement Alternat Med 2010;7(4):409–18.

149. Vitetta L, et al. Mind-body medicine: stress and its impact on overall health and longevity. Ann N Y Acad Sci 2005;1057:492–505.

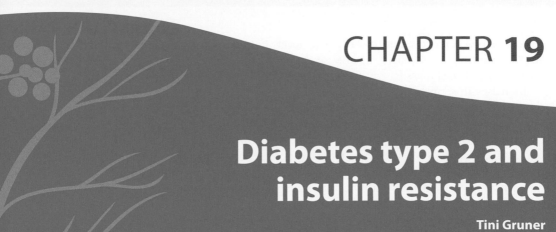

CHAPTER 19

Diabetes type 2 and insulin resistance

Tini Gruner
ND, MSc, PhD

OVERVIEW

Diabetes type 2, in contrast to type 1, is a lifestyle disease. Abdominal obesity leads to altered glucose tolerance (where glucose tissue uptake is impaired), which in turn leads to insulin resistance, hyperinsulinaemia, diabetes type 2 and cardiovascular abnormalities such as hypertension, hypertriglyceridaemia, low high-density lipoproteins (HDL), microvascular lesions and atherosclerosis.[1,2] It is also a risk factor for polycystic ovarian syndrome, sleep apnoea and some hormone-sensitive cancers.[3] It has been aptly called the 'hyperactive fork and hypoactive foot, a "deadly duet" '.[4] It is considered an epidemic and urgent action is called for.

Australian Government statistics show that the prevalence of diabetes has tripled from 1990 to 2015, with more than 85% of those people being diagnosed with diabetes type 2 and 12.4% with type 1. The overall proportion of people with diabetes is 4.7% (excluding gestational diabetes) and the highest incidence is in the 65–74 age group. Men are affected 40% more than women, and people in the lowest socioeconomic group are twice as likely to have diabetes as those in the highest socioeconomic group. However, it is estimated that there are equally as many cases of diabetes that are undiagnosed. Even then these figures may be conservative, considering the high prevalence of obesity.[5]

It is estimated that approximately 40% of Europeans above the age of 60 have metabolic syndrome (the precursor of diabetes type 2), with rates in the American population climbing to approximately two-thirds.[1,6] While in the past diabetes type 2 was a disease of older people it now affects people of all ages, including children and adolescents.[7] In the United States one-third of children are overweight or obese.[8] The cost of this disease to the individual (increased premature morbidity and mortality, comorbidities, reduced quality of life) and the public (higher taxes, overburdened healthcare system) are enormous, with about 18% of total healthcare expenditure in Europe due to diabetes alone. Since this is a preventable disease, even small changes in diet and lifestyle can have great beneficial effects, both to the patient and on the financial impact to the healthcare system.[7,9] However, particularly with diabetes type 2 in children, more research is needed regarding the benefits of behaviour modification.[10]

Two commonly encountered mechanisms seem to underlie the development of insulin resistance, leading to metabolic syndrome: high cortisol levels and adiposity.

Excessive blood glucose and/or fatty acid levels ('glucolipotoxicity') promote oxidative stress, resulting in impaired insulin secretion, decreased glucokinase expression and reduction in β-cell mass.[11]

Increases in serum cortisol, such as is seen in stress, leads to gluconeogenesis (often derived from protein, leading to progressive muscle wasting) and therefore increased glucose levels in blood.[12,13] The interconnection of cortisol and glucose could therefore be the cause for the progressive nature of the disease.[14] Up-regulation of cortisol due to stress (see also Chapter 18 on stress and fatigue) increases glucose and very-low-density lipoprotein (VLDL) secretion from the liver while inhibiting their reuptake, thus promoting hyperinsulinaemia, insulin resistance and storage of energy in the form of visceral fat.[15,16] A similar process is observed in ageing, promoted by ghrelin, where thermogenesis in brown fat cells is impaired while fat storage increases in white fat cells.[17]

Disturbances in the hypothalamic–pituitary–adrenal (HPA) axis not only increase cortisol levels but also enhance immune activation.[18] These disturbances exert their influence on other steroid hormones. Assaying these may give a better understanding of underlying wider ranging pathology; it may also give clues as to their possible treatment.[19] Increased inflammatory markers have been noted, linking the signs and symptoms of metabolic syndrome to an inflammatory process.[20] One study[18] hypothesises that the pathoaetiology of metabolic syndrome results from pro-inflammatory cytokines (IL-1, IL-6, TNF-α), due to inflammatory processes or emotional stress, enhancing sympathetic nervous system (SNS) activity and leading to obesity from enhanced feeding activity and increased leptin levels due to neuropeptide Y. A further indicator of inflammation in insulin resistance is an elevation in C-reactive protein (CRP).[21] Genetic links have also been suggested, with glucocorticoid receptor polymorphism.[22]

Research echoes all of the above.[23] Chronic elevations in blood glucose result in glycosylation of red blood cells and other biological substances, leading to oxidative tissue damage and mitochondrial impairment.[24] It is suggested that excessive production of hydrogen peroxide and increased activation of NADPH oxidase is the underlying mechanism that results in the common, late complications of diabetes, such as microvascular damage in the blood vessels, eyes and kidneys. However, it has been suggested[25,26] that oxidative stress could also be the cause, not just the result, of this syndrome.[27,28]

Sorbitol, chemically classed as a sugar alcohol and used as a sweetener in foods, is also produced in small amounts from glucose or fructose in the body.[29] In diabetes this production is enhanced as a result of enhanced aldose reductase activity, as seen in an increased sorbitol to glucose ratio. Sorbitol then accumulates in the cells, giving rise to diabetic complications.[30]

High dietary saturated fat (in particular *trans* fat) intake, low omega-3 and other polyunsaturated fatty acids use, alcohol consumption, sedentary lifestyle and mental stress are all promoters of metabolic syndrome (Figure 19.1). Certain personality types have enhanced sympathetic nervous system activity, with increased secretion of catecholamines, cortisol and serotonin, which all appear to be involved in the pathogenesis of metabolic syndrome.[6,31]

Metabolism of glucose uptake into the cells and the role of insulin

In most tissues, except hepatic tissue, glucose relies on a transport system called GLUT4 to be able to enter the cell. This system requires insulin for optimal uptake of glucose by muscle and adipose tissue, where insulin enhances the translocation of GLUT4 from the intracellular pool to the cell membrane.[33] The putative metabolic cause for diabetes type 2 lies in suboptimal functioning of these glucose transporters due to insulin resistance.[32]

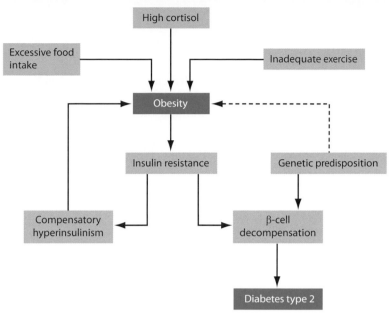

Figure 19.1
Overview of diabetes type 2 aetiology

Source: Gropper et al. 2009[32]

It has been found that insulin is more effective in the presence of chromium. The mechanism is not entirely elucidated, but it is suggested that chromium (Cr^{3+}), bound to transferrin, enters the cells via transferrin receptors. Once inside the cell, chromium is released and four chromium ions bind with apochromodulin, forming holochromodulin (often simply called 'chromodulin'). Chromodulin then binds to the insulin receptor, which increases receptor activity.[32] Figures 19.2a and 19.2b illustrate the initial phase of insulin uptake (Figure 19.2a) and the resultant uptake of glucose into the cell (Figure 19.2b), and the role of chromodulin.

Testing for diabetes type 2 and metabolic syndrome

In-house testing comprises blood glucose, urinalysis (dipstick), blood pressure and anthropometric measurements. The latter includes body mass index (BMI*), waist circumference,† and body composition measured through skinfold thickness or bioimpedance.[2]

Metabolic syndrome is confirmed when there are abnormalities in three or more of the following:

- elevated fasting glucose
- elevated glucose tolerance test (GTT)
- elevated insulin
- increased waist circumference or BMI

---

* Calculated as weight (in kg)/(height (m)^2). Ideal range is 18.5–25, with values > 30 indicating obesity.
† Ideal range for males is < 102 cm and for females < 88 cm. Measurements above these values constitute abdominal obesity.

- high blood pressure (> 130/85)
- high triglycerides
- low HDL.

Since multiple parameters are involved in diabetes type 2 and metabolic syndrome the combined results of in-house and pathology testing can give conclusive evidence. Table 19.1 shows information on each of the laboratory tests involved. Figure 19.3 shows a hypothetical glucose tolerance test with hyperglycaemia and delayed glucose clearance, elevated insulin levels (high fasting insulin with more than eightfold rise following glucose loading), insulin resistance (insulin peaks later than glucose) and hypercortisolism.

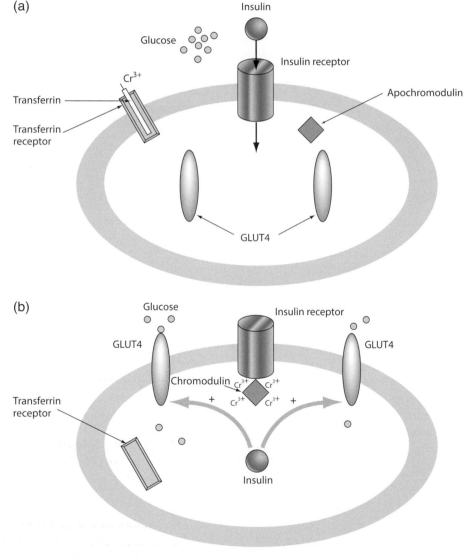

Figure 19.2
(a) Cell activation for glucose uptake (b) Glucose uptake into the cell
Source: Adapted from Devlin[33] and Gropper et al.[32]

Table 19.1
Pathology tests recommended for suspected diabetes type 2 and metabolic syndrome

Test	Tissue	Comments
Fasting glucose	Serum	Values > 5.5 or 6 mmol/L are indicative of diabetes type 2 or metabolic syndrome.
Fasting insulin	Serum	Normal values are 4–10 mU/L.
GTT	Serum	Commonly, the test is done over two hours, with blood samples taken pre-glucose loading and two hours after. Values > 7.8 mmol/L post-loading are indicative of diabetes type 2. However, this test will not show insulin and cortisol levels or the finer details of glucose control. Thus, a three-hour test with half-hourly measurements of glucose, insulin and cortisol is recommended. Insulin should not rise more than eightfold after glucose loading. A hypothetical glucose tolerance test result is shown in Figure 19.3.
Glycosylated haemoglobin (HbA$_{1c}$)	Serum	HbA$_{1c}$ measures long-term glucose control and is an indicator of how well diabetics are managing their disease. Non-diabetic: 2.2–4.8% Good diabetic control: 2.5–5.9% Fair diabetic control: 6–8% Poor diabetic control: > 8%
Sorbitol and/or fructosamine	Saliva, serum	Diagnostic tests for diabetes, monitoring effectiveness of therapy.[34]
Cortisol	Serum, urine, saliva	Cortisol is subject to diurnal variations, being highest in the morning and lowest at night. The best time for measuring cortisol levels in serum are early morning and again around 4 pm. Night-time or 24- hour urinary cortisol, or repeat salivary samples, may even be more advantageous.[35]
Lipid studies	Serum	Triglycerides > 1.81 and 1.52 mmol/L, and HDL < 0.75 and 0.91 mmol/L in males and females, respectively, are indicative of diabetes type 2 or metabolic syndrome.
Liver profile	Serum	Elevations in alanine aminotransferase (ALT) have been found in insulin resistance and metabolic syndrome.[36]
CRP, erythrocyte sedimentation rate (ESR) (inflammatory markers)	Serum	The ideal range for CRP and ESR is < 1. Elevation, even if still within the normal range, is indicative of inflammation, with the level of these markers proportional to the degree of inflammation.
Homocysteine	Serum	Homocysteine is an inflammatory amino acid produced in the methylation cycle. It is commonly elevated in metabolic and heart diseases.[37] Ideal range is < 10.
Active B12	Serum	Active B12 (holotranscobalamin) has been termed the best and earliest indicator of impending vitamin B12 deficiency.[38] It needs to be > 35 pmol/L.
Folate	RBC	Folate and vitamin B12 are both needed in the homocysteine-methionine (methylation) cycle. Values differ markedly between laboratories.
Vitamin D	Serum	Despite the high amount of sunshine, vitamin D deficiency is high in Australia. It is needed for insulin secretion and found to be low in people not receiving much sunlight on their skin.[39] Both the inactive (25-hydroxyvitamin D) and the active (1,25-dihydroxyvitamin D) forms can be measured. Ideal values for vitamins are in the upper half of the reference range. For 25-hydroxyvitamin D ideally values should be above 100 nmol/L.
Thyroid-stimulating hormone (TSH)	Serum	Hypothyroidism is present when THS is elevated. It may explain some people's inability to lose weight. However, subtle elevations (> 2.5 mIU/L) within the reference range (0.4–5.0 mIU/L) could indicate a 'labouring' thyroid or a subclinical hypothyroid state.[40,41]

Source: Pagana & Pagana 2006[42]

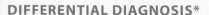

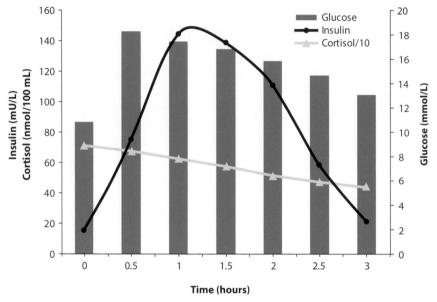

Figure 19.3

Hypothetical three-hour glucose tolerance test with hyperglycaemia, hyperinsulinaemia, insulin resistance and hypercortisolism

RISK FACTORS

Although diabetes type 2 is currently predominantly a disease of the developed nations it is estimated that the largest rise is expected in the developing economies[45] due to a trend towards Western-type foods.[46] A diet high in refined and simple carbohydrates and human-modulated fats, and low in fibre, antioxidants and polyunsaturated fatty acids, especially omega-3 (due to increased availability and affordability of convenience and snack food), stress and a sedentary lifestyle have contributed to the increase in obesity and, with that, insulin resistance and metabolic syndrome.[47] Further, as a result of the 'fat-free fad', carbohydrate-based substances (such as olestra) have been added to food to make it more palatable, adding to the overall carbohydrate load. And the more carbohydrates are consumed the more insulin is required for its metabolism.

Gestational diabetes is not only a major risk factor for developing diabetes type 2 later in life[48] but also for birth defects and infant mortality.[49] Low blood levels of vitamin D has been found in children with diabetes type 2, with increased markers of cardio-metabolic risks.[50] Peripheral neuropathy and retinopathy are common in diabetes and have been associated with vitamin D deficiency.[51,52] The former is also linked to vitamin B12 deficiency.[53] Low vitamin D and calcium[54] as well as magnesium[55] have also been associated with higher risk of diabetes type 2.

This disease process brings with it a number of other risk factors, notably in cardio-vascular health. Hypertension and dyslipidaemia are commonly encountered and in fact are part of metabolic syndrome. The derangement of steroid hormones, including sex hormones and dehydroepiandrosterone (see Figure 18.3 in Chapter 18 on stress and fatigue), can lead to lack of libido, erectile dysfunction and prostate problems in men, and menstrual irregularities, infertility and exacerbation of hormonal symptoms in women. Non-alcoholic fatty liver disease[56] and decreased lung function[57] are also commonly encountered in this condition.

Another concomitant effect of obesity and insulin resistance is changes in body composition, with increased fat-mass and decreased lean body mass, leading to sarcopenia. Although a condition of old age, it has been shown that diabetics are more prone to sarcopenia than non-diabetics.[58] It has been suggested that insulin resistance is responsible for the inability to increase lean muscle mass from protein intake and synthesis.[59] Due to the reduced life quality that accompanies any chronic health problem and possibly the decreased feelings of self-worth from being overweight, depression and anxiety should also be considered. Yet depression may play a role in the aetiology of stress and metabolic syndrome, too (see also Chapter 15 on depression).

CONVENTIONAL MEDICATION

It is now commonly accepted that diet and lifestyle need to be considered in order to control this disease.[40] A number of diets have been recommended; however, no definitive dietary approach has been established (see later this chapter).

Medications

In addition, medical treatment aims to regulate blood sugar to gain control of diabetes type 2. The drugs mentioned here are only suitable if there is some function left in the pancreatic β-cells; otherwise insulin needs to be given. In the first instance, biguanides (such as metformin) will be prescribed. The supposed mechanisms include reduced gluconeogenesis and increased insulin sensitivity. A possible side effect of this drug is pernicious anaemia. Therefore, vitamin B12 (active B12) should be measured regularly, and if found to decline or be low, vitamin B12 treatment via monthly intramuscular injections should be initiated.[60]

Sulphonylureas are recommended to enhance the secretion of insulin in response to blood glucose. However, care needs to be taken in patients with liver or kidney disease. They also promote weight gain and are therefore not ideal in metabolic syndrome.

Another treatment option is α-glucosidase inhibitors. This class of drugs reduces the breakdown of carbohydrates in the intestines by inhibiting the enzymes involved in this process, thus reducing the rise in blood sugar levels following a meal. They are therefore useful in obesity. However, the remaining carbohydrates are likely to be fermented in the gastrointestinal tract, leading to unwelcome side effects such as bloating and flatulence. The glitazones (thiazolidinediones) reduce hyperinsulinaemia but have no direct effect on glucose. Their beneficial action in diabetes type 2 may be the lowering of free fatty acids, therefore increasing muscular glucose usage.

Various combinations of these drugs, notably metformin with sulphonylureas, are currently used, particularly when good glucose control (as assessed by HbA_{1c} levels) is not achieved by one drug alone. Only as a last resort will insulin be used for diabetes type 2. Cardiovascular risk factors are commonly controlled by blood pressure and lipid-lowering medication (see Chapters 11–13 on the cardiovascular system).

Additional support

Diabetes type 2 is a disease where patients need to not only take medications but also be actively involved in their treatment in order to achieve optimal glycaemic control and reduce the risk of comorbidities. Prerequisites for this are the patients' understanding and willingness to cooperate. A range of wellness literature has been produced to educate patients on managing their disease. The internet provides a plethora of guidelines and suggestions regarding lifestyle and dietary changes, glucose control, available medications and self-monitoring of progress.[61–63] Diabetes educators do their best to motivate and encourage, and various programs and initiatives have been implemented.[9,64] However, in

---

Diabetes type 1

Pathogenesis and conventional treatment for diabetes type 1

Diabetes type 1 is primarily an autoimmune disease where the β-cells of the pancreas, which produce insulin, are destroyed by leucocyte infiltration.[69] The starting age is usually during childhood or adolescence. The disease is characterised mainly by ketoacidosis with the typical acetone-breath, polyuria with resultant thirst, postural hypotension and anorexia due to uncontrolled hyperglycaemia, which interferes with electrolyte and osmotic balance. This is a catabolic disease with elevated glucagon and muscle wasting due to gluconeogenesis, and can lead to coma and death if untreated. Lifelong exogenous insulin by injection is the usual treatment. In recent years the transplant of a whole pancreas or pancreatic islet cells has been trialled, with several patients not requiring insulin for some time after the procedure, but cytotoxic drugs are then needed for life.[40] This treatment is still in its infancy and not yet common practice. Diagnosis is made from either urine or fasting blood glucose levels. Reference ranges are the same as for diabetes type 2. A glucose tolerance test may be performed to corroborate the results of the urine or blood test. To ascertain long-term control, HbA_{1c} will be measured every three to six months.

Acute diabetic complications include hypoglycaemia due to too much insulin administration, which can lead to coma. Long-term complications involve damage to the micro- and macrovascular systems, nervous tissue, skin and eyes and are the result of fluctuations in blood sugar levels that are part of the disease picture. Common conditions include cataracts, retinopathy leading to blindness, nephropathy leading to renal failure, neuropathy, myocardial infarction and stroke and gangrene of the feet leading to amputations.

Treatment protocols and potential adjunctive interventions for diabetes type 1*

A nutritious, balanced diet with regular meals is recommended. Sugar needs to be restricted. The use of artificial sweeteners, so often recommended as sugar substitutes and considered safe for people with diabetes, may have harmful effects long term and should be avoided or at least limited. Vitamin D deficiency has been linked to the pathogenesis of autoimmune diseases, including diabetes type 1.[13,70] Early intervention with vitamin D may be able to arrest the pro-inflammatory cytokine production and therefore avoid or alleviate the disease if supplementation is commenced early (although not currently proven). Oxidative stress is part of diabetes type 1 and its complications, and antioxidants should be considered.[71,72] Lipoic acid is particularly beneficial for preventing and treating diabetic complications.[73] It has also been used, in conjunction with vitamin E, in diabetic neuropathy.[74] For glaucoma and raised intraocular pressure, high-dose vitamin C, lipoic acid, vitamin B12, magnesium, melatonin, *Ginkgo biloba* and *Coleus forskohlii* have been suggested.[75] Essential fatty acids (EFAs) have also been shown to play a role in diabetes type 1.[72,76]

*In conjunction with insulin, not as a replacement

Sources: Gropper et al. 2009[32] and Manders et al. 2012[59]

---

order to stay focused on treatment goals such as diet and exercise, emotional and social support from family and peers is paramount.[65] Individual and cultural preferences need to be catered for in order to make lasting changes.[66–68]

KEY TREATMENT PROTOCOLS

Management of diabetes 2 (or metabolic syndrome) needs to be a multipronged approach, including stress management, dietary and lifestyle changes, exercise and nutritional and herbal supplements. Although several specific diets have been examined in diabetic patients, diets are always more clinically effective if individualised to the patient,[77] so the focus should be on dietary improvement rather than strict and inflexible recommendations for any particular diet. Patients are more motivated to use self-care and more likely to seek alternative treatments, including the ones described below, if medication alone is not able to satisfactorily control the disease.[78] Those under naturopathic care tend to have greater motivation for implementing lifestyle and diet changes as well as improved self-monitoring, leading to better overall metabolic control (and therefore quality of life).[79,80]

Modify lifestyle and diet

Fat-weight loss, even if it is small, is paramount and has resulted in greater insulin sensitivity, lower blood pressure and improved lipid profile, thus reducing risk factors for both diabetes type 2 and heart disease.[1] A hypocaloric diet rather than a total fast has been advocated, together with physical exercise and reduction in alcohol consumption.[6] With calorie restriction, a vegetarian diet has been shown to be superior to a conventional diabetic diet regarding reductions in visceral fat, diabetic medication, adiponectin and insulin resistance and increases in leptin and antioxidant status.[81] These lifestyle changes, although superior to drug treatment, are sometimes difficult to achieve and an extensive healthcare program needs to be initiated to prevent relapse.[6] A slow reduction in weight seems to be better than rapid weight-loss diets for lasting success as the weight is more likely to stay off. **Protein** needs to be emphasised as there is often a reduction in lean body mass due to the gluconeogenic effects of raised cortisol.

There has been much debate regarding the best diet for this condition: high complex-carbohydrate/low-fat (HC/LF) or high-protein/low-carbohydrate diet (HP/LC), or anything in between.[82–84] It is posited that the HP/LC diet may be too high in saturated fats due to its high meat content and hence contribute to increased calorie consumption. Although weight loss after one year seems to be the same on either diet, the HC/LF dieters tend to have a better low-density lipoprotein (LDL) profile. However, the HP/LC diet has led to greater fat loss, reduced blood glucose levels and improved triglyceride, HDL and blood pressure values.[82,85–87] Another advantage of a **low-carbohydrate diet** lies in its reduced insulin requirements. Further, there is evidence that some animal fats (in dairy and meat), particularly conjugated linoleic acid, can have a protective effect on obesity, diabetes, heart disease and cancer.[88–90] With the low-fat diet recommendations, apparently people now consume less than half the amount of conjugated linoleic acid needed to reap the benefits.[91]

The beneficial effects of **fish consumption**, especially those with high omega-3 content, on cardiovascular risk factors are well known. However, one recent research publication suggests that long-chain omega-3 fatty acids in amounts greater than 200 mg or two serves of fish per day may expose people to an increased risk of diabetes type 2.[92] Monounsaturated fatty acids (MUFA—such as those found in olive oil) have also drawn attention in conjunction with the Mediterranean diet. A systematic review of diets high in MUFA found significant differences in HbA_{1c} in overweight, insulin-resistant and diabetes type 2 patients compared with controls.[93]

Care needs to be taken, too, with low-fat products as the fat is often replaced with carbohydrates or a 'fat substitute' that may have other nutritional consequences (e.g. reducing the absorption of fat-soluble vitamins).[94] Believing that this is a low-fat (= 'healthy') food, people may tend to eat more, thus making up the calories. Yet fat ingestion as part of the normal diet serves another purpose: cholecystokinin is released in response to fat in the meal, creating a feeling of satiety.

Fasting may be another option to improve glucose control, with small trials indicating clinical benefit for patients with diabetes.[95] Studies of diabetics during Ramadan indicate that most diabetic patients observe clinical improvement during fasting, though a small minority may have adverse events due to fluctuating blood glucose levels.[96,97] As such, fasting can be considered a clinically useful recommendation, though appropriate monitoring should be ensured.

In order to achieve a feeling of satiety without overindulging in calorie-rich foods, **fibre** needs to be an essential dietary constituent of every person attempting to lose weight.[83] Fibre will bind fats and lower the absorption of glucose through delaying gastric emptying. Studies with psyllium hulls (***Plantago ovata***) have shown significant reductions in fasting plasma glucose, cholesterol, LDL and triglycerides, and elevations in HDL.[98,99] Similar results have been achieved with flax seed powder (***Linum usitatissimum***).[100] However, care needs to be taken as too much of it will reduce nutrient absorption and can lead to flatulence.

Data from the Nurses' Health Study indicate that higher intake of bioflavonoids, in particular **anthocyanidin**-containing foods such as blueberries, have a protective effect regarding the development of diabetes type 2.[101]

Artificial sweeteners have been used extensively in the food industry for several decades to replace sugar in food items as their metabolism does not depend on insulin. These products have therefore been advocated to people with diabetes as safe to use. However, evidence suggests that the use of fructose (particularly high-fructose corn syrup) and sorbitol are involved in diabetic complications. This has been known for at least 35 years and yet these sweeteners are still in use today.[30,102,103] It is also known that countries, like the United States, that have high consumption of high-fructose corn syrup have higher incidence of diabetes type 2.[104] These substances should therefore be avoided.

Since modern foods play a big role in obesity people may not be knowledgeable regarding food choice and its impact on health.[105] **Diet plans**[106] and **education via cooking classes**[107] have shown to improve nutrient intake for type 2 diabetics. There is evidence that the Mediterranean diet can reduce the incidence of diabetes type 2 and favourably affect cardiovascular profile, even without influencing weight.[108–110] The DASH (Dietary Approaches to Stop Hypertension) diet has been suggested to decrease the risk of cardiovascular complications in young people with diabetes.[111]

Overall, the current recommendations still lean towards a high carbohydrate (45–60%) with up to 10% as sucrose, moderate fat (up to 35%) and low protein (10–20%) intake. Additional micronutrient intake (other than from food) is not recommended.[112] The reason for such an approach is that apparently high-quality research does not exist for other interventions. This approach disregards any scientific evidence collected in ways other than large clinical trials.

Increase physical activity and exercise

The positive influence of exercise on glucose control cannot be over-emphasised,[6] as a plethora of literature on this topic testifies. It facilitates the uptake of glucose into the cells and lowers insulin resistance, apart from the beneficial effect on body composition. Even small daily tasks, such as getting up to change the TV channel or taking the stairs rather than the lift, will be beneficial.[113]

In insulin resistance and diabetes type 2, high levels of fatty acids are stored in skeletal muscle, with exercise being able to reduce this through β-oxidation (fat burning), thus lowering triglycerides and improving glucose control.[114] For people with impaired fasting glucose, before the development of diabetes type 2, even greater benefits can be achieved, as seen in improvements in glycolysis, aerobic metabolism, β-oxidation and mitochondrial biogenesis.[115]

In particular, strength training maximises fat loss and minimises the loss of lean body mass, which usually accompanies weight loss diets.[2] Sarcopenia is common in people with diabetes, particularly in the elderly.[116] Since it is the muscles that utilise glucose to produce energy, lack of muscle mass further promotes the disease process. Low-volume high-intensity interval training also appears to be one of the most effective forms of exercise for diabetic patients.[117]

Tai Chi has been shown to significantly improve glycaemic control and lower triglyceride levels in Chinese diabetic women.[118] In a six-month trial in Korea those people adhering to the activity schedule experienced much better glucose control and quality of life.[119] Similarly, **Qi-Gong** has helped with diabetes control by improving psychological, physiological and metabolic markers.[120,121] However, as with any lifestyle modification in general, and exercise in particular, it is important that people make a commitment and adhere to it long term. As these changes usually have a glucose-lowering effect, blood glucose needs to be monitored carefully regarding possible hypoglycaemia, and medication may need to be adjusted.[116]

Diabetic foot care

'Diabetic foot' is the umbrella term for the numerous foot problems in people with diabetes that arise from arterial complications and peripheral neuropathy. This combination can lead in turn to poor circulation, poor wound healing and eventual ulcer development. Therapies such as corrective footwear, diabetic socks and regular podiatrist review are encouraged, as well as hyperbaric oxygen and various wound management techniques when or if ulceration does occur. However, one of the best patient recommendations may simply be that of increased vigilance—studies suggest that increasing awareness of the issue is effective in reducing serious lesions. Simple tips such as testing shoe tightness with the fingers to reduce pressure—which many patients may not be aware of, due to neuropathy—may stave off serious issues in the future. Improving circulation may also reduce the possibility of ulcer formation by improving wound-healing ability. Considering that 10–15% of people with diabetes can expect complications, that over half of diabetic hospital admissions are related to foot complications and that diabetes is the most common reason for medical amputation, these recommendations need to be an integral part of diabetic patient management.

Sources: Giurini & Lyons 2005[122] and Watkins 2003[123]

Reduce risk factors, increase insulin release and receptor sensitivity and reduce hyperinsulinaemia

The precursor to diabetes type 2 is insulin resistance and compensatory hyperinsulinaemia. Although insulin is overproduced and secreted by the pancreas it is not facilitating glucose uptake into the cell. Fat loss has increased insulin sensitivity and should be pursued.[58] Certain nutrients and herbs can aid insulin sensitivity, therefore reducing hyperinsulinaemia.

Nutritional interventions

A whole range of vitamins, minerals, amino acids and bioactive substances have been explored in the treatment of diabetes type 2 and insulin resistance. Nutrients that have shown a positive effect include **vitamins** A, B1, B3 and biotin, the **minerals** calcium, potassium, zinc and manganese, and fructo-oligosaccharides. Some **amino acids**, such as taurine (needed for liver detoxification pathways and control of heart rhythm and blood pressure) and L-arginine (for nitric oxide production to maintain endothelial function) may also help.[3,4,32,72,83] However, there are nutrients that are very specific for diabetes type 2, as demonstrated below.

Most animals produce their own **vitamin C** from glucose. The two molecules are structurally similar, and competition for cellular uptake between vitamin C and glucose has been suggested as a possible mechanism by which this vitamin exerts its positive influence on glucose metabolism. Further, vitamin C is needed to stimulate the release of insulin following glucose ingestion. As little as 500 mg a day has been shown to be effective. Vitamin C also acts as an antioxidant, reduces blood pressure and protects blood vessels.[4]

Chromium is needed to facilitate the entry of glucose into the cells by stimulating insulin uptake and enhancing its activity (Figure 19.2).[32] Supplementation has had a beneficial effect on metabolic syndrome by lowering fasting blood glucose (FBG), postprandial glucose (PPG) and corresponding insulin levels, and by improving insulin sensitivity, HbA_{1c} values and lipid profiles. Increased benefits have been noted with higher doses.[83,124] Another possible effect of chromium is its action on down-regulating pancreatic β-cell activity, thus increasing glucagon levels.[125] However, in other research daily chromium (as picolinate) supplementation of up to 1000 μg for six months has failed to show any improvement in risk factors for insulin resistance and impaired glucose tolerance.[126]

Magnesium is essential for all reactions requiring energy as it is needed to stabilise *adenosine triphosphate* (ATP). Low levels have been found in cardiovascular disease and diabetes, and in people with high alcohol intake. Normalisation through supplementation of up to 400 mg/day has enhanced insulin sensitivity, reduced fasting glucose and improved HbA_{1c}.[32,127] Trials with small amounts of magnesium have yielded mixed results. However, reductions in FBG and HbA_{1c}, and increases in postprandial insulin, glucose uptake and glucose oxidation have been noted.[124]

Urinary (and with that whole body) **zinc** losses have been noticed in diabetes type 1 and 2, presumably due to hyperglycaemia and accompanying polyuria. Zinc is needed for insulin metabolism as well as intracellular antioxidant systems, and hence its lack has been associated with diabetic complications.[128] To increase its effectiveness as oral agent a novel complex with a garlic extract has been trialled in mice, which led to significant improvements in diabetic and cardiovascular parameters, together with an increase in adiponectin.[129]

Enhanced insulin sensitivity with reductions in FBG, HbA_{1c} and hepatic glucose production and better insulin-mediated glucose uptake have been found with **vanadium**.[124] Vanadium mimics the action of insulin, as seen by its similar effects on the translocation of GLUT4 to the cell membrane.[32] Care needs to be taken as high doses are toxic. **Coenzyme Q10** has been shown to reduce blood glucose, hyperinsulinaemia, high blood pressure, triglycerides and lipid peroxidation.[4] It is particularly important for people on statin drugs as some of these have a depleting effect on this nutrient.[130] **N-acetyl carnitine**, made from lysine by methylation, is instrumental in the transport of fatty acids across the mitochondrial membrane for β-oxidation. It is therefore essential for energy production from fat burning.[72] Administration of this nutrient has enhanced glucose uptake, storage and utilisation and insulin sensitivity.[124] A relatively high amount, above 3 g/day, is needed to achieve these effects.

Vitamin E tends to decrease HbA_{1c}, FBG and PPG.[124] There may be benefit in **vitamin D** supplementation, especially in children, to reduce cardiometabolic risk factors.[48] High-dose vitamin D supplementation has been shown to improve insulin sensitivity in people with impaired fasting glucose and thus delay the onset of diabetes.[131] The bioactive nutrient α-**lipoic acid** is both water and fat soluble and has been shown to enhance cellular glucose uptake and utilisation. In conjunction with exercise, this nutrient has been shown to enhance glucose transport and insulin signalling in skeletal muscle cells.[132] As little as 300 mg per day over eight weeks has reduced fasting and post-prandial glucose, insulin resistance and glutathione peroxidase significantly in diabetes type 2 patients.[133]

Supplementing with branched-chain amino acids, especially **leucine**, may counteract the catabolic effects of insulin resistance due to its insulinotropic action and therefore increase muscle protein synthesis and improve glycaemic control. More research is needed to confirm these findings.[57,134]

Herbal medicines

In diabetes type 2, insulin resistance and metabolic syndrome, a range of herbal supplements have been proven to be of help in blood glucose and insulin regulation.[135] In particular, bitters have been indicated.[136] *Galega officinalis* allegedly increases the action of insulin. Its active ingredient, galegine, was used as a model for metformin.[124,137] *Coccinia indica* (ivy gourd) seems to mimic the action of insulin, *Bauhinia forficata* (Pata de Vaca) has been dubbed 'vegetable insulin', *Allium sativum* and *Allium cepa* can decrease fasting serum glucose as well as exerting a beneficial effect on cardiovascular risk factors, *Opuntia streptacantha* (prickly pear) has reportedly insulin sensitising properties and *Aloe vera* juice has hypoglycaemic effects.[124,137] **Berberis-containing herbs** have shown regulatory effects not only on glucose control but also on cardiovascular pathology.[136] *Coleus forskohlii* has putative beneficial effects on insulin resistance and diabetes type 2. *Inula racemosa* has shown increased insulin sensitivity in an animal model,[3] and *Ocimum sanctum* is effective in lowering FBG, PPG and glucosuria.[124,137] The use of *Cinnamomum cassia* can potentiate the action of insulin.[138]

Gymnema sylvestre has glucose-lowering ability without causing hypoglycaemia. Decreases in FBG, HbA_{1c} and urinary glucose excretion have been found, leading to a reduced need for conventional medication. *Gymnema sylvestre* is thought to delay glucose uptake in the small intestines, and through its restorative action on β-cells the release of insulin from the pancreas has been increased.[124,139] Lipid studies have also shown favourable effects.[140] If given at least 30 minutes before eating, it reduces appetite and the cravings for sweets by anaesthetising the taste buds (1–2 mL). Therefore it may aid in weight loss.[137] *Gymnema sylvestre* therefore has the ability to affect a number of factors linked to the aetiology and pathophysiology of diabetes type 2 simultaneously, something that no other single hypoglycaemic agent is able to exert.[140]

The various forms of **ginseng** (*Panax ginseng*, *Panax quinquefolium* and *Eleuthero-coccus senticosus*) have beneficial effects in diabetes type 2.[124] Decreases in PPG, FBG and HbA$_{1c}$ have been noted with *Panax quinquefolium*.[124,141] Supplementation with **Trigonella foenum-graecum** has led to lowered FBG, PPG, postprandial insulin, urine glucose and carbohydrate absorption, with modulation of peripheral glucose utilisation, thus increasing glycaemic control.[124,137] **Momordica charantia** (bitter melon) has hypoglycaemic (both for PPG and FBG) and antidiabetic effects. It has the ability to: stimulate the pancreas to release insulin; increase glucose uptake, glycogen synthesis and glucose oxidation; and decrease hepatic gluconeogenesis.[124,137,139]

Tinospora cordifolia can avert blood sugar elevation by reducing glycogenolysis (the breakdown of glycogen to form free glucose) from liver and muscle, therefore preventing excess lactic acid being converted to glucose in the liver and increasing glucose utilisation in muscle tissue.[139] The Indian herb **Salacia oblonga** has been used in trials to treat diabetes and it was found to be as effective as prescription drugs.[142] Apart from working as an antioxidant by restoring glutathione levels, **Silybum marianum** can lower blood and urinary glucose and HbA$_{1c}$. It also has beneficial effects on insulin, lowering its requirement.[124] In other studies, the positive effect was mainly on diabetic complications and lipid parameters.[136]

Reduce immune system activation and inflammation

Inflammation plays an important part in the pathophysiology of chronic and lifestyle-induced diseases such as diabetes type 2, and **polyunsaturated fatty acids** (PUFAs) play an important role in regulating pro-inflammatory cytokines.[143,144] Not only the omega-3 but also the omega-6 series have positive effects, leading to anti-inflammatory prostaglandin E$_3$ and E$_1$, respectively. Low levels of γ-linolenic acid have been found in type 2 diabetics due to the reduced activity of the enzymes delta 5 and delta 6 desaturase,[143,145] as insulin is needed for their activation.[146] Research has therefore focused on the beneficial effects of fish oils to bypass these enzymes. In addition to the triglyceride-lowering and anti-inflammatory effects that have been noted with the administration of fish oils,[31,83] reductions in serum lipids, lipoproteins, platelet aggregation and blood pressure and increases in cell membrane fluidity have been found.[144,147]

Due to the inflammatory component of metabolic syndrome, antioxidants are paramount. **Vitamin E** has been investigated with mixed results regarding its effects on inflammation, diabetes and heart disease.[83] However, antioxidants need to be administered in conjunction with each other due to their mutual recycling. It is important, too, to use mixed tocopherols, not the synthetic d-α-tocopherol.

Oxidative stress is increased postprandially, and **antioxidant** supplementation, consisting of **N-acetylcysteine** (NAC) and vitamin E and C, has exerted endothelial protection in people with impaired glucose tolerance.[148] NAC has beneficial effects in insulin resistance due to its antioxidant properties[149] and being a cofactor for glutathione production. Cysteine, complexed with chromium, has shown superior anti-inflammatory and insulin resistance-lowering properties as well as regulation of various metabolic markers than either of these nutrients on their own. Vitamin C further enhances this effect.[150,151]

Vitamin D plays a role in immune modulation and insulin secretion. There are correlations between insulin resistance, diabetes type 2 and heart disease, and supplementation of 1000 IU/day or more (regardless of body status) has shown to improve these parameters.[13,39,72,152] Chronic immune activation, as is the case in obesity, increases **tryptophan** breakdown, potentially leading to serotonin deficit and symptoms of mood disorder, depression and impaired satiety. The latter increases caloric intake, especially from carbohydrates, perpetuating a vicious circle.[153]

Reduce stress

Stress increases cortisol through HPA axis activation (see Chapter 18 on stress and fatigue). Elevated cortisol promotes visceral adiposity, insulin resistance and loss of glycaemic control,[154,155] therefore contributing to metabolic syndrome.[23,156] The vicious cycle of visceral fat storage, gluconeogenesis from muscle protein and increased demand for insulin with resultant increase in cortisol promotes carbohydrate cravings, which in turn leads to further abdominal fat gain. To break this cycle stress management is paramount. The following herbs not only have adaptogenic properties with balancing effects on stress hormones, they also have shown direct benefits in treating insulin resistance and diabetes type 2.

Eleutherococcus senticosus is known for its adaptogenic properties during stress. It is used during periods of fatigue and debility. It has shown positive effects on blood pressure, total and LDL cholesterol, triglycerides and glucose. There may be reduction of stress-related symptoms and faster recovery in chronic illness due to increased aerobic metabolism.[157] Due to its potential hypoglycaemic effects, people with diabetes should monitor their blood glucose levels when taking this herb.[141] *Panax ginseng* is another adaptogen used in stress, in chronic diseases and to replenish depleted energy stores.[136] The rate of carbohydrate absorption is reduced, with increased glucose uptake, transport and storage in the form of glycogen. Insulin secretions can be modulated.[124] Although small drops in blood glucose have been reported, Mills and Bone[136] claim that further results in diabetes can only be achieved when the herb has been injected.

Prevent/address diabetic complications

Despite medication, chronic elevations and fluctuations in blood glucose in both diabetes type 1 and 2 cannot be avoided entirely. Oxidative stress and inflammation have been found not only in people with diabetes but also in obese people and those with insulin resistance. This, plus the increase in free fatty acids, and possibly other metabolites, is responsible for the oxidative stress that leads to diabetic complications such as damage to the nerves, the vascular endothelium and the kidneys. Various antioxidant treatments have been used to alleviate oxidative damage and thus delay or prevent these complications.[71,149,158]

Nutritional interventions

EFAs, including **evening primrose oil**, can alleviate diabetic complications due to their anti-inflammatory properties (as outlined earlier).[136,147] **NAC** has been recommended as being useful to alleviate oxidative stress.[149,158] It is the limiting amino acid for glutathione production, and whey is an excellent source of this nutrient.[159] Supplementation with either whey or NAC may therefore increase the availability of the endogenous antioxidant glutathione.

Vitamin E improves the action of other antioxidants, especially vitamin C and glutathione. It reduces LDL and the risk of cardiovascular complications of insulin resistance. It may help to preserve pancreatic β-cells. Since vitamin E works closely with **selenium** in endogenous antioxidant systems, the combined use has resulted in greater benefits.[4] Its use in nephropathy has resulted in decreased microalbuminaemia due to reductions in thromboxane A_2.[160]

The renin-angiotensin system is crucial in the development of diabetic nephropathy. It is negatively regulated by **vitamin D**, which suppresses renin expression. Research on mice has shown a protective effect of vitamin D on the renal system by modulating the renin-angiotensin system.[161] The active form of vitamin B6, **pyridoxal 5'-phosphate**, has been shown in rats to prevent advanced glycation endproducts being formed, thus favourably influencing diabetic nephropathy. This may yet prove to be a valuable treatment in this condition for people with diabetes.[162]

The mechanism by which α-**lipoic acid** exerts its benefits in diabetes is thought to be due to its ability to facilitate the translocation of GLUT4 to the cell membrane, in readiness for glucose uptake into the cell.[73] It also prevents or reduces diabetic complications resulting from oxidative damage,[163] such as cataract formation, polyneuropathy and damage to blood vessels. As an antioxidant it also helps to recycle other antioxidants, such as vitamins C and E, and glutathione.[4,73,124]

Diabetic neuropathy is characterised by demyelinisation with resultant reductions in nerve conduction velocity.[164] A review[74] found that α-lipoic acid in conjunction with vitamin E reduced diabetic neuropathy and corrected nerve conduction velocity. Although some conflicting data exists regarding what exactly α-lipoic acid improves in diabetic neuropathy, there is no doubt that it does have a beneficial effect in this condition.[165] Its application is safe and effective.[166]

Sorbitol accumulation in cells is known to contribute to diabetic complications. **Vitamin C** at 1000 mg per day has shown to have a beneficial effect by reducing aldose reductase activity and therefore positively influencing the development or progression of any diabetic complications, despite fasting plasma glucose levels remaining unchanged.[167] One of the most troublesome symptoms of diabetic neuropathy is pain. **Acetyl-L-carnitine** at a daily dose of 1000 mg has been effective in regenerating nerve fibres and significantly reducing pain.[168] Vitamin B12, in its coenzyme form of **methylcobalamin**, has been injected intrathecally (injection into the subarachnoid space) with dramatic improvements in leg pain, heaviness and paresthesia (tingling, numbness and pins and needles).[169] This suggests that vitamin B12 deficiency plays a role in diabetic neuropathy.

Herbal medicines

Silybum marianum has been trialled in diabetes type 2 due to its antioxidant profile and beneficial effects on diabetes. An improvement in glycaemic control has been found which could reduce the risk of diabetic complications.[170] *Gymnema sylvestre* has wide-ranging actions on blood glucose metabolism and is therefore able to alleviate a range of diabetic complications, including cardiovascular risk factors such as hypertension, hyperlipidaemia and atherosclerosis, and the diabetic complications trio nephropathy, neuropathy and retinopathy, as well as susceptibility to infection and erectile dysfunction.[140] Not only blood glucose levels but also endogenous antioxidants were normalised and lipid peroxidation reduced in diabetic rats following administration of an ethanolic gymnema extract.[171] In diabetic patients with nephropathy, *Curcuma longa* has shown to reduce proteinuria.[172]

Leg ulcers are a common complication of diabetes and are often difficult to heal. *Aesculus hippocastanum*, due to its venous toning, antioxidant and anti-inflammatory effects, has been used to treat this condition.[173] Significant improvements have been noted in wound slough and in reduced necessity to change wound dressings.[174,175] Diabetic retinopathy has been treated with traditional Chinese medicine and antioxidants.

Chinese 'yin-nourishing, kidney-tonifying and blood-activating' herbs have been used to enhance blood flow to the eyes, resulting in improved visual acuity.[176] However, there have been no conclusive trials as yet on the use of antioxidants in this condition,[177–179] although it would be reasonable to concur that antioxidants are called for since this condition is the result of oxidative damage.

Similarly, nephropathy is thought to be a result of oxidative stress. Several combinations of **traditional Chinese herbal medicine** remedies to nourish Qi, together with Western medicine, have been used with good results.[180,181] A traditional Chinese medicine formulation to remove blood stasis, stomach heat and heart fire, while supporting the stomach and kidneys, has proven superior to drug treatment.[182] Another study[183] used a combination of *Fructus arctii* and *Astragalus membranaceus,* which reduced proteinuria and albuminuria and improved blood glucose and lipids. ***Ginkgo biloba*** is known as an antioxidant, circulatory stimulant and neuroprotectant,[136] and its use in diabetic nephropathy seems therefore logical. In the early stages of the disease *Ginkgo biloba* has been found to be effective in increasing renal function with resultant decreased albuminuria and other improvements.[184,185] Benefits have also been shown with *Ginkgo biloba* in respect to intercellular and vascular adhesion molecules.[186]

Address comorbidities

Insulin resistance, diabetes type 2, heart disease and metabolic syndrome are closely related. Due to insulin resistance, the risk of heart disease is increased in diabetes type 2 as part of the metabolic syndrome.[37] Hypertension and dyslipidaemia (high triglycerides, high LDL and low HDL) are part of the symptom picture in metabolic syndrome and need to be addressed conjointly with insulin resistance and diabetes type 2.[1,2] Refer to Chapters 11–13 on the cardiovascular system for more detailed interventions.

Nutritional interventions

EFAs prevent organ damage in diabetes type 2[76] through their effect on dyslipidaemia and the ability to lower triglycerides, blood pressure and atherogenesis.[144] Dietary omega-3 polyunsaturated fatty acids (fish oils) have exerted beneficial effects in dyslipidaemia and cardiovascular disease.[187] Brain function has been improved on omega-3 fatty acids,[31] evidenced by the fact that people with diabetes type 2 have reported less depression when supplementing with omega-3 fatty acids. This may be linked to the beneficial effects that omega-3 fatty acids have on cardiovascular disease.[188]

Vitamin B12 and **folate** are both needed for the remethylation of homocysteine to methionine (the universal methyl group donor). **Vitamin B6** facilitates the breakdown of homocysteine via the transsulphuration pathway.[32] Together, they are needed to reduce homocysteine levels, which can pose an independent risk factor for heart disease and diabetes type 2.[37] Some research has cast doubt on the link of homocysteine to heart disease. However, the fact remains that it is also linked to reduced bioavailability of nitric oxide, therefore indirectly effecting cardiovascular disease.[189]

A derivative of vitamin B5, **pantethine**, has shown promising results in preventing diabetes-induced angiopathy due to its triglyceride, lipid and apolipoprotein-lowering effects.[190] It is particularly useful in dyslipidaemia when this is not amenable to dietary or other means.[191] **Broccoli sprouts** powder at 10 g/day has favourably influenced lipid profiles in diabetes type 2 patients by significantly decreasing serum triglycerides, the ratio of oxidised LDL to LDL and the atherogenic index of plasma (calculated from triglycerides, cholesterol and HDL).[192]

Herbal medicines

One of the early manifestations of heart disease is hypertension. This can be improved by ***Crataegus monogyna***. This herb has also shown benefits in other areas of heart disease, such as congestive heart failure[136] and decreased cardiac output, circulatory disturbances and arrhythmias.[141] ***Coleus forskohlii*** has blood pressure lowering as well as platelet-inhibiting effects.[136] ***Trigonella foenum-graecum***, apart from its beneficial effects on blood glucose, has been shown to lower atherosclerotic parameters.[136] Similarly, ***Cynara scolymus*** can reduce hyperlipidaemic parameters such as cholesterol and triglycerides.[136] A *Rosa* spp. fruit drink, given to obese individuals, has resulted in significantly improved systolic blood pressure, cholesterol and LDL.[193] ***Portulaca oleracea*** (purslane) has reduced insulin resistance by lowering body weight, fasting and postprandial glucose, insulin, cholesterol, triglycerides and LDL, while increasing HDL.[194]

Novel treatments

Considering the side effects of conventional treatment, new and innovative approaches to diabetes type 2 are being explored. It has been suggested to target insulin resistance and metabolic syndrome by modulating appetite, inflammation, lipid and energy metabolism, and fat storage, for instance through ablation of the ghrelin receptor[17] or nicotinic acetylcholine receptor selective antagonist.[195] NADPH oxidase inhibitors such as phycocyanobilin (derived from spirulina) may decrease diabetes risk.[11] Stearidonic acid (found in the seed oils of hemp, blackcurrant, corn Cromwell and spirulina), an alternative source to fish of omega-3 fatty acids, may have therapeutic efficacy.[8] Aldose reductase activity has been linked to increased risk of diabetic complications, and various natural substances have been trialled in vivo, such as *Ganoderma lucidum*,[196] bitter gourd, curry leaves, black pepper, cumin, fenugreek, fennel, basil, lemon, orange and spinach[197] exhibiting high aldose reductase inhibition. Some of these have already been incorporated into some diabetic supplements on the market. It is important to note that the evidence for these novel interventions are mostly derived from trials where single substances have been used. As is the case with antioxidants, combinations of the above may yield even better results. Nutrients and herbs that match the individual patient's profile best need to be chosen.

INTEGRATIVE MEDICAL CONSIDERATIONS

Relaxation exercises such as meditation have shown beneficial effects not only on mood and depression but also on insulin receptors and the HPA axis.[31] Since metabolic syndrome is a multifaceted disease a whole range of parameters need to be considered and attended to. Therefore, a close working relationship with the patient's general practitioner would be advisable.

Hydrotherapy may be a useful adjunct to exercise recommendations, with one small American study showing daily hot-tub therapy over six weeks improved blood glucose management, reduced reliance on insulin and reduced weight in diabetic patients.[198] Heat therapies have shown the most effect in patients with diabetes.[199] A systematic review has also shown **yoga** to be associated with significant improvements in lipid profile, blood pressure, body mass index, waist/hip ratio and cortisol levels in diabetic patients.[200]

The Indian system of Ayurveda has a wide range of herbal medicines for many diseases. In diabetes type 2, **Pterocarpus marsupium** (kino tree) has decreased elevated blood glucose and glycosylated haemoglobin levels.[201] Traditional Chinese medicine, in combination with Western medicine, has resulted in better glycaemic control.[202] Other useful modalities and therefore referrals include acupuncture, fitness training (gym), grief counselling and creativity (art and music). Considering that this disease is preventable the collaboration of multiple sectors in our society is paramount. Not only the healthcare system, healthcare providers and diabetes educators but also the food industry, politicians, the media and various other organisations are all indispensable in achieving changes in this epidemic. Lastly, people need to be able and willing to make changes in their lives and access the support that is available to them.[7,203,204]

CLINICAL SUMMARY

Diabetes is a disease characterised by high blood glucose levels due to low or absent insulin. While in diabetes type 1 the insulin-producing pancreatic β-cells are destroyed due to auto-immunity, and patients are dependent on insulin injections for life, type 2 is predominantly a lifestyle disease. Being overweight, leading a sedentary lifestyle and eating a diet high in refined carbohydrates and sugars leads to hyperinsulinaemia, insulin resistance and ultimately to diabetes type 2. Due to the macro- and microvasular damage caused by elevated blood glucose, heart disease, nephropathy, retinopathy and neuropathy are common comorbidities. This is known as metabolic syndrome. Medical treatment mainly focuses on increasing insulin secretion and sensitivity, and reducing carbohydrate absorption. Comorbidities are treated symptomatically. Medications used all have various adverse effects that need to be considered.

In order to achieve lasting effects, underlying issues need to be identified and addressed, such as stress, high cortisol and the risk of diabetic complications and comorbidities. Naturo-pathic medicine is based on diet and lifestyle changes with supporting nutrients and herbs. Exercise is paramount, together with a low carbohydrate (or at least low glycaemic index) diet with sufficient protein to counteract gluconeogenesis and reductions in lean body mass. Care needs to be taken with low-fat products as the fat may be replaced by carbohydrates. Nutritional interventions include magnesium, chromium, N-acetyl carnitine, α-lipoic acid and others. Herbally, *Gymnema sylvestre*, *Galega officinale*, *Trigonella foenum-graecum*, the various ginsengs and a number of other herbs have shown beneficial effects (Figure 19.4).

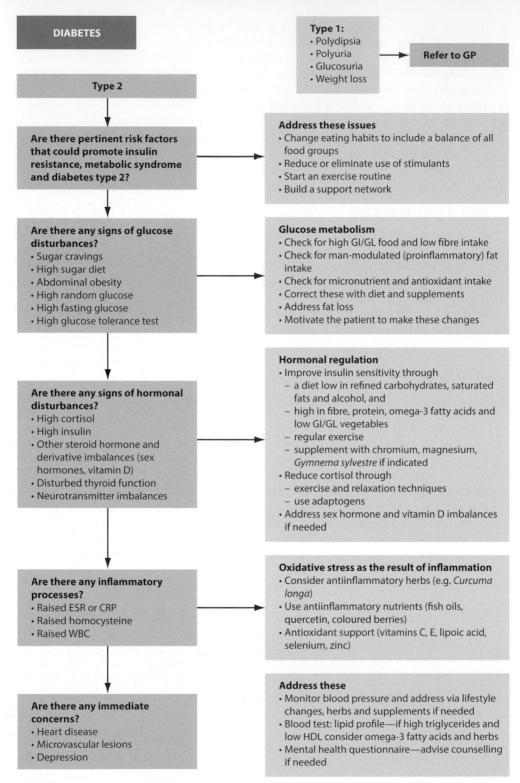

Figure 19.4
Naturopathic treatment decision tree—diabetes

Table 19.2
Review of the major evidence

Intervention	Mechanisms of action*	Key literature	Summary of results	Comment
Diet and exercise	Facilitates cellular glucose uptake Lowers insulin resistance and reduces insulin requirements Reduces blood glucose Improves body composition	Khazrai et al. 2014[77]	Reductions in total and saturated fat intake, and obesity Increase in physical activity, insulin sensitivity and glucose tolerance	This trial confirms that lifestyle, diet and exercise play a major role in reducing the risk factors for diabetes type 2
Calorie-restricted diet and exercise	Improves insulin sensitivity Lowers blood pressure Improves lipid profile Promotes fat-weight loss	Kahleova & Matoulek 2011[81]	Vegetarian diet increased insulin sensitivity, decreased oxidative stress markers, adiponectin, visceral and subcutaneous fat, leptin	It is not only the type of food but also the amount that is important
Tai Chi	Improves glycaemic control Lowers triglyceride levels	Meta-analysis: Chao et al. 2018[205]	Greater decline in fasting glucose and HbA_{1c}, increased quality of life in adherence group	Even gentle exercise is sufficient to improve diabetes type 2 parameters
Gymnema sylvestre	Decreases FBG and HbA_{1c} Delays glucose uptake in small intestine Restorative action on pancreatic β-cells Decreases sweet cravings and appetite	Systematic review: Pothuraju et al. 2014[206]	Blood glucose on active arm normalised Lipid peroxidation was decreased in serum, liver and kidney	Note: most research has been conducted in animal studies or with polyherbal formulations. Further human trials of *Gymnema* specifically are necessary
Trigonella foenum-graecum	Lowers FBG, PPG, postprandial insulin, urine glucose, carbohydrate absorption Modulates peripheral glucose utilisation Lowers atherosclerotic parameters	Meta-analysis: Gong et al. 2016[207]	Significant reductions in FBG, 24-hour urinary glucose, total cholesterol, VLDL, LDL, triglycerides in the treated group HDL remained unchanged	More research is needed to corroborate results and test for diabetes type 2. The evidence is strongest for lipid modification over glucose modification

Table 19.2
Review of the major evidence (continued)

Intervention	Mechanisms of action*	Key literature	Summary of results	Comment
Chromium	Stimulates insulin uptake Facilitates entrance of glucose into cells Lowers FBG, PPG, HbA$_{1c}$ Improves lipid profile Down-regulates pancreatic β-cells activity	Pooled analyses: Huang et al. 2018[208] Meta-analyses: Costello et al. 2016[209] Suksomboon et al. 2014[210]	Chromium dinocysteinate (CDNC) lowers insulin resistance by reducing blood levels of TNF-α, insulin and oxidative stress in type 2 diabetic subjects. Chromium chloride and chromium picolinate reduce fasting glucose levels, HbA1c and triglyceride levels, and increase HDL cholesterol	While trending towards benefit in diabetic patients (particularly as an adjunct treatment), results are variable
Magnesium	Stabilises ATP production Enhances insulin sensitivity Reduces FBG, HbA$_{1c}$ and hepatic glucose production Increases proton-pump inhibitors, glucose uptake and glucose oxidation	Rodríguez-Morán et al. 2011[55]	Evidence from epidemiological studies consistently shows a strong inverse relationship between dietary magnesium intake and the risk of developing diabetes type 2	Although observational studies routinely show deficiency in diabetic patients, more human trials are needed to establish effectiveness of magnesium supplementation in diabetic patients

*References available in key treatment protocols

KEY POINTS

- Contributors to diabetes type 2 include stress/high cortisol, sedentary lifestyle and unbalanced diet.
- Treatment should have dietary and lifestyle modifications as a foundation, supplementing with chromium, magnesium and lipoic acid, utilising herbs that help balance blood glucose such as *Gymnema sylvestre* and *Trigonella foecum-gracum*, exercise and stress management if indicated.
- Waist control can be more important than weight control in diabetic patients, as it is the fat stored around the waist that is most linked to diabetic risk factors.

FURTHER READING

Esser N, Legrand-Poels S, Piette J, et al. Inflammation as a link between obesity, metabolic syndrome and type 2 diabetes. Diabetes Res Clin Pract 2014;105(2):141–50.

Kirwan JP, Sacks J, Nieuwoudt S. The essential role of exercise in the management of type 2 diabetes. Cleve Clin J Med 2017;84(7 Suppl. 1):S15.

Ríos JL, Francini F, Schinella GR. Natural products for the treatment of type 2 diabetes mellitus. Planta Med 2015;81(12/13):975–94.

Via MA, Mechanick JI. Nutrition in type 2 diabetes and the metabolic syndrome. Med Clin 2016;100(6):1285–302.

Acknowledgement: Thanks are extended to Alina Porojan for assisting Dr Gruner with the resubmission. This chapter has been updated by Jon Wardle, based on Tini Gruner's original work.

REFERENCES

1. Mota M, Pănuş C, Mota E, et al. The metabolic syndrome—a multifaced disease. Rom J Intern Med 2004;42(2):247–55.

2. Shils ME, Shike M, Ross AC, et al. Modern nutrition in health and disease. Philadelphia: Lippincott Williams & Wilkins; 2006.

3. Kelly GS. Insulin resistance: lifestyle and nutritional interventions. Altern Med Rev 2000;5(2):109–32.

4. Roberts K, Dunn K, Jean SK, et al. Syndrome X: medical nutrition therapy. Nutr Rev 2000;58(5):154–60.

5. Australian Institute of Health and Welfare. Diabetes Snapshot. AIHW: Canberra. 2019. Available at: https://www.aihw.gov.au/reports/diabetes/diabetes-snapshot/contents/how-many-australians-have-diabetes.

6. Wirth A. Non-pharmacological therapy of metabolic syndrome. Herz 1995;20(1):56–69.

7. Lindström J, Neumann A, Sheppard KE, et al. Take action to prevent diabetes–the IMAGE toolkit for the prevention of type 2 diabetes in Europe. Horm Metab Res 2010;42(Suppl. 1):S37–55.

8. Banz WJ, Davis JE, Clough RW, et al. Stearidonic acid: is there a role in the prevention and management of type 2 diabetes mellitus? J Nutr 2012;142(3):635S–40S.

9. Katula JA, Vitolins MZ, Rosenberger EL, et al. Healthy Living Partnerships to Prevent Diabetes (HELP PD): design and methods. Contemp Clin Trials 2010;31(1):71–81.

10. Johnson ST, Newton AS, Chopra M, et al. In search of quality evidence for lifestyle management and glycemic control in children and adolescents with type 2 diabetes: a systematic review. BMC Pediatr 2010;10:97–104.

11. McCarty MF, Barroso-Aranda J, Contreras F. NADPH oxidase mediates glucolipotoxicity-induced beta cell dysfunction–clinical implications. Med Hypotheses 2010;74(3):596–600.

12. Khani S, Tayek JA. Cortisol increases gluconeogenesis in humans: its role in the metabolic syndrome. Clin Sci 2001;101(6):739–47.

13. Holick MF. Diabetes and the vitamin D connection. Curr Diab Rep 2008;8(5):393–8.

14. Vinson GP. Angiotensin II, corticosteroids, type II diabetes and the metabolic syndrome. Med Hypotheses 2007;68(6):1200–7.

15. Brindley DN. Role of glucocorticoids and fatty acids in the impairment of lipid metabolism observed in the metabolic syndrome. Int J Obes Relat Metab Disord 1995;19(Suppl. 1):S69–75.

16. Ginsberg HN, Zhang Y-L, Hernandez-Ono A. Regulation of plasma triglycerides in insulin resistance and diabetes. Arch Med Res 2005;36(3):232–40.

17. Lin L, Saha PK, Ma X, et al. Ablation of ghrelin receptor reduces adiposity and improves insulin sensitivity during aging by regulating fat metabolism in white and brown adipose tissues. Aging Cell 2011;10(6):996–1010.

18. Hristova M, Aloe L. Metabolic syndrome–neurotrophic hypothesis. Med Hypotheses 2006;66(3):545–9.

19. Walker BR. Steroid metabolism in metabolic syndrome X. Best Pract Res Clin Endocrinol Metab 2001;15(1):111–22.

20. Pickup JC, Mattock MB, Chusney GD, et al. NIDDM as a disease of the innate immune system: association of acute-phase reactants and interleukin-6 with metabolic syndrome X. Diabetologia 1997;40(11):1286–92.

21. Clifton PM. Diet and C-reactive protein. Curr Atheroscler Rep 2003;5(6):431–6.

22. Rosmond R. The glucocorticoid receptor gene and its association to metabolic syndrome. Obes Res 2002;10(10):1078–86.

23. Björntorp P, Rosmond R. The metabolic syndrome—a neuroendocrine disorder? Br J Nutr 2000;83(Suppl. 1):S49–57.

24. Hernandez-Mijares A, Rocha M, Apostolova N, et al. Mitochondrial complex I impairment in leukocytes from type 2 diabetic patients. Free Radic Biol Med 2011;50(10):1215–21.

25. Henriksen EJ, Diamond-Stanic MK, Marchionne EM. Oxidative stress and the etiology of insulin resistance and type 2 diabetes. Free Radic Biol Med 2011;51(5):993–9.

26. Folli F, Corradi D, Fanti P, et al. The role of oxidative stress in the pathogenesis of type 2 diabetes mellitus micro- and macrovascular complications: avenues for a mechanistic-based therapeutic approach. Curr Diabetes Rev 2011;7(5):313–24.

27. Sebeková K, Boor P, Valachovicová M, et al. Association of metabolic syndrome risk factors with selected markers of oxidative status and microinflammation in healthy omnivores and vegetarians. Mol Nutr Food Res 2006;50(9):858–68.

28. Wu C-H, Huang H-W, Huang S-M, et al. AGE-induced interference of glucose uptake and transport as a possible cause of insulin resistance in adipocytes. J Agric Food Chem 2011;59(14):7978–84.

29. Kohlmeier M. Nutrient metabolism. Amsterdam, The Netherlands: Academic Press, Elsevier; 2003.

30. Aida K, Tawata M, Shindo H, et al. Clinical significance of erythrocyte sorbitol-blood glucose ratios in type II diabetes mellitus. Diabetes Care 1990;13(5):461–7.

31. Singh RB, Pella D, Mechirova V, et al. Can brain dysfunction be a predisposing factor for metabolic syndrome? Biomed Pharmacother 2004;58(Suppl. 1):S56–68.

32. Gropper S, Smith J, Groff J. Advanced nutrition and human metabolism. 5th ed. Australia: Wadsworth, Cengate Learning; 2009.

33. Devlin TM. Textbook of biochemistry with clinical correlations. 5th ed. New York: Wiley-Liss; 2002.

34. Morenkova SA. Comparative analysis of dependence of saliva sorbitol and fructosamine levels on blood glucose level in patients with diabetes. Biomed Khim 2004;50(6): 612–14.

35. Pasquali R, Vicennati V, Cacciari M, et al. The hypothalamic-pituitary-adrenal axis activity in obesity and the metabolic syndrome. Ann N Y Acad Sci 2006;1083:111–28.

36. Schindhelm RK, Diamant M, Bakker SJL, et al. Liver alanine aminotransferase, insulin resistance and endothelial dysfunction in normotriglyceridaemic subjects with type 2 diabetes mellitus. Eur J Clin Invest 2005;35(6):369–74.

37. Hayden MR, Tyagi SC. Homocysteine and reactive oxygen species in metabolic syndrome, type 2 diabetes mellitus, and atherosclerOPathy: the pleiotropic effects of folate supplementation. Nutr J 2004;3:4.

38. Herbert V, Fong W, Gulle V, et al. Low holotranscobalamin II is the earliest serum marker for subnormal vitamin B12 (cobalamin) absorption in patients with AIDS. Am J Hematol 1990;34:132–9.

39. Boucher BJ. Inadequate vitamin D status: does it contribute to the disorders comprising syndrome 'X'? Br J Nutr 1998;79(4):315–27.

40. Kumar P, Clark M. Clinical medicine. 7th ed. Edinburgh: Elsevier/Saunders; 2009.

41. Dickey RA, Wartofsky L, Feld S. Optimal thyrotropin level: normal ranges and reference intervals are not equivalent. Thyroid 2005;15(9):1035–9.

42. Pagana KD, Pagana TJ. Mosby's manual of diagnostic and laboratory tests. 3rd ed. USA: Mosby; 2006.

43. Crowley LV. An introduction to human disease: pathology and pathophysiology correlations. 6th ed. Sudbury, Massachusetts: Jones and Bartlett Publishers; 2004.

44. Tierney LM, McPhee SJ, Papadakis MA. Medical diagnosis and treatment. 44th ed. New York: McGraw-Hill; 2005.

45. Haque N, Salma U, Nurunnabi TR, et al. Management of type 2 diabetes mellitus by lifestyle, diet and medicinal plants. Pak J Biol Sci 2011;14(1):13–24.

46. Misra A, Singhal N, Khurana L. Obesity, the metabolic syndrome, and type 2 diabetes in developing countries: role of dietary fats and oils. J Am Coll Nutr 2010;29(3 Suppl.): 289S–301S.

47. Pegklidou K, Nicolaou I, Demopoulos VJ. Nutritional overview on the management of type 2 diabetes and the prevention of its complications. Curr Diabetes Rev 2010;6(6):400–9.

48. Nicklas JM, Zera CA, Seely EW, et al. Identifying postpartum intervention approaches to prevent type 2 diabetes in women with a history of gestational diabetes. BMC Pregnancy Childbirth 2011;11:23.

49. Reece EA. Diabetes-induced birth defects: what do we know? What can we do? Curr Diab Rep 2012;12(1): 24–32.

50. Ganji V, Zhang X, Shaikh N, et al. Serum 25-hydroxyvitamin D concentrations are associated with prevalence of metabolic syndrome and various cardiometabolic risk factors in US children and adolescents based on assay-adjusted serum 25-hydroxyvitamin D data from NHANES 2001–2006. Am J Clin Nutr 2011;94(1):225–33.

51. Shehab D, Al-Jarallah K, Mojiminiyi OA, et al. Does Vitamin D deficiency play a role in peripheral neuropathy in Type 2 diabetes? Diabet Med 2012;29(1):43–9.

52. Payne JF, Ray R, Watson DG, et al. Vitamin D insufficiency in diabetic retinopathy. Endocr Pract 2012;18(2):185–93.

53. Jawa AA, Akram J, Sultan M, et al. Nutrition-related vitamin B12 deficiency in patients in Pakistan with type 2 diabetes mellitus not taking metformin. Endocr Pract 2010;16(2):205–8.

54. Mitri J, Dawson-Hughes B, Hu FB, et al. Effects of vitamin D and calcium supplementation on pancreatic β cell function, insulin sensitivity, and glycemia in adults at high risk of diabetes: the Calcium and Vitamin D for Diabetes Mellitus (CaDDM) randomized controlled trial. Am J Clin Nutr 2011;94(2):486–94.

55. Rodríguez-Morán M, Simental Mendía LE, Zambrano Galván G, et al. The role of magnesium in type 2 diabetes: a brief based-clinical review. Magnes Res 2011;24(4): 156–62.

56. Smith BW, Adams LA. Nonalcoholic fatty liver disease and diabetes mellitus: pathogenesis and treatment. Nat Rev Endocrinol 2011;7(8):456–65.

57. Dharwadkar AR, Dharwadkar AA, Banu G, et al. Reduction in lung functions in type-2 diabetes in Indian population: correlation with glycemic status. Indian J Physiol Pharmacol 2011;55(2):170–5.

58. Morley JE. Diabetes, sarcopenia, and frailty. Clin Geriatr Med 2008;24(3):455.

59. Manders RJ, Little JP, Forbes SC, et al. Insulinotropic and muscle protein synthetic effects of branched-chain amino acids: potential therapy for type 2 diabetes and sarcopenia. Nutrients 2012;4(11):1664–78.

60. MIMS Annual. Australian Edition edn: CMPMedica; June 2006.

61. Chomutare T, Fernandez-Luque L, Arsand E, et al. Features of mobile diabetes applications: review of the literature and analysis of current applications compared against evidence-based guidelines. J Med Internet Res 2011;13(3):e65.

62. Ramadas A, Quek KF, Chan CKY, et al. Web-based interventions for the management of type 2 diabetes mellitus: a systematic review of recent evidence. Int J Med Inform 2011;80(6):389–405.

63. Arsand E, Tatara N, Østengen G, et al. Mobile phone-based self-management tools for type 2 diabetes: the few touch application. J Diabetes Sci Technol 2010;4(2):328–36.

64. Cohen LB, Taveira TH, Khatana SAM, et al. Pharmacist-led shared medical appointments for multiple cardiovascular risk reduction in patients with type 2 diabetes. Diabetes Educ 2011;37(6):801–12.

65. Riddell MA, Renwick C, Wolfe R, et al. Cluster randomized controlled trial of a peer support program for people with diabetes: study protocol for the Australasian Peers for Progress study. BMC Public Health 2012;12:843.

66. Mechanick JI, Marchetti AE, Apovian C, et al. Diabetes-specific nutrition algorithm: a transcultural program to optimize diabetes and prediabetes care. Curr Diab Rep 2012;12(2):180–94.

67. Wang Y, Chuang L, Bateman WB. Focus group study assessing self-management skills of Chinese Americans with type 2 diabetes mellitus. J Immigr Minor Health 2012;14(5):869–74.

68. Wolever RQ, Dreusicke M, Fikkan J, et al. Integrative health coaching for patients with type 2 diabetes: a randomized clinical trial. Diabetes Educ 2010;36(4):629–39.

69. Giarratana N, Penna G, Amuchastegui S, et al. A vitamin D analog down-regulates proinflammatory chemokine production by pancreatic islets inhibiting T cell recruitment and type 1 diabetes development. J Immunol 2004;173(4):2280–7.

70. Lips P. Vitamin D physiology. Prog Biophys Mol Biol 2006;92(1):4–8.

71. Chertow B. Advances in diabetes for the millennium: vitamins and oxidant stress in diabetes and its complications. Medgenmed 2004;6(3 Suppl.):4.

72. Triggiani V, Resta F, Guastamacchia E, et al. Role of antioxidants, essential fatty acids, carnitine, vitamins, phytochemicals and trace elements in the treatment of diabetes mellitus and its chronic complications. Endocr Metab Immune Disord Drug Targets 2006;6(1): 77–93.

73. Packer L, Kraemer K, Rimbach G. Molecular aspects of lipoic acid in the prevention of diabetes complications. Nutrition 2001;17(10):888–95.

74. van Dam PS. Oxidative stress and diabetic neuropathy: pathophysiological mechanisms and treatment perspectives. Diabetes Metab Res Rev 2002;18(3):176–84.

75. Head KA. Natural therapies for ocular disorders, part two: cataracts and glaucoma. Altern Med Rev 2001;6(2):141–66.

76. Das UN. Essential fatty acids in health and disease. J Assoc Physicians India 1999;47(9):906–11.

77. Khazrai YM, Defeudis G, Pozzilli P. Effect of diet on type 2 diabetes mellitus: a review. Diabetes Metab Res Rev 2014;30(S1):24–33.

78. Bradley R, Sherman KJ, Catz S, et al. Survey of CAM interest, self-care, and satisfaction with health care for type 2 diabetes at group health cooperative. BMC Complement Altern Med 2011;11:121.

79. Bradley R, Sherman KJ, Catz S, et al. Adjunctive naturopathic care for type 2 diabetes: patient-reported and clinical outcomes after one year. BMC Complement Altern Med 2012;12:44.

80. Oberg EB, Bradley RD, Allen J, et al. CAM: naturopathic dietary interventions for patients with type 2 diabetes. Complement Ther Clin Pract 2011;17(3):157–61.

81. Kahleova H, Matoulek M, Malinska H, et al. Vegetarian diet improves insulin resistance and oxidative stress markers more than conventional diet in subjects with Type 2 diabetes. Diabet Med 2011;28(5):549–59.

82. Brehm BJ, D'Alessio DA. Weight loss and metabolic benefits with diets of varying fat and carbohydrate content: separating the wheat from the chaff. Nat Clin Pract Endocrinol Metab [serial online] 2008;4(3):Available from: http://www.medscape.com/viewprogram/8640_pnt. [cited July 2, 2008].

83. Neff LM. Evidence-based dietary recommendations for patients with type 2 diabetes mellitus. Nutr Clin Care 2003;6(2):51–61.

84. de Koning L, Fung TT, Liao X, et al. Low-carbohydrate diet scores and risk of type 2 diabetes in men. Am J Clin Nutr 2011;93(4):844–50.

85. Pelkman CL, Fishell VK, Maddox DH, et al. Effects of moderate-fat (from monounsaturated fat) and low-fat weight-loss diets on the serum lipid profile in overweight and obese men and women. Am J Clin Nutr 2004;79(2):204–12.

86. Clifton P. Effects of a high protein diet on body weight and comorbidities associated with obesity. Br J Nutr 2012;108(Suppl. 2):S122–9.

87. Hussain TA, Mathew TC, Dashti AA, et al. Effect of low-calorie versus low-carbohydrate ketogenic diet in type 2 diabetes. Nutrition 2012;28(10):1016–21.

88. Belury MA, Mahon A, Banni S. The conjugated linoleic acid (CLA) isomer, t10c12-CLA, is inversely associated with changes in body weight and serum leptin in subjects with type 2 diabetes mellitus. J Nutr 2003;133(1): 257S–60S.

89. Belury MA. Dietary conjugated linoleic acid in health: physiological effects and mechanisms of action. Annu Rev Nutr 2002;22:505–31.

90. Gaullier J-M, Halse J, Hoye K, et al. Supplementation with conjugated linoleic acid for 24 months is well tolerated by and reduces body fat mass in healthy, overweight humans. J Nutr 2005;135(4):778–84.

91. Dhiman TR, Nam S-H, Ure AL. Factors affecting conjugated linoleic acid content in milk and meat. Crit Rev Food Sci Nutr 2005;45(6):463–82.

92. Djoussé L, Gaziano JM, Buring JE, et al. Dietary omega-3 fatty acids and fish consumption and risk of type 2 diabetes. Am J Clin Nutr 2011;93(1):143–50.

93. Schwingshackl L, Strasser B, Hoffmann G. Effects of monounsaturated fatty acids on glycaemic control in patients with abnormal glucose metabolism: a systematic review and meta-analysis. Ann Nutr Metab 2011;58(4):290–6.

94. Abboud L, Carrns A. Even a diet of fat-free foods can pose a weighty problem. Wall Street Journal. 2002 New York, N.Y.: Jun 11:D.4.

95. Li C, Sadraie B, Steckhan N, et al. Effects of a one-week fasting therapy in patients with type-2 diabetes mellitus and metabolic syndrome—a randomized controlled explorative study. Exp Clin Endocrinol Diabetes 2017;125(9):618–24.

96. Bener A, Yousafzai MT. Effect of Ramadan fasting on diabetes mellitus: a population-based study in Qatar. J Egypt Public Health Assoc 2014;89(2):47–52.

97. Bener A, Al-Hamaq AOA, Öztürk M, et al. Effect of ramadan fasting on glycemic control and other essential variables in diabetic patients. Ann Afr Med 2018;17(4):196.

98. Rodríguez-Morán M, Guerrero-Romero F, Lazcano-Burciaga G. Lipid- and glucose-lowering efficacy of Plantago Psyllium in type II diabetes. J Diabetes Complications 1998;12(5):273–8.

99. Bajorek SA, Morello CM. Effects of dietary fiber and low glycemic index diet on glucose control in subjects with type 2 diabetes mellitus. Ann Pharmacother 2010;44(11):1786–92.

100. Mani UV, Mani I, Biswas M, et al. An open-label study on the effect of flax seed powder (Linum usitatissimum) supplementation in the management of diabetes mellitus. J Diet Suppl 2011;8(3):257–65.

101. Wedick NM, Pan A, Cassidy A, et al. Dietary flavonoid intakes and risk of type 2 diabetes in US men and women. Am J Clin Nutr 2012;95(4):925–33.

102. Hatano M, Katsu K, Fuda H, et al. Studies on clinical markers of diabetes mellitus. 6. Red blood cell sorbitol and diabetic complications. Meikai Daigaku Shigaku Zasshi 1990;19(2):230–3.

103. Brunzell JD. Use of fructose, xylitol, or sorbitol as a sweetener in diabetes mellitus. Diabetes Care 1978;1(4):223–30.

104. Kmietowicz Z. Countries that use large amounts of high fructose corn syrup have higher rates of type 2 diabetes. BMJ 2012;345:e7994.

105. Kline GA, Pedersen SD. Errors in patient perception of caloric deficit required for weight loss–observations from the Diet Plate Trial. Diabetes Obes Metab 2010;12(5):455–7.

106. Azadbakht L, Surkan PJ, Esmaillzadeh A, et al. The Dietary Approaches to Stop Hypertension eating plan affects C-reactive protein, coagulation abnormalities, and hepatic function tests among type 2 diabetic patients. J Nutr 2011;141(6):1083–8.

107. Archuleta M, Vanleeuwen D, Halderson K, et al. Cooking schools improve nutrient intake patterns of people with type 2 diabetes. J Nutr Educ Behav 2012;44(4):319–25.

108. Díez-Espino J, Buil-Cosiales P, Serrano-Martínez M, et al. Adherence to the Mediterranean diet in patients with type

2 diabetes mellitus and HbA1c level. Ann Nutr Metab 2011;58(1):74–8.

109. Salas-Salvadó J, Bulló M, Babio N, et al. Reduction in the incidence of type 2 diabetes with the Mediterranean diet: results of the PREDIMED-Reus nutrition intervention randomized trial. Diabetes Care 2011;34(1):14–19.

110. Itsiopoulos C, Brazionis L, Kaimakamis M, et al. Can the Mediterranean diet lower HbA1c in type 2 diabetes? Results from a randomized cross-over study. Nutr Metab Cardiovasc Dis 2011;21(9):740–7.

111. Liese AD, Bortsov A, Günther ALB, et al. Association of DASH diet with cardiovascular risk factors in youth with diabetes mellitus: the SEARCH for Diabetes in Youth study. Circulation 2011;123(13):1410–17.

112. Dämon S, Schätzer M, Höfler J, et al. Nutrition and diabetes mellitus: an overview of the current evidence. Wien Med Wochenschr 2011;161(11–12):282–8.

113. Just do it: diabetes and exercise. Clin Diab 2008;26(3):140–1.

114. Turcotte LP, Fisher JS. Skeletal muscle insulin resistance: roles of fatty acid metabolism and exercise. Phys Ther 2008;88(11):1279–96.

115. Earnest CP. Exercise interval training: an improved stimulus for improving the physiology of pre-diabetes. Med Hypotheses 2008;71(5):752–61.

116. Gulve AE. Exercise and glycemic control in diabetes: benefits, challenges, and adjustments to pharmacotherapy. Phys Ther 2008;88(11):1297–321.

117. Little JP, Gillen JB, Percival ME, et al. Low-volume high-intensity interval training reduces hyperglycemia and increases muscle mitochondrial capacity in patients with type 2 diabetes. J Appl Physiol 2011;111(6):1554–60.

118. Ying Z, Fu FH. Effects of 14-week tai ji quan exercise on metabolic control in women with type 2 diabetes. Am J Chin Med 2008;36(4):647–54.

119. Song R, Ahn S, Roberts BL, et al. Adhering to a T'ai Chi program to improve glucose control and quality of life for individuals with type 2 diabetes. J Altern Complement Med 2009;15(6):627–32.

120. Liu X, Miller YD, Burton NW, et al. A preliminary study of the effects of Tai Chi and Qigong medical exercise on indicators of metabolic syndrome, glycaemic control, health-related quality of life, and psychological health in adults with elevated blood glucose. Br J Sports Med 2010;44(10):704–9.

121. Putiri AL, Lovejoy JC, Gillham S, et al. Psychological effects of Yi Ren Medical Qigong and progressive resistance training in adults with type 2 diabetes mellitus: a randomized controlled pilot study. Altern Ther Health Med 2012;18(1):30–4.

122. Giurini JM, Lyons TE. Diabetic foot complications: diagnosis and management. Int J Low Extrem Wounds 2005;4(3):171–82.

123. Watkins PJ. ABC of diabetes: the diabetic foot. BMJ 2003;326(7396):977–9.

124. Yeh GY, Eisenberg DM, Kaptchuk TJ, et al. Systematic review of herbs and dietary supplements for glycemic control in diabetes. Diabetes Care 2003;26(4):1277–94.

125. McCarty MF. Chromium and other insulin sensitizers may enhance glucagon secretion: implications for hypoglycemia and weight control. Med Hypotheses 1996;46(2):77–80.

126. Ali A, Ma Y, Reynolds J, et al. Chromium effects on glucose tolerance and insulin sensitivity in persons at risk for diabetes mellitus. Endocr Pract 2011;17(1):16–25.

127. Neff LM. Evidence-based dietary recommendations for patients with type 2 diabetes mellitus. Nutr Clin Care 2003;6(2):51–61.

128. Chausmer AB. Zinc, insulin and diabetes. J Am Coll Nutr 1998;17(2):109–15.

129. Adachi Y, Yoshida J, Kodera Y, et al. Oral administration of a zinc complex improves type 2 diabetes and metabolic syndromes. Biochem Biophys Res Commun 2006;351(1):165–70.

130. Hargreaves IP, Duncan AJ, Heales SJR, et al. The effect of HMG-CoA reductase inhibitors on coenzyme Q10: possible biochemical/clinical implications. Drug Saf 2005;28(8):659–76.

131. Nazarian S, St Peter JV, Boston RC, et al. Vitamin D3 supplementation improves insulin sensitivity in subjects with impaired fasting glucose. Transl Res 2011;158(5):276–81.

132. Henriksen EJ, Saengsirisuwan V. Exercise training and antioxidants: relief from oxidative stress and insulin resistance. Exerc Sport Sci Rev 2003;31(2):79–84.

133. Ansar H, Mazloom Z, Kazemi F, et al. Effect of alpha-lipoic acid on blood glucose, insulin resistance and glutathione peroxidase of type 2 diabetic patients. Saudi Med J 2011;32(6):584–8.

134. van Loon LJC. Leucine as a pharmaconutrient in health and disease. Curr Opin Clin Nutr Metab Care 2012;15(1):71–7.

135. Gloria YY, David ME, Ted JK, et al. Systematic review of herbs and dietary supplements for glycemic control in diabetes. Diabetes Care 2003;26(4):1277.

136. Mills S, Bone K. Principles and practice of phytotherapy. 2nd ed. Sydney: Churchill Livingstone; 2013.

137. Bone K. Phytotherapy for diabetes and the key role of Gymnema. Mod Phytother 2002;7(1):7–11.

138. Davis PA, Yokoyama W. Cinnamon intake lowers fasting blood glucose: meta analysis. J Med Food 2011;14(9):884–9.

139. Gormley JJ. Gymnema sylvestre: providing new hope for those with diabetes. Better Nutr 1996;58(4):42.

140. Leach MJ. Gymnema sylvestre for diabetes mellitus: a systematic review. J Altern Complement Med 2007;13(9):977–83.

141. Blumenthal M. The ABC clinical guide to herbs. Austin, Texas: American Botanical Council; 2003.

142. Anonymous. Diabetes herb as effective as drugs. Better Nutr 2005;67(5):12.

143. Kapoor R, Huang YS. Gamma linolenic acid: an antiinflammatory omega-6 fatty acid. Curr Pharm Biotechnol 2006;7(6):531–4.

144. Braun L, Cohen M. Herbs & natural supplements. 3rd ed. Sydney: Churchill Livingstone; 2010.

145. König D, Berg A, Halle M, et al. Mehrfach ungesattigte Fettsauren, koronare Herzerkrankung und Diabetes mellitus Typ II—Hinweise fur den Stellenwert von Gamma-Linolensäure. Forsch Komplementmed 1997;4(2):94.

146. Brenner RR. Hormonal modulation of delta6 and delta5 desaturases: case of diabetes. Prostaglandins Leukot Essent Fatty Acids 2003;68(2):151–62.

147. Malasanos TH, Stacpoole PW. Biological effects of omega-3 fatty acids in diabetes mellitus. Diabetes Care 1991;14(12):1160–79.

148. Neri S, Calvagno S, Mauceri B, et al. Effects of antioxidants on postprandial oxidative stress and endothelial dysfunction in subjects with impaired glucose tolerance and type 2 diabetes. Eur J Nutr 2010;49(7):409–16.

149. Evans JL, Maddux BA, Goldfine ID. The molecular basis for oxidative stress-induced insulin resistances. Antioxid Redox Signal 2005;7(7–8):1040–52.

150. Jain SK, Croad JL, Velusamy T, et al. Chromium dinicocysteinate supplementation can lower blood glucose,

CRP, MCP-1, ICAM-1, creatinine, apparently mediated by elevated blood vitamin C and adiponectin and inhibition of NFkappaB, Akt, and Glut-2 in livers of zucker diabetic fatty rats. Mol Nutr Food Res 2010;54(9):1371–80.

151. Jain SK, Kahlon G, Morehead L, et al. Effect of chromium dinicocysteinate supplementation on circulating levels of insulin, TNF-α, oxidative stress, and insulin resistance in type 2 diabetic subjects: randomized, double-blind, placebo-controlled study. Mol Nutr Food Res 2012;56(8):1333–41.

152. Coyne DW. Vitamin D and the Diabetic Patient. Medscape Nephrology [serial online]. 2008. Available from: http://www.medscape.com/viewarticle/573383_print. [cited August 5, 2008].

153. Brandacher G, Hoeller E, Fuchs D, et al. Chronic immune activation underlies morbid obesity: is IDO a key player? Curr Drug Metab 2007;8(3):289–95.

154. Mechanick JI. Metabolic mechanisms of stress hyperglycemia. JPEN J Parenter Enteral Nutr 2006;30(2):157–63.

155. Vanitallie TB. Stress: a risk factor for serious illness. Metabolism 2002;51(6 Suppl. 1):40–5.

156. Nieuwenhuizen AG, Rutters F. The hypothalamic-pituitar y-adrenal-axis in the regulation of energy balance. Physiol Behav 2008;94(2):169–77.

157. Szolomicki S, Samochowiec L, Wojcicki J, et al. The influence of active components of Eleutherococcus senticosus on cellular defence and physical fitness in man. Phytother Res 2000;14(1):30.

158. Evans JL, Goldfine ID, Maddux BA, et al. Oxidative stress and stress-activated signaling pathways: a unifying hypothesis of type 2 diabetes. Endocr Rev 2002;23(5):599–622.

159. Bounous G. Whey protein concentrate (WPC) and glutathione modulation in cancer treatment. Anticancer Res 2000;20(6C):4785–92.

160. Hirnerová E, Krahulec B, Strbová L, et al. Effect of vitamin E therapy on progression of diabetic nephropathy. Vnitr Lek 2003;49(7):529–34.

161. Li YC. Vitamin D and diabetic nephropathy. Curr Diab Rep 2008;8(6):464–9.

162. Nakamura S, Li H, Adijiang A, et al. Pyridoxal phosphate prevents progression of diabetic nephropathy. Nephrol Dial Transplant 2007;22(8):2165–74.

163. Ruhe RC, McDonald RB. Use of antioxidant nutrients in the prevention and treatment of type 2 diabetes. J Am Coll Nutr 2001;20(5 Suppl.):363S–9S, discussion 381S–3S.

164. Tong HI. Influence of neurotropic vitamins on the nerve conduction velocity in diabetic neuropathy. Ann Acad Med Singapore 1980;9(1):65–70.

165. Foster TS. Efficacy and safety of alpha-lipoic acid supplementation in the treatment of symptomatic diabetic neuropathy. Diabetes Educ 2007;33(1):111–17.

166. Becić F, Kapić E, Rakanović-Todić M. Pharmacological significance of alpha lipoic acid in up to date treatment of diabetic neuropathy. Med Arh 2008;62(1):45–8.

167. Wang H, Zhang ZB, Wen RR, et al. Experimental and clinical studies on the reduction of erythrocyte sorbitol-glucose ratios by ascorbic acid in diabetes mellitus. Diabetes Res Clin Pract 1995;28(1):1–8.

168. Sima AAF, Calvani M, Mehra M, et al. AcetyL-L-carnitine improves pain, nerve regeneration, and vibratory perception in patients with chronic diabetic neuropathy. Diabetes Care 2005;28(1):89–94.

169. Ide H, Fujiya S, Asanuma Y, et al. Clinical usefulness of intrathecal injection of methylcobalamin in patients with diabetic neuropathy. Clin Ther 1987;9(2):183–92.

170. Huseini HF, Larijani B, Heshmat R, et al. The efficacy of Silybum marianum (L.) Gaertn. (silymarin) in the treatment of type II diabetes: a randomized, double-blind, placebo-controlled, clinical trial. Phytother Res 2006;20(12):1036–9.

171. Kang M-H, Lee MS, Choi M-K, et al. Hypoglycemic activity of Gymnema sylvestre extracts on oxidative stress and antioxidant status in diabetic rats. J Agric Food Chem 2012;60(10):2517–24.

172. Khajehdehi P, Pakfetrat M, Javidnia K, et al. Oral supplementation of turmeric attenuates proteinuria, transforming growth factor-β and interleukin-8 levels in patients with overt type 2 diabetic nephropathy: a randomized, double-blind and placebo-controlled study. Scand J Urol Nephrol 2011;45(5):365–70.

173. Leach M. Aesculus hippocastanum. Aust J Med Herb 2001;13(4):136–40.

174. Leach MJ. Evidence-based practice: a framework for clinical practice and research design. Int J Nurs Pract 2006;12(5):248–51.

175. Leach MJ. Integrative health care: a need for change? J Complement Integr Med 2006;3(1):1–11.

176. Deng YP, Xie XJ. Preliminary study on the treatment of diabetic retinopathy utilizing with nourishing yin, tonifying kidney and blood-activating herbs. Zhongguo Zhong Xi Yi Jie He Za Zhi 1992;12(5):270.

177. Lopes de Jesus C, Atallah A, Valente O, et al. Vitamin C and superoxide dismutase (SOD) for diabetic retinopathy. Cochrane Database Syst Rev 2008;(1):CD006695.

178. Millen AE, Gruber M, Klein R, et al. Relations of serum ascorbic acid and alpha-tocopherol to diabetic retinopathy in the Third National Health and Nutrition Examination Survey. Am J Epidemiol 2003;158(3):225–33.

179. Millen AE, Klein R, Folsom AR, et al. Relation between intake of vitamins C and E and risk of diabetic retinopathy in the Atherosclerosis Risk in Communities Study. Am J Clin Nutr 2004;79(5):865–73.

180. Zou LH, Zhang JH, Liu PF. Clinical observation on Qidi Yiqi Yangyin Huoxue Recipe in treating diabetic nephropathy at stage III and IV. Zhongguo Zhong Xi Yi Jie He Za Zhi 2006;26(11):1023–6.

181. Zhao L, Lan LG, Min XL, et al. Integrated treatment of traditional Chinese medicine and western medicine for early- and intermediate-stage diabetic nephropathy. Nan Fang Yi Ke Da Xue Xue Bao 2007;27(7):1052–5.

182. Wu S, Han Y, Li J. Treatment of incipient diabetic nephropathy by clearing away the stomach-heat, purging the heart fire, strengthening the spleen and tonifying the kidney. J Tradit Chin Med 2000;20(3):172–5.

183. Wang HY, Chen YP. Clinical observation on treatment of diabetic nephropathy with compound fructus arctii mixture. Zhongguo Zhong Xi Yi Jie He Za Zhi 2004;24(7):589–92.

184. Lu J, He H. Clinical observation of gingko biloba extract injection in treating early diabetic nephropathy. Chin J Integr Med 2005;11(3):226 8.

185. Zhu HW, Shi ZF, Chen YY. Effect of extract of ginkgo biloba leaf on early diabetic nephropathy. Zhongguo Zhong Xi Yi Jie He Za Zhi 2005;25(10):889–91.

186. Li XS, Fu XJ, Lang XJ. Effect of extract of Ginkgo biloba on soluble intercellular adhesion molecule-1 and soluble vascular cell adhesion molecule-1 in patients with early diabetic nephropathy. Zhongguo Zhong Xi Yi Jie He Za Zhi 2007;27(5):412–14.

187. Rudkowska I. Fish oils for cardiovascular disease: impact on diabetes. Maturitas 2010;67(1):25–8.

188. Pouwer F, Nijpels G, Beekman AT, et al. Fat food for a bad mood. Could we treat and prevent depression in Type 2 diabetes by means of omega-3 polyunsaturated

fatty acids? A review of the evidence. Diabet Med 2005;22(11):1465–75.

189. Romerio SC, Linder L, Nyfeler J, et al. Acute hyperhomocysteinemia decreases NO bioavailability in healthy adults [see comment]. Atherosclerosis 2004;176(2):337–44.

190. Eto M, Watanabe K, Chonan N, et al. Lowering effect of pantethine on plasma beta-thromboglobulin and lipids in diabetes mellitus. Artery 1987;15(1):1–12.

191. Arsenio L, Bodria P, Magnati G, et al. Effectiveness of long-term treatment with pantethine in patients with dyslipidemia. Clin Ther 1986;8(5):537–45.

192. Bahadoran Z, Mirmiran P, Hosseinpanah F, et al. Broccoli sprouts powder could improve serum triglyceride and oxidized LDL/LDL-cholesterol ratio in type 2 diabetic patients: a randomized double-blind placebo-controlled clinical trial. Diabetes Res Clin Pract 2012;96(3):348–54.

193. Andersson U, Berger K, Högberg A, et al. Effects of rose hip intake on risk markers of type 2 diabetes and cardiovascular disease: a randomized, double-blind, cross-over investigation in obese persons. Eur J Clin Nutr 2012;66(5):585–90.

194. El-Sayed M-IK. Effects of Portulaca oleracea L. seeds in treatment of type-2 diabetes mellitus patients as adjunctive and alternative therapy. J Ethnopharmacol 2011;137(1):643–51.

195. Marrero MB, Lucas R, Salet C, et al. An alpha7 nicotinic acetylcholine receptor-selective agonist reduces weight gain and metabolic changes in a mouse model of diabetes. J Pharmacol Exp Ther 2010;332(1):173–80.

196. Fatmawati S, Kurashiki K, Takeno S, et al. The inhibitory effect on aldose reductase by an extract of Ganoderma lucidum. Phytother Res 2009;23(1):28–32.

197. Saraswat M, Muthenna P, Suryanarayana P, et al. Dietary sources of aldose reductase inhibitors: prospects for alleviating diabetic complications. Asia Pac J Clin Nutr 2008;17(4):558–65.

198. Hooper PL. Hot-tub therapy for type 2 diabetes mellitus. N Engl J Med 1999;341(12):924–5.

199. Krause M, Ludwig MS, Heck TG, et al. Heat shock proteins and heat therapy for type 2 diabetes: pros and cons. Curr Opin Clin Nutr Metab Care 2015;18(4):374–80.

200. Thind H, Lantini R, Balletto BL, et al. The effects of yoga among adults with type 2 diabetes: a systematic review and meta-analysis. Prev Med 2017;105:116–26.

201. Lodha R, Bagga A. Traditional Indian systems of medicine. Ann Acad Med Singapore 2000;29(1):37–41.

202. Hung J-Y, Chiou C-J, Chang H-Y. Relationships between medical beliefs of superiority of Chinese or Western medicine, medical behaviours and glycaemic control in diabetic outpatients in Taiwan. Health Soc Care Community 2012;20(1):80–6.

203. Wolever RQ, Webber DM, Meunier JP, et al. Modifiable disease risk, readiness to change, and psychosocial functioning improve with integrative medicine immersion model. Altern Ther Health Med 2011;17(4):38–47.

204. Uusitupa M, Tuomilehto J, Puska P. Are we really active in the prevention of obesity and type 2 diabetes at the community level? Nutr Metab Cardiovasc Dis 2011;21(5):380–9.

205. Chao M, Wang C, Dong X, et al. The effects of Tai Chi on type 2 diabetes mellitus: a meta-analysis. J Diabetes Res 2018.

206. Pothuraju R, Sharma RK, Chagalamarri J, et al. A systematic review of Gymnema sylvestre in obesity and diabetes management. J Sci Food Agric 2014;94(5):834–40.

207. Gong J, Fang K, Dong H, et al. Effect of fenugreek on hyperglycaemia and hyperlipidemia in diabetes and prediabetes: a meta-analysis. J Ethnopharmacol 2016;194:260–8.

208. Huang H, Chen G, Dong Y, et al. Chromium supplementation for adjuvant treatment of type 2 diabetes mellitus: results from a pooled analysis. Mol Nutr Food Res 2018;62(1):1700438.

209. Costello RB, Dwyer JT, Bailey RL. Chromium supplements for glycemic control in type 2 diabetes: limited evidence of effectiveness. Nutr Rev 2016;74(7):455–68.

210. Suksomboon N, Poolsup N, Yuwanakorn A. Systematic review and meta-analysis of the efficacy and safety of chromium supplementation in diabetes. J Clin Pharm Ther 2014;39(3):292–306.

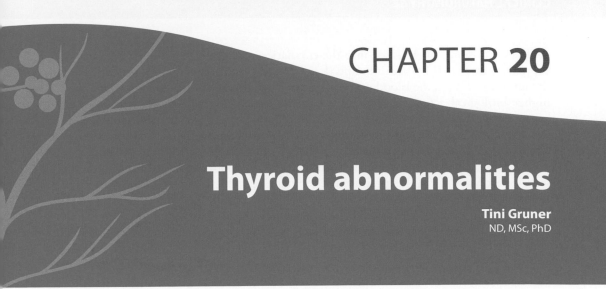

CHAPTER 20

Thyroid abnormalities

Tini Gruner
ND, MSc, PhD

OVERVIEW

The main function of the thyroid is to produce hormones that control the metabolic rate of all cells as well as energy, cell growth and tissue differentiation.[1-3] This is regulated by thyrotrophin-releasing hormone (TRH), secreted by the hypothalamus, which activates thyroid-stimulating hormone (TSH), secreted by the pituitary gland, to produce thyroxine (T_4) and triiodothyronine (T_3) (Figure 20.1).[2]

The precursors for thyroid hormone production are tyrosine and iodine. Iodine is oxidised to iodide (I^-) via hydrogen peroxide and actively transported into the thyroid gland where it accumulates (~60 mg/day). This leads to a much higher concentration in this gland than elsewhere in the body. It is then attached to the tyrosyl residues on thyroglobulin to produce T_4 and some T_3.[4]

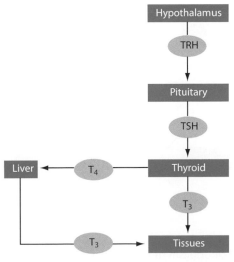

Figure 20.1
Thyroid hormone stimulation

These hormones are released into the circulation where most are bound to transport proteins. Less than 0.1% are unbound (free T_3 and T_4) and active as hormones. Although the amount of T_4 in the blood exceeds that of T_3 nearly 50-fold, it is T_3 that has much higher biological activity.[5,6] Zinc seems to be needed to facilitate the uptake of the hormone by the cells[7] and favorably affects T_3.[8] Some organs and tissues can convert T_4 to T_3 (mainly liver, kidneys, brain, muscle and brown adipose tissue), with most of the circulating T_3 having been produced peripherally[9] or in the liver. The conversion of T_4 to T_3 is accomplished by 5'-deiodinase, which is selenium dependent.[6,10] In the absence of selenium, reverse T_3 (rT_3) is produced at cellular level, which is metabolically inactive.[11] Figure 20.2 shows the metabolic pathways of T_4 conversion.[6]

Thyroid function not only depends on sufficient precursors (such as iodine and tyrosine) but also on hormone synthesis regulation and the demand for these hormones. Synthesis of T_3 and T_4 depends on negative feedback from TSH levels as well as the amount of iodine within the thyroid gland.[4]

Disturbances in any of these hormones or cofactors can lead to increased TSH production by the pituitary gland with subsequent (non-toxic) goitre formation. This increased thyroid tissue is an attempt to produce sufficient thyroid hormones in order to maintain normal blood levels (Figure 20.3). However, if the enlarged thyroid gland overproduces thyroid hormones, leading to hyperthyroidism, it is called a 'toxic goitre'.[12]

Thyroid antibodies (to thyroglobulin, peroxidase or thyroid receptor) are only raised in the autoimmune forms of hypothyroidism (Hashimoto's disease) and hyperthyroidism (Graves' disease). Before manifesting in its hypothyroid phase, Hashimoto's disease presents temporarily in a hyperthyroid phase with low TSH, high or normal free T_3, high free T_4 and rT_3. Gastrointestinal pathogens, through 'molecular mimicry', could be partly responsible for this.[2,13] See Chapter 31 on autoimmunity for further details.

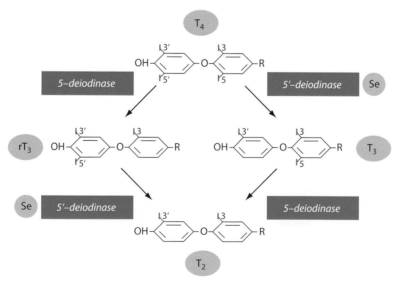

Figure 20.2
Conversion of T_4 to T_3 and catabolism to T_2*

*The selenium-dependent 5'-deiodinase converts T_4 to the more potent T_3 and further degrades this to T_2. In the absence of selenium the inactive rT3 is produced, which then accumulates.

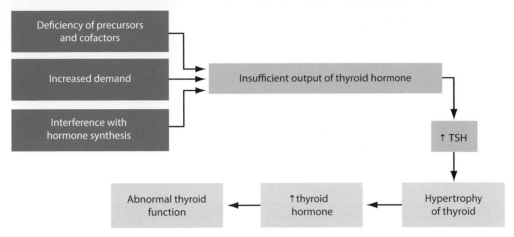

Figure 20.3
Development of goitre
Adapted from Crowley 2004[12]

Hypothyroidism

In hypothyroidism a disturbance in glucose tolerance has been found to be due to decreased sensitivity to insulin, and raised cortisol and free fatty acids.[14] This is not surprising considering that insulin resistance, diabetes type 2, stress (hypercortisolism and hyperadrenalism) and hypothyroidism share a number of common signs and symptoms, taking into account the link between the hormones involved in these conditions. Raised cortisol levels with impaired glucagon response were noted when hypoglycaemia was induced in hypothyroid patients.[15] Insulin and glucose control was regained when these patients were given thyroid hormone replacement therapy.[16] Further, hypothyroidism, like insulin resistance and diabetes type 2, leads to inhibition of delta 5 and 6 desaturase, impeding the utilisation of dietary omega-3 and omega-6 fatty acids.[2] A rise in blood pressure has been noted in the hypothyroid state, which normalised on thyroid treatment.[17] Conversely, impaired extrathyroidal conversion of T_4 to T_3 has been found in diseases such as heart and liver disease and diabetes type 2, where there is high plasma free fatty acid concentration with no obvious thyroid pathology.[2]

Sick euthyroid syndrome, also called low T_3 syndrome or rT_3 dominance, an underfunctioning thyroid with apparently normal test results, can occur as part of a number of health problems. It has been found, for a variety of reasons, to be part of virtually all severe systemic illnesses, fasting and major operations, affecting T_3, T_4 and rT_3.[18] Treating obese people with hypocaloric diets leads to similar thyroid hormone changes as in anorexia, namely decreases in T_3 and T_4 and increases in rT_3. These hormones will normalise with weight normalisation.[19] Certain medications also influence thyroid hormone status by either increasing or decreasing T_4.[9] The secondary hypothyroidism arises from an inability of the pituitary gland to secrete TSH, possibly due to low TRH, while tertiary hypothyroidism results from a malfunction of the hypothalamus. Therefore, when there is indication from the symptom picture that thyroid function could be compromised, not only TSH but also T_3 and T_4 should be measured in order to determine treatment options.[20]

Hyperthyroidism

In hyperthyroidism T_3 and T_4 are elevated, leading to suppression of TSH. The most common cause is Graves' disease where the body overproduces thyroid-stimulating immunoglobulin, an antibody that activates TSH receptors but does not undergo negative feedback. Less common causes are hypothalamic or anterior pituitary oversecretion (example of TRH) or a hypersecreting thyroid tumour. The result is uninhibited thyroid hormone production and resultant increase in basal metabolic rate. A goitre is usually present in this condition.[21,22] Manifestations of hyper- and hypothyroidism are listed in Table 20.1.

Table 20.1
Manifestations of hyper- and hypothyroidism[5,12,13]

Clinical effects	Hypothyroidism	Hyperthyroidism
General features	Goitre, myxoedema, deep voice, impaired growth	Exophthalmos, lid lag, decreased blinking
Metabolic effects	Decreased basal metabolic rate, weight gain, cold intolerance, hypothermia	Increased basal metabolic rate, weight loss, heat intolerance, borderline hyperthermia
Mental/emotional	Mental and physical sluggishness, somnolence, placid and phlegmatic personality, depression	Hyperkinesis, wakefulness, restlessness, irritability, emotional lability
Gastrointestinal effects	Constipation, decreased appetite	Diarrhoea, increased appetite
Cardiovascular effects	Increased cholesterol, decreased cardiac output, bradycardia	Decreased cholesterol, increased cardiac output, tachycardia and palpitations
Respiratory effects	Hypoventilation	Dyspnoea
Metabolic syndrome effects	Sluggish muscle tone and reflexes	Increased muscle tone and reflexes, tremor, twitching, accelerated bone loss and risk of fractures, myopathy
Skin and hair	Course, cold, dry, myxoedema	Thin and silky, warm, moist

Testing for thyroid function

Table 20.2 gives an overview of the laboratory parameters for each condition, and Table 20.3 shows the reference ranges (currently 0.3–5.0 mU/L with some variations between laboratories) and the ideal ranges of these parameters. By measuring TSH only, thyroid conditions can be missed or misinterpreted. (Further information regarding tests commonly employed to assess thyroid (dys)function can be found in the review by Shivaraj et al.[23]) In addition, the thyroid should be checked for goitre and nodules by palpation and the latter, if needed, by ultrasound or biopsy.[9]

Laboratory reference values for these parameters encompass 95% of the 'healthy' population, and generally only when individual values are outside this range will further investigations and possibly therapy be instigated by the doctor. However, the upper limit of current reference ranges has been deemed too high, with high-normal values potentially including people with subclinical (occult) hypothyroid (SCH) or the risk of developing this condition.[24–26] It is believed that with high-normal TSH values the thyroid is labouring (as in SCH). Yet some researchers still believe that the upper limit of the reference range should be maintained.[27–29] Although people with diagnosed anti-thyroid peroxidase antibodies (antiTPO) and overt thyroid disease were excluded,

Table 20.2
Thyroid test results for common thyroid disorders*

Condition	TSH	Total T$_4$	Free T$_4$	T$_3$
Hyperthyroidism	Suppressed	Increased	Increased	Increased
Hypothyroidism (primary)	Increased	Low/low-normal	Low/low-normal	Normal or low
TSH deficiency (secondary or tertiary hypothyroid)	Low/low-normal	Low/low-normal	Low/low-normal	Normal or low
Sick euthyroid syndrome	Low/low-normal	Slightly low	Slightly low	Slightly low, with increased rT$_3$

*Adapted from Kumar and Clark[13] and Sherwood 2013[21]

Table 20.3
Reference ranges and ideal ranges of thyroid parameters[3]

Parameter	Reference range	Ideal range
TSH	0.3–5 mU/L	0.4–2.5 mU/L
T$_3$	2.6–6.0 pmol/L	4–5 pmol/L
T$_4$	9–19 pmol/L	14–19 pmol/L
rT$_3$	140–540 pmol/L	< 240 pmol/L
Thyroglobulin Ab	< 4 IU/mL	< 1 IU/mL
Peroxidase Ab	< 6 IU/mL	< 1 IU/mL
Thyroid hormone receptor Ab	< 1 IU/L	< 1 IU/L

Ab = antibodies

subjects with SCH may still have been included in some of these studies. Further, it should be taken into account that TSH levels, at least in hypothyroid patients taking T$_4$, are subject to circadian variability, which influences not only the reference range but also the time of day of blood sampling.[30]

The reference ranges and/or upper limits for TSH suggested by various researchers are listed in Table 20.4. Åsvold et al.[31] found that the risk of developing hypothyroidism gradually increased from TSH of 0.5–1.4 mU/L to TSH of 4.0–4.5 mU/L, and the risk of developing hyperthyroidism was higher in women with a TSH of 0.2–0.49 mU/L. Bar-Andziak et al.[32] surveyed more than 4000 elderly people in Poland and found that around 80% had SCH, with women being more likely to develop this condition than men. The overall incidence in Australia is estimated at 5 in 1000 in males and 27 in 1000 in females. Approximately 10–12 million people in the United States have hypothyroidism.[33] High-normal TSH was also associated with metabolic syndrome.[34] In a healthy thyroid the actual hormones (T$_3$ and T$_4$) should ideally be in the high-normal range. The ratio of T$_4$ to T$_3$ has been estimated as 4:1 in healthy thyroid function.[2] Antibodies should be absent and rT$_3$ should be low. In both hyper- and hypothyroidism, despite the best treatment measures, symptoms can persist, leading to compromised quality of life. It would therefore be prudent to assess thyroid function not only through laboratory testing and temperature readings, but also through a comprehensive interview or questionnaire that takes the patient's symptoms and overall health status into account.[35]

Table 20.4
Suggested TSH reference ranges

Reference range	Authors	Study type
1.0–1.9 mU/L	Guan et al. 2008[36]	Five-year follow-up population study (China)
1.18 mU/L	Wartofsky & Dickey[24] Dickey & Wartofsky[26]	Laboratory data from people with low incidence of thyroid disease
1.95 mU/L	Völzke et al. 2009,[37] 2010[38]	Population study (Pomerania – SHIP)
2.0 mU/L	Walter et al. 2012[39]	Cross-sectional study
2.5–4 mU/L	Walsh et al. 2010[40]	Busselton Health Surveys (Australia)
2.93–3.38 mU/L	Žrković et al. 2011[41]	Cohort study
3.0–3.5 mU/l	Moncayo et al. 2007[42]	Intravenous TRH stimulation
~3.5 mU/L	Rosario et al. 2010[43]	Population study (Brazil)
3.6 mU/L	Schalin-Jäntti et al. 2011[44]	Population study (Finland)

RISK FACTORS

Hypothyroidism

Subclinical hypothyroidism

SCH has been characterised by elevated TSH with normal T_3 and T_4.[45,46] There is still debate regarding the significance and possible treatment of SCH. Although treatment with T_4 and/or T_3 has apparently not been shown to provide benefits,[47] withholding treatment may be ill advised. Subtle improvements with early hormonal intervention have been observed, thus warranting thyroid hormone replacement in subclinical manifestations.[48,49] Most at risk are the elderly and women over the age of 60 years, with increased risk of developing overt hypothyroidism.[46] It is therefore recommended that this population group, people with autoimmune disease and anybody with suggestive symptoms of hypo-thyroidism be screened.[50] TSH values ranging between 4.5 and 10 mU/L, particularly if antibodies or symptoms are present, may indicate the need for commencement of low-dose T_4 treatment.[51] However, some researchers consider a TSH range up to 20 mU/L (well above the upper limit of the reference range) as the cut-off before instigating therapy.[33] It is interesting to note that the upper limit of normal for TSH has been reduced from 10 mU/L to between 4 and 5 mU/L during the last decade,[33] with suggestions that this may be further reduced to 2.5 mU/L in the near future. This is based on the observa-tion that 95% of people with normal thyroid function have values under 2.5 mU/L.[24] Suboptimal thyroid function may be due to latent Hashimoto's disease, which could lead, if not addressed early, to overt hypothyroidism.[24,26,33,46]

Patients with SCH tend to have higher readings of blood pressure, C-reactive protein (CRP) homocysteine, cholesterol and low-density lipoprotein (LDL), and therefore may be presenting with cardiovascular risk factors or disease, including congestive heart failure. Endothelial dysfunction[37] and arterial stiffness[52] have been found with high-normal TSH levels, suggestive of increased risk of heart disease. TSH below 2 mU/L has been associated with lower levels of homocysteine and CRP.[53] In addition, TSH levels over 2.5 mU/L have been associated with increased multiple sclerosis (MS),[54] with MS parameters correlating with T_3 and T_4.[55] Weight loss in obese children and adolescents resulted in reduced TSH in relation to insulin levels.[56]

Early treatment is therefore recommended[33]; this will also improve long-term life quality by preventing the development of overt hypothyroidism and also reducing the risk factors for cardiovascular disease, not to mention the benefits to the healthcare system. Low T_4 has been attributed to decreases in thyrotropin as well as T_4-binding globulins. Supplementation with T_3, not T_4, has resulted in improvements. The effect of severe systemic illness on thyroid function has been termed 'nonthyroidal illness syndrome' (NTIS).[18] Further, a low T_3 syndrome has been described with increased pro-inflammatory cytokines, notably IL-6, which inhibits 5'-deiodinase. This is commonly seen in congestive heart failure, and T_3 has been shown to be a stronger indicator of all-cause and congestive heart failure mortality than age or dyslipidaemia.[33]

Stress

Stress seems to play a crucial part in thyroid dysregulation and interference with hormone synthesis by triggering the release of corticotrophin-releasing hormone, noradrenaline and cortisol. These hormones have an inhibitory influence on TSH secretion and suppress 5'-deiodinase, thus contributing to the suppression of thyroid function[57] (see Chapter 18 on stress and fatigue). Cortisol also impacts thyroid receptor and T_4 to T_3 conversion. Walter et al.[39] suggest that cortisol and TSH are positively correlated.

The thyroid, and the adrenal glands, require tyrosine for thyroid hormone and catecholamine synthesis, respectively. Low protein intake and/or impaired protein digestion/use may lead to low tyrosine stores, resulting in low thyroid hormones, especially if this amino acid is required to preferentially produce stress hormones (dopamine, noradrenaline and adrenaline). Urinary cortisol metabolite levels have also been linked to thyroid disorders, both in hyper- and hypothyroidism, indicative of the influence of stress on thyroid function.[58]

Iodine deficiency

Iodine is a common deficiency worldwide, leading to hypothyroidism.[13,21] It is estimated that two billion people worldwide do not get sufficient iodine in their diet.[59] Various parts of Australia and New Zealand[60,61] have been found to be deficient. Often the first visible sign is the development of a goitre. Congenital hypothyroidism, caused by maternal iodine deficiency, leads to mental and physical retardation in infants known as cretinism.[9,62] Iodine reference values, according to the World Health Organization/-International Council for the Control of Iodine Deficiency Disorders (WHO/ICCIDD), are given in Table 20.5. These reference ranges should be adhered to and excessive iodine intake avoided because this may lead to either hyper- or hypothyroidism.[63–65] Although salt iodisation led to a decline in goitre, an increase in autoimmune thyroiditis has also been noted.[66,67] In patients presenting with thyroid dysfunction without a known cause iodine excess should therefore be considered.[68] Adequate selenium status is protective of iodine excess.[69]

Medical alert
Acute exacerbation of hyperthyroid symptoms can occur, called a 'thyroid storm'. It can be brought on by major internal or external stressful events or if hyperthyroidism is inadequately controlled. This condition requires urgent medical attention.[13]

Table 20.5
24-hour urinary iodine reference values[1,2]

Urinary iodine (µg/L)	Iodine nutritional status
< 20	Severe deficiency
20–49	Moderate deficiency
50–99	Mild deficiency
100–199	Optimal status
≥ 200	Risk of adverse effects (e.g. hyperthyroidism)

Selenium deficiency

Like iodine, the thyroid gland contains the highest amount of selenium of any tissue.[70] It is needed for the conversion of T_4 to T_3 (Figure 20.2) as part of several (but not all) deiodinases where it is incorporated as selenocysteine. If selenium is low, the result is not only reduced active thyroid hormone (T_3) but the resultant accumulation of rT_3. Further, rT_3 is also known to block the action of thyroid hormone, thus contributing to hypothyroidism. It is therefore important to measure rT_3, especially with normal T_4 and low T_3 results. Hence, when T_3 is low selenium deficiency should be considered as rT_3 could be elevated.[18] Trauma from injury affects thyroid metabolism with lowered selenium levels, and supplementation with selenium has led to faster normalisation of T_4 and reductions in rT_3. In congenital hypothyroidism, selenium (as selenomethionine) was found to lower TSH and thyroglobulin. It was suggested that the mechanism involved feedback to the hypothalamus–pituitary, therefore reducing the stimulation of thyroid tissue and increasing intracellular conversion of T_4 to T_3.

Similarly, in critically ill patients low selenium and T_3 and elevated rT_3 have been found, in addition to low TSH and T_4. However, not only low selenium but also increased cytokine production during inflammation in these patients are responsible for low 5'-deiodinase; this may explain the elevated rT_3. The abnormalities in these parameters have been found to correlate with the severity of the disease.[71] Kandhro et al.[72] postulated an important role for selenium in reducing the severity of hypothyroidism related to iodine deficiency. However, iodine needs to be replenished prior to selenium supplementation.[69] Selenium deficiency plays a role in autoimmune thyroid disease,[70] and supplementation with selenium has shown some beneficial effect on both hyper- and hypothyroidism.[73]

Pregnancy

Thyroid hormone production increases during pregnancy to accommodate the needs of the developing fetus. However, in areas where iodine is marginal or insufficient a woman's thyroid function may become compromised when pregnant. Thyroid dysfunction are common in women of childbearing age,[74] with an estimated 4–15% having overt or latent autoimmune thyroiditis,[75] even when test results indicate euthyroid.[76] Going undiagnosed and untreated into a pregnancy there is an increased risk of miscarriage, preterm delivery and fetal neurological impairment (such as is seen in cretinism)[77–79] as well as postpartum thyroid disease.[80,81] It is therefore important to identify and, if necessary, to treat these women as otherwise it can have adverse effects on fertility and pregnancy outcome, apart from fetal growth and brain development.[77,82,83] Thyroid issues should also be ruled out in women who fail to conceive[84] or who miscarry.[81]

During pregnancy, a 50% increase in iodine intake is recommended in order to meet the requirements of both mother and child.[85] A study of pregnant women in

New Zealand found urinary iodine concentrations well below the recommended sufficiency level; however, most had TSH and free T_4 levels still within the reference range,[78] begging the question whether reference ranges need to be adjusted for pregnancy.[86] Indeed, Skeaff[85] found improved neurodevelopment in children whose mothers had been supplemented with iodine during early pregnancy, but Rebagliato et al.[87] warns that excess iodine intake can also lead to maternal thyroid dysfunction (both hyper- and hypothyroidism). Elevated TSH could possibly be a transient stunning effect of the thyroid due to a sudden increase in iodine intake. Women are therefore recommended to start iodine supplementation well before pregnancy, especially in iodine-deficient areas.[88,89] A systematic review on intervention with thyroxine and selenomethionine for hypothyroidism or SCH found beneficial effects with treatment.[90]

A correlation between iron deficiency and goitre has been found in iodine and selenium depleted children, which requires further investigations regarding possible cause and effect relationship.[91] Zinc levels have also been negatively correlated with thyroid volume in nodular goitre and with autoimmune thyroid disorders, and positively correlated with free T_3.[92]

Toxins and drugs

Workers exposed to mercury vapours had a higher risk of hypothyroidism with decreased T_3 and increased rT_3 values, especially if they were also low in iodine.[93] Various chemicals can disrupt thyroperoxidase activity, leading to reduced iodine incorporation into thyroid hormone.[94] Endocrine-disrupting chemicals in the environment, specifically organochlorides such as polychlorinated biphenyls, pesticides and dioxin[95,96] and additives in plastics,[97] impact on thyroid hormones. Chlorinated and fluoridated drinking water may also contribute to thyroid dysfunction.[98,99] Interestingly, smoking was inversely related to SCH.[100]

Amiodarone, a commonly prescribed antiarrhythmic drug, has been associated with thyroid dysfunction[101,102] due to a potential iodine excess.[67] Children on antiepileptic medication, namely carbamazepine (Tegretol) and valproate (Epilim), have shown decreased T_4 levels and their thyroid function should therefore be assessed regularly.[103]

Hyperthyroidism

Molecular mimicry

In hyperthyroidism thyroid hormones are high, suppressing TSH. The increases in T_3 and T_4 are evidently due to an antithyroid autoantibody thyroid-stimulating immunoglobulin, which acts like TSH but is not controlled by the same negative feedback mechanism.[12]

DIFFERENTIAL DIAGNOSIS[9,13]

Hyperthyroidism
- Anxiety
- General elevated stress
- Insomnia
- Addison's disease

Hypothyroidism
- Cushing's syndrome
- Depression
- Psychosis
- Chronic fatigue
- Diabetes type 2
- Dementia
- Cognitive decline in older patients (especially women)
- Thyroid carcinoma

Certain gram-negative bacteria, such as *Yersinia enterocolitica* and *Escherichia coli*, have been shown to contain TSH binding sites. It could therefore be possible that infection with these organisms could initiate hyperthyroidism through 'molecular mimicry'.[13]

CONVENTIONAL TREATMENT

Hyperthyroidism

Whether hyperthyroidism should be treated or not depends on the clinical assessment and the risk of consequences of untreated disease.[104] Depending on the severity of the disease, hyperthyroidism is treated with drugs that suppress the production of thyroid hormones, radioactive iodine to destroy part or all of the thyroid gland or surgery to remove some or the entire thyroid. The latter two are likely to require thyroid hormone replacement for life.[13]

In order to make treatment effective but not detrimental to health, in total thyroid-ectomy a replacement dose of T_4 is usually given at 1.6 µg/kg body weight, with an absorption rate of approximately 65%, resulting in a daily dose of 100–200 µg. It takes four to six weeks for hormone levels to adjust to treatment.[42]

Hypothyroidism

The aim of treatment is to normalise thyroid function, and the treatment of choice for hypothyroidism is levothyroxine sodium (L-T_4). It is best taken one hour prior to or two to three hours after meals as the absorption of T_4 is altered by food intake. Absorption of thyroxine also depends on various factors such as gastric acid secretion, gastric atrophy and *Helicobacter pylori* infection.[105]

In primary hypothyroidism, optimisation is achieved when TSH levels are 0.5–2 mU/L,[42,106] and in secondary hypothyroidism (where TSH is low) with T_4 and T_3 levels in the upper normal range. It is therefore important not to rely on TSH levels alone. However, even with normalisation of TSH and thyroid hormones many people's life quality is not optimised.[107] A German study (SHIP) found that treatment needs to be monitored carefully as close to 30% of patients on thyroxine still had TSH levels outside the reference range (below or above).[108] It has therefore been recommended to treat so that thyroxine is in the upper range of normal.[109]

When two doses of L-T_4 were compared, one to bring T_4 into the middle and the other into the upper range of normal, the higher dose resulted in lower body mass index, cholesterol and LDL. When the high dose of L-T_4 was combined with liothyronine (L-T_3) at a ratio of 9:1, further benefits were obtained.[42] In contrast, Walsh et al.[110] found no difference in symptoms when T_4 was aimed at getting TSH into the lower reference range.

This indicates that in certain situations L-T_4 alone is insufficient to return thyroid function to normal.[111] It is estimated that in 10–20% of hypothyroid patients symptoms will persist. This could be due to impaired conversion of T_4 to T_3 (see earlier under *Selenium*), a polymorphism in the enzyme 5'-deiodinase,[42] plus several others.[112] Treatment with L-T_3 should therefore be considered when T_4 alone does not improve symptoms or laboratory parameters.[18,42] This is particularly the case in secondary hypothyroidism due to other ill health where there is impaired conversion from T_4 to T_3. In vivo, however, T_3 has a short half-life, leading to supraphysiological peaks without normalisation of TSH. Slow-release formulations are therefore needed.[42] To overcome the problem regarding when to give T_4 and when T_3, combination preparations are available. However, apart from using the L-T$_3$ with its half-life problems, the studies done on this have not included measures that indicated the need for T$_3$.[113] To overcome the instability of T$_3$, desiccated extract of bovine or porcine thyroid have been used.[42,106] (Desiccated bovine or porcine thyroid extract is contained in some natural formulations currently on the market and which are available to naturopaths.) This was the standard treatment before L-T$_4$ was available commercially, but reproducible results were difficult, if not impossible, to obtain due to the variability of thyroid hormone content in these preparations.[42]

In younger people diagnosed with hypothyroidism, treatment with T$_4$ should be instigated at the highest calculated dose, whereas in older people the dose should be conservative and slowly titrated up to avoid complications, particularly in those people with coronary artery disease. However, long-term treatment above the optimal dose can lead to osteoporosis and atrial fibrillation and should therefore be avoided.[42,106]

In autoimmune hypothyroid women planning pregnancy, TSH levels should be kept below 2.5 mU/L, with a 30% increase in L-T$_4$ dosage once pregnancy has been confirmed.[33] Table 20.6 lists the treatments currently employed to treat hyper- and hypothyroidism.

Table 20.6
Conventional treatment for hyper- and hypothyroidism

Condition	Drug	Action
Hyperthyroidism	Propylthiouracil carbimazole (active metabolite: methimazole)	Antithyroid drugs: inhibit formation of thyroid hormone; immunosuppressive
	Propranolol	Beta-blocker: ↓ sympathetic nervous system activity ↓ peripheral T$_4$ to T$_3$ conversion
	Radioactive iodine	Radiation destroys part or all of thyroid gland (could lead to hypothyroidism)
	Surgery	Partial or total thyroidectomy (could lead to hypothyroidism)
Hypothyroidism	Oroxine (thyroxine) (L-T$_4$)	Replacement of thyroid hormone (T$_4$)
	In some cases, liothyronine (L-T$_3$) has been added to T$_4$	Replacement of thyroid hormones (T$_3$ and T$_4$)
	Desiccated extract of beef or pork thyroid	Replacement of thyroid hormones (T$_3$ and T$_4$)

KEY TREATMENT PROTOCOLS

General considerations

Diagnostic aids

Accurate diagnosis is vital for an effective treatment protocol. In the early stages of thyroid disorders the symptoms can be quite general (such as loose stools or constipation, and changes in energy) and part of a multitude of disease entities. When the prominent signs and symptoms of hyper- and hypothyroidism appear the disease is quite advanced. It is therefore imperative to find early markers so intervention can be started to prevent the manifestation of advanced disease states.

Temperature regulation

One such marker is body temperature. Ideally, a temperature reading needs to be taken at the same time each day in the morning, straight after waking and before getting out of bed. The reason for taking the temperature in the morning is the influence melatonin exerts on thyroid hormones.[107] The thermometer should be placed under the tongue until it beeps (for digital thermometers) or for a minimum of five minutes (if using a mercury one). Ear thermometers or taking the temperature under arm is too inaccurate for this purpose (although the latter has been advocated for decades). This should be repeated for four consecutive days and an average taken of the readings. For a woman of childbearing age, the temperature should be taken in

> ### Naturopathic Treatment Aims
>
> - Reduce stress.
> - Support stressed systems with adaptogens and anxiolytics (if indicated).
> - Enhance optimal thyroid function.
> - Increase quality of life.
> - Hyperthyroidism:
>   - Support overactive metabolic pathways, organs and systems through nutrient-dense foods, antioxidants, energy-production cofactors and other specific nutrients as indicated.
>   - Slow down thyroid function using phytotherapy.
> - Hypothyroidism:
>   - Ensure precursors (tyrosine, iodine) and cofactors (selenium, zinc) for thyroid hormone production are replete.
>   - Stimulate thyroid function using phytotherapy.

the first half of her cycle, ideally the days straight after menses, as there is a natural rise in temperature at ovulation and throughout the second half of the cycle.

A normal reading is 36.5–37.0°C. Low readings have been linked to thyroid under-function, and values above this range to hyperthyroidism. Research in elderly hospitalised patients revealed a link between low core (rectal) temperature, low T_3 and high rT_3 and mortality. Further, low serum albumin and weight loss (as indicators of malnutrition) have also been linked to hypothermia (defined as a core temperature between 35.0 and 36.5°C). Interestingly, TSH was not significantly different in these patients.[108] However, when healthy males were subjected to different sleep temperatures a significant increase was found in plasma cortisol and TSH with lowered body temperature.[109] Likewise, a rise in TSH and drop in T_3 and T_4 were noted in cold climates and winter months, especially in people above the age of 40 years.[110] In some subjects with fever, rT_3 was found to be directly correlated, whereas T_3 was inversely correlated to body temperature at 40°C reducing to levels seen only in severe hypothyroidism.[111] It seems that the thyroid gland is very sensitive to either heat or cold stress as a result of the hypothalamus–pituitary–thyroid axis dysregulation, and reacts by reducing its hormone production.[107,110] Considering the function of the thyroid in regulating metabolism, these results are not surprising.

A number of factors can interfere with the accuracy of the temperature method. Late nights, lack of sleep, infections and acute illnesses will alter the readings. Antidepressant medication has also been linked to lower body temperature. A significant rise in TSH and a drop in T_3 and T_4 have been noted after administration of antidepressants such as tricyclics and selective serotonin reuptake inhibitors (SSRIs) but also after lithium and electroshock treatment. In some patients a blunted TSH response to TRH has been found.[112] This begs the question whether these treatments interfere with negative feedback loops (such as between T_3 and TSH or TSH and TRH) or whether tyrosine was needed preferentially to produce adrenaline.

A low morning temperature may be the first indicator of suboptimal thyroid function. If this is the case it should be followed by a blood test. However, with no prior thyroid

---

Addressing underlying pathology

Treatment depends on the findings as a result of case taking, dietary analysis and pathology tests. If stress is a major contributor, adaptogens (e.g. *Withania somnifera, Rhodiola rosea, Panax ginseng, Eleutherococcus senticosus*) or anxiolytics (e.g. *Piper methysticum, Passiflora incarnata, Ziziphus spinosa*) could be of use.[113–116] If autoimmunity is present, anti-inflammatory (e.g. bioflavonoids,[117] enzymes[117] and *Curcuma longa*)[113] and immuno-suppressant (e.g. *Tylophora indica* and *Hemidesmus indicus*)[113] agents may be indicated.

---

pathology it is unlikely that a medical practitioner will order anything other than TSH. Yet it is obvious from the research discussed here that a TSH reading alone will not always reflect the actual functioning of the thyroid. If there is suspicion of thyroid pathology despite a low-normal TSH, T_3, T_4, thyroid antibodies and ideally rT_3 should be assessed. Currently, rT_3 is an out-of-pocket expense to the patient but worth doing if there is good clinical indication for this.

Manage mental health complications

In hypothyroidism there is an increased risk for depression. Comparisons between hypothyroid and euthyroid people revealed higher rates of depression in the former.[118]

Older people with SCH are more likely to visit a doctor for depression than people with normal thyroid function.[119] A thorough psychological examination is therefore warranted in people with SCH.[120] Being depressed can also have a negative influence on regular medication intake (for hypothyroid) as noncompliance with medication is more likely and perpetuates the depression.[121] See also Chapter 15 on depression.

Anxiety is common in hyperthyroid patients, which is not always easy to differentiate and hyperthyroidism should be ruled out.[122] Pathology testing is therefore recommended to rule out thyroid disease. However, thorough investigation regarding symptoms can reveal differences by which to determine the diagnosis. However, this should be rechecked if there is suggestive symptomatology.[123] See also Chapter 18 on stress and fatigue.

Hyperthyroidism

Managing increased metabolic rate

Nutritional treatment

In hyperthyroidism, metabolic rate and, as a result, energy production is increased. The overactive metabolism needs to be supported through nutrient-dense foods with ample amounts of fruit and vegetables for **antioxidant support**. Further, supplementation with Krebs cycle and oxidative phosphorylation nutrients, notably B vitamins, magnesium, coenzyme Q10 and carnitine (Table 20.7) is highly advisable.[2,6,22] See Table 20.9 for a summary of evidence.

The higher metabolic rate also affects bone growth, mineralisation and remodelling, which are determined by TSH and T_3. This is particularly the case in thyrotoxicosis. Supplementing with calcium and vitamin D may be needed.[124] L-carnitine, an amino acid often depleted in hyperthyroid patients, has been shown to be of benefit in both reducing the severity of the disease (including thyroid storm) as well as positively affecting bone density.[125,126]

Further, an increased metabolic rate brings with it increases in inflammation and oxidative stress, particularly if autoimmunity is also present.[127] The best cellular defence

Table 20.7
Nutraceuticals for hyperthyroidism

Supplement	Dosage	Rationale
B complex	1 b.i.d.	High quality, high dose, preferably in their activated (phosphorylated) forms, for ready use in energy production in the Krebs cycle
Coenzyme Q10	100 mg/day	Essential for energy production in the electron transport chain
Magnesium	100–400 mg/day	Needed in Krebs cycle and for any adenosine triphosphate (ATP)-dependent reactions
Antioxidants	1 b.i.d.	Broad-spectrum, high dose, to dampen the oxidative damage occurring through the higher metabolic rate and autoimmunity (if present)[59]
Vitamin C	1000 mg/day	Shown to benefit hyperthyroidism Best taken in small frequent doses
Leonurus cardiaca	15–40 mL/wk	To reduce iodine metabolism and thyroid hormone production[54,56]
Lycopus virginicus	15–25 mL/wk	Adjuvant therapy for thyroid hyperfunction. Inhibition of peripheral deiodination of T_4 to T_3[113,115]

includes broad-spectrum antioxidants (including the vitamins A, C and E, the minerals zinc and selenium and the bioactive substances α-lipoic acid, N-acetylcysteine and coenzyme Q10), as well as intracellular antioxidant support (notably glutathione and superoxide dismutase).[128] **Essential fatty acids** are also needed. **Vitamin C** at 1000 mg per day has been shown to give beneficial effects in hyperthyroidism.[22,129]

Herbal treatment
In order to dampen thyroid hormone production herbs such as *Lycopus virginicus* and *Leonurus cardiaca* are useful.[113,115] In a rat model, oral administration of *Lycopus virginicus* has reduced T_3 levels; this is thought to be the result of decreased peripheral T_4 conversion to T_3.[130] *Leonurus cardiaca* is used for nervous cardiac disorders such as palpitations,[115] and since these symptoms also occur in hyperthyroidism this herb has been used as an adjuvant for this condition.[113] Other herbs with thyroid-blocking action include *Melissa officinalis* and *Lithospermum* spp.[131,132]

Interfering factors
Dietary goitrogens (see the box below) or smoking can have an inhibitory effect on thyroid function by interfering with iodine uptake and thyroid hormone production. Paradoxically, excess iodine intake can also impede thyroid hormone production.[1,133]

Goitrogen sources

Regular intake of any substance containing thiocyanate, such as:

- raw brassica (coleslaw or cassava)
- tobacco

Others:
- millet
- soy
- catechins from tea

Sources: Danzi & Klein 2008,[1] Higdon 2003,[133] Doerge & Sheehan 2002,[134] Teas et al. 2007,[135] Messina & Redmond 2066,[136] Chandra 2013,[137] Sathyapalan et al. 2011[138] and Milerová et al. 2006.[139]

However, this is not recommended as a treatment as increased production of thyroid hormones could be the result, at least initially, therefore contributing to the problem.

Hypothyroidism

General considerations

Other autoimmune conditions, food allergies/intolerances and *Candidiasis* have been found to play a role in hypothyroid, especially Hashimoto's. They should be ruled out or, if present, addressed for optimal outcome of treatment.[22]

Cofactors for hormone production

For hypothyroidism, hormone precursors and cofactors, such as combinations of **tyrosine**, **iodine**, **selenium** and **zinc**, are recommended to support the thyroid (Table 20.8). However, hyperthyroidism can develop as a result of recent supplementation with iodine (or T_4) to correct a hypothyroid state. Commonly, nodules develop on the thyroid gland, secreting thyroid hormones that are not regulated by TSH. If this should occur iodine supplementation needs to cease and treatment as for hyperthyroidism instigated.[1]

Table 20.8
Nutraceuticals for hypothyroidism

Nutrient	Dosage	Rationale
Iodine[1,133,140,141]	150 µg/day	Constituent of thyroid hormone
Tyrosine[141]	1000–3000 mg/day	Constituent of thyroid hormone Needs to be taken between meals
Selenium[133,141]	100–200 µg/day	Facilitates the conversion from T_4 to the active form T_3
Zinc[7,8]	25 mg 1–2/day	Supports thyroid hormone regulation
Withania somnifera[142,143*]	5–13 mL/day 1:2 extract	Increasing T_3 and T_4
Bacopa monnieri[144*]	5–13 mL/day 1:2 extract	Increasing T_4
Fucus vesiculosus[113]	4.5–8.5 mL/day 1:1 extract	Contains iodine
Desiccated thyroid extract[33]		Contains T_3 and T_4

*Animal model research

Iodine

Iodine from dietary sources is usually well absorbed (close to 100%) but most of this is excreted in the urine (~90%). Adult requirements are ~150 µg/d. High calcium as well as salt intake reduces iodine absorption, which may play a role for people with marginal iodine status.[22]

Foods rich in iodine include seaweed products, seafood, eggs and products where iodine has been added to the feed. It has been noted that populations living in coastal areas with low iodine soils but an abundance of seaweed can maintain adequate iodine status, presumably through inhaling it.[145]

In the past, iodine has been used to sterilise milking equipment, resulting in iodine-rich milk. But in recent years iodine has been replaced by other methods of sterilisation (notably chlorine), so dairy is not a good source of iodine any longer.[146] The health risks involved with iodine deficiency have led to food fortifications by adding iodine to table salt in certain parts of the world, such as Australia, New Zealand and the United Kingdom where goitre used to be prevalent.[133] On one hand the decreasing use of salt has further contributed to lowered iodine status.[146] On the other hand, excess iodine intake due to food fortification also poses risks. Some of the soy formulations, such as Bonsoy milk, contain seaweed, and therefore caution should be exerted as to the dangers of giving soy to infants and affecting their thyroid function. Close monitoring is therefore indicated.[147]

Available iodine supplements include potassium iodide and potassium iodate, iodised vegetable oil, nascent (atomic) iodine and Lugol's solution. When treating iodine deficiency it was noted that simultaneously correcting other nutrient deficiencies, notably iron and vitamin A, produced significantly better results.[1,6,69,148] In pregnancy the requirement for thyroid hormone increases; this needs to be met by adequate iodine status. Therefore, additional iodine at about 125–150 µg/day should be supplied to allow for the increase in metabolic demand,[149–151] especially in vegans.[140]

When considering the body's status of any nutrient, including iodine, factors such as digestion, absorption, tissue uptake and metabolism need to be considered in addition to intake.[152] For instance, goitrogens (see the box on p. 424) in large amounts, particularly raw, interfere with iodine uptake and should be avoided, especially if iodine status is already compromised.[1,133]

As detailed in Table 20.8 certain herbs, such as **Withania somnifera**, **Bacopa monnieri** and **Fucus vesiculosus**, may be beneficial in hypothyroidism.[120,142–144] *Withania somnifera* has also been shown to cause a decrease in hepatic lipid peroxidation and may thus be useful in concomitant heart and liver disease.[143]

Nutraceuticals in thyroid disorders

It should be noted that currently there is a scarcity of evidence from robust human studies for the use of nutritional and herbal interventions to treat thyroid disorders. More studies are required to firmly endorse these interventions.

INTEGRATIVE MEDICAL CONSIDERATIONS

In mild cases of hyper- and hypothyroidism diet and lifestyle changes and nutritional and herbal supplements may be sufficient. If TSH or thyroid hormones show severe disturbances or do not normalise (or at least show a trend towards normal) with natural treatment within six months, medication should be considered. A careful balance needs to be reached where medication and supplements enhance each other without causing imbalances in the opposite direction. This needs to be done in conjunction with the patient's general practitioner.

Since the HPA axis is often involved in thyroid disorders other hormones, such as cortisol and insulin, and imbalanced physiological processes could be at the root of the condition. It may therefore be prudent to test for these hormones as well and treat any resultant imbalances. Any therapies that help reduce stress are of value, such as bodywork, mind therapies and relaxation techniques. The homeopathic remedy Thyroidinum has been given in cases of thyroid dysfunction[153]; however, data does not firmly support this treatment.

CLINICAL SUMMARY

Stress and chronic illness promote both hyper- and hypothyroidism and need to be addressed. Since temperature regulation is dependent on thyroid function, taking morning temperature readings can give initial clues regarding the gland's function. See also Figure 20.4 (naturopathic treatment decision tree).

In hyperthyroidism, usually as the result of autoimmunity, the metabolic rate is increased, and the clinical symptom picture is one of restlessness, including weight loss, increased nutrient turnover with resultant weight loss and heat intolerance. Its diagnosis is made on below-normal TSH levels with high T_3 and T_4. Treatment includes suppressing thyroid hormone levels with drugs/herbs and supporting the increased nutrient demand with nutritional supplements.

In contrast, in hypothyroidism the metabolic rate is decreased. The clinical symptom picture is one of sluggishness, including lethargy, tiredness, slow nutrient turnover with resultant weight gain, and cold intolerance. It is diagnosed by raised TSH and low T_3 and T_4. Treatment includes thyroid hormone replacement and prescribing precursors, cofactors and stimulants for thyroid hormone synthesis.

Less obvious (and therefore often missed), but nonetheless clinically relevant, forms of hypothyroidism are subclinical and secondary hypothyroidism. In subclinical hypothyroidism TSH is still within the normal range but tends towards the higher end of normal, with T_3 and T_4 being low-normal. In secondary hypothyroidism (usually as part of chronic illness) TSH as well as T_3 and T_4 are low or low-normal. It is therefore important to test for T_3 and T_4 in addition to TSH if the symptom picture or case history is suggestive of either of these conditions. Treatment is the same as for hypothyroidism.

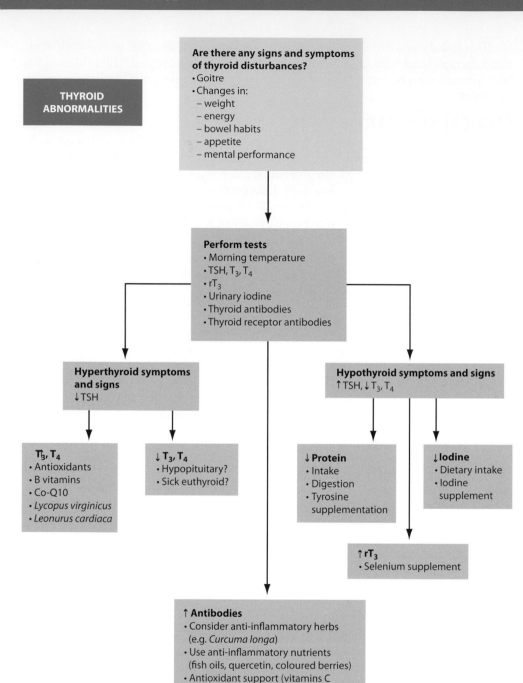

THYROID
ABNORMALITIES

Are there any signs and symptoms of thyroid disturbances?
• Goitre
• Changes in:
– weight
– energy
– bowel habits
– appetite
– mental performance

Perform tests
• Morning temperature
• TSH, T_3, T_4
• rT_3
• Urinary iodine
• Thyroid antibodies
• Thyroid receptor antibodies

Hyperthyroid symptoms and signs
↓TSH

Hypothyroid symptoms and signs
↑TSH, ↓T_3, T_4

T_3, T_4
• Antioxidants
• B vitamins
• Co-Q10
• *Lycopus virginicus*
• *Leonurus cardiaca*

↓ T_3, T_4
• Hypopituitary?
• Sick euthyroid?

↓ Protein
• Intake
• Digestion
• Tyrosine supplementation

↓Iodine
• Dietary intake
• Iodine supplement

↑rT_3
• Selenium supplement

↑Antibodies
• Consider anti-inflammatory herbs (e.g. *Curcuma longa*)
• Use anti-inflammatory nutrients (fish oils, quercetin, coloured berries)
• Antioxidant support (vitamins C and E, lipoic acid, selenium, zinc)

Figure 20.4
Naturopathic treatment decision tree—thyroid abnormalities

Table 20.9
Review of the major evidence*

Intervention	Mechanisms of action	Key literature	Summary of results	Comment
Iodine	Constituent of thyroid hormone Combats thyroid goitre by competing for absorption and receptor binding with other halides (bromine, fluoride, chlorine) Iodinated lipids regulate and promote apoptosis in cancer cells Deficiency in pregnancy can lead to neural and mental impairment in infants	Zimmermann 2011[59] Thomson et al. 2011[65] Harding et al. 2017[154]	Median iodine excretion indicated mild iodine deficiency, with up to one-quarter of children showing moderate to severe deficiency Girls had significantly lower values than boys No goitre was detected in any of the children Excess iodate intake led to hypothyroidism in some people and hyperthyroidism in others which reversed in most after cessation of supplementation	These results are indicative of a widespread mild to moderate iodine deficiency in Australia This may already show in childhood with impaired growth and cognitive dysfunction Supplementary iodine intake needs to be monitored
Selenium	Facilitates conversion from T_4 to active T_3 Is part of the glutathione peroxidase enzyme which keeps hydrogen peroxidase reduced to water after conversion of iodide into iodine Deficiency of selenium can lead to impaired thyroid cellular defence	Kandhro et al. 2011[72] Zheng et al. 2018[155]	Faster and higher increase in T_3 and T_4, rT_3 rising less in active group and earlier normalisation Selenium deficiency exacerbates hypothyroidism in iodine deficiency	Not only selenium deficiency but also inflammatory cytokines, present in critically ill patients, interfere with thyroid hormone synthesis Selenium not only increases conversion of T_4 to T_3, it also reduces antibody production This shows the intricate interplay between these two nutrients
Carnitine	L-carnitine is a peripheral antagonist of thyroid hormone action Role in energy production by facilitating transport of fatty acids into mitochondria Hyperthyroidism depletes the body of L-carnitine	Benvenga et al. 2004[125] Benvenga 2005[126]	L-carnitine has been proven effective in improving as well as preventing some forms of hyperthyroidism as well as in thyroid storm It also beneficially affects bone mineralisation	This non-toxic amino acid may be very useful in hyperthyroidism

*Certain nutrients involved in thyroid function

KEY POINTS

- Stress may induce both hyper- and hypothyroidism.
- Both hyper- and hypothyroidism can be the result of deranged autoimmunity.
- In hyperthyroidism the increased metabolic activity needs to be supported through nutrient-dense diet and supplements, notably B vitamins and antioxidants.
- Nutritional deficiencies, particularly iodine and selenium, are indicated in hypothyroidism.
- Subclinical hypothyroidism is often under diagnosed and therefore not treated.

FURTHER READING

Chaker L, Bianco AC, Jonklaas J, et al. Hypothyroidism. Lancet 2017;390(10101):1550–6.

Eastman CJ. Screening for thyroid disease and iodine deficiency. Pathology 2012;44(2):153–9.

Garber JR, Cobin RH, Gharib H, et al. Clinical practice guidelines for hypothyroidism in adults: cosponsored by the American Association of clinical endocrinologists and the American Thyroid Association. Thyroid 2012;22(12):1200–35.

Rosen JE, Gardiner P, Lee SL. Complementary and integrative treatments: thyroid disease. Otolaryngol Clin North Am 2013;46(3):423–35.

Acknowledgement: Thanks are extended to Alina Porojan for assisting Dr Gruner with the edition 2 resubmission. Jerome Sarris performed a minor update on this chapter for edition 3.

REFERENCES

1. Shils ME, Shike M, Ross AC, et al. Modern nutrition in health and disease. Philadelphia: Lippincott Williams & Wilkins; 2006.
2. Lord RS, Alexander BJ. Laboratory evaluations for integrative and functional medicine. 2nd ed. Duluth, Georgia: Metametrix Institute; 2008.
3. Thibodeau G, Patton K. Anatomy and physiology. 5th ed. Mosby; 2003.
4. Mansourian AR. Metabolic pathways of tetraidothyronine and triiodothyronine production by thyroid gland: a review of articles. Pak J Biol Sci 2011;14(1):1–12.
5. Woolever DR, Beutler AI. Hypothyroidism: a review of the evaluation and management. Family Practice Recertification 2007;29(4):45–52.
6. Guinea pigs can synthesize ascorbic acid when injected with L-gulonolactone oxidase. Nutr Rev 1982;40(10): 310–11.
7. Ganapathy S, Volpe SL. Zinc, exercise, and thyroid hormone function. Crit Rev Food Sci Nutr 1999;39(4):369–90.
8. Maxwell C, Volpe SL. Effect of zinc supplementation on thyroid hormone function. A case study of two college females. Ann Nutr Metab 2007;51(2):188–94.
9. Tierney LM, McPhee SJ, Papadakis MA. Medical diagnosis and treatment. 44th ed. New York: McGraw-Hill; 2005.
10. Brown KM, Arthur JR. Selenium, selenoproteins and human health: a review. Public Health Nutr 2001;4(2B):593–9.
11. Leonard JL. Non-genomic actions of thyroid hormone in brain development. Steroids 2008;73(9–10):1008–12.
12. Crowley LV. An introduction to human disease: pathology and pathophysiology correlations. 6th ed. Sudbury, Massachusetts: Jones and Bartlett Publishers; 2004.
13. Kumar P, Clark M. Clinical medicine. 7th ed. Edinburgh: Elsevier/Saunders; 2009.
14. Kosovskiĭ MI, Katkova SP, Nugmanova LB, et al. [Glucose tolerance disorders in patients with hypothyroidism]. Probl Endokrinol (Mosk) 1992;38(2):26–9.
15. Clausen N, Lins PE, Adamson U, et al. Counterregulation of insulin-induced hypoglycaemia in primary hypothyroidism. Acta Endocrinol (Copenh) 1986;111(4):516–21.
16. Stanická S, Vondra K, Pelikánová T, et al. Insulin sensitivity and counter-regulatory hormones in hypothyroidism and during thyroid hormone replacement therapy. Clin Chem Lab Med 2005;43(7):715–20.
17. Fommei E, Lervasi G. The role of thyroid hormone in blood pressure homeostasis: evidence from short-term hypothyroidism in humans. J Clin Endocrinol Metab 2002;87(5):1996–2000.
18. Chopra IJ. Nonthyroidal illness syndrome or euthyroid sick syndrome? Endocr Pract 1996;2(1):45–52.
19. Douyon L, Schteingart DE. Effect of obesity and starvation on thyroid hormone, growth hormone, and cortisol secretion. Endocrinol Metab Clin North Am 2002;31(1):173–89.
20. Ochi Y, Kajita Y. [Determination of thyroid hormone]. Nippon Rinsho 1999;57(8):1794–9.
21. Sherwood L. Human physiology: from cells to systems. 8th ed. Australia: Cengage Learning; 2013.
22. Gaby AR. Nutritional medicine. Concord, NH: Fritz Perlberg Publishing; 2011.
23. Shivaraj G, et al. Thyroid function tests: a review. Eur Rev Med Pharmacol Sci 2009;13(5):341–9.
24. Wartofsky L, Dickey RA. The evidence for a narrower thyrotropin reference range is compelling. J Clin Endocrinol Metab 2005;90(9):5483–8.
25. Spencer CA, Hollowell JG, Kazarosyan M, et al. National Health and Nutrition Examination Survey III thyroid-stimulating hormone (TSH)-thyroperoxidase antibody relationships demonstrate

that TSH upper reference limits may be skewed by occult thyroid dysfunction. J Clin Endocrinol Metab 2007;92(11):4236–40.

26. Dickey RA, Wartofsky L, Feld S. Optimal thyrotropin level: normal ranges and reference intervals are not equivalent. Thyroid 2005;15(9):1035–9.

27. Brabant G, Beck-Peccoz P, Jarzab B, et al. Is there a need to redefine the upper normal limit of TSH? Eur J Endocrinol 2006;154(5):633–7.

28. Schlienger JL, Sapin R, Vinzio S, et al. What is an elevated TSH level? [Qu'est ce qu'un taux de TSH élevé?]. Immuno-Analyse et Biologie Specialisee 2007;22(3):160–6.

29. Eskelinen SI, Vahlberg TJ, Isoaho RE, et al. Associations of thyroid-stimulating hormone and free thyroxine concentrations with health and life satisfaction in elderly adults. Endocr Pract 2007;13(5):451–7.

30. Sviridonova MA, Fadeyev VV, Sych YP, et al. Clinical significance of TSH circadian variability in patients with hypothyroidism. Endocr Res 2013;38(1):24–31.

31. Åsvold BO, Vatten LJ, Midthjell K, et al. Serum TSH within the reference range as a predictor of future hypothyroidism and hyperthyroidism: 11-Year follow-up of the HUNT study in Norway. J Clin Endocrinol Metab 2012;97(1):93–9.

32. Bar-Andziak E, Milewicz A, Jędrzejuk D, et al. Thyroid dysfunction and thyroid autoimmunity in a large unselected population of elderly subjects in Poland—The 'PolSenior' multicentre crossover study. Endokrynol Pol 2012;63(5):346–55.

33. Danzi S, Klein I. Recent considerations in the treatment of hypothyroidism. Curr Opin Investig Drugs 2008;9(4):357–62.

34. Lee YK, Kim JE, Oh HJ, et al. Serum TSH level in healthy Koreans and the association of TSH with serum lipid concentration and metabolic syndrome. Korean J Intern Med 2011;26(4):432–9.

35. Razvi S, McMillan CV, Weaver JU. Instruments used in measuring symptoms, health status and quality of life in hypothyroidism: a systematic qualitative review. Clin Endocrinol (Oxf) 2005;63(6):617–24.

36. Guan H, Shan Z, Teng X, et al. Influence of iodine on the reference interval of TSH and the optimal interval of TSH: results of a follow-up study in areas with different iodine intakes. Clin Endocrinol (Oxf) 2008;69(1):136–41.

37. Völzke H, Robinson DM, Spielhagen T, et al. Are serum thyrotropin levels within the reference range associated with endothelial function? Eur Heart J 2009;30(2): 217–24.

38. Völzke H, Schmidt CO, John U, et al. Reference levels for serum thyroid function tests of diagnostic and prognostic significance. Horm Metab Res 2010;42(11):809–14.

39. Walter KN, Corwin EJ, Ulbrecht J, et al. Elevated thyroid stimulating hormone is associated with elevated cortisol in healthy young men and women. Thyroid Res 2012;5:13.

40. Walsh JP, Bremner AP, Feddema P, et al. Thyrotropin and thyroid antibodies as predictors of hypothyroidism: a 13-year, longitudinal study of a community-based cohort using current immunoassay techniques. J Clin Endocrinol Metab 2010;95(3):1095–104.

41. Žrković M, Ciri J, Beleslin B, et al. Further studies on delineating thyroid-stimulating hormone (TSH) reference range. Horm Metab Res 2011;43(13):970–6.

42. Moncayo H, Dapunt O, Moncayo R. Diagnostic accuracy of basal TSH determinations based on the intravenous TRH stimulation test: an evaluation of 2570 tests and comparison with the literature. BMC Endocr Disord 2007;7:5.

43. Rosario PW, Xavier ACM, Calsolari MR. TSH reference values for adult Brazilian population [Valores de referência

do TSH para a população Brasileira adulta]. Arq Bras Endocrinol Metabol 2010;54(7):603–6.

44. Schalin-Jäntti C, Tanner P, Välimäki MJ, et al. Serum TSH reference interval in healthy Finnish adults using the Abbott Architect. 2000i analyzer. Scand J Clin Lab Invest 2011;71(4):344–9.

45. Krysiak R, Marek B, Okopień B. [Subclinical hypothyroidism]. Wiad Lek 2008;61(4–6):139–45.

46. Papi G, Uberti ED, Betterle C, et al. Subclinical hypothyroidism. Curr Opin Endocrinol Diabetes Obes 2007;14(3):197–208.

47. Villar H, Saconato H, Valente O, et al. Thyroid hormone replacement for subclinical hypothyroidism. Cochrane Database Syst Rev 2007;(3):CD003419.

48. Abu-Helalah M, Law MR, Bestwick JP, et al. A randomized double-blind crossover trial to investigate the efficacy of screening for adult hypothyroidism. J Med Screen 2010;17(4):164–9.

49. Gharib H. Commentary: review: Available evidence does not support a benefit for thyroid hormone replacement in adult with subclinical hypothyroidism. ACP J Club 2008;6.

50. Tchong L, Veloski C, Siraj ES. Hypothyroidism: management across the continuum. J Clin Outcomes Manag 2009;16(5):231–5.

51. Arrigo T, Wasniewska M, Crisafulli G, et al. Subclinical hypothyroidism: the state of the art. J Endocrinol Invest 2008;31(1):79–84.

52. Lambrinoudaki I, Armeni E, Rizos D, et al. High normal thyroid-stimulating hormone is associated with arterial stiffness in healthy postmenopausal women. J Hypertens 2012;30(3):592–9.

53. Gursoy A, Ozduman Cin M, Kamel N, et al. Which thyroid-stimulating hormone level should be sought in hypothyroid patients under L-thyroxine replacement therapy? Int J Clin Pract 2006;60(6):655–9.

54. Ruhla S, Weickert MO, Arafat AM, et al. A high normal TSH is associated with the metabolic syndrome. Clin Endocrinol (Oxf) 2010;72(5):696–701.

55. Tarcin O, Abanonu GB, Yazici D, et al. Association of metabolic syndrome parameters with TT3 and FT3/FT4 ratio in obese Turkish population. Metab Syndr Relat Disord 2012;10(2):137–42.

56. Aeberli I, Jung A, Murer SB, et al. During rapid weight loss in obese children, reductions in TSH predict improvements in insulin sensitivity independent of changes in body weight or fat. J Clin Endocrinol Metab 2010;95(12):5412–18.

57. Tsigos C, Chrousos GP. Hypothalamic-pituitary-adrenal axis, neuroendocrine factors and stress. J Psychosom Res 2002;53(4):865–71.

58. Taniyama M, Honma K, Ban Y. Urinary cortisol metabolites in the assessment of peripheral thyroid hormone action: application for diagnosis of resistance to thyroid hormone. Thyroid 1993;3(3):229–33.

59. Zimmermann MB. The role of iodine in human growth and development. Semin Cell Dev Biol 2011;22(6):645–52.

60. Mann JI, Aitken E. The re-emergence of iodine deficiency in New Zealand? N Z Med J 2003;116(1170):U351–U.

61. Thomson CD. Selenium and iodine intakes and status in New Zealand and Australia. Br J Nutr 2004;91(5): 661–72.

62. Boucai L, Hollowell JG, Surks MI. An approach for development of age-, gender-, and ethnicity-specific thyrotropin reference limits. Thyroid 2011;21(1):5–11.

63. Cerqueira C, Knudsen N, Ovesen L, et al. Doubling in the use of thyroid hormone replacement therapy in

Denmark: association to iodization of salt? Eur J Epidemiol 2011;26(8):629–35.

64. Sang Z, Wang PP, Yao Z, et al. Exploration of the safe upper level of iodine intake in euthyroid Chinese adults: a randomized double-blind trial. Am J Clin Nutr 2012;95(2):367–73.

65. Thomson CD, Campbell JM, Miller J, et al. Minimal impact of excess iodate intake on thyroid hormones and selenium status in older New Zealanders. Eur J Endocrinol 2011;165(5):745–52.

66. Zaletel K, Gaberscek S, Pirnat E. Ten-year follow-up of thyroid epidemiology in Slovenia after increase in salt iodization. Croat Med J 2011;52(5):615–21.

67. Teng W, Shan Z, Teng X, et al. Effect of iodine intake on thyroid diseases in China. N Engl J Med 2006;354(26):2783–93.

68. Leung AM, Braverman LE. Iodine-induced thyroid dysfunction. Curr Opin Endocrinol Diabetes Obes 2012;19(5):414–19.

69. Zimmermann MB, Köhrle J. The impact of iron and selenium deficiencies on iodine and thyroid metabolism: biochemistry and relevance to public health. Thyroid 2002;12(10):867–78.

70. Duntas LH. Selenium and the thyroid: a close-knit connection. J Clin Endocrinol Metab 2010;95(12):5180–8.

71. Gärtner R. Selenium and thyroid hormone axis in critical ill states: an overview of conflicting view points. J Trace Elem Med Biol 2009;23(2):71–4.

72. Kandhro GA, Kazi TG, Sirajuddin, et al. Effects of selenium supplementation on iodine and thyroid hormone status in a selected population with goitre in Pakistan. Clin Lab 2011;57(7–8):575–85.

73. Drutel A, Archambeaud F, Caron P. Selenium and the thyroid gland: more good news for clinicians. Clin Endocrinol (Oxf) 2013;78(2):155–64.

74. Glinoer D, Spencer CA. Serum TSH determinations in pregnancy: how, when and why? Nat Rev Endocrinol 2010;6(9):526–9.

75. Kennedy RL, Malabu UH, Jarrod G, et al. Thyroid function and pregnancy: before, during and beyond. J Obstet Gynaecol 2010;30(8):774–83.

76. Chen L, Hu R. Thyroid autoimmunity and miscarriage: a meta-analysis. Clin Endocrinol (Oxf) 2011;74(4):513–19.

77. Mönig H, Hensen J, Lehnert H. [Thyroid disorders and pregnancy]. Internist (Berl) 2010;51(5):620–4.

78. Pettigrew-Porter A, Skeaff S, Gray A, et al. Are pregnant women in New Zealand iodine deficient? A cross-sectional survey. Aust N Z J Obstet Gynaecol 2011;51(5):464–7.

79. Thangaratinam S, Tan A, Knox E, et al. Association between thyroid autoantibodies and miscarriage and preterm birth: Meta-analysis of evidence. BMJ 2011;342(7806):1–8.

80. Azizi F. The occurrence of permanent thyroid failure in patients with subclinical postpartum thyroiditis. Eur J Endocrinol 2005;153(3):367–71.

81. Janssen OE, Benker G. Thyroid gland: aspects of reproductive medicine—Update 2011. Schilddrüse: Reproduktionsmedizinische aspekte—Update 2011 2011;8(1):22–31.

82. Budenhofer BK, Ditsch N, Jeschke U, et al. Thyroid (dys-) function in normal and disturbed pregnancy. Arch Gynecol Obstet 2013;287(1):1–7.

83. Yazbeck CF, Sullivan SD. Thyroid disorders during pregnancy. Med Clin North Am 2012;96(2):235–56.

84. Sato PH, Walton DM. Glutaraldehyde-reacted immunoprecipitates of L-gulonolactone oxidase are suitable for administration to guinea pigs. Arch Biochem Biophys 1983;221(2):543–7.

85. Skeaff SA. Iodine deficiency in pregnancy: the effect on neurodevelopment in the child. Nutrients 2011;3(2):265–73.

86. Costeira MJ, Oliveira P, Ares S, et al. Parameters of thyroid function throughout and after pregnancy in an iodine-deficient population. Thyroid 2010;20(9):995–1001.

87. Rebagliato M, Murcia M, Espada M, et al. Iodine intake and maternal thyroid function during pregnancy. Epidemiology 2010;21(1):62–9.

88. Moleti M, Di Bella B, Giorgianni G, et al. Maternal thyroid function in different conditions of iodine nutrition in pregnant women exposed to mild-moderate iodine deficiency: an observational study. Clin Endocrinol (Oxf) 2011;74(6):762–8.

89. Marco A, Vicente A, Castro E, et al. Patterns of iodine intake and urinary iodine concentrations during pregnancy and blood thyroid-stimulating hormone concentrations in the newborn progeny. Thyroid 2010;20(11):1295–9.

90. Reid SM, Middleton P, Cossich MC, et al. Interventions for clinical and subclinical hypothyroidism in pregnancy. Cochrane Database Syst Rev 2010;(7):CD007752.

91. Das S, Bhansali A, Dutta P, et al. Persistence of goitre in the post-iodization phase: micronutrient deficiency or thyroid autoimmunity? Indian J Med Res 2011;133:103–9.

92. Ertek S, Cicero AF, Caglar O, et al. Relationship between serum zinc levels, thyroid hormones and thyroid volume following successful iodine supplementation. Hormones (Athens) 2010;9(3):263–8.

93. Ellingsen DG, Efskind J, Haug E, et al. Effects of low mercury vapour exposure on the thyroid function in chloralkali workers. J Appl Toxicol 2000;20(6):483–9.

94. Song M, Kim Y-J, Park Y-K, et al. Changes in thyroid peroxidase activity in response to various chemicals. J Environ Monit 2012;14(8):2121–6.

95. Langer P. The impacts of organochlorines and other persistent pollutants on thyroid and metabolic health. Front Neuroendocrinol 2010;31(4):497–518.

96. Langer P, Tajtáková M, Kočan A, et al. Thyroid ultrasound volume, structure and function after long-term high exposure of large population to polychlorinated biphenyls, pesticides and dioxin. Chemosphere 2007;69(1):118–27.

97. Andra SS, Makris KC. Thyroid disrupting chemicals in plastic additives and thyroid health. J Environ Sci Health C Environ Carcinog Ecotoxicol Rev 2012;30(2):107–51.

98. Trumbo PR. Perchlorate consumption, iodine status, and thyroid function. Nutr Rev 2010;68(1):62–6.

99. Keith M. The effects of municipal water fluoridation: are we watering down thyroid function? Alive: Canada's Natural Health & Wellness Magazine 2010;331:104.

100. Cho NH, Choi HS, Kim KW, et al. Interaction between cigarette smoking and iodine intake and their impact on thyroid function. Clin Endocrinol (Oxf) 2010;73(2):264–70.

101. Padmanabhan H. Amiodarone and thyroid dysfunction. South Med J 2010;103(9):922–30.

102. Ghosh R. Thyroid dysfunction in long-term amiodarone therapy. GM: Midlife & Beyond 2010;40(10):547–9.

103. Aggarwal A, Rastogi N, Mittal H, et al. Thyroid hormone levels in children receiving carbamazepine or valproate. Pediatr Neurol 2011;45(3):159–62.

104. Mai VQ, Burch HB. A stepwise approach to the evaluation and treatment of subclinical hyperthyroidism. Endocr Pract 2012;18(5):772–80.

105. Centanni M, Franchi A, Santaguida MG, et al. Oral thyroxine treatment: towards an individually tailored dose [La terapia tiroxinica: dall'empirismo al dosaggio individualizzato]. Recenti Prog Med 2007;98(9):445–51.

106. Clarke N, Kabadi UM. Optimizing treatment of hypothyroidism. Treat Endocrinol 2004;3(4):217–21.

107. Mazzoccoli G, Giuliani A, Carughi S, et al. The hypothalamic-pituitary-thyroid axis and melatonin in humans: possible interactions in the control of body temperature. Neuro Endocrinol Lett 2004;25(5):368–72.

108. Nogues R, Sitges-Serra A, Sancho JJ, et al. Influence of nutrition, thyroid hormones, and rectal temperature on in-hospital mortality of elderly patients with acute illness. Am J Clin Nutr 1995;61(3):597–602.

109. Beck U, Reinhardt H, Kendel K, et al. Temperature and endocrine activity during sleep in man. Activation of cortisol and thyroid-stimulating hormone, inhibition of human growth hormone secretion by raised or decreased ambient and body temperatures. Arch Psychiatr Nervenkr 1976;222(2–3):245–56.

110. Reed HL. Circannual changes in thyroid hormone physiology: the role of cold environmental temperatures. Arctic Med Res 1995;54(Suppl. 2):9–15.

111. Ljunggren JG, Kallner G, Tryselius M. The effect of body temperature on thyroid hormone levels in patients with non-thyroidal illness. Acta Med Scand 1977;202(6):459–62.

112. Höflich G, Kasper S, Danos P, et al. Thyroid hormones, body temperature, and antidepressant treatment. Biol Psychiatry 1992;31(8):859–62.

113. Bone K. A clinical guide to blending liquid herbs. USA: Elsevier; 2003.

114. Blumenthal M. The ABC clinical guide to herbs. Austin, Texas: American Botanical Council; 2003.

115. Blumenthal M. The complete German commission E monographs—Therapeutic guide to herbal medicines. Austin, Tex.: American Botanical Council; 1999.

116. Mills S, Bone K. Principles and practice of phytotherapy. 2nd ed. Sydney: Churchill Livingstone; 2013.

117. Pizzorno J, Murray M. Textbook of natural medicine. 3rd ed. USA: Churchill Livingstone; 2006.

118. Demet MM, Ozmen B, Deveci A, et al. Depression and anxiety in hypothyroidism. West Indian Med J 2003;52(3):223–7.

119. Chueire VB, Romaldini JH, Ward LS. Subclinical hypothyroidism increases the risk for depression in the elderly. Arch Gerontol Geriatr 2007;44(1):21–8.

120. Demartini B, Masu A, Scarone S, et al. Prevalence of depression in patients affected by subclinical hypothyroidism. Panminerva Med 2010;52(4):277–82.

121. Sevinc A, Savli H. Hypothyroidism masquerading as depression: the role of noncompliance. J Natl Med Assoc 2004;96(3):379–82.

122. Kathol RG, Delahunt JW. The relationship of anxiety and depression to symptoms of hyperthyroidism using operational criteria. Gen Hosp Psychiatry 1986;8(1):23–8.

123. Iacovides A, Fountoulakis KN, Grammaticos P, et al. Difference in symptom profile between generalized anxiety disorder and anxiety secondary to hyperthyroidism. Int J Psychiatry Med 2000;30(1):71–81.

124. Jammula S, Sunil Kumar K, Siva Krishna K, et al. Effect of thyroid disorders on skeletal health. Turk J Endocrinol Metab 2012;16(1):19–25.

125. Benvenga S, Amato A, Calvani M, et al. Effects of carnitine on thyroid hormone action. Ann N Y Acad Sci 2004;1033:158–67.

126. Benvenga S. Effects of L-carnitine on thyroid hormone metabolism and on physical exercise tolerance. Horm Metab Res 2005;37(09):566–71.

127. Gershwin M, Nestel P, Keen CE. Handbook of nutrition and immunity. Totowa, New Jersey: Humana Press; 2004.

128. Ma A, Qi S, Chen H. Antioxidant therapy for prevention of inflammation, ischemic reperfusion injuries and allograft rejection. Cardiovasc Hematol Agents Med Chem 2008;6(1):20–43.

129. Seven A, Taşan E, Inci F, et al. Biochemical evaluation of oxidative stress in propylthiouracil treated hyperthyroid patients. Effects of vitamin C supplementation. Clin Chem Lab Med 1998;36(10):767–70.

130. Winterhoff H, Gumbinger HG, Vahlensieck U, et al. Endocrine effects of Lycopus europaeus L. following oral application. Arzneimittelforschung 1994;44(1):41–5.

131. Yarnell E, Abascal K. Botanical medicine for thyroid regulation. Alternat Complement Therapies 2006;12(3):107.

132. Auf'mkolk M, Ingbar JC, Kubota K, et al. Extracts and auto-oxidized constituents of certain plants inhibit the receptor-binding and the biological activity of Graves' immunoglobulins. Endocrinology 1985;116(5): 1687–93.

133. Higdon J. An evidence-based approach to vitamins and minerals. New York: Thieme; 2003.

134. Doerge DR, Sheehan DM. Goitrogenic and estrogenic activity of soy isoflavones. Environ Health Perspect 2002;3:349–53.

135. Teas J, Braverman LE, Kurzer MS, et al. Seaweed and soy: companion foods in Asian cuisine and their effects on thyroid function in American women. J Med Food 2007;10(1):90.

136. Messina M, Redmond G. Effects of soy protein and soybean isoflavones on thyroid function in healthy adults and hypothyroid patients: a review of the relevant literature. Thyroid 2006;16(3):249–58.

137. Chandra AK, De N. Catechin induced modulation in the activities of thyroid hormone synthesizing enzymes leading to hypothyroidism. Mol Cell Biochem 2013;374(1–2):37–48.

138. Sathyapalan T, Manuchehri AM, Thatcher NJ, et al. The effect of soy phytoestrogen supplementation on thyroid status and cardiovascular risk markers in patients with subclinical hypothyroidism: a randomized, double-blind, crossover study. J Clin Endocrinol Metab 2011;96(5):1442–9.

139. Milerová J, Cerovská J, Zamrazil V, et al. Actual levels of soy phytoestrogens in children correlate with thyroid laboratory parameters. Clin Chem Lab Med 2006;44(2):171–4.

140. Leung AM, Lamar A, He X, et al. Iodine status and thyroid function of Boston-area vegetarians and vegans. J Clin Endocrinol Metab 2011;96(8):E1303–7.

141. Braun L, Cohen M. Herbs & natural supplements. 3rd ed. Sydney: Churchill Livingstone; 2010.

142. Panda S, Kar A. Changes in thyroid hormone concentrations after administration of ashwagandha root extract to adult male mice. J Pharm Pharmacol 1998;50(9):1065–8.

143. Panda S, Kar A. Withania somnifera and Bauhinia purpurea in the regulation of circulating thyroid hormone concentrations in female mice. J Ethnopharmacol 1999;67(2):233–9.

144. Kar A, Panda S, Bharti S. Relative efficacy of three medicinal plant extracts in the alteration of thyroid hormone concentrations in male mice. J Ethnopharmacol 2002;81(2):281.

145. Smyth PPA, Burns R, Huang RJ, et al. Does iodine gas released from seaweed contribute to dietary iodine intake? Environ Geochem Health 2011;33(4):389–97.

146. Li M, Ma G, Boyages SC, et al. Re-emergence of iodine deficiency in Australia. Asia Pac J Clin Nutr 2001;10(3):200–3.

147. Charlton K, Skeaff S. Iodine fortification: why, when, what, how, and who? Curr Opin Clin Nutr Metab Care 2011;14(6):618–24.

148. Zimmermann MB, Adou P, Torresani T, et al. Effect of oral iodized oil on thyroid size and thyroid hormone metabolism in children with concurrent selenium and iodine deficiency. Eur J Clin Nutr 2000;54(3):209–13.

149. Glinoer D. Feto-maternal repercussions of iodine deficiency during pregnancy. An update. Ann Endocrinol (Paris) 2003;64(1):37–44.

150. Glinoer D. Pregnancy and iodine. Thyroid 2001;11(5):471–81.

151. Glinoer D. What happens to the normal thyroid during pregnancy? Thyroid 1999;9(7):631–5.

152. Moss J. A perspective on high dose iodine supplementation—Part VI—Basics concerning iodine absorption, metabolism and their impact on thyroid function. Nutritional Perspectives: Journal of the Council on Nutrition 2011;34(2):15–24.

153. Tarkas PI. Thyroidinum. Indian J Homoeopathic Med 1989;24(1):67.

154. Harding KB, Peña-Rosas JP, Webster AC, et al. Iodine supplementation for women during the preconception, pregnancy and postpartum period. Cochrane Database Syst Rev 2017;(3):CD011761.

155. Zheng H, Wei J, Wang L, et al. Effects of selenium supplementation on Graves' disease: a systematic review and meta-analysis. Evid Based Complement Alternat Med 2018.

CHAPTER 21

Dysmenorrhoea and menstrual complaints

Jon Wardle
ND, MPH, PhD

OVERVIEW

Menstrual complaints are often broadly—and sometimes incorrectly—categorised under the broad moniker of premenstrual syndrome (PMS). PMS is defined as a recurrent set of physical and behavioural symptoms occurring cyclically 7–14 days before menstruation (the luteal phase) and are troublesome enough to interfere with some aspects of the female's life.[1] In common clinical usage this has also extended to symptoms (such as dysmenorrhoea) that occur during menstruation and cease by the end of the full flow of menses. Despite its high prevalence PMS remains poorly understood and often not prioritised in medical treatment.[1] Multiple aetiologies have been proposed, most prominently those in Table 21.1. In reality a number of these may be responsible for underlying imbalances, even in the same patient. PMS is a highly controversial diagnosis, and numerous proposed aetiologies for PMS mean that more than 150 individual symptoms have been associated with the condition. The most common are listed in Table 21.2.[1]

Although diagnosis is difficult given the broad range of possible aetiologies and symptoms, premenstrual dysphoric disorder (PMDD), a more severe form of PMS, is a recent addition to the *Diagnostic and Statistical Manual of Mental Disorders* (DSM-5).[2] To be diagnosed with PMDD a woman must have *one* or more symptoms including: marked affective lability, irritability, depressed mood or anxiety; in combination with *one* or more symptoms including decreased interest in usual activities, concentration difficulties, lethargy, change in appetite, sleep issues, a sense of being out of control or physical symptoms such as bloating. A total of *five* of these criteria must be met for a diagnosis of PMDD, though the diagnosis and medicalisation of PMDD is somewhat controversial.

Patients fulfilling the diagnostic criteria for PMDD also fulfil medical diagnostic criteria for PMS but not necessarily vice versa. However, it may be viewed as disturbing that behavioural aspects form the focus of diagnosis in PMDD, when in clinical practice a vast array of hormonal and physiological interactions take place within a woman's body around the time of menstruation, resulting in a variety of broader symptoms and forming a more complex basis of underlying aetiology.

Table 21.1
Proposed aetiologies of premenstrual syndrome

Category	Example
Fluid and electrolyte balance	Aldosterone excess High sodium:potassium ratio Renin/angiotensin abnormalities
Hereditary factors	Genetic risk
Hormonal factors	Oestrogen deficiency Oestrogen excess High oestrogen:progesterone ratio Progesterone deficiency High prolactin
Inflammatory mediators	Prostaglandin excess Prostaglandin deficiency
Psychological factors	Poor coping skills Poor self-esteem Beliefs about menstrual cycle
Social factors	Current and former marital and sexual relationships Stress Cultural and societal attitudes about PMS Poor social networks
Biochemical factors	Various vitamin and mineral deficiencies Dopamine deficiency

Source: Edmonds 2007[1]

Table 21.2
The most common symptoms of premenstrual syndrome

Abdominal bloating	Depression	Lethargy
Anxiety	Dizziness	Low self-esteem
Back pain	Fatigue	Mood swings
Breast tenderness	Headache	Nervousness
Change in appetite	Insomnia	Social isolation
Clumsiness	Irritability	Sugar cravings
Constipation	Joint pain	Water retention

Dysmenorrhoea

While PMS is often used as an all-encompassing term of convenience for menstrual complaints, menstrual symptoms do not occur only prior to menstruation. Dysmenorrhoea is painful menstruation and is the most common menstrual complaint, as well as having the most potential to substantially interfere with patients' lives. In fact, dysmenorrhoea is the most frequent gynaecological problem in adolescent girls (the prevalence is 80–90%).[1] Daily activities are frequently affected and it is the most common cause of regular absenteeism in young women.

Primary dysmenorrhoea classically presents as a cramping lower abdominal pain that usually begins during the day before menstruation. The pain gradually eases after the start of menstruation and is sometimes gone by the end of the first day of bleeding.

Primary dysmenorrhoea occurs in a high percentage of young women only in ovulatory cycles and the pain is normally limited to the first 48–72 hours of menstruation.[1]

Secondary dysmenorrhoea may occur during other parts of the menstrual cycle and can be either relieved or worsened by menstruation. Pain from secondary dysmenorrhoea is often described as dull and aching rather than being spasmodic or cramping in nature. It can occur before menstruation (up to one week) or get worse once menstruation starts.

Hormonal and biochemical influences

Endocrine studies suggest that PMS is *not* the result of a simple excess or deficiency in certain hormone levels.[3] Low progesterone,[4] excessive oestrogen[5] or normal levels of both[6] have not been associated with increasing incidence of PMS. Though prolactin levels have been associated with several symptoms of PMS there has been little hard evidence to suggest that elevated prolactin levels are present in women with PMS.[6,7] Similarly while aldosterone is thought to be at least partly responsible for the congestive symptoms of PMS there have been no reports of significant differences between women with and without PMS.[5] It has been postulated that PMS is not associated with abnormal hormone levels but rather an abnormal response to sex hormones[8] that may be exacerbated during episodes of stress.[9] High blood flow is also associated with an increased instance of dysmenorrhoea.[10]

It is thought that deviations from normal ovarian function—rather than hormone levels per se—are associated with changes to other body systems (such as neurotransmitters) seen in PMS.[11] Serotonin is thought to be particularly affected by changes in hormone levels and responsible for many mood change symptoms associated with PMS.[12]

It has also been hypothesised that women with PMS may have lower levels of circulating endogenous opiates (or serotonin) or a more sudden withdrawal after the postovulation surge, leaving them more susceptible to depression and more sensitive to pain in the luteal phase.[13–15] Prostaglandins are also associated with the PMS symptoms of breast pain, fluid retention, abdominal cramping, headaches, irritability and depression.[16] The high levels of the leukotrienes that increase uterine muscle spasm (C4 and D4) in the menstrual blood of women with dysmenorrhoea also support the hypothesis that prostaglandins are an important part of the aetiology.[17] Anti-inflammatory prostaglandins may also be associated with reducing the exaggerated effects of prolactin.[18]

Psychosocial factors can also influence the menstrual cycle. Emotional and physical stressors such as travel, illness, stress, weather changes and other environmental factors can influence the length of the menstrual cycle, ovulation and severity of PMS.[19] One study found that 75% of women receiving care for PMS had another diagnosis that could account for their symptom complex—predominantly depression and other mood disorders.[20]

DIFFERENTIAL DIAGNOSIS

- Endometriosis
- Ovarian cysts
- Irritable bowel syndrome
- Inflammatory bowel disease
- Urinary tract infection
- Pelvic inflammatory disease

RISK FACTORS

Epidemiological data observe a strong relationship between smoking or exposure to tobacco products and a higher incidence of dysmenorrhoea.[21–23] Obesity is also a risk factor for menstrual disturbances, with women who have a body mass index (BMI) over 30 incurring a threefold risk of developing them.[24] Approximately three-quarters of women have a separate diagnosis—particularly mood disorders or other hormone-mediated diagnoses—that contribute significantly to their symptoms.[20] High levels of caffeine may be associated with increased prevalence and severity of PMS symptoms,[25,26] though this may be due to an additive relationship of sugar with caffeine.[27] Many women may medicate themselves with caffeine during PMS symptoms, which may exacerbate their symptoms.[28]

CONVENTIONAL TREATMENT

The basic aim of treatment of menstrual disorders in conventional medicine focuses on symptomatic relief and coping strategies in line with the hormonal dysfunction rather than reliance on medication. Conventional treatment of primary dysmenorrhoea is usually associated with pain management (such as ibuprofen) or a combined oral contraceptive pill. Secondary dysmenorrhoea is more complex and may be associated with other conditions such as pelvic infection or endometriosis. Common symptomatic relief for dysmenorrhoea with analgesics (such as paracetamol or ibuprofen) or antiprostaglandin agents (such as indomethacin or mefenamic acid) may also be recommended. In cases of secondary dysmenorrhoea the conventional treatment is to identify and treat the cause.

Various pharmaceutical agents are used in conventional treatment, including diuretics (such as spironolactone—particularly with fluid retention), vitamins (such as B6), serotonin-specific reuptake inhibitor (SSRI) agents or danazol (particularly with severe mastalgia).[29] Hormone therapy is also common, and consists of hormonal agents such as the oral contraceptive pill, progestogens or implants. However, these have little evidence of efficacy in PMS.[30] Progesterone treatment is increasingly popular, particularly among integrative medical practitioners; however, the evidence for effective treatment with progesterone alone is unclear.[31]

KEY TREATMENT PROTOCOLS

Although various diagnoses can often present in menstrual disorders, naturopathic treatment focuses not on treatment of particular disorders but rather the restoration of a normal menstrual cycle. Other chapters in the reproductive section (Chapters 21–24) focus on various aspects of hormone normalisation, so this chapter focuses on specific symptoms associated with PMS, particularly dysmenorrhoea as

> ### Naturopathic Treatment Aims
>
> - Remove risk factors.
> - Regulate HPO axis function and normalise hormones.
> - Reduce inflammation and inflammatory mediators.
> - Treat menstrual pain symptomatically.
> - Address psychological factors (causations and clinical manifestations).

it is often the most encountered symptom in clinical practice. A normal menstrual cycle should be free of the discomfort associated with pathological conditions such as PMS, PMDD or dysmenorrhoea. This return to normalcy can be sought through a number of mechanisms, most commonly hormonal regulation via the hypothalamic–pituitary–ovarian (HPO) axis. Inflammation is also a key focus of treatment, as prostaglandins are required to stimulate contraction of the uterine muscle as part of a normal menstrual cycle. However, the presence of too many prostaglandins can cause pain, and as such modulation of inflammation is also a key aspect of treatment.

HPO axis regulation

As opposed to conditions specifically linked to certain hormone excesses such as endometriosis (oestrogen) and polycystic ovarian syndrome (androgen), treatment of broader menstrual disorders focuses on hormone normalisation, often through modulation of the HPO axis. In this sense naturopathic treatments are not necessarily associated with specific actions on hormones but rather work to restore the appropriate function of the body's own natural processes that regulate these hormones. For example, while *Vitex agnus-castus* was initially thought to work on increasing progesterone levels or decreasing prolactin, research is suggesting it has a role even further upstream on the HPO axis due to its dopaminergic action.

In addition to prescriptive naturopathic medicines, many of which are explored in more detail in other reproductive chapters, a number of different lifestyle factors, discussed below, can disrupt the functioning of the HPO axis.

Abraham's classifications

In 1983 Dr Guy Abraham publicised a system for classifying of PMS into four distinct subgroups.[32] These subtypes have since had a major influence on naturopathic practice internationally. However, while they may be somewhat clinically useful in a broad sense they should be treated as guidelines only as they have not been confirmed by research and patients rarely fit neatly into one group. The subtypes are discussed below.

PMS-A (anxiety)

This is thought to be related to high levels of oestrogen and a deficiency of progesterone. Its symptom complex is irritability, anxiety and emotional lability.

PMS-C (carbohydrate craving)

This is thought to be caused by enhanced intracellular binding of insulin though its exact mechanism is unclear. The symptom complex of this category is increased appetite, carbo-hydrate craving, headache and heart palpitations.

PMS-D (depression)

This is thought to be due to low levels of oestrogen leading to excessive breakdown of neurotransmitters and could be due to symptoms related to enhanced androgen or progesterone production.

PMS-H (hyperhydration)

This is thought to be caused by elevations of aldosterone due to excessive oestrogen, sodium consumption, adrenal stress or magnesium deficiency. The symptom complex of this subtype is weight gain, breast tenderness and fullness, peripheral swelling and abdominal bloating.

Dietary factors

Dietary factors may also play a significant role. Women with PMS typically consume more dairy products, refined sugar and high-sodium foods than women without PMS.[32] Fish, eggs and fruit have been associated with less dysmenorrhoea while wine is associated with more.[33] Women following a low-fat, vegetarian diet also had lower incidence of dysmenorrhoea.[22,23,34] This is thought to be due to increased sex hormone-binding globulin (which was measured in the study) and its effects on oestrogen or arachidonic acid. A diet high in oily fish and avoidance of foods with significant arachidonic acid content reduces the severity of dysmenorrhoea, possibly through improving the synthesis of anti-inflammatory prostaglandins and leukotrienes. Higher amounts of fibre have been associated with lower levels of menstrual pain.[35] High intakes of total and saturated fats and low unrefined carbohydrate and fibre consumption were also associated with dysmenorrhoea.[36]

Regulating blood sugar levels may be important in modulating hormonal status. It has been observed that PMS symptoms are worse in women with abnormal glucose tolerance.[37] The body appears more sensitive to insulin during the luteal phase; this has led some researchers to theorise that hypoglycaemia may account for some premenstrual symptoms. Consumption of foods high in sugar content—particularly chocolate—may also increase the severity of menstrual symptoms.[27] Regulating eating patterns may therefore help to improve dysmenorrhoea—eating breakfast was associated with a lower incidence of dysmenorrhoea[38] as was a history of calorie-restrictive dieting.[39] This relationship was also observed irrespective of BMI.[40]

Other lifestyle factors

Increased or regular exercise is associated with lower incidence of dysmenorrhoea and most other premenstrual symptoms.[41–46] This may be due in part to the apparent hormone normalisation role of exercise or increased physical activity,[47] or its effects on stress reduction in women with dysmenorrhoea.[48] More detailed information on the effects of stress on reproductive function can be found in Chapter 23 on polycystic ovarian syndrome and Chapter 34 on fertility.

A study of 380 women found that those with higher levels of stress were twice as likely to experience dysmenorrhoea in their cycle.[49] Relaxation therapy through various meditative or relaxation techniques has been demonstrated to improve premenstrual symptoms and dysmenorrhoea.[50,51]

PMS supplements

Herbal medicines

Vitex agnus-castus has had demonstrated effect in treating a variety of premenstrual symptoms.[52–55] *Vitex agnus-castus* reduces prolactin through its action on dopamine receptors.[52,55–59] However, other studies have suggested a dose-dependent effect, as lower doses (120 mg) were found to increase dopamine secretion while higher doses (240–480 mg) were found to decrease secretion.[60] *Vitex agnus-castus* may also have effects on progesterone levels; one study has shown it can normalise progesterone levels in women with hyperprolactinaemia within three months,[58] while another has suggested it can stimulate progesterone receptor expression.[61] Recent research has suggested that *Vitex agnus-castus* may exert activity in the opiate system, and the activation of mood regulatory and analgesic pathways via this system may be at least partly responsible for its efficacy in menstrual disorders.[62]

Actaea racemosa is thought to modulate oestrogen levels by reducing luteinising hormone secretion.[63,64] Although no clinical studies are available it has a strong tradition of use in dysmenorrhoea and menstrual disorders and has been approved by Commission E for use in these conditions.[65]

Tea from the leaves of *Rosa gallica* has also been demonstrated to mildly improve dysmenorrhoea and other menstrual symptoms in women.[66] *Psidii guajava folium* has been demonstrated to be effective in dysmenorrhoea[67] as has *Matricaria recutita*.[68] Uterine tonic herbs may also be used in PMS treatment.

Hypericum perforatum may be useful in women displaying irritability or depression in PMS, and one small pilot trial has demonstrated a significant reduction in PMS symptom scores.[69] A more recent study found *Hypericum perforatum* to improve PMS scores above placebo but not those related to mood or pain.[70] Other **nervine herbs** such as *Valeriana officinalis*, *Piper methysticum*, *Passiflora incarnata* and *Melissa officinalis* have also been traditionally used in PMS for similar circumstances.[71] ***Ginkgo biloba*** has also shown demonstrable improvement in psychosocial aspects of PMS, though it is most effective at reducing congestive symptoms such as breast pain, tenderness and fluid retention.[72]

Nutritional medicines

Calcium supplementation has been shown to reduce PMS symptoms.[73,74] Women who had 1000–1200 mg calcium reported that their menstrual pain reduced by half.[74] **Magnesium** has also been shown to reduce PMS mood and fluid retention symptoms.[75,76] Although serum magnesium levels are often normal in women with PMS, they can have lower red blood cell magnesium levels than women without and levels are known to fluctuate throughout the cycle.[77–79] **Vitamin E** can be useful for breast symptoms, tension, irritability and lack of coordination in PMS.[80–82] **Vitamin A** also has a long history of use in PMS treatment.[83] **Zinc** levels have also been demonstrated to be low in women with PMS.[84] Depleted levels of **tryptophan** have been associated with increased aggression in women during the premenstrual phase,[85] which may indicate a potential use for supplementation by diet or by medication.

Relieving symptomatic pain in dysmenorrhoea

Topical application of warmth

There may be an element of clinical truth in the traditional habit of curling up with a **hot water bottle**. Application of heat to the abdomen has also been demonstrated to be at least as effective as ibuprofen or paracetamol in clinical studies.[86,87] **Massage** with liniments or warming salves (e.g. *Zingiber officinale*) or moxibustion may also offer relief.

Herbal smooth muscle relaxants

Herbs with demonstrated ability to relax smooth muscle, such as ***Valeriana officinalis***,[88] ***Lavandula angustifolia***,[89] ***Matricaria recutita***,[90] ***Achillea millefolium***[91] and ***Foeniculum vulgare***[92] may be used to treat dysmenorrhoea, usually beginning a few days before menstruation and continuing until bleeding stops. ***Zingiber officinale*** has been shown to be equally effective as the nonsteroidal anti-inflammatory drugs (NSAIDs) ibuprofen and mefenamic acid in the symptomatic treatment of menstrual pain[93] and a systematic review suggest that 750–2000 mg in the first 3–4 days of the menstrual cycle is effective at reducing menstrual pain. This may be particularly useful in women who experience nausea in conjunction with menstrual pain. It can be taken as an infusion or several preparations—often sold for travel sickness or nausea—are available. *Foeniculum vulgare* was found to reduce the severity of dysmenorrhoea when taken (20 drops of liquid tincture five times per day) during the first three days of menses and is thought to be as effective as commonly used conventional analgesics.[94] Two RCTs have also shown Trigonella foenum-graecum to be effective at reducing the severity of dysmenorrhoea.[95,96]

   Viburnum opulus and ***Viburnum prunifolium*** both have a strong tradition of use as uterine relaxants[71] in addition to many early case reports,[97,98] though they are yet to be clinically studied. While these are not symptomatic in the sense that they immediately resolve symptoms, they are effective only in treating the symptoms of dysmenorrhoea and do not address the underlying cause.

Endocrine interactions

In addition to high blood sugar or cortisol, low thyroid function may exacerbate PMS symptoms and low thyroid function has been found in women with PMS.[99–101] The menstrual cycle appears to have an effect on thyroid function, with reverse triiodothyronine concentrations found to be higher in the luteal as opposed to follicular phase.[100] Given the complex interactions that exist between hormonal systems this is not unusual. Thyroid treatment is expanded in Chapter 20 on thyroid abnormalities.

INTEGRATIVE MEDICAL CONSIDERATIONS

Oral contraceptive use

Hormone supplementation is also commonly used in conventional medicine to treat menstrual symptoms and may affect levels of vitamins A, B2, B3, B5, B12 and folate. Vitamin B6 supplementation can restore biochemical values and treat PMS symptoms in women taking oral contraception.[102] OCP use may also reduce the action of *Vitex agnus-castus*.[103]

Traditional Chinese medicine

Acupressure has been demonstrated to be an effective treatment for dysmenorrhoea.[104,105] Although methodological flaws were found to be present in many trials, a systematic review of **acupuncture** also found promising results for acupuncture for improvement in PMS symptoms.[106] This was best seen in patients who committed to weekly treatments and was most effective when combined with herbal and dietary treatments.

Traditional Chinese herbal medicine was found to be more effective than acupuncture in the treatment of dysmenorrhoea[107] and a variety of effective herbal treatments are available.[108] Chinese exercise therapy or **Qi gong** has also had documented encouraging success in alleviating various premenstrual symptoms.[109,110] As prescription is usually determined by a physical state diagnosis based on a classical Chinese understanding of the human body, a comprehensive knowledge of traditional Chinese medicine theory is required to appropriately prescribe many of these herbal formulations. However, a recent Cochrane review of Chinese herbal medicine for PMS did not find sufficient evidence to recommend Chinese herbal medicine for PMS.[111]

Other allied health modalities

A systematic review of spinal manipulation in dysmenorrhoea found **spinal manipulation** to be no better than sham manipulation, though did suggest it was more effective than no treatment.[112]

Transcutaneous electrical nerve stimulation (TENS) has been demonstrated as a non-invasive, clinically significant intervention for dysmenorrhoea.[113,114] TENS may also reduce cortisol and prolactin levels through the opioid-modulating analgesia system.[113]

Topical application of a 2 : 1:1 mixture of the **aromatherapy oils** *Lavandula officinalis*, *Salvia sclarea* and *Rosa centifolia* was demonstrated to be effective in symptomatic treatment of dysmenorrhoea in one small study.[115] Other aromatherapy treatments may also be suitable.

Regular **massage** may be a useful adjunct therapy in severe perimenstrual disorders. One small trial has demonstrated positive effects on pain and water retention in the

Traditional herbal reproductive medicine

Naturopathy, and herbal medicine specifically, has a rich history in treating disorders of the female reproductive system and it would be remiss from a historical and clinical context to ignore this component. Herbal medicine in particular has a long tradition. Some herbs, such as *Vitex agnus-castus, Paeonia lactiflora* and *Actaea racemosa*, have been used as generalist reproductive herbs, and are thought to work predominantly as hormonal regulators rather than having specific activity (it is now thought that they act directly on HPO regulation).

Fluid retention

Diuretics such as *Taraxacum officinale* have traditionally been used for symptoms of fluid retention.

Oestrogen modulation

Some herbs have been traditionally considered 'oestrogenic' in nature, in that they support oestrogen function in the body, though they may not be intrinsically oestrogenic themselves. Some examples are *Chamaelirium luteum* and *Dioscorea villosa*.

Spasmolytic activity

Spasmolytic herbs have been used traditionally for menstrual cramping. These include *Angelica sinensis*, *Viburnum* spp., *Ligusticum wallichii* and *Rubus idaeus*. *Achillea millefolium* is specifically used as a spasmolytic that also reduces bleeding.

Antihaemorrhagic

Antihaemorrhagics include *Achillea millefolium, Equisetum arvense, Alchemilia vulgaris, Lamium album, Panax notoginseng* and uterine antihaemorrhagics such as *Capsella bursa-pastoris* and *Trillium erectum*.

Anodyne

Corydalis ambigua, Piscidia erythrina, Tanacetum parthenium and *Anemone pulsatilla* have been traditionally used for pain management in reproductive disorders.

Uterine tonics

Uterine tonics are herbs that have traditionally been used for their normalising effect on the uterus and assisting with normal uterine function. They include *Rubus idaeus, Angelica sinensis, Chamaelirium luteum, Aletris farinosa, Caulophyllum thalictroides* and, more recently, *Tribulus terrestris*.

Emmenagogues

Emmenagogues—or uterine stimulants—are traditionally used when there is a desire to increase the strength of uterine contractions. They are traditionally prescribed to initiate menstruation caused by hormonal irregularities or when the period is slow or delayed. Due to their action they are also contraindicated in pregnancy. Examples are *Ruta graveolens, Artemesia vulgaris, Salvia officinalis* and *Mentha pulegium*. Emmenagogues have also been prescribed for certain conditions associated with heavy bleeding due to 'poor uterine tone', usually indicated by heavy flow, little pain and significant clotting. They are also used in combination with uterine tonics after miscarriage to adequately expel tissue and promote healing and regeneration.

Circulatory stimulants

Another concept often discussed in various humoral medicines (including traditional Chinese medicine, traditional naturopathy and Ayurvedic medicine) is the concept of warming herbs being used in reproductive conditions that are cold or stagnant in nature. They are used to promote circulation and blood flow and to remove obstruction. Examples are *Zingiber officinale* and *Cinnamomum verum*. Pain is often related to 'blood or *Qi*' stagnation in traditional Chinese medicine and equivalent ancient naturopathic humoral tradition.

In practice naturopathy is a holistic modality, and also makes use of other various herbal action—nervines, adaptogens and so on—as deemed appropriate for the individual patient. Treatment very rarely makes use of reproductive herbs alone.

longer term but only short-term benefit for mood and anxiety.[116] Another small trial of abdominal massage using traditional Chinese medicine (TCM) meridian theory has also shown benefit in regard to perimenstrual symptoms such as pain and bloating.[117]

CLINICAL SUMMARY

Every woman will experience her menstrual cycle differently. Although often viewed as 'hormonal issues', menstrual problems are not associated with simple hormone excess or deficiency, but rather a complex interconnection of factors that interfere with the HPO axis. This may be far removed from the female reproductive system (e.g. gastrointestinal function or stress). PMS symptoms are often treated successfully through amelioration of underlying causes with dietary and lifestyle modification—half the world's population was not designed to 'malfunction' once a month. Ultimately, rather than a focus on labels or diagnoses, naturopathic treatment of menstrual irregularities should focus on restoration of a regular menstrual cycle, whatever that may look like.

Although naturopathic philosophy dictates finding the underlying cause for dysmenorrhoea, there is little likelihood of patient compliance (and therefore ultimately clinical success) without addressing symptomatic complaints. This may necessitate either an integrated approach to treatment with conventional medications or a separate prescription for purely symptomatic naturopathic medications. The patient should also be counselled on appropriate or sensible dressing to cope with breast tenderness or abdominal bloating (such as loose-fitting clothes around the abdomen or a firm-fitting bra to wear during episodes of PMS).

Symptomatic treatment is very important. However, smooth muscle relaxants or analgesics should be considered only a temporary solution and treatment of the underlying factors should be prioritised. Treatment of primary dysmenorrhoea should see positive results within the first one or two cycles. Secondary dysmenorrhoea requires treatment of its causative aetiology and is often more complex (see Chapter 22 on endometriosis).

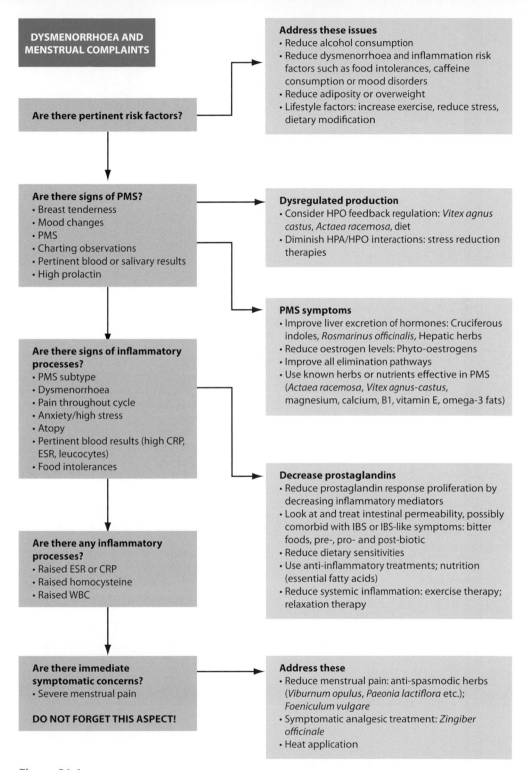

Figure 21.1
Naturopathic treatment decision tree—dysmenorrhoea and menstrual complaints

Table 21.3
Review of the major evidence

Intervention	Mechanisms of action	Key literature	Summary of results	Comment
Thiamine	Currently unknown	RCT: Gokhale 1996[118] Three-month RCT (n = 556) crossover design with women with moderate to severe spasmodic dysmenorrhoea; 100 mg thiamine versus placebo	Thiamine significantly increased the proportion of women with no pain before crossover after 60 days compared with placebo (51% versus 0%) After completion of the RCT, 87% of all women experienced no pain	No analysis was made to determine differences between levels of dysmenorrhoea
Vitamin E	Thought to be via prostaglandin regulation	RCTs: Butler & McKnight 1955,[119] Ziaei et al. 2005[120] Four menstrual cycle RCT (n = 278) with women aged 15–17 years with primary dysmenorrhoea; 400 IU vitamin E versus placebo	Vitamin E group had lower visual analogue scale (VAS) pain scores at two months (3 versus 5; $p \leq 0.001$) and four months (0.5 versus 6; $p \leq 0.001$); shorter pain duration at two months (4.2 hours versus 15 hours; $p \leq 0.001$) and four months (1.6 hours versus 17 hours; $p \leq 0.001$); and lower blood loss at two months (54 versus 70; $p \leq 0.001$) and four months (46 versus 70; $p \leq 0.001$) than placebo group	The form of vitamin E was not made known Blood loss was also self-measured using a 'staining score' of menstrual pads
Omega-3 fatty acids	Prostaglandin regulation assisting in reducing inflammatory factors Neurochemical modulation	RCTs: Harel et al. 1996[121] Deutch 1995[122] four-month RCT (n = 42) Crossover design with adolescents with dysmenorrhoea Fish oil (1080 mg EPA; 720 mg DHA) 1.5 mg vitamin E versus placebo	Reduction in Cox Menstrual Symptom Scale Score of 69.9–44.0 ($p \leq 0.001$) for fish oil group versus placebo	Omega-3 containing oils have encouraging evidence for reducing menstrual symptoms
Magnesium	Inhibition of biosynthesis of PGF_2 alpha smooth muscle relaxant	Systematic review: Wilson & Murphy 2001[123] Cochrane systematic review found seven randomised trials	Magnesium was more effective than placebo for pain relief and resulted in less extra medication being required	Only three trials were considered to be suitable for inclusion in analysis: Seifert et al. 1989[124], Fontana-Kleiber & Hogg 1990[125], Benassi et al. 1992[126]

Table 21.3
Review of the major evidence (continued)

Intervention	Mechanisms of action	Key literature	Summary of results	Comment
Psidii guajavae folium extract	Unknown action thought to be facilitated and associated with action resulting in reduction of menstrual blood volume	RCT: Doubova et al. 2007[67] Four-month RCT (n = 197) Women with dysmenorrhoea were assigned to one of four groups: 3 mg *Psidii guajavae folium* extract; 6 mg guava extract; 1200 mg ibuprofen; or placebo	Reduction in VAS pain score consistently over three cycles (p ≤ 0.001) though was slightly less than ibuprofen group	Although study showed reduction in pain scores from baseline in all groups, results were inconsistent over three cycles except for 6 mg and ibuprofen groups
Zingiber officinale	Prostaglandin regulation and strong anti-inflammatory Warming-rubefacient properties	Systematic reviews: Chen et al. 2016[127] Daily et al. 2015[128]	Significant reduction in pain scores across all groups Seven RCTs of varying quality, but consistently show that 750–2000 mg of Zingiber in first 3–4 days of menstrual cycle reduce primary dysmenorrhoea	No significant difference occurred between interventions when conventional anti-inflammatories used as a comparator
Foeniculum vulgare (fennel)	Unknown but thought to be facilitated by the action on uterine prostaglandins	RCTs: Modaress & Asidipour 2006[94] Namovar et al. 2003[129] Two-cycle RCT (n = 110) in adolescent women with dysmenorrhoea assigned to take either 250 mg mefenamic acid every six hours or 30 drops of fennel extract every six hours Namovar et al. 2003[129] (n = 30) Adolescent women with moderate to severe dysmenorrhoea were given no treatment in first cycle, 250 mg mefenamic acid every six hours in second cycle, and 25 drops fennel extract in third cycle	80% of girls in the fennel group and 73% of girls in the mefenamic acid group showed complete pain relief or pain decrease, while 80% in the fennel group and 62% in the mefenamic acid group no longer needed to rest Both mefenamic acid and fennel extract reduced menstrual pain (p ≤ 0.001) No significant difference was observed during first day though mefenamic acid was significantly superior on second and third days There was no significant difference in time taken to enact effect between mefenamic acid and fennel extract	No significant difference in pain relief between the two groups Study design and methodological flaws may reduce validity
Pycnogenol (standardised extract of *Pinus pinaster*)	Antioxidant Reduction of factors associated with the growth and adhesion of endometrial tissue (via oxidative stress)	RCT: Kohama et al. 2004[130] Three-cycle open CT (n = 47) in women with dysmenorrhoea assigned to take 60 mg Pycnogenol	Abdominal pain was reduced in first cycle (p ≤ 0.05) and further in second cycle (p ≤ 0.01)	No significant reduction in back pain nor days experiencing pain

FURTHER READING

Hudson T. Women's encyclopedia of natural medicine. New York: McGraw-Hill; 2008.

Iacovides S, Avidon I, Baker FC. What we know about primary dysmenorrhea today: a critical review. Hum Reprod Update 2015;21(6):762–78.

Pattanittum P, Kunyanone N, Brown J, et al. Dietary supplements for dysmenorrhoea. Cochrane Database Syst Rev 2016;(3):Art. No.: CD002124, doi:10.1002/14651858.CD002124.pub2.

Pellow J, Nienhuis C. Medicinal plants for primary dysmenorrhoea: a systematic review. Complement Ther Med 2018;37:13–26.

Trickey R. Women, hormones and the menstrual cycle: herbal and medical solutions from adolescence to menopause. Melbourne: MHHG; 2012.

REFERENCES

1. Edmonds K, editor. Obstetrics & gynaecology. London: Blackwell; 2007.

2. American Psychiatric Association. Diagnostic and statistical manual of mental disorders. 5th ed. Arlington: American Psychiatric Association; 2013.

3. Roca C, Schmidt P, Bloch M, et al. Implications of endocrine studies of premenstrual syndrome. Psychiatr Ann 1996;26:576–80.

4. Backstrom T, Carstensen H. Estrogen and progesterone in plasma in relation to premenstrual tension. J Steroid Biochem 1974;5:257–60.

5. Munday M, Brush M, Taylor R. Correlations between progesterone, estradiol, and aldosterone levels in the premenstrual syndrome. Clin Endocrinol (Oxf) 1981;14(1):1–9.

6. Rubinow D, Hoban M, Grover G. Changes in plasma hormones across the menstrual cycle in patients with menstrually related mood disorders and in control subjects. Am J Obstet Gynecol 1988;158:5–11.

7. O'Brien P, Symonds E. Prolactin levels and the premenstrual syndrome. Br J Obstet Gynaecol 1982;89:306–8.

8. Dalton K. The aetiology of premenstrual syndrome is with the progesterone receptors. Med Hypotheses 1990;31:323–7.

9. Nock B. Nordrenergic regulation of progestin receptors: new findings. Ann N Y Acad Sci 1986;415–22.

10. Sundell G, Milsom I, Andersch B. Factors influencing the prevalence and severity of dysmenorrhoea in young women. Br J Obstet Gynaecol 1990;97:588–94.

11. Rubinow D, Schmidt C. The treatment of premenstrual syndrome—forward into the past. N Engl J Med 1995;332:1574–5.

12. Kessel B. Premenstrual syndrome: advances in diagnosis and treatment. Obstet Gynecol Clin North Am 2000;27(3):625–39.

13. Chuong C, Coulam C, Kao P, et al. Neuropeptide levels in the premenstrual syndrome. Fertil Steril 1985;44: 760–5.

14. Rapkin A. The role of serotonin in the premenstrual syndrome. Clin Obstet Gynecol 1992;35(3):629–36.

15. Steiner M, Pearlstein T. Premenstrual dysphoria and the serotonin system: pathophysiology and treatment. J Clin Psychiatry 2000;61(12):S17–21.

16. Budoff P. The use of prostaglandin inhibitors for the premenstrual syndrome. J Reprod Med 1983;28:465–8.

17. Nigam S, Benedetto C, Zonca M. Increased concentrations of eicosanoids and platelet-activating factor in menstrual blood from women with primary dysmenorrhoea. Eicosanoids 1991;4(3):137–41.

18. Horrobin D. The role of essential fatty acids and prostaglandins in the premenstrual syndrome. J Reprod Med 1983;28(7):465–8.

19. Hamilton J, Parry B, Algna S, et al. Premenstrual mood changes: a guide to evaluation and treatment. Psychiatr Ann 1984;30:474–82.

20. DeJong R, Rubinow D, Roy-Byrne P, et al. Premenstrual mood disorder and psychiatric illness. Am J Psychiatry 1985;142:1359–61.

21. Chen C, Cho S, Damokosh AI, et al. Prospective study of exposure to environmental tobacco smoke and dysmenorrhea. Environ Health Perspect 2000;108(11):1019–22.

22. Hornsby P, Wilcox A, Weinberg C. Cigarette smoking and disturbance of menstrual function. Epidemiology 1998;9(2):193–8.

23. Parazzini F, Tozzi L, Mezzopane R, et al. Cigarette smoking, alcohol consumption, and risk of primary dysmenorrhea. Epidemiology 1994;5(4):469–72.

24. Masho S, Adera T, South-Paul J. Obesity as a risk factor for premenstrual syndrome. J Psychosom Obstet Gynaecol 2005;26(1):33–9.

25. Rossignol A, Bonnlander H. Caffeine-containing beverages, total fluid consumption, and premenstrual syndrome. Am J Public Health 1990;80(9):1106–10.

26. Rossignol A, Zhang J, Chen Y, et al. Tea and premenstrual syndrome in the People's Republic of China. Am J Public Health 1989;79(1):67–9.

27. Rossignol A, Bonnlander H. Prevalence and severitry of the premenstrual syndrome. Effects of foods and beverages that are sweet or high in sugar content. J Reprod Med 1991;36:131–6.

28. Rossignol A, Bonnlander H, Song L, et al. Do women with premenstrual symptoms self-medicate with caffeine? Epidemiology 1991;2(6):403–8.

29. Murtagh J. General practice. Sydney: McGraw-Hill; 2007.

30. Wyatt K. Premenstrual syndrome. Clin Evid 2000;9:2125–44.

31. Ford O, Lethaby A, Roberts H. Progesterone for premenstrual syndrome. Cochrane Database Syst Rev 2006;(4):CD003415.

32. Abraham G. Nutritional factors in the etiology of the premenstrual syndrome. J Reprod Med 1983;28:446–64.

33. Balbi C, Musone R, Menditto A, et al. Influence of menstrual factors and dietary habits on menstrual pain in adolescence age. Eur J Obstet Gynecol Reprod Biol 2000;91(2):143–8.

34. Barnard N, Scialli A, Hurlock D, et al. Diet and sex-hormone binding globulin, dysmenorrhea, and premenstrual symptoms. Obstet Gynecol 2000;95(2):245–50.

35. Nagata C, Hirokawa K, Shimuzu N, et al. Associations of menstrual pain with intakes of soy, fat and dietary fiber in Japanese women. Eur J Clin Nutr 2005;59(1):88–92.

36. Nagata C, Hirokawa K, Shimizu N, et al. Soy, fat and other dietary factors in relation to premenstrual symptoms in Japanese women. Br J Obstet Gynaecol 2004;111(6):594–9.

37. Roy S, Ghosh B, Bhattacharjee S. Changes in glucose oral tolerance during normal menstrual cycle. J Indian Med Assoc 1971;57(6):210–14.

38. Fujiwara T. Skipping breakfast is associated with dysmenorrhoea in young women in Japan. Int J Food Sci Nutr 2003;54(6):505–9.

39. Fujiwara T. Diet during adolescence is a trigger for subsequent development of dysmenorrhea in young women. Int J Food Sci Nutr 2007;58(6):437–44.

40. Montero P, Bernis C, Fernandez V. Influence of body mass index and slimming habits on menstrual pain and cycle irregularity. J Biosoc Sci 1996;28(3):315–23.

41. Aganoff J, Boyle G. Aerobic exercise, mood states and menstrual cycle symptoms. J Psychosom Res 1994;38:183–92.

42. Choi P, Salmon P. Symptom changes across the menstrual cycle in competitive sportswomen, exercisers and sedentary women. Br J Clin Psychol 1995;34(3):447–60.

43. Golomb L, Solidum A, Warren M. Primary dysmenorrhea and physical activity. Med Sci Sports Exerc 1998;30(6):906–9.

44. Jahromi M, Gaeini A, Rahimi Z. Influence of a physical fitness course on menstrual cycle characteristics. Gynecol Endocrinol 2008;24(11):659–62.

45. Prior J, Vigna Y. Conditioning exercise and premenstrual symptoms. J Reprod Med 1987;32:423–8.

46. Pullon S, Reinken J, Sparrow MJ. Treatment of premenstrual symptoms in Wellington women. N Z Med J 1989;102(862):72–4.

47. Stoddard J, Dent C, Shames L, et al. Exercise training effects on premenstrual distress and ovarian steroid hormones. Eur J Appl Physiol 2007;99(1):27–37.

48. Lustyk M, Widman L, Paschane A, et al. Stress, quality of life and physical activity in women with varying degrees of premenstrual symptomatology. Women Health 2004;39(3):35–44.

49. Wang L, Wang X, Wang W, et al. Stress and dysmenorrhoea: a population based prospective study. Occup Environ Med 2004;61(12):1021–6.

50. Arias A, Steinberg K, Banga A, et al. Systematic review of the efficacy of meditation techniques as treatments for medical illness. J Altern Complement Med 2008;12(8):817–23.

51. Goodale I, Domar A, Benson H. Alleviation of premenstrual syndrome with the relaxation response. Obstet Gynecol 1990;75(4):649–55.

52. Berger D, Schaffner W, Schrader E, et al. Efficacy of Vitex agnus castus L. extract Ze 440 in patients with pre-menstrual syndrome (PMS). Arch Gynecol Obstet 2000;264(3):150–3.

53. Loch E, Selle H, Boblitz N. Treatment of premenstrual syndrome with a phytopharmaceutical formulation containing Vitex agnus castus. J Womens Health Gend Based Med 2000;9(3):315–20.

54. Schellenberg R. Treatment for the premenstrual syndrome with agnus castus fruit extract: prospective, randomised, placebo controlled study. BMJ 2001;322(7279):134–7.

55. Wuttke W, Jarry H, Christoffel V, et al. Chaste tree (Vitex agnus-castus)—pharmacology and clinical indications. Phytomedicine 2003;10(4):348–57.

56. Jarry H, Leonhardt S, Gorkow C, et al. In vitro prolactin but not LH and FSH release is inhibited by compounds in extracts of Agnus castus: direct evidence for a dopaminergic principle by the dopamine receptor assay. Exp Clin Endocrinol 1994;102(6):448–54.

57. Meier B, Berger D, Hoberg E, et al. Pharmacological activities of Vitex agnus-castus extracts in vitro. Phytomedicine 2000;7(5):373–81.

58. Milewicz A, Gejdel E, Sworen H, et al. Vitex agnus castus extract in the treatment of luteal phase defects due to latent hyperprolactinemia. Results of a randomized placebo-controlled double-blind study. Arzneimittelforschung 1993;43(7):752–6, [in German].

59. Sliutz G, Speiser P, Schultz A, et al. Agnus castus extracts inhibit prolactin secretion of rat pituitary cells. Horm Metab Res 1993;25(5):253–5.

60. Merz P, Gorkow C, Schrödter A, et al. The effects of a special Agnus castus extract (BP1095E1) on prolactin secretion in healthy male subjects. Exp Clin Endocrinol Diabetes 1996;104(6):447–53.

61. Liu J. Evaluation of estrogenic activity of plant extracts for the potential treatment of menopausal symptoms. J Agric Food Chem 2001;49(5):2472–9.

62. Webster D, Lu J, Chen S, et al. Activation of the mu-opiate receptor by Vitex agnus-castus methanol extracts: implication for its use in PMS. J Ethnopharmacol 2006;106(2):216–21.

63. Duker E, Kopanski L, Jarry H, et al. Effects of extracts from cimicifuga racemosa on gonadotrophin release in menopausal women and ovariectomized rats. Planta Med 1991;57(5):420–4.

64. Seidlova-Wuttke D, Hesse O, Jarry H, et al. Evidence for selective estrogen receptor modulator activity in a black Cohosh (Cimicifuga racemosa) extract: comparison with estradiol-17 beta. Eur J Endocrinol 2003;149:351–62.

65. Blumenthal M, Goldberg A, Brinckmann J, editors. Herbal medicine: expanded Commission E monographs (English translation). Austin: Integrative Medicine Communications; 2000.

66. Tseng Y, Chen C, Yang Y. Rose tea for relief of primary dysmenorrhea in adolescents: a randomized controlled trial in Taiwan. J Midwifery Womens Health 2005;50(5):51–7.

67. Doubova S, Morales H, Hernández S, et al. Effect of a Psidii guajavae folium extract in the treatment of primary dysmenorrhea: a randomized clinical trial. J Ethnopharmacol 2007;110(2):305–10.

68. Banikarim C, Chacko M, Kelder S. Prevalence and impact of dysmenorrhea on Hispanic female adolescents. Arch Pediatr Adolesc Med 2000;154:1226–9.

69. Stevinson C, Ernst E. A pilot study of Hypericum perforatum for the treatment of premenstrual syndrome. Br J Obstet Gynaecol 2000;107(7):870–6.

70. Canning S, Waterman M, Orsi N, et al. The efficacy of Hypericum perforatum (St John's wort) for the treatment of premenstrual syndrome: a randomized, double-blind, placebo-controlled trial. CNS Drugs 2010;24(3):207–25.

71. Mills S, Bone K. Principles and Practice of Phytotherapy. Edinburgh: Churchill Livingstone; 2000.

72. Tamborini A, Taurelle R. Value of standardized Ginkgo biloba extract (EGb 761) in the management of congestive symptoms of premenstrual syndrome. Rev Fr Gynecol Obstet 1993;88(7–9):447–57.

73. Thys-Jacobs S, Ceccarelli S, Bierman A, et al. Calcium supplementation and the premenstrual syndrome. J Gen Intern Med 1989;4:183–9.

74. Thys-Jacobs S, Starky P, Bernstein D, et al. Calcium carbonate and the premenstrual syndrome: effects on premenstrual and menstrual symptoms. Am J Obstet Gynecol 1998;179(2):444–52.

75. Facchinetti F, Borella P, Sances G, et al. Oral magnesium successfully relieves premenstrual mood changes. Obstet Gynecol 1991;78:177–81.

76. Walker A, De Souza M, Vickers M, et al. Magnesium supplementation alleviates premenstrual symptoms of fluid retention. J Womens Health 1998;7:1157–65.

77. Abraham G, Lubran M. Serum and red cell magnesium levels in patients with PMT. Am J Clin Nutr 1981;34:2364–6.

78. Facchinetti F, Borella P, Valentini M, et al. Premenstrual increase of intracellular magnesium levels in women with ovulatory, asymptomatic menstrual cycles. Gynecol Endocrinol 1988;2:249–56.

79. Sherwood R, Rocks B, Stewart A, et al. Magnesium and the premenstrual syndrome. Ann Clin Biochem 1986;23:667–70.

80. London R, Murphy L, Kitlowski K, et al. Efficacy of alpha-tocopherol in the treatment of the premenstrual syndrome. J Reprod Med 1987;32(6):400–4.

81. London R, Sundaram G, Murphy L, et al. The effect of alpha-tocopherol on premenstrual symptomatology: a double-blind study. J Am Coll Nutr 1983;2(2):115–22.

82. London R, Sundaram G, Schultz M, et al. Evaluation and treatment of breast symptoms in women with the premenstrual syndrome. J Reprod Med 1981;28:503–8.

83. Argonz J, Abinzano C. Premenstrual tension treated with vitamin A. J Clin Endocrinol Metab 1950;10(12):1579–90.

84. Chuong C, Dawson E. Zinc and copper levels in premenstrual syndrome. Fertil Steril 1994;62:313–20.

85. Bond A, Wingrove J, Critchlow D. Tryptophan depletion increases aggression in women during the premenstrual phase. Psychopharmacology (Berl) 2001;156(4):477–80.

86. Akin M, Price W, Rodriguez G, et al. Continuous, low-level, topical heat wrap therapy as compared to acetaminophen for primary dysmenorrhea. J Reprod Med 2004;49(9):739–45.

87. Akin M, Weingand K, Hengehold D, et al. Continuous low-level topical heat in the treatment of dysmenorrhea. Obstet Gynecol 2001;97(3):343–9.

88. Mirabi P, Dolatian M, Mojab F, et al. Effects of valerian on the severity and systemic manifestations of dysmenorrhea. Int J Gynaecol Obstet 2011;115(3):285–8.

89. Lis-Belchin M, Hart S. Studies on the mode of action of the essential oil of lavender (Lavandula angustifolia). Phytother Res 1999;13(6):540–2.

90. Achterrath-Tuckermann U, Kunde R, Flaskamp E, et al. Pharmacological investigations with compounds of chamomile. V: investigations on the spasmolytic effect of compounds of chamomile and Kamillosan on the isolated guinea pig ileum. Planta Med 1980;39(1):38–50.

91. Jenabi E, Fereidoony B. Effect of Achillea millefolium on relief of primary dysmenorrhea: a double-blind randomized clinical trial. J Pediatr Adolesc Gynecol 2015;28(5): 402–4.

92. Ostad S, Soodi M, Shariffzadeh M, et al. The effect of fennel essential oil on uterine contraction as a model for dysmenorrhea, pharmacology and toxicology study. J Ethnopharmacol 2001;76(3):299–304.

93. Ozgoli G, Goli M, Moattar F. Comparison of effects of ginger, mefenamic acid, and ibuprofen on pain in women with primary dysmenorrhea. J Altern Complement Med 2009;15(2):129–32.

94. Modaress Nejad V, Asadipour M. Comparison of the effectiveness of fennel and mefenamic acid on pain intensity in dysmenorrhoea. East Mediterr Health J 2006;12(3–4):423–7.

95. Inanmdar W, Sultana A, Mubeen U, et al. Clinical efficacy of Trigonella foenum graecum (Fenugreek) and dry cupping therapy on intensity of pain in patients with primary dysmenorrhea. Chin J Integr Med 2016; 1–8.

96. Younesy S, Amiraliakbari S, Esmaeili S, et al. Effects of fenugreek seed on the severity and systemic symptoms of dysmenorrhea. J Reprod Infertil 2014;15(1):41.

97. Jarboe C, Schmidt C, Nicholson J, et al. Uterine relaxant properties of Viburnum. Nature 1966;212:837.

98. Munch J, Pratt H. The uterine-sedative action of authentic Viburnum. XI. Bioassay methods. Pharmaceut Arch 1941;12:88–91.

99. Brayshaw N, Brayshaw D. Thyroid hypofunction in premenstrual syndrome. N Engl J Med 1986;315: 1486–7.

100. Girdler S, Pedersen C, Light K. Thyroid axis function during the menstrual cycle in women with premenstrual syndrome. Psychoneuroendocrinology 1995;20(4):395–403.

101. Schmidt P, Grover G, Roy-Byrne P, et al. Thyroid function in women with premenstrual syndrome. J Clin Endocrinol Metab 1993;76(3):671–4.

102. Bermond P. Therapy of side effects of oral contraceptive agents with vitamin B6. Acta Vitaminol Enzymol 1982;4(1–2):45–54.

103. Braun L, Cohen M. Herbs and natural supplements: an evidence-based guide. Melbourne: Churchill Livingstone; 2007.

104. Pouresmail Z, Ibrahimzadeh R. Effects of acupressure and ibuprofen on the severity of primary dysmenorrhea. J Tradit Chin Med 2002;22:205–10.

105. Smith CA, Armour M, Zhu X, et al. Acupuncture for dysmenorrhoea. Cochrane Database Syst Rev 2016;(4):Art. No.: CD007854, doi:10.1002/14651858.CD007854. pub3.

106. Kim S, Park H, Lee H, et al. Acupuncture for premenstrual syndrome: a systematic review and meta-analysis of randomised controlled trials. BJOG 2011;118(8):899–915.

107. Zhu X, Proctor M, Bensoussan A, et al. Chinese herbal medicine for primary dysmenorrhoea. Cochrane Database Syst Rev 2008;(2):CD005288.

108. Jia W, Wang X, Xu D, et al. Common traditional Chinese medicinal herbs for dysmenorrhea. Phytother Res 2006;20(10):819–24.

109. Jang H, Lee M. Effects of qi therapy (external qigong) on premenstrual syndrome: a randomized placebo controlled study. J Altern Complement Med 2004;10:456–62.

110. Jang H, Lee M, Kim M, et al. Effects of qi-therapy on premenstrual syndrome. Int J Neurosci 2004;114:909–21.

111. Jing Z, Yang X, Ismail K, et al. Chinese herbal medicine for premenstrual syndrome. Cochrane Database Syst Rev 2009;(1):CD006414.

112. Abaraogu UO, Igwe SE, Tabansi-Ochiogu CS, et al. A systematic review and meta-analysis of the efficacy of manipulative therapy in women with primary dysmenorrhea. Explore (NY) 2017;13(6):386–92.

113. Akinbo S, Tella B, Olisah A, et al. Effect of transcutaneous electric nerve stimulation (TENS) on hormones profile in subjects with primary dysmenorrhoea—a preliminary study. S Afr J Physiother 2007;63(3):45–8.

114. Proctor M, Smith C, Farquhar C, et al. Transcutaneous electrical nerve stimulation and acupuncture for primary dysmenorrhoea. Cochrane Database Syst Rev 2002;(1):CD002123.

115. Han S, Hur M, Buckle J, et al. Effect of aromatherapy on symptoms of dysmenorrhea in college students: a randomized placebo-controlled clinical trial. J Altern Complement Med 2006;12(6):535–41.

116. Hernandez-Reif M, Martinez A, Field T, et al. Premenstrual symptoms are relieved by massage therapy. J Psychosom Obstet Gynaecol 2000;21(1):9–15.

117. Kim J, Jo Y, Hwang S. The effects of abdominal meridian massage on menstrual cramps and dysmenorrhea in full-time employed women. Taehan Kanho Hakhoe Chi 2005;35(7):1325–32.

118. Gokhale L. Curative treatment of primary (spasmodic) dysmenorrhoea. Indian J Med Res 1996;103:227–31.

119. Butler E, McKnight E. Vitamin E in the treatment of primary dysmenorrhoea. Lancet 1955;268(6869):844–7.

120. Ziaei S, Zakeri M, Kazemnejad A. A randomised controlled trial of vitamin E in the treatment of primary dysmenorrhoea. Br J Obstet Gynaecol 2005;112(4):466–9.

121. Harel Z, Biro F, Kottenhahn R, et al. Supplementation with omega-3 polyunsaturated fatty acids in the management of dysmenorrhea in adolescents. Am J Obstet Gynecol 1996;174(4):1335–8.

122. Deutch B. Menstrual pain in Danish women correlated with low n-3 polyunsaturated fatty acid intake. Eur J Clin Nutr 1995;49(7):508–16.

123. Wilson M, Murphy P. Herbal and dietary therapies for primary and secondary dysmenorrhoea. Cochrane Database Syst Rev 2001;(3):CD002124.

124. Seifert B, Wagler P, Dartsch S, et al. Magnesium-a new therapeutic alternative in primary dysmenorrhea. Zentralbl Gynakol 1989;111(11):755–60.

125. Fontana-Klaiber H, Hogg B. Therapeutic effects of magnesium in dysmenorrhea. Schweiz Rundsch Med Prax 1990;79(16):491–4.

126. Benassi L, Barlette F, Baroncini L, et al. Effectiveness of Magnesium Pidolate in the prophylactic treatment of primary dysmenorrhoea. Clin Exp Obstet Gynecol 1992;19(3):176–9.

127. Chen CX, Barrett B, Kwekkeboom KL. Efficacy of oral ginger (Zingiber officinale) for dysmenorrhea: a systematic review and meta-analysis. Evid Based Complement Alternat Med 2016;6295737.

128. Daily JW, Zhang X, Kim DS, et al. Efficacy of ginger for alleviating the symptoms of primary dysmenorrhea: a systematic review and meta-analysis of randomized clinical trials. Pain Med 2015;16(12):2243–55.

129. Namavar Jahromi B, Tartifizadeh A, Khabnadideh S. Comparison of fennel and mefenamic acid for the treatment of primary dysmenorrhea. Int J Gynaecol Obstet 2003;80(2):153–7.

130. Kohama T, Suzuki N, Ohno S, et al. Analgesic efficacy of French maritime pine bark extract in dysmenorrhea: an open clinical trial. J Reprod Med 2004;49(10):828–32.

CHAPTER **22**

Endometriosis

Jon Wardle
ND, MPH, PhD

OVERVIEW

Endometriosis is the abnormal growth of endometrial tissue in areas other than the wall of the uterus.[1] The exact cause of endometriosis is unknown, although a number of theories do exist. It is one of the more common causes of infertility in Western societies. However, sufferers may experience combinations of many underlying causes and no two people are identical in their symptoms or causes. Theories in naturopathic medicine include the following (see Figure 22.1).

- Excessive oestrogens may promote the proliferation of endometrial tissue. Oestrogen levels may be higher for a number of reasons, including increased production or decreased excretion, or may be dominated by oestrogen metabolites that are more proliferative, inflammatory and genotoxic.[2,3]
- Environmental toxins may mimic hormones in the body, exacerbating endometriosis symptoms.[4]

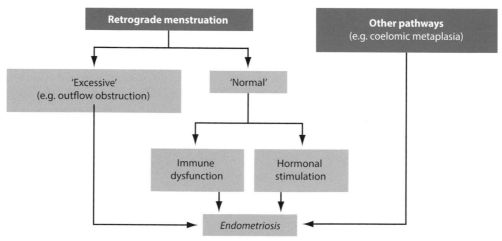

Figure 22.1
Postulated theories for the development of endometriosis

- Although retrograde menstruation is present in most cycling women, not all these women have endometriosis. It is thought inflammatory mediators may cause endometrial tissue to adhere to other tissues[5]; an autoimmune component has also been linked to endometriosis, with endometriosis fulfilling the criteria for autoimmune disease (based on the presence of inflammatory cytokines and tissue-specific antibodies). More information on treatment protocols for autoimmune disease can be found in Chapter 31.[6]
- There may be a genetic component. Endometriosis has been linked to dysfunctions in embryonic development.
- Other theories suggest that endometriosis does not represent transplanted endometrial tissue but starts de novo from local stem cells. This process has been referred to as *coelomic metaplasia*. Various triggers, such as excessive oestrogen levels, menses, toxins or immune factors, may be necessary to start this process. This would explain the rare instances of endometriosis in men.[7,8]

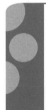

DIFFERENTIAL DIAGNOSIS
- Primary or secondary dysmenorrhoea
- Benign or malignant neoplasms (both gynaecological and non-gynaecological)
- Pelvic inflammatory disease
- Appendicitis
- Urinary tract infections
- Venereal diseases

RISK FACTORS
Several risk factors need to be addressed in patients with endometriosis. Although often hormonal or inflammatory in nature, removal of these risk factors may not be enough to significantly reduce symptoms. Lack of exercise can increase levels of both oestrogen and inflammatory mediators as well as reduce oestrogen excretion.[9] However, strenuous physical activity during menstruation may increase the risk of adhesion. Epidemiological data also suggest that positive correlations of symptoms and occurrence are seen with: increased cigarette smoking; increased carbohydrate, alcohol and coffee intake; stress; and low body mass index.[10] Aromatase found in adipose tissue may also increase the formation of oestrogen.[11] Therefore weight loss may be indicated in some patients.

CONVENTIONAL TREATMENT
Conventional medical treatment aims to reduce the symptoms of endometriosis and improve fertility. This can be done surgically (most often laparoscopic to remove tissue, although occasionally hysterectomy is required) or medically. Medical interventions focus predominantly on reducing excessive oestrogen levels, which include: those androgenic in nature, such as danazol or progesterone supplementation; inducing hypo-oestrogenic states by decreasing follicle-stimulating hormone (FSH) and luteinising hormone (LH) through the use of gonadotrophin-releasing hormone agonists (GnRH agonists); continuous hormonal contraception to stop bleeding; or aromatase inhibitors to block the formation of oestrogens, particularly in adipose tissue.[1]

KEY TREATMENT PROTOCOLS

In naturopathic treatment, endometriosis is most often considered a disorder of hormonal imbalance (usually related to oestrogen) or inflammation and may have a number of underlying factors.

Oestrogen modulation

Hypothalamic–pituitary–ovarian axis modulation

Oestrogen levels in the body may be affected by disruptions of the hypothalamic–pituitary–ovarian (HPO) axis. The anterior pituitary releases FSH and LH, which encourages oestrogen release from growing ovarian follicles. Ordinarily feedback loops regulate hormone release from the HPO axis, but in some reproductive disorders this may be disrupted. Herbal medicines such as **Vitex agnus-castus**[12] and **Actaea racemosa**[13] may help restore proper functioning of the HPO axis through direct and indirect means. Exercise has been shown to both reduce oestrogen production and increase oestrogen excretion[10] (see Chapter 21 on dysmenorrhoea and menstrual complaints).

> ### Naturopathic Treatment Aims
>
> - Address risk and exacerbating factors.
> - Modulate oestrogen levels.
> - Decrease inflammation.
> - Address secondary aims and symptoms.
> - Address dietary and lifestyle issues affecting the condition.

Aromatase

Aromatase is an enzyme of the cytochrome P450 superfamily, the function of which is to aromatise androgens, thereby producing oestrogens. It is normally found in the ovaries and, to a much lesser extent, in the skin and fat. Aromatase is not present in the normal endometrium but is expressed aberrantly in endometriosis.[1]

Prostaglandin E2 (PGE_2) was found to be the most potent known inducer of aromatase activity in endometrial cells.[14,15] Inflammation may not only increase aromatase but also make endometrial tissue more sensitive to its effects.[16] Factors known to increase aromatase activity are hyperinsulinaemia, increased adiposity, obesity and ageing.[17]

Aromatase activity may be decreased by increased consumption of dietary phyto-oestrogens[18] in addition to reduction in adiposity and inflammation.

Oestrogen-like compounds and oestrogen receptor activity

Many compounds—both natural and synthetic—may mimic endogenous sex hormones.[4,19,20] Several chemicals in current industrial use may interfere with the body's hormone responses. Compounds such as dioxins, polychlorinated biphenyls (PCBs) and bisphenols (found in pesticides, petrochemicals and plastics) may bind to and activate endogenous oestrogen receptor sites. However, unlike natural hormones these xeno-oestrogens (literally 'foreign oestrogens') may exert effects many times more potent than endogenous oestrogens.[21] **Phyto-oestrogens** (literally 'plant oestrogens') also bind to and activate these oestrogen receptor sites, although they are often much less powerful than regular oestrogen and therefore act as oestrogen modulators by preventing the more powerful compounds—endogenous hormones and the xeno-oestrogens— binding in excess oestrogen conditions but binding to empty sites in oestrogen-deficient conditions.[22] A compound exhibiting this activity is known as a selective oestrogen

Table 22.1
Relative phyto-oestrogenic content (μg/100 g) of commonly used therapeutic supplements

Trifolium pratense	1 767 000
Flaxseed (crushed)	546 000
Soybeans	103 920
Tofu	27 150
Sesame seed	8 008
Flax bread	7 540
Multigrain bread	4 798
Pumpkin	3 870
Chickpeas	3 600
Lentils	3 370
Soy milk	2 457

Sources: Mazur & Adlercreutz 1998,[2] Lea & Whorwell 2003,[14] Noble et al. 1997,[15] Petterson & Kiesling 1984,[24] Dalessandri et al. 2004[25] and McAlindon et al. 2001[26]

receptor modulator (SORM)—similar in effect to the pharmaceutical compound tamoxifen. The isoflavones (such as genistein and daidzein) from soy products, lignans from lentils and flaxseed, coumestans from *Trifolium pratense* and flavonoids found in a variety of sources are examples of phyto-oestrogens. Sources of phyto-oestrogens are listed in Table 22.1. Although most research has focused on phyto-oestrogenic compounds from soy products, most dietary consumption of these compounds in Western diets occurs from lignans.[23] Different soy products may also vary in their phyto-oestrogenic content: soybeans, tofu and tempeh are good sources, while soy milk is generally not. Studies suggest that *Actaea racemosa* may contain negligible amounts of phyto-oestrogenic compounds while still exerting strong oestrogen modulating ability.[13] This is thought to be related more to its effects on LH. *Vitex agnus-castus* has also shown significant competitive binding to oestrogen receptors in vitro.[12]

The generalisation that all phyto-oestrogens are inherently weaker than endogenous oestrogen is not correct. The herbs *Trifolium pratense* and *Humulus lupulus* actually exert stronger activity in the body than endogenous oestrogen. This may make them therapeutically useful in oestrogen-deficient conditions—those associated with menopause, for example—but may potentially exacerbate symptoms of oestrogen-dependent disorders and render their use inappropriate in high doses in conditions such as endometriosis.[27,28] It is also prudent to avoid herbs known to promote oestrogenic symptoms, such as *Chamaelirium luteum* and *Dioscorea villosa*. Studies suggest that long-term treatment with high-dose phyto-oestrogenic compounds (in excess of 150 mg of soy isoflavones daily for five years) can lead to endometrial hyperplasia.[29] This suggests a role for lower doses associated with modified dietary intake for long-term management. **Cruciferous indoles**, in addition to their activity on oestrogen excretion and conversion, may also directly inhibit stimulation of oestrogen receptors by oestrogen or oestrogen-like compounds,[30,31] though the particular mechanism is unknown at this time.

Promoting oestrogen excretion

Inadequate oestrogen excretion may result in excess circulating oestrogens, sometimes contributing as much as excessive production of endogenous oestrogens. The main route of elimination of excess oestrogens is the liver. The major pathways of elimination are the phase II liver pathways glucuronidation, sulfation and methylation.[32] These pathways bind the used hormones with a water-soluble substance, which can then be eliminated through bile and eventually faeces, as well as via sweat, urine and the lungs. All elimination pathways should be encouraged in naturopathic practice. Liver support is discussed in more detail in Chapter 7, but there are some therapies that specifically support oestrogen excretion.

Cruciferous indoles, such as indole-3-carbinol (I3C) and di-indolyl-methane (DIM), found in brussels sprouts, broccoli, cabbage, garlic and other 'sulfurous' vegetables,[33] are particularly useful for the oestrogen-specific pathways as they induce enzyme reactions that assist with detoxification and conversion of 17β-oestradiol to less active forms (2-hydroxyoestrone as opposed to 16α-hydroxyestrone).[25,26,34–38] Although trials have been largely based on direct supplementation (of 300–400 mg/day of I3C or 100 mg/day of DIM), some studies do suggest food supplementation may also be effective.[26,33,39] Herbs such as ***Silybum marianum*** and ***Bupleurum falcatum*** can also improve liver enzyme activity in regard to oestrogen clearance.[40] ***Rosmarinus officinalis*** has been found to directly increase hepatic metabolism of oestrogens and reduce their uterotropic action in animal studies.[41] **Vitamin B complexes** may increase the inactivation of oestrone in the body.[42] See Chapter 7 on liver disease for further information on detoxification enzyme reactions involving common natural products.

Phase I liver detoxification processes convert oestrogens to either 2-hydroxyoestrone (2OH oestrone), 16- or 4-hydroxyoestrone. 2OH oestrone is a 'cancer-protective' metabolite (oestrogen antagonist) and the latter two are 'pro-carcinogenic' (oestrogen agonists).[43] Each of the enzymes involved are subject to genetic polymorphisms that are measurable in more complex cases. Other factors can also affect this oestrogen conversion (see Figure 22.2).[43]

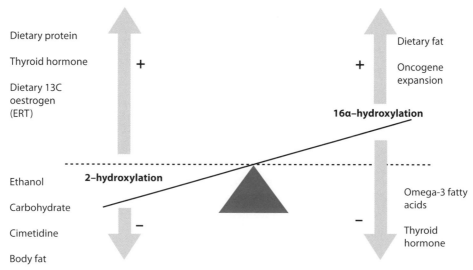

Figure 22.2
Factors affecting oestrogen conversion pathways

The liver is not the only organ associated with oestrogen excretion. The enterohepatic circulatory system will recycle sex hormones if intestinal transit time is sufficiently slow. If there is not enough fibre in the diet, the oestrogens will be recirculated before they are excreted. Increased fibre consumption has been associated with lower oestrogen metabolites.[44] Fibre is also required to increase dioxin, PCB and other oestrogen-like molecules from the body in animal models.[45,46]

The liver in traditional medicine gynaecology

The reproductive section (Chapters 21–24) of the book may seem a strange place to discuss liver pathology, but the liver has long played a key role in gynaecology diagnosis and treatment in traditional medicine. In Western humoral theory most gynaecological complaints were caused by an 'excess of yellow bile' (hot womb—fiery and red menstrual loss) or a deficiency resulted in too little menses and a feeling of coldness or heaviness on the area ('damp'). In traditional Chinese medicine the liver has long been associated with common gynaecological complaints such as premenstrual syndrome (PMS), irregular menses, amenorrhoea, infertility and dysmenorrhoea. Both systems related the mental symptoms often associated with PMS to 'liver disharmony'. These broader concepts have had a great influence on contemporary naturopathic practice. Detoxification of hormones is still a key treatment aim in gynaecological disorders such as PMS, dysmenorrhoea, fibroids and endometriosis.

Regulating inflammation

Inflammatory cytokines

Endometriosis is a chronic inflammatory disease, characterised by altered function of immune-related cells, an increased number of activated macrophages and their secreted products, such as growth factors, cytokines and angiogenic factors in the peritoneal environment.[6,47–54] The presence of inflammatory mediators may actually encourage endometrial tissue ordinarily found in retrograde menstruation to adhere to tissue.[5] Pain reduction is often the most commonly sought treatment. This is thought to be due to underlying excessive cytokine levels.[55]

Endometriosis, irritable bowel syndrome and intestinal permeability

Endometriosis and irritable bowel syndrome (IBS) exhibit markedly similar symptoms and one is, in fact, quite commonly misdiagnosed for the other.[16,56] IBS is often associated with marked increases in inflammatory mediated cytokines IL-6, IL-10 and TNF-α. These inflammatory mediators are associated with altered bowel bacteria.[57] These same cytokines are implicated in encouraging endometrial tissue to adhere to other tissue when in excess amounts in the peritoneal fluid. This is thought to be in some part due to the migration from these cells in dysbiosis (see the 'leaky gut' theory in Chapter 4 on IBS). Positive correlations have been observed between dysbiosis and endometriosis in rhesus monkeys,[58] and successful treatment of IBS with probiotics has been demonstrated to improve endometriosis outcomes.[16]

IL-6, IL-8 and TNF-α appear to be most associated with this phenomenon though others may also play a role. These specific cytokines are also linked to IBS and intestinal dysbiosis (see the box above). One theory is that these cytokines migrate to nearby areas, and in this case encourage endometrial tissue to adhere. High oestrogen levels may exacerbate this role by modulating immune response on macrophages and monocytes through their functional receptors.[59] Higher oestrogen levels have also been associated with increased intestinal permeability and promotion of gram-negative intestinal bacteria.[60] Probiotics, increasing fibre (and in particular the immune-regulating fibres such as fructo-oligosaccharides), anti-inflammatory foods such as fish oils, garlic and ginger, and herbs such as ***Viburnum opulus*** and ***Boswellia serrata*** can also reduce inflammation in endometriosis.[61] Even subclinical inflammation has been associated with progression of endometriosis indicating that even mild anti-inflammatory approaches may prove clinically useful.[62]

Angiogenesis and apoptosis

Excessive endometrial angiogenesis is proposed as an important mechanism in the pathogenesis of endometriosis and is thought to play an underlying role in the proliferation seen in the condition.[63] Nuclear factor-kappa B (NF-κB) is thought to play an integral role in this increased proliferation. In endometriosis cells NF-κB appears to be continuously activated, and suppression of NF-κB activity by NF-κB inhibitors or proteasome inhibitors suppresses proliferation of endometrial cells in vitro.[64] Various inflammatory mediators, growth factors and oxidative stress are thought to be responsible for this activation. **Curcumin** has been demonstrated to reduce angiogenesis and induce apoptosis in endometrial cells in vitro and inactivates NF-κB.[65] Other therapeutic agents specifically indicated to reduce angiogenesis and proliferation—although they have not been specifically studied in endometriosis—include **vitamin D** and foods rich in **flavonoids**, **cruciferous indoles** and **resveratrol** (see the box below).[33,61] Correction of exacerbating factors, particularly inflammatory mediators, may also reduce proliferation.

Vitamin D in endometriosis

Vitamin D analogues, such as danazol, have long been used in the treatment of endometriosis. However, vitamin D itself, and the vitamin D system, is thought to play a role in the immune complex changes observed in endometriosis, and plays a large role in the endometrium.[66,67] The active D_3 form has been described as a potent regulator of cell growth and differentiation in endometriosis.[68] Variations in vitamin D binding protein (DBP) have also been found in patients with endometriosis.[69] It is thought that DBP may influence inflammatory mediators in the body. Only 5% of DBP is actually bound to vitamin D and its metabolites. The remainder has several important functions, including conversion to a powerful macrophage activating factor involved in increasing inflammatory processes in the body. Vitamin D is also associated with increased high-density lipoprotein cholesterol levels,[70] which are associated with reductions in symptoms of endometriosis.[71]

An experimental treatment protocol using aromatase inhibitors given concomitantly with supplemental vitamin D has achieved promising results in the treatment of endometriosis.[72] Research has also demonstrated reduced lesion weight in endometriosis cells with vitamin D.[73]

Some evidence suggests that endometriotic tissue may not have enhanced proliferative abilities, but rather reduced apoptosis.[74–76] Therapeutic interventions that may increase apoptosis, such as ***Curcuma longa***, ***Scutellaria baicalensis***, zinc, selenium and foods rich in a broad range of various phytochemicals (including **flavonoids**, **cruciferous indoles** and **isothiocyanates**), may be useful in treating endometriosis.[33,61]

Prostaglandin regulation

Oestrogen is also reported to increase PGE_2 formation by stimulating cyclooxygenase type 2 (COX-2) enzymes in endometrial stromal cells,[77,78] thereby producing a positive feedback loop for continuous local production of oestrogen and prostaglandins; this favours the proliferative and inflammatory characteristics of endometriosis.

The prostaglandins series 1 and 3 have anti-inflammatory effects that may help patients with endometriosis.

Animal studies have found reduced production levels of inflammatory prostaglandins PGE_2 and $PGF_2\alpha$, and decreased endometrial implant diameter in those animals treated with eicosapentaenoic acid (EPA) and docosahexaenoic acid (DHA) of marine origin.[79] In vitro studies have also found that **omega-3 fatty acids** found in fish oils reduced survival rates of endometrial cells when compared with omega-6, mixed polyunsaturated fats (PUFA) or control groups.[80] Epidemiological data of essential fatty acid consumption in women with endometriosis have shown reduced symptoms with increased consumption.[81,82] However, increased consumption of other inflammatory polyunsaturated fats, particularly of the omega-6 series, was also linked with an increase in symptoms.[83] Exercise, increasing water consumption and eliminating food allergies will also reduce inflammatory mediators.

Addressing endometrial tissue damage

Adhesions

Adhesions increase when women have endometriosis. Vitamin E has been specifically demonstrated to reduce adhesion formation.[84–86] This action is thought to be primarily through reduction of series 2 prostaglandins and better removal of pelvic debris by white blood cells.[87] Italian research has demonstrated a reduction in adhesion weight when treated with **vitamin D** compounds.[77,88] Curcuma longa may reduce the size and activity of adhesions.[89] **Zinc**, *Calendula officinalis* and **vitamin C** are also traditionally used.

Surgery

It is accepted that in specific patients endometriosis can spread directly. The risk of endometrial implantation is increased by surgery, particularly surgery to remove endometrial tissue.[3] This is due to the increase of inflammatory mediators to the area.[6] Reducing inflammation and encouraging appropriate healing responses can reduce the risk of recurring endometrial growths after surgery.

INTEGRATIVE MEDICAL CONSIDERATIONS

Traditional Chinese medicine

Acupuncture may have success in relieving the pain of dysmenorrhoea in endometriosis.[90] In traditional Chinese medicine endometriosis is seen as a disorder of Qi, blood and liver stagnation, an approach that has had documented success in the literature.[91,92] Gui Zhi Fu Ling Wan is indicated to move blood, transform stagnation and remove masses—particularly in lower abdominal areas. Its modern integrated naturopathic application extends to dysmenorrhoea, endometriosis and fibroids (see Chapter 21 on dysmenorrhoea), in particular the emperor herbs *Cinnamomum verum*, *Poria cocos* and *Paeonia lactiflora*.[93] Chinese exercise therapy (**Qi gong**) referral may also be appropriate in this condition. One study of Chinese herbal medicine found it effective in preventing the recurrence of endometrial adhesions after surgery.[94]

Oral contraceptive pill

Hormone supplementation is commonly used in conventional medicine to reduce endometriosis symptoms. Women taking contraceptive agents therapeutically may become deficient in vitamins B2, B3, B5, B12 and folate and may experience raised levels of vitamin A.[61] Hormone use may reduce the effects of *Vitex agnus-castus* and increase the hypertensive side effects associated with *Glycyrrhiza glabra*. Any treatment that aims to increase liver function will reduce the effectiveness of the hormonal drugs.[61]

Specific diets

Although there has been little study into specific diets for endometriosis patients, several guidelines recommend the FODMAPs diet for patients.[95] This is largely due to the success of this diet in IBS, which has a large overlap with endometriosis. One small trial has shown improvement in endometriosis symptoms after 12 months on a gluten-free diet.[96] Dietary intolerances may be a major cause of underlying inflammation and may warrant further examination in endometriosis.

CLINICAL SUMMARY

Although often classified as a single pathology, from a naturopathic perspective it may have a number of underlying causes and possible treatments. These could be inflammatory, hormonal or even unrelated to reproductive system (e.g. the link between IBS and endometriosis). As the end result of longstanding process, endometrial growths can take some time to resolve, and adjunctive and preventive treatment with surgery may be appropriate for quicker symptomatic relief.

Endometriosis shares many properties with autoimmune conditions. Examine the inflammatory status of the patient and do not rely on hormonal modulation alone. Endometriosis is also an oestrogen-dependent condition. Look at the factors that may influence this, including liver function, HPO function and nervous system function.

Endometriosis is a complex condition with many interconnecting systems. It is likely that the condition is multifactorial and a number of treatment approaches are required. Do not fall into the temptation of over-focusing on one factor (such as hormones). Many of these factors have underlying nutritional or lifestyle aetiologies. Do not over-complicate things. Studies suggest that sometimes simple dietary modifications may be enough to significantly improve outcomes.

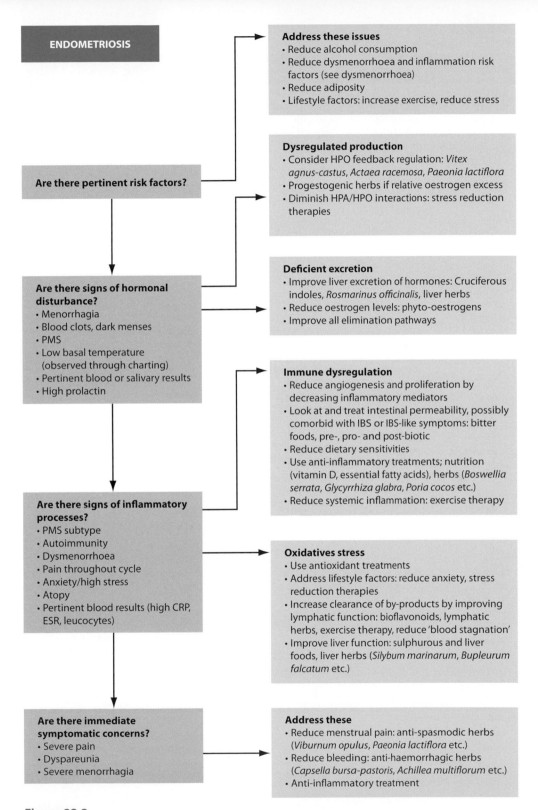

Figure 22.3
Naturopathic treatment decision tree—endometriosis

Table 22.2
Review of the major evidence

Intervention	Mechanisms of action	Key literature	Summary of results	Comment
Antioxidant dietary therapy	Reduction of factors associated with the growth and adhesion of endometrial tissue (via oxidative stress)	RCT: Sesti et al. 2007[97] Six-month study of 222 consecutive women undergoing conservative surgery to remove endometriosis	Post-surgical ingestion of supplement had no significant effect on the recurrence rate of ovarian endometriosis when compared with placebo	Supplement consisted of vitamins (B6, A, C, E), minerals (calcium, magnesium, selenium, zinc, iron), probiotics (of *Bifidobacteria, Lactobacillus* and *Streptococcus* strains) and omega-3 and omega-6 fatty acids
Pycnogenol (an extract of *Pinus pinaster*)	Reduction of factors associated with the growth and adhesion of endometrial tissue (via oxidative stress)	RCT: Kohama et al. 2007[98] 48-week trial of 50 women who had undergone conservative surgery to remove endometriosis	Pycnogenol reduced symptom scores more slowly than conventional GnRHa although recurrence occurred after 28 weeks in GnRHa group CA-125 was reduced though no change was observed in E_2 levels	Patients with smaller endometriomas responded more profoundly than patients with larger endometriomas
Acupuncture	Opioid pathway modulation Other unknown mechanisms	Systematic review: Zhu et al. 2011[90] 24 studies, only one of good methodological quality	Dysmenorrhoea scores were lower by 4.8 points in acupuncture group	Overall most studies included had poor methodology Focused on associated dysmenorrhoea rather than changes on endometrial tissue
Chinese herbal medicine (CHM)	Unknown mechanism, prescribed in accordance with traditional theory	Systematic review: Flower et al. 2012[99] Two RCTs involving 158 women	Both groups displayed improvement in symptom scores Symptomatic relief and pregnancy rate with CHM was not significantly different to gestrinone, but CHM with herbal enema was significantly better than danazol for symptom improvement	Post-surgical administration of CHM may have fewer side effects than conventional medications with equal efficacy

KEY POINTS

- Endometriosis shares many properties with autoimmune conditions. Examine the inflammatory status of the patient and do not rely on hormonal modulation alone.

- Endometriosis is an oestrogen-dependent condition. Look at the factors that may influence this, including liver function, HPO function and nervous system function.

- Endometriosis is a complex condition with many interconnecting systems. It is likely that the condition is multifactorial and a number of treatment approaches are required. Do not fall into the temptation of over-focusing on one factor (such as hormones).

- Many of these factors have underlying nutritional or lifestyle aetiologies. Do not overcomplicate things. Studies suggest that sometimes simple dietary modifications may be enough to significantly improve outcomes.

FURTHER READING

Fjerbaek A, Knudsen UB. Endometriosis, dysmenorrhea and diet—what is the evidence? Eur J Obstet Gynecol Reprod Biol 2007;132(2):140–7.

Hudson T. Women's encyclopedia of natural medicine. New York: McGraw-Hill; 2008.

Trickey R. Women, hormones and the menstrual cycle. Melbourne: MHHG; 2012.

Viganò D, Zara F, Usai P, et al. Irritable bowel syndrome and endometriosis: new insights for old diseases. Dig Liver Dis 2018;50(3):213–322.

Weiss G, et al. Inflammation in reproductive disorders. Reprod Sci 2009;16(2):216–29.

Zhang T, De Carolis C, Gene CWM, et al. The link between immunity, autoimmunity and endometriosis: a literature update. Autoimmun Rev 2018;17:945–55.

REFERENCES

1. Edmonds K, editor. Obstetrics & gynaecology. London: Blackwell; 2007.

2. Mazur W, Adlercreutz H. Naturally occurring estrogens in food. Pure Appl Chem 1998;70:1759–76.

3. Guidice L, Kao L. Endometriosis. Lancet 2004;364(9447):1789–99.

4. Rier S. The potential role of exposure to environmental toxicants in the pathophysiology of endometriosis. Ann N Y Acad Sci 2002;955:201–12.

5. Halme J, White C, Kauma S, et al. Peritoneal macrophages from patients with endometriosis release growth factor activity in vitro. J Clin Endocrinol Metab 1988;66: 1044–9.

6. Eisenberg VH, Zolti M, Soriano D. Is there an association between autoimmunity and endometriosis? Autoimmun Rev 2012;11(11):806–14.

7. Martin J, Hauck A. Endometriosis in the male American Surgeon. Am Surg 1985;51(7):426–30.

8. Schrodt G, Alcorn M, Ibanez J. Endometriosis of the male urinary system: a case report. J Urol 1980;124(5):722–3.

9. Westerlind K, Williams N. Effect of energy deficiency on estrogen metabolism in premenopausal women. Med Sci Sports Exerc 2007;39(7):1090–7.

10. Missmer S, Hankinson S, Spiegelman D, et al. Incidence of laparoscopically confirmed endometriosis by demographic, anthropometric, and lifestyle factors. Am J Epidemiol 2004;160(8):784–96.

11. Wake D, Elferink C, Rask E, et al. Increased aromatase expression in human subcutaneous adipose tissue in obesity. Endocr Abstr 2004;7:60.

12. Wuttke W, Jarry H, Christoffel V, et al. Chaste tree (Vitex agnus-castus) pharmacology and clinical indications. Phytomedicine 2003;10(4):348–57.

13. Seidlova-Wuttke D. Evidence for selective estrogen receptor modulator activity in a black Cohosh (Cimicifuga racemosa) extract: comparison with estradiol-17 beta. Eur J Endocrinol 2003;149:351–62.

14. Lea R, Whorwell P. Irritable bowel syndrome or endometriosis, or both? Eur J Gastroenterol Hepatol 2003;15(10):1131–3.

15. Noble L, Takayama K, Zeitoun K, et al. Prostaglandin E2 stimulates aromatase expression in endometriosis-derived stromal cells. J Clin Endocrinol Metab 1997;82:600–6.

16. Bukulmez O, Hardy D, Carr B, et al. Inflammatory status influences aromatase and steroid receptor expression in endometriosis. Endocrinology 2008;149(3): 1190–204.

17. Simpson E, Clyne C, Rubin G, et al. Aromatase—a brief overview. Annu Rev Physiol 2002;64:93–127.

18. Brooks J, Thompson L. Mammalian lignans and genistein decrease the activities of aromatase and 17beta-hydroxysteroid dehydrogenase in MCF-7 cells. J Steroid Biochem Mol Biol 2005;94(5):461–7.

19. Birnbaum L, Cummings A. Dioxins and endometriosis: a plausible hypothesis. Environ Health Perspect 2002;110(1):15–21.

20. Foster W, Agarwhal S. Environmental contaminants and dietary factors in endometriosis. Ann N Y Acad Sci 2002;955:213–29.

21. Tsutumi O. Assessment of human contamination of estrogenic endocrine-disrupting chemicals and their risk for human reproduction. J Steroid Biochem Mol Biol 2005;93(2–5):325–30.

22. Wang L. Mammalian phytoestrogens: enterodiol and enterolactone. J Chromatogr B Analyt Technol Biomed Life Sci 2002;777(1–2):289–309.

23. Valsta L, Kilkkinen A, Mazur W. Phyto-oestrogen database of foods and average intake in Finland. Br J Nutr 2003;89:S31–8.

24. Petterson H, Kiessling K. Liquid chromatographic determination of the plant estrogens coumestrol and isoflavones in animal feed. J Assoc Off Anal Chem 1984;67(3):503–6.

25. Dalessandri K, Firestone G, Fitch M, et al. Pilot Study: effect of 3,3'-diindolyl-methane supplements on urinary hormone metabolites in postmenopausal women with a history of early stage breast cancer. Nutr Cancer 2004;50(2):161–7.

26. McAlindon T, Gulin J, Chen T, et al. Indole-3-carbinol in women with SLE: effect on estrogen metabolism and disease activity. Lupus 2001;10(11):779–83.

27. Beck V, Unterrieder E, Krenn L, et al. Comparison of hormonal activity (estrogen, androgen and progestin) of standardized plant extracts for large scale use in hormone replacement therapy. J Steroid Biochem Mol Biol 2003;84(2–3):259–68.

28. Zava D, Dollbaum C, Blen M. Estrogen and progestin bioactivity of foods, herbs, and spices. Proc Soc Exp Biol Med 1998;217(3):369–78.

29. Unfer V, Casini M, Costabile L, et al. Endometrial effects of long-term treatment with phytoestrogens: a randomized, double-blind, placebo-controlled study. Fertil Steril 2004;82:145–8.

30. Ashok B, Chen Y, Liu X, et al. Abrogation of oestrogen-mediated cellular and biochemical effects by indole-3-carbinol. Nutr Cancer 2001;41(1–2):180–7.

31. Meng Q, Yuan F, Goldberg I, et al. Indole-3-carbinol is a negative regulator of estrogen receptor-alpha signalling in human tumour cells. J Nutr 2000;130(12):2927–31.

32. Voet D. Biochemistry. 3rd ed. New York: Wiley & Sons; 2004.

33. Higdon J. An evidence-based approach to dietary phytochemicals. Stuttgart: Thieme; 2007.

34. Bradlow H, Michnovicz J, Halper M, et al. Long-term responses of women to indole-3-carbinol or a high fibre diet. Cancer Epidemiol Biomarkers Prev 1994;3(7):591–5.

35. Michnovicz J. Increased estrogen 2-hydroxylation in obese women using oral indole-3-carbinol. Int J Obes Relat Metab Disord 1998;22(3):227–9.

36. Michnovicz J, Adlercreutz H, Bradlow H. Changes in levels of urinary estrogen metabolites after oral indole-3-carbinol treatment in humans. J Natl Cancer Inst 1997;89(10):718–23.

37. Michnovicz J, Bradlow H. Altered oestrogen metabolism and excretion in humans following consumption of indoile-3-carbinol. Nutr Cancer 1991;16:59–66.

38. Wong G, Bradlow L, Sepkovic D, et al. Dose-ranging study of indole-3-carbinol for breast cancer prevention. J Cell Biochem Suppl 1997;28–29(Suppl. 1):S111–16.

39. Parrazini F, Chiaffarino F, Surace M, et al. Selected food intake and risk of endometriosis. Hum Reprod 2004;19(8):1755–9.

40. Morazzoni P, Bombardelli E. Silybum marianum (Carduus marianus). Fitoterapia 1995;66:3–42.

41. Zhu B, Loder D, Cai M, et al. Dietary administration of an extract from rosemary leaves enhances the liver microsomal metabolism of endogenous estrogens and decreases their uterotropic action in CD-1 mice. Carcinogenesis 1998;19(10):1821–7.

42. Zondek B, Finkerlstein M. Effect of Vitamin B Complex on inactivation of estrone in vivo and in vitro. Science 1947;105(2723):259–60.

43. Sepkovic D, Bradlow H. Estrogen hydroxylation—the good and the bad. Ann N Y Acad Sci 2009;1155:57–67.

44. Thompson L, Boucher B, Lui Z, et al. Phytoestrogen content of foods consumed in Canada, including isoflavones, lignans and coumestan. Nutr Cancer 2006;54(2):184–201.

45. Kimura Y, Nagata Y, Buddington R. Some dietary fibers increase elimination of orally administered polychlorinated biphenyls but not that of retinol in mice. J Nutr 2004;134:135–42.

46. Aozasa O, Ohta S, Nakao T, et al. Enhancement in fecal excretion of dioxin isomer in mice by several dietary fibers. Chemosphere 2001;45(2):195–200.

47. Braun D, Gebel H, House R, et al. Spontaneous and induced synthesis of cytokines by peripheral blood monocytes in patients with endometriosis. Fertil Steril 1996;65:1125–9.

48. Bullimore D. Endometriosis is sustained by tumour necrosis factor α. Med Hypotheses 2003;60:84–8.

49. Gurgan T, Bukulmez O, Yarali H, et al. Serum and peritoneal fluid levels of IGF I and II and insulinlike growth binding protein-3 in endometriosis. J Reprod Med 1999;44:450–4.

50. Kim J, Suh C, Kim S, et al. Insulin-like growth factors (IGFs), IGF-binding proteins (IGFBPs), and IGFBP-3 protease activity in the peritoneal fluid of patients with and without endometriosis. Fertil Steril 2000;73:996–1000.

51. Koninckx P, Kennedy S, Barlow D. Endometriotic disease: the role of peritoneal fluid. Hum Reprod Update 1998;4:741–51.

52. Punnonen J, Teisala K, Ranta H, et al. Increased levels of interleukin-6 and interleukin-10 in the peritoneal fluid of patients with endometriosis. Am J Obstet Gynecol 1996;174:1522–6.

53. Rana N, Braun D, House R, et al. Basal and stimulated secretion of cytokines by peritoneal macrophages in women with endometriosis. Fertil Steril 1996;65:925–30.

54. Richter O, Mallmann P, van der Ven H, et al. TNF-α secretion by peritoneal macrophages in endometriosis. Zentralbl Gynakol 1998;120:332–6.

55. Thomson J, Redwine D. Chronic pelvic pain associated with autoimmunity and systemic and peritoneal inflammation and treatment with immune modification. J Reprod Med 2005;50:745–58.

56. Viganò D, Zara F, Usai P, et al. Irritable bowel syndrome and endometriosis: new insights for old diseases. Dig Liver Dis 2018;50(3):213–322.

57. Tamboli C, Neut C, et al. Dysbiosis in inflammatory bowel disease. Gut 2004;53(1):1–4.

58. Bailey M, Coe C. Endometriosis is associated with an altered profile of intestinal microflora in female rhesus monkeys. Hum Reprod 2002;17(7):1704–8.

59. Capellino S, Montagna P, Villaggio B, et al. Role of estrogens in inflammatory response: expression of estrogen receptors in peritoneal fluid macrophages from endometriosis. Ann N Y Acad Sci 2006;1069:263–7.

60. Enomoto N, Ikejima K, Bradford B, et al. Role of Kupffer cells and gut-derived endotoxins in alcoholic liver injury. J Gastroenterol Hepatol 2000;15:S20–5.

61. Braun L, Cohen M. Herbs and Natural Supplements: an evidence based guide. 3rd ed. Melbourne: Churchill Livingstone; 2010.

62. Agic A, Xu H, Finas D, et al. Is endometriosis associated with systemic subclinical inflammation? Gynecol Obstet Invest 2006;62:139–47.

63. Healy DL, et al. Angiogenesis: a new theory for endometriosis. Hum Reprod Update 1998;4(5):736–40.

64. Guo S. Nuclear factor-κB (NF-κB): an unsuspected major culprit in the pathogenesis of endometriosis that is still at large? Gynecol Obstet Invest 2007;63(2):71–97.

65. Wieser F, Yu J, Park J, et al. Curcumin suppresses angiogenesis, cell proliferation and induces apoptosis in

an in vitro model of endometriosis [Poster]. Fertil Steril 2007;88:S204–5.

66. Vigano P, Lattuada D, Mangioni S, et al. Cycling and early pregnant endometrium as a site of regulated expression of the vitamin D system. J Mol Endocrinol 2006;36(3):415–24.

67. Cermisoni G, Alteri A, Corti L, et al. Vitamin D and endometrium: a systematic review of a neglected area of research. Int J Mol Sci 2018;19(8):2320.

68. Agic A, Xu H, Altgassen C, et al. Relative expression of 1,25-dihydroxyvitamin D3 receptor, vitamin D 1 alpha-hydroxylase, vitamin D 24-hydroxylase, and vitamin D 25-hydroxylase in endometriosis and gynecologic cancers. Reprod Sci 2007;14(5):486–97.

69. Ferroro S, Gillot D, Anserini P, et al. Vitamin D binding protein in endometriosis. J Soc Gynecol Investig 2005;12(4):272–7.

70. Moyad M. The potential benefits of dietary and/or supplemental calcium and vitamin D. Urol Oncol 2003;21(5):384–91.

71. Choktanasiri W, Boonkasemsanti W, Sittisomwong T, et al. Long-acting triptorelin for the treatment of endometriosis. Int J Gynaecol Obstet 1996;54(3):237–43.

72. Ailawadi R, Jobanputra S, Kataria M, et al. Treatment of endometriosis and chronic pelvic pain with letrozole and norethindrone acetate: a pilot study. Fertil Steril 2004;81(2):290–6.

73. Panina P, inventor Bioxil SpA & Panina, P, assignee. Use of Vitamin D compounds to treat endometriosis. Italy: 2006.

74. Beliard A, Noel A, Foidart J. Reduction of apoptosis and proliferation in endometriosis. Fertil Steril 2004;82:80–5.

75. Gebel H, Braun D, Tambur A, et al. Spontaneous apoptosis of endometrial tissue is impaired in women with endometriosis. Fertil Steril 1998;69:1042–7.

76. Scotti S, Regidor P, Schindler A, et al. Reduced proliferation and cell adhesion in endometriosis. Mol Hum Reprod 2000;6:610–17.

77. Kluft C, Gevers-Leuven J, Helmerhorst F, et al. Pro-inflammatory effects of oestrogens during use of oral contraceptives and hormone replacement treatment. Vascul Pharmacol 2002;39(3):149–54.

78. Tamura M, Deb S, Sebastian S, et al. Estrogen up-regulates cyclooxygenase-2 via estrogen receptor in human uterine microvascular endothelial cells. Fertil Steril 2004;81(5):1351–6.

79. Covens A, Christopher P, Casper R. The effect of dietary supplementation with fish oil on surgically-induced endometriosis in rabbits. Fertil Steril 1988;49(4):698–703.

80. Gazvani M, Smith L, Haggarty P, et al. High w-3:w-6 fatty acids ratios in culture medium reduce endometrial-cell survival in combined endometrial gland and stromal cell cultures from women with and without endometriosis. Fertil Steril 2001;76(4):717–22.

81. Fjerbaek A, Knudsen U. Endometriosis, dysmenorrhea and diet–what is the evidence? Eur J Obstet Gynecol Reprod Biol 2007;132(2):140–7.

82. Missmer S, Chavarro J, Malspeis S, et al. A prospective study of dietary fat consumption and endometriosis risk. Hum Reprod 2010;25(6):1528–35.

83. Britton J, Westhoff C, Howe G, et al. Diet and benign ovarian tumours (United States). Cancer Causes Control 2000;11(5):389–401.

84. Hemedah O, Chilikuri S, Bonet V. Prevention of adhesions by administration of sodium carboxymethyl cellulose and Vitamin E. Surgery 1993;114(5):907–10.

85. Kagoma P, Burger S, Seifter N. The effect of vitamin E on experimentally induced peritoneal adhesions in mice. Arch Surg 1985;120(8):949–51.

86. Kalferentzos F, Spiliotis J, Kaklamanis L. Prevention of peritoneal adhesion formation in mice by Vitamin E. J R Coll Surg Edinb 1987;32(5):288–90.

87. Meydani M. Vitamin E. Lancet 1995;345(8943):170–5.

88. Perez-Fernandez R, Seoane S, Garcia-Caballero T, et al. Vitamin D, Pit-1, GH, and PRL: possible roles in breast cancer development. Curr Med Chem 2007;14(29):3051–8.

89. Arablou T, Kolahdouz-Mohammadi R. Curcumin and endometriosis: review on potential roles and molecular mechanisms. Biomed Pharmacother 2018;97:91–7.

90. Zhu X, Hamilton K, McNicol E. Acupuncture for pain in endometriosis. Cochrane Database Syst Rev 2011;(9):CD007864.

91. Li J, Zheng J, Wang D. [Clinical observation on treatment of endometriosis by tonifying qi and promoting blood circulation to remove stasis and purgation principle] article in Chinese. Zhongguo Zhong Xi Yi Jie He Za Zhi 1999;19(9):533–5.

92. Wang R, Zhou L. [Clinical observation on treatment of endometriosis with principle of activating blood circulation to remove stasis]. [Chinese]. Zhongguo Zhong Xi Yi Jie He Za Zhi 2004;24(3):258–9.

93. Shan J, Cheng W, Zhai DX, et al. Meta-analysis of Chinese traditional medicine bushen huoxue prescription for endometriosis treatment. Evid Based Complement Alternat Med 2017;5416423.

94. Zhao R, Hao Z, Zhang Y, et al. Controlling the recurrence of pelvic endometriosis after a conservative operation: comparison between Chinese herbal medicine and western medicine. Chin J Integr Med 2013;19(11):820–5.

95. Jacobson T. Potential cures for endometriosis. Ann N Y Acad Sci 2011;1221:70–4.

96. Marziali M, Venza M, Lazzaro S, et al. Gluten-free diet: a new strategy for management of painful endometriosis related symptoms? Minerva Chir 2012;67(6):499–504.

97. Sesti F, Pietropolli A, Capozzolo T, et al. Hormonal suppression treatment or dietary therapy versus placebo in the control of painful symptoms after conservative surgery for endometriosis stage III-IV. A randomized comparative trial. Fertil Steril 2007;88(6):1541–7.

98. Kohama T, Herai K, Inoue M. Effect of French maritime pine bark extract on endometriosis as compared with leuprorelin acetate. J Reprod Med 2007;52(8):703–8.

99. Flower A, Liu J, Lewith G, et al. Chinese herbal medicine for endometriosis. Cochrane Database Syst Rev 2012;(5):CD006568.

CHAPTER 23

Polycystic ovarian syndrome

Jon Wardle
ND, MPH, PhD

OVERVIEW

Polycystic ovarian syndrome (PCOS) is a term used to describe a constellation of clinical and biochemical features. For many of these the aetiology remains poorly understood. Several factors also preclude difficulties in diagnosis of PCOS. PCOS is not a single disease, but a symptom that can include a heterogeneous range of symptoms that can change over time and the lack of a precise and uniform consensus on diagnosis. In fact, PCOS as a term does not always accurately represent the clinical picture experienced by patients, and for this reason there are increasing calls to develop a more accurate diagnostic term, though lack of consensus on replacement terms means PCOS is likely to remain current for some time.[1]

In 2003 a consensus workshop indicated PCOS to be present if two out of three criteria are met: oligo-ovulation and/or anovulation; excess androgen activity (as determined by elevated free androgen index); and polycystic ovaries (by gynaecological ultrasound). In 2006, the Androgen Excess PCOS Society suggested a tightening of the diagnostic criteria to all of the following: excess androgen activity; oligoovulation/anovulation and/or polycystic ovaries; and exclusion of other entities (e.g. hyperprolactinaemia) that would cause excess androgen activity.[2] Elevated fasting insulin or high insulin levels in glucose tolerance tests may also be used to suggest diagnosis. Other blood tests may be suggestive but not diagnostic—for example, if the luteinising hormone (LH) to follicle-stimulating hormone (FSH) ratio is greater than 1:1, or if there are low levels of sex-hormone binding globulin. The presence of ovarian cysts does not automatically imply a diagnosis of PCOS. The prevalence of PCOS is thought to be 5–10% of women and is one of the main causes of infertility in Western women.[3,4]

The symptoms of PCOS usually appear upon menarche, and are associated with early puberty brought about by early secretion of androgens.[5] This may also be associated with low birthweight. However, the condition can develop a considerable time after menarche in the presence of other environmental factors such as weight gain and subsequent insulin resistance.

Increased ovarian androgen biosynthesis in the PCOS results from abnormalities at all levels of the hypothalamic–pituitary–ovarian (HPO) axis. Androgen excess in women with PCOS may be of either ovarian or adrenal origin. It is also thought that insulin may induce overactivity of 11b-hydroxysteroid dehydrogenase, resulting in excessive adrenal androgen production.[6] Androgens may be converted to oestrone in fatty tissue, causing blood oestrone and ultimately stimulating LH production, which triggers ovarian androgen production. Increased frequency of LH pulses in PCOS may result from an increased frequency of hypothalamic gonadotrophin-releasing hormone (GnRH) pulses, resulting in higher production of LH compared with FSH. The increase in pituitary secretion of LH can lead to an increase in androgen production by ovarian theca cells. Increased efficiency in the conversion of androgenic precursors in theca cells leads to enhanced production of androstenedione, which can then be converted by 17-beta-hydroxysteroid dehydrogenase (17β-OHSD) to form testosterone or aromatised by the aromatase enzyme to form oestrone, which can be further converted to oestradiol by 17β-OHSD (Figure 23.1).[6]

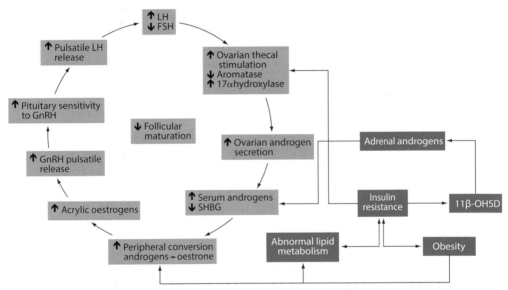

Figure 23.1
Hormonal interactions in PCOS

SHBG = sex hormone-binding globulin, LH = luteinising hormone, FSH = follicle-stimulating hormone, GnRH = gonadotrophin-releasing hormone, 11β-OHSD = 11β-hydroxysteroid dehydrogenase

Insulin acts synergistically with LH to enhance androgen production. Insulin also inhibits hepatic synthesis of sex hormone-binding globulin (which ordinarily binds to testosterone) and therefore increases the proportion of testosterone that is biologically available. Testosterone inhibits and oestrogen stimulates hepatic synthesis of sex hormone-binding globulin.[6]

Polycystic ovaries in PCOS develop when the ovaries are stimulated to produce excessive amounts of androgens—particularly testosterone—through the release of excessive LH by the anterior pituitary gland or through high levels of insulin in the blood.[7] This causes the follicle to begin maturation but the lack of LH surge results in anovulation, meaning the ovum does not release, and ultimately a cyst is formed (Figure 23.2).

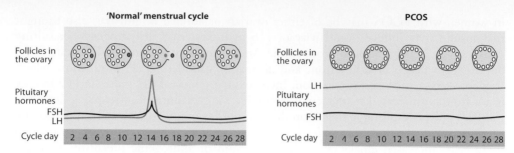

Figure 23.2
Hormonal and reproductive changes in PCOS compared with normal menstruation

DIFFERENTIAL DIAGNOSIS

- Environmental disruptions
- Hyperprolactinaemia
- Cushing's syndrome

- Thyroid disorders
- Amenorrhoea
- Ovarian tumours

RISK FACTORS

A majority of, though not all, patients in Western settings with PCOS have insulin resistance and are often overweight.[8] Elevated insulin levels contribute to or cause the abnormalities seen in the HPO axis that lead to PCOS. Hyperinsulinaemia may increase GnRH pulse frequency, LH dominance over FSH, increased ovarian androgen production, decreased follicular maturation and decreased sex hormone-binding globulin (SHBG) binding—all of which can lead to the development of PCOS.[6] Insulin resistance is a common finding among patients of normal weight as well as overweight patients.

It is easy to view a typical PCOS patient with insulin hypersensitivity as the conventional overweight type. However, insulin resistance is also common in lean women with PCOS.[9] It is also easy to view PCOS as a primarily androgen-dependent disorder; however, oestrogen dominance is also commonly present in women with PCOS. Although weight loss is generally associated with good clinical effect and being overweight is common in women with PCOS, it should never be assumed that women with PCOS will always be overweight. This trend should be noted to prevent misdiagnosing the condition in women who are not overweight.

Thyroid problems may make PCOS symptoms worse[10] and women with PCOS also have a high prevalence of autoimmune thyroid conditions.[11] Thyroid function should therefore also be checked in patients with PCOS (see Chapter 20 on thyroid abnormalities).

Liver support may also be required in women with PCOS. Approximately 30% of women with PCOS have raised liver enzymes, and diabetes and insulin resistance also increase the risk of non-alcoholic liver disease.[12,13] Hyperinsulinaemia may inhibit the production of SHBG in the liver.

The presence of higher levels of inflammatory mediators has been observed in women with PCOS.[14] The presence of low-grade inflammation is hypothesised to damage hormone receptors, suppress ovulation, stimulate androgen production and exacerbate insulin resistance, though this link does remain controversial.[15]

CONVENTIONAL TREATMENT

Due to the functional nature of diagnosis, conventional treatment in PCOS is generally focused on a number of goals including: reducing hyperinsulinaemia; restoring normal menstruation, reproductive function and fertility; and reducing associated symptoms such as hirsutism.[7]

Weight reduction and exercise are generally seen as first-line treatments in managing PCOS. Primary treatment of insulin resistance with metformin or thiazolidinediones is used if the former interventions have had little success.

Anovulation can be treated with ovulation-induction drugs such as clomiphene, bromocriptine, gonadotrophin or GnRH. This treatment has a relatively high risk profile and most often reserved to force ovulation when the patient is trying to conceive. When conception is still not achieved assisted reproductive techniques such as in vitro fertilisation are commonly recommended.

Exclude pregnancy

It is always important to exclude pregnancy in women of any age presenting with amenorrhoea. It is not unknown in clinical practice to see a patient who has unknowingly become pregnant, despite denying the possibility, or in someone who has previously been labelled 'infertile'.

The treatment of hirsutism and acne in PCOS generally focuses on reducing androgen levels. Electrolysis, as well as more temporary measures such as waxing and bleaching, is recommended for hirsutism.

If pregnancy is desired, assisted reproductive techniques, including radical drug therapy with clomiphene or a similar agent, or in vitro fertilisation techniques, are also commonly prescribed (see Chapter 34 on fertility).[7]

DIAGNOSTIC TEMPERATURE CHARTING

Due to the often significant timeframes encountered when treating patients with PCOS (or other gynaecological disorders), tools such as charting may be employed to observe hormonal status changes over time. Menstrual cycle charting based on basal body temperature (BBT) has been traditionally used in naturopathic practice to ascertain changes in hormone levels in women of reproductive age (Figure 23.3). It is thought to reflect the menstrual cycle in two ways: within two days before LH surge there should be a low point in BBT; and following ovulation women should generally see a sustained increase in BBT of between 0.2 and 0.5°C.[16] This rise is most likely due to the thermogenic effect of a metabolite of progesterone.

There has been some contention as to the effectiveness of BBT charting in pregnancy outcomes; however, its use in naturopathy has been extended more broadly to the menstrual cycle in general.

It should be noted that focusing on individual components of charting is very often inadequate.[16] However, when integrated they can form a useful clinical tool that provides a broad overview of reproductive function and actively involves patients in their treatment. Despite the fact that more specific and accurate investigations currently exist, charting may still have a role to play in clinical practice because it is inexpensive,

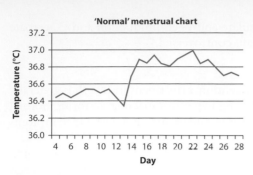
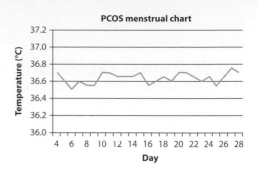

Figure 23.3
'Normal' versus PCOS menstrual charts

The 'normal' chart (left) shows a concordance in temperature with expected levels of progesterone and an immediate strong rise in temperature, giving a strong indication of ovulation. The PCOS chart (right) shows an anovular cycle with no pattern differentiating follicular and luteal phases. Mucus changes may be evident in this case and may represent follicular activity and surges in oestrogen that do not result in ovulation.

non-invasive and generally reliable. It also actively involves the patient in the therapeutic and diagnostic process. However, interpretation can be subjective and difficult and in more complex cases other investigative techniques may be more appropriate (see Chapter 2 for other diagnostic techniques).

Temperature should be taken (sublingually) immediately upon rising. Several factors—including alcohol consumption the night before, restless sleep, variations in waking time and illness—may affect temperature and should be noted on the chart.

Sustained temperature rise shows the most likely day of ovulation (the actual rise begins 12 hours before ovulation during the LH surge).

Consistently low temperature (under 36.5°C) may indicate a hypothyroid condition, which may play a role in poor reproductive function (see Chapter 20 on thyroid abnormalities).

Progesterone

Adequate progesterone levels will result in a sustained, noticeable and prompt rise in BBT. A small or unsustained rise with dips in temperature will be indicative of poor progesterone levels. However, temperature levels alone do not confirm appropriate levels of progesterone. The luteal phase needs to be at least 11 days to indicate adequate progesterone levels. Progesterone levels need to peak approximately seven days after ovulation to ensure adequate uterine lining for implantation.

Follicular phase length

Long or short follicular phase length (less than 11 days) is indicative of oestrogen imbalances. In short follicular phases this may be further compounded by effects on the corpus luteum, resulting in inadequate progesterone production.

Mucus

Ovarian follicular activity combined with surges in oestrogen that do not result in ovulation are a common occurrence in PCOS. Mucus changes may be evident in these women.

KEY TREATMENT PROTOCOLS

There is emerging evidence that naturopathic treatment approaches to PCOS are successful. For example, an Australian trial using combination herbal medicines in conjunction with lifestyle advice from a naturopath significantly improved BMI, insulin and LH levels, reduced the incidence of oligomenorrhoea by 32% and saw improvements in quality of life and depression and anxiety scores in women with PCOS.[17] While such

> **Naturopathic Treatment Aims**
>
> - Reduce underlying issues such as overweight or insulin resistance.
> - Reduce androgen excess.
> - Regulate and balance hormones more generally.
> - Promote ovulation.
> - Reduce inflammation.
> - Encourage lifestyle changes.

emerging evidence shows that naturopathic care overall seems to be effective in PCOS, other naturopathic treatments are also known to have specific effects in the management of PCOS.[17]

Follicle-stimulating hormone and luteinising hormone regulation

The management of insulin resistance, particularly via diet and lifestyle changes, should be prioritised above pharmacological management. However, some herbal medicines may affect levels of FSH and LH and may therefore proffer some benefit in the treatment of PCOS. Despite its status as a phyto-estrogen, *Actaea racemosa* does not seem to affect the release of prolactin and FSH, though it does reduce LH, in the limited research currently conducted.[18] This central effect is thought to be due to its role on dopaminergic regulation of reproductive hormones rather than its effects on oestrogen receptors.[18,19] This is also supported by traditional use: the *British Herbal Pharmacopeia* lists *Actaea racemosa*'s main actions as being useful in ovarian dysfunction and ovarian insufficiency.[20]

Vitex agnus-castus has had conflicting results, with some studies showing no change in FSH or LH, and another suggesting increased LH release,[21–23] though no studies have focused specifically on women with PCOS. Its use may actually worsen PCOS, and its use may be more suited to conditions such as hypothalamic amenorrhoea instead. *Vitex agnus-castus* is thought to have antiandrogenic properties. However, as an HPO-regulating agent *Vitex agnus-castus* may be useful for treating PCOS patients, who often have altered responses to progesterone[24] or elevated levels of prolactin.[25] *Humulus lupulus* also reduces LH with continued use and may therefore be useful to reduce androgens in PCOS.[26] A review of **soy** studies suggests that soy consumption has no effect on FSH or thyroid-stimulating hormone (TSH).[27]

Unpublished (though publicly available) data suggest that supplementation with the herb *Tribulus terrestris* for three months may normalise ovulation and result in pregnancy in women with endocrine infertility.[28] *Mentha spicata* (via tea therapy— two cups per day for five days) use has been associated with increases in LH, FSH and oestrogen levels in women with PCOS.[29]

Glycyrrhiza glabra is a commonly used herb in the treatment of PCOS. Though trials for its stand-alone treatment in PCOS are lacking, there exists a theoretical basis behind its use. *Glycyrrhiza glabra* has been demonstrated to reduce testosterone levels in healthy women.[30] Various forms of *Glycyrrhiza* spp. have been used in a combination product (as the key ingredient with *Paeonia lactiflora*) to treat PCOS in some small trials that showed reduction in FSH:LH ratio, ovarian testosterone production and improvements in ovulation.[31,32] However, the situation in the combination product has been confused further by the fact that while this research has focused on *Glycyrrhiza uralensis*, clinical application is still dominated by *Glycyrrhiza glabra*. The clinical effects of these minor differences are unknown. *Glycyrrhiza* spp. may also exert further potent phyto-oestrogenic activity independent of these effects.[33] *Glycyrrhiza glabra* is also demonstrated to reduce body fat mass in normal weight subjects.[34] A *Paeonia lactiflora* and *Glycyrrhiza glabra* combination has been found to have numerous effects on PCOS, including regulating FSH:LH ratios (possibly through stimulation of pituitary dopamine receptors),[31] lowering testosterone levels and improving oestradiol to testosterone ratios.[32,35]

Exogenous **melatonin** has been demonstrated to enhance LH secretion, LH pulse amplitude and LH sensitivity to GnRH.[36–39] This was thought to be the result of melatonin supplementation mimicking the effects of PCOS—possibly due to the effects of melatonin on increasing cortisol levels. This effect is known to increase in hypo-oestrogenic states.[39] However, while most studies have been in postmenopausal or older women, melatonin supplementation in younger women has been associated with return to menstrual regularity, as well as the reduction of LH levels in younger women with high baseline levels, in clinical settings.[40,41] This has led to calls for a possible role of melatonin in the treatment of PCOS and, despite its popularity in some streams of naturopathic medicine, it remains unclear at this stage what role it may play; further research is required.[42] Other factors known to affect melatonin levels should also be considered (see Chapter 16 on insomnia).

Other factors may also affect LH levels. Various human studies have suggested that inadequate nutrition or short periods of fasting reduces LH pulsing, though not always LH levels.[43–45] This is thought to be due to relative increases in cortisol caused by these states.[46] Animal studies seem to suggest that increased endotoxin load can reduce plasma LH levels.[47]

HPO and hypothalamic–pituitary–adrenal (HPA) axis interaction

It is well known that women with PCOS exhibit abnormalities in cortisol metabolism as well as higher levels than controls.[48] It is also known that a return to states of normal cortisol from high cortisol levels in women with amenorrhoea or menstrual disturbances often precedes the resumption of normal ovarian activity.[49] These findings further support the role for stress reduction in regulating LH and FSH function in the treatment of reproductive disorders such as PCOS.

The reproductive axis is inhibited at all levels by various components of the HPA axis. Corticotrophin-releasing hormone (CRH) can either directly or indirectly (through β-endorphin) suppress gonadotrophin-releasing hormone. Glucocorticoids may also exert inhibitory effects by rendering target tissues resistant to reproductive hormones, inhibiting GnRH and LH secretion and inhibiting ovarian oestrogen and progesterone biosynthesis.[6] The effects of the HPA axis interaction with the female reproductive system can result in idiopathic or hypothalamic amenorrhoea (e.g. that associated with stress, depression, anxiety or eating disorders) in its own right, or result in the hypogonadism associated with Cushing's syndrome,[6] though it may also result in further indirect complication of other disorders of hormonal dysregulation like PCOS.

However, these interactions can also be bidirectional (Figure 23.4). CRH, for example, is regulated to some extent in reproductive tissue by oestrogen. CRH is responsible for a number of functions in reproductive tissue (Table 23.1) and disorders; events (such as

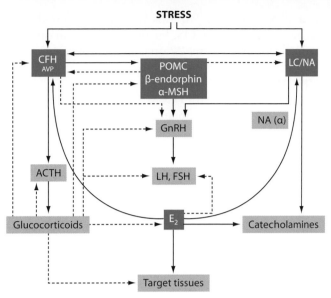

Figure 23.4
Interactions of the HPO and HPA axis

CRH = corticotrophin-releasing hormone; GnRH = gonadotrophin-releasing hormone; LH = luteinising hormone; E_2 = ovarian oestradiol; α-MSH = melanocyte-stimulating hormone; ACTH = adrenocorticotrophic hormone; AVP = arginine-vasopressin; FSH = follicle stimulating hormone; NA (α) = norepinephrine stimulation via α-noradrenergic receptors; POMC = proopiomelanocortin; solid line = stimulation; dotted line = inhibition; LC = locus coeruleus

Table 23.1
Reproductive corticotrophin-releasing hormone, potential physiological roles and potential pathogenic effects

Reproductive CRH	Potential physiological roles	Potential pathogenic effects
Ovarian CRH	Follicular maturation Ovulation Luteolysis Suppression of female sex steroid production	Premature ovarian failure (↑ secretion) Anovulation (↓ secretion) Corpus luteum dysfunction (↓ secretion) Ovarian dysfunction (↓ secretion)
Uterine CRH	Decidualisation	Infertility (↓ secretion)
	Blastocyst implantation	Recurrent spontaneous abortion (↓ secretion)
	Early maternal tolerance	
Placental CRH	Labour	Premature labour (↑ secretion)
	Maternal hypercortisolism Fetoplacental circulation Fetal adrenal steroidogenesis	Delayed labour (↓ secretion) Pre-eclampsia and eclampsia (↑ secretion)

Source: van der Spuy 2004[50]

chronic stress adaptation) that affect these levels may also have clinically relevant effects on reproductive function. Due to this bidirectional activity, a multifaceted approach to disorders, focusing on regulation of both reproductive and adrenal hormones, may be more successful in conditions such as PCOS rather than targeting one system alone, particularly considering PCOS may often be a disorder of oestrogen excess (via adipose tissue) as well as androgen excess. For this reason, generalised hormone-balancing protocols may also be beneficial in PCOS. Further information on balancing reproductive hormones can be found in Chapter 22 on endometriosis.

Weight management

Although not all people presenting with PCOS are overweight, in those who are, weight loss is an essential part of PCOS treatment, and improvement is unlikely to be seen in the absence of dietary and lifestyle changes. Obesity appears to have both PCOS-independent and PCOS-synergistic effects on metabolic and endocrinological profiles, particularly related to central adiposity.[50] Not only can realistic weight loss result in dramatic improvement in the condition, but being overweight can also make pharmacological treatment less effective.[51,52] Obese women with PCOS are less likely to conceive than lean women with PCOS.[50]

Hyperinsulinaemia is the main mechanism by which adiposity appears to affect ovarian function in PCOS.[50] Weight loss also proffers more effectiveness than current medication for insulin resistance and related disorders, which suggests high relevance for prioritising this approach in naturopathic management of PCOS.[53]

Specific individual pharmacotherapy of any kind—including that of dietary and herbal supplements—is generally clinically ineffective in weight loss in an insulin-resistant person[54] and therefore therapy should focus on an integrated approach to weight management. Weight management is discussed in more detail in Chapter 3, and specific strategies for reducing hyperinsulinaemia are further discussed in Chapter 19; however, there have been some specific studies exploring dietary and lifestyle management of PCOS.

As little as 2–5% reduction in weight can be enough to improve metabolic and reproductive indices in women with PCOS.[55] This modest improvement can restore ovulatory function and improve insulin sensitivity by over 70%.[56] A 5–10% reduction in weight can reduce central fat stores by 30% and weight loss also increases SHBG concentration, reduces testosterone concentration and androgenic stimulation of the skin (resulting in reduction in hirsutism), improves menstrual function and conception rates and reduces miscarriage rates in women with PCOS.[57–63]

High-protein diets are typically associated with excellent weight loss results in insulin-resistant and PCOS women.[64,65] Protein supplementation with whey protein powder has also been found to improve biomarkers in PCOS patients.[66] Although high-protein or low-carbohydrate diets are often successful in weight loss in women with PCOS, this weight loss may not automatically equate to improvements in insulin parameters or ovarian function.[67] However, Mediterranean-style diets have been associated with both weight loss and improved insulin parameters in both generic insulin resistant and PCOS patients.[68,69]

Long-term modest weight loss is far more important in PCOS than acute weight loss. In fact drastic weight loss in women with PCOS could potentially have negative effects on reproductive function.[70] Patient compliance may be improved in low-carbohydrate or high-protein diets compared with low-fat diets,[71] and in patients who have consistent eating habits as opposed to stricter, variable or inflexible diet.[72]

Although short-term trials do not seem to indicate macronutrient composition is as important as caloric restriction in short-term weight loss in women with PCOS,[73] the improved longer term outcomes and compliance suggest a role for Mediterranean-style or high-protein dietary changes. However, rather than advocating drastic low-carbohydrate measures in diet, a more prudent approach is to increase protein, which can improve satiety and reduce carbohydrate intake by default.

Dietary counselling and exercise may result in a trend towards normalisation of hormone levels (as observed by LH:FSH ratio) in PCOS patients, even in the absence of weight loss.[74] In overweight, infertile women with amenorrhoea or anovulation, 12 weeks of exercise and diet therapy were also associated with development of menstrual regularity and normalisation of O1/O2 ratio.[75]

Associated risks of overweight and hyperinsulinaemia also need to be considered in PCOS; for example, there is a high incidence of non-alcoholic fatty acid liver disease in PCOS (see Chapter 7 for more details on NAFLD). Supplementation of omega-3 fatty acids has been studied specifically in women with PCOS and found to reduce liver fat, triglycerides and blood pressure.[76]

Fatness or fitness?

It is easy to assume that all that is required to treat PCOS is to reduce the weight of the patient. However, improving physical fitness may often be more effective than crude weight loss in PCOS management. Similarly, an assumption should not be made that leanness equates to fitness and improvement in reproductive symptom management (e.g. endometriosis is far more common in lean women, and female athlete triad syndrome is a common cause of amenorrhoea in women participating in sports that emphasise leanness). It may be prudent to aim for goals that more accurately reflect fitness levels (stamina in daily tasks and energy levels) rather than crude measurements. Weight management should focus on achieving a healthy weight and not some arbitrary number. Some women will never acquire an 'athletic' body type even at peak fitness. Holistic treatment may in these cases extend to reducing the psychological effect of body issues as well as physical considerations, and encouraging the patient to be comfortable with their healthy body. This may require referral to non-clinical resources (e.g. advice on flattering clothing choices) as much as clinical ones.

The role of leptin

Leptin is a hormone secreted by adipocytes and regulates body weight via not only its effects on metabolism and satiety but also the fact that elevated leptin levels may decrease aromatase activity in granulosa cells.[50] However, levels of this hormone appear to be related to the overweight status of the patient, as elevated leptin levels are observed in overweight women with and without PCOS (Figure 23.5).[77,78] However, leptin does act directly on ovarian function through specific receptors.[80–83] Generally, leptin inhibits the HPA axis and stimulates the reproductive system, which may result in ovarian over-production of androgens.

Impaired postprandial cholecystokinin (CCK) secretion, possibly associated with increased levels of testosterone, may also play a role in the greater frequency of binge eating and being overweight in women with PCOS.[84] The hormone ghrelin—implicated in appetite regulation—was also found to be lower in PCOS women than in controls, indicating alterations in satiety.[85] In overweight women with PCOS a dysfunctional leptin resistance may be observed and this may be one reason weight loss is a successful intervention in PCOS.[86,87]

Reducing insulin resistance

The treatment of insulin resistance is covered in more depth in Chapter 19 on diabetes, though some advances have been made specifically in relation to PCOS. **Inositol** appears to have the ability to increase ovulation and reduce hyperandrogenism in

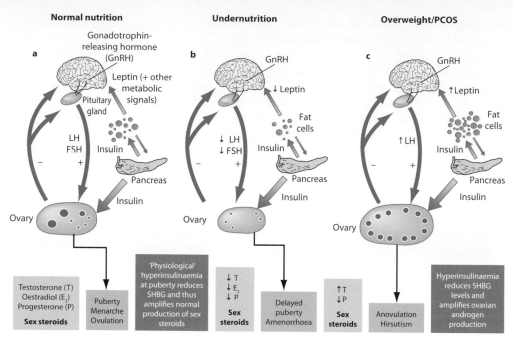

Figure 23.5

Leptin and insulin interactions with sex hormones in normal nutrition, undernutrition and overweight/PCOS

Sources: Takeuchi & Tsutsumi 2000,[77] Telli et al[78] and Sharpe & Franks 2002[79]

women with PCOS, including those without weight issues, as well as improving insulin parameters.[88–90] **Alpha-lipoic acid** has also been found to increase insulin sensitivity in lean women with PCOS.[91] **Vitamin D** may sensitise insulin receptors and promote maturation of ovarian follicles in women with PCOS.[92] **Magnesium** is a nutrient that has a significant role in insulin resistance more generally, and in PCOS specifically.[93]

Galega officinalis is traditionally used to treat insulin resistance and contains chromium salts as well as guanidines.[94,95] Early research established hypoglycaemic activity in these guanidine compounds.[96] The drug metformin, used successfully in conventional treatment of PCOS, is a synthetic guanidine derivative. **Berberine**-containing herbs up-regulate insulin receptors and stimulate uptake of glucose into cells, and can block testosterone production in the ovaries.[97] One small study has shown berberine to outperform metformin on metabolic characteristics of PCOS.[98,99] Other herbs that may show promise in treating insulin resistance more generally include *Momordica indica*, *Gymnema sylvestre* and *Aloe vera*.[100] Interventions useful in insulin resistance are covered in more depth in Chapter 19. **Chromium** was found to improve insulin resistance parameters, though not ovulation, in women with PCOS.[101,102] Insulin resistance may be associated with higher aromatase activity.[103] This is explored further in Chapter 22 on endometriosis.

Reducing hirsutism

Hirsutism is common in women with PCOS and often weight loss alone has been associated with reducing the effects of hirsutism.[59,62,63] An infusion of *Mentha spicata* was found to lower free testosterone, while not lowering total testosterone or didehydroepiandrosterone (DHEA), in a small study of women with PCOS and hirsutism.[29,104] *Serenoa repens* has also been found to reduce the severity of androgenic dermatological conditions (alopecia) in both men and women and may therefore be useful in PCOS.[105] **Zinc** may also be of some value in reducing androgenic activity in skin.[106] Hormonal modulation more generally will also assist with skin conditions associated with excess androgens, and are discussed in more detail in Chapter 27 on acne.

INTEGRATIVE MEDICAL CONSIDERATIONS

Acupuncture and Asian herbal medicine

Women with PCOS treated with acupuncture have shown improvements in hormone levels, ovulation and BBT.[107] This is thought to be particularly related to the effects of acupuncture on the sympathetic nervous system in PCOS. However, a recent Cochrane review noted that as no truly randomised trials existed, it was not possible to make comment on the effectiveness of acupuncture for PCOS.[108]

There has been much discussion surrounding the successful treatment of PCOS with the herbs *Paeonia lactiflora* and *Glycyrrhiza glabra*. This is based on successful treatment of PCOS in a series of small uncontrolled studies in a combination herbal product of which these two herbs were only two components of many.[31,32] A Japanese combination (*unkei-to*) has also demonstrated some effect in women with PCOS,[109,110] as have a variety of other combinations of herbal products.[111,112]

These remedies have a strong tradition of use in PCOS, which is being reinforced through modern research; however, they need to be properly prescribed in accordance with traditional Chinese medicine or *kampo* principles. It should also be remembered that, due to the difficulties in developing a uniform diagnosis of PCOS, these formulations may not be applicable to all populations with or manifestations of PCOS. It is known, for example, that the metabolic characteristics and responses to treatment of Asian women with PCOS may be significantly different to those seen in Western populations.[112] Their use in contemporary naturopathic practice needs to take these principles into consideration.

Fertility treatment

Many patients ignore PCOS until they unsuccessfully attempt to conceive. Even once PCOS has been resolved these patients may require further preconception care on a more individual basis. Referral to a fertility program or specialist may be warranted. Fertility treatment is discussed in more detail in Chapter 34.

Homeopathy

A case series has found that individualised homeopathic treatment may be successful at restoring ovulation in women with amenorrhoea.[113] However, it is difficult to ascertain whether this is due to homeopathic treatment itself or to other lifestyle factors—such as improvements in diet and exercise—addressed or encouraged during these consultations.

Psychotherapeutic options

Some women with PCOS fail to fall within social norms regarding outer appearance and may feel stigmatised and feel a loss of feminine identity—this may affect mood, sexual function and quality of life more generally.[114] Appropriate counselling and psychotherapeutic options may help lessen the impact on quality of life in PCOS patients.

CLINICAL SUMMARY

PCOS is a notoriously difficult condition to manage, and requires ongoing commitment by both the practitioner and the patient. Treatment for PCOS needs to be looked at long term. It may be months before the initial menstrual bleeding (which may seem 'excessive' in both volume and timeframe by normal standards once it does finally arrive). PCOS treatment can be a long journey. Patients need to be counselled on this before embarking on treatment to ensure they know what to expect and to ensure they do not get disheartened by the lack of immediate results. Ensure the patient is appropriately counselled as to this and employ them in their treatment for better compliance.

Charting can be a useful tool to indicate changes in hormone levels that are getting closer to those required for ovulation, even when menstrual changes are not apparent. Patients with amenorrhoea may also require a change in their prescription at the point of their first menstrual bleed to assist their cycle to become regular. Reduction of hirsutism also requires long-term management. Hair follicles will often take at least three months (their life cycle) before effects are observed in women with PCOS. It may be prudent to counsel patients to make cosmetic adjustments until then if this is a big concern, in addition to counselling them on the long timeframe of treatment.

PCOS treatment needs to focus on dietary and lifestyle modification, which is more effective than medication. It is unlikely that there will be any clinical improvement without dietary and lifestyle management, and neglecting to make clinical improvements in weight management or insulin resistance will also render possible pharmacological interventions less effective. Part of the role of a naturopath in weight management is to identify appropriate foods and exercises that will ensure patient compliance.

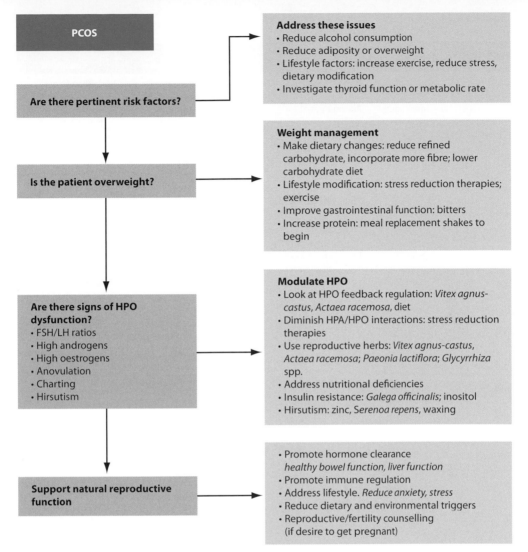

Figure 23.6
Naturopathic treatment decision tree—PCOS

Table 23.2
Review of the major evidence

Intervention	Mechanisms of action	Key literature	Summary of results	Comment
Mentha spicata	Ingestion has effects on androgen receptors	Non-randomised trial: Akdoğan et al. 2007[29] Twenty-one women with hirsutism were given one cup of Mentha spicata infusion b.d. for five days	There was a significant decrease in free testosterone and increase in LH, FSH and oestradiol. No significant decreases in total testosterone or dehydroepiandrostenedione sulfate levels were observed	*Mentha spicata* may have anti-androgenic effects in PCOS
Unkei-to	Potentially through stimulation of pituitary dopamine receptors	RCTs: Takahashi et al. 1988, 1994 Twenty-four week RCTs of 34 women with PCOS given 7.5 g of TJ-68 (unkei-to)	Significant reductions in FSH:LH ratio, ovarian testosterone production and improvements in ovulation	These small trials used a combination herbal medicine prescribed according to traditional Chinese medicine or kampo principles Their use in naturopathic prescription may not mirror this
Inositol	Reduction of metabolic risk factors	RCTs: Two six to eight week trials of inositol versus placebo in both obese ($n = 44$) and lean ($n = 20$) women with PCOS	Women in inositol group ovulated more than placebo group. Serum triglycerides, insulin, free testosterone and blood pressure all increased significantly when compared with placebo	Inositol increases the action of insulin in patients with polycystic ovary syndrome, thereby improving ovulatory function and decreasing serum androgen concentrations, blood pressure and plasma triglyceride concentrations
Whey protein	Reduction of metabolic risk factors	RCT: Kasim-Karakas et al. 2007[66] Measured changes in hormone levels of women with PCOS ($n = 28$) after acute glucose (oral five-hour glucose challenge test) and acute protein intakes (with whey protein) Protein suppressed ghrelin significantly more than glucose and had more satietogenic effect	Glucose ingestion caused significantly more hyperinsulinaemia and stimulated cortisol and DHEA more than protein	Study represents short-term effects only, though provides some mechanistic support for increasing protein and decreasing simple sugars in PCOS treatment

Table 23.2
Review of the major evidence (continued)

Intervention	Mechanisms of action	Key literature	Summary of results	Comment
Chinese herbal medicine (CHM)	Unknown, prescribed in accordance with traditional theory	Systematic review: Zhang et al. 2010[115] Four RCTs involving 344 women	There were no significant differences between CHM treatment and clomiphene or laparoscopic drilling for ovulation and pregnancy	An additive effect to clomiphene was observed to improve pregnancy rates
Naturopathic herbal medicine and lifestyle intervention	Various	RCT: Arentz et al. 2017[116] Three-month trial of lifestyle and herbal medicine (2 tablets) intervention overseen by a naturopathic practitioner (n = 122)	At three months, women in the combination group recorded a reduction in oligomenorrhoea of 33%. Significant improvements were found for body mass index; insulin and luteinising hormone; blood pressure; quality of life; depression, anxiety and stress; and pregnancy rates	The herbal intervention consisted of two tablets. Tablet 1 contained *Cinnamomum verum, Glycyrrhiza glabra, Hypericum perforatum* and *Paeonia lactiflora*. Tablet 2 contained *Tribulus terrestris*

KEY POINTS

- Use dietary and lifestyle modification first—these approaches are far more effective than any medication, and any medication is unlikely to work until these are addressed.
- Address the other risk factors that are associated with PCOS (e.g. cardiovascular).
- Part of the role of a naturopath in weight management is to identify appropriate foods and exercises that will ensure patient compliance.
- PCOS can be an intractable condition and PCOS treatment can be a long process. Ensure the patient is appropriately counselled as to this and employ them in their treatment for better compliance.

FURTHER READING

Arentz S, Smith CA, Abbott J, et al. Nutritional supplements and herbal medicines for women with polycystic ovary syndrome; a systematic review and meta-analysis. BMC Complement Altern Med 2017;17(1):500.

Giallauria F, et al. Androgens in polycystic ovary syndrome: the role of exercise and diet. Semin Reprod Med 2009;27(4):306–15.

Huang S, Chen A. Traditional Chinese medicine and infertility. Curr Opin Obstet Gynecol 2008;20(3):211–15.

Trickey R. Women, hormones and the menstrual cycle: herbal and medical solutions from adolescence to menopause. Melbourne: MHHG; 2012.

Wilkes S, Murdoch A. Obesity and female fertility: a primary care perspective. J Fam Plann Reprod Health Care 2009;35(3):181–5.

REFERENCES

1. Khadilkar SS. Polycystic ovarian syndrome: is it time to rename PCOS to HA-PODS? J Obstet Gynecol India 2016;66(2):81–7.
2. Azziz R, Carmina E, Dewailly D, et al. Task force on the phenotype of the polycystic ovary syndrome of the Androgen Excess and PCOS Society. The Androgen Excess and PCOS Society criteria for the polycystic ovary syndrome: the complete task force report. Fertil Steril 2009;91:456–88.
3. Asuncion M, Calvo R, San Millan J, et al. A prospective study of the prevalence of the polycystic ovary syndrome in unselected Caucasian women from

Spain. J Clin Endocrinol & Metabol 2000;85: 2434–8.

4. Knochenhauer E, Key T, Kahsar-Miller M, et al. Prevalence of the polycystic ovary syndrome in unselected black and white women of the southeastern United States: a prospective study. J Clin Endocrinol & Metabol 1998;83:3078–82.

5. Ibanez L, Valls C, Potau N, et al. Polycystic ovary syndrome after precocious pubarche: ontogeny of the low-birthweight effect. Clin Endocrinol 2001;55:667–72.

6. Speroff L, Fritz M. Clinical gynecologic endocrinology and infertility. 7th ed. Philadelphia: Lippincott Williams & Wilkins; 2005.

7. Kovacs G, Norman R, editors. Polycystic ovarian syndrome. Cambridge: Cambridge University Press; 2008.

8. Wilkes S, Murdoch A. Obesity and female fertility: a primary care perspective. J Fam Plann Reprod Health Care 2009;35(3):181–5.

9. Altuntas Y, Bilir M, Ucak S, et al. Reactive hypoglycemia in lean young women with PCOS and correlations with insulin sensitivity and with beta cell function. Eur J Obstet Gynecol Reprod Biology 2005;119(2):198–205.

10. Ghosh S, Kabir S, Pakrashi A, et al. Subclinical hypothyroidism: a determinant of polycystic ovary syndrome. Horm Res 1993;39(1):61–6.

11. Jannsen O, Mehlmauer N, Hahn S, et al. High prevalence of autoimmune thyroiditis in patients with polycystic ovary syndrome. Eur J Endocrinol 2004;150:363–9.

12. El-Serag H, Tran T, Everhart J. Diabetes increases the risk of chronic liver disease and hepatocellular carcinoma. Gastroenterology 2004;126:460–8.

13. Schwimmer J, Khorram O, Chiu V, et al. Abnormal aminotransferase activity in women with polycystic ovary syndrome. Fertil Steril 2005;83:494–7.

14. Diamanti-Kandarakis E, Paterakis T, Kandarakis HA. Indices of low-grade inflammation in polycystic ovary syndrome. Ann NY Acad Sci 2006;1092:175–86.

15. Duleba AJ, Dokras A. Is PCOS an inflammatory process? Fertil Steril 2012;97:7–12.

16. Martinez A, van Hooff M, Schoute E, et al. The reliability, acceptability and applications of basal body-temperature (BBT) records in the diagnosis and treatment of infertility. Eur J Obstet Gynecol Reprod Biology 1992;47:121–7.

17. Arentz S, Smith CA, Abbott J, et al. Combined lifestyle and herbal medicine in overweight women with polycystic ovary syndrome (PCOS): a randomized controlled trial. Phytother Res 2017;31(9):1330–40.

18. Duker E, Kopnski L, Jarry H, et al. Effects of extracts from cimicifuga racemosa on gonadotrophin release in menopausal women and ovariectomized rats. Planta Med 1991;57:420–4.

19. Borrelli F, Izzo A, Ernst E. Pharmacological effects of cimicifuga racemosa. Life Sci 2003;73:1215–29.

20. Scientific Committee of the British Herbal Medical Association. British herbal pharmacopoeia. 1st ed. Bournemouth: British Herbal Medicine Association; 1983.

21. Jarry H, Leonhardt S, Gorkow C, et al. In vitro prolactin but not LH and FSH release is inhibited by compounds in extracts of Agnus castus: direct evidence for a dopaminergic principle by the dopamine receptor assay. Exp Clin Endocrinol 1994;102(6):448–54.

22. Laurintzen C, Reuter H, Repges R, et al. Treatment of premenstrual tension with Vitex agnus castus: controlled, double blind study versus pyroxidin. Phytomed 1997;4:183–9.

23. Milewicz A, Gejdel E, Sworen H, et al. [Vitex agnus castus extract in the treatment of luteal phase defects due to latent hyperprolactinaemia. Results of a randomized

24. Shayya R, Chang R. Reproductive endocrinology of adolescent polycystic ovary syndrome. BJOG 2010;117(2):150–5.

25. Bracero N, Zacur H. Polycystic ovary syndrome and hyperprolactinemia. Obstet Gynecol Clin North Am 2001;28(1):77–84.

26. Okamato R, Kumai A. Antigonadotrophic activity of hop extract. Acta Endocrinol 1992;127(4):371–7.

27. Balk E, Chung M, Chew P, et al. Effects of soy on health outcomes. Evid Rep Technol Assess (Summ) 2005;126:1–8.

28. Tabakova P, Dimitrov M, Ogynyanov K, et al. Clinical study of Tribestan® in females with endocrine sterility. Sofia: Bulgarian Pharmacology Group; 2000.

29. Akdoğan M, Tamer M, Süre E, et al. Effect of spearmint (Mentha spicata Labiatae) teas on androgen levels in women with hirsutism. Phytother Res 2007;21(5):444–7.

30. Armanini D, Mattarello M, Fiore C, et al. Licorice reduces serum testosterone in healthy women. Steroids 2004;69(11–12):763–6.

31. Takahashi K, Kitao M. Effects of TJ-68 (shakuyaku-kanzo-to) on polycystic ovarian disease. Int J Fertil Menopausal Stud 1994;39(2):69–76.

32. Takahashi K, Yoshino K, Shirai T, et al. [Effects of traditional medicine (Shakuyaku-kanzo-to) on testosterone secretion in patients with polycystic ovarian syndrome detected by ultrasound] in Japanese. Nippon Sanka Fujinka Gakkai Zasshi 1988;40(6):789–96.

33. Setchell K, Cassidy A. Dietary isoflavones: biological effects and relevance to human health. J Nutr 1999;129:758S–767S.

34. Armanini D, De Palo C, Mattarello M, et al. Effect of licorice on the reduction of body fat mass in healthy subjects. J Endocrinol Invest 2003;26(7):646–50.

35. Yaginuma T, Izumi R, Yasui H, et al. [Effects of traditional herbal medicines on serum testosterone levels and its induction of regular ovulation in hyperandrogenic and oligomenorrheic women] in Japanese. Nippon Sanka Fujinka Gakkai Zasshi 1998;34(7):939–44.

36. Cagnacci A, Arangino S, Renzi A, et al. Influence of melatonin administration on glucose tolerance and insulin sensitivity of postmenopausal women. Clin Endocrinol 2001;54:339–46.

37. Cagnacci A, Paoletti A, Soldani R, et al. Melatonin enhances the luteinizing hormone and follicle-stimulating hormone response to gonadotropin-releasing hormone in the follicular, but not in the luteal menstrual phase. J Clin Endocrinol Metab 1995;80:1095–9.

38. Cagnacci A, Soldani R, Yen S. Exogenous melatonin enhances luteinizing hormone levels of women in the follicular but not in the luteal menstrual phase. Fertil Steril 1995;63:996–9.

39. Cagnacci A, Soldani R, Yen S. Melatonin enhances cortisol levels in aged women: reversible by estrogens. J Pineal Res 1997;22(2):81–5.

40. Bellipanni G, Bianchi P, Pierpaoli W, et al. Effects of melatonin in perimenopausal and menopausal women: a randomized and placebo controlled study. Exp Gerontol 2001;36(2):297–310.

41. Bellipanni G, Di Marzo F, Blasi F, et al. Effects of melatonin in perimenopausal and menopausal women: our personal experience. Ann N Y Acad Sci 2005;1057:393–402.

42. Cagnacci A, Volpe A. A role for melatonin in PCOS? Fertil Steril 2002;77(5):1089.

43. Alvero R, Kimzey L, Sebring N, et al. Effects of fasting on neuroendocrine function and follicle development in lean women. J Clin Endocrinol Metab 1998;83:76–80.

placebo-controlled double-blind study] (in German). Arzneimittelforschung 1993;43(7):752–6.

44. Loucks A, Heath E. Dietary restriction reduces luteinizing hormone (LH) pulse frequency during waking hours and increases LH pulse amplitude during sleep in young menstruating women. J Clin Endocrinol Metab 1994;78:910–15.

45. Olson B, Cartledge T, Sebring N, et al. Short-term fasting affects luteinizing hormone secretory dynamics but not reproductive function in normal-weight sedentary women. J Clin Endocrinol Metab 1995;80:1187–93.

46. Bergendahl M, Evans WS, Pastor C, et al. Short-term fasting suppresses leptin and (conversely) activates disorderly growth hormone secretion in midluteal phase women – a clinical research center study. J Clin Endocrinol Metab 1999;84(3):883–94.

47. Daniel JA, Whitlock BK, Wagner CG, et al. Regulation of the growth hormone and luteinizing hormone response to endotoxin in sheep. Domest Anim Endocrinol 2002;23(1–2):361–70.

48. Yildiz B, Azziz R. Adrenocortical dysfunction in polycystic ovary syndrome. In: Kovacs G, Norman R, editors. Polycystic ovary syndrome. 2nd ed. Cambridge: Cambridge University Press; 2007.

49. Kondoh Y, Uemura T, Murase M, et al. A longitudinal study of disturbances of the hypothalamic-pituitary-adrenal axis in women with progestin-negative functional hypothalamic amenorrhea. Fertil Steril 2001;76(4):748–52.

50. van der Spuy ZM, Dyer SJ. The pathogenesis of infertility and early pregnancy loss in polycystic ovrian syndrome. Best Pract Res Clin Obstet Gynaecol 2004;18(5):755–71.

51. Dale O, Tanbo T, Haug E, et al. The impact of insulin resistance on the outcome of ovulation induction with low-dose FSH in women with polycystic ovarian syndrome. Hum Reprod 1998;13:567–70.

52. Homburg R. Adverse effect of luteinizing hormone on fertiltiy: fact or fantasy. Baillere's Clin Obstet Gynecol 1998;12:555–63.

53. Knowler W, Barrett-Connor E, Fowler S, et al. Reduction in the incidence of type 2 diabetes with lifestyle intervention or metformin. N Engl J Med 2002;346:393–403.

54. Norris S, Zhang X, Avenell A, et al. Efficacy of pharmacotherapy for weight loss in adults with type 2 diabetes mellitus: a meta-analysis. Arch Int Med 2004;164(13):1395–404.

55. Moran L, Brinkworth G, Noakes M, et al. Effects of lifestyle modification in polycystic ovarian syndrome. Reprod Biomed Online 2006;12:569–78.

56. Huber-Buchholz M, Carey D, Norman R. Restoration of reproductive potential by lifestyle modification in obese polycystic ovary syndrome: role of insulin sensitivity and luteinizing hormone. J Clin Endocrinol Metab 1999;84:1470–4.

57. Clark A, Ledger W, Gallerty C, et al. Weight loss results in significant improvement in pregnancy ovulation and outcome rates in anovulatory obese women. Hum Reprod 1995;10:2705–12.

58. Crosignani P, Colombo M, Vegetti W, et al. Overweight and obese anovulatory patients with polycystic ovaries: parallel improvements in anthropometric indices, ovarian physiology and fertility rate induced by diet. Hum Reprod 2003;18:1928–32.

59. Kiddy D, Hamilton-Fairley S, Bush A. Improvement in endocrine and ovarian function during dietary treatment of obese women with polycystic ovary syndrome. Clin Endocrinol 1992;36:105–11.

60. Moran L, Noakes M, Clifton P, et al. Dietary composition in restoring reproductive and metabolic physiology in overweight women with polycystic ovary syndrome. J Clin Endocrinol Metab 2003;88:812–19.

61. Pasquali R, Gambineri A, Biscotti D, et al. Effect of long-term treatment with metformin added to hypocaloric diet on body composition, fat distribution, and androgen and insulin levels in abdominally obese women with and without the polycystic ovary syndrome. J Clin Endocrinol Metab 2000;85:2767–74.

62. Piacquadio D, Rad F, Spellman M, et al. Obesity and female androgenic alopecia: cause and effect? J Am Acad Dermatol 1994;30:1028–30.

63. Ruutiainen K, Erkkola R, Gronroos M, et al. Influence of body mass index and age on the grade of hair growth and hormonal parameters of hirsute women. Int J Gynecol Obstet 1988;24:361–8.

64. Mathers J, Daly M. Dietary carbohydrates and insulin sensitivity. Curr Opin Clin Nutr Metab Care 1998;1:553–7.

65. Skov A, Toubro S, Ronn B. Randomized trial on protein vs. carbohydrate in ad libitum fat reduced diet for the treatment of obesity. Int J Obes Relat Metab Disord 1999;23:528–36.

66. Kasim-Karakas S, Cunningham W, Tsodikov A. Relation of nutrients and hormones in polycystic ovary syndrome. Am J Clin Nutr 2007;85(3):688–94.

67. Stamets K, Taylor D, Kunselman A, et al. A randomized trial of the effects of two types of short term hypocaloric diets on weight loss in women with polycystic ovarian syndrome. Fertil Steril 2004;81:630–7.

68. Carmina E, Legro R, Stamets K, et al. Difference in body weight between American and Italian women with polycystic ovarian syndrome: influence of diet. Hum Reprod 2003;18:2289–93.

69. Esposito K, Marfella R, Ciotola M, et al. Effect of a mediterranean-style diet on endothelial dysfunction and markers of vascular inflammation in the metabolic syndrome: a randomized trial. J Am Med Assoc 2004;292:1440–6.

70. Tsagareli V, Noakes M, Norman R. Effect of a very-low-calorie diet on in vitro fertilization outcomes. Fertil Steril 2006;86:227–9.

71. Hession M, Rolland C, Kulkarni U, et al. Systematic review of randomized controlled trials of low-carbohydrate vs. low-fat/low-calorie diets in the management of obesity and its comorbidities. Obes Rev 2009;10(1):36–50.

72. Wing R, Phelan S. Long-term weight loss maintenance. Am J Clin Nutr 2005;82(Suppl. 1):222–5.

73. Moran L, Noakes M, Clifton P, et al. Short-term meal replacements followed by dietary macronutrient restriction enhance weight loss in polycystic ovarian syndrome. Am J Clin Nutr 2006;84(1):77–87.

74. Bruner B, Chad K, Chizen D. Effects of exercise and nutritional counseling in women with polycystic ovary syndrome. Appl Physiol Nutr Metab 2006;31(4):384–91.

75. Miller P, Forstein D, Styles S. Effect of short-term diet and exercise on hormone levels and menses in obese, infertile women. J Reprod Med 2008;53(5):315–19.

76. Cussons A, Watts G, Mori T, et al. Omega-3 fatty acid supplementation decreases liver fat content in polycystic ovary syndrome: a randomized controlled trial employing proton magnetic resonance spectroscopy. J Clin Endocrinol Metab 2009;94(10):3842–8.

77. Takeuchi T, Tsutsumi O. Basal leptin concentrations in women with normal and dysfunctional ovarian conditions. Int J Gynecol Obstet 2000;69(2):127–33.

78. Telli M, Yildirm M, Noyan V. Serum leptin levels in women with polycystic ovarian syndrome. Fertil Steril 2002;77(5):932–5.

79. Sharpe R, Franks S. Environment, lifestyle and infertility—an inter-generational issue. Nat Cell Biol 2002;4(Suppl.): s33–40.

80. Brannian J, Hansen K. Leptin and ovarian folliculogenesis: implications for ovulation induction and ART outcomes. Semin Reprod Med 2002;20(2):103–12.

81. Cioffi J, Van Blerkom J, Antczak M, et al. The expression of leptin and its receptors in pre-ovulatory human follicles. Mol Hum Reprod 1997;3(6):467–72.

82. Finn P, Cunningham M, Pau K, et al. The stimulatory effect of leptin on the neuroendocrine reproductive axis of the monkey. Endocrinology 1998;139(11):4652–62.

83. Mitchell M, Armstrong D, Robker R, et al. Adipokines: implications for female fertility and obesity. Reproduction 2005;130(5):583–97.

84. Hirschberg A, Naessen S, Stridsberg M, et al. Impaired cholecystokinin secretion and disturbed appetite regulation in women with polycystic ovary syndrome. Gynecol Endocrinol 2004;19(2):79–87.

85. Moran L, Noakes M, Clifton P, et al. Ghrelin and measures of satiety are altered in polycystic ovarian syndrome but not differentially affected by diet composition. J Clin Endocrinol Metab 2004;89:3337–44.

86. Moschos S, Chan J, Mantzoros C. Leptin and reproduction: a review. Fertil Steril 2002;77(3): 433–44.

87. Spritzer P, Poy M, Wiltgen D, et al. Leptin concentrations in hirsute women with polycystic ovary syndrome or idiopathic hirsutism: influence on LH and relationship with hormonal, metabolic, and anthropometric measurements. Hum Reprod 2001;16(7):1340–6.

88. Gerli S, Mignosa M, DiRenzo G. Effects of inositol on ovarian function and metabolic factors in women with PCOS: a randomized double-blind placebo controlled trial. Eur Rev Med Pharmacol Sci 2003;7:151–9.

89. Iuorno M, Jakubowicz D, Baillargeon J, et al. Effects of d-chiro-inositol in lean women with the polycystic ovary syndrome. Endocr Pract 2002;8(6):417–23.

90. La Marca A, Grisendi V, Dondi G, et al. The menstrual cycle regularization following D-chiro-inositol treatment in PCOS women: a retrospective study. Gynecol Endocrinol 2015;31(1):52–6.

91. Masharani U, Gjerde C, Evans J, et al. Effects of controlled-release alpha lipoic acid in lean, nondiabetic patients with polycystic ovary syndrome. J Diabetes Sci Technol 2010;4(2):359–64.

92. Thomson RL, Spedding S, Buckley JD. Vitamin D in the aetiology and management of polycystic ovary syndrome. Clin Endocrinol 2012;77(3):343–50.

93. Sharifi F, Mazloomi S, Hajihosseini R, et al. Serum magnesium concentrations in polycystic ovary syndrome and its association with insulin resistance. Gynecol Endocrinol 2012;28(1):7–11.

94. Neef H, Augustijns P, Declercq P, et al. Inhibitory effects of Galega officinalis on glucose transport across monolayers of human intestinal epithelial cells (Caco-2). Pharm Pharmacol Lett 1996;6(2):86–9.

95. Neef H, Declercq P, Laekeman G. Hypoglycaemic activity of selected European plants. Phytother Res 1995;6(2):45–8.

96. Muller H, Reinwein H. Pharmacology of galegin. Arch Expll Path Pharm 1927;125:212–28.

97. Orio F, Muscogiuri G, Palomba S, et al. Berberine improves reproductive features in obese Caucasian women with polycystic ovary syndrome independently of changes of insulin sensitivity. ESPEN J 2013;8(5):e200–4.

98. An Y, Sun Z, Zhang Y, et al. The use of berberine for women with polycystic ovary syndrome undergoing IVF treatment. Clin Endocrinol 2014;80(3):425–31.

99. Wei W, Zhao H, Wang A, et al. A clinical study on the short-term effect of berberine in comparison to metformin on the metabolic characteristics of women with polycystic ovary syndrome. Eur J Endocrinol 2012;166(1):99–105.

100. Yeh G, Eisenber D, Kaptchuk T, et al. Systematic review of herbs and dietary supplements for glycemic control in diabetes. Diabetes Care 2003;26:1277–94.

101. Lucidi R, Thyer A, Easton C, et al. Effect of chromium supplementation on insulin resistance and ovarian and menstrual cyclicity in women with polycystic ovary syndrome. Fertil Steril 2005;84(6):1755–77.

102. Lydic M, McNurlan M, Bembo S, et al. Chromium picolinate improves insulin sensitivity in obese subjects with polycystic ovary syndrome. Fertil Steril 2006;86(1):243–6.

103. La Marca A, Morgante G, Palumbo M, et al. Insulin-lowering treatment reduces aromatase activity in response to follicle-stimulating hormone in women with polycystic ovary syndrome. Fertil Steril 2002;78(6):1234–9.

104. Grant P. A randomised clinical trial of the effects of spearmint herbal tea on hirsutism in females with polycystic ovarian syndrome. Endoce Abst 2008;15:P282.

105. Prager N, Bickett K, French N, et al. A randomized, double-blind, placebo-controlled trial to determine the effectiveness of botanically derived inhibitors of 5-alpha-reductase in the treatment of androgenetic alopecia. J Altern Complement Med 2002;8(2):143–52.

106. Stamatiadis D, Bulteau-Portois M, Mowszowicz I. Inhibition of 5 alpha-reductase activity in human skin by zinc and azelaic acid. Br J Dermatol 1988;119:627–33.

107. Stener-Victorin E, Jedel E, Mannerås L. Acupuncture in polycystic ovary syndrome: current experimental and clinical evidence. J Neuroendocrinol 2008;20(3):290–8.

108. Lim D, Chen W, Cheng L, et al. Acupuncture for polycystic ovarian syndrome. Cochrane Database Syst Rev 2011;(8):CD007689.

109. Ushiroyama T, Hosotani T, Mori K, et al. Effects of switching to wen-jing-tang (unkei-to) from preceding herbal preparations selected by eight-principle pattern identification on endocrinological status and ovulatory induction in women with polycystic ovary syndrome. Am J Chin Med 2006;34(2):177–87.

110. Ushiroyama T, Ikeda A, Sakai M, et al. Effects of unkei-to, an herbal medicine, on endocrine function and ovulation in women with high basal levels of luteinizing hormone secretion. J Reprod Med 2001;46(5):451–6.

111. Huang S, Chen A. Traditional Chinese medicine and infertility. Curr Opin Obstet Gynecol 2008;20(3):211–15.

112. Yu Ng E, Ho P. Polycystic ovary syndrome in asian women. Semin Reprod Med 2008;26(1):14–21.

113. Cardigno P. Homeopathy for the treatment of menstrual irregularities: a case series. Homeopathy 2009;98(2):97–106.

114. Janssen O, Hahn S, Tan S, et al. Mood and sexual function in polycystic ovary syndrome. Semin Reprod Med 2008;26(1):45–52.

115. Zhang J, Li T, Zhou L, et al. Chinese herbal medicine for subfertile women with polycystic ovarian syndrome. Cochrane Database Syst Rev 2010;(9):CD007535.

116. Arentz S, Smith CA, Abbott J, et al. Nutritional supplements and herbal medicines for women with polycystic ovary syndrome; a systematic review and meta-analysis. BMC Complement Altern Med 2017;17(1):500.

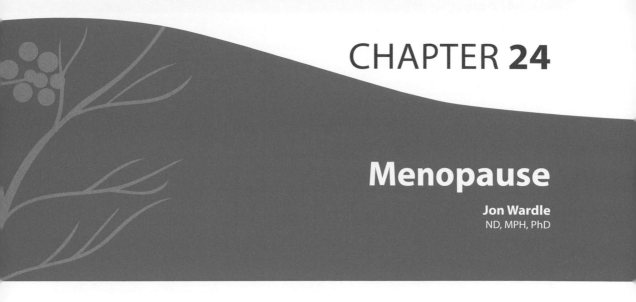

CHAPTER 24

Menopause

Jon Wardle
ND, MPH, PhD

OVERVIEW

Menopause represents the natural transition from fertility to age-related non-fertility. The term 'menopause' specifically means the cessation of menstruation, and most often occurs between the ages of 45 and 55 years, with the average age for the last period being 51 years.

All healthy women will transition from a reproductive (premenopausal) period—marked by regular ovulation and cyclic menstrual bleeding—to a postmenopausal period marked by amenorrhoea. The onset of the menopausal transition is marked by changes in the menstrual cycle and in the duration or amount of menstrual flow (Figure 24.1). Subsequently, cycles are missed, but the pattern is often erratic early in the menopausal transition. Therefore the menopause is defined retrospectively after 12 months of continued amenorrhoea.

The term 'perimenopause' is most often used to describe the time leading up to and directly following menopause.[2] During perimenopause, hormone levels fluctuate and women may experience a variety of symptoms including vasomotor symptoms (hot flushes and night sweats), vulvovaginal atrophy, emotional fluctuations and cognitive decline (memory problems). Some women experience very little in the way of these symptoms; for others this time is particularly debilitating. Low oestrogen levels post-menopause also increase the risk of a number of other physical conditions including osteoporosis and cardiovascular disease. The various symptoms of the menopausal transition are associated with a variety of physiological changes and the responses to these changes. Figure 24.1 shows the symptoms associated with changes in hormone levels.

In the postmenopausal phase FSH rise to levels 10–15 times the level that can be expected during the follicular phase of a reproductive cycle, while LH levels increase to around three times that experienced during menstruation. The ovaries do continue to excrete minimal amounts of oestrogens, and continue to excrete significant amounts of androgens.[2]

It should also be noted that individual women will experience the menopausal transition differently, with prevalence rates of the main symptoms varying greatly across the different stages of menopause.[3]

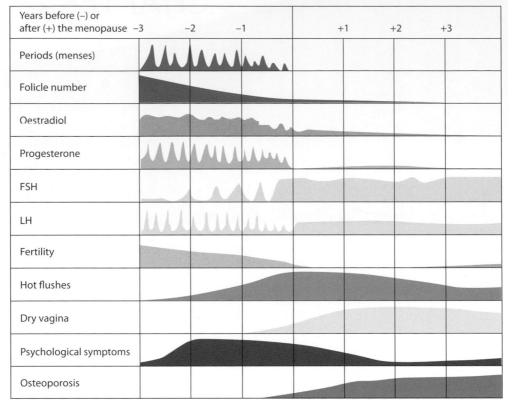

Cessation of menses

Years before (–) or after (+) the menopause	–3	–2	–1		+1	+2	+3
Periods (menses)							
Folicle number							
Oestradiol							
Progesterone							
FSH							
LH							
Fertility							
Hot flushes							
Dry vagina							
Psychological symptoms							
Osteoporosis							

Figure 24.1
Menopausal symptom and hormone changes over time

Source: Reeves et al. 2007[1]

DIFFERENTIAL DIAGNOSIS

- Other sources of hot flushes (diabetes, panic attacks, hyperthyroidism)
- General gynaecological hormone imbalances (particularly in women aged under 40)
- Medication side effects
- Every woman aged over 55 will undergo the menopausal transition; differential diagnosis should instead be used for individual symptomology rather than 'menopause'

RISK FACTORS

Although much focus tends to be drawn towards the effect that hormone therapy (HT) can have on increasing breast cancer risk, other modifiable lifestyle factors such as little exercise, smoking, postmenopausal weight gain and high alcohol consumption may increase the risk of not only breast cancer but exacerbate other menopausal symptoms as well.[4]

Risk factors for severity of symptoms during perimenopause include genetics (symptoms experienced by the mother may give a guide) and body mass index

(BMI)—women with a higher BMI may experience a lower level of perimenopause symptoms due to the production of oestrogen by aromatase in adipose tissue (see Chapter 22 on endometriosis).

The duration of symptoms appears independent of HT but is less in those groups with higher physical activity.[5] Other lifestyle factors, such as increased alcohol and caffeine use and smoking, are also associated with worsened menopausal symptoms.[6] It should also be noted that after undergoing the menopausal transition, the protective effects of oestrogen on some physiological process (such as cardiovascular disease) will no longer be present.

CONVENTIONAL TREATMENT

Conventional treatment for menopause focuses largely on attempts to alleviate associated symptoms. Much controversy has raged during recent years over what is termed the 'medicalisation' of naturally occurring life stages, of which the most publicised is menopause. Conventional practice has often viewed menopause as a condition of oestrogen deficiency, and treatment is based on the use of supplemental hormones (commonly referred to as HT).

There is much conjecture and controversy surrounding the use of HT in menopause. There are definite benefits to using HT. HT is effective for vasomotor symptoms, vulvo-vaginal atrophy symptoms and osteoporosis-related fracture prevention, and benefits cardiovascular and central nervous systems.[1] However, continued use of HT can increase the risk for venous thromboembolism and increases the risk of developing breast cancer.[1]

Bioidentical hormone therapy: safer, more effective?

Most of the data suggesting risks associated with HT have been conducted using equine or synthetic hormones, and there is little evidence of the safety or efficacy of bioidentical or natural hormones. Theoretically they are suggested to proffer advantage in that they are more closely aligned with the innate hormones seen in the body and can be individually tailored (when compounded), but they should not automatically be considered the safer option. Both the Therapeutic Goods Administration of Australia and The Federal Drug Administration in the United States consider the adverse effects of HT as reported to be a 'class effect'—that is, that bioidentical hormones can be considered to have the same risks and benefits as conventional HT. In fact most conventional HT used in Australia already uses oestradiol and other forms considered to be bioidentical. However, progestin is known to have very different, often contradictory, physiological actions to natural progesterone in many women. Regardless, focusing solely on direct hormone replacement does not address the underlying causes of the symptoms experienced by perimenopausal women and therefore when used alone may not be reflective of naturopathic or holistic best practice. While HT use is ultimately a matter for discussion between doctor and patient, it should form only part of the treatment strategy in the naturopathic management of menopause.

HT may be recommended in certain circumstances—specifically, distressing symptoms or significant osteoporosis.[1] Longer term use of HT is generally considered a matter for discussion between doctor and patient, with risks taken into account in addition to potential benefit to bone health and quality of life. Generally, long-term use is discouraged and doctors are encouraged to use lower therapeutic doses.

Various forms of oestrogen have been used for many years as a hormonal supplement to treat menopausal symptoms and are generally thought to be the most effective treatment for vasomotor symptoms. Oestrogen is therefore no longer recommended for preventing chronic conditions, although it is effective and approved for osteoporosis prevention.[3] Women with an intact uterus are usually prescribed the 'opposed' regimen (when oestrogen is combined with a progestin to avoid the development of endometrial hyperplasia and endometrial cancer). Testosterone may also be given to women. Examples of commonly used HT in Australia are listed in Tables 24.1 and 24.2.

However, much conventional medical treatment of menopause is comprised of educational and lifestyle management of symptoms. Several other classes of prescription medications are also used to treat menopausal symptoms, including antihypertensive medications such as clonidine for hot flushes and various antidepressants or anxiolytics

Table 24.1
Common forms of oestrogens prescribed in menopause

Generic name	Proprietary name(s) (examples)	Daily dose range	Usual daily protective dose
Oral			
Conjugated equine oestrogen	Premarin	0.3–2.5 mg	0.625 mg
Oestradiol valerate	Progynova	1.0–4.0 mg	2.0 mg
Oestriol	Ovestin	1.0–4.0 mg	2.0 mg
Piperazine oestrone sulphate	Ogen	0.625–5 mg	1.25 mg
Implants			
Oestradiol	Oestradiol implants	20–100 mg	50 mg
Skin patch			
Oestradiol	Various	25–100 µg every 3½ to 7 days	50 µg
Topical gel			
Oestradiol 0.1%	Sandrena	0.5–1.5 mg	1 mg
Nasal spray			
Oestradiol	Aerodiol	150–600 µg	300 µg
Vaginal preparations			
Creams			
Oestriol 1 mg/g	Ovestin	0.5 g	0.5 g
Pessaries			
Oestradiol	Vagifem	25 µg	1 pessary (25 µg)
Oestriol	Ovestin ovula	0.5 mg	0.5 mg

Source: Society of Obstetricians and Gynaecologists of Canada 2009[1]

Table 24.2
Progestogens often used in menopause

Generic name	Daily dose range	Usual daily protective dose
Dydrogesterone	10–20 mg	10 mg
Medroxyprogesterone acetate	2.5–20 mg	10 mg
Norethisterone	1.25–5 mg	2.5 mg

for psychological symptoms. Much of this research has come from the treatment of menopausal women with breast cancer, in whom hormone therapy is contraindicated.

KEY TREATMENT PROTOCOLS

Perimenopause is a natural stage of life and not a disease or a disorder. Therefore it does not in-and-of itself require medical intervention or treatment. However, this natural transition is not always a smooth one and in certain cases the physical, mental and emotional effects associated with peri-menopause can be quite severe and may significantly disrupt the lives of women experiencing them. Naturopathic treatment therefore focuses on reducing these effects and ensuring quality of life throughout this

> ### Naturopathic Treatment Aims
>
> - Improve quality of life.
> - Reduce symptoms (hot flushes, psychological symptoms and fatigue).
> - Maintain ideal weight and health parameters (for cardiovascular and bone health).
> - Manage stress.
> - Address sexual health.
> - Modify diet to improve symptoms and to reduce osteoporosis and cardiovascular risk.

transition. Various lifestyle and dietary habits can have significant effects on the severity of menopausal symptoms, so treatment should otherwise focus on ensuring optimal health.

Naturopathic treatment focuses on general improvement in physiology as opposed to correction or counteracting the effects of menopause with oestrogen supplementation. Many clinicians make the assumption that only climacteric symptoms are of concern in menopausal patients. As naturopathic treatment of a perimenopausal patient is focused on supportive care throughout the process, rather than correction of an aetiological or pathological condition, a broader clinical enquiry that extends beyond symptoms relating to oestrogen deficiency needs to be undertaken. Enquiries need to be made about mental state—anger and irritability, depression, moodiness, loss of self-esteem and sleeping difficulties. Sexual function and urinary function also need to be explored in depth.

Ameliorating hot flushes

Because **exercise** has demonstrated effects on sex steroids, it may moderate at least the severity, if not the frequency, of hot flushes.[5,7–9] One epidemiological study found that women who belonged to a gymnasium club reported lower incidence of hot flushes than those who were not, although their individual exercise regimens were unreported.[10] However, studies on exercise, while generally demonstrating reduced severity and incidence of hot flushes, suggest it has had the greatest effect on quality-of-life scores.

A 2007 systematic review of 17 trials of which 11 could be included showed a demonstrated effect of *Trifolium pratense* in reducing hot flush symptoms in menopause.[22]

A 2005 review of trials found 12 clinical trials of *Actaea racemosa* (black cohosh: BC) in vasomotor symptoms, all but one of which demonstrated benefit,[27] and a later non-specific review found significant benefit also.[28]

Actaea racemosa may act through a number of pathways independent of its activity as a phyto-oestrogen. Recent evidence suggests that it may have an effect on opiate receptors.[29] BC extract has also been demonstrated to exert dopaminergic activity in vitro.[30] This may in part also explain the effects of BC in menopause as dopaminergic drugs are often used to treat menopausal symptoms such as hot flushes. Some studies have suggested that BC has an equipotent effect to oestrogen,[31] although this does not

The importance of empathy

Improving health parameters more generally will improve symptoms. Patients should be moved towards a general health program as soon as possible as this will ultimately improve their symptoms and lessen their duration. It should also be noted that the menopausal transition is experienced differently by each woman, and what works in one patient may not be suitable for another. Much of the distress associated with perimenopause can be exacerbated by cultural stigma or confusion. Patients may need to be reminded that the transition is not 'the end' of anything and may need to be reassured through the process.

Many practitioners, both naturopathic and allopathic, tend to underestimate the effects of perimenopausal symptoms on their patients.[11] However, fewer than 25% of women experience a (relatively) symptom-free menopause and over 25% of women experience debilitating symptoms.[12] The importance of support, empathy and education in treatment should not be ignored in patients undergoing the menopausal transition, as many women turn to practitioners for explanation and reassurance rather than treatment.[13] This is particularly true in complementary medicine practice. Women undergoing the menopause transition turn to complementary medicines not only to seek effective treatment but also to gain greater control over their symptoms.[14] It is therefore essential that a strong participatory relationship is encouraged during treatment and that the naturopath does not fall into the habit of product-prescribing only.

When looking at the literature there seems to be little relation to gross product sales (i.e. the most commonly sold complementary therapies for menopause) and evidence for specific clinical effectiveness in the menopause. However, these therapies may be working on broader improvements or act on a psychosomatic level by offering the patients the opportunity to take control of their condition. For example, while acupuncture does not seem to have specific effects on menopausal symptoms such as hot flushes[15] it does seem to offer improvements to quality of life scores in perimenopausal women overall.[16]

Oestrogen-like compounds and oestrogen receptor activity

Many compounds—both natural and synthetic—may mimic endogenous sex hormones.[15-17] **Phyto-oestrogens** may bind to and activate these oestrogen receptor sites. Given the use of hormone replacement therapy in conventional treatment, these compounds are gaining popularity amongst both the public and practitioners for relieving menopausal symptoms.

For example, the phyto-oestrogenic isoflavones found in *Trifolium pratense* and soy are thought to have beneficial effects on cognitive abilities, bone mineral density and plasma lipid concentrations in menopausal women.[18] Phyto-oestrogenic activity may also be utilised in traditional Chinese medicine. *Astragalus membranaceus* and *Scutellaria baicalensis* are traditionally used to treat menopausal symptoms in traditional Chinese medicine and exert oestrogenic activity in vivo.[19]

Dietary intake of phyto-oestrogens and an increased consumption of wholegrain foods may also be associated with a reduction in vasomotor symptoms.[20] A 12-week study of perimenopausal women consuming a phyto-oestrogen-rich diet (miso, flax and tofu) observed better improvement in hot flushes and vaginal dryness than women consuming a regular diet.[21]

Many compounds exerting oestrogenic activity will be discussed in relation to symptoms. Although many of these compounds have not been studied specifically for menopausal symptoms, phyto-oestrogens are discussed in more detail in Chapter 22 on endometriosis.

seem reflective of the entirety of the data.[32,33] It should be noted, however, that significant heterogeneity exists in the results for differing formulations, suggesting that quality issues need to be considered before prescribing.

Angelica sinensis and **Matricaria recutita** in combination has been demonstrated to reduce hot flushes and improve sleep in menopausal women,[34] but other trials have failed to demonstrate these results when *Angelica sinensis* was used alone.[35,36]

> ## Black cohosh safety
>
> Although concerns relating to the hepatotoxicity of *Actaea racemosa* have been raised, systematic reviews have suggested it can be generally thought to be a safe medicine, with the main side effects being mild and reversible, and no direct causal link to BC was found in cases of severe hepatotoxicity.[23] In the most recent trial, long-term supplementation of BC for a period of one year was found to have no effects on hepatic blood flow or liver function.[24] However, an association does exist as hepatotoxicity has occurred in several people taking supplements containing BC, though the causative relationship remains highly controversial.[25] This is thought to be related to issues of product quality, concomitant medications or individual genetic susceptibility. Although the specific mechanism relating to hepatotoxicity associated with BC use is unknown, one theory gaining credence is an immunological reaction to triterpene glycosides in the plant in susceptible individuals, rather than the direct result of inherent toxicity.[26] Therefore these issues should be considered when advising or treating patients using these therapies, as they should be for any other pharmacological intervention.

Humulus lupulus supplementation over 12 weeks was found to reduce discomforting symptoms of menopause, particularly hot flushes, even at low doses.[37] This is thought to be due to the oestrogenic nature of *Humulus lupulus*.[38] ***Salvia officinalis*** was also demonstrated to improve symptoms of hot flushes and nights sweats in perimenopausal women.[39]

Several trials have shown that **relaxation training** can have positive effects on hot flush symptoms.[40–43] These include biofeedback, breathing exercises and meditation. **Yoga** may also be beneficial in reducing menopausal symptoms exacerbated by mental stress.[44,45]

Addressing psychological symptoms

Panax ginseng has been demonstrated to improve psychological symptoms, particularly fatigue, insomnia and depression, in menopausal women.[46] In menopausal women with psychological and psychosomatic symptoms, sole therapy using ***Hypericum perforatum*** demonstrated significant improvement (76.4% self-evaluation and 79.2% clinician evaluation), including improved sexual wellbeing.[47] ***Piper methysticum*** as an adjuvant treatment has been demonstrated to reduce anxiety in perimenopausal women.[48] It may also be useful in treating sleep disorders not associated with vasomotor symptoms that are often experienced by perimenopausal women (see Chapter 16 on insomnia).

Treatment with a combination *Hypericum perforatum* and BC product for 16 weeks resulted in a 50% reduction in menopause rating scale (MRS) scores, with a 41.8% reduction in the Hamilton depression rating scale.[49] Although BC may be effective in treating neurovegetative symptoms of depression in menopausal women, combination treatment was more effective than BC treatment alone.[18] These changes seem more significant than the effects on vasomotor symptoms alone. And while *Hypericum perforatum* does not seem to exert a significant effect on hot flush symptoms, it does proffer significant improvement on quality-of-life scales due to its effect on other symptoms associated with the menopause.[50] BC also has positive effects on overall quality-of-life scales and other broader menopause rating scales when used alone in addition to its effects on individual symptoms.[51,52] Several relaxation therapies have also proven to be effective in alleviating or reducing a number of perimenopausal symptoms, rather than having specific outcomes.

Addressing urogenital symptoms

Improving sexual function and libido

Women undergoing the perimenopausal transition often experience changes in libido or dyspareunia, which can be influenced by a number of physiological or psycho-social ways. Hormone changes may influence sexual function in a number of ways. Low levels of oestrogens and androgens seem to be directly related to libido, as do low levels of testosterone.[53] Physical changes enacted by alterations in hormone levels—for example, vaginal dryness associated with lower levels of oestrogen—will have a signifi-cant negative effect on sexual response. Lack of lubrication can result in soreness and tenderness, and ultimately less enjoyment during sexual encounters for these reasons. Anticipation of painful sex due to lack of lubrication after a negative experience may further decrease desire. Patients need to be counselled adequately on the practical impli-cations of the menopausal transition as many women may not have previously needed to apply measures such as endogenous lubrication. Oestrogens also have a vasodilatory effect that can result in increased blood flow in vaginal, clitoral and urethral areas; this may reduce during menopause, and loss of oestrogen is also associated with relaxation of vaginal tissue and muscle tone in genital areas. Encouraging circulation and tone in these areas—for example, through **pelvic floor exercises** or more general regimens such as exercise, yoga or Tai chi—may also be useful.

Physical changes alone are not solely responsible for the negative effects of the peri-menopausal transition on sexual function and libido. Psychological changes such as depression, anxiety and low self-esteem can all affect sexual desire and enjoyment, as can many of the medicines prescribed for these conditions. Conversely, the effects of menopausal changes on a woman's sex life can also precipitate psychological changes. The social construct of menopause in modern society can also have a deleterious effect in this regard. Menopause in Western societies is often viewed negatively, particularly in relation to the loss of femininity. This is in stark contrast to many traditional cultures, who often view the transition as a positive one that affords them respect as elders and relief from child-bearing. Patients need to be counselled appropriately throughout this period, encouraged to explore their femininity and sexual selves and reminded that these aspects of themselves need not diminish once menstruation ceases. One study has shown that while yoga therapy did not increase general self-esteem, it was significant in improving esteem relating to perceived sexual attractiveness.[54]

Many **herbal medicines** have been used to increase libido. *Asparagus racemosus* is colloquially referred to as 'she with one thousand husbands' in the Ayurvedic tradition in reference to its effects on sexual function and has demonstrated positive results in animal studies, but is yet to be tested through human trials.[55] This situation is also true of other traditionally used aphrodisiac herbs such as *Turnera diffusa* and *Tribulus terrestris*. A product containing *Panax ginseng*, *Turnera diffusa*, *Ginkgo biloba* and L-arginine has been found to significantly increase libido in women at all stages of the menopausal transition compared with placebo in two small trials.[56,57]

Treating the psychological symptoms associated with menopause may also improve libido. *Hypericum perforatum*—a herb commonly used to treat the psychosocial problems associated with menopause—was found to improve libido when used to treat seasonal affective disorder[58] and improved sexual wellbeing in 80% of perimenopausal women when prescribed for psychosocial symptoms.[51] *Trigonella foenum-graecum* has been used for postmenopausal vaginal dryness in the North American naturopathic tradition.[59]

Vaginal atrophy and incontinence

After menopause the vaginal lining may thin due to lower oestrogen levels. This may result in painful intercourse and a greater susceptibility to vaginal infections. Regular intercourse may be beneficial as it increases blood flow to the genitalia, but adequate lubrication is required—natural or supplemental. Naturopathic treatment options for recurrent bladder infections are covered in Chapter 30.

Vitamin D may have a role in reducing vaginal atrophy. Supplementation with vitamin D has reduced vaginal atrophy in one small trial.[60]

Incontinence incidence may increase in postmenopausal women. Many women may resign themselves to this being a normal part of the ageing process, but there are several therapeutic options available. **Pelvic floor exercises** may reduce the incidence of incontinence in postmenopausal women and improve quality of life.[61] Increased **physical exercise** more generally may also be beneficial in reducing the incidence or severity of urinary incontinence.[62]

Urinary tract infections

Approximately 15% of menopausal women will experience frequent bladder infections.[2] General recommendations for urinary tract infections are discussed in Chapter 30 on urinary tract infection, but there are several factors to take into consideration when treating urinary tract infections in perimenopausal women, such as decreased acidity of the urine and loss of bladder elasticity, due to lower oestrogen levels and the fact that urinary tract infections are often symptomless during the menopause. A trial of oral lactobacilli supplementation was found to improve vaginal flora in peri- and postmenopausal women, highlighting its importance for promoting urogenital health.[63]

Long-term considerations

Although much focus tends to be drawn towards the association between hormone therapy and increasing breast cancer, other modifiable lifestyle factors such as little exercise, smoking, postmenopausal weight gain and high alcohol consumption have similar rates of increased risk of breast cancer.[4] And although fat intake alone is not associated with increased risk of breast cancer, attention to this lifestyle factor can help to improve the cardiovascular outcomes usually associated with the menopausal transition.[64] Attention needs to be paid to the long-term consequences of the menopausal transition as well as short-term symptomatic treatment.

Dietary modification is an essential part of treating a perimenopausal patient. Not only are long-term risks such as osteoporosis and cardiovascular health significantly affected by dietary intakes but dietary factors also have important effects on symptom severity during the menopausal transition. No consultation is complete without investigation of the dietary component. The two key long-term issues that clinicians should consider concern osteoporosis and cardiovascular disease.

Mitigating potential osteoporosis

In a clinical setting osteoporosis is often addressed in the context of menopausal treatment because it is found in postmenopausal women and can be largely prevented by correcting oestrogen deficiency. Approximately 30% of postmenopausal women are estimated to have osteoporosis.[58] The hypo-oestrogenic state leads to loss of bone density in postmenopausal women by activation of the bone remodelling units with an excess of bone resorption compared with bone formation.[65]

Adequate dietary intakes are necessary for prevention and treatment of osteoporosis. Diets high in calcium-rich foods, leafy vegetables and some phyto-oestrogens and low in refined carbohydrates and acidic foods should be encouraged, as well as increased sun exposure for vitamin D. Another dietary intervention that may be beneficial for osteoporosis in postmenopausal women is **omega-3 fatty acids**. Several human and animal studies have shown significant decreases in bone resorption and a protective effect on bone with omega-3 fatty acids.[66–68]

Adequate **calcium** and **vitamin D** consumption are essential in the treatment of osteoporosis. It is generally recommended that 1500 mg of calcium and 800 IU per day of vitamin D are recommended for postmenopausal women.[1] Dietary sources of calcium are listed in Table 24.3. However, dietary intake of calcium alone may not be sufficient, particularly in women who have undergone early menopause.[69] Sunlight exposure of 5–10 minutes per day may be required, particularly considering that older people may synthesise vitamin D less well over time. Supplementation of both calcium and vitamin D may be necessary. However, large studies such as the Women's Health Initiative have shown that reliance on supplementation can be fraught, as compliance can be low—only 59% of women were taking more than 80% of their recommended supplementation towards the study's end.[70] Dietary modification should therefore form

Table 24.3
Calcium content of foods

Food	Amount	Calcium content (mg)
Yoghurt	200 g (1 small tub)	520
Calcium-enriched milk	250 mL (1 mug)	475
Skim milk	250 mL (1 mug)	400
Tahini	20 g	310
Full-fat milk	250 mL (1 mug)	300
Calcium-enriched soy milk	250 mL (1 mug)	290
Sardines	5 whole	286
Cheddar cheese	30 g (1 slice)	232
Parmesan cheese	20 g	230
Salmon (tinned)	½ cup with bones	220
Prawns	1 cup	132
Mussels	6 whole	120
Dried figs	3	108
Tofu	80 g	96
Ice-cream	60 g (2 scoops)	90
Soy beans, chickpeas or kidney beans	½ cup	70
Dried apricots	10 halves	42
Silverbeet or spinach	½ cup	38
Oranges	1 whole	35
Broccoli	1 cup	25

Source: Reeves et al. 2007[4]

the basis of treatment. More dietary recommendations for bone health can be found in Chapter 25 on osteoarthritis.

Phyto-oestrogenic food therapy may offer a limited protective role.[71] Considering that HT and SORM therapy are both used to prevent the effects of osteoporosis, this is worth exploring. Increased soy consumption may inhibit bone resorption and stimulate bone formation[72,73] and population studies indicate that the incidence of osteoporosis is lower in countries with higher soy consumption.[21]

Regular exercise can increase bone density in postmenopausal women.[70] However, high impact exercise may be counterproductive as more severe forms of exercise may result in micro-damage, increasing the risk of fracture.[74] Regular Tai chi exercise may improve bone density scores and offer protection against fracture in postmenopausal women.[75] Further benefits of specific exercises are discussed in Chapter 25 on osteoarthritis.

Improving cardiovascular health

Women are afforded a higher degree of protection against cardiovascular disease before menopause due to higher oestrogen levels. However, reductions in oestrogen levels postmenopause result in women having the same incidence of cardiovascular disease as men by the age of 70 years.[76] Despite this protective mechanism it is still estimated that 94% of adverse cardiovascular risk in women is associated with modifiable risk factors such as type 2 diabetes, hypertension, diet, stress, smoking and obesity.[77] Therefore women who have previously not had to consider cardiovascular health implications may need to investigate this issue in more depth (see Chapters 11–13 on the cardiovascular system).

INTEGRATIVE MEDICAL CONSIDERATIONS

Acupuncture and osteopathy

Acupuncture does offer specific effects on menopausal symptoms such as hot flushes,[22,78] but demonstrates significantly greater improvements to quality of life scores in perimenopausal women more broadly.[16] Traditional Chinese medicine has a long history of treating menopausal symptoms and, typically, acupuncture would not be used alone.[79] However, to be effective these treatments need to be prescribed according to traditional Chinese medicine theory. One small trial of osteopathic manipulations has demonstrated improvements in menopausal symptoms.[80]

Exercise

As well as the benefits of regular exercise in treating specific menopausal symptoms such as hot flushes previously outlined, exercise confers a number of other benefits in perimenopausal patients. These benefits include decreased bone loss and improved circulation, cardiovascular function, mental wellbeing, endurance and energy. Perimenopausal patients usually comprise an older demographic than the typical patient, and encouraging healthy behaviours can ensure healthy ageing and protection against many age-related conditions. Although the evidence for yoga in menopausal hot flushes is equivocal,[81] yoga has been shown to improve broader menopausal symptoms such as quality of life[82] and psychological outcomes associated with the menopausal transition,[83] or may proffer improvements in specific symptoms such as insomnia in menopausal patients.[84]

CLINICAL SUMMARY

Perimenopause is a natural part of the lifecycle and therefore symptoms are not necessarily indicative of pathology. As a natural process the patient needs to be supported, not treated. The changes will result in symptoms and these can be expected to continue for some time (one year or more). Naturopathic treatments will not be instantaneous; for example, *Actaea racemosa* treatment will require two weeks to observe its effect and three months before optimal benefit can be observed.[62]

It is important to note that empowerment of patients is particularly useful for managing perimenopausal symptoms. Patients should be involved in the treatment process as much as is practicable, and a shift towards self-care modalities is encouraged and some effort spent on developing a positive and empathetic therapeutic relationship with the patient.

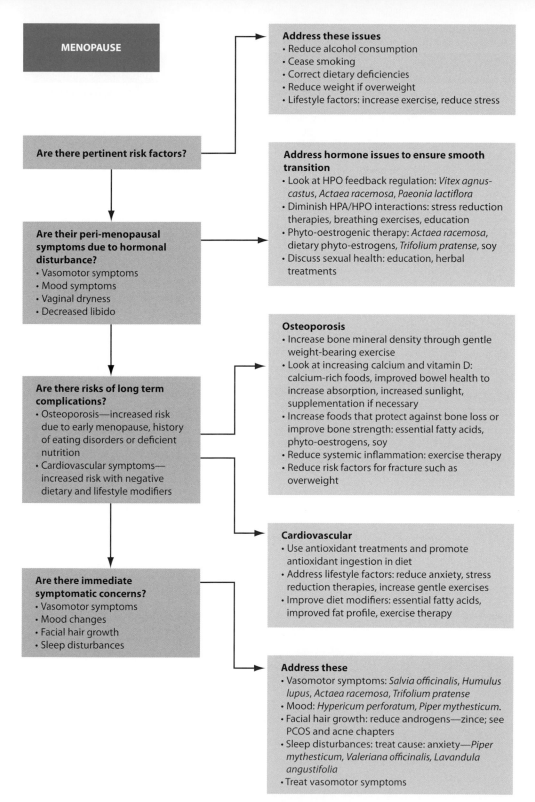

MENOPAUSE

Address these issues
- Reduce alcohol consumption
- Cease smoking
- Correct dietary deficiencies
- Reduce weight if overweight
- Lifestyle factors: increase exercise, reduce stress

Are there pertinent risk factors?

Address hormone issues to ensure smooth transition
- Look at HPO feedback regulation: *Vitex agnus-castus*, *Actaea racemosa*, *Paeonia lactiflora*
- Diminish HPA/HPO interactions: stress reduction therapies, breathing exercises, education
- Phyto-oestrogenic therapy: *Actaea racemosa*, dietary phyto-estrogens, *Trifolium pratense*, soy
- Discuss sexual health: education, herbal treatments

Are their peri-menopausal symptoms due to hormonal disturbance?
- Vasomotor symptoms
- Mood symptoms
- Vaginal dryness
- Decreased libido

Osteoporosis
- Increase bone mineral density through gentle weight-bearing exercise
- Look at increasing calcium and vitamin D: calcium-rich foods, improved bowel health to increase absorption, increased sunlight, supplementation if necessary
- Increase foods that protect against bone loss or improve bone strength: essential fatty acids, phyto-oestrogens, soy
- Reduce systemic inflammation: exercise therapy
- Reduce risk factors for fracture such as overweight

Are there risks of long term complications?
- Osteoporosis—increased risk due to early menopause, history of eating disorders or deficient nutrition
- Cardiovascular symptoms—increased risk with negative dietary and lifestyle modifiers

Cardiovascular
- Use antioxidant treatments and promote antioxidant ingestion in diet
- Address lifestyle factors: reduce anxiety, stress reduction therapies, increase gentle exercises
- Improve diet modifiers: essential fatty acids, improved fat profile, exercise therapy

Are there immediate symptomatic concerns?
- Vasomotor symptoms
- Mood changes
- Facial hair growth
- Sleep disturbances

Address these
- Vasomotor symptoms: *Salvia officinalis*, *Humulus lupus*, *Actaea racemosa*, *Trifolium pratense*
- Mood: *Hypericum perforatum*, *Piper mythesticum*.
- Facial hair growth: reduce androgens—zince; see PCOS and acne chapters
- Sleep disturbances: treat cause: anxiety—*Piper mythesticum*, *Valeriana officinalis*, *Lavandula angustifolia*
- Treat vasomotor symptoms

Figure 24.2
Naturopathic treatment decision tree—menopause

Table 24.4
Review of the major evidence*

Intervention	Mechanisms of action	Key literature	Summary of results	Comment
Actaea racemosa	Dopaminergic stimulation Opiate receptor stimulation Oestrogen receptor stimulation	Systematic review, meta-analysis: Geller & Studee 2005[21] Leach & Moore 2012[27] 16 RCTs with 2027 women	A majority of trials do support the use of *Actaea racemosa* in vasomotor symptoms; however, these are not confirmed by meta-analysis, which shows *Actaea racemosa* to have no demonstrated benefit above placebo	Although *Actaea racemosa* has been demonstrated to improve vasomotor symptoms and menopause and quality of life scores, there are marked differences between various formulations, suggesting quality issues need to be appropriately explored when prescribing
Humulus lupulus	Phyto-oestrogenic modulation Hypothermic effects	RCT: Heyerick et al. 2003[40] 12-week RCT ($n = 67$) Groups received either 100 mg or 250 mg *Humulus lupulus* extract	Hot flush frequency was significantly decreased at six weeks but not 12 weeks Results were not dose-dependent, with lower dose achieving better results at both six and 12 weeks	Although promising, this trial is hampered by its small study size Given that it affirms traditional use, further studies are warranted
Trifolium pratense	Phyto-oestrogenic modulation	Systematic review, meta-anlaysis: Coon et al. 2007[26] Lethaby et al. 2007[85]	A 2007 systematic review of 17 trials of which 11 could be included showed a demonstrated effect of *Trifolium pratense* in reducing hot flush symptoms in menopause. Meta-analysis indicated a weighted mean reduction of 1.5 hot flushes in the treatment group against placebo Another review analysed fewer trials and found no significant effect beyond placebo	There is significant heterogeneity between trial methodologies and product quality

Table 24.4
Review of the major evidence* (continued)

Intervention	Mechanisms of action	Key literature	Summary of results	Comment
Salvia officinalis and *Medicago sativa*	Mechanisms of action currently unknown	Open trial: De Leo et al. 1998[52] Open trial of 30 women	Twenty women had vasomotor symptoms completely disappear, four women had significantly reduced symptoms and six women showed some reduction in symptom scores	While affirming traditional use, this study suffers from poor design and further trials are necessary
Exercise	Modulates neuroendocrine system Mood-elevating effect	Systematic review Daley et al. 2011[82]	Exercise did not improve vasomotor symptoms better than HT and though there was a trend for improvements in vasomotor symptoms, these were not always significant	The existing studies provided insufficient evidence to determine the effectiveness of exercise as a treatment for vasomotor menopausal symptoms, or whether exercise is more effective than HT or yoga
Acupuncture	Unknown from a Western medicine perspective, thought to be focused on traditional theory of 'clearing heat' and 'nourishing Yin'	Cochrane review: Dodin et al. 2013[86]	Hot flush frequency was significantly reduced in acupuncture versus control group Hot flush intensity in acupuncture group versus control group also significantly better	Acupuncture has no improvement over sham acupuncture, but does have significant treatment over no treatment
Phyto-oestrogen-rich diet	Selective oestrogen receptor modulator	RCT: Murkies et al. 2008[8] Six-week RCT ($n = 58$) Groups randomised to diets supplemented with soy or wholegrain wheat flour	Significant reduction in vasomotor symptoms in soy ($\downarrow$ 40%) and wheat groups ($\downarrow$ 25%) ($p \leq 0.001$) Significant reductions also observed in menopause scores and FSH levels	More rapid reduction observed in soy group

*As menopause is not a defined medical condition but rather a collection of symptoms associated with a transitional stage through life, many of the treatments are covered in other relevant chapters.

KEY POINTS

- Menopause is a natural process and patients need to be supported through it, not 'treated'.
- Improving health parameters more generally will improve symptoms.
- Menopause is experienced differently by each woman; what works in many of your patients may not work in your current patient. Particular care in this regard needs to be undertaken when developing a herbal or nutritional prescription.
- Much of the distress of perimenopause is associated with stigma or confusion. Remind your patients that this is not 'the end' of anything and provide reassurance.
- Involve patients in treatment processes—encourage a shift towards self-care modalities.

FURTHER READING

Hudson T. Women's encyclopedia of natural medicine. New York: McGraw-Hill; 2008.

Leach M, Moore V. Black cohosh (Cimicifuga spp.) for menopausal symptoms. Cochrane Database Syst Rev 2012;(9):CD007244.

Moore TR, Franks RB, Fox C. Review of efficacy of complementary and alternative medicine treatments for menopausal symptoms. J Midwifery Womens Health 2017;62(3):286–97.

Roberts H, Hickey M. Managing the menopause: an update. Maturitas 2016;86:53–8.

Tonob D, Melby MK. Broadening our perspectives on complementary and alternative medicine for menopause: a narrative review. Maturitas 2017;99:79–85.

REFERENCES

1. Society of Obstetricians and Gynaecologists of Canada. Menopause and osteoporosis update. J Obstet Gynaecol Can 2009;31(1):S27–30.
2. Edmonds K, editor. Obstetrics & gynaecology. London: Blackwell; 2007.
3. Nelson H. Menopause. Lancet 2008;371(9614):760–70.
4. Reeves G, Pirie K, Beral V, et al. Million Women Study Collaboration. Cancer incidence and mortality in relation to body mass index in the Million Women Study: cohort study. BMJ 2007;335:1134.
5. Col N, Guthrie J, Politi M, et al. Duration of vasomotor symptoms in middle-aged women: a longitudinal study. Menopause 2009;16(3):453–7.
6. Greendale G, Gold E. Lifestyle factors: are they related to vasomotor symptoms and do they modify the effectiveness or side effects of hormone therapy? Am J Med 2005;118(12):148–54.
7. Zhang C, Wang S, Zhang Y, et al. In vitro estrogenic activities of Chinese medicinal plants traditionally used for the management of menopausal symptoms. J Ethnopharmacol 2005;98(3):295–300.
8. Murkies A, Lombard C, Strauss B, et al. Dietary flour supplementation decreases post-menopausal hot flushes: effect of soy and wheat. Maturitas 2008;61(1–2):27–33.
9. Brzezinski A, Adlercreutz H, Shaoul R, et al. Short-term effects of phytoestrogen-rich diet on postmenopausal women. Menopause 1997;4(2):89–94.
10. Ivarsson T, Spetz A, Hammar M. Physical exercise and vasomotor symptoms in postmenopausal women. Maturitas 1998;29(2):139–46.
11. Ghali W, Freund K, Boss R, et al. Menopausal hormone therapy: physician awareness of patient attitudes. Am J Med 1997;103:3.
12. Porter M, Penney G, Russell D, et al. A population based survey of women's experience of the menopause. Br J Obstet Gynaecol 2002;103:1025–8.
13. Murtagh J. General practice. Sydney: McGraw-Hill; 2007.
14. Gollschewski S, Kitto S, Anderson D, et al. Women's perceptions and beliefs about the use of complementary and alternative medicines during menopause. Complement Ther Med 2008;16(3):163–8.
15. Lee M, Shin B, Ernst E. Acupuncture for treating menopausal hot flushes: a systematic review. Climacteric 2009;12(1):16–25.
16. Ailfhaily F, Ewies A. Acupuncture in managing menopausal symptoms: hope or mirage? Climacteric 2007;10(5):371–80.
17. Poluzzi E, Piccinni C, Raschi E, et al. Phytoestrogens in postmenopause: the state of the art from a chemical, pharmacological and regulatory perspective. Curr Med Chem 2014;21(4):417–36.
18. Briese V, Stammwitz U, Friede M, et al. Black cohosh with or without St. John's wort for symptom-specific climacteric treatment–results of a large-scale, controlled, observational study. Maturitas 2007;57(4):405–14.
19. Al-Akoum M, Maunsell E, Verreault R, et al. Effect of Hypericum perforatum (St John's Wort) on hot flashes and quality of life in perimenopausal women: a randomized pilot trial. Menopause 2009;16(2):307–14.
20. Mollá M, García-Sánchez Y, Sarri A, et al. Cimicifuga racemosa treatment and health related quality of life in post-menopausal Spanish women. Gynecol Endocrinol 2009;25(1):21–6.
21. Geller S, Studee L. Soy and red clover for mid-life and aging. Climacteric 2006;9(4):245–63.
22. Lindh-Astrand L, Nedstrand E, Wyon Y, et al. Vasomotor symptoms and quality of life in previously sedentary postmenopausal women randomised to physical activity or estrogen therapy. Maturitas 2004;48(2):97–105.
23. Thurston R, Joffe H, Soares C, et al. Physical activity and risk of vasomotor symptoms in women with and without a history of depression: results from the Harvard Study of Moods and Cycles. Menopause 2006;13:553–60.

24. Hammar M, Berg G, Lindgren R. Does physical exercise influence the frequency of postmenopausal hot flushes? Acta Obstet Gynecol Scand 1990;69(5):409–12.

25. Teschke R. Black cohosh and suspected hepatotoxicity: inconsistencies, confounding variables, and prospective use of a diagnostic causality algorithm. A critical review. Menopause 2010;17(2):426–40.

26. Coon J, Pittler M, Ernst E. Trifolium pratense isoflavones in the treatment of menopausal hot flushes: a systematic review and meta-analysis. Phytomedicine 2007;14(2–3):153–9.

27. Leach M, Moore V. Black cohosh (Cimicifuga spp.) for menopausal symptoms. Cochrane Database Syst Rev 2012;(9):CD007244.

28. Nasr A, Nafeh H. Influence of black cohosh (Cimicifuga racemosa) use by postmenopausal women on total hepatic perfusion and liver functions. Fertil Steril 2009;92(5):1780–2.

29. Chitturi S, Farrell G. Hepatotoxic slimming aids and other herbal hepatotoxins. J Gastrolenterol Hepatol 2008;23:366–73.

30. Geller S, Studee L. Botanical and dietary supplements for menopausal symptoms: what works, what does not. J Womens Health (Larchmt) 2005;14(7):634–49.

31. Cheema D, Coomarasamy A, El-Toukhy T. Non-hormonal therapy of post-menopausal vasomotor symptoms: a structured evidence-based review. Arch Gynecol Obstet 2007;276(5):463–9.

32. Reame N, Lukacs J, Padmanabhan V, et al. Black cohosh has central opioid activity in postmenopausal women: evidence from naloxone blockade and positron emission tomography neuroimaging. Menopause 2008;15(5):832–40.

33. Jarry H, Metten M, Spengler B, et al. In vitro effects of the Cimicifuga racemosa extract BNO 1055. Maturitas 2003;44(Suppl. 1):31–8.

34. Wuttke W, Seidlová-Wuttke D, Gorkow C. The Cimicifuga preparation BNO 1055 vs. conjugated estrogens in a double-blind placebo-controlled study: effects on menopause symptoms and bone markers. Maturitas 2003;44(Suppl.): S67–77.

35. Borrelli F, Ernst E. Black cohosh (Cimicifuga racemosa) for menopausal symptoms: a systematic review of its efficacy. Pharmacol Res 2008;58(1):8–14.

36. Low Dog T. Menopause: a review of botanical dietary supplements. Am J Med 2005;118(Suppl12B):98–108.

37. Kupfersztain C, Rotem C, Fagot R, et al. The immediate effect of natural plant extract, Angelica sinensis and Matricaria chamomilla (Climex) for the treatment of hot flushes during menopause. A preliminary report. Clin Exp Obstet Gynecol 2003;30(4):203–6.

38. Haines CJ, Lam PM, Chung TK, et al. A randomized, double-blind, placebo-controlled study of the effect of a Chinese herbal medicine preparation (Dang Gui Buxue Tang) on menopausal symptoms in Hong Kong Chinese women.[see comment]. Climacteric 2008;11(3):244–51.

39. Hirata J, Swiersz L, Zell B, et al. Does dong quai have estrogenic effects in postmenopausal women? A double-blind, placebo-controlled trial. Fertil Steril 1997;68(6):981–6.

40. Heyerick A, Vervarcke S, Depypere H, et al. A first prospective, randomized, double-blind, placebo-controlled study on the use of a standardized hop extract to alleviate menopausal discomforts. Maturitas 2006;54(2):164–75.

41. Chadwick L, Pauli G, Farnsworth N. The pharmacognosy of Humulus lupulus L. (hops) with an emphasis on estrogenic properties. Phytomedicine 2006;13(1–2):119–31.

42. De Leo V, Lanzetta D, Cazzavacca R, et al. Treatment of neurovegetative menopausal symptoms with a phytotherapeutic agent. Minerva Ginecol 1998;50(5):207–11.

43. Carmody J, Crawford S, Churchill L. A pilot study of mindfulness-based stress reduction for hot flashes. Menopause 2006;13(5):760–9.

44. Freedman R, Woodward S. Behavioral treatment of menopausal hot flushes: evaluation by ambulatory monitoring. Am J Obstet Gynecol 1992;167(2):436–9.

45. Irvin J, Domar A, Clark C, et al. The effects of relaxation response training on menopausal symptoms. J Psychosom Obstet Gynaecol 1996;17(4):202–7.

46. Nedstrand E, Wijma K, Wyon Y, et al. Applied relaxation and oral estradiol treatment of vasomotor symptoms in postmenopausal women. Maturitas 2005;51(2):154–62.

47. Booth-LaForce C, Thurston R, Taylor M. A pilot study of a Hatha yoga treatment for menopausal symptoms. Maturitas 2007;57(3):286–95.

48. Chattha R, Raghuram N, Venkatram P, et al. Treating the climacteric symptoms in Indian women with an integrated approach to yoga therapy: a randomized control study. Menopause 2008;15(5):862–70.

49. Uebelhack R, Blohmer J, Graubaum H, et al. Black cohosh and St. John's wort for climacteric complaints: a randomized trial. Obstet Gynecol 2006;107(2.1):247–55.

50. Tode T, Kikuchi Y, Hirata J, et al. Effect of Korean red ginseng on psychological functions in patients with severe climacteric syndromes. Int J Gynaecol Obstet 1999;67(3):169–74.

51. Grube B, Walper A, Wheatley D. St. John's Wort extract: efficacy for menopausal symptoms of psychological origin. Adv Ther 1999;16(4):177–86.

52. De Leo V, la Marca A, Morgante G, et al. Evaluation of combining kava extract with hormone replacement therapy in the treatment of postmenopausal anxiety. Maturitas 2001;39(2):185–8.

53. Gracia C, Sammel M, Freeman E, et al. Predictors of decreased libido in women during the late reproductive years. Menopause 2004;11(2):144–50.

54. Elavsky S, McAuley E. Exercise and self-esteem in menopausal women: a randomized controlled trial involving walking and yoga. Am J Health Promot 2007;22(2):83–92.

55. Mills S, Bone K. Principles and practice of phytotherapy. 2nd ed. Edinburgh: Churchill Livingstone; 2013.

56. Ito T, Polan M, Whipple B, et al. The enhancement of female sexual function with ArginMax, a nutritional supplement, among women differing in menopausal status. J Sex Marital Ther 2006;32(5):369–78.

57. Ito T, Trant A, Polan M. A double-blind placebo-controlled study of ArginMax, a nutritional supplement for enhancement of female sexual function. J Sex Marital Ther 2001;27(5):541–9.

58. Bonaiuti D, Shea B, Iovine R, et al. Exercise for preventing and treating osteoporosis in postmenopausal women. Cochrane Database Syst Rev 2002;(3):CD000333.

59. Braun L, Cohen M. Herbs and natural supplements: an evidence-based guide. 3rd ed. Sydney: Elsevier; 2010.

60. Yildirim B, Kaleli B, Düzcan E, et al. The effects of postmenopausal vitamin D treatment on vaginal atrophy. Maturitas 2004;49(4):334–7.

61. Borello-France D, Downey P, Zyczynski H, et al. Continence and quality-of-life outcomes 6 months following an intensive pelvic-floor muscle exercise program for female stress urinary incontinence: a randomized trial comparing low- and high-frequency maintenance exercise. Phys Ther 2008;88(12):1545–53.

62. Peterson J. Minimize urinary incontinence: maximize physical activity in women. Urol Nurs 2008;28(5):351–6.

63. Petricevic L, Unger F, Viernstein H, et al. Randomized, double-blind, placebo-controlled study of oral lactobacilli to improve the vaginal flora of postmenopausal women. Eur J Obstet Gynecol Reprod Biol 2008;141(1):54–7.

64. Prentice R, Caan B, Chlebowski R, et al. Low-fat dietary pattern and risk of invasive breast cancer: the Women's Health Initiative randomized controlled dietary modification trial. JAMA 2006;295:629–42.

65. Bjarnason N. Postmenopausal bone remodelling and hormone replacement. Climacteric 1998;1(1):72–9.

66. Fernandes G, Lawrence R, Sun D. Protective role of n-3 lipids and soy protein in osteoporosis. Prostaglandins Leukot Essent Fatty Acids 2003;68(6):361–72.

67. Griel A, Kris-Etherton P, Hilpert K, et al. An increase in dietary n-3 fatty acids decreases a marker of bone resorption in humans. Nutr J 2007;6:2.

68. Sun D, Krishnan A, Zaman K, et al. Dietary n-3 fatty acids decrease osteoclastogenesis and loss of bone mass in ovariectomized mice. J Bone Miner Res 2003;18(7):1206–16.

69. Bischoff-Ferrari H, Willett W, Wong J, et al. Fracture prevention with vitamin D supplementation: a meta-analysis of randomized controlled trials. JAMA 2005;293:2257–64.

70. Jackson R, LaCroix A, Gass M, et al. Women's Health Initiative Investigators. Calcium plus vitamin D supplementation and the risk of fractures. N Engl J Med 2006;354:669–83.

71. Potter S, Baum J, Teng H, et al. Soy protein and isoflavones: their effects on blood lipids and bone density in postmenopausal women. Am J Clin Nutr 1998;83(Suppl.):1375S–1379S.

72. Ma D, Qin L, Wang P, et al. Soy isoflavone intake increases bone mineral density in the spine of menopausal women: meta-analysis of randomized controlled trials. Clin Nutr 2008;27(1):57–64.

73. Ma D, Qin L, Wang P, et al. Soy isoflavone intake inhibits bone resorption and stimulates bone formation in menopausal women: meta-analysis of randomized controlled trials. Eur J Clin Nutr 2008;62(2):155–61.

74. Rittweger J. Can exercise prevent osteoporosis? J Musculoskelet Neuronal Interact 2006;6(2):162–6.

75. Wayne P, Kiel D, Krebs D, et al. The effects of Tai Chi on bone mineral density in postmenopausal women: a systematic review. Arch Phys Med Rehabil 2007;88(5):673–80.

76. Tunstall-Pedoe H. Myth and paradox of coronary risk and menopause. Lancet 1998;351(9113):1425–7.

77. Yusuf S, Hawken S, Ounpuu S, et al. INTERHEART Study Investigators. Effect of potentially modifiable risk factors associated with myocardial infarction in 52 countries (the Interheart study): case-control study. Lancet 2004;364:937–52.

78. Borud E, Alraek T, White A, et al. The Acupuncture on Hot Flushes Among Menopausal Women (ACUFLASH) study, a randomized controlled trial. Menopause 2009;16(3):484–93.

79. Maciocia G. Obstetrics & gynecology in Chinese medicine. Edinburgh: Churchill Livingstone; 1997.

80. Cleary C, Fox J. Menopausal symptoms: an osteopathic investigation. Complement Ther Med 1994;2:181–6.

81. Daley A, Stokes-Lampard H, Macarthur C. Exercise for vasomotor menopausal symptoms. Cochrane Database Syst Rev 2011;(5):CD006108.

82. Joshi S, Khandwe R, Bapat D, et al. Effect of yoga on menopausal symptoms. Menopause Int 2011;17(3):78–81.

83. Cramer H, Lauche R, Langhorst J, et al. Effectiveness of yoga for menopausal symptoms: a systematic review and meta-analysis of randomized controlled trials. Evid Based Complement Alternat Med 2012;2012:863905.

84. Afonso R, Hachul H, Kozasa E, et al. Yoga decreases insomnia in postmenopausal women: a randomized clinical trial. Menopause 2012;19(2):186–93.

85. Lethaby A, Brown J, Marjoribanks J, et al. Phytoestrogens for vasomotor menopausal symptoms. Cochrane Database Syst Rev 2007;(4):CD001395.

86. Dodin S, Blanchet C, Marc I, et al. Acupuncture for menopausal hot flushes. Cochrane Database Syst Rev 2013;(7):Art. No.: CD007410, doi:10.1002/14651858. CD007410.pub2.

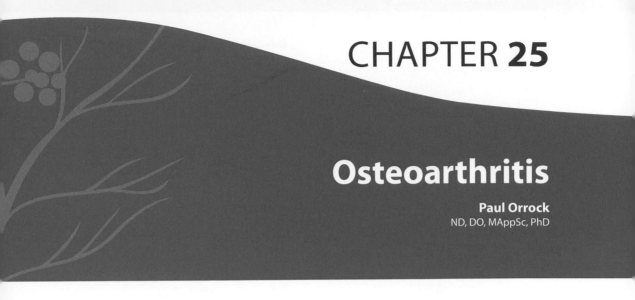

CHAPTER 25

Osteoarthritis

Paul Orrock
ND, DO, MAppSc, PhD

OVERVIEW

Osteoarthritis, also called degenerative joint disease, is primarily a disease of ageing, as 90% of all people have radiographic features of it in the weight-bearing joints by the age of 40 years.[1-3] It is defined by degeneration of the cartilage and subsequent hypertrophy of the bone surrounding the articulations. There are no systemic signs of disease with this condition. Typically the pain is localised to joints in a non-symmetrical pattern, and is usually relieved by rest and gentle motion. There are hereditary and mechanical risk factors involved in this condition, with obesity and repetitive mechanical loading especially provocative in the lower limb articulations. Degeneration in a joint can be primary by 'wear and tear' or secondary to an articular injury—for example a fracture, or metabolic diseases like hyperparathyroidism.[2,3]

Arthritis and musculoskeletal conditions are large contributors to illness, pain and disability.[3] Accounting for more than 4% of the overall disease burden, measured in terms of disability-adjusted life years (DALY), these conditions account for a significant proportion of healthy years of life lost. More than 6.1 million Australians are reported to have arthritis or a musculoskeletal condition.[4] Most commonly reported conditions are back pain and various forms of arthritis. Further, more than one million Australians are reported to have disability associated with arthritis and related disorders, with mobility limitation the major feature. These conditions are the second most common reason for presentation to a general practitioner,[3,4] and the third leading cause of health expenditure.[5] In view of this large disease burden—the number of people affected and the high disability impact—arthritis and musculoskeletal conditions were declared a National Health Priority Area (NHPA) in July 2002. The 2004–05 National Health Survey (NHS) suggests that about 1.3 million Australians (almost 7% of the population) have doctor-diagnosed osteoarthritis. Females (8%) are more likely than males (5%) to have osteoarthritis, and it is much more common among older Australians.[3]

Diagnostic considerations

Radiological changes on x-ray are useful to identify some of the key signs of the osteo-arthritic joint (Figure 25.1): the narrowing of the joint space, marginal osteophyte

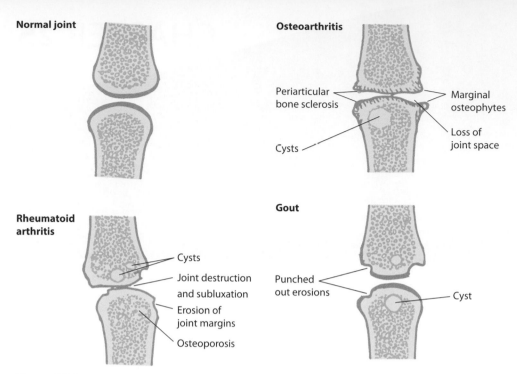

Figure 25.1
Demonstrating contrasting radiological findings between common arthrides

formation, subchondral sclerosis and the hypertrophy of the periarticular bones. However, radiological changes are not always observed in people with joint symptoms, and people with radiological changes do not always have symptoms. Cartilage is not seen on x-ray as it is not radio-opaque, so ultrasound and magnetic resonance imaging (MRI) and visualisation under arthroscopy might be necessary to clarify the joint changes.[2,3]

In clinical research studies, the diagnosis and severity of osteoarthritis is commonly measured using the Western Ontario and McMaster Universities Osteoarthritis Index (WOMAC). The WOMAC evaluates three clinical domains including pain, stiffness and physical function in people with osteoarthritis of the hip and knee, and assesses change in symptoms of patients who have received therapeutic intervention. Ordinal Likert scales are used to grade the severity of each domain, and the instrument has been extensively evaluated for validity.[6,7]

The differential diagnosis of osteoarthritis from other forms of arthritde, like rheumatoid arthritis and gout, should include a consideration of the pattern of joint involvement and whether signs of inflammation are present (Table 25.1 and Figure 25.2). If the patient has a recent history of infection or fever, is younger than 40 years old or presents with abnormal routine blood tests, other forms of arthritis (such as rheumatoid or septic) should be considered (see Chapter 31 on autoimmunity). Laboratory tests (e.g. erythrocyte sedimentation rate [ESR], rheumatoid factor and synovial fluid analysis) may be used to rule out alternative diagnoses.[2,3,8]

Table 25.1
Differential diagnosis of joint patterns

Characteristic	Status	Disease
Inflammation	Present	Rheumatoid arthritis, systemic lupus erythematosus, gout
	Absent	Osteoarthritis
Number of involved joints	Monoarticular	Gout, trauma, septic arthritis, Lyme disease, osteoarthritis
	Oligoarticular (two to four joints)	Reiter's disease, psoriatic arthritis, inflammatory bowel disease
	Polyarticular (five or more)	Rheumatoid arthritis, systemic lupus erythematosus
Site of joint involvement	Distal interphalangeal	Osteoarthritis, psoriatic arthritis (not rheumatoid arthritis)
	Metacarpophalangeal, wrists	Rheumatoid arthritis, systemic lupus erythematosus (not osteoarthritis)
	First metatarsophalangeal	Gout, osteoarthritis

Source: Adapted from Papadakis & McPhee 2009[2]

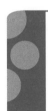

DIFFERENTIAL DIAGNOSIS

- Type: osteo/rheumatoid/psoriatic arthritis
- General pain
- Muscular trauma or stiffness
- Reiter's disease
- Gout
- Crepitus
- Systemic lupus erythematosus
- Lyme disease

Source: Australian Institute of Health and Welfare 2007[3]

RISK FACTORS

The risk factors for osteoarthritis have been categorised into a succinct list of modifiable and unmodifiable factors.[9]

Modifiable

The first and most obvious factor is injury to a joint complex, and this is especially true in men. Trauma to the meniscus and cruciate ligament tears are particularly provocative in the development of osteoarthritis, and this relationship remains despite surgical repair.[2,3,9]

Obesity is a major risk factor in both the development of weight-bearing joint osteoarthritis and its severity and subsequent disability.[3,5,9,10] Women are particularly susceptible in this factor, and obesity appears to be predisposing to osteoarthritis, and not just secondary to becoming sedentary because of it.

The link between occupational overuse and the development of osteoarthritis has been shown in many different work activities, particularly when the knee is involved in repeated bending, kneeling, squatting or climbing,[3,9] and this effect is exacerbated by the addition of heavy-load lifting.[11]

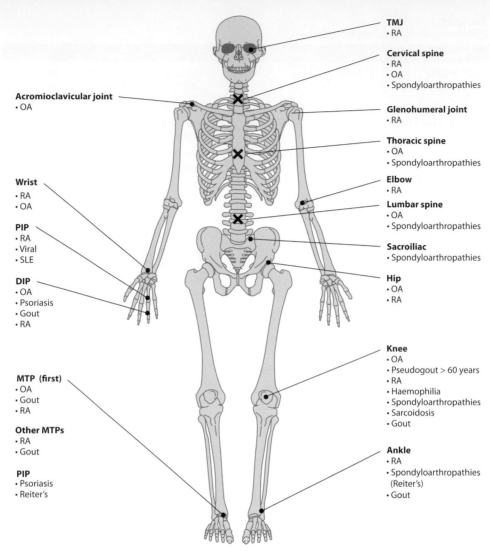

Figure 25.2
Differential diagnosis in arthritis based on patterns of regional joint presentations

Unmodifiable

The prevalence of osteoarthritis has an interesting age and gender relationship. Men more commonly have the radiological signs of the condition before the age of 50 years, and conversely women have it after that age. Women are more likely to have bilateral knee osteoarthritis as well as hand osteoarthritis. The disease increases in incidence and severity with age.[9]

In terms of family history, there is an inherited tendency towards osteoarthritis, with the heritability component estimated in twin studies at 60–65% for hip and hand osteoarthritis, and 40–50% for knee osteoarthritis, although there has been no single gene defect identified.[12] There is also evidence that race is involved as a risk factor. For example, there is evidence that Chinese subjects have a lower incidence of hand and hip osteoarthritis.[10] These risk factors can compound, as in obesity with occupational bending and twisting. There is some evidence that recreational overuse is a risk, specifically in elite sports.[9]

CONVENTIONAL TREATMENT

The exercise program and weight-loss strategies are elements of the self-help management plan that all health practitioners would support—see the discussion below regarding the evidence. Prescription of nonsteroidal anti-inflammatory drugs (NSAIDs) is included as the first choice for pain and inflammation control, with the addition of analgesics where necessary. The prescription should be accompanied by an assessment of the presence of risk factors for NSAIDs including age, hypertension, upper gastrointestinal events and cardiovascular, renal or liver disease. Other issues to be considered are aspirin allergy and polypharmacy (e.g. concurrent use of diuretics, angiotensin-converting enzyme inhibitors [ACEI] and/or anticoagulants).[2,3,13,14]

In Australia, the percentage of people with osteoarthritis using the common medications are: 8.0% use celecoxib (NSAID), 6.6% paracetamol, 5.3% meloxicam (NSAID) and 3.9% diclofenac sodium (NSAID).[3]

The foundations of conventional treatment can be summarised as[2,3,14,15]:

- a supervised exercise program
- weight loss
- NSAID medication
- intraarticular injection with steroids
- total joint replacement.

KEY TREATMENT PROTOCOLS

The goals in the naturopathic treatment of people with osteoarthritis are to attenuate inflammation, enhance joint integrity and repair damage, improve joint mobility and strength, reduce pain, address oxidation and remove metabolic waste products.

This schedule of therapeutic aims has a large number of individualised permutations based on the many pieces of information that are gleaned from the personal history and lifestyle analysis of each person with osteoarthritis. In naturopathic medicine, this is a vital component of the management of a multifactorial condition such as osteoarthritis. As in any naturopathic approach to case reasoning, the therapeutic order is useful to prioritise management, and to ensure the naturopathic principles are followed.[16] The following is a summary of modalities that may be used within naturopathic medicine that have been investigated for this condition.

The naturopathic approach to managing this condition reflects the evidence-based

Naturopathic Treatment Aims
• Remove obstacles to joint health
– obesity
– sedentary lifestyle
– pro-inflammatory diet.
• Support joint healing
– nutrient support for joint complexes
– physical medicine for circulation and drainage.
• Reduce pain
– improve sleep
– reduce medication intake.
• Improve functional capabilities
– range of motion (ROM)
– activities of daily living.
• Limit progression of degeneration.
• Address comorbidities of chronic pain such as depression.
• Improve daily functioning.
• Encourage beneficial lifestyle changes.

guidelines of a number of mainstream groups. The Osteoarthritis Research Society International (OARSI) has published practice guidelines for managing hip and knee osteoarthritis.[17] The guidelines state that optimal management requires a combination of non-pharmacological and pharmacological approaches. The first priority is education of the patient about the condition and the importance of changes in lifestyle, exercise and weight reduction in order to unload the damaged joints. The initial focus should be on self-help and patient-driven treatments rather than on passive therapies delivered by health professionals.[18] The focus on self-help in obesity and exercise management is also a key element of the guidelines from both the Royal Australian College of General Practitioners[19] and the National Arthritis and Musculoskeletal Conditions Advisory Group.[8]

Treat the whole patient

Although clinical treatment will inevitability focus on amelioration of pain, degeneration and inflammation in arthritis patients, it is also important to consider how this affects their day-to-day lives.

Qualitative studies of patients with rheumatoid arthritis suggested that fatigue, not pain, was the factor associated with their condition that affected their life the most.[20] Similar findings have since been observed in osteoarthritis patients as well.[21] Fatigue may be associated with pain, pain medication, poor sleeping patterns or any number of factors. Arthritis may also affect the patient's ability to perform daily tasks and interact socially or with their partner, and has other psychosocial or emotional ramifications, all of which need to be appropriately addressed in the naturopathic treatment of arthritis.

The approach in naturopathic medicine to 'address weakened or dysfunctioning systems or organs' coincides with the clinical approach of looking for the existence of comorbidities that may be linked to the primary problem (Figure 25.3).[23] This is clear in the management of osteoarthritis, where assessment and treatment may be necessary in the (among others):

- nutritional/dietary domain—especially regarding obesity and weight control
- cardiovascular system—limiting the ability to exercise
- psychoemotional aspect—the effects of chronic pain and disability
- gastrointestinal system—absorption of nutrients, food sensitivities and reactions to conventional medications.[18,22]

Attenuate inflammation

The process of inflammation (Figure 25.4) plays a central role in many disorders, especially those in the musculoskeletal system. Like many processes in the body, there can be positive outcomes from a resolution or there can be uncontrolled and damaging results. The activators of inflammation can include injury, radiation, infection, oxidative stress and certain foods. Tissue injury stimulates the release of inflammatory signalling molecules such as bradykinin and the release of inflammatory cytokines such as IL-1, TNF and IL-6. Cells that respond to infection or injury include macrophages and mast cells.[23] Macrophages and other immune cells secrete chemokines that recruit leucocytes from the circulation to the site of inflammation. Mast cells release histamine, prostaglandins and leukotrienes that act as chemokines, increase vascular permeability and act on the vascular endothelium to increase tissue recruitment of leucocytes.[23] Cyclooxygenase (COX) is an enzyme that is responsible for the formation of pro-inflammatory prostaglandins, prostacyclins and thromboxanes from the omega-6 arachidonic acid (see Chapter 31 on autoimmunity for further detail).

Omega-3 essential fatty acids compete with the omega-6, thereby moderating the inflammatory effect (Figure 25.4). There is evidence that omega-3 oils containing

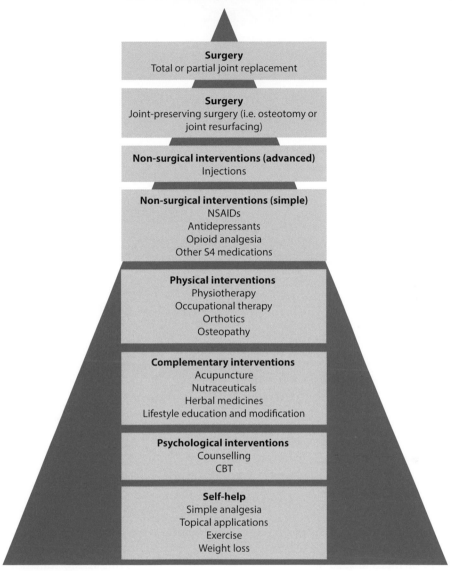

Figure 25.3
Integrative treatment of osteoarthritis

Adapted from Dieppe & Lohmander 2005[23]

eicosapentaenoic acid (EPA) and docosahexaenoic acid (DHA) have anti-inflammatory actions,[24–26] but clinical data are lacking in regard to the treatment of osteoarthritis.[24] The most widely available sources of EPA and DHA are cold water oily fish such as salmon, herring, mackerel, anchovies and sardines.

Harpagophytum procumbens, a South African herb, has been reviewed for efficacy and safety in treating osteoarthritis with favourable results, especially in reducing pain.[25,27] The mechanism of action has not been established, but is thought to be the anti-inflammatory activity of harpagoside.[28]

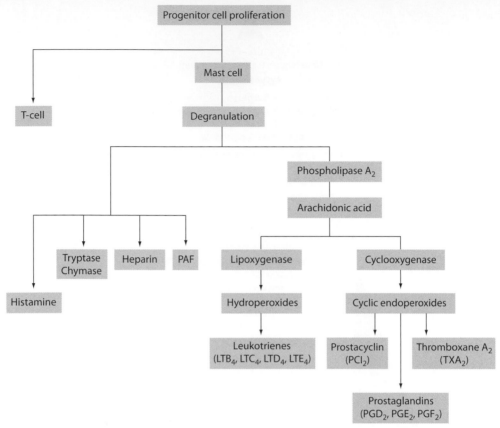

Figure 25.4
The inflammatory cascade

Source: Pearlman 1999[29]

A proprietary blend of ***Solidago virgaurea***, ***Populus tremula*** and ***Fraxinus excelsior*** has been demonstrated to be effective in reducing pain and inflammation in arthritis via a variety of mechanisms. While most of the 43 studies justifying the formulation's use have focused on pain measures, many have also uncovered various anti-inflammatory mechanisms, with efficacy often comparable to conventional anti-inflammatory medication.[30,31] The gum resin extracted from the herb ***Boswellia serrata*** has some evidence as a potent anti-inflammatory, antiarthritic and analgesic agent.[32] Standardised preparations of the bark of ***Salix* spp**. have shown positive effects in a number of trials in musculoskeletal conditions.[25,33] ***Uncaria* spp**. is known to have anti-inflammatory activity in vitro, possibly by inhibiting the production of the pro-inflammatory cytokine, TNF-α,[25] but clinical trials have been inconclusive.[26] ***Zingiber officinale*** has been found to have anti-inflammatory actions,[25,34] and has some clinical trial evidence.[35]

An interesting pilot study using a real practice model showed that **individualised herbal medicine formulas** resulted in improvement of symptoms of osteoarthritis of the knee.[36] Twenty adults, previously diagnosed with osteoarthritis of the knee, were recruited into this randomised, double-blind, placebo-controlled, pilot study carried out in a primary care setting. All subjects were seen in consultation three times by a herbal practitioner who was blinded to the randomisation coding. Each subject was prescribed treatment and given lifestyle advice according to usual practice: continuation of conventional medication where applicable, healthy-eating advice and nutrient supplementation. Individualised herbal medicine was prescribed for each patient but only dispensed for those randomised to active treatment—the remainder were supplied with a placebo. At baseline and outcome (after 10 weeks of treatment), subjects completed a food frequency questionnaire and the WOMAC knee health and Measure Yourself Outcome Profile (MYMOP) wellbeing questionnaires. There was significant improvement in the active group ($n = 9$) for the mean WOMAC stiffness subscore at week 5 and week 10, but not in the placebo group ($n = 5$). Also the mean WOMAC total and subscores all showed clinically significant improvement (20%) in knee symptoms at weeks 5 and 10 compared with baseline. Moreover, the mean MYMOP symptom 2 subscore, mostly relating to osteoarthritis, showed significant improvement at week 5 and week 10 compared with baseline for the active, but not for the placebo, group. This pilot study showed that herbal medicine prescribed for the individual by a herbal practitioner resulted in improvement of symptoms of osteoarthritis of the knee. This methodology mirrors normal clinical procedures, and should encourage similar larger clinical trials that have more relevance to naturopathic practice.

Enhance joint integrity and repair damage

Primary and secondary prevention are the main foci of naturopathic medicine, and maintaining and repairing articular and periarticular tissue is a foundation for managing osteoarthritis. Developing, maintaining and repairing collagen-based connective tissue requires optimal tissue levels of the essential amino acids, as well as vitamin C and iron as cofactors. Bone and cartilage are built on a matrix of minerals, mainly calcium and phosphorus, and an extracellular ground substance of proteoglycans (Figure 25.5).

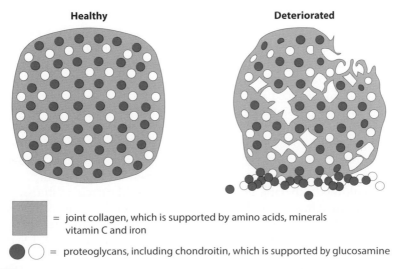

Healthy   **Deteriorated**

= joint collagen, which is supported by amino acids, minerals vitamin C and iron

= proteoglycans, including chondroitin, which is supported by glucosamine

Figure 25.5
Healthy and deteriorated collagen matrices

Proteoglycans are glycoproteins that have a core protein with glycosaminoglycan (GAG) chains.

Glucosamine and **chondroitin** are both natural components of proteoglycans, the building blocks of cartilage, and are thought to increase its synthesis when taken orally. Glucosamine is manufactured from oyster and crab shells, and chondroitin from bovine or shark cartilage. There are conflicting results in the research findings for both symptom relief and limiting the progression of the disease.

The large Glucosamine/Chondroitin Arthritis Intervention Trial (GAIT) trials[37,38] have found varying positive and negative results in both domains of clinical effect, and one study[26] puts forward a list of concerns that may explain why the body of evidence remains equivocal, including:

- the tendency of industry-sponsored trials to have positive results
- poor supplement quality
- varying dosing methods
- trials too brief to allow slow therapeutic effect
- underpowered trials.[26]

A recent trial of chondroitin sulfate suggests that it could be a disease-modifying agent.[39]

Methylsulfonylmethane (**MSM**) has been used as a sulfur-based nutritional supplement in conditions with joint pain, but a recent systematic review of clinical trials was unable to reach a firm conclusion on its usefulness because of methodological flaws and despite a number of positive trial findings.[40–42]

Improving joint mobility

The result of inflammation and fibrosis in osteoarthritis is limited joint motion, and this interferes with activities of daily living and has the global effect of reducing fitness and compliance to exercise therapy.

Massage and physical therapy provide viable options for managing osteoarthritis. There have been some trials using massage for osteoarthritis, but methodological quality is lacking, particularly regarding the difficulties of blinding and control. A trial of standard Swedish massage found statistical improvements in the WOMAC global scores, pain, stiffness and physical function domains.[43] Objective improvements in knee strength (47%), reduced pain (76%) and ROM (53%) have been observed in studies using manual physiotherapy for osteoarthritis.[44] Other adjunctive therapies such as balneotherapy,[45] pulsed electromagnetic fields[46] and transcutaneous electrical nerve stimulation (TENS)[47] may also provide short-term relief and improvement in function,[48] although more studies of better methodological quality are needed. Further studies investigating orthotics and braces have also shown minor benefit.[49]

The term 'multimodal therapy' generally includes ROM exercise, soft tissue mobilisation and muscle strengthening and stretching—all within the scope of the naturopath inclined to physical medicine.[50] Studies suggest that patients with osteoarthritis receive moderate short-term (up to eight weeks) clinical impact measured on WOMAC global and pain scores.

Adding therapeutic oils (such as *Zingiber officinale* or *Citrus* spp.) to the massage appears to have potential as an alternative method for short-term knee pain relief.[51]

Reduce pain

Our physiological understanding of the source of pain, especially in osteoarthritis, is not well understood,[52] yet seems to encompass a wide range of contributing local and systemic factors. Examples of such mechanisms include the loss of hyaline articular cartilage and subsequent joint space narrowing, inflammatory mediators (such as bradykinin, histamine, prostaglandins, lactic acid, substance P, vasoactive intestinal peptide and calcitonin gene-related peptide), nerve innervation, pain sensitisation and the cortical experience[53] of pain.

With such a mixture of factors potentially implicated in the pain response, both orthodox and complementary management plans use multiple treatment options. This provides a unique opportunity for collaboration and integration between both systems of medicine to provide the best patient outcomes. Benefits of such an approach include the potential to reduce current workloads on general practitioners (for mild to moderate patient presentations) and lessen the side effects experienced by many patients limited to drug therapy alone.

Plasters of *Capsicum* spp. have been applied topically for centuries, with modern research now identifying the proposed mechanism of action. Capsaicin, an alkaloidal constituent in the chilli plant, is able to reversibly deplete C-fibre afferent neurons of the neuropeptide substance P,[54] which leads to subsequent nerve desensitisation in amounts of just 0.025% in topical creams.

Preparations of **Phytodolor** (an alcohol-based formulation containing *Populus tremula*, *Fraxinus excelsior* and *Solidago virgaurea*),[55,56] *Harpagophytum procumbens*, *Zingiber officinale*, *Rosa canina* and avocado/soy bean unsaponifiables[55,56] have all shown benefit in the symptomatic management of osteoarthritis.

Clinical evidence suggests **acupuncture**, in combination with primary care when required, is associated with marked clinical improvement in patients with chronic osteoarthritis-associated pain of the knee or hip.[57] Improvement in WOMAC scores, increase in joint mobility and function[58,59] and quality-of-life improvements have all been identified through clinical studies.[59,60] One review,[61] however, suggests that acupuncture requires more evidence of effectiveness in osteoarthritis and what evidence exists is dubious. The most recent Cochrane review[62] concluded that sham-controlled trials show small statistically significant benefits; however, the authors add that the benefits are small and may be due to placebo or incomplete blinding.

Thermotherapy may reduce the pain associated with osteoarthritis. It involves the application of heat or cold (such as a heat or ice pack and ice massage) to treat symptoms of osteoarthritis. This could be applied by a massage therapist, physical therapist or naturopath in an integrated setting. The application of cold is known to have an effect by reducing swelling and inflammation, numbing pain and blocking nerve impulses and muscle spasms to the joint (see Chapter 40 on pain management for more detail on this).

A Cochrane systematic review[63] found that thermotherapy is most effective in an acute stage of osteoarthritis when minor joint inflammation is present and is administered through the application of an ice pack wrapped in a towel for 20 minutes, five days a week for two weeks.

Cautious evidence supporting **balneotherapy** (mineral baths) for relief of pain and stiffness in osteoarthritis has been reported in a Cochrane systematic review.[64]

Vitamin D deficiency appears to be prevalent in people with chronic musculoskeletal pain.[65–68] The mechanism appears to be related to a decrease in calcium absorption leading to dysfunctional collagen deposition in the periosteum, which generates painful stimuli. Oral supplementation with vitamin D in deficient subjects leads to a reduction in pain.[68]

The Framingham study data[69] link vitamin D deficiency to osteoarthritis. In a study of 556 subjects, dietary and supplement intake of vitamin D and serum levels of 25-hydroxyvitamin D were evaluated. Osteoarthritis was measured using knee radiographs. The authors concluded that low intake and low serum levels of vitamin D each appeared to be associated with an increased risk for progression of osteo-arthritis of the knee.[69] These conclusions have been supported in a more recent review.[70]

Quality matters

As with many nutraceuticals, quality and dosing variances can affect the therapeutic application and efficacy of treatment in trials. Glucosamine comes in a variety of forms which, though they theoretically can be hydrolysed in the stomach into equivalent forms, may have effects on therapeutic dosing require-ments. Additionally, quality issues may also arise. Some formulations are demonstrated to be consistently more effective than placebo or other formulations in clinical trials.[1,71] Although concerns have been raised that these positive results may be related to industry sponsorship, it has been deemed equally likely that these results may also be due to the stricter quality controls of some formulations.[72] In clinical practice recommending any generic complementary medicine can be fraught; it is recommended that practi-tioners make specific recommendations for products they know to have high standards of quality and efficacy.

Address oxidation

When inflammation is present, the breakdown of cells and tissues creates a burden of products of oxidation. The process of oxidation (producing reactive oxygen species) is a key factor in conditions of ageing, and the extracellular space depends on trace elements for antioxidation.

The Framingham study demonstrated a reduction in risk of cartilage loss and knee pain over eight years, with possible effects from vitamin E 8–10 mg/day in patients with knee osteoarthritis.[70] This early promise has not been supported in trials since, with two systematic reviews finding very limited evidence for vitamin C or E.[42,73]

Remove metabolic waste products

A traditional naturopathic protocol used to treat osteoarthritis involves stimulation of the body's detoxification pathways to clear metabolic waste. While this philosophy has not yet been scientifically tested via rigorous studies, traditional evidence does support this practice.[74,75] The traditional use of **herbal 'alteratives'** and **'diuretics'** such as *Apium graveolens*, *Taraxacum officinale* or *Urtica dioica* to treat rheumatism, appears to be predicated upon these herbs' abilities to stimulate the removal of metabolic waste by increasing diuresis and potentially reducing blood composition of metabolic by-products. This protocol may be potentially beneficial in treating gout (see the box on gout on the next page).

Gout

Overview

- Acute onset of pain, usually in the evening
- Primarily male population
- Usually presents as monoarticular joint pain in the metatarsophalangeal joint
- High serum uric acid, urate crystals in the joint
- Genetic causations, triggered by increased alcohol and poor diet

Protocols

- Modify diet (reduce/avoid alcohol, high-purine foods, excess refined carbohydrates, saturated fats)
- Encourage hydration: 2.5 L per day keeps uric acid in solution and promotes excretion. Reversing dehydration also important
- Reduce weight and exercise in moderation
- Remove/reduce uric acid (via herbal diuretics and aquaretics, folic acid)
- Reduce inflammation via botanical and nutrient prescription

Complementary and alternative medicine interventions

- Dietary advice (low purines and alcohol, healthy carbs/protein/fats balance, increase anthocyanidin-rich fruits such as cherries, blueberries)
- Folic acid has a similar mechanism of action to conventional gout medications such as allopurinol (it reduces xanthine oxidase) but requires large doses—over 5 mg—to be therapeutically effective—a trial of 10–20 mg daily should be considered
- Give lifestyle advice (exercise, reduced weight if required)
- Anti-inflammatories (such as bromelain, quercetin, omega-3, *Glycyrrhiza glabra*, *Harpagophytum procumbens*, *Boswellia serrata*)
- Diuretics/aquaretics (such as *Taraxacum officinale*, *Urtica dioica*, *Apium graveolens*)

Source: Demio 2008[76]

INTEGRATIVE MEDICAL CONSIDERATIONS

Self-management

Self-management education programs have an important role to play in managing chronic conditions such as osteoarthritis, and suit an integrative model of shared care between conventional and complementary medicine practitioners. Self-management education programs are interventions designed to educate patients in self-care activities that promote health and the management of chronic diseases, increasing their motivation and decreasing the negative effects the condition has on their daily function.[77] The National Health Priority Action Council states that, by taking the behavioural approach to the management of the psychosocial aspects of chronic disease, patients have outcomes of decreased pain and improved quality of life.[77] This approach matches the holistic underpinning of naturopathic medicine.

Weight loss

Obesity is clearly a risk factor for developing osteoarthritis, particularly for women. There is very strong evidence that people who are obese (with a body mass index [BMI] of over 30) are at higher risk of their osteoarthritis being symptomatic and progressing than those with a BMI under 30. The relationship between obesity and osteoarthritis is thought to be because of the increased stress on articular surfaces in the weight-bearing joints.[2,3,7] Reducing obesity in the patient with osteoarthritis should be considered as both a primary and a secondary prevention strategy. The condition is multifactorial, and is best managed in a multidisciplinary team including naturopaths.

The Arthritis, Diet and Activity Promotion Trial (ADAPT) was a randomised, single-blind controlled clinical trial that demonstrated that weight loss was central to the improvement in WOMAC physical function, pain and stiffness scores; these results were enhanced when combined with a moderate exercise program.[78]

Exercise therapy

Exercise guidance is a foundation of a naturopathic approach to wellness, and in the management of osteoarthritis coincides with the mainstream evidence-based guidelines. Exercise is important both as a treatment of symptoms and to prevent the development of osteoarthritis. Increasing physical activity improves general physical health and assists in the management of obesity, both vital risk factors for osteoarthritis, as mentioned.

Enhancing muscular strength is an outcome of exercise programs, and muscular weakness and dysfunction can cause joint instability and subsequent injury. To prevent this injury and resultant degeneration, and to prevent further injury in the degenerative joint, exercise programs must be a central component of the management plan in osteoarthritis.

Physical exercise of a light-to-moderate intensity increases muscle strength as well as range of motion, aerobic capacity and endurance that contributes to improved physical functioning and pain reduction. Various programs (Table 25.2) offer different benefits and no specific type of exercise regimen has been shown to be superior.[2,3,17,19] A number of Cochrane reviews support the application of therapeutic exercise in the management of osteoarthritis,[79–81] with evidence for moderate intensity[81] and aquatic programs.[79]

An interesting systematic review looked at **Tai Chi**, a traditional Chinese martial art style, which has been one of the most researched therapeutic exercises. The authors report that there is evidence suggesting that Tai Chi may be effective for pain control in patients with knee osteoarthritis, but the evidence is not as convincing for pain reduction or improvement of physical function.[82]

CLINICAL SUMMARY

The fact that osteoarthritis is common in society and causes disability means that it is vital that naturopathic practitioners become knowledgeable and coherent in their management of this group of patients. The main clinical consequences of osteoarthritis are pain, immobility and subsequent sleep and mood disturbances, and each of these should be assessed at the initial consultation. Depending on the severity and chronicity of these presenting complaints, a decision about naturopathic management should be made based on the available evidence, and the need for referral to a multidisciplinary team—see the decision tree at Figure 25.6. There is evidence for naturopathic intervention to reduce inflammation and pain in order to optimise functional capability, but as the disease becomes more severe and disabling orthodox medical and surgical intervention becomes more likely. The naturopathic evidence-based approach involves dietary modifications as well as nutritional, herbal and physical medicine. Finally, any patient with chronic pain requires integrative management, as the consequences progress to affecting other systems beyond the musculoskeletal.

Table 25.2
Exercise interventions in osteoarthritis

Name	Description	Indications	Cautions/ contraindications	Comments
ROM exercise	Active movement within range	Maintain joint ROM, ↑ joint nutrition, prevent soft tissue shortening[83]	If there is painful ROM, then this can aggravate—find ranges that are comfortable	Foundation of rehabilitation for painful musculoskeletal conditions
Myofascial stretching	Static loading or proprioceptive neuromuscular facilitation (PNF—use of contract and release)	↑ muscle length and flexibility— optimise ROM[83]	A lack of patient comprehension will limit the use of active participation	Good evidence basis[83]
Yoga asanas	Full ROM postures with adjunctive breathing exercises	General ROM maintenance and optimisation; strengthening; painful musculoskeletal conditions, balance and coordination, anxiety, depression[84]	Yoga can take articulations to an end-range, so when instability is present, care must be taken Instructors have to be well trained to provide safety	Evidence is inconclusive— large number of low-quality RCTs
Resistance training	Repetitive weight resisted motion within ROM	↑ muscle strength and endurance; ↑ BMR, ↑ muscle mass; ↑ BMD; improved glucose metabolism[83]	Soft tissue injury/ inflammation; instability of articulations	Exercise professional required to set form and progression
Aerobic conditioning	Varied exercise aiming to increase oxygen demand and use	Obesity, general conditioning to prevent disease, depression[83]	Cardiac/respiratory disease, painful weight-bearing conditions	Requires careful grading in intensity, excellent evidence profile
Tai Chi	Chinese system of slow movements	Painful musculoskeletal conditions[85]	Nil known	Traditional use in aged population group
Aquatic	Variety of exercises in water	↑ coordination, flexibility and strength,[79,83] for painful conditions	Wounds/infection	Decreases load on weight-bearing tissues
Pilates	Resisted movement system with apparatus and floor exercises	↑ muscle strength and control— trunk/lumbar/ pelvic[86] Injury rehabilitation	Overuse of abdominal musculature may increase intra-abdominal pressure and theoretically aggravate intervertebral disc conditions	Requires careful guidance to establish muscle control

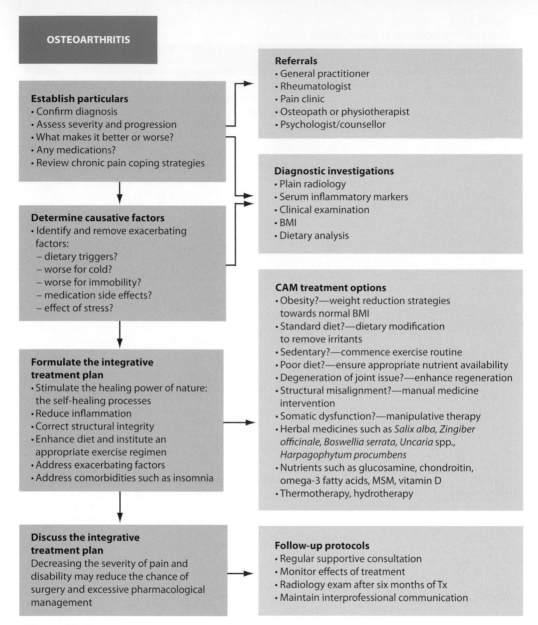

OSTEOARTHRITIS

Establish particulars
- Confirm diagnosis
- Assess severity and progression
- What makes it better or worse?
- Any medications?
- Review chronic pain coping strategies

Determine causative factors
- Identify and remove exacerbating factors:
  – dietary triggers?
  – worse for cold?
  – worse for immobility?
  – medication side effects?
  – effect of stress?

Formulate the integrative treatment plan
- Stimulate the healing power of nature: the self-healing processes
- Reduce inflammation
- Correct structural integrity
- Enhance diet and institute an appropriate exercise regimen
- Address exacerbating factors
- Address comorbidities such as insomnia

Discuss the integrative treatment plan
Decreasing the severity of pain and disability may reduce the chance of surgery and excessive pharmacological management

Referrals
- General practitioner
- Rheumatologist
- Pain clinic
- Osteopath or physiotherapist
- Psychologist/counsellor

Diagnostic investigations
- Plain radiology
- Serum inflammatory markers
- Clinical examination
- BMI
- Dietary analysis

CAM treatment options
- Obesity?—weight reduction strategies towards normal BMI
- Standard diet?—dietary modification to remove irritants
- Sedentary?—commence exercise routine
- Poor diet?—ensure appropriate nutrient availability
- Degeneration of joint issue?—enhance regeneration
- Structural misalignment?—manual medicine intervention
- Somatic dysfunction?—manipulative therapy
- Herbal medicines such as *Salix alba*, *Zingiber officinale*, *Boswellia serrata*, *Uncaria* spp., *Harpagophytum procumbens*
- Nutrients such as glucosamine, chondroitin, omega-3 fatty acids, MSM, vitamin D
- Thermotherapy, hydrotherapy

Follow-up protocols
- Regular supportive consultation
- Monitor effects of treatment
- Radiology exam after six months of Tx
- Maintain interprofessional communication

Figure 25.6
Naturopathy treatment decision tree—osteoarthritis

Table 25.3
Review of the major evidence

Intervention	Mechanisms of action	Key literature	Summary of results	Comment
Omega-3 (EPA, DHA)	Anti-inflammatory effects via leukotriene modulation	Setty et al. 2005[25]	Review article: Inconclusive results	Weak in vivo evidence in osteoarthritis
Harpagophytum procumbens	Anti-inflammatory activity of harpagoside[28]	Brien et al. 2006[27] Warnock et al. 2007[87]	Systematic review: Two high-quality RCTs; ($n = 211$) osteoarthritis multiple sites; ↓ pain Single group open study; ($n = 259$) ↓ pain, stiffness, function ($p < 0.0001$); ↑ QOL SF-12; 60% patients ↓ medications Adverse effects have been described as no different to placebo[87]	Some evidence as a chondroprotective[25] Contra-indicated in duodenal ulcers[25] Concluded useful for mild to moderate degenerative rheumatic disorders[87]
Boswellia serrata	Anti-inflammatory, antiarthritic and analgesic activities from the boswellic acids	Ernst 2009[32] Sangupta et al. 2008[88]	Systematic review: Three RCTs ($n = 171$) knee osteoarthritis; ↓ pain, WOMAC scores Double-blind RCT: ($n = 75$) with osteoarthritis: extract of *Boswellia serrata* (5-Loxin); statistically significant improvements in pain scores and physical function scores[88]	Individual trials have small sample sizes 5-Loxin is an extract enriched with 30% 3-O-acetyl-11-keto-beta-boswellic acid (AKBA)
Salix alba	Anti-inflammatory and analgesic activity from the active constituent salicin	Chrubasik et al. 2001[33] Beer et al. 2008[89]	Open randomised study: ($n = 93$) low back pain; ↓ pain; equal effect to NSAID group Open observational study: ($n = 128$) knee and hip osteoarthritis; ↓ clinical symptoms and WOMAC scores	Encouraging evidence to support a botanical with strong traditional use Further rigorous studies needed
Zingiber officinale	Anti-inflammatory effects from compounds such as gingerol[25,34] Warming rubefacient	Altman 2001[35]	Double-blind RCT: ($n = 247$) knee osteoarthritis pain on standing; ↓ pain ($p < 0.043$)	Traditionally combines well with *Salix* spp.

Table 25.3
Review of the major evidencem (continued)

Intervention	Mechanisms of action	Key literature	Summary of results	Comment
Glucosamine and chondroitin	Chondro-protective, enhancing repair of joint tissue	Sawitzke et al. 2008[38] Kahan et al. 2009[39]	Double-blind RCT: ($n = 572$) knee osteoarthritis; joint space width not different to control Double-blind RCT: ($n = 622$) knee osteoarthritis; ↓ joint space width ($p < 0.0001$)	Glucosamine and chondroitin sulfate combined Used chondroitin sulfate alone Difference between quality of products should be noted
Methylsulfonyl-methane (MSM)	Scavenge hydroxyl free radicals, rectify dietary deficiencies of sulfur improving cartilage formation	Brien et al. 2008[40]	Systematic review: ($n = 168$) mild/moderate knee osteoarthritis; ↓ pain (p value not reported)	Systematic review of RCTs that noted methodological flaws
Antioxidants	Inhibit oxidation	McAlindon et al. 1996[69] McAlindon et al. 2005[90]	Framingham cohort: ($n = 640$); vitamin C, beta-carotene and vitamin E ↓ knee osteoarthritis progression and cartilage loss	No effect on primary prevention
Massage and physical therapy	Enhance mobility, and increases Circulatory stimulation	Perlman et al. 2006[43]	Quasi-RCT: ($n = 68$) knee osteoarthritis; Swedish massage for eight weeks; WOMAC pain, stiffness ($p < 0.001$), ROM ($p = 0.03$)	Underpowered, not full blinding of assessors
Thermotherapy	Drainage of oedema analgesic	Brosseau et al. 2003[63]	Systematic review: Three RCTs, knee osteoarthritis; improved function and knee strength, decreased swelling	Potentially beneficial adjunctive therapy
Acupuncture	Pain reduction via modulation of opiate pathways; improves mobility	Manheimer et al. 2007[62]	Meta-analysis: Nine RCTs; knee osteoarthritis; pain, function compared with usual care	Sham-controlled; have variation in design

> ## KEY POINTS
>
> - The presence of pain, immobility, sleep and mood disturbances should be assessed at the initial consultation.
> - As osteoarthritis becomes more severe and disabling, orthodox medical and surgical intervention becomes more likely.
> - Patients with chronic pain require integrative management.
> - Beyond chronic pain management, it is important to address lifestyle factors and the underlying factors that contribute to the pathogenesis of osteoarthritis.

FURTHER READING

Liu X, Machado GC, Eyles JP, et al. Dietary supplements for treating osteoarthritis: a systematic review and meta-analysis. Br J Sports Med 2018;52(3):167–75. doi:10.1136/bjsports-2016-097333. [Epub 2017 Oct 10]; Review.

Manheimer E, Cheng K, Wieland LS, et al. Acupuncture for hip osteoarthritis. Cochrane Database Syst Rev 2018;(5):CD013010, doi:10.1002/14651858.CD013010. Review.

Wang Y, Lu S, Wang R, et al. Integrative effect of yoga practice in patients with knee arthritis: a PRISMA-compliant meta-analysis. Medicine (Baltimore) 2018;97(31):e11742. doi:10.1097/MD.0000000000011742.

Acknowledgment: The author would like to acknowledge Justin Sinclair for his assistance with the integrative approaches for the treatment of osteoarthritis.

REFERENCES

1. Reginster J, et al. Current role of glucosamine in the treatment of osteoarthritis. Rheumatology (Oxford) 2007;46(5):731–5.
2. 2009 Current medical diagnosis and treatment. 48th cd. New York: McGraw Hill Medical; 2009.
3. Australian Institute of Health and Welfare. Australia's health 2014. Australia's health series no. 14. Canberra: AIHW; 2014. Cat. no. AUS 178.
4. Britt H, Miller G, Henderson J, et al. General practice activity in Australia 2012–13. General practice series no. 33. Sydney: Sydney University Press; 2013.
5. Australian Institute of Health and Welfare. Health expenditure Australia 2015–16. Health and welfare expenditure series no. 58. Canberra: AIHW; 2017. Cat. no. HWE 68.
6. Bellamy NB, et al. Validation study of WOMAC: a health status instrument for measuring clinically important patient relevant outcomes to anti-rheumatic drug therapy in patients with osteoarthritis of the hip or knee. J Rheumatol 1988;15:1833–40.
7. Auw Yang KR, et al. Validation of the short-form WOMAC function scale for the evaluation of osteoarthritis of the knee. J Bone Joint Surg 2007;89-B(1):50–6.
8. National Arthritis and Musculoskeletal Conditions Advisory Group. Evidence to support the national action plan for osteoarthritis, rheumatoid arthritis and osteoporosis: opportunities to improve health-related quality of life and reduce the burden of disease and disability. Canberra: Department of Health and Ageing; 2004.
9. March LB, Bagga H. Epidemiology of osteoarthritis in Australia. Med J Aust 2004;180(5 Suppl.):SS6–10.
10. Hart DS, Spector TD. The relationship of obesity, fat distribution and osteoarthritis in women in the general population: the Chingford study. J Rheumatol 1993;20:331–5.
11. Coggon DC, et al. Occupational activity and osteoarthritis of the knee. Arthritis Rheum 2000;43:1443–9.
12. Spector TC, et al. Genetic influences on osteoarthritis in women: a twin study. BMJ 1996;312:940–3.
13. RACGP. Guideline for the non-surgical management of hip and knee osteoarthritis. Melbourne: The Royal Australian College of General Practitioners; 2009.
14. Jordan KA, et al. EULAR Recommendations 2003: an evidence based approach to the management of knee osteoarthritis: report of a Task Force of the Standing Committee for International Clinical Studies Including Therapeutic Trials (ESCISIT). Ann Rheum Dis 2003;62(12):1145–55.
15. Recommendations for the medical management of osteoarthritis of the hip and knee: 2000 update American College of Rheumatology Subcommittee on Osteoarthritis guidelines. Arthritis Rheum 2000;43:1905–15.
16. Zeff J, et al. A hierarchy of healing: the therapeutic order. The unifying theory of naturopathic medicine. In: Pizzorno JE, Murray MT, editors. Textbook of natural medicine. 3rd ed. Edinburgh: Churchill Livingstone; 2006.
17. Zhang WM, et al. OARSI recommendations for the management of hip and knee osteoarthritis, part II: OARSI evidence-based, expert consensus guidelines. Osteoarthritis Cartilage 2008;16(2):137e–162e.
18. Hart J. Osteoarthritis and complementary therapies. Altern Complement Ther 2008;14(3):116–20.
19. Royal Australian College of General Practitioners. Osteoarthritis Working Group: Guideline for the non-surgical management of hip and knee osteoarthritis. 2009. Online. Available: http://

www.nhmrc.gov.au/PUBLICATIONS/synopses/_files/cp117-hip-knee-osteoarthritis.pdf. 1 Nov 2013.

20. Hewlett S, et al. Patients' perceptions of fatigue in rheumatoid arthritis: overwhelming, uncontrollable, ignored. Arthritis Rheum 2005;53(5):697–702.

21. Power J, et al. Fatigue in osteoarthritis: a qualitative study. BMC Musculoskelet Disord 2008;1(9):63.

22. Kelly A. Managing osteoarthritis pain. Nursing 2006;36(11):20–1.

23. Laufer S, et al. Inflammation and rheumatic diseases: the molecular basis of novel therapies. Stuttgart: Thieme; 2008.

24. Calder P. Dietary modification of inflammation with lipids. Proc Nutr Soc 2002;61:345–58.

25. Setty AS, Sigal LH. Herbal medications commonly used in the practice of rheumatology: mechanisms of action, efficacy, and side effects. Semin Arthritis Rheum 2005;34(6):773–84.

26. Tancred J. Joint care. J Complement Med 2009;8(2):12–19.

27. Brien SL, et al. Devil's claw (Harpagophytum procumbens) as a treatment for osteoarthritis: a review of efficacy and safety. J Altern Complement Med 2006;12(10):981–93.

28. Braun L, Cohen M. Herbs and natural supplements. An evidence-based guide. Sydney: Elsevier; 2005.

29. Pearlman DS. Pathology of the inflammatory response. J Allergy Clin Immunol 1999;104:S132–7.

30. Ernst E. The efficacy of Phytodolor for the treatment of musculoskeletal pain—a systematic review of randomized clinical trials. Nat Med J 1999;2(1):14–16.

31. Gundermann K, Müller J. Phytodolor—effects and efficacy of a herbal medicine. Wien Med Wochenschr 2007;157(13–14):343–7.

32. Ernst E. Frankincense: a systematic review. BMJ 2009;337:a2813.

33. Chrubasik SK, et al. Treatment of low-back pain with a herbal or synthetic anti-rheumatic: a randomized controlled study. Willow bark extract for low-back pain. Rheumatology (Oxford) 2001;40:1388–93.

34. Tjendraputra ET, et al. Effect of ginger constituents and synthetic analogues on cyclooxygenase-2 enzyme in intact cells. Bioorg Chem 2001;29(3):156–63.

35. Altman RM, Marcussen KC. Effects of a ginger extract on knee pain in patients with osteoarthritis. Arthritis Rheum 2001;44(11):2531–8.

36. Hamblin LL, et al. Improved arthritic knee health in a pilot RCT of phytotherapy. J R Soc Promot Health 2008;128(5):255–62.

37. Clegg DR, et al. Glucosamine, chondroitin sulfate, and the two in combination for painful knee osteoarthritis. N Engl J Med 2006;354(8):795–808.

38. Sawitzke AS, et al. The effect of glucosamine and/or chondroitin sulfate on the progression of knee osteoarthritis: a report from the Glucosamine/chondroitin Arthritis Intervention Trial. Arthritis Rheum 2008;58(10):3183–91.

39. Kahan AU, et al. Long-term effects of chondroitins 4 and 6 sulfate on knee osteoarthritis: the study on osteoarthritis progression prevention, a two-year, randomized, double-blind, placebo-controlled trial. Arthritis Rheum 2009;60(2):524–33.

40. Brien SP, et al. Systematic review of the nutritional supplements dimethyl sulfoxide (DMSO) and methylsulfonylmethane (MSM) in the treatment of osteoarthritis. Osteoarthritis Cartilage 2008;16(11):1277–88.

41. Kim LA, et al. Efficacy of methylsulfonylmethane (MSM) in osteoarthritis pain of the knee: a pilot clinical trial. Osteoarthritis Cartilage 2006;14(3):286–94.

42. Ameye LG, Chee WS. Osteoarthritis and nutrition: from nutraceuticals to functional foods: a systematic review of the scientific evidence. Arthritis Res Ther 2006;8(4):R127.

43. Perlman AS, et al. Massage therapy for osteoarthritis of the knee: a randomized controlled trial. Arch Intern Med 2006;166(22):2533–8.

44. Marks R, Cantin D. Symptomatic osteoarthritis of the knee: the efficacy of physiotherapy. Physiotherapy 1997;83(6):306–12.

45. Verhagen A, et al. Balneotherapy for osteoarthritis. Cochrane Database Syst Rev 2003;(4):CD000518.

46. Hulme J, et al. Electromagnetic fields for the treatment of osteoarthritis. Cochrane Database Syst Rev 2002;(1):CD003523.

47. Osiri M, et al. Transcutaneous electrical nerve stimulation for knee osteoarthritis. Cochrane Database Syst Rev 2000;(4):CD002823.

48. Fransen M. When is physiotherapy appropriate? Best Pract Res Clin Rheumatol 2004;18(4):477–89.

49. Brouwer R, et al. Braces and orthoses for treating osteoarthritis of the knee. Cochrane Database Syst Rev 2005;(1):CD004020.

50. Orrock P. Naturopathic physical medicine. In: Chaitow L, editor. Naturopathic physical medicine. Edinburgh: Elsevier; 2008.

51. Yip YB, Tam ACY. An experimental study on the effectiveness of massage with aromatic ginger and orange essential oil for moderate-to-severe knee pain among the elderly in Hong Kong. Complement Ther Med 2008;16(13):131–8.

52. Hunter DJ, et al. The symptoms of osteoarthritis and the genesis of pain. Med Clin North Am 2008;93(1):83–100.

53. Treede R-D, et al. The cortical representation of pain. Pain 1998;79:105–11.

54. Hayman M, Kam PC. Capsaicin: a review of its pharmacology and clinical applications. Curr Anaesth Crit Care 2008;19(5–6):338–43.

55. Hochberg M. Non-conventional treatment of osteoarthritis by herbal medicine. Osteoarthritis Cartilage 2008;16(Suppl. 1):S2–4.

56. Chrubasik J, et al. Evidence of effectiveness of herbal antiinflammatory drugs in the treatment of painful osteoarthritis and chronic low back pain. Phytother Res 2007;21:675–83.

57. Witt CM, et al. Acupuncture in patients with osteoarthritis of the knee or hip: a randomized, controlled trial with an additional nonrandomized arm. Rev Int Acupuntura 2007;1(1):40–1.

58. Witt C, et al. Acupuncture in patients with osteoarthritis of the knee: a randomised trial. Lancet 2005;366(9480):136–43.

59. Berman BM, et al. The evidence for acupuncture as a treatment for rheumatologic conditions. Rheum Dis Clin North Am 2000;26(1):103–15.

60. Ezzo J, et al. Acupuncture for osteoarthritis of the knee: a systematic review. Arthritis Rheum 2001;44(4):819–25.

61. Ernst E. Acupuncture: what does the most reliable evidence tell us? J Pain Symptom Manage 2009;37(4):709–14.

62. Manheimer E, Cheng K, Linde K, et al. Acupuncture for peripheral joint osteoarthritis. Cochrane Database Syst Rev 2010;(1):Art. No.: CD001977, doi:10.1002/14651858. CD001977.pub2.

63. Brosseau LY, et al. Thermotherapy for treatment of osteoarthritis. Cochrane Database Syst Rev 2003;(4):CD004259.

64. Verhagen AP, Bierma-Zeinstra SMA, Boers M, et al. Balneotherapy for osteoarthritis. Cochrane Database Syst Rev 2007;(4):Art. No.: CD006864, doi:10.1002/14651858. CD006864.

65. Thomas ML-J, et al. Hypovitaminosis D in medical inpatients. N Engl J Med 1998;338(12):777–83.

66. Nesby-O'Dell SS, et al. Hypovitaminosis D prevalence and determinants among African American and white women of reproductive age: third National Health and Nutrition Examination Survey. 1988–1994. Am J Clin Nutr 2002;79:187–92.

67. Plotnikoff GA, Quigley JM. Prevalence of severe hypovitaminosis D in patients with persistent, nonspecific musculoskeletal pain. Mayo Clin Proc 2003;78(12):1463–70.

68. Holick M. Vitamin D deficiency: what a pain it is. Mayo Clin Proc 2003;78(12):1457–9.

69. McAlindon TF, et al. Relation of dietary intake and serum levels of vitamin D to progression of osteoarthritis of the knee among participants in the Framingham Study. Ann Intern Med 1996;125(5):353–9.

70. Holick M. Vitamin D deficiency: medical progress. N Engl J Med 2007;357(3):266.

71. Pavelka K, et al. Glucosamine sulfate use and delay of progression of knee osteoarthritis: a 3-year, randomised, placebo-controlled, double-blind study. Arch Intern Med 2002;162:2113–23.

72. Towheed T, et al. Glucosamine therapy for treating osteoarthritis. Cochrane Database Syst Rev 2006;(2):CD002946.

73. Wang YP, et al. The effect of nutritional supplements on osteoarthritis. Altern Med Rev 2004;9(3):275–96.

74. Chaitow L, editor. Naturopathic physical medicine. Edinburgh: Elsevier; 2008.

75. Mills S, Bone K. Principles and practice of phytotherapy. Edinburgh: Churchill Livingstone; 2000.

76. Demio P. Gout. In: Rakel D, editor. Integrative medicine. 2nd ed. Philadelphia: Saunders Elsevier; 2008.

77. National Health Priority Action Council. National service improvement framework for osteoarthritis, rheumatoid arthritis and osteoporosis. Canberra: Department of Health and Ageing; 2006.

78. Messier SL, et al. Exercise and dietary weight loss in overweight and obese older adults with knee osteoarthritis. Arthritis Rheum 2004;50(5):1501–10.

79. Bartels EL, et al. Aquatic exercise for the treatment of knee and hip osteoarthritis. Cochrane Database Syst Rev 2007;(4):CD005523.

80. Fransen MM, et al. Exercise for osteoarthritis of the hip or knee. Cochrane Database Syst Rev 2003;(3):CD004376.

81. Brosseau LM, et al. Intensity of exercise for the treatment of osteoarthritis. Cochrane Database Syst Rev 2003;(3):CD004376.

82. Soo Lee MP, et al. Tai Chi for osteoarthritis: a systematic review. Clin Rheumatol 2008;27(2):211–18.

83. Bandy WD, Sanders B. Therapeutic exercise: techniques for intervention. 1st ed. Philadelphia: Lippincott Williams and Wilkins; 2001.

84. Lipton L. Using yoga to treat disease: an evidence based review. JAAPA 2008;21(2):34–41.

85. Lee M, et al. Tai Chi for osteoarthritis: a systematic review. Clin Rheumatol 2008;27(2):211–18.

86. Bernardo L. The effectiveness of Pilates training in healthy adults: an appraisal of the research literature. J Bodyw Mov Ther 2007;11:106–10.

87. Warnock MM, et al. Effectiveness and safety of devil's claw tablets in patients with general rheumatic disorders. Phytother Res 2007;21(12):1228–33.

88. Sengupta KA, et al. A double blind, randomized, placebo controlled study of the efficacy and safety of 5-Loxin® for treatment of osteoarthritis of the knee. Arthritis Res Ther 2008;10(4):R85.

89. Beer A-MT. Willow bark extract (Salicis cortex) for gonarthrosis and coxarthrosis—results of a cohort study with a control group. Phytomedicine 2008;15:907–13.

90. McAlindon TJ, et al. Do antioxidant micronutrients protect against the development and progression of knee osteoarthritis? Arthritis Rheum 2005;39(4):648–56.

CHAPTER 26

Fibromyalgia

Leslie Axelrod
ND

OVERVIEW

Fibromyalgia (FM) is a syndrome based on widespread pain in the absence of a known aetiology, along with multiple somatic symptoms such as increased frequency of fatigue, non-restorative sleep, irritable bowel syndrome (IBS), headache, impaired cognition and mood.[1] This condition is more prevalent in women aged 20–50 years, but has also been seen in paediatric and geriatric populations. It affects 0.5% to 5.8% of the population in North America and Europe.[2,3] Updated criteria are likely to increase the reported incidence of this condition.[1]

The 2010 guidelines have been modified to include the wide array of symptoms experienced by FM patients. Previously, the diagnosis was primarily based on positive identification of 11 out of 18 tender points on physical exam, using digital palpation by the clinician (Figure 26.1).[4] These recent criteria are based solely on subjective reporting. Physical exam is only performed to rule out other conditions. The patient is encouraged to identify areas of pain, throughout the body, using a widespread pain index (WPI). In addition, somatic symptoms are identified and quantified using a symptom severity (SS) scale. A tally is made of these two indices and a diagnosis is made accordingly. A patient is diagnosed with FM if WPI > 7 and SS > 5 or WPI 4–6 and SS > 9[1]. Criteria state that the pain should be generalised pain, meaning present in at least four of five regions. Symptoms should be present for at least three months. Also, fibromyalgia may also be diagnosed in the presence of other valid diagnoses. The 2016 criteria increases sensitivity and specificity while reducing misdiagnoses of regional pain disorders.

The aetiology of FM is not fully understood, but ongoing research has been elucidating some possible mechanisms for this syndrome. Studies have revealed abnormal cytokine levels in response to stimulated peripheral mononuclear cells compared to controls, which has led to the development of newer lab testing for FM.[5,6] Biochemical, metabolic and cellular changes have been demonstrated in multiple systems including mitochondrial dysfunction with aberrations in adenosine-5'-triphosphate (ATP) synthesis and use, central nervous system (CNS) changes affecting cerebral blood flow, neurotransmitter synthesis and function and increased pain perception.[8]

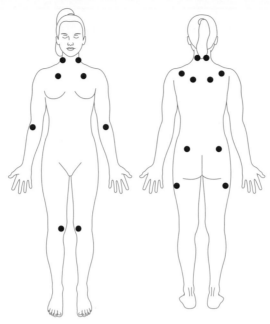

Figure 26.1
1990 criteria: fibromyalgia diagnostic tender points

Differential diagnosis*		
Condition	**Similarities**	**Confirmatory findings**
Vitamin D deficiency	Symptoms: widespread myalgias, depression, cognitive changes and fatigue	Lab: Low serum 25(OH)D
Hypothyroidism	Symptoms: myalgias,[11,12] fatigue, cognitive and mood changes	PE: possible thyromegaly Lab: Low TSH, Free T_3, FT_4 or Total T_3, TT4, and T_3 uptake
Inflammatory myalgias (polymyalgia rheumatica, polymyositis)	Symptoms: localised myalgias, fatigue, mood changes	History: severe pain localised to the proximal muscles (pelvic and shoulder girdle) Lab: possibly elevated CRP, ESR and elevated aldolase, creatine kinase in polymyositis
Rheumatoid arthritis	Symptoms: pain, sleep disturbances, fatigue and mood changes[13]	History: morning stiffness > one hour PE: joint effusion present Lab: possible positive RF, anti-CCP, elevated ESR and CRP
Myofascial pain syndrome (MPS) and trigger points (TrPs)	Symptoms: musculoskeletal pain with shared locations between TrP and tender points of FM[14] Autonomic dysfunction and sleep disturbances[15]	PE: referred pain with pressure, palpation of a taut band or tender nodules, stretch ROM limitation, elicited local twitch[16] Labs: Negative lab findings for both

*A variety of conditions present with non-specific myalgia, in the presences of somatic symptoms, similar to FM
CCP = cyclic citrullinated peptide; CRP = C-reactive protein; ESR = erythrocyte sedimentation rate; ROM = range of motion; RF = rheumatoid factor; 25(OH)D = 25-hydroxyvitamin D

Fibromyalgia diagnostic criteria

1) WPI: Note the number of areas in which the patient has had pain over the last week. In how many areas has the patient had pain? Score will be between 0 and 19.

Put a tick to indicate a painful region.

☐ Shoulder, L ☐ Shoulder, R	☐ Upper Leg, L ☐ Upper Leg, R	☐ Lower Back ☐ Upper Back ☐ Neck
☐ Hip, L ☐ Hip, R	☐ Lower Leg, L ☐ Lower Leg, R	
☐ Upper Arm, L ☐ Upper Arm, R	☐ Jaw, L ☐ Jaw, R	☐ No pain in any of these areas
☐ Lower Arm, L ☐ Lower Arm, R	☐ Chest ☐ Abdomen	

WPI score _____

2) SS scale score:

_____ Fatigue

_____ Waking unrefreshed

_____ Cognitive symptoms

For each of the 3 symptoms above, indicate the level of severity over the past week using the following scale:

    0 = no problem

    1 = slight or mild problems, generally mild or intermittent

    2 = moderate, considerable problems often present and/or at a moderate level

    3 = severe: pervasive, continuous, life-disturbing problems

Considering somatic symptoms in general, indicate whether the patient has:*

    0 = no symptoms

    1 = few symptoms

    2 = a moderate number of symptoms

    3 = a great deal of symptoms

The SS scale score is the sum of the severity of the 3 symptoms (fatigue, waking unrefreshed, cognitive symptoms) plus the extent (severity) of somatic symptoms in general. The final score is between 0 and 12.

_____ SS Scale Score

Criteria

A patient satisfies diagnostic criteria for fibromyalgia if the following 3 conditions are met:

1) Widespread pain index (WPI) ≥7 and symptom severity (SS) scale score ≥5 or WPI 4–6 and SS scale score ≥9.

2) Symptoms have been present at a similar level for at least 3 months.

3) The patient does not have a disorder that would otherwise explain the pain.

* Somatic symptoms that might be considered: muscle pain, irritable bowel syndrome, fatigue/tiredness, thinking or remembering problem, muscle weakness, headache, pain, cramps in the abdomen, numbness/tingling, dizziness, insomnia, depression, constipation, pain in the upper abdomen, nausea, nervousness, chest pain, blurred vision, fever, diarrhoea, dry mouth, itching, wheezing, Raynaud's phenomenon, urticaria/welts, ringing in ears, vomiting, heartburn, oral ulcers, loss of/change in taste, seizures, dry eyes, shortness of breath, loss of appetite, rash, sun sensitivity, hearing difficulties, easy bruising, hair loss, frequent urination, painful urination and bladder spasms.

Figure 26.2
Fibromyalgia diagnostic criteria sheet

Source: National Data Bank for Rheumatic Diseases 2013[7]

Hypothalamic–pituitary–adrenal (HPA) axis function is affected, resulting in a hyporesponsiveness of the adrenals and circadian rhythm abnormalities.[9] Somatic and visceral alterations have also been demonstrated in the literature.[10] The result of these changes contributes to the high incidence of comorbidities associated with this syndrome.

RISK FACTORS

There are a variety of risk factors associated with FM patients, including emotional, physical and genetic influences (Table 26.1). FM has comorbidities with multiple other rheumatological conditions. These findings combined with the high incidence of mood disorders, decreased pain threshold and non-restorative sleep predispose FM patients to irregularities in the HPA axis that are common in this cohort.[17,18] This spectrum of systemic changes along with aberrations in the health of the gastrointestinal tract contribute to this cascade via alterations in serotonin synthesis and use, nutritional deficiencies and immune dysfunction and must be differentiated from other disease patterns presenting with myalgias.[3]

Table 26.1
Predictive risks factors for developing fibromyalgia[18,19]

Age 20–50 years	Female > male (9:1)[2]
Lower education level and socioeconomic status	Comorbidity and outcome with other rheumatic diseases, such as rheumatoid arthritis, lupus and chronic fatigue syndrome (CFS) (see Chapter 38 on CFS)
Increased incidence of anxiety, depression and somatisation	Non-restorative sleep Poor social support system Previous history of domestic abuse and emotional trauma
Abnormal stress response	High prevalence of gastrointestinal dysfunction Inherited enzyme defects and familial link

CONVENTIONAL TREATMENT

A variety of allopathic medications have been used in the treatment of FM, including muscle relaxants, antidepressants, nonsteroidal anti-inflammatory drugs (NSAIDs), opioids, steroids and anti-convulsants with mixed and inconsistent results.[20]

Presently the United States Food and Drug Administration has approved three drugs for FM, serotonin–noradrenaline reuptake inhibitors (SNRIs) duloxetine and milnacipran and the gamma-aminobutyric acid (GABA) analogue, pregabalin. These SNRI medications have been found to be superior to other antidepressant classes including SSRIs and monoamine oxidase (MAO) medications[21,22] (Table 26.2). The tricyclic antidepressant (TCA) amitriptyline was also found be more effective than most SSRIs and MAOs and is widely used.[20] Interestingly, depression is commonly unaffected in FM patients using these regimens, possibly due to the low doses employed. In addition, suicidal ideations are 'black box warning' for many of these medications.[23]

The mechanism of action for pregabalin, an antiepileptic medication, is reduced levels of substance P, glutamate and noradrenaline, via modulation of calcium uptake.[24] Pain and sleep were most improved with its use but not fatigue, depressed mood or anxiety. Limitations of most of these studies include the short-term length of six months, absence of comorbidities and the exclusion of patients with severe somatic issues.[25,26] Comparison of these three approved drugs reveals no statistically significant difference for most parameters, except for pregabalin being superior to milnacipran for sleep.[27] Multiple

Table 26.2
Medication efficacy based on *p* values*

Symptom	SSRIs (fluoxetine and paroxetine)	SNRIs (duloxetine, milnacipran)	MAOs (moclobemide, pirlindole)	TCAs (amitriptyline)
Pain	0.04	< 0.001	0.03	< 0.001
Fatigue	0.25	0.23	0.66	0.003
Sleep	0.18	< 0.001	0.19	< 0.001
Depressed mood	0.02	0.001	0.88	0.76

*Meta-analysis of 18 randomised controlled trials (RCTs),[14] *p* < 0.05 significant

other pharmacological agents are being studied with promising results but presently lack adequate research. The opioid agonist naltrexone, given in low dosages (4.5 mg), showed a 30% reduction of symptoms, including pain and fatigue in a placebo-controlled study of 10 women. Side effects of insomnia and vivid dreams were considered transient.[28] A study of 26 patients using medical cannabis, 26 ± 8.3 g per month over approximately 11 months revealed significant improvement in the Revised Fibromyalgia Impact Questionnaire. A reported 50% of patients stopped taking other medications.[29] The synthetic cannabinoid, nabilone, recently approved in the United States, revealed significant improvement in pain relief and functional improvement in a randomised double-blind study of 40 FM patients. A double-blind, placebo-controlled, four-way crossover study with 20 FM patients using pharmaceutical-grade cannabis revealed a 30% decrease in pain scores with application of pressure. Patients used a vaporiser and were monitored for three hours after use. The more effective cannabis product included THC 13.4 mg and CBD 17.8 mg.[30,31]

Overall, the present pharmacological agents used do not address the full spectrum of FM and better, long-term, quality studies and scientific evidence is needed.

KEY TREATMENT PROTOCOLS

Metabolic changes occur at the cellular level, causing functional aberrations in FM patients. These include changes in glycolysis and isoenzyme production and reduction of energy reserves. Increased lactate production and decreased lactate dehydrogenase isoenzymes were present in the muscle tissue of FM patients.[32] A small study using magnetic resonance spectroscopy revealed decreased phosphocreatine, an essential

> **Naturopathic Treatment Aims**
>
> - Reduce pain.
> - Improve sleep.
> - Address mood and cognitive changes.
> - Address any digestive dysfunction.
> - Improve daily functioning.
> - Address underlying mitochondrial and cellular changes

muscle energy storage form, and reduced ATP levels in the quadriceps of FM patients compared with controls during rest. Total oxidative capacity and phosphorylation potential was also reduced during rest and exercise.[33] Increased oxidative DNA damage, along with a reduction of enzymatic activities of glutathione peroxidase, superoxide dismutase and catalase, were found in FM patients compared to controls.[34] Physical and mental impairment scores were correlated to the DNA oxidative damage. Another study found decreased platelet ATP, along with higher calcium and magnesium levels, implying irregularities in the calcium–magnesium pump mechanisms at the cellular level.[35] These biochemical aberrations contribute to the fatigue, weakness and exercise intolerance associated with FM.

Inconsistencies in the levels of magnesium are evident in the various blood components. Increased platelet magnesium and calcium levels have been found, low serum and red blood cell magnesium levels are noted.[36,37] Reduced serum magnesium levels correlate with fatigue but not to the number of tender points.[38] Studies of **malic acid** in combination with magnesium revealed dose dependent improvement with significant reductions in pain and tenderness measures in those taking 600/2400 mg compared with 300/1200 mg for at least two months.[37,39] A randomised, double-blind, placebo-controlled eight-week study using an intravenous (IV) micronutrient therapy (IVMT), **Myers' cocktail** (which contains magnesium) thiamine, vitamin C, calcium and B vitamins) demonstrated statistically significant improvement in tender points, pain, depression and quality of life in the IVMT group at eight weeks, while the placebo group of IV lactated Ringer's solution showed statistically significant improvement in tender points. The dramatic response of the placebo group negated a statistical significance between the groups. The response persisted for four weeks post-treatment for both groups.[40] Another eight-week uncontrolled case study of seven previously non-responsive patients by Massey revealed a 60% decrease in pain and 80% reduction in fatigue.[41]

The irregularities of the calcium–magnesium pump mechanism as suggested by Bazzichi may play a role in the muscle pain attributed to FM.[35] Other aberrations in calcium absorption and use may exist in the patient presenting with widespread pain. **Vitamin D** in the form of 1 alpha, 25-hydroxyvitamin D (25[OH]D3) promotes the calcium-dependent exocytotic activities of the cell when coupled with ATP, potentiating the bone anabolic effects of this nutrient.[42,43] A deficiency of vitamin D may masquerade as a generalised non-specific pain, depression and poor FM assessment scores.[44,45]

In multiple studies of patients presenting with persistent non-specific muscle pain as well as FM, 25(OH)D levels were frequently depressed.[46,47] Supplementation of vitamin D_2, 50 000 IU weekly for eight weeks, yielded significant clinical improvement in mild to moderately (10–25 µg/mL) deficient patients, but not severely deficient patients.[44] However, this regimen of supplementation has not consistently yielded pain reduction in moderately deficient patients, even after three months.[48] The most benefit was achieved when serum 25(OH)D levels were raised to over 50 µg/mL in FM patients with supplementation.[49] Armas et al. found supplemental vitamin D_3 prolonged 25(OH)D levels over time compared with vitamin D_2.[50]

Correction of vitamin D deficiency has not consistently yielded improvement in FM but may improve cognitive performance and mood disorders, especially anxiety and depression.[51,52] Evaluation of 25(OH)D levels and correction of low serum levels are warranted in all patients presenting with widespread pain.[53]

Phosphorylated **D-ribose** is a component of ATP and nicotinamide adenine dinucleotide (NADH) as D-ribose-5-phosphate, and may be helpful to FM patients. A small uncontrolled trial of 41 patients with FM and/or CFS, given 5 g of ribose three times daily, revealed significant improvement in energy and wellbeing according to a visual analogue scale.[53] Another supplement involved in ATP production via fatty acid transport into the mitochondria is **acetyl L-carnitine** (ALC). A randomised placebo-controlled study of 122 patients with FM taking three 500 mg capsules of ALC daily compared with placebo revealed significant improvement in musculoskeletal pain, number of tender points and depression as the 10-week study progressed past the sixth week.[54]

Modifying neurotransmission

The concept of 'somatisation' has been associated with FM secondary to the increased reporting of hypersensitivity to pain, cognitive dysfunction, depression, anxiety, social isolation and insomnia.[55] There is an increased incidence of adverse life events and psychological distress common to this primarily female cohort.[17] In addition to psychosocial stressors, the biochemical changes associated with neurotransmitter synthesis and use have been implicated and may contribute to the mental and emotional state of these patients (see Chapters 14–17 on the nervous system).

There is a genetic correlation of FM in families secondary to a defect in neurotransmitter metabolism. This polymorphic rate defect displays itself in catecholamine turnover secondary to catecholamine-O-methyl transferase enzyme and is linked to dopaminergic, adrenergic/non-adrenergic neurotransmission and the mu-opioid system.[56] This aberration has been associated with increased nociceptive response to painful stimuli. In addition to dopamine and adrenaline metabolism, reduced levels of serotonin and its precursors, **tryptophan** and **5-hydroxytryptophan** (5-HTP), are seen.[57,58] Low levels of plasma and serum serotonin (5-HT) have been highlighted in the literature and pharmacological treatment has focused on the use of antidepressants, most recently SSRIs and SNRIs, for treatment of pain, sleep and mood disturbances.[59] In FM patients, low levels of serotonin in combination with elevated levels of substance P, a neurotransmitter that has been associated with enhanced pain perception secondary to normal stimuli, has been considered to be a precipitating factor for the increased pain hypersensitivity found in FM.[60]

The conversion of tryptophan to serotonin involves the intermediary, 5-HTP. This biochemical pathway may be inhibited by stress, insulin resistance, tetrahydrobiopterin, pyridoxal 5-phosphate and magnesium deficiency.[61] Supplementation with 5-HTP alone has shown significant improvement in the number of tender points, anxiety, fatigue, pain intensity and quality of sleep during a 90-day trial of patients with primary FM syndrome. Mild transient side effects were reported in 30% of the patients.[61,62]

Another metabolic pathway utilises **S-adenosyl methionine (SAMe)** in the conversion of 5-HT to melatonin. It has been shown to be an effective antidepressant in psychiatric populations.[63] Two separate six-week trials of oral SAMe revealed improvement in pain, fatigue, mood and sleep, but not tender point count[64,65] (see Chapter 15 on depression). Longer studies are warranted to realise the potential benefits.

Herbal medicines specifically for treating FM have not been well documented in the scientific literature. Since combination formulas are the traditional mode of herbal dispensing, a balanced combination of herbal medicines would most likely best address the complex nature of an FM patient. However, single herbal medicines addressing the separate components of this syndrome will be presented, allowing the naturopathic practitioner to develop an individualised compound to best suit the needs of their patients (Table 26.3).[66,67]

Rhodiola rosea was found to increase 5-HT levels in the hippocampus of depressive rats to normal levels using 1.5 g/kg, 3 g/kg and 6 g/kg dosages.[68] A randomised placebo-controlled double-blind study of ***Hypericum perforatum*** (St John's wort: SJW) in the treatment of depressive patients with somatic complaints including depression, fatigue and disturbed sleep resulted in 70% of the patients being symptom-free after four weeks.[69] A rat study revealed a decrease in tryptophan, an increase in corticosterone and lower 5-HT in the hippocampus and amygdala under stressful physical conditions. When SJW was given to the stressed rats, serum 5-HT levels increased more than

Table 26.3
Fibromyalgia: summary of herbal medicine actions and examples

Adaptogens/tonics	*Withania somnifera, Panax ginseng, Rhodiola rosea, Eleutherococcus senticosus*
Antispasmodics	*Viburnum opulus, Piper methysticum, Piscidia erythrina, Scutellaria lateriflora*
Nervines	*Scutellaria lateriflora, Passiflora incarnata, Matricaria recutita, Melissa officinalis*
Thymoleptics	*Hypericum perforatum, Avena sativum, Lavandula angustifolia, Turnera diffusa*
Hypnotics	*Humulus lupulus, Passiflora incarnata, Valeriana* spp.
Analgesics	*Corydalis ambigua, Eschscholzia californica*
Digestives (aromatics, bitters, mucilages)	*Zingiber officinale, Taraxacum officinale, Ulmus fulva*
Circulatory stimulants	*Zingiber officinale, Ginkgo biloba, Cinnamomum zeylanicum, Zanthoxylum* spp.

Sources: Bone 2003[66] and Grieves 1973[67]

110%, 163% and 172% in the hypothalamus, amygdala and hippocampus respectively ($p < 0.01$), but corticosterone or tryptophan were not altered, demonstrating an adaptive response to stress.[70] In addition, a meta-analysis, including the Cochrane database, comparing SJW to key SSRIs revealed that there was a similar efficacy between the medications but fewer side effects with the HP.[71,72]

Regulation of circadian rhythm

Dysregulated circadian rhythms, manifesting as poor sleep patterns, non-restorative sleep and chronic fatigue, have been reported in FM patients.[73] Elevation of late evening cortisol and alterations in melatonin levels may contribute to the poor sleep patterns seen in this cohort.[74] Normal basal circadian rhythm is typically evidenced by a sharp rise in serotonin synthesis and a release of 5-HT in the early evening, preceding an elevation in melatonin production. There are conflicting data regarding melatonin secretion in FM patients. Decreased urinary melatonin secretion levels were found between the hours of 11 pm and 7 am[75–77] Meanwhile, in another study, plasma melatonin levels were elevated in FM patients between the hours of 11 pm and 6.50 am compared with controls, but secretory patterns remained similar.[78] This discrepancy between urinary and plasma melatonin levels was not demonstrated in non-depressed patients.[78] Despite the discrepancy and different methods of evaluation, it was found that administration of 3 mg of **melatonin** at bedtime in a small uncontrolled study revealed significant improvement in tender point count, pain severity and sleep after four weeks.[77]

HPA axis modulation

Another contributing factor to the non-restorative sleep, low energy and heightened pain perception may be associated with abnormalities in the HPA axis.[79] Dexamethasone suppression tests in FM patients show statistically significant increased release of ACTH with no resulting change in cortisol, indicating a hyporesponsiveness of the adrenal function to stimuli.[79] The increased ACTH:cortisol ratios, compared with controls, correlate to increased stress and anxiety measures. Also, the percentage of cortisol suppression is related to pain and fatigue as reported by patients.[80] Corticoid response to acute exercise is also impaired in FM patients.[81] In addition to lower basal plasma and urinary cortisol levels, there is a decreased expression of corticosteroid receptors, all of these contributing to the abnormal glucocorticoid response.[82] The combined dysfunction associated with the HPA axis and the adrenal response contributes to the aetiopathology and symptomology of FM.

A combination of *Eleutherococcus senticocus*, *Schisandra chinensis* and *Rhodiola rosea* revealed improved exercise endurance and tolerance to stress.[83,84] In addition, a single administration of *Panax ginseng* up-regulated the release of ACTH and corticosteroid initially but did not maintain this effect after seven days of *Panax ginseng* administration. However, *Panax ginseng* was shown to modulate the effect of hydrocortisone administration on the pituitary adrenocortical system even after seven days.[85]

Digestive disorders and dysbiosis

It is estimated that 30–70% of patients with FM have IBS concurrently.[86,87] In addition to altered visceral and somatic perception, both patient subsets have decreased serotonin synthesis and use, which may contribute to increased sensitivity to abdominal pain (see Chapter 4 on IBS).[87,88] In addition, the low levels of serotonin may alter motor and secretory function that can result in diarrhoea or constipation, both manifestations of IBS.[88] Increased intestinal and gastroduodenal permeability is associated with FM. In addition increased incidence of dysbiotic changes, as evidenced by the lactulose hydrogen breath test, implicates the prevalence of small intestinal bowel overgrowth (SIBO) in both these groups. The proximal small intestine typically has low levels of colonic type bacteria, but issues such as dysmotility and lack of gastric acid may exacerbate SIBO. The intensity of abdominal pain in FM patients with SIBO appears to correlate to the degree of bacterial overgrowth found in the small intestine.[89] In a double-blind randomised placebo-controlled trial, FM patients identified with SIBO were treated to achieve full eradication of the pathogenic flora compared with a non-eradicated group. The group that achieved complete eradication of dysbiotic flora had a significant improvement in pain and depression, in comparison to the non-eradicated group.[90] Eradication with antibiotics is standard allopathic treatment for SIBO, but recurrence rate is high, especially in populations using proton-pump inhibitors, which decrease gastric secretions.[91] A variety of natural agents, including allium sativa, grapefruit seed extract and berberine containing botanicals have been shown effective against *Staphylococcus*, *Escherichia coli* and *Klebsiella*, organisms associated with SIBO.[92–94] In addition, use of the probiotic *Lactobacillus plantarum* helps delay or prevent symptom recurrence after antibiotic therapy of SIBO.[95]

Studies using **glutamine** and **fibre** in animal studies demonstrated a reduction of bacterial translocation into lymph nodes, along with improvement in gut barrier function secondary to glutamine.[96–98] A nutrient solution of **L-arginine** alone at levels of 300 and 600 mg or in combination with nucleotides and omega-3 fatty acids showed a reduction in bacterial translocation.[99] In addition the **omega-3 fatty acids** may improve the outcome of FM patients over time by modulating inflammatory cytokines[100] (see Chapter 31 on autoimmunity). Strong consideration should also be given to normalise intestinal motility, gastric secretions, secretory immunoglobulin A (IgA), bile and pancreatic secretions, which help prevent SIBO.[101] The modification of SIBO and bacterial translocation may decrease the inflammatory response that appears to develop with longstanding FM.

Consider immune alteration

Immune activation was apparent in dermal biopsies of FM patients that revealed significantly elevated levels of IgG deposits in the dermis. In addition there was higher mean number of mast cells and an association between degranulated mast cells and the individual IgG immunofluorescence scores.[102] This IgG correlation may account, in part, for the prevalence of rhinitis in this cohort (70%) in the absence of positive skin allergy tests in 50–65% of this population.[103] Both IBS and migraines, common manifestations associated with FM, also demonstrate elevated IgG levels.[104,105] In a study of IBS patients, food antigen-specific IgE antibodies were not significantly different between FM patients and controls. IgG4 antibodies were significantly elevated in one study but did not significantly correlate with the severity of symptoms.[106]

IBS and migraines may both benefit by eliminating IgG positive foods, and reduction of circulating IgG may be beneficial in the treatment of FM patients. In addition to the role of IgG in functional bowel disturbances, IBS and migraines, it is possible that dermal IgG may contribute to sensory alterations and widespread pain. It appears that IgG plays a more significant role than IgE in the pathogenesis of a variety of co-existing complaints and that standard scratch testing and IgE titres are not the most accurate method of testing for this cohort. Also, since the severity of symptoms does not always correlate with the antibody titres, it is important to eliminate all reactive foods, even low-scoring ones.[106] Enzyme-linked immunosorbent assay (ELISA) testing of food antigens and subsequent trial elimination would be justified in this population.

Circulatory disturbances

It has been hypothesised that circulatory changes may be partially responsible for the pain, presence of tender points, exercise intolerance, Raynaud's phenomenon and cognitive changes present in FM.[107] Alterations in microcirculation and temperature were at the level of tender points, resulting in lower skin temperature. A lack of blood flow was implicated by decreased erythrocyte velocity and increased concentration of erythrocytes at tender points.[107] Muscle biopsy revealed increased dialysate lactate secondary to alterations in nitric oxide pathways; this may contribute to the reported exercise intolerance and exertion fatigue reported during aerobic exercise in these patients.[108] Impaired cerebral perfusion flow is also evident by brain single photon emission computed tomography (SPECT) and clinically correlated with the severity and associated disability of the small group evaluated.[109]

The correlation between circulatory and oxygenation disturbances with FM may explain the beneficial effect of **coenzyme Q10 (co-Q10)** and *Ginkgo biloba*. A small, uncontrolled study of 200 mg daily of both co-Q10 and *Ginkgo biloba* showed promise for improving quality-of-life measures.[110] Increased tissue perfusion was demonstrated by both substances. CoQ10 is present primarily in the mitochondria and assists in the generation of ATP via cellular respiration but also has been shown to be protective against lipid peroxidation secondary to cerebral hypo/hyperperfusion in rats.[111,112] Co-Q10 is also effective in the treatment of fatigue and migraines.[111,113] *Ginkgo biloba* increased blood flow velocity cerebrally, as well as having an effect on promoting vasculogenesis capacity, via endothelial progenitor cells stimulation in the peripheral blood, resulting in improved perfusion of the peripheral tissues.[114,115]

INTEGRATIVE MEDICAL CONSIDERATIONS

The FM patient is complex with irregularities in a multitude of processes including, but not limited to, cellular, neuroendocrine, digestive, vascular and emotional alterations.

The ubiquitous nature of this condition would benefit by a combination of energetic medicine, supplements, lifestyle and mind–body interventions. Table 26.4 summarises the primary naturopathic treatments for general muscle injury and pain (though it should be noted, these studies are not specific to fibromyalgia or myofascial pain syndrome).

Dry needling and injection therapy

Dry needling, considered '**Western' or 'medical' acupuncture**, is the use of acupuncture needles inserted into myofascial trigger points (MTrPs) (Figure 26.3). MTrPs have been found in patients with and without FM and appear to contribute to the pain associated with FM.[128,129] This method differs from traditional acupuncture in that it

Table 26.4
Example of naturopathic treatments for general muscle injury and pain

Intervention	Agent	Results	Comment
Homoeopathy	Homoeopathic: *Arnica montana* 6cH[116,117]	Animal studies pre and post showed a reduction in oedema, increased local blood and lymph flow to inflamed region Pre-treatment of carrageenan-induced oedema had a 30% inhibition (< 0.05)	Pre-treatment was more effective than after induction agent The succussed placebo was equal to the *Arnica* in some instances Results varied with induction agent used
	Traumeel ointment and injection (acute sprains, arthrosis, epicondylitis and local inflammation)[118–120]	Decreased IL6 and significant reduction of oedema Improved healing time in rats Large-scale human retrospective questionnaire assessed 79–87% 'good' or 'very good' results	The retrospective questionnaire study group was large but not very reliable due to subjectivity
Herbal medicine	*Boswellia carterii* or *serrata* (oral and topical)[121,122] *Boswellia carterii* in combination with *Commiphora myrrha*[122]	Anti-inflammatory action via inhibition of pro-inflammatory prostaglandins and increased analgesic activity when given separately or in combination (*Boswellia carterii* and myrrh combined) Results superior when combined	In vivo small rat study revealed topical application of *Boswellia* spp. extracts equally effective as oral using plant isolates versus whole plant Statistically significant results on inflammation for combined plant isolates
	Curcuma longa[123,124]	Anti-inflammatory action included reduction of paw swelling and inhibition of granulomatous tissue formation in rats	Oral absorption is an issue and is significantly increased when bound to piperine[125]
Enzymes	Bromelain[126,127]	Decreased traumatically induced oedema and lowered PG_2 and substance P levels in rats	Proteolytic activity, stability and resistance to trypsin inactivation varies among products Better results > 50 mg/mL Poor oral absorption Concentrated bolus better than time release

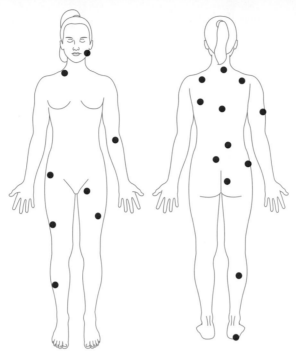

Figure 26.3
Common trigger points

Adapted from Simons 1998[16]

does not typically treat systemic conditions and is primarily confined to local treatment. The training between practitioners can vary significantly which may affect outcome of treatment. Baldry proposes that the needle should be inserted 5–10 mm, left in for 30 seconds for patients with MPS and then withdrawn and re-inserted for two to three minutes if the pain persists with pressure. FM patients are treated with fewer points, leaving the needles in for 5–10 seconds due to the increased sensitivity to pain in these patients. Baldry advises superficial dry needling, 2–3 mm depth, to deep dry needling, to reduce post-treatment soreness. Repeated treatments are typically necessary for both MPS and FM.[129] It is recommended that the practitioner elicit a 'twitch response' upon insertion, thought to be a rapid depolarisation of the muscle fibres, for superior results.[15] Deep versus superficial needling appears controversial. Ceccherelli et al. found improvement in the three-month follow-up of myofascial pain in patients who received deep needling versus superficial compared with minimal change initially post-treatment.[130]

Numerous studies have shown no significant difference between injection therapy or dry needling. Various agents have been used for injection therapy including anaesthetic, saline and sterile water with conflicting results in pain reduction for all agents. Some studies state there is no difference between saline and anaesthetic, while others state that anaesthetic is more effective.[131,132] There does not appear to be a significant difference between using saline or sterile water in pain reduction. However, sterile water injections were reported to be much more painful.[133]

Use of anaesthetic, usually lidocaine, xylocaine or procaine, was found to have prolonged results, past the expected duration of the anaesthetic effect. Injection into TrPs proved effective for pain relief for patients with myofascial pain, with and without FM, two weeks post-injection.[15]

A comparison of needle sizing, 21-, 23-, 25-gauge, all one inch, revealed no significant difference in effectiveness using a visual analogue score and local disability rating. In addition reported pain level elicited during the treatment was comparable between needle sizes.[134]

Technique is important and it may be recommended for the patient to be recumbent with the chosen needle length being long enough to reach the TrP.[16] Vapocoolant spray or distraction technique such as stretching or pinching can be employed to decrease needle insertion pain. Localisation of the TrP is essential and achieved by gentle palpation of a nodule in the taut band, eliciting a local twitch response with palpation or needle insertion. The TrP is isolated by mild superficial stretching between two fingers and the needle tip accurately inserted into the TrP. Multiple sites, typically 5–10, may be injected each visit, with 0.2 mL solution injected into each TrP or tender spot. Active stretch post-injection with full ROM is strongly encouraged with strenuous exercise discouraged for two to three days following.[15]

Traditional Chinese medicine

Acupuncture diagnosis commonly assesses pain as 'blood and Qi [energy] stagnation' and focuses on movement of these vital substances.[135] One study demonstrated an elevated number of erythrocytes in conjunction with a decrease in regional blood flow at the level of tender points of FM patients; this correlates to the Chinese theory of blood stagnation. Lower skin temperature was also found.[107] A follow-up study measured these indices pre- and post-acupuncture treatment. The therapeutic effect of acupuncture revealed a significant increase in blood flow and temperature at the level of the tender points after treatment.[136] Acupuncture has been shown to increase serotonin levels in rats with the insertion of a bilateral acupoint, Urinary Bladder 23. Elevated levels began after 20 minutes and maintained for 60 minutes post-treatment.[137] Substance P levels were reduced using electroacupuncture of local and distal points in a rat model.[138]

Acupuncture may have an adaptogenic response on cortisol levels. Animal studies on horses and rabbits using electroacupuncture showed an increase in cortisol levels post-treatment.[139-141] The inconsistencies of positive results with acupuncture, specifically on FM patients, may be based in part on the techniques used. In a meta-analysis of five randomised controlled studies, out of 11 evaluated, results were based on variables including reduction of pain, number of tender points and improvement in quality of life and sleep. The studies involving electroacupuncture overall achieved the best results. In addition, most of the positive studies used individualised treatments.[140] The negative studies used manual therapy, which may not have had sufficient stimulation to 'obtain Qi' in a population that has sensory perception alterations.

Cupping and moxibustion techniques, which were not addressed in the meta-analysis, may also have beneficial effects when included in acupuncture treatment.[142] The validity of sham acupuncture continues to be controversial, especially in a population with widespread pain. In acupuncture, insertion of needles into a painful point, termed an 'ashi' point, which is not otherwise considered a standard acupuncture point, is considered to be an effective treatment strategy for pain reduction. Meanwhile, the US National Institutes of Health consensus stance is that acupuncture is a sufficient adjuvant therapy to treat FM patients.[143]

Homeopathy

A double-blind, randomised, parallel-group, placebo-controlled study using individualised homeopathic medicine with daily LM potency over a three-month period was shown to be effective in treating FM. The number of tender points, pain on palpation and quality of health all improved significantly.[118] Another study using individualised homeopathic prescriptions revealed more significant improvement on fatigue and function with less effect on pain.[144]

Exercise and manual therapy

Exercise intolerance is a common manifestation in FM patients. Multiple studies, including a meta-analysis of eight studies, showed that **aerobic-only exercise training** programs revealed significant improvement in outcome measures, including physical function and global wellbeing while reducing pain, tender points and FM impact scores. Stretching and relaxation exercises did not yield the same effect. Improvement was seen as early as six weeks and maintained with exercise up to 12 months in some studies.[145–147] A review of pool exercise studies yielded improvement in mood and sleep as well as physical function and pain. The improvements, as reviewed in follow-up studies, showed a positive response for up to two years.[148]

Manual therapies have revealed positive results for a variety of parameters. A small study of FM patients receiving twice-weekly 30-minute massage treatments revealed a decrease of substance P and reduction in pain and anxiety, in addition to improvement in quality and number of sleep hours.[149] A small study of combined therapy of ultrasound and interferential current compared with sham procedure proved effective in reducing the pain intensity and tender point count while improving sleep in FM patients.[150] Low-dose ultrasound also significantly improved pain threshold in patient with MTrPs.[151,152]

Hydrotherapy

Hydrotherapy has been studied in various forms, with and without other physical therapy modalities. A warm-water pool-based exercise program revealed immediate improvement in pain indices in FM patients.[153] When a pool-based exercise therapy was compared with balneotherapy, 35 minutes three times per week, there was statistically significant improvement seen in morning stiffness, sleep, pain, tender points and global evaluation by the FM patient and the clinician in both groups. Pool-based exercise results maintained longer for most indices but overall did not show a significant superiority over balneotherapy alone.[154] Evcik revealed that 20 minutes of bathing alone once per day five days per week for three weeks significantly reduced the number of tender points and improved visual analogue scores, Fibromyalgia Impact Questionnaire score and Beck depression index.[155] All of these improvements were still statistically significant at the six-month follow-up, except for the Beck depression index.[156] When inflammatory mediators were measured in patients on a similar regimen, a significant reduction in IL-1 and leukotriene B_4 (LTB_4) was found in the FM patients.[156]

Mind–body therapy

The psychological component of FM in this primarily female population has been explored. Violence against women is epidemic as demonstrated in a cross-sectional, self-administered, anonymous survey of 1952 female patients. Physical, sexual and alcohol abuse and emotional status were all investigated among a diverse community-based population. The results of the survey indicated that one in 20 women had experienced domestic violence in the past year, one in five in their adult life and one in three as either a child or an adult. Participants that had experienced abuse within the past year were more likely to have depression, anxiety and somatisation.[157] Findings of another large case-controlled study of 574 women revealed an increased prevalence of abuse among FM patients over controls. There was a significant correlation between frequency of abuse and FM.[17] A Spanish epidemiological and quality-of-life study revealed low educational level, low social class and self-reported depression are much more prevalent in this FM population.[158] Depression co-existing with FM appears to decrease the pain threshold in these patients.[159] Effective treatment of FM must address the psychological impact as well as the biochemical changes to effect a longstanding improvement (see Chapter 15 on depression).

The prognosis for FM patients is partially dependent on social support and self-efficacy, which has been shown to predict positive lifestyle changes in FM patients.[159] A randomised controlled study of 91 patients with FM using mindfulness training during eight weekly sessions of 2.5 hours revealed alleviation of depressive symptoms, as assessed by the Beck Depression Inventory.[160] The effect of a six-week guided imagery program was to improve functional status and self-efficacy in the management of pain. Actual pain level did not change significantly.[161]

CLINICAL SUMMARY

FM is a complex syndrome that must be addressed on a physical, as well as psychological level (Figure 26.4). Aberrations occur in most body systems resulting in endocrine, circulatory, digestive and sleep disturbances. Pain perception is a result of some of these disturbances and influences the social and psychological abilities of the FM patient. A small array of allopathic medications appears helpful for some of the symptoms but also has unwanted side effects. Supplements, including nutritional and botanical, are promising; however, studies are typically small and uncontrolled (Table 26.5). Physical therapies including needling techniques, exercise and manual therapies have also been shown to be helpful.

Due to the complexity of this syndrome, a multidimensional approach should be taken to achieve the best results for patients experiencing the wide array of symptoms that are associated with FM.

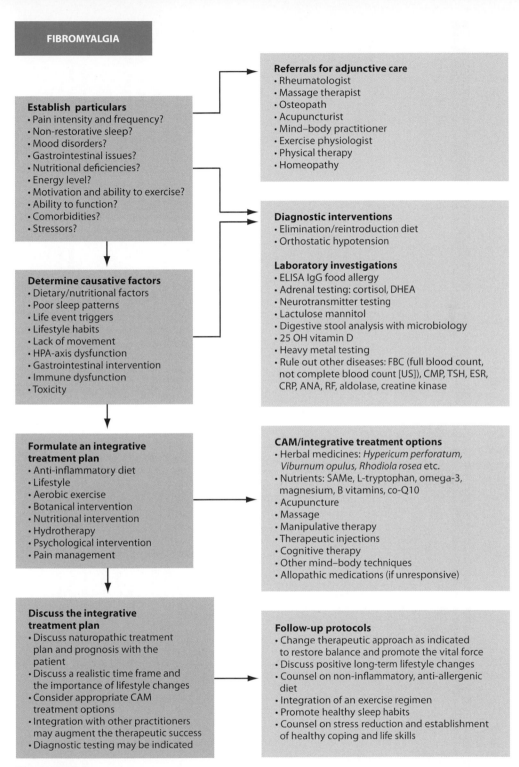

FIBROMYALGIA

Establish particulars
- Pain intensity and frequency?
- Non-restorative sleep?
- Mood disorders?
- Gastrointestinal issues?
- Nutritional deficiencies?
- Energy level?
- Motivation and ability to exercise?
- Ability to function?
- Comorbidities?
- Stressors?

Referrals for adjunctive care
- Rheumatologist
- Massage therapist
- Osteopath
- Acupuncturist
- Mind–body practitioner
- Exercise physiologist
- Physical therapy
- Homeopathy

Determine causative factors
- Dietary/nutritional factors
- Poor sleep patterns
- Life event triggers
- Lifestyle habits
- Lack of movement
- HPA-axis dysfunction
- Gastrointestinal intervention
- Immune dysfunction
- Toxicity

Diagnostic interventions
- Elimination/reintroduction diet
- Orthostatic hypotension

Laboratory investigations
- ELISA IgG food allergy
- Adrenal testing: cortisol, DHEA
- Neurotransmitter testing
- Lactulose mannitol
- Digestive stool analysis with microbiology
- 25 OH vitamin D
- Heavy metal testing
- Rule out other diseases: FBC (full blood count, not complete blood count [US]), CMP, TSH, ESR, CRP, ANA, RF, aldolase, creatine kinase

Formulate an integrative treatment plan
- Anti-inflammatory diet
- Lifestyle
- Aerobic exercise
- Botanical intervention
- Nutritional intervention
- Hydrotherapy
- Psychological intervention
- Pain management

CAM/integrative treatment options
- Herbal medicines: *Hypericum perforatum, Viburnum opulus, Rhodiola rosea* etc.
- Nutrients: SAMe, L-tryptophan, omega-3, magnesium, B vitamins, co-Q10
- Acupuncture
- Massage
- Manipulative therapy
- Therapeutic injections
- Cognitive therapy
- Other mind–body techniques
- Allopathic medications (if unresponsive)

Discuss the integrative treatment plan
- Discuss naturopathic treatment plan and prognosis with the patient
- Discuss a realistic time frame and the importance of lifestyle changes
- Consider appropriate CAM treatment options
- Integration with other practitioners may augment the therapeutic success
- Diagnostic testing may be indicated

Follow-up protocols
- Change therapeutic approach as indicated to restore balance and promote the vital force
- Discuss positive long-term lifestyle changes
- Counsel on non-inflammatory, anti-allergenic diet
- Integration of an exercise regimen
- Promote healthy sleep habits
- Counsel on stress reduction and establishment of healthy coping and life skills

Figure 26.4
Naturopathic treatment decision tree—fibromyalgia

Table 26.5
Review of the major evidence

Intervention	Mechanisms of action	Key literature	Summary of results	Comment
5-HTP **Dosage:** 100 mg 1–3 × day	Serotonin precursor Low serotonin and tryptophan levels associated with increased pain via elevated substance P, mood changes and insomnia	Caruso et al. 1990[61] Sarzi et al. 1992[62]	Two clinical trials Improvement in most parameters, ranging good to fair	Most improvement with co-existing sleep and mood disturbances
SAMe **Daily dosage:** 800 mg	Methyl donor involved in neurotransmitter synthesis, including serotonin	Jacobsen et al. 1991[64] Grasetto & Varotto 1994[162]	Clinical trial ($n = 44$) revealed improvement in clinical disease activity ($p = 0.04$), pain ($p = 0.002$), fatigue ($p = 0.02$), morning stiffness ($p = 0.03$) and mood ($p = 0.006$) Uncontrolled study ($n = 47$) Improvement in sleep ($p < 0.05$) and tender point count ($p < 0.01$)	Improved sleep, depression and tender point count, particularly after week 6
Magnesium/malic acid **Daily dosage:** Magnesium 600 mg Malic acid 2400 mg	Involved in glycolysis and mitochondrial function	Abraham 1992[37] Russell et al. 1995[39]	Clinical trial ($n = 15$) Significant reduction in tender point score ($p < 0.001$) Clinical trial ($n = 24$): Significant reduction in pain and tenderness after two months	Small, placebo-controlled studies, appear to be dose-dependent with better results at two months
Micronutrient IV	Supplies nutrients including magnesium (see above) and B vitamins involved in neurotransmitter synthesis Malabsorption of nutrients may be a result of FM related to digestive dysfunction	Ali et al. 2009[40]	Double-blind RCT ($n = 31$): Relief of symptoms for most patients compared with base line Both IVMT and placebo had statistically significant results, but not compared with each other	Lactated Ringer's solution was the placebo providing rehydration and electrolytes, which may be responsible for the improvement in the placebo group; this contributed to the absence of statistical significance of the study
D-ribose **Dosage:** 5 g 3 × day	Increase in cellular energy synthesis, especially in cardiac and skeletal muscle	Teitelbaum et al. 2006[53]	Clinical trial ($n = 41$): Significant improvement in visual analogue scale for energy (45%) and reported wellbeing ($p < 0.0001$)	Uncontrolled study with coexisting chronic fatigue syndrome in many of the patients

Table 26.5
Review of the major evidence (continued)

Intervention	Mechanisms of action	Key literature	Summary of results	Comment
Acetyl L-carnitine Dosage: 500 mg 3 × day	Decreases lactate production from glucose Increases phosphocreatinine, noradrenaline and serotonin[163]	Rossini et al. 2007[54]	Double-blind RCT ($n = 122$): Significant improvement in pain, tender points and depression	Most significant improvement after six weeks
Co-Q10/*Ginkgo biloba* Daily dosage: CoQ10 200 mg Gingko 200 mg	Co-Q10 assists in cellular respiration *Ginkgo biloba* increases cerebral and peripheral circulation	Lister 2002[110]	Uncontrolled study ($n = 25$) Progressive improvement of quality of life for 64%; 9% claimed to be worse	Questionnaire-based study showed promise for helping somatic symptoms of migraines and cognition, fatigue
Vitamin D Dosage: Vitamin D2 50 000 IU/week[44] Studies indicate better absorption with D3 compared to D2[164]	Deficiency associated with muscle weakness and increased pain levels in FM[45,46]	Arvold et al. 2009[44] Matthana 2011[49] Makrani 2017[45]	Studies showed short-term improvement of overall FM score but did not significantly improve musculoskeletal symptoms	Valuable for patients with widespread pain, but inconsistent improvement with FM patients Symptoms improved most when 25(OH)D serum levels > 50 μg/mL
Homeopathy	Unknown mechanism of action	Bell et al. 2004[118] Relton et al. 2009[144]	Individualised homeopathy significantly better than placebo	Results highly dependent on individualised treatment and practitioner skill
Acupuncture, dry needling, injection	Increases oxygenation and blood flow to tender points Increases endorphins, serotonin and cortisol	Mayhew & Ernst 2007[163] Li et al. 2006[142] Chang-Zern Hong et al. 2001[13] Cummings & White 2001[165] Ga et al. 2007[166]	Meta-analysis of five acupuncture RCTs revealed mixed results for FM Review of 23 randomised controlled studies of dry needling for MTrP revealed mixed results No significant difference between dry needling and injection	Pain reduction appears more dependent on technique and type of sham acupuncture for all methods Significantly better results using electroacupuncture than acupuncture alone Treatment of MTrP in FM patients decreased tender point count
Physical therapies, balneotherapy, exercise, manual therapy (massage, ultrasound, interferential)	Increased circulation and oxygenation to skeletal muscle Increased cerebral circulation with exercise	Busch et al. 2008[145] Gowans et al. 2007[148] Richards 2002[146] Almeida 2003[150] Altan et al. 2004[154] Evcik et al. 2002[155]	Studies show reduction of tender point counts Improvement in sleep, pain threshold and tender point counts	Aerobic exercise was consistently more effective than stretching and relaxation exercises Improvement in pain threshold is found with various manual therapies

FURTHER READING

Bontle, et al. A diagnostic biomarker profile for fibromyalgia syndrome based on an NMR metabolomics study of selected patients and controls. BMC Neurol 2017;17:88.

Chaitow L. Fibromyalgia syndrome, a practitioner's guide to treatment. 3rd ed. Churchill Livingstone; 2010.

Wolfe F, et al. 2016 Revisions to the 2010/2011 fibromyalgia diagnostic criteria. Semin Arthritis Rheum 2016;46(3):319–29.

REFERENCES

1. Wolfe F, et al. The American College of Rheumatology preliminary diagnostic criteria for fibromyalgia and measurement of symptom severity. Arthritis Care Res (Hoboken) 2010;62(5):600–10.
2. Gran JT. The epidemiology of chronic generalized musculoskeletal pain. Best Pract Res Clin Rheumatol 2003;17(4):547–61.
3. Dadabhoy D, et al. Biology and therapy of fibromyalgia. Evidence-based biomarkers for fibromyalgia syndrome. Arthritis Res Ther 2008;10(4):211.
4. Wolfe F, et al. The American College of Rheumatology 1990 criteria for the classification of fibromyalgia. Report of the Multicenter Criteria Committee. Arthritis Rheum 1990;33(2):160–72.
5. Behm FG, Gavin IM, Karpenko O, et al. Unique immunologic patterns in fibromyalgia. BMC Clin Pathol 2012;12:25.
6. Behm FG, Gavin IM, Karpenko O, et al. Cytokine and chemokine profiles in fibromyalgia, rheumatoid arthritis and systemic lupus erythematosus: a potentially useful tool in differential diagnosis. Rheumatol Int 2015;35:991–6.
7. National Data Bank for Rheumatic Diseases. 2013. Fibromyalgia diagnostic criteria. Online. Available: http://www.arthritis-research.org/sites/default/files/FM%20Criteria%20Work%20Sheet.pdf. 18 Feb 2013.
8. Sprott H, et al. Increased DNA fragmentation and ultrastructural changes in fibromyalgic muscle fibres. Ann Rheum Dis 2004;63(3):245–51.
9. Korszun A, et al. Melatonin levels in women with fibromyalgia and chronic fatigue syndrome. J Rheumatol 1999;26(12):2675–80.
10. Mayer EA, Raybould HE. Role of visceral afferent mechanisms in functional bowel disorders. Gastroenterology 1990;99(6):1688–704.
11. Pillai MG, et al. Prevalence of musculoskeletal manifestations in thyroid disease. Thyroid Res Pract 2009;6(1):12–16.
12. Kole AK, et al. Rheumatic manifestations in primary hypothyroidism. Indian J Rheumatol 2013;8(1):8–13.
13. Nicassio PM, et al. The contribution of pain and depression to self-reported sleep disturbance in patients with rheumatoid arthritis. Pain 2012;153(1):107–12.
14. Hong C, et al. Difference in pain relief after trigger point injections in myofascial pain patients with and without fibromyalgia. Arch Phys Med Rehabil 1996;77(11):1161–6.
15. Molodofsky H. The contribution of sleep-wake physiology to fibromyalgia. In: Advances in Pain Research and Therapy, vol. 17. New York: Raven Press; 1990. p. 227–50, [Chapter 13].
16. Simons D, et al. Travell & Simons' Myofascial pain and dysfunction: the trigger point manual, vol. 1. 2nd ed. Philadelphia: Lippincott, Williams & Wilkins; 1998. p. 21–2, 155–69.
17. Sarzi-Puttini P, et al. Dysfunctional syndromes and fibromyalgia: a 2012 critical digest. Clin Exp Rheumatol 2012;30(6 Suppl. 74):143–51.
18. Gur A, Oktayoglu P. Central nervous system abnormalities in fibromyalgia and chronic fatigue syndrome: new concepts in treatment. Curr Pharm Des 2008;14(13):1274–94.
19. Ruiz-Perez I, et al. Risk factors for fibromyalgia: the role of violence against women. Clin Rheumatol 2009;28(7):777–86.
20. Lautenschlager J. Present state of medication therapy in fibromyalgia syndrome. Scand J Rheumatol Suppl 2000;113:32–6.
21. Tofferi JK. Treatment of fibromyalgia with cyclobenzaprine: a meta-analysis. Arthritis Rheum 2004;51(1):9–13.
22. Hauser W, et al. Treatment of fibromyalgia syndrome with antidepressants: a meta-analysis. JAMA 2009;301(2):198–209.
23. Food and Drug Administration News. FDA proposes new warnings about suicidal thinking, behavior in young adults

who take antidepressant medications, in P07–77. 2 May 2007.

24. Häuser W, et al. Treatment of fibromyalgia syndrome with gabapentin and pregabalin—a meta-analysis of randomized controlled trials. Pain 2009;145(1–2):69–81.

25. Smith MT, et al. Pregabalin for the treatment of fibromyalgia. Expert Opin Pharmacother 2012;10: 1527–33.

26. Choy E, et al. A systematic review and mixed treatment comparison of the efficacy of pharmacological treatments for fibromyalgia. Semin Arthritis Rheum 2011;41(3):335–45.

27. Russell IJ, et al. The effects of pregabalin on sleep disturbance symptoms among individuals with fibromyalgia syndrome. Sleep Med 2009;10(6):604–10.

28. Younger J, et al. Low-dose naltrexone reduces the primary symptoms of fibromyalgia. J Pain 2009;10(4):S41.

29. Habib G, Artul S. Medical cannabis for the treatment of fibromyalgia. J Clin Rheum 2018.

30. Skrabek R, et al. Nabilone for the treatment of pain in fibromyalgia. J Pain 2008;9(2):164–73.

31. van de Donk T, Niesters M, Kowal MA, et al. An experimental randomized study on the analgesic effects of pharmaceutical-grade flowers of cannabis sativa in chronic pain patients with fibromyalgia. Pain 2019;160(4):860–9.

32. Anonymous. Is fibromyalgia caused by a glycolysis impairment? Nutr Rev 1994;52(7):248–50.

33. Park JH, et al. Use of P-31 magnetic resonance spectroscopy to detect metabolic abnormalities in muscles of patients with fibromyalgia. Arthritis Rheum 1998;41(3):406–13.

34. La Rubia M, Rus A, et al. Is fibromyalgia-related oxidative stress implicated in the decline of physical and mental health status? Clin Exp Rheumatol 2013;31(6 Suppl. 79):S121–7.

35. Bazzichi L, et al. ATP, calcium and magnesium levels in platelets of patients with primary fibromyalgia. Clin Biochem 2008;41(13):1084–90.

36. Eisinger J, et al. Selenium and magnesium status in fibromyalgia. Magnes Res 1994;7(3–4):285–8.

37. Abraham GE. Management of fibromyalgia: rationale for the use of magnesium and malic acid. J Nutr Med 1992;3:49–59.

38. Sendur OF, et al. The relationship between serum trace element levels and clinical parameters in patients with fibromyalgia. Rheumatol Int 2008;28(11): 1117–21.

39. Russell IJ, et al. Treatment of fibromyalgia syndrome with Super Malic: a randomized, double blind, placebo controlled, crossover pilot study. J Rheumatol 1995;22(5):953–8.

40. Ali A, et al. Intravenous micronutrient therapy (Myers' Cocktail) for fibromyalgia: a placebo-controlled pilot study. J Altern Complement Med 2009;15(3):247–57.

41. Massey PB. Reduction of fibromyalgia symptoms through intravenous nutrient therapy: results of a pilot clinical trial. Altern Ther Health Med 2007;13(3):32–4.

42. Xiaoyu Z, et al. 1alpha, 25(OH)2-vitamin D3 membrane-initiated calcium signaling modulates exocytosis and cell survival. J Steroid Biochem Mol Biol 2007;103(3–5):457–61.

43. Biswas P, Zanello LP. 1alpha, 25(OH)(2) vitamin D(3) induction of ATP secretion in osteoblasts. J Bone Miner Res 2009;24(8):1450–60.

44. Arvold DS, et al. Correlation of symptoms with vitamin D deficiency and symptom response to cholecalciferol treatment: a randomized controlled trial. Endocr Pract 2009;15(3):203–12.

45. Makrani AH, et al. Vitamin D and fibromyalgia: a meta-analysis. Korean J Pain 2017;30(4):250–7.

46. Plotnikoff GA, Quigley JM. Prevalence of severe hypovitaminosis D in patients with persistent, nonspecific musculoskeletal pain. Mayo Clin Proc 2003;78(12):1463–70.

47. Badsha H. Myalgias or non-specific muscle pain in Arab or Indo-Pakistani patients may indicate vitamin D deficiency. Clin Rheumatol 2009;28(8):971–3.

48. Warner AE, Arnspiger SA. Diffuse musculoskeletal pain is not associated with low vitamin D levels or improved by treatment with vitamin D. J Clin Rheumatol 2008;14(1):12–16.

49. Matthana MH. The relation between vitamin D deficiency and fibromyalgia syndrome in women. Saudi Med J 2011;32(9):925–9.

50. Armas LA, et al. Vitamin D2 is much less effective than vitamin D3 in humans. J Clin Endocrinol Metab 2004;89(11):5387–91.

51. Wilkins CH, et al. Vitamin D deficiency is associated with worse cognitive performance and lower bone density in older African Americans. J Natl Med Assoc 2009;101(4):349–54.

52. Armstrong DJ, et al. Vitamin D deficiency is associated with anxiety and depression in fibromyalgia. Clin Rheumatol 2007;26(4):551–4.

53. Teitelbaum JE. The use of D-ribose in chronic fatigue syndrome and fibromyalgia: a pilot study. J Altern Complement Med 2006;12(9):857–62.

54. Rossini M, et al. Double-blind, multicenter trial comparing acetyl L-carnitine with placebo in the treatment of fibromyalgia patients. Clin Exp Rheumatol 2007;25(2):182–8.

55. Schochat T, Raspe H. Elements of fibromyalgia in an open population. Rheumatology (Oxford) 2003;42(7):829–35.

56. Zubieta JK, et al. COMT val158met genotype affects mu-opioid neurotransmitter responses to a pain stressor. Science 2003;299(5610):1240–3.

57. Russell IJ, et al. Serum amino acids in fibrositis/fibromyalgia syndrome. J Rheumatol Suppl 1989;19:158–63.

58. Yunus MB, et al. Plasma tryptophan and other amino acids in primary fibromyalgia: a controlled study. J Rheumatol 1992;19(1):90–4.

59. Wolfe F, et al. Serotonin levels, pain threshold, and fibromyalgia symptoms in the general population. J Rheumatol 1997;24(3):555–9.

60. Russell IJ, et al. Elevated cerebrospinal fluid levels of substance P in patients with the fibromyalgia syndrome. Arthritis Rheum 1994;37(11):1593–601.

61. Caruso I, et al. Double-blind study of 5-hydroxytryptophan versus placebo in the treatment of primary fibromyalgia syndrome. J Int Med Res 1990;18(3):201–9.

62. Sarzi P, Caruso I. Primary fibromyalgia syndrome and 5-hydroxy-L-tryptophan: a 90-day open study. J Int Med Res 1992;20(2):182–9.

63. Kagan BL, et al. Oral S-adenosylmethionine in depression: a randomized, double-blind, placebo-controlled trial. Am J Psychiatry 1990;147(5):591–5.

64. Jacobsen S, et al. Oral S-adenosylmethionine in primary fibromyalgia. Double-blind clinical evaluation. Scand J Rheumatol 1991;20(4):294–302.

65. Grassetto M, et al. Primary fibromyalgia is responsive to S-adenosyL-L-methionine. Current Therapeutic Research. 1994;55(7):797–806.

66. Bone K. A clinical guide to blending liquid herbs: herbal formulations for the individual patient. St Louis: Churchill Livingstone; 2003.

67. Grieves B. A modern herbal. Chatham: Jonathan Cape Ltd; (1931). 1973.

68. Chen QG, et al. The effects of Rhodiola rosea extract on 5-HT level, cell proliferation and quantity of neurons at cerebral hippocampus of depressive rats. Phytomedicine 2009;16(9):830–8.

69. Hubner WD. Hypericum treatment of mild depressions with somatic symptoms. J Geriatr Psychiatry Neurol 1994;7(Suppl. 1):S12–14.

70. Ara I, Bano S. St. John's Wort modulates brain regional serotonin metabolism in swim stressed rats. Pak J Pharm Sci 2009;22(1):94–101.

71. Rahimi R. Efficacy and tolerability of Hypericum perforatum in major depressive disorder in comparison with selective serotonin reuptake inhibitors: a meta-analysis. Prog Neuropsychopharmacol Biol Psychiatry 2009;33(1):118–27.

72. Linde K. St John's wort for major depression. Cochrane Database Syst Rev 2008;(4):CD000448.

73. Korszun A. Sleep and circadian rhythm disorders in fibromyalgia. Curr Rheumatol Rep 2000;2(2):124–30.

74. Crofford LJ, et al. Basal circadian and pulsatile ACTH and cortisol secretion in patients with fibromyalgia and/or chronic fatigue syndrome. Brain Behav Immun 2004;18(4):314–25.

75. Klein DC, et al. The melatonin rhythm-generating enzyme: molecular regulation of serotonin N-acetyltransferase in the pineal gland. Recent Prog Horm Res 1997;52:307–57, discussion 357–8.

76. Wikner J, et al. Fibromyalgia—a syndrome associated with decreased nocturnal melatonin secretion. Clin Endocrinol (Oxf) 1998;49(2):179–83.

77. Citera G, et al. The effect of melatonin in patients with fibromyalgia: a pilot study. Clin Rheumatol 2000;19(1):9–13.

78. Matthews CD. Human plasma melatonin and urinary 6-sulphatoxymelatonin: studies in natural annual photoperiod and in extended darkness. Clin Endocrinol (Oxf) 1991;35(1):21–7.

79. Griep EN. Altered reactivity of the hypothalamic-pituitary-adrenal axis in the primary fibromyalgia syndrome. J Rheumatol 1993;20(3):469–74.

80. Wingenfeld K, et al. The low-dose dexamethasone suppression test in fibromyalgia. J Psychosom Res 2007;62(1):85–91.

81. Paiva ES, et al. Impaired growth hormone secretion in fibromyalgia patients: evidence for augmented hypothalamic somatostatin tone. Arthritis Rheum 2002;46(5):1344–50.

82. Macedo JA, et al. Glucocorticoid sensitivity in fibromyalgia patients: decreased expression of corticosteroid receptors and glucocorticoid-induced leucine zipper. Psychoneuroendocrinology 2008;33(6):799–809.

83. Sun LJ, et al. [Effects of schisandra on the function of the pituitary-adrenal cortex, gonadal axes and carbohydrate metabolism in rats undergoing experimental chronic psychological stress, navigation and strenuous exercise]. Zhonghua Nan Ke Xue 2009;15(2):126–9.

84. Panossian A, et al. Adaptogens exert a stress-protective effect by modulation of expression of molecular chaperones. Phytomedicine 2009;16(6–7):617–22.

85. Filaretov AA, et al. Role of pituitary-adrenocortical system in body adaptation abilities. Exp Clin Endocrinol 1988;92(2):129–36.

86. Almansa C, et al. Prevalence of functional gastrointestinal disorders in patients with fibromyalgia and the role of psychologic distress. Clin Gastroenterol Hepatol 2009;7(4):438–45.

87. Wallace DJ, Hallegua DS. Fibromyalgia: the gastrointestinal link. Curr Pain Headache Rep 2004;8(5):364–8.

88. Crowell MD. Role of serotonin in the pathophysiology of the irritable bowel syndrome. Br J Pharmacol 2004;141(8):1285–93.

89. Goebel A, et al. Altered intestinal permeability in patients with primary fibromyalgia and in patients with complex regional pain syndrome. Rheumatology (Oxford) 2008;47(8):1223–7.

90. Pimentel M. Eradication of small intestinal bacterial overgrowth reduces symptoms of irritable bowel syndrome. Am J Gastroenterol 2000;95(12):3503–6.

91. Lauritano EC, et al. Small intestinal bacterial overgrowth recurrence after antibiotic therapy. Am J Gastroenterol 2008;103(8):2031–205.

92. Ankri S, et al. Antimicrobial properties of allicin from garlic. Microbes Infect 1999;1(2):125–9.

93. Freile ML, et al. Antimcrobial activity of aqueous extracts of berberine isolated from Berberis heterophylla. Fitoterapia 2003;74(7–8):702–5.

94. Drozdowicz D, et al. Gastroprotective activity of grapefruit (Citrus paradisi) seed extract against gastric lesions. In: Nuts and seeds in health and disease prevention. Academic Press; 2011. p. 553–60, [Chapter 66].

95. Quigley EM, et al. Small intestinal bacterial overgrowth: roles of antibiotics, prebiotics, and probiotics. Gastroenterology 2006;130(2 Suppl):S78–90.

96. Spaeth G. Fibre is an essential ingredient of enteral diets to limit bacterial translocation in rats. Eur J Surg 1995;161(7):513–18.

97. Evans MA, Shronts EP. Intestinal fuels: glutamine, short-chain fatty acids, and dietary fiber. J Am Diet Assoc 1992;92(10):1239–46, 1249.

98. Xu D. Elemental diet-induced bacterial translocation associated with systemic and intestinal immune suppression. JPEN J Parenter Enteral Nutr 1998;22(1):37–41.

99. Aydogan A, et al. Effects of various enteral nutrition solutions on bacterial translocation and intestinal morphology during the postoperative period. Adv Ther 2007;24(1):41–9.

100. Kang JX, Weylandt KH. Modulation of inflammatory cytokines by omega-3 fatty acids. Subcell Biochem 2008;49:133–43.

101. Bures J, et al. Small intestinal bacterial overgrowth syndrome. World J Gastroenterol 2010;16(24):2978–90.

102. Enestrom S. Dermal IgG deposits and increase of mast cells in patients with fibromyalgia—relevant findings or epiphenomena? Scand J Rheumatol 1997;26(4):308–13.

103. Baraniuk JN, et al. Nasal secretion analysis in allergic rhinitis, cystic fibrosis, and nonallergic fibromyalgia/chronic fatigue syndrome subjects. Am J Rhinol 1998;12(6):435–40.

104. Zuo XL, et al. Alterations of food antigen-specific serum immunoglobulins G and E antibodies in patients with irritable bowel syndrome and functional dyspepsia. Clin Exp Allergy 2007;37(6):823–30.

105. Arroyave H. Food allergy mediated by IgG antibodies associated with migraine in adults. Rev Alerg Mex 2007;54(5):162–8.

106. Zar S, et al. Food-specific IgG4 antibody-guided exclusion diet improves symptoms and rectal compliance in irritable bowel syndrome. Scand J Gastroenterol 2005;40(7):800–7.

107. Jeschonneck M, et al. Abnormal microcirculation and temperature in skin above tender points in patients with fibromyalgia. Rheumatology (Oxford) 2000;39(8):917–21.

108. McIver KL, et al. NO-mediated alterations in skeletal muscle nutritive blood flow and lactate metabolism in fibromyalgia. Pain 2006;120(1–2):161–9.

109. Guedj E, et al. Clinical correlate of brain SPECT perfusion abnormalities in fibromyalgia. J Nucl Med 2008;49(11):1798–803.

110. Lister RE. An open, pilot study to evaluate the potential benefits of coenzyme Q10 combined with Ginkgo biloba extract in fibromyalgia syndrome. J Int Med Res 2002;30(2):195–9.

111. Mizuno K, et al. Antifatigue effects of coenzyme Q10 during physical fatigue. Nutrition 2008;24(4):293–9.

112. Tsukahara Y. Antioxidant role of endogenous coenzyme Q against the ischemia and reperfusion-induced lipid peroxidation in fetal rat brain. Acta Obstet Gynecol Scand 1999;78(8):669–74.

113. Sandor PS, et al. Efficacy of coenzyme Q10 in migraine prophylaxis: a randomized controlled trial. Neurology 2005;64(4):713–15.

114. Zhang J, et al. The therapeutic effect of Ginkgo biloba extract in SHR rats and its possible mechanisms based on cerebral microvascular flow and vasomotion. Clin Hemorheol Microcirc 2000;23(2–4):133–8.

115. Chen J, et al. Effects of Ginkgo biloba extract on number and activity of endothelial progenitor cells from peripheral blood. J Cardiovasc Pharmacol 2004;43(3):347–52.

116. Macêdo S, et al. Anti-inflammatory activity of Arnica montana 6cH: preclinical study in animals. Homeopathy 2004;93(2):84–7.

117. Kawakami A, et al. Inflammatory process modulation by homeopathic Arnica montana 6CH: the role of individual variation. Evid Based Complement Alternat Med 2011;2011.

118. Bell IR, et al. Improved clinical status in fibromyalgia patients treated with individualized homeopathic remedies versus placebo. Rheumatology (Oxford) 2004;43(5):577–82.

119. Zenner S, et al. Therapy experience with a homeopathic ointment: results of drug surveillance conducted on 3,422 patients. Biol Ther 1994;12(3):204–11.

120. Lussignoli S, et al. Effect of Traumeel S, a Homeopathic formulation, on blood-induced inflammation in rats. Complement Ther Med 1999;7(4):225–30.

121. Singh S, et al. Boswellic acids: a leukotriene inhibitor also effective through topical application in inflammatory disorders. Phytomedicine 2008;15(6–7):400–7.

122. Shulan S, et al. Evaluation of the anti-inflammatory and analgesic properties of individual and combined extracts from Commiphora myrrha, and Boswellia carterii. J Ethnopharmacol 2012;139(2):649–56.

123. Mukhopadhyay A. Anti-inflammatory and irritant activities of Curcumin analogues in rats. Agents Actions 1982;12(4):508–15.

124. Lorenzo D, et al. Plant food supplements with anti-inflammatory properties: a systematic review (II). Crit Rev Food Sci Nutr 2013;53(5):507–16.

125. Shaikh J, et al. Nanoparticle encapsulation improves oral bioavailability of curcumin by at least 9-fold when compared to curcumin administered with piperine as absorption enhancer. Eur J Pharm Sci 2009;37(3–4):223–30.

126. Gaspani L. In vivo and in vitro effects of bromelain on PGE_2 and SP concentrations in the inflammatory exudate in rats. Pharmacology 2002;65:83–6.

127. Hale LP, et al. Proteinase activity and stability of natural bromelain preparations. Int Immunopharmacol 2005;5(4):783–93.

128. Chaitow L, et al. Acupuncture treatment of fibromyalgia and myofascial pain. In: Fibromyalgia syndrome: a practitioner's guide to treatment. 2nd ed. Edinburgh: Churchill Livingstone; 2003. p. 113–27, [Chapter 6].

129. Baldry PE, Thompson JW. Treatment of Myofascial trigger point pain and fibromyalgia syndromes. In: Acupuncture, trigger points and musculoskeletal pain. 3rd ed. Churchill Livingstone; 2005. p. 127–48, [Chapter 10].

130. Ceccherelli F, et al. Comparison of superficial and deep acupuncture in the treatment of lumbar myofascial pain: a double-blind randomized controlled study. Clin J Pain 2002;18(3):149–55.

131. Hameroff SR, et al. Comparison of bupivacaine, etidocaine, and saline for trigger-point therapy. Anesth Analg 1981;60(10):752–5.

132. Hanten WP. Effectiveness of a home program of ischemic pressure followed by sustained stretch for treatment of myofascial trigger points. Phys Ther 2000;80(10):997–1003.

133. Wreje U, et al. A multicenter randomized controlled trial of injections of sterile water and saline for chronic myofascial pain syndromes. Pain 2005;61(3):441–4.

134. Yoon S, et al. Comparison of 3 needle sizes for trigger point injection in myofascial pain syndrome of upper- and middle-trapezius muscle: a randomized controlled trial. Arch Phys Med Rehabil 2009;90(8):1332–9.

135. Maciocia G. The practice of Chinese medicine: the treatment of diseases with acupuncture and Chinese herbs. London: Churchill Livingstone; 1994.

136. Sprott H, et al. [Microcirculatory changes over the tender points in fibromyalgia patients after acupuncture therapy (measured with laser-Doppler flowmetry)]. Wien Klin Wochenschr 2000;112(13):580–6.

137. Yoshimoto K, et al. Acupuncture stimulates the release of serotonin, but not dopamine, in the rat nucleus accumbens. Tohoku J Exp Med 2006;208(4):321–6.

138. Tu WZ, et al. [Effect of electroacupuncture of local plus distal acupoints in the same segments of spinal cord on spinal substance P expression in rats with chronic radicular pain]. Zhen Ci Yan Jiu 2008;33(1):7–12.

139. Schneider A, et al. Neuroendocrinological effects of acupuncture treatment in patients with irritable bowel syndrome. Complement Ther Med 2007;15(4): 255–63.

140. Cheng R, et al. Electroacupuncture elevates blood cortisol levels in naive horses; sham treatment has no effect. Int J Neurosci 1980;10(2–3):95–7.

141. Liao YY, et al. Effect of acupuncture on adrenocortical hormone production: I. Variation in the ability for adrenocortical hormone production in relation to the duration of acupuncture stimulation. Am J Chin Med 1979;7(4):362–71.

142. Li CD, et al. [Clinical study on combination of acupuncture, cupping and medicine for treatment of fibromyalgia syndrome]. Zhongguo Zhen Jiu 2006;26(1):8–10.

143. Acupuncture. NIH Consensus Statement 1997;15(5):1–34.

144. Relton C, et al. Healthcare provided by a homeopath as an adjunct to usual care for fibromyalgia (FMS): results of a pilot randomised controlled trial. Homeopathy 2009;98(2):77–82.

145. Busch AJ, et al. Exercise for fibromyalgia: a systematic review. J Rheumatol 2008;35(6):1130–44.

146. Richards SC, Scott DL. Prescribed exercise in people with fibromyalgia: parallel group randomised controlled trial. BMJ 2002;325(7357):185.

147. Valim V, et al. Aerobic fitness effects in fibromyalgia. J Rheumatol 2003;30(5):1060–109.

148. Gowans SE, deHueck A. Pool exercise for individuals with fibromyalgia. Curr Opin Rheumatol 2007;19(2):168–73.

149. Field T, et al. Fibromyalgia pain and substance P decrease and sleep improves after massage therapy. J Clin Rheumatol 2002;8(2):72–6.

150. Almeida T. The effect of combined therapy (ultrasound and interferential current) on pain and sleep in fibromyalgia. Pain 2003;104(3):665–72.

151. Srbely JZ. Stimulation of myofascial trigger points with ultrasound induces segmental antinociceptive effects: a randomized controlled study. Pain 2008;139(2):260–6.

152. Falconer J. Therapeutic ultrasound in the treatment of musculoskeletal conditions. Arthritis Care Res 1990;3(2):85–91.

153. Segura-Jiménez V, et al. A warm water pool-based exercise program decreases immediate pain in female fibromyalgia patients: uncontrolled clinical trial. Int J Sports Med 2013;34(7):600–5.

154. Altan L. Investigation of pool based exercise on fibromyalgia syndrome. Rheumatol Int 2004;24(5): 272–7.

155. Evcik D. The effects of balneotherapy on fibromyalgia patients. Rheumatol Int 2002;22(2):58–9.

156. Ardic F, et al. Effects of balneotherapy on serum IL-1,PGE2 and LTB4 levels in Fibromyalgia patients. Rheumatol Int 2007;27(5):441–6.

157. McCauley J, et al. The 'battering syndrome': prevalence and clinical characteristics of domestic violence in primary care internal medicine practices. Ann Intern Med 1995;123(10):737–46.

158. Mas AJ, et al. Prevalence and impact of fibromyalgia on function and quality of life in individuals from the general population: results from a nationwide study in Spain. Clin Exp Rheumatol 2008;26(4):519–26.

159. Beal CC, Stuifbergen AK, Brown A. Predictors of a health promoting lifestyle in women with fibromyalgia syndrome. Psychol Health Med 2009;14(3):343–53.

160. Sephton SE, et al. Mindfulness meditation alleviates depressive symptoms in women with fibromyalgia: results of a randomized clinical trial. Arthritis Rheum 2007;57(1):77–85.

161. Menzies V. Effects of guided imagery on outcomes of pain, functional status, and self-efficacy in persons diagnosed with fibromyalgia. J Altern Complement Med 2006;12(1):23–30.

162. Grassetto M, Varotto A, et al. Primary fibromyalgia is responsive to S-adenosyl-L-methionine. Curr Ther Res 1994;55(7):797–806.

163. Mayhew E, Ernst E. Acupuncture for fibromyalgia—a systematic review of randomized clinical trials. Rheumatology (Oxford) 2007;46(5):801–4.

164. Autier P, et al. A systematic review: influence of vitamin D supplementation on serum 25-hydroxy-vitamin D concentration. J Clini Endocrinol Metab 2012;97(8):2606–13.

165. Cummings T, White A. Needling therapies in the management of myofascial trigger point pain: a systematic review. Arch Phys Med Rehabil 2001;82(7):986–92.

166. Ga H. Acupuncture needling versus lidocaine injection of trigger points in myofascial pain syndrome in elderly patients—a randomised trial. Acupunct Med 2007;25(4):130–6.

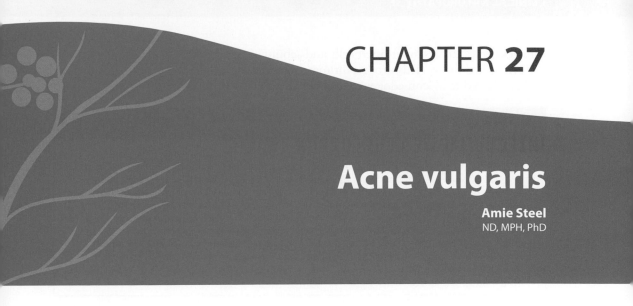

CHAPTER 27

Acne vulgaris

Amie Steel
ND, MPH, PhD

OVERVIEW

Acne vulgaris is a condition typified by inflammation of the pilosebaceous follicles in the skin.[1] It is characterised by a variety of lesions including nodules, papules, pustules and open and closed comedones. The global prevalence of acne vulgaris is estimated at 9.4% of the general population[2] while moderate to severe acne affects approximately 20% of adolescents and young adults and the severity of the symptoms is associated with pubertal maturity.[3] However, the sequence of the pathophysiological development of these lesions is still unclear. The dominant hypothesis at this stage focuses on increased circulating androgens stimulating sebaceous gland activity, and the resulting sebum production triggering hyperkeratosis. This process blocks the follicle and results in dilation and the ultimate formation of a comedone.[1] The transition from a comedone to a lesion such as a pustule, papule or nodule is believed to be due to a bacterium, called *Propionibacterium acnes*, colonising the follicle and triggering an inflammatory response within the follicle wall.[1] This cascade involves T helper cells (CD4+), most likely subtype T helper 1, and macrophages, which infiltrate the local area, possibly as a result of antigenic stimulation. The antigen identified as the most likely initiator of inflammation is *Propionibacterium acnes*. This trigger is believed to develop due to weakness in the follicular basement membranes, associated with reduced linoleic acid levels in the follicular wall. This has been explained through increased sebum production depleting local fatty acid stores. Once an inflammatory cascade has begun, hyperproliferation of

DIFFERENTIAL DIAGNOSIS

- Acne conglobata
- Acne fulminans
- Acne keloidalis nuchae
- Acneiform eruptions
- Acne rosacea
- Cutaneous sarcoidosis
- Folliculitis

- Perioral dermatitis
- Sebaceous hyperplasia
- Polycystic ovarian syndrome
- Underlying medical conditions (e.g. Cushing's syndrome)
- Drug therapy (steroid, anticonvulsants)

follicles can occur. As keratinised cells and sebum compact within the follicular lumen, a 'horny plug' forms. This process ultimately results in the development of a comedone and is referred to as 'comedogenesis'.[1]

Propionibacterium acnes

Propionibacterium acnes was initially considered the cause of acne vulgaris following its identification in acne lesions in 1896. This has been supported by evidence of a failure of antibiotic treatment of acne due to erythromycin-resistant strains of *P. acnes*. However, more recent research has determined that *P. acnes* may trigger or exacerbate acne vulgaris, but it is not the only factor. In fact, some acne lesions do not have any sign of bacterial infection. It is now considered that *P. acnes* is not the primary cause of acne, although it is still considered a significant contributor to the inflammation.[1,3] *P. acnes* is more commonly connected with the appearance of pustules, rather than the least severe comedones. This occurs due to the bacteria breaking down sebum into specific fatty acids, which trigger an inflammatory response. The inflammation weakens the dermal layer and opportunistic staphylococcal organisms invade, forming a pustule.[1] *P. acnes* has also been proposed to initiate the transformation of naive CD4 cells into T helper (TH)17 cells, resulting in the production of interleukin-17.[2]

RISK FACTORS

Predisposing and exacerbating factors relating to the development of acne vulgaris include hereditary predisposition, premenstrual hormonal fluctuations, increased androgen levels, heavy or irritating clothing, backpacks or helmets, the application of oily creams, the use of certain drugs and exposure to increased heat and humidity.[1] Recent advancements in genomic research has identified an association between severe teenage acne and the chromosomal locus of 8q24 (also associated with a range of cancers) and with the upregulation of androgen receptors.[4] Some dietary and lifestyle factors, such as smoking,[1] exposure to dioxins,[1] dairy intake[5] or glycaemic load,[1,5] may also increase the risk of acne; however, specific attributable risk in this area remains unclear until further research is conducted.

CONVENTIONAL TREATMENT

Treatment of acne vulgaris focuses on the bacterial and hormonal aetiology of the condition. The hormonal mainstays of medical intervention include oral contraceptives and antiandrogen medication (spironolactone, cyproterone acetate or flutamide), often combined with steroidal anti-inflammatory medication in instances of severe inflammation or hyperandrogenism.[6–8] Approaching acne management through hormonal regulation is justified through the presence of androgen receptors in the basal layer of sebaceous glands and in the outer root sheath keratinocytes in the hair follicle. Oral contraceptives interfere with the stimulation of these receptors by reducing ovarian production of androgens, while the other antiandrogen medications act as receptor blockers. Topical management through the use of peeling agents (benzoyl peroxide, tretinoin or isotretinoin) and antibacterial agents (tetracycline) are also commonly used to control lesions.[1,8]

The most common drug used in severe, chronic acne vulgaris is isotretinoin. Isotretinoin affects epidermis health through a number of mechanisms, including promotion of epidermal cell differentiation, stimulation of keratinocyte proliferation and reduction of sebaceous gland size (by suppressing the proliferation of basal sebocytes and sebum production). Immunomodulatory and anti-inflammatory properties have also been identified. Isotretinoin is usually prescribed on average for 20 weeks, with a starting dose of 0.5–1 mg/kg/day and concomitant prescription of oral antibiotics for the first four weeks of treatment.[8]

Naturopathic management of patients taking this medication needs to be approached carefully due to potential side effects of oral retinoid therapy. Individuals who have been prescribed isotretinoin should avoid pregnancy, due to potential congenital malformations associated with the drug. There is also a risk of psychiatric conditions such as depression, psychoses and suicidal thoughts. It is also worth noting that, however rare, liver conditions such as acute hepatitis can be triggered through isotretinoin therapy and, because of this, hepatoprotective interventions may be worth considering. At the very least ethanol extracts of herbs may need to be modified to reduce potentially compounding the impact upon liver health. Most commonly, however, isotretinoin affects mucous membranes and can cause cheilitis, dry eyes, dry mouth, dry skin and desquamation of lips.[9] Recent research has identified elevated serum homocysteine levels in patients with cystic acne undergoing isotretinoin therapy; however, no differences in vitamin B12, folic acid or liver function tests were observed.[10] The health implications of this result is discussed in more detail in Chapters 11–13 on the cardiovascular system. An additional study has found isotretinoin to decrease free triiodothyronine (T_3), thyroid-stimulating hormone and thyroid-stimulating hormone receptor antibodies alongside luteinising hormone, prolactin, testosterone, cortisol and adrenocortiocotrophic hormone.[11] Some possible complementary prescriptions that may support those taking isotretinoin include zinc, methionine, arginine, vitamin E, soy protein, fish oil and L-carnitine. However, any inclusion of these interventions in the treatment plan would require careful and close monitoring as research in this area is still preliminary.[12]

Potential side effects of isotretinoin therapy

The side effects of isotretinoin therapy are essentially the same as vitamin A toxicity (hyper-vitaminosis A syndrome) and include:

- hepatoxicity
- musculoskeletal disorders
- transient hyperlipidaemia
- cheilitis

- teratogenicity
- pseudotumor cerebri (benign intracranial hypertension)
- psychiatric effects.

Source: Desai et al. 2007[13]

KEY TREATMENT PROTOCOLS

The understanding of acne vulgaris from a naturopathic perspective focuses on the factors that can contribute to androgen excess and inflammatory responses. As there are a number of underlying factors that can be involved, depending on the individual, the treatment will centre on those that have been identified to be relevant to the patient. However, more general management of inflammation and androgen excess is also an important component of the naturopathic approach to treatment.

Naturopathic Treatment Aims

- Increase detoxification through all channels of elimination.
- Reduce oxidative load and improve antioxidant status.
- Regulate blood sugar levels.
- Reduce production of inflammatory compounds.
- Regulate sympathetic and parasympathetic nervous system activity.
- Reduce serum androgen levels.
- Reduce sebum production and sebocyte proliferation.

Hormone modulation

The sebaceous glands, and the skin in general, are sites for androgen synthesis within the human body. In fact, prior to puberty, the sebaceous glands, particularly in the face and scalp, are the primary sites of androgen conversion from adrenal precursor hormones such as DHEA-S. All key enzymes required to convert cholesterol to androgens, particularly testosterone, are locally present within the sebaceous gland. Androgens, specifically dihydrotestosterone, are understood to be involved in both the regulation of cell proliferation and lipogenesis. In contrast, oestrogens are understood to inhibit excessive sebaceous gland activity, possibly by increasing androgen binding to its binding globulin.[14,15]

Management of acne focusing specifically on the elevated androgen levels includes the application of herbs such as ***Serenoa repens***. This plant medicine acts to reduce the conversion of testosterone to dihydrotestosterone through inhibition of the enzyme responsible, 5-α-reductase. However, there are two subtypes of 5-α-reductase and *Serenoa repens* is only confirmed to inhibit type II (which occurs in the prostate). While its effects on type I (which occurs elsewhere) remains unexamined. The clinical effectiveness of *Serenoa repens* for acne vulgaris is not certain. Although no research is apparently specifically related to acne vulgaris, preliminary research reports successful outcomes when using this herb in a range of other androgen-dominant conditions.[16–18] An additional approach to the herbal management of hormone modulation often considered in acne vulgaris is ***Vitex agnus-castus***.[19] *Vitex agnus-castus* has been traditionally used for the regulation of hormonal conditions particularly focusing on sexual and reproductive functions,[20] and this has been supported through more recent research identifying dopaminergic and oestrogenic compounds extracted from the herb,[21] although much of this research has focused on female reproductive complaints.[22] Another herbal intervention to be considered is a *kampo* (traditional Japanese medicine) combination formula of ***Paeonia* spp.** and ***Glycyrrhiza* spp.**, which has been found to reduce testosterone and improve oestrogen:testosterone ratio in women with polycystic ovarian syndrome.[23] Although the exact mechanism is unclear, it has been argued that this occurs due to an increased aromatase activity, thereby converting testosterone to 17β-oestradiol, and/or central nervous system activity resulting in an increase in pituitary secretion of follicle-stimulating hormone and luteinising hormone.[23] Preliminary research also suggests a possible benefit when combining spironolactone and *Glycyrrhiza* spp. for the management of hyperandrogenism.[24]

Similarly, other natural substances may be used in managing acne vulgaris, although not yet specifically investigated for the condition, based upon their known activity within the body. For example, enterolactone, a phyto-oestrogenic compound derived from flaxseed, has been found to reduce the Free Androgen Index (FAI).[25] However, this substance is activated from precursors found in flaxseed by the microflora found in the human colonic intestinal tract; this microflora may be affected by the use of oral antibiotics.[26]

Free Androgen Index

The FAI (sometimes called the Testosterone Free Index or TFI) is determined by calculating the ratio of the total testosterone concentration to the concentration of sex hormone binding globulin. It often increases in severe acne, hirsutism, polycystic ovarian syndrome and male androgenic alopecia (male-pattern baldness).[27]

The effects of stress: androgens and inflammation

The symptoms of acne vulgaris are worse in times of psychological stress.[1] Physiological adaptation to stress may be a contributing factor to acne vulgaris due to the hormonal cascade this produces. In particular, increased physiological stress results in hypothalamic secretion of noradrenaline and thereby corticotrophic-releasing hormone (CRH). CRH then stimulates release of adrenocorticotrophic hormone (ACTH) from the anterior pituitary. The primary target of ACTH is the adrenal cortex through which it affects adrenal androgen secretion.[28] CRH also inhibits secretion of gonadotrophic releasing hormone, resulting in lower gonadic hormones, thereby further exacerbating the androgen:oestrogen imbalance often seen in acne vulgaris.[28]

In addition to the hormonal repercussions of stress, cutaneous tissue is the site of a complex system of autocrine and paracrine functions that are stimulated by prostaglandins. Increased inflammatory response stimulates a cascade of stress hormone release, which begins with CRH and culminates in the release of cortisol, thereby generating an anti-inflammatory response. The expression of CRH receptors is modulated by hormones such as testosterone and oestrogen.[14]

These dual effects of stress support the potential benefits associated with **adaptogenic herbs** (see Chapter 8 on respiratory disorders) including *Rhodiola rosea*,[29] *Panax ginseng* and *Withania somnifera*.[30] It also suggests that herbs with both anti-inflammatory and adrenal tonic activity such as *Glycyrrhiza glabra*[31] may be beneficial.

Androgen metabolism and clearance

Naturopathically, the skin has been referred to as 'the third kidney'. The rationale behind this statement is the role the skin plays in detoxification of the system. Both phase I and phase II detoxification enzymes are found in human skin. The phase I enzymes in integumentary tissue are mostly represented by alcohol dehydrogenase; however, CYP450 enzymes are also present although at much lower levels.[32] The subtypes of CYP450 found in the skin are generally involved in hydroxylation of a number of compounds, including retinoids, prostanoids, inflammatory mediators, arachidonic acid and cholesterol. In contrast, the phase II enzymes are expressed in high concentrations. These include glutathione-*S*-transferase, catechol-O-methyltransferase and steroid sulfotransferase.[32] Likewise, aromatase has been found in high concentrations in sebaceous glands and may act to clear excess androgens.[33] This implies that the skin does have an important role in detoxification, particularly through phase II enzymes. It also suggests that compromised or stressed liver detoxification may place further burden on the skin, thereby aggravating dermal conditions such as acne vulgaris. With this in mind, it may be more accurate to refer to the skin as the 'second liver' rather than the third kidney.

Androgens and diet

A potential confounding factor within hormone imbalances related to acne may come from the diet.[38] For example, milk intake as a teenager has been associated with an increased incidence of acne. These results were not found to be linked to saturated fat intake as skim milk consumption had a higher association and it has been hypothesised that the hormonal content of the milk may be a contributing factor, particularly for adolescent females. Alternatively, the higher glycaemic index (GI) load of skim milk compared with full cream milk may be a contributing factor.[39]

A diet with a high glycaemic load can result in increased plasma levels of glucose, insulin and insulin-like growth factor-1 (IGF-1), all of which have been associated with

---

Alteratives and depuratives

Historically, naturopaths have emphasised the importance of detoxification to manage a number of conditions including renal, urinary, hepatic, endocrine and skin disease.[34] It is explained by Benedict Lust in his seminal text that 'the origin of all is again to be readily explained by accumulations of foreign matter; and here we have especially to do with the accumulations affecting the normal function of those organs so important for the secretion of waste matter from the body: the kidneys and the skin'.[34] This is the foundation upon which the herbal medicine management of skin disorders was originally based: the use of alteratives and depuratives. An alterative or depurative has been defined as a herb that 'improves detoxification and aids elimination to reduce the accumulation of metabolic waste products within the body'.[31] Herbs that are traditionally considered to have this action include (but are by no means limited to): *Iris versicolor*, *Arctium lappa*, *Galium aparine*, *Echinacea* spp., *Chionanthus virginicus*, *Berberis aquifolium*, *Smilax ornata* and *Rumex crispus*. However, it is interesting to note that no current research validating the empirical use of these herbs has been found. This is an important area within naturopathic management of skin diseases, and such research would provide great benefit to evidence-based naturopathic practice.

Clearance of excess hormones and other aggravating substances has historically been managed naturopathically using depurative herbs. These herbs are associated with improved detoxification and elimination of metabolic wastes.[31] There are a number of herbs that have been traditionally used for chronic skin disorders (see above for more information). However, very little modern research has been undertaken investigating the benefits of these herbs in acne vulgaris.[19] More recently, naturopaths have been using an extract from cruciferous vegetables, known as indole-3-carbinol, to stimulate hepatic metabolism of excess steroidal hormones, including androgens.[35] Like the depurative herbs, however, there is no specific research linking this compound with acne vulgaris, but understanding its mechanism of action does suggest some potential clinical benefit.

In contrast to these beneficial interventions, cigarette smoking and tobacco-related products have been found to inhibit aromatase activity,[36] and as such may exacerbate acne vulgaris, but this has not yet been supported through epidemiological research.[37]

---

an increased FAI. By following a low-glycaemic load and high-protein diet, researchers have found reduced lesion count, reduced FAI and increased IGF-binding protein-1.[40] However, research in this area is still inconclusive due to conflicting results.[41]

Inflammation, infection and topical management

Immune modulation to reduce inflammation and bacterial infection of the acne lesions is another important component of the naturopathic management of acne vulgaris. This is often achieved through minimising oxidation, decreasing physiological stress and reducing inflammatory triggers such as elevated blood glucose levels and bacterial infection of the lesion. However, more direct anti-inflammatory approaches may also be included in the treatment of acne vulgaris. One such option is **quercetin**, a compound synthesised by plants, with a known anti-inflammatory effect through inhibition of TNF-α, NFκB, IL-2 and IFNγ.[42] Another commonly used compound is **bromelain**, derived from pineapples. Bromelain is an enzyme complex that acts to reduce inflammation through inhibiting cyclo-oxygenase-2 expression and inactivating NFκB.[43]

Oxidative stress and inflammatory mediators

Oxidative stress has been found to be increased in patients with acne vulgaris, although it is unclear whether this is a cause or symptom.[44,45] However, as oxidative stress has been linked to inflammatory responses, it is an important factor to address when managing this condition.

Dietary intake of *trans*-fatty acids, found in margarines, spreads, frying and cooking oils,[46] has been associated with increased inflammatory markers such as C-reactive protein (CRP),[47] TNF receptor-1 and TNF receptor-2.[48] For this reason, it is recommended that dietary intake of processed and deep-fried foods be reduced in people with acne vulgaris.

Furthermore, compromised levels of dietary antioxidants have been linked with acne vulgaris. One study identified a strong relationship between low levels of vitamin A and vitamin E and acne. In fact, it was found that levels in the lower quintile were associated with the severity of the condition.[49] The link between oxidative stress and acne vulgaris also suggests that medicinal herbs with known antioxidant activity, such as **Rosmarinus officinalis**[50] and **Camellia sinensis**,[51] may be beneficial. However, beyond some interest in *Camellia sinensis* as a cosmetic ingredient,[51] it must be noted that no known clinical research has been undertaken investigating the oral use of these herbs in acne vulgaris.

Nutrients such as **selenium**[52] and **zinc**[53] also have known antioxidant activity and may be beneficial in reducing oxidative stress in acne vulgaris. Selenium has undergone clinical trials for patients with acne vulgaris and has been found to improve the antioxidant profile of people with acne[54] as well as reduce the number of inflammatory lesions (Figure 27.1).[56] The clinical significance of this research is not yet clear, although it is known that lower glutathione peroxidase levels are found in patients with acne compared with controls.[57] Clinical research for oral zinc supplements in acne vulgaris has also been undertaken, and found to result in statistically significant improvements.[58] Combining zinc with other anti-inflammatory nutrients such as vitamin E and lactoferrin—an iron-binding milk-derived protein—has also been found to produce a clinical improvement in acne vulgaris symptoms.[59] As mentioned in the previous section, *P. acnes* has been found to induce Th17 ad Th1 responses in mononucleocytes, but vitamin A (all-*trans* retinoic acid) and vitamin D (1,25-dihydroxyvitamin D3) may inhibit this action.[60]

Topical treatments and antimicrobial activity

Medical management of acne vulgaris usually incorporates an aspect of antibacterial and topical treatments, and naturopathic approaches are no different. Essential oils are often used topically on acne lesions, with the main focus of such treatments being antimicrobial activity. A range of **essential oils** including *Thymus vulgaris* L., *Rose damascena* Mill. and *Cinnamomum zeylanicum* N. have recently been identified through in vitro research to exert antimicrobial activity on *Propionibacterium acnes*.[61] Another study compared **Melaleuca alternifolia** essential oil with benzoyl peroxide, a common topical antibacterial treatment.[62] This study found both treatments to be effective; although the *Melaleuca alternifolia* had a slower response rate it also had fewer side effects. In fact, in vitro research[63] has found that *Propionibacterium acnes* is susceptible to *Melaleuca alternifolia* at concentrations as low as 0.25%. Additional in vitro research has found *Juglans regia* to be more effective than *Melaleuca alterniflolia* as an antimicrobial for acne-related organisms.[64]

Topical application of **Camellia sinensis** has also been investigated in relation to sebum production. A recent animal study[65] found that a number of green tea catechins (including epigallocatechin-3-gallate) reduced sebocyte proliferation, and other compounds such as kaempferol reduce sebocyte lipogenesis. This potential treatment has been further explored using patients with acne vulgaris and a 2% 'tea lotion'[66]; however, the exact formula of the tea lotion was not defined and as such the clinical relevance is unclear. Preliminary research has identified a polysaccharide found in *Camellia sinensis* extracts that reduces *Propionibacterium acnes* adhesion to human cutaneous tissue.[67] This

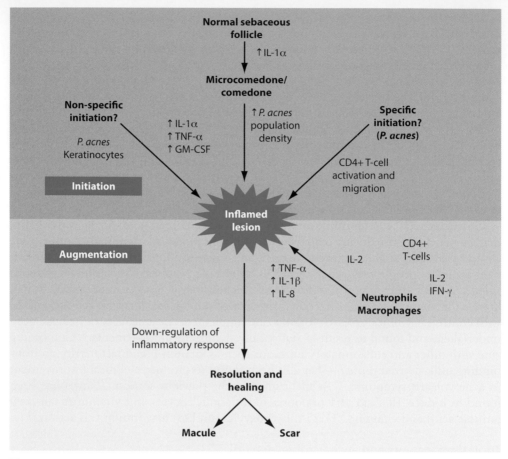

Figure 27.1
Events in the evolution of an inflammatory acne lesion
Source: Farrar & Ingham 2004[55]

research needs to be expanded further to explore the application of green tea extract on topical acne lesions, but the implications are promising.

Other emerging research indicates the topical application of resveratrol, an antioxidant compound occurring in grapes, may reduce the severity of acne but the mechanism of action has not been explored.[68] In contrast, a small human study investigating the effect of topical application of *Curcuma longa* in reducing acne inflammation found no benefit.[69]

INTEGRATIVE MEDICAL CONSIDERATIONS

Beyond the naturopathic treatments already considered, there are a number of other therapies that may be considered when developing an integrative medical treatment plan.

Psychotherapy

One such consideration is psychotherapy. Given the physiological impact of stress on the pathogenesis of acne and the importance of emotional health to overall wellbeing, it is important to consider counselling as an important therapy adjunctive to acne management. The basic acknowledgment of emotional responses such as embarrassment and low self-image is an important part of this process and can be implemented from the first consultation.[70]

Phototherapy

Phototherapy is another method of treatment to be considered. Blue light phototherapy has been examined for acne management,[71] and was found to reduce lesions (although not to affect *Propionibacterium acnes* colonies). A similar result has also been found for red light phototherapy.[72] The combination of both red and blue light phototherapy is also showing some promise.[73]

Hygiene considerations

Skin hygiene is a controversial consideration within a treatment regimen associated with the management of acne vulgaris. Some preliminary research has found that the difference between showering immediately after exercise-induced sweating and waiting four hours before showering made no statistically significant difference to the symptoms of acne.[74] Similar research was conducted regarding face-washing and acne, comparing groups using a standard mild cleanser and washing once, twice and four times a day for six weeks.[75] The group washing twice per day had improvements in both open comedones and non-inflammatory lesions; however, there appeared to be no real advantage to washing more frequently than this. Hygiene considerations more generally—such as higher environmental bacterial levels on floors, bedding and so on— have been implicated in other skin conditions such as atopic dermatitis and therefore could be considered.[76]

Acupuncture treatment for acne vulgaris has been examined through a meta-analysis of 10 RCTs. The findings suggest that acupuncture may be as effective as standard conventional treatments but with fewer side effects.[77]

Ayurvedic herbs

Ayurvedic herbal medicine may also provide some support in managing acne vulgaris. An in vitro study was undertaken to explore the effect of a number of Ayurvedic herbs on inflammatory mediators associated with *Propionibacterium acnes* infection and the pathogenesis of acne vulgaris.[78] Of the herbs studied, **Rubia cordifolia**, **Curcuma longa**, **Hemidesmus indicus**, **Azadirachta indica** and **Sphaeranthus indicus** were found to reduce the inflammatory mediators interleukin-8 and tumour necrosis factor-α, and to inhibit reactive oxygen species (free radicals). **Curcuma longa** and **Hemidesmus indicus** are often used in Western herbal medicine, but it is worth noting that the extraction process for the herbs used was reflective of practices used in Ayurvedic medicine and may not directly correspond with ethanol-based extracts as used in Western herbal medicine.

CLINICAL SUMMARY

The management of acne vulgaris requires a thorough evaluation of physiology beyond the skin including the endocrine, gastrointestinal and immune systems. While these factors can be seen as underlying mechanisms and therefore treatment of these systems may be treating the cause, it is also important to address the root issues. As outlined in the naturopathic treatment decision tree (Figure 27.2), addressing endocrine imbalance may involve treating glucose metabolism, supporting hormone clearance, adjusting hormone regulation or controlling sympathetic nervous system function, or all of these combined. The application of naturopathic philosophy requires the practitioner to consider each of these elements when developing an individualised treatment plan. Such a treatment plan also needs to extend outside of ingested medicines and even topical treatments to focus heavily on dietary and lifestyle practices. Without taking this thorough and holistic approach to treatment relief from symptoms will be much more difficult to achieve and less likely to be sustained.

Skin conditions such as acne vulgaris can be frustrating to treat; it is important to counsel patients on the treatment process. Flare-ups can happen, and can potentially be managed sporadically by the judicious immunosuppressant herbs. Stress levels need to be managed in addition to monitoring and adjusting the diet where needed. Hormonal fluctuations in a female's cycle also should be considered. In conclusion, it is important to always approach the treatment of acne vulgaris with compassion and an understanding that it may be affecting the self-esteem and mood of the sufferer.

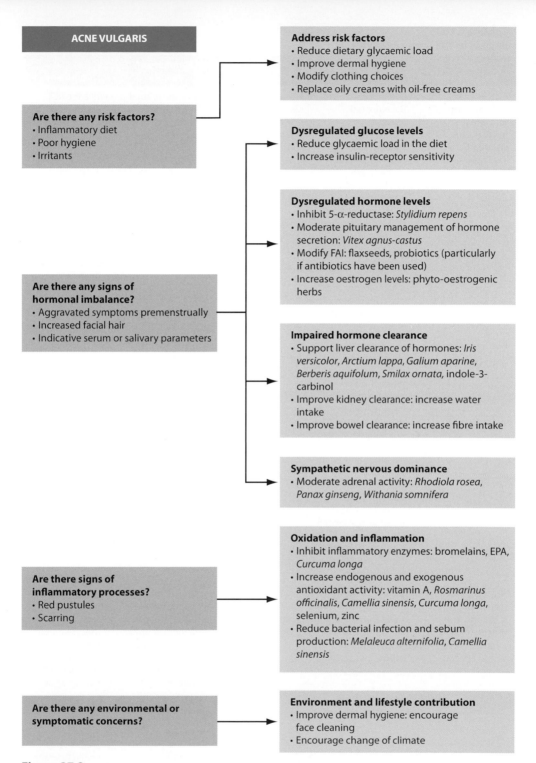

Figure 27.2
Naturopathic treatment decision tree—acne vulgaris

Table 27.1
Review of the major evidence

Intervention	Mechanisms of action	Key literature	Summary of results	Comment
Anti-inflammatory nutrients (lactoferrin, vitamin E and zinc)	Lactoferrin: Bacteriostatic effects via the peptide lactoferricin[79] Vitamin E: Inhibit multiple pro-inflammatory pathways[80] and levels are lower in patients with acne[81] Zinc: Potential mechanisms range from genomic, metabolomic, anti-inflammatory and direct inhibition of 5-alpha-reductase and *P. acnes*[82]	Review: Cervantes et al. 2017[82] Randomised controlled trial: Chan et al. 2017[83]	Reduction in total lesions from two weeks Maximum reduction in lesions and comedones by 10 weeks Improved sebum scores	While the RCT examined a combination of three nutrients, the role of each individually needs closer attention, particularly as the evidence for zinc in acne is much more advanced than the other two treatments.
Dietary change	High glycaemic diet: Potentiates a change in sebum production, stimulates inflammation, reduces levels of sex hormone-binding globulin, and increases androgen levels[84] Cow's milk intake: Contributes to raised IGF-I and postprandial insulin IGF-I acts indirectly to block transcription factor that regulates acne genes[85]	Review: Spencer et al. 2009[86]	Acne prevalence increases with Westernisation of diets Associated with cow's milk intake and high glycaemic foods Inconclusive association with chocolate and saturated fatty acids No association with salt and iodine intake	The studies included in this review were heterogenous and included cross-sectional, cohort and clinical intervention studies so meta-analysis was not possible
Antioxidants (selenium, silymarin and n-acetylcysteine)	Lipid peroxidation as caused by oxidative stress may be an early trigger for the pathophysiology of acne[87]	Double-blind RCT: Ahmed et al. 2012[11] ($n = 84$)	Improved markers of antioxidant status (reduced malondialdehyde levels, increased serum glutathione) and reduced acne lesions over the eight weeks compared with placebo	This study draws on a small sample and uses treatments that may have multiple activities in managing acne It cannot be concluded from this study that any antioxidants would have the same effect on acne lesions

Table 27.1
Review of the major evidence (continued)

Intervention	Mechanisms of action	Key literature	Summary of results	Comment
Topical tea tree oil water-based gel	Bactericidal action against *Propionibacterium acnes*[63]	Positive-controlled randomised study: Basset et al. 1990[62] (n = 124)	Comparison between a 5% tea tree oil water-based gel and a 5% benzoyl peroxide lotion found both reduced number of inflamed and non-inflamed lesions Onset was slower with tea tree oil gel	No placebo group was included in this study; blinding was difficult due to the distinctive odour of tea tree oil

KEY POINTS

- Hormonal imbalance, particularly androgen excess, plays a large role in the pathophysiology of acne vulgaris.
- Inflammation is a key consideration in the management of acne vulgaris and can be affected by bacterial infection, dietary choices, stress response or hormonal imbalance.
- Managing acne vulgaris can be achieved with little steps, but it is always important to address dietary and lifestyle factors, however slowly.
- Consider the psychological impact of acne vulgaris, thus sensitivity, compassion and patience are needed during the treatment process.

FURTHER READING

Cervantes J, Eber AE, Perper M, et al. The role of zinc in the treatment of acne: a review of the literature. Dermatol Ther 2017.

Mansu SS, Liang H, Parker S, et al. Acupuncture for acne vulgaris: a systematic review and meta-analysis. Evid Based Complement Alternat Med 2018.

Tan JKL, Bhate K. A global perspective on the epidemiology of acne. Br J Dermatol 2015;172(S1):3–12.

Williams HC, Dellavalle RP, Garner S. Acne vulgaris. Lancet 2012;379(9813):361–72.

REFERENCES

1. Williams HC, Dellavalle RP, Garner S. Acne vulgaris. Lancet 2012;379(9813):361–72.
2. Tan JK, Bhate K. A global perspective on the epidemiology of acne. Br J Dermatol 2015;172(S1):3–12.
3. Bhate K, Williams HC. Epidemiology of acne vulgaris. Br J Dermatol 2013;168(3):474–85.
4. Zhang M, Qureshi AA, Hunter DJ, et al. A genome-wide association study of severe teenage acne in European Americans. Hum Genet 2014;133:259–64.
5. Ismail NH, Manaf ZA, Azizan NZ. High glycemic load, milk and ice cream consumption are related to acne vulgaris in Malaysian young adults: a case control study. BMC Dermatol 2012;12(1):13.
6. George R, Clarke S, Thibutot D. Hormonal therapy for acne. Semin Cutan Med Surg 2008;27:188–96.
7. Arowojolu AO, Gallo MF, Lopez LM, et al. Cochrane Review: combined oral contraceptive pills for treatment of acne. Evid Based Child Health 2011;6(5):1340–433.
8. Zaenglein AL, et al. Guidelines of care for the management of acne vulgaris. J Am Acad Dermatol 2016;74(5):945–73.
9. Rademaker M. Adverse effects of isotretinoin: a retrospective review of 1743 patients started on isotretinoin. Australas J Dermatol 2010;51(4):248–53.
10. Kamal M, Polat M. Effect of different doses of isotretinoin treatment on the levels of serum homocysteine, vitamin B 12 and folic acid in patients with acne vulgaris: a prospective controlled study. J Pak Med Assoc 2015;65(9):950–3.
11. Karadag AS, Ertugrul DT, Tutal E, et al. Isotretinoin influences pituitary hormone levels in acne patients. Acta Derm Venereol 2011;91(1):31–4.

12. Hanson N, Leachman S. Safety issues in isotretinoin therapy. Semin Cutan Med Surg 2001;20(3):166–83.

13. Desai A, Kartono F, Del Rosso JQ. Systemic retinoid therapy: a status report on optimal use and safety of long-term therapy. Dermatol Clin 2007;25(2):185–93.

14. Zouboulis CC. Acne and sebaceous gland function. Clin Dermatol 2004;22:360–6.

15. Tan JK, Bhate K. A global perspective on the epidemiology of acne. Br J Dermatol 2015;172(S1):3–12.

16. Prager N, Bickett K, French N, et al. A randomized, double-blind, placebo-controlled trial to determine the effectiveness of botanically derived inhibitors of 5-alpha-reductase in the treatment of androgenetic alopecia. J Altern Complement Med 2002;8(2):143–52.

17. Wadsworth TL, Worstell TR, Greenbery NM, et al. Effects of dietary saw palmetto on the prostate of transgenic adenocarcinoma of the mouse prostate model (TRAMP). Prostate 2007;67(6):661–73.

18. Champault G, Patel J, Bonnard A. A double-blind trial of an extract of the plant Serenoa repens in benign prostatic hyperplasia. Br J Clin Pharmacol 2012;18(3):461–2.

19. Yarnell E, Abascal K. Herbal medicine for acne vulgaris. Altern Complement Therap 2006;12(6):303–9. %R. doi:10.1089/act.2006.12.303.

20. Felter HW, Lloyd JU. King's American dispensary. 18th ed. Portland: Eclectic Medical Publications; 1905. reprinted 1983.

21. Jarry H, Spengler B, Wuttke W, et al. In vitro assays for bioactivity-guided isolation of endocrine active compounds in Vitex agnus-castus. Maturitas 2006;55(Suppl. 1):S26–36.

22. van Die MD, Burger HG, Teede HJ, et al. Vitex agnus-castus extracts for female reproductive disorders: a Systematic Review of Clinical Trials. Planta Med 2013;79(7):562–75.

23. Takahashi K, Kitao M. Effect of TJ-68 (Shakuyaku-Kanzo-To) on polycystic ovarian disease. Int J Fertil 1994;39(2):69–76.

24. Armanini D, Castello R, Scaroni C, et al. Treatment of polycystic ovary syndrome with spironolactone plus licorice. Eur J Obstet Gynecol Reprod Biol 2007;131(1):61–7. 10.1016/j.ejogrb.2006.10.013.

25. Demark-Wahnefried W, Price D, Polascik T, et al. Pilot study of dietary fat restriction and flaxseed supplementation in men with prostate cancer before surgery: exploring the effects on hormonal levels, prostate-specific antigen, and histopathologic features. Urology 2001;58(1):47–52.

26. Kilkkinen A, Pietinen P, Klaukka T, et al. Use of oral antimicrobials decreases serum enterolactone concentration. Am J Epidemiol 2002;155(5):472–7.

27. Vankrieken L. Testosterone and the Free Androgen Index. www.diagnostics.siemens.com: Siemens Diagnostic; 2000.

28. Charmandari E, Tsigos C, Chrousos G. Endocrinology of the stress response. Annu Rev Physiol 2005;67(1):259–84. doi:10.1146/annurev.physiol.67.040403.120816.

29. Spasov AA, Wikman GK, Mandrikov VB, et al. A double-blind, placebo-controlled pilot study of the stimulating and adaptogenic effect of Rhodiola rosea SHR-5 extract on the fatigue of students caused by stress during an examination period with a repeated low-dose regimen. Phytomedicine 2000;7(2):85–9.

30. Bhattacharya SK, Muruganandam AV. Adaptogenic activity of Withania somnifera: an experimental study using a rat model of chronic stress. Pharmacol Biochem Behav 2003;75(3):547–55.

31. Bone K. A clinical guide to blending liquid herbs. Missouri: Churchill Livingstone; 2003.

32. Luu-The V, Duche D, Ferraris C, et al. Analysis of phases 1 and 2 metabolism enzymes in human skin suggests important role of phase 2 enzymes in the detoxification. Toxicol Lett 2008;180S:s121.

33. Chen W, Thiboutot D, Zouboulis CC. Cutaneous androgen metabolism: basic research and clinical perspectives. J Invest Dermatol 2002;119(5):992–1007.

34. Lust B. Universal buyer's guide naturopathic encyclopaedia directory and yearbook for drugless therapy 1918–1919. New York: Lust and Butler; 1918.

35. Jellinck PH, Newcombe A-M, Gek Forkert P, et al. Distinct forms of hepatic androgen 6β-hydroxylase induced in the rat by indole-3-carbinol and pregnenolone carbonitrile. J Steroid Biochem Mol Biol 1994;51(3–4):219–25.

36. Osawa Y, Tochigi B, Tochigi M, et al. Aromatase inhibitors in cigarette smoke, tobacco leaves and other plants. J Enzyme Inhib Med Chem 1990;4(2):187–200.

37. Firooz A, Sarhangnejad R, Davoudi SM, et al. Acne and smoking: is there a relationship? BMC Dermatol 2005;5(1):2.

38. Adebamowo CA, Speigelman D, Danby FW, et al. High school dietary dairy intake and teenage acne. J Am Acad Dermatol 2005;52:207–14.

39. Tan JK, Bhate K. A global perspective on the epidemiology of acne. Br J Dermatol 2015;172(S1):3–12.

40. Smith RN, Mann NJ, Braue A, et al. The effect of a high-protein, low glycemic-load diet versus a conventional, high glycemic-load diet on biochemical parameters associated with acne vulgaris: a randomized, investigator-masked, controlled trial. J Am Acad Dermatol 2007;57:247–56.

41. Kaymak Y, Adisen E, Ilter N, et al. Dietary glycemic index and glucose, insulin, insulin-like growth factor-I, insulin-like growth factor binding protein 3, and leptin levels in patients with acne. J Am Acad Dermatol 2007;57:819–23.

42. Sun Yu E, Jung Min H, Yeon An S, et al. Regulatory mechanisms of IL-2 and IFN[gamma] suppression by quercetin in T helper cells. Biochem Pharmacol 2008;76(1):70–8.

43. Bhui K, Prasad S, George J, et al. Bromelain inhibits COX-2 expression by blocking the activation of MAPK regulated NF-kappa B against skin tumor-initiation triggering mitochondrial death pathway. Cancer Lett 2009;282(2):167–76.

44. Arican O, Kurutas EB, Sasmaz S. Oxidative stress in patients with acne vulgaris. Mediators Inflamm 2005;6(2005):380–4.

45. Sarici G, Cinar S, Armutcu F, et al. Oxidative stress in acne vulgaris. J Eur Acad Dermatol Venereol 2010;24(7):763–7.

46. Menaa F, Menaa A, Menaa B, et al. Trans-fatty acids, dangerous bonds for health? A background review paper of their use, consumption, health implications and regulation in France. Eur J Nutr 2012;1–14.

47. Lopez-Garcia E, Schulze MB, Meigs JB, et al. Consumption of trans fatty acids is related to plasma biomarkers of inflammation and endothelial dysfunction. J Nutr 2005;135(3):562–6.

48. Mozaffarian D, Pischon T, Hankinson SE, et al. Dietary intake of trans fatty acids and systemic inflammation in women. Am J Clin Nutr 2004;79(4):606–12.

49. El-akawi Z, Abdel-Latif N, Abdul-Razzak K. Does the plasma level of vitamins A and E affect acne condition? Clin Exp Dermatol 2006;31(3):430–4.

50. Albayrak S, Aksoy A, Albayrak S, et al. In vitro antioxidant and antimicrobial activity of some Lamiaceae species. Iran J Sci Technol 2013;A1:1–9.

51. Gianeti MD, Mercurio DG, Maia Campos PM. The use of green tea extract in cosmetic formulations: not only an antioxidant active ingredient. Dermatol Ther 2013;26(3):267–71.

52. Elango N, Samuel S, Chinnakkannu P. Enzymatic and non-enzymatic antioxidant status in stage (III) human oral squamous cell carcinoma and treated with radical radio therapy: influence of selenium supplementation. Clin Chim Acta 2006;373(1–2):92–8.

53. Mariani E, Mangialasche F, Feliziani FT, et al. Effects of zinc supplementation on antioxidant enzyme activities in healthy old subjects. Exp Gerontol 2008;43(5):445–51.

54. Michaelsson G, Edqvist LE. Erythrocyte glutathione peroxidase activity in acne vulgaris and the effect of selenium and vitamin E treatment. Acta Derm Venereol 1984;64(1):9–14.

55. Farrar MD, Ingham E. Acne: inflammation. Clin Dermatol 2004;22:380–4.

56. Ahmed SS. Effects of oral antioxidants on lesion counts associated with oxidative stress and inflammation in patients with papulopustular acne. J Clin Exp Dermatol Res 2012;3:163.

57. Aybey B, Ergenekon G, Hekim N, et al. Glutathione peroxidase (GSH-Px) enzyme levels of patients with acne vulgaris. J Eur Acad Dermatol Venereol 2005;19(6):766–7.

58. Sardana K, Garg VK. An observational study of methionine-bound zinc with antioxidants for mild to moderate acne vulgaris. Dermatol Ther 2010;23(4):411–18.

59. Chan H, Chan G, Santos J, et al. A randomized, double-blind, placebo-controlled trial to determine the efficacy and safety of lactoferrin with vitamin E and zinc as an oral therapy for mild to moderate acne vulgaris. Int J Dermatol 2017;56(6):686–90.

60. Agak GW, Qin M, Nobe J, et al. Propionibacterium acnes induces an IL-17 response in acne vulgaris that is regulated by vitamin A and vitamin D. J Invest Dermatol 2014;134(2):366–73.

61. Zu Y, Yu H, Liang L, et al. Activities of ten essential oils towards Propionibacterium acnes and PC-3, A-549 and MCF-7 cancer cells. Molecules 2010;15(5):3200–10.

62. Bassett IB, Pannowitz DL, Barnetson RSC. A comparative study of tea-tree oil versus benzoylperoxide in the treatment of acne. Med J Aust 1990;153(8):455–8.

63. Carson CF, Riley TV. Susceptibility of Propionibacterium acnes to the essential oil of Melaleuca alternifolia. Lett Appl Microbiol 1994;19(1):24–5.

64. Qa'dan F, Thewaini A-J, Ali DA, et al. The antimicrobial activities of Psidium guajava and Juglans regia leaf extracts to acne-developing organisms. Am J Chin Med 2005;33(02):197–204.

65. Kim JK, Shin HJ, Lee BG, et al. Evaluation of skin sebosuppression by components of total green tea (Camellia sinensis) extracts. Food Sci Biotechnol 2008;17(3):464–9.

66. Sharquie KE, Noaimi AA, Al-Salih MM. Topical therapy of acne vulgaris using 2% tea lotion in comparison with 5% zinc sulphate solution. Saudi Med J 2008;29(12):1757–61.

67. Lee J-H, Sun Shim J, Sun Lee J, et al. Inhibition of pathogenic bacterial adhesion by acidic polysaccharide from green tea (Camellia sinensis). J Agric Food Chem 2006;54:8717–23.

68. Fabbrocini G, Staibano S, Giuseppe De R, et al. Resveratrol-containing gel for the treatment of acne vulgaris: a single-blind, vehicle-controlled, pilot study. Am J Clin Dermatol 2011;12(2):133–41.

69. Shaffrathul JH, Karthick PS, Rai R, et al. Turmeric: role in hypertrichosis and acne. Indian J Dermatol 2007;52(2):116.

70. Panconesi E, Hautmann G. Psychotherapeutic approach in acne treatment. Dermatology 1998;196(1):116.

71. Ammad S, Gonzales M, Edwards C, et al. An assessment of the efficacy of blue light phototherapy in the treatment of acne vulgaris. J Cosmet Dermatol 2008;7(3):180–8.

72. Aziz-Jalali MH, Tabaie SM, Djavid GE. Comparison of red and infrared low-level laser therapy in the treatment of acne vulgaris. Indian J Dermatol 2012;57(2):128.

73. Bae JY, Lee JI, Kim HL, et al. Comparative study of 595 nm pulsed-dye laser (V-beam) monotherapy and blue and red LED combination phototherapy in the treatment of acne vulgaris. 프로그램북 (구 초록집) 2017;69(2):336.

74. Short RW, Agredano YZ, Choi JM, et al. A single-blinded, randomized pilot study to evaluate the effect of exercise-induced sweat on truncal acne. Pediatr Dermatol 2008;25(1):126–8.

75. Choi JM, Lew VK, Kimball AB. A single-blinded, randomized, controlled clinical trial evaluating the effect of face washing on acne vulgaris. Pediatr Dermatol 2006;23(5):421–7.

76. Leung A, Schiltz A, Hall C, et al. Severe atopic dermatitis is associated with a high burden of environmental Staphylococcus aureus. Clin Exp Allergy 2008;38(5): 789–93.

77. Mansu SS, Liang H, Parker S, et al. Acupuncture for acne vulgaris: a systematic review and meta-analysis. Evid Based Complement Alternat Med 2018.

78. Jain A, Basal E. Inhibition of Propionibacterium acnes-induced mediators of inflammation by Indian herbs. Phytomedicine 2003;10:34–8.

79. Mohanty D, Jena R, Choudhury PK, et al. Milk derived antimicrobial bioactive peptides: a review. Int J Food Prop 2016;19(4):837–46.

80. Jiang Q. Natural forms of vitamin E: metabolism, antioxidant, and anti-inflammatory activities and their role in disease prevention and therapy. Free Radic Biol Med 2014;72:76–90.

81. El-akawi Z, Abdel-Latif N, Abdul-Razzak K. Does the plasma level of vitamins A and E affect acne condition? Clin Exp Dermatol 2006;31(3):430–4.

82. Cervantes J, Eber AE, Perper M, et al. The role of zinc in the treatment of acne: a review of the literature. Dermatol Ther 2017.

83. Chan H, Chan G, Santos J, et al. A randomized, double-blind, placebo-controlled trial to determine the efficacy and safety of lactoferrin with vitamin E and zinc as an oral therapy for mild to moderate acne vulgaris. Int J Dermatol 2017;56(6):686–90.

84. Pappas A. The relationship of diet and acne. Dermatoendocrinol 2009;1(5):262–7.

85. Melnik BC. In: Clemens R, Hernell O, Michaelsen KF, editors. Evidence for acne-promoting effects of milk and other insulinotropic dairy products. Karger: Milk and Milk Products in Human Nutrition; 2011.

86. Spencer EH, Ferdowsian HR, Barnard ND. Diet and acne: a review of the evidence. Int J Dermatol 2009;48(4):339–47.

87. Bowe W, Patel N, Logan A. Acne vulgaris: the role of oxidative stress and the potential therapeutic value of local and systemic antioxidants. J Drugs Dermatol 2012;11(6):742.

CHAPTER **28**

Inflammatory skin disorders— atopic eczema and psoriasis

Amie Steel
ND, MPH, PhD

OVERVIEW

Atopic dermatitis (eczema) is most frequently diagnosed in infancy but may continue through the adult years.[1] It represents the highest burden of skin diseases globally[2] and involves an inherited tendency towards type 1 hypersensitivity reactions. Individuals with eczema may also present with other allergic conditions (such as allergic rhinitis and asthma) in their family history.[1] The physiological response to the allergen causes chronic inflammation and requires pathology testing for conclusive diagnosis. In particular, a full blood count to identify elevated eosinophil levels and a serum IgE test are both important, and emphasise the allergenic basis of the disease.[1] The presentation of atopic dermatitis may vary depending on the life stage of the individual. Infantile eczema tends to involve lesions that are moist, red, vesicular and covered with crusts. They will tend to occur on the face, neck, buttocks and extensor surfaces of the arms and legs.[1] Adults may also present with some moist, red lesions; however, these will mainly be concentrated in flexor regions of the arms and legs. More commonly, adults will present with dry, scaling lesions and with lichenification (thick, leathery patches) in the other areas. Pruritus (itching) is a commonly reported symptom irrelevant of the age.[1] Over time, affected regions may become more sensitive to irritants such as soaps, fabrics and changes in climate (temperature and humidity).[1] These irritants impair skin barrier function by damaging the stratum corneum intercellular bilayers, through either the lipid organisation or removing the lipids overall.[3] The prevalence of eczema in children in countries such as United Kingdom, New Zealand and Australia is increasing by more than 14% per year.[4]

In contrast, the prevalence of psoriasis is much lower (< 3%) psoriasis and the mean age of onset is estimated to be 33 years.[5] The pathophysiology of psoriasis is complex and involves immunological pathways and genetic susceptibility.[5] It has been mostly linked with increased cellular proliferation and hyperkeratinisation of the dermal layer although this feature is believed to be preceded by leucocyte infiltration by CD4+ and CD8+ T-cells alongside high levels of cytokines associated with the T helper subtype 1 pathway (interferon-γ, interleukin 2 and interleukin 12)[5] and tumour necrosis factor-α.[6] It is believed that these T-cells remain activated and cause the skin to constantly regenerate and for this reason psoriasis is categorised as an autoimmune condition.[5]

Like eczema, psoriasis also begins with small red papules, but lesions eventually develop a silvery plaque (although the basal layer remains red and inflamed). Most commonly, psoriatic lesions are seen on the face, scalp, elbow and knees.[4] Another potentially important intracellular compound is cyclic-AMP (cAMP), which is understood to regulate cellular proliferation, although the precise mechanism and resulting effect on psoriasis are still unclear.[7]

Another observation that may, over time, assist in the understanding of psoriasis pathophysiology is the comorbidity of psoriasis with other conditions such as obesity, diabetes mellitus (type 2), metabolic syndrome, depression, heart disease, bowel disorders and cancer.[5] Potential mechanisms to explain these comorbidities have been proposed as: lipid abnormalities; inflammatory cascade associated with obesity; and the effects of lifestyle behaviours (dietary habits or a decrease in physical activity).[6] It has also been argued, although unconfirmed, that the connection between bowel disorders and skin may be due to autointoxication through intestinal absorption of microbial antigens.[7] However, these hypotheses are still unproven and as such the cause and development of psoriasis require further exploration.

A key consideration in the clinical management of psoriasis and eczema is the potential similarity in presentation and sometimes treatment principles of the two conditions, contrasted by the very different pathophysiological nature. Eczema is an atopic, allergic condition, while psoriasis has autoimmune features. With this in mind, it is important to confirm the accuracy of the diagnosis before initiating a treatment plan (see the box on testing for atopy and Figure 28.1 for the comparative features of eczema and psoriasis). Generic autoimmune considerations can be found in Chapter 31 on autoimmunity.

DIFFERENTIAL DIAGNOSIS*

- Eczema (atopic and contact dermatitis)
- Psoriasis
- Tinea
- Stevens-Johnson syndrome
- Toxic epidermal necrolysis
- Erythema multiforme major
- Drug rash with eosinophilia and systemic symptoms
- Candidal intertrigo
- Erythrasma
- Dermatophyte infection
- Annular erythemas
- Lupus erythematosus
- Lichen planus
- Pityriasis rosea and versicolor

*For dermatitis

RISK FACTORS

The most important identified risk factor associated with both eczema and psoriasis is heredity; this link is much stronger in atopic eczema. The potential to develop an atopic condition of any kind is much more likely if it is already present within the family.[1] Further contributing factors worth considering in eczema rely on the identification of irritants. Common examples include strong detergents, wool, specific allergenic foods (eggs, dairy, fish and nuts), psychological stress and scratching.[1] Change in climate can also be an ongoing aggravating factor in eczema.[8] Psoriasis has more lifestyle risk factors such as smoking, alcohol consumption, stress and obesity.[5]

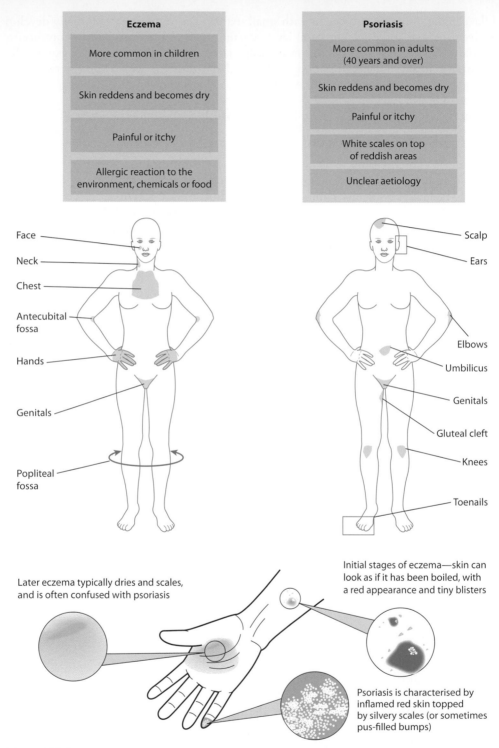

Eczema

More common in children

Skin reddens and becomes dry

Painful or itchy

Allergic reaction to the environment, chemicals or food

Psoriasis

More common in adults (40 years and over)

Skin reddens and becomes dry

Painful or itchy

White scales on top of reddish areas

Unclear aetiology

Face
Neck
Chest
Antecubital fossa
Hands
Genitals
Popliteal fossa

Scalp
Ears
Elbows
Umbilicus
Genitals
Gluteal cleft
Knees
Toenails

Later eczema typically dries and scales, and is often confused with psoriasis

Initial stages of eczema—skin can look as if it has been boiled, with a red appearance and tiny blisters

Psoriasis is characterised by inflamed red skin topped by silvery scales (or sometimes pus-filled bumps)

Figure 28.1
Comparative features of eczema and psoriasis

CONVENTIONAL TREATMENT

Conventional management of eczema ideally involves identification of the allergens and perhaps also any aggravating factors. Beyond this, pharmaceutical treatment relies heavily upon topical glucocorticoids to reduce chronic inflammation, and antihistamine to reduce pruritus.[1]

Common food allergens in atopy

Foods commonly identified as allergens in atopic dermatitis include:

- cow's milk
- egg white
- peanut
- wheat
- nuts
- fish

Source: Host & Halken 2003[9]

Testing for atopy

Testing for allergies in atopic conditions can include the following elements:

- *Case history*. This should include factors such as triggers, family history, environmental factors and onset/duration/frequency/severity of symptoms.
- *Skin prick test*. This requires standardised extracts and methods to be accurate, and as such should be performed only by trained professionals. Smaller children may have smaller wheals than older children. The test may not be effective if dermatitis is active at the site of testing or the person is on immunosuppressive creams. Anti-histamines should be avoided for at least three days before testing.
- *A specific IgE test*. This will identify specific reactive IgE from the serum allergen challenge. To confirm the allergy, the identified allergen (via the above tests) should be excluded from the diet for one to four weeks and should result in a marked reduction in symptoms. Introduction of the proposed allergen (known as a 'challenge') should then be conducted. (If there is unequivocal evidence of reactivity from the case history that supports the skin prick test or specific IgE test, the challenge may not be necessary.) If there are concerns of anaphylaxis, the challenge should be undertaken in the presence of a health professional.
- *Patch test*. This has been used for delayed hypersensitivity reactions.

Source: Host & Halken 2003[9]

Management of psoriasis mostly focuses on interventions to reduce cellular proliferation, including glucocorticoids, tar preparations and ultraviolet light. Severe cases may result in the use of methotrexate.[1]

KEY TREATMENT PROTOCOLS

Provide gastrointestinal support

The gastrointestinal system is considered to be an important consideration in managing skin disorders such as atopic eczema and psoriasis. The principle behind this connection focuses on intestinal hyperpermeability as an important factor in pathogenesis. It is proposed that weakness in

Naturopathic Treatment Aims

- Reduce dermal inflammation.
- Improve hydrochloric acid secretion.
- Investigate and address potential dysbiosis.
- Regulate blood sugar levels.
- Improve fat digestion and absorption.
- Improve stool consistency and frequency.

gap junctions between enterocytes in the jejunum and lower duodenum allows toxins to migrate into the circulation from the intestinal lumen. As these are processed and excreted through the skin they contribute to the dermal physiological changes associated with skin conditions.[7] For this reason, a focus of naturopathic treatment in eczema and psoriasis is gastrointestinal support to promote healthy permeability, and reduce the absorption of undigested peptides and food antigens.

Address dysbiosis and immune function

Dysbiosis, or imbalance in the gastrointestinal bacterial population, has been associated with the development of atopic disease. It is suggested that an incorrect balance of bacteria results in inflammatory damage and reduced mucous membrane function throughout the digestive tract, thereby contributing to the pathogenesis of the condition. Growing interest in the microbiome research has uncovered an inverse relationship between microbiota diversity and the severity of atopic disease.[10]

GALT and the hygiene hypothesis

The gut-associated lymphoid tissue (GALT) consists of Peyer's patches, lymphoid nodules and the appendix. To induce an allergenic response from a food-based antigen, such as casein in cow's milk, the compound must be transported into Peyer's patches from the intestinal lumen.[11] However, a healthy intestinal cell is lined with epithelial cells constituting a thick layer of glycoproteins. In addition to this, further protection is provided by mucins, digestive enzymes and secretory IgA (sIgA). The process of developing immune reactivity to specific antigens is quite complex and involves many types of immune cells within the GALT, and is explained in more detail in Chapter 31 on autoimmunity. However, it has been suggested that larger particles being processed in the B-cells within the Peyer's patches may result in the development of T helper 2 cell dominance, while immune response to microbes will stimulate T helper 1 cells (Figure 28.2).[11] If this occurs at an early age, it exacerbates the T helper 2 dominance that naturally occurs during gestation as a way of protecting the developing fetus from maternal immunity, and may contribute to the development of atopy.[12] It is upon this understanding that the foundations for the hygiene hypothesis are laid. Initially, the rationale behind the hygiene hypothesis was linked to the epidemiological evidence that people in developed countries with improved sanitary practices had higher prevalence of atopic conditions. It was argued that this was due to a lack of provocation of the GALT, resulting in a maintenance of T helper 2 dominance.[12] However, more recent researchers now suggest that, although this may be true, the same benefit can be achieved by ensuring exposure to commensal gut microbiota, rather than relying on pathogenic infections to stimulate T helper 1 cells and redress the balance.[13]

Research in this field has evolved in recent years beyond confirmation that maternal probiotic supplementation during pregnancy and breastfeeding reduces the risk of eczema,[14] to examine the optimal dosage regimen for maximum benefit. Current evidence suggests a combination of *Lactobacillus rhamnosus* LPR and *Bifidobacterium longum* BL999 or *Lactobacillus paracasei* ST11 and *Bifidobacterium longum* BL999 achieved similar risk reduction in developing eczema although neither appear to affect atopic sensitisation.[15] It is, however, important to acknowledge that no other combinations were examined in this study and as such it is not clear whether these results are unique to these formulas or are simply reflective of the use of probiotics. This may be explained by other research, which found that a similar dose of *Lactobacillus rhamnosus* also resulted in a decrease in eczema symptoms.[16] The difference in this study was the measurement of objective pathology markers such as CRP and interleukin-6. Interestingly, the levels of CRP were markedly higher in the group given *Lactobacillus rhamnosus* than the placebo group. From this, it is suggested that the probiotic bacteria result in an inflammatory

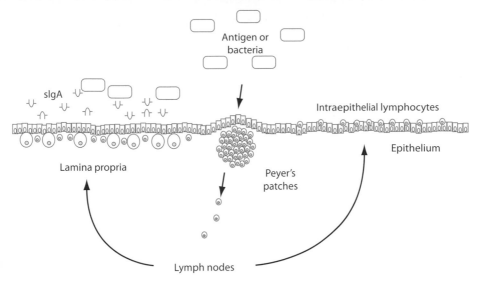

Figure 28.2
Overview of intestinal immune responses

Source: Rautava et al. 2005[12]

response being generated from within the intestinal epithelial cells, contributing to the healing of eczema. As CRP inhibits the production of a range of inflammatory cytokines and chemokines, this may contribute to the explanation. Furthermore, interleukin-6 (also increased in the intervention group) stimulates mucosal protein synthesis and IgA production, thereby reducing intestinal permeability and counteracting elevated IgE levels.[16] The rationale behind using probiotics to prevent atopy has been reviewed through meta-analyses focusing on infants and was found to confirm the benefit of this intervention.[17,18] A further meta-analysis examining probiotics for the treatment rather than prevention of eczema reported benefits for children and adults but not infants. Interestingly, probiotics containing a mixture of different bacterial species or of *Lactobacillus* species showed greater benefit than treatment with *Bifidobacterium* species alone.[19] Emerging evidence suggests the lack of success in treating eczema with probiotics may in fact be linked to a vitamin D deficiency due to a proposed function for vitamin D to facilitate signalling between gut microbiota and the host individual.[20]

In conjunction with possible probiotics use, some medicinal herbs may be useful, due to their antimicrobial properties; however, research into this approach for the management of eczema has not been undertaken. In particular, using herbs such as ***Ocimum basilicum*,**[21] ***Allium sativum***[22] and ***Hydrastis canadensis***[23] may help to reduce the growth of pathogenic organisms prior to reinoculation with beneficial flora via probiotic supplementation.

Reduce intestinal permeability

Intestinal permeability has been proposed to be an important component within the underlying pathophysiology of atopic conditions such as eczema. The concept of intestinal permeability is structured upon the tight junctions that exist between intestinal cells. These tight junctions are built from a number of membrane proteins. A number of factors proposed to increase intestinal permeability such as oxidative stress and inflammatory cytokines are also linked with atopy. This suggests that the relationship between intestinal permeability and eczema may be bilateral. Similarly, psoriasis has been described as a non-specific manifestation of bowel pathology in which undigested peptides and antigens from food and microbes are absorbed into the intestinal portal system and are eventually transported to the skin for elimination.[7] This viewpoint is congruent with the traditional naturopathic approach for skin conditions (see the box on alteratives and depuratives in the previous chapter). For more information on the pathophysiology of intestinal permeability and poor food digestion, see Chapter 6 on food allergy and intolerance.

Probiotics are the most validated approach to managing intestinal permeability in eczema. For example, a probiotic mix (*Lactobacillus rhamnosus* 19070-2 and *Lactobacillus reuteri* DSM 12246) was found to reduce intestinal hyperpermeability.[24] However, the same study also found that there was a direct correlation between the lactulose:mannitol ratio (a measure of intestinal permeability) and the severity of eczema (see the box on birth, breastfeeding and atopy below). Another probiotic organism, *Saccharomyces boulardii*, has also been found to reduce intestinal hyperpermeability.[25] However, neither of these treatments has been evaluated for the management of psoriasis.

Another important consideration when addressing intestinal permeability is to ensure the adequate digestion of food and therefore prevent large undigested food particles being absorbed. With this in mind, herbs containing **bitter principles** are often used to provide vagal stimulation of gastric acid. Such herbs include *Gentiana lutea*, *Andrographis paniculata*, *Taraxacum officinale* and *Cynara scolymus*.[26] A similar effect has also been traditionally achieved through diet, by the ingestion of foods such as dandelion leaves and **lemon juice in warm water**. An example of a nutrient that may be useful in this situation is **zinc** due to its role as a cofactor to carbonic anhydrase.[27]

Birth, breastfeeding and atopy

Breastfeeding is promoted by the World Health Organization (WHO) as an important factor in infant health.[28] WHO recommends exclusive breastfeeding up to six months, and nutritionally sound complementary feeding starting from six months and continuing up to two years old and later if appropriate. One rationale behind this stance is the potential risk associated with feeding infants products other than breast milk in developing atopic conditions, among other acute and chronic health risks. Breast milk contains a number of physiological factors that benefit the infant, beyond its nutrient composition, and may be important in preventing atopy. These include a range of immune factors designed to reduce the likelihood of bacterial infection, and epidermal growth factor, which assists in the development of the intestinal lining, thereby improving nutrient absorption and reducing sensitisation to foreign particles.[28] Colostrum is also provided to breastfeeding infants in the first few days of life, and provides an immune protection to the infant while it becomes accustomed to the newly developing colony of gut microbiota.[28] Inoculation with the strains of microbes that constitute the colony is achieved at birth through vaginal delivery. In contrast, infants birthed through caesarean section have a different profile of microbiota, and an increased risk of atopy, suggesting the composition of flora is vital to healthy immune induction.[29] Furthermore, preventive supplementation with probiotics given to women in late stages of pregnancy only benefited infants born through caesarean section.[30]

Modulate immune response

Modulating immune response is inevitably involved in the management of inflammatory conditions such as atopic dermatitis and psoriasis. This can occur on two levels. Superficial management, such as reducing histamine release, can still provide some beneficial results. This can be achieved through the use of **antiallergy** herbs such as

Albizia lebbeck,[31] or nutrients such as **vitamin C**,[32] **magnesium**,[33] **zinc**, copper and **vitamin B6**.[34] On a deeper level, regulating T-cell activity and reducing oxidative stress may also be important. See Chapter 31 on autoimmune disease for more discussion.

Reduce inflammation

Inflammation is a key feature of the pathogenesis of atopic dermatitis.[35] This is associated with an overproduction of IgE antibodies, which is linked to an inherited sensitivity and dysregulation of T- and B-cells. Through its effects on eicosanoid production, the arachidonic acid cascade is considered to be an additional potential trigger to the onset of atopic dermatitis, and to be involved in the ongoing modification of symptoms.[35] For example, it is understood that histamine contributes to itching, but it has been suggested that the itching threshold is lowered by products of the arachidonic acid cascade such as PGE_1, PGE_2 and PGH_2.[35] Considering the role that essential fatty acids such as gamma-linolenic acid and docosahexaenoic acid play in regulating this cascade, it is unsurprising that research has found a strong connection between **essential fatty acid** deficiency, essential fatty acid supplementation and eczema management (see the box on EFA deficiency and eczema). Other anti-inflammatory interventions as proposed in Chapter 27 on acne vulgaris may also be indicated in eczema. Although a small clinical trial without placebo was undertaken to investigate the benefit of oral curcuminoids (from ***Curcuma longa***) in patients with psoriasis with inconclusive results,[36] larger and better designed studies are still needed in this area.

Current understanding of immune function indicates that T helper 2 cells promote IgE production.[37] An imbalance between T helper 1, which is induced by infection, and T helper 2 cells, associated with allergic reactions, is evident in atopic eczema.[38] This knowledge has led to the development of the 'hygiene hypothesis' as an explanation of the aetiology of atopy (see the box on GALT and the hygiene hypothesis). More recently, however, molecular research has identified the association between genetic predisposition to the development of atopy with polymorphisms in receptors to bacterial endotoxins, thereby reducing an individual's T helper 1 response. This does not necessarily mean the 'hygiene hypothesis' is untrue, but it may indicate that the underlying process is somewhat complex.[39] As such, herbs that have been traditionally

---

EFA deficiency and eczema

The most abundant fatty acid in the skin is linoleic acid (omega-6).[40] Gamma-linolenic acid is known to be converted to arachidonic acid through a series of enzymatic reactions. However, the enzyme required to convert the GLA metabolite, dihomo-γ-linolenic acid (DGLA), to arachidonic acid, delta-5-desaturase, is not present in skin epidermis (Figure 28.3). Furthermore, the enzymes 15-lipoxygenase and cyclo-oxygenase are both still active, and act upon DGLA to form the anti-inflammatory compound 15-hydroxyeicosatraenoic acid (15-HETrE). In fact, 15-HETrE may have a more potently anti-inflammatory effect than similar metabolites of 15-lipoxygenase activity from omega-3 fats such as docosahexaenoic acid (DHA) and eicosapentaenoic acid (EPA).[40]

However, GLA supplementation does not seem to prevent the development of eczema; rather its benefits appear to focus on ameliorating the symptoms.[41] A pilot study found that supplementation with DHA (5.4 g/day) still reduced the symptoms of atopic dermatitis.[42]

In both eczema and psoriasis, leukotriene B4 and 15-HETrE, by-products of arachidonic acid metabolism, are elevated. Furthermore, it has been suggested that people with atopic dermatitis may have a defect in the conversion of linoleic acid to γ-linolenic acid (via delta-6 desaturase). This may also explain why no therapeutic benefit has been associated with flaxseed oil supplementation, as it has with fish oil.[40]

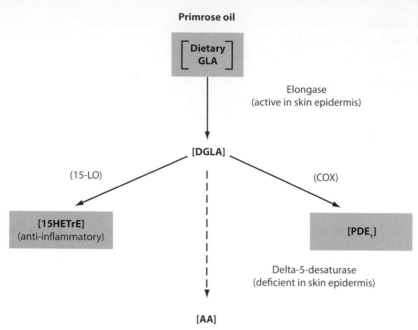

Figure 28.3
The anti-inflammatory role of evening primrose oil in skin tissue

Source: Kurd et al. 2008[36]

defined as immunomodulatory, such as ***Withania somnifera***, ***Echinacea angustifolia*** and ***Eleutherococcus senticosus***,[26] are often used. Recent in vitro research has also found that the equivalent of 10 mg of zinc per day increases levels of interferon-γ, which is primarily associated with T helper 1 activity; however, the clinical significance of this activity is still unclear.

An interesting contrast to atopic eczema in the T helper story is psoriasis. Psoriatic conditions are generally associated with elevated T helper 1 levels. The T helper 1 response that occurs in psoriasis is most commonly associated with a previous streptococcal or staphylococcal throat infection. The sensitised T helper 1 cells that result from this infection then migrate to the dermal layer, and produce cytokines such as interferon-γ. These cytokines contribute to hyperproliferation, a key feature of psoriasis.[43] A substantial amount of evidence suggests that a key intervention in managing T helper 1 dominant conditions such as psoriasis is **vitamin D**, which acts by promoting T helper 2 responses while blocking T helper 1. Similarly, retinoic acid (**vitamin A**) has also been found to reduce T helper 1 cell cytokines while increasing T helper 2 transcription.[44] Although this implies that both vitamins A and D may be beneficial in psoriasis, and are to be avoided in atopic dermatitis, this may not be the case. Vitamin A deficiency still appears to increase the severity of atopic conditions. It has been suggested that this is due to an important link between vitamin A and atopy, encompassing its role in the maintenance and repair of the lamina propria, and the resulting gut-associated lymphoid tissue function.[44]

Attenuate oxidation

As atopic dermatitis is an inflammatory condition, oxidative stress is a potential side effect to be considered. Although at this stage it is not considered to be a causative factor, oxidative load may be placing a further burden on immunity and contributing to later problems. In support of this, impaired nitrogen and oxygen radical quenching has been suggested in preliminary research.[45] Similarly, psoriatic patients have also been linked with increased oxidative stress.[46] With this in mind, antioxidant nutrients such as **vitamin C**, selenium and zinc may be indicated,[27] although no known research focused on eczema has been conducted in this area. Antioxidant herbs, although they have not yet been researched for eczema specifically, may also be beneficial.

Manage stress

Stress has been found to enhance humoral immunity, at the expense of cell-mediated immunity, resulting in T helper 2 cell dominance and thereby favouring the production of IgE and creating a predisposition to allergy.[38] In support of this, increased activity of the hypothalamus–pituitary–adrenal (HPA) axis and consequent inflammatory reactions have been associated with people with diagnosed atopic dermatitis, including changes in eosinophil counts and serum IgE levels.[37] This may be explained by the effect of glucocorticoids in suppressing T helper 1 and promoting T helper 2 activity. Further evidence of this is seen in patients undergoing corticosteroid therapy resulted in increased serum IgE levels.[38] As such, it has been suggested that stress hormones in early life may generate Th2 cell predominance.[37] Stress may also affect the pathophysiology of atopic dermatitis by contributing to intestinal dysbiosis (as discussed earlier). This may occur through increased bacterial adherence and decreased luminal lactobacilli.[37]

Asthma and eczema

One of the most common examples used to explain the naturopathic principle tolle causam, or 'treat the cause', is the link between eczema and asthma, known medically as the atopic march. One in three children who develop atopic dermatitis in the first four years of life develop asthma[47] and this risk persists through to adult life.[48] The rationale behind this, from a naturopathic perspective, is that the dysfunctional physiological process that contributes to the development of atopic dermatitis is not addressed at its roots by conventional therapy such as topical emollients, topical steroid creams and antihistamines. Instead, the immune dysfunction such as T helper 2 cell predominance develops into cellular memory[48] and may result in other compounds, such as inhaled antigens, becoming allergenic, thereby resulting in atopic rhinitis or asthma.

Based upon this knowledge, herbal interventions that have immune and HPA-modulating activity, such as ***Eleutherococcus senticosus*** and ***Rhodiola rosea***, are recommended.[49] Similarly, nutrients that support parasympathetic nervous system activity, such as **choline**, **magnesium**, **vitamin B1** and **vitamin B5**,[27] may also be indicated (see Chapter 18 on stress and fatigue for more information).

Connective tissue function

Maintaining dermal barrier function is an important component in minimising the damage caused by atopic dermatitis. It is generally understood that most of the issues surrounding disturbed barrier function are due to disturbed lipid composition in the stratum corneum layer of the epidermis.[9] It was upon this knowledge that the rationale for essential fatty acid supplementation in atopic dermatitis was initially based. It was identified that low levels of long-chain fatty acids were found in the serum and the cell membranes of people with atopic dermatitis, and that this state contributed to increased inflammation and transepidermal water loss.[50] Following on from this, a range of studies have investigated the effect of essential fatty acids status and the consequent benefit of supplementation in atopic dermatitis; however, the outcomes of these studies have been mixed.[51–53] Although this area has not been particularly well researched, nutrients that support collagen synthesis, such as **vitamin C**, **lysine**, **proline**, **copper** and **iron**, may also be considered.[27] Likewise, herbs that promote collagen synthesis, such as ***Centella asiatica***,[54] could be beneficial, and have been shown to have potential benefit in psoriatic conditions.[55]

INTEGRATIVE MEDICAL CONSIDERATIONS

Homeopathy

Homeopathy may be used in managing atopic dermatitis; however, as is the nature of classical homeopathy, it is difficult to identify a specific remedy as it is very focused on the individual. An interesting study[56] that used a comparative cohort design to review the efficacy of homeopathic treatment of eczema compared with conventional treatment was conducted. Although there were some flaws in the study, it identified an equal benefit for younger children taking the homeopathic remedy compared with conventional treatment.

Psychotherapeutic treatment

Psychotherapeutic treatment may also provide support when managing patients with atopic dermatitis.[57] The rationale behind this may be multifaceted. It has been suggested that, as atopic dermatitis is known to be exacerbated during circumstances of perceived stress, relaxation techniques and cognitive behavioural exercises may assist the person in managing their response, and as such reduce its physiological impact. Furthermore, behavioural interventions can reduce the habit of scratching displayed by people with atopic dermatitis, and as such have a favourable effect on the itch–scratch cycle. There are a number of interventions that have been investigated, and the overall outcome seems promising.[57]

Environment

Climatic change may also be a beneficial intervention to consider in managing atopic dermatitis. In particular, moving to subtropical climates from subarctic or temperate climates, even for a period of four weeks, can incur benefits to patients for up to three years. The benefit may be due to a number of reasons, including exposure to sea water and increased ultraviolet A and B radiation.[58] **Climatotherapy** and **balneotherapy**— whereby patients with skin conditions such as psoriasis and atopic dermatitis attend spas, exposing themselves to mineral waters and sun for periods of a few weeks—can also offer improvement in these conditions, particularly for those who have responded poorly to treatment.[59,60]

Adjuvant topical treatments

One small trial has shown improvement in psoriasis using **topically applied caffeine**.[61] This is thought to be due to the actions of caffeine on increasing intracellular cAMP. Caffeine cream can be quite easily prepared by crushing caffeine tablets available from pharmacies together with a cream base. A small study of patients with mild psoriasis also found improvement in symptoms with *Aloe vera*, though care needs to be taken in case the patient is sensitive to this treatment.[62] Glycyrrhetinic acid, found in ***Glycyrrhiza glabra***, may potentiate the action of hydrocortisone in skin by inhibiting the enzyme 11β-hydroxysteroid dehydrogenase.[63]

Traditional Chinese medicine

A Cochrane review of Chinese herbal medicine for atopic eczema suggested that it may be an effective treatment option for atopic eczema.[64] A later trial has indicated that acupuncture combined with Chinese herbal medicine is more effective in the treatment of atopic dermatitis than herbal medicine alone.[65]

CLINICAL SUMMARY

The management of inflammatory skin disorders requires a systemic approach. It is vital that the practitioner investigates the predisposing risk factors and triggers while also addressing any gastrointestinal dysfunction and concomitant immune dysregulation (Figure 28.3). However, it is also important that the management of any underlying systems is undertaken on an individual level. Treating gastrointestinal function will only benefit the client if their gastrointestinal system is under-functioning. Likewise, removal of common allergens will only reduce the inflammatory response if those allergens are actually relevant to the person.

An individualised treatment plan which considers the person's predisposition, triggers and underlying systemic factors will, once implemented, result in improvement in symptoms fairly quickly (sometimes within days). However, full resolution will often take longer and often relies on the person's ability to avoid exposure to allergens that trigger the symptoms.

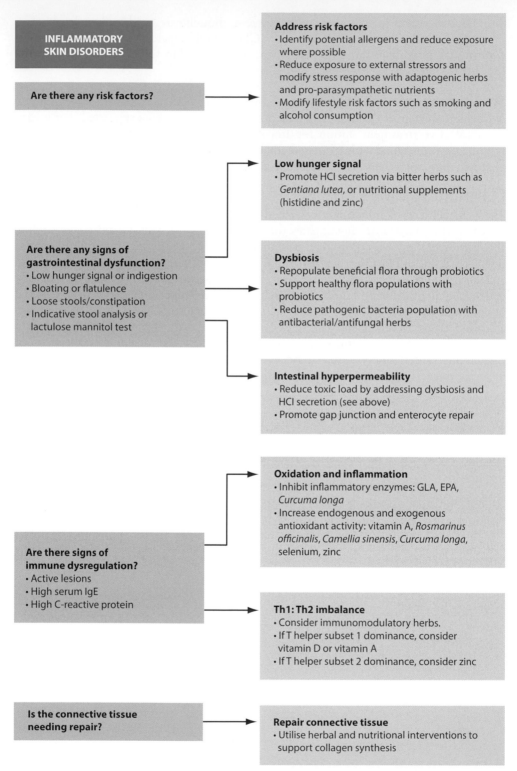

Figure 28.4
Naturopathic treatment decision tree—inflammatory skin disorders

Table 28.1
Review of the major evidence

Intervention	Mechanisms of action	Key literature	Summary of results	Comment
Gamma-linolenic acid	Gamma-linolenic acid inhibits the synthesis of inflammatory prostaglandins,[66] which may contribute to the pathogenesis of atopic dermatitis[50]	RCT: Wright, 1982[53] Takwale et al. 2003[52]	Atopic dermatitis: Dose-dependent response from evening primrose seed oil superior to placebo with regard to itch, scaling and general impression of sensitivity Eczema: not effective	All participants were using concomitant mild topical steroids, emollients and systemic antihistamines No objective measurements were used The study did not investigate the essential fatty acid baseline status Furthermore, olive oil was used actively in the 'control' arm
Probiotics	Probiotics are hypothesised to modulate the innate and adaptive immune responses through interactions with the gut-associated lymphoid tissue[29]	Meta-analysis: Kim et al. 2014[19]	Atopic dermatitis: Benefits observed in children (1–18 years) and adults. Benefits to infants not clear. Mixture of species more effective than single bacterium.	Studies were only included if they used the Scoring of Atopic Dermatitis as a primary outcome measure
Psychological intervention	Through psychological interventions it is proposed that a person's response to internal and external stressors will diminish and as such the pathophysiological implications to the physical response to stress are not as severe[57]	Systematic review: Chida et al. 2007[57]	Eczema: inconclusive	The meta-analysis included heterogenous range of interventions, thus a true meta-analysis was not possible The inclusion of aromatherapy failed to consider the potential physiological effect of the essential oils
Glycyrrhiza glabra topical gel	Glycyrrhiza glabra may be reducing the symptoms of eczema through anti-inflammatory activity[26]	RCT: Saeedi et al. 2003[67]	Eczema: Dose-dependent reduction in symptoms with the most effective result from 2% topical gel (60–84% reduction in symptoms)	The researchers did not use any standardised measurements tools, only a Likert scale Also, the placebo was not described However, a high level of detail pertaining to the sourcing and processing of the herbal extract and gel
Narrow band ultraviolet B phototherapy	Penetrates the dermal layer and slows the growth of skin	RCT: Reynolds et al. 2001[68]	Psoriasis: Mean reduction in total disease activity and extent of disease was significant compared with visible light	Difficult to maintain true placebo as fluorescent light has some visibility so technicians would have known it was placebo

FURTHER READING

Daley D. The evolution of the hygiene hypothesis: the role of early-life exposures to viruses and microbes and their relationship to asthma and allergic diseases. Curr Opin Allergy Clin Immunol 2014;14(5):390–6.

DaVeiga SP. Epidemiology of atopic dermatitis: a review. Allergy Asthma Proc 2012;33(3):227–34.

Harvima IT, Nilsson G. Stress, the neuroendocrine system and mast cells: current understanding of their role in psoriasis. Expert Re Clin Immunol 2012;8:235–41.

Muehleisen B, Gallo RL. Vitamin D in allergic disease: shedding light on a complex problem. J Allergy Clin Immunol 2013;131(2):324–9.

Preedy VR, editor. Handbook of diet, nutrition and the skin. Wageningen: Wageningen Academic Publishers; 2012.

REFERENCES

1. Gould BE. Pathophysiology for the health professional. 3rd ed. Philadelphia: Saunders Elsevier; 2006.
2. Hay RJ, Johns NE, Williams HC, et al. The global burden of skin disease in 2010: an analysis of the prevalence and impact of skin conditions. J Invest Dermatol 2014;134(6):1527–34.
3. Boguniewicz M, Leung DY. Atopic dermatitis: a disease of altered skin barrier and immune dysregulation. Immunol Rev 2011;242(1):233–46.
4. Williams H, Stewart A, von Mutius E, et al. Is eczema really on the increase worldwide? J Allergy Clin Immunol 2008;121:947–54.
5. Griffiths CEM, Barker JNWN. Pathogenesis and clinical features of psoriasis. Lancet 2007;370(9583):263–71.
6. Gottlieb AB, Chao C, Dann F. Psoriasis comorbidities. J Dermatolog Treat 2008;19(1):5–21.
7. McMillin DL, Richards DG, Mein EA, et al. Systemic aspects of psoriasis: an integrative model based on intestinal etiology. Integr Med 2000;2:105–13.
8. Proksch E, Folster-Holst R, Jensen J-M. Skin barrier function, epidermal proliferation and differentiation in eczema. J Dermatol Sci 2006;43:159–69.
9. Host A, Halken S. Practical aspects of allergy-testing. Paediatr Respir Rev 2003;4(4):312–18.
10. Nylund L, Nermes M, Isolauri E, et al. Severity of atopic disease inversely correlates with intestinal microbiota diversity and butyrate-producing bacteria. Allergy 2015;70(2):241–4.
11. Simecka JW. Mucosal immunity of the gastrointestinal tract and oral tolerance. Adv Drug Deliv Rev 1998;34:235–59.
12. Rautava S, Kalliomaki M, Isolauri E. New therapeutic strategy for combating increasing burden of allergic disease: probiotics—a Nutrition, Allergy, Mucosal Immunology and Intestinal Microbiota (NAMI) Research Group report. J Allergy Clin Immunol 2005;116:31–7.
13. Adlerberth I, Wold AE. Establishment of the gut microbiota in Western infants. Acta Paediatr 2009;98(2):229–38.
14. Wickens K, Black PN, Stanley TV, et al. A differential effect of 2 probiotics in the prevention of eczema and atopy: a double-blind, randomized, placebo-controlled trial. J Allergy Clin Immunol 2008;122:788–94.
15. Rautava S, Kainonen E, Salminen S, et al. Maternal probiotic supplementation during pregnancy and breast-feeding reduces the risk of eczema in the infant. J Allergy Clin Immunol 2012;130(6):1355–60.
16. Viljanen M, Pohjavuori E, Haahtela T, et al. Induction of inflammation as a possible mechanism of probiotic effect in atopic eczema-dermatitis syndrome. J Allergy Clin Immunol 2005;115:1254–9.
17. Pelucchi C, Chatenoud L, Turati F, et al. Probiotics supplementation during pregnancy or infancy for the prevention of atopic dermatitis: a meta-analysis. Epidemiology 2012;23(3):402–14.
18. Zuccotti G, Meneghin F, Aceti A, et al. Probiotics for prevention of atopic diseases in infants: systematic review and meta-analysis. Allergy 2015;70(11):1356–71.
19. Kim SO, Ah YM, Yu YM, et al. Effects of probiotics for the treatment of atopic dermatitis: a meta-analysis of randomized controlled trials. Ann Allergy Asthma Immunol 2014;113(2):217–26.
20. Ly NP, Litonjua A, Gold DR, et al. Gut microbiota, probiotics, and vitamin D: interrelated exposures influencing allergy, asthma, and obesity? J Allergy Clin Immunol 2011;127(5):1087–94.
21. Colivet J, Marcano G, Belloso G, et al. Antimicrobial effect of ethanolic extracts from basil (Ocimum basilicum L.) on growth of Staphylococcus aureus. Rev Venez de Cienc y Tecnología de Alimentos 2011;2(2):313–20.
22. Iciek M, Kwiecien I, Wlodek L. Biological properties of garlic and garlic-derived organosulfur compounds. Environ Mol Mutagen 2009;50(3):247–65.
23. Hwang BY, Roberts SK, Chadwick LR, et al. Antimicrobial constituents from goldenseal (the Rhizomes of Hydrastis canadensis) against selected oral pathogens. Planta Med 2003;69(7):623–7.
24. Rosenfeldt V, Benfeldt E, Valerius NH, et al. Effect of probiotics on gastrointestinal symptoms and small intestinal

permeability in children with atopic dermatitis. J Pediatr 2004;145:612–16.

25. Vilela GE, De Abreu Ferrari DLM, da Gama Torres OH, et al. Influence of Saccharomyces boulardii on the intestinal permeability of patients with Crohn's disease in remission. Scand J Gastroenterol 2008;43(7):842–8.

26. Blumenthal M. British herbal pharmacopoeia. London: BHMA Publishing; 1996.

27. Gropper SS, Smith JL, Groff JL. Advanced nutrition and human metabolism. 5th ed. Belmont: Wadsworth; 2009.

28. World Health Organization. Infant and young child feeding: model chapter for textbooks for medical students and allied health professionals. Geneva: World Health Organization; 2009. p. 1–99.

29. Bager P, Wohlfahrt J, Westergaard T. Caesarean delivery and risk of atopy and allergic disease: meta-analyses. Clin Exp Allergy 2008;38:634–42.

30. Kuitunen M, Kukkonen K, Juntunen-Backman K, et al. Probiotics prevent IgE-associated allergy until 5 years in caesarean-delivered children but not in the total cohort. J Allergy Clin Immunol 2009;123:335–41.

31. Tripathi RM, Sen PC, Das PK. Studies on the mechanism of action of Albizia lebbeck, an Indian indigenous drug used in the treatment of atopic allergy. J Ethnopharmacol 1979;1(4):385–96.

32. Clemetson CAB. Histamine and ascorbic acid in human blood. J Nutr 1980;110(4):662–8.

33. Bois P, Gascon A, Beaulnes A. Histamine-liberating effect of magnesium deficiency in the rat. Nature 1963;197(4866):501–2.

34. Maintz L, Benfadal S, Allam J, et al. Evidence for a reduced histamine degradation capacity in a subgroup of patients with atopic eczema. J Allergy Clin Immunol 2006;117(5):1106–12.

35. Ikai K, Imamura S. Role of eicosanoids in the pathogenesis of atopic dermatitis. Prostaglandins Leukot Essent Fatty Acids 1993;48:409–16.

36. Kurd SK, Smith N, VanVoorhees A, et al. Oral curcumin in the treatment of moderate to severe psoriasis vuglaris. A prospective clinical trial. J Am Acad Dermatol 2008;58:625–31.

37. Wright RJ, Cohen RT, Cohen S. The impact of stress on the development and expression of atopy. Curr Opin Allergy Clin Immunol 2005;5:23–9.

38. Marshall GD, Roy SR. Stress and allergic diseases. Psychoneuroimmunology. Elsevier; 2007.

39. Prescott SL, Dunstan JA. Immune dysregulation in allergic respiratory disease: the role of T regulatory celss. Pulm Pharmacol Ther 2005;18:217–28.

40. Ziboh VA, Miller CC, Cho Y. Significance of lipoxygenase-derived fatty acids in cutaneous biology. Prostaglandins Other Lipid Mediat 2000;63:3–13.

41. Kitz R, Rose MA, Schonborn H, et al. Impact of early dietary gamma-linolenic acid supplementation on atopic eczema in infancy. Pediatr Allergy Immunol 2006;17:112–17.

42. Koch C, Dolle S, Metzger M, et al. Docosahexaenoic acid (DHA) supplementation in atopic eczema: a randomised, double-blind, controlled trial. Br J Dermatol 2008;158:786–92.

43. Baker BS, Powles A, Fry L. Peptidoglycan. A major aetiological factor for psoriasis. Trends Immunol 2006;27(12):545–52.

44. Mora JR, Iwata M, von Andrian UH. Vitamin effects on the immune system: vitamins A and D take centre stage. Nat Rev Immunol 2008;8:685–98.

45. Omata N, Tsukahara H, Ito S, et al. Increased oxidative stress in childhood atopic dermatitis. Life Sci 2001;69:223–8.

46. Kokcam I, Naziroglu M. Antioxidants and lipid peroxidation status in the blood of patients with psoriasis. Clin Chim Acta 1999;289:23–31.

47. van der Hulst AE, Klip H, Brand PLP. Risk of developing asthma in young children with atopic eczema: a systematic review. J Allergy Clin Immunol 2007;120:565–9.

48. Burgess JA, Dharmage SC, Byrnes GB, et al. Childhood eczema and asthma incidence and persistence: a cohort study from childhood to middle age. J Allergy Clin Immunol 2008;122(2):280–5.

49. Safonova GM, Shilov YI, Perevozchikov AB. Protective effects of plant polyphenols on the immune system in acute stress. Dokl Biol Sci 2001;378(1–6):223–35.

50. Wright S. Essential fatty acids and the skin. Prostaglandins Leukot Essent Fatty Acids 1989;38:229–36.

51. Newson RB, Shaheen SO, Henderson AJ, et al. Umbilical cord and maternal blood red cell fatty acids and early childhood wheezing and eczema. J Allergy Clin Immunol 2004;114:531–7.

52. Takwale A, Tan E, Agarwal S, et al. Efficacy and tolerability of borage oil in adults and children with atopic eczema: randomised, double blind, placebo controlled parallel group trial. BMJ 2003;327:1–4.

53. Wright S. Oral evening primrose seed oil improves atopic eczema. Lancet 1982;2:1120–2.

54. Shukla A, Rasik AM, Jain GK, et al. In vitro and in vivo wound healing activity of asiaticoside isolated from Centella asiatica. J Ethnopharmacol 1999;65(1):1–11.

55. Sampson JH, Raman A, Karlsen G, et al. In vitro keratinocyte antiproliferant effect of Centella asiatica extract and triterpenoid saponins. Phytomedicine 2001;8(3):230–5.

56. Keil T, Witt CM, Roll S, et al. Homoeopathic versus conventional treatment of children with eczema: a comparative cohort study. Complement Ther Med 2008;16:15–21.

57. Chida Y, Steptoe A, Hirakawa N, et al. The effects of psychological intervention on atopic dermatitis. Int Arch Allergy Immunol 2007;144:1–9.

58. Byremo G, Rod G, Carlsen KH. Effect of climatic change in children with atopic eczema. Allergy 2006;61:1403–10.

59. Kazandjieva J, Grozdev I, Darlenski R, et al. Climatotherapy of psoriasis. Clin Dermatol 2008;26(5):477–85.

60. Matz H, Orion E, Wolf R. Balneotherapy in dermatology. Dermatol Ther 2003;16(2):132–40.

61. Vali A, Asilian A, Khalesi E, et al. Evaluation of the efficacy of topical caffeine in the treatment of psoriasis vulgaris. J Dermatolog Treat 2005;16(4):234–7.

62. Paulsen E, Korsholm L, Brandrup F. A double-blind, placebo-controlled study of a commercial Aloe vera gel in the treatment of slight to moderate psoriasis vulgaris. J Eur Acad Dermatol Venereol 2005;19(3):326–31.

63. Teelucksingh S, Mackie A, Burt D, et al. Potentiation of hydrocortisone activity in skin by glycyrrhetinic acid. Lancet 1990;335(8697):1060–3.

64. Zhang W, Leonard T, Bath-Hextall F, et al. Chinese herbal medicine for atopic eczema. Cochrane Database Syst Rev 2004;(4):CD002291.

65. Salameh F, Perla D, Solomon M, et al. The effectiveness of combined Chinese herbal medicine and acupuncture in the treatment of atopic dermatitis. J Altern Complement Med 2008;14(8):1043–8.

66. Kohlmeier M. Nutrient metabolism. San Diego: Academic Press; 2003.

67. Saeedi M, Morteza-Semnani K, Ghoreishi M-R. The treatment of atopic dermatitis with licorice gel. J Dermatolog Treat 2003;14:153–7.

68. Reynolds NJ, Franklin V, Gray JC, et al. Narrow-band ultraviolet B and broad-band ultraviolet A phototherapy in adult atopic eczema: a randomised controlled trial. Lancet 2001;357:2012–16.

CHAPTER 29

Benign prostatic hypertrophy

Kieran Cooley
ND

OVERVIEW

While benign prostatic hypertrophy (BPH) of the prostate (or more accurately benign prostatic *hyperplasia*) and erectile dysfunction (ED) are typically seen in the ageing male, these can occur at any age. Current understanding of the disease involves imbalanced states of androgens (particularly dihydrotestosterone [DHT]), oestrogens, insulin and insulin-like growth factor (IGF) and detrusor dysfunction of the bladder neck.[1] The chief complaint of patients with BPH is urinary frequency, urgency, nocturia, decreased and intermittent force of stream and the sensation of incomplete emptying of the bladder, although these symptoms are neither specific nor necessary for the diagnosis of BPH and do not correlate with the extent or degree of hypertrophy of the prostate.[1] One study suggests that 20% of men in their 40s and 90% of men in their 70s have varying degrees of BPH,[2] although incidence rates for age groups vary depending on population demographics (some suggest 50% of men older than 60, and 80% of men over 80 years).[3] Increasing age is the predominant factor associated with prevalence of BPH. Likewise, the incidence and prevalence of ED are also linked to age, with American data suggesting a tripling of the incidence occurring between the ages of 40 and 70 years, and up to 66% of men having suffered from some ED (mild to complete) by the age of 70 years.[4] Worldwide estimates suggest up to 330 million men could be affected by this disorder,[5] although criticism exists pertaining to the over-medicalisation and resulting prescription rates for drugs providing only symptomatic relief for some age-associated disorders like ED.[6] Conversely, both ED and BPH may suffer from under-diagnosis due to the symptomatic nature and psychological stigma associated with each of these diseases.[7]

Previously, diagnosis of BPH was thought to involve solely lower urinary tract symptoms (LUTS) syndrome; however, recent evidence suggests that LUTS is often due to anatomical disorders (detrusor muscle dysfunction)[8,9] and that symptoms of BPH do not correlate well with prostate size. However, an enlarged prostate could contribute to detrusor dysfunction and urinary retention, often termed 'LUTS-BPH'. Clinicians should note that not all men with BPH have LUT symptoms and LUTS is not specific or exclusive to BPH.

There is little certainty surrounding the exact pathogenesis of BPH. It is characterised by periurethral prostate tissue proliferation, which is indicated by an increase in the number (not size) of epithelial and stromal cells.[10] This has been posited to be a relatively normal (or at least highly pervasive) process of ageing, often linked to the prostate tissue response to increase in DHT androgens that occurs in the ageing male. Environmental exposure to hormone disruptors like xeno-oestrogens may result in a cascade of events that influence the development of dysfunctional regulation of testosterone, 17β-oestradiol and DHT (Figure 29.1).[10] The enzymes aromatase and 5-alpha reductase are involved in hormone regulation and these are often targets of both conventional as well as naturopathic treatment. Other evidence suggests that increased exposure to growth factors (insulin and IGF) initiates the onset of hyperproliferation, ultimately leading to decreased urinary and vascular flow and an increased risk for ED, LUTS, prostatitis and prostate cancer, all of which can be associated disorders.[1] As the prostate enlarges, it causes discomfort in the groin and increased pressure on the bladder, leading to variable urine flow rates, frequent urination, nocturia and a sense of incomplete voiding. With chronicity or severity of enlargement, blockage of the urethra can occur, increasing the risk for urinary tract infections, bladder stones or infection and possible kidney damage.

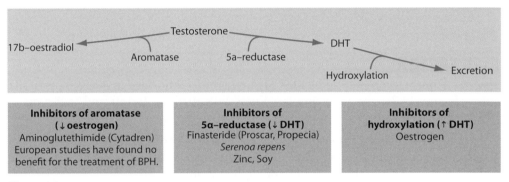

Figure 29.1
Hormonal factors in BPH
Source: Rakel 2007[11]

In 2001 a landmark paper suggested a link between ED, BPH, cardiovascular disease and depression in ageing males,[12] supporting earlier suggestions linking some of these disorders to vascular function.[13] Since then, further evidence has confirmed a strong correlation among these disorders, with significantly higher prevalence rates of any of the listed conditions when a comorbidity from any of the other disorders exists. The correlation is particularly strong between BPH and ED, possibly due to a shared vasculogenic pathophysiology, revolving around atherosclerosis and endothelial dysfunction or injury, in production of nitric oxide (NO).[14] Other factors associated with cardiovascular disease and/or depression (such as central obesity, increased circulating levels of insulin, diabetes, decreased physical activity, hypertension and increased oxidative stress) are also implicated in the state that promotes the hyperproliferation of prostatic tissue and decreased functioning of circuitry relating to achieving an erection.[15,16] Most recently, metabolic syndrome has been added to the list of comorbid disorders predictive of BPH, with a significant association being demonstrated between any number of criteria for metabolic syndrome and the risk of progression to clinical BPH even while adjusting for age and serum testosterone levels (odds ratio 1.423, 95% confidence interval 1.020–1.986).[17]

A thorough history and appropriately directed diagnostic studies are essential to appropriate diagnosis of BPH. The 2012 Canadian guidelines for management of BPH outline a diagnostic algorithm for LUTS, which may be useful given that these symptoms are often non-specific to BPH.[18]

DIFFERENTIAL DIAGNOSIS

- Carcinoma of the bladder
- Cystitis (infection or radiation induced)
- Foreign bodies in the bladder (stones or retained stents), bladder trauma or infection
- Pelvic floor dysfunction or chronic pelvis pain (prostatodynia)
- Prostatitis or prostatic abscess
- Prostate cancer
- Overactive bladder (OAB) or neurogenic bladder
- Urethral stricture due to trauma or a sexually transmitted disease
- Urinary tract infection

RISK FACTORS[1,3,19]

Several factors may promote BPH/LUTS, whereas other influences may have a protective effect (Figure 29.2). The following is a list of potential risk factors and indicators of BPH.

- Urethral stricture as a result of recurrent urinary tract infection, prostatitis, bladder infection/trauma or bladder neck contractions (congenital or acquired) can induce LUTS and stimulate the onset of hyperproliferation.
- Comorbid conditions such as cardiovascular disease, metabolic syndrome, ED and depression are also implicated in increased incidence or potential for earlier onset of BPH.
- Increased serum prostate-specific antigen (PSA) can be indicative of BPH, but it is neither sensitive nor specific to BPH, although monitoring change in this marker over time gives some small clinically relevant indication of prostate status or change. Suggested PSA levels that may indicate a hyperproliferative prostate are higher than 1.6 µg/mL for men in their 50s, higher than 2.0 µg/mL for men in their 60s and higher than 2.3 µg/mL for men in their 70s. Guidelines differ across regions with respect to the utility of PSA as well as the exact values or ranges that may be concerning.
- A positive digital rectal exam is the strongest indicator of BPH and regular screening is recommended in men over 50 years old or those exhibiting symptoms. Some guidelines suggest that a digital rectal exam is not recommended as a screening exam for men older than 75 years of age as this may prompt invasive therapy that ultimately does not improve overall mortality and quality of life. The extent to which BPH may increase the risk of prostate cancer is relatively controversial and speculative in nature, in part due to limitations in the existing research.

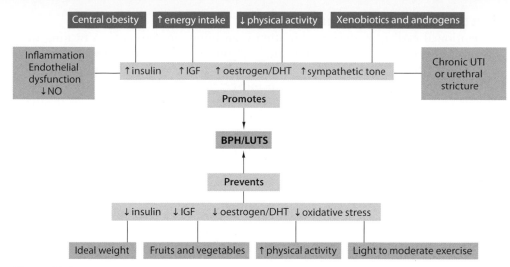

Figure 29.2
Factors affecting BPH or LUTS

CONVENTIONAL TREATMENT

Conventional treatment of BPH varies but often begins with 'watchful waiting' if the symptoms are mild. Alpha-blockers (alfuzosin and tamsulosin) are often selected for decreasing sympathetic tone with minimal change in blood pressure to give LUTS relief and are often employed in those without significantly raised levels of PSA.[1,19,20] 5-alpha reductase inhibitors (finasteride or dutasteride) inhibit the conversion of testosterone to DHT and are the most frequently prescribed treatment, sometimes in conjunction with alpha-blockers with greater success.[21] If symptoms are severe (there is a long history of smoking or risk factors for cancer) or PSA levels are relatively high, surgical removal of the prostate (transurethral resection of the prostate or TURP) may be indicated. Less invasive surgical therapies procedures such as laser prostectomy, transurethral microwave therapy (TUMT) and transurethral needle ablation (TUNA) may be options for younger patients, although in general these therapies have not been shown to be superior to TURP in terms of long-term outcomes.[20,22]

KEY TREATMENT PROTOCOLS

A comprehensive strategy addressing cardio-vascular risk and reduction of inflammation is required to address the underlying vascular cause. Additional strategies to provide symptomatic relief from LUTS are necessary for short-term management of this debilitating disorder. The initial approach in treating this disorder is always to assess the lifestyle of the patient and recommend judicious and achievable adjustments when required (Figure 29.3).

Naturopathic Treatment Aims

- Address risk factors including achievement of healthy weight and increased physical activity.
- Regulate hormones, particularly through aromatase and 5-alpha reductase as well as environmental sources of hormones.
- Address symptom relief and quality-of-life issues.
- Protect endothelial function through decreasing inflammation and improving NO production.
- Address latent, recurrent or chronic infection and sources of oxidative stress.

Lifestyle and exercise modification

As mentioned earlier, lifestyle modification is an important protocol in treating BPH and ED. Observational studies indicate there is a positive association between abdominal obesity and BPH,[23,24] and an inverse association between physical activity and BPH.[19,20] Diets high in fats or in calories may encourage abdominal obesity and sympathetic nervous system activity, both of which can increase the risk of BPH. Sympathetic nervous system activation (which is the 'fight or flight' arm of the autonomic nervous system) may cause the prostate smooth muscle to contract, resulting in a worsening of LUTS. Studies suggest that there is no increased risk of BPH with higher caloric intake when accompanied by increased physical activity.[24] With respect to ED, weight loss, physical activity, smoking cessation and decreased sympathetic activity (relaxation) have also been suggested as beneficial treatments.[25] Dietary sources of caffeine and other diuretics should be reduced, and fluid intake monitored to reduce nocturia and urinary output to the bladder from the kidneys.

Three potential mechanisms for physical activity and decreased risk for BPH and ED may be proposed.

- It may increase blood flow to the area, allowing the body to remove wastes efficiently.
- It may decrease sympathetic stress responses, thus relaxing prostatic tissue.
- It may reduce excess abdominal weight, increasing overall lower body pressure, thus relaxing the prostate and rectal region and improving blood flow into and out of the area.

Nutritional hormonal modulation

Clinicians should consider dietary strategies to modulate hormones, hydroxylation of DHT and maintain healthy cholesterol and cardiovascular states; these strategies include avoiding sources of pesticides,[26] increasing fruit consumption, increasing the intake of zinc and essential fatty acid, decreasing butter consumption, avoiding margarine,[27] decreasing coffee consumption[28] and keeping cholesterol levels below 200 mg/dL.[29]

Inconclusive evidence exists regarding protein intake and BPH. Some research demonstrates that a **high-protein diet** (total calories made up of 44% protein, 35% carbohydrate and 21% fat) can inhibit 5-alpha reductase, while a low-protein diet (10% protein, 70% carbohydrate and 20% fat) may stimulate the enzyme.[30] Contrary to this evidence, a large eight-year observational study of 3523 men with BPH suggests that total protein intake is positively associated with BPH, with the association being slightly stronger for animal protein intake than for vegetable protein intake.[24] A second epidemiological study based in China also revealed a correlation between higher animal intake and the incidence of BPH (91.1% in those eating high animal diets as opposed to 11.8% in those not eating animal protein).[31]

Authors of these studies suggest that a high protein intake may result in a greater osmolar load, which may be one possible mechanism for its detrimental effects on symptoms of BPH. This will increase urinary output and therefore impose undue extra burden on an already partially obstructed or strained elimination system.[24] Consistent with an anti-inflammatory approach, a diet high in quality, plant-derived and coldwater fish-based protein sources in moderate amounts seems prudent, given the current evidence.

Zinc supplementation has reduced the size of the prostate (confirmed by rectal palpation, radiography and endoscopy) and reduced overall symptomatology in the majority of patients with BPH in studies conducted in the 1970s as well as recently.[32] The clinical efficacy of zinc is probably due to its critical involvement in many aspects of androgen metabolism. High amounts of oestrogen can inhibit intestinal uptake of zinc, whereas elevated androgens increase absorption. Because oestrogen levels are increased in men with BPH, zinc uptake may be low, suggesting a higher functional need for this nutrient and begging the need for additional supplementation.[33,34] However, one case-control study suggested a positive association between zinc levels and BPH.[35] This deviation from other research may be partially explained by dietary confounding factors.

The relationship between zinc levels and 5-alpha reductase activity in hyperplastic prostates is inconsistent; however, zinc has been shown to inhibit the activity of 5-alpha reductase, and decreases the conversion of testosterone to DHT.[36–39] Zinc can also inhibit specific binding of androgens to the cytosol and nuclear androgen receptors present in high amounts in prostatic tissue.[36] These mechanisms suggest that zinc has more of a preventive role by maintaining a nutritional status that discourages prostate hypertrophy. No interventional studies investigating the use of zinc for BPH exist, although observational studies suggest it has a safe and effective role in diminishing the size of the prostate, particularly for prostate cancer, although one study suggests it can increase urinary symptoms.[40–44]

Zinc is also involved in the regulation of prolactin secretion, leading to increased uptake of testosterone and subsequent rise in DHT in the prostate.[45–47] Natural (from beer, stress and tryptophan)[48,49] and pharmaceutical prolactin antagonists (bromocriptine)[50] have been shown to reduce many of the symptoms of prostatic hyperplasia. However, this strategy can have severe side effects, particularly pertaining to cardiovascular and neurological systems, including severe changes in mood.[50,51]

A 100-g serving of soybeans or **soy** products contains 90 mg of **beta-sitosterol**, which has been shown to decrease cholesterol; this is a potential mechanism for soy's effect on BPH. The cholesterol-lowering effects of phytosterols are well documented,[52,53] while also showing an effect on treating BPH.[9] One double-blind study[54] in 200 men using beta-sitosterol (20 mg) or placebo three times daily demonstrated an increase in the maximum urine flow rate from a baseline of 9.9 mL/s to 15.2 mL/s and a decrease in mean residual urinary volume of 30.4 mL from 65.8 mL in the beta-sitosterol group. No changes were observed in the placebo group. An increased consumption of soy and soy foods is associated with a decrease in the risk of prostate cancer,[55,56] which is associated with the incidence of BPH. Phyto-estrogens in soy (isoflavonoids, genistein and daidzein) as well as *Trifolium pratense* are implicated due to their effect on oestrogen receptors[55,57] and inhibition of 5-alpha reductase.[58] Other sources of beta-sitosterols such as *Hypoxis hemerocallidea* may also be of benefit, although many of these studies are lacking in the rigour of reporting including dose and method of extraction as well as adverse-event reporting.[59] Clinical use of these substances may be most appropriate for men with BPH in the 'watchful waiting' stage of the condition,[60] with clinically effecting doses of beta-sitosterol ranging from 60–130 mg daily.[61,62]

One study[63] suggested that 60 mg twice daily of the dried, ground flowers of *Opuntia* **spp.** over two to six months was effective at reducing urinary urgency and the sensation of a full bladder, although this remains to be repeated in other studies and stands as preliminary evidence.

The diet should be as free as possible from environmental toxins such as pesticides and other contaminants because many of these compounds (such as dioxin, polyhalogenated biphenyls, hexachlorobenzene and dibenzofurans) increase 5-alpha reduction of steroids.[30] Diethylstilboestrol produces changes in rat prostates histologically similar to BPH.[64] While cadmium is a known antagonist of zinc and can influence testosterone levels through effects on the activity of 5-alpha reductase, its concentration in, and effects on, the prostate are unclear. Several studies have produced conflicting results.[65,66]

Herbal hormonal modulation

During the 1990s, botanical medicine in Germany and Australia were considered 'first-line' treatments for BPH and accounted for greater than 90% of all drugs in the medical management of BPH.[67] In Italy plant extracts accounted for roughly 50% of all medications prescribed for BPH, while alpha-blockers and 5-alpha reductase inhibitors account for only 5.1% and 4.8%, respectively.[68]

Clinical success with any of the botanical treatments of BPH may be determined by the degree of obstruction as indicated by the residual urine content.[1,26] For mild LUTS and residual urine levels less than 50 mL, the results are usually excellent. For levels between 50 and 100 mL, the results are usually quite good. Residual urine levels greater than 100 mL will be more difficult to produce significant improvements in the customary four- to six-week period without co-management using other therapies including pharmaceuticals, and with botanical medicine adding little to the overall reduction in symptoms within a four- to six-week period. One small ($n = 40$) but well-designed clinic-based research study investigating the open use of phytotherapy for LUTS/BPH demonstrated a statistically significant superiority of phytotherapy use (as both adjuvant to pharmacological treatment or as a stand-alone) over use of alpha-blockers to reduce urinary retention, and improve erectile and ejaculatory dysfunction.[69] Adulteration and/ or contamination in herbal products for ED is relatively widespread,[70,71] particularly in 'commercial' natural health products in some countries. As with usual prescriptions, clinicians should ensure that patients are accessing high-quality products.

The liposterolic extract of the fruit of ***Serenoa repens*** (Saw palmetto: SP), native to Florida in the United States, has been commonly used for the signs and symptoms of BPH, as well as investigated in numerous clinical studies. The mechanism of action is postulated to be related to inhibition of DHT binding to both the cytosolic and the nuclear androgen receptors, inhibition of 5-alpha reductase, interference with intraprostatic oestrogen receptors and an anti-inflammatory effect.[10] As a result of this multitude of effects, positive results have been produced in numerous double-blind clinical studies. However, different extracts of SP (permixon) may have more of an anti-inflammatory mechanism of action in modulating BPH[67,70–75]; clinicians should be mindful of these differences in therapeutic action from the myriad extraction methods used in natural health products and the multifaceted effects of herbal medicines, particularly SP.[72]

Synthesis research, including systematic reviews of clinical trials, has previously reported excellent results using SP while noting that discrepancies exist.[69,70] One early examination of 21 randomised controlled trials (RCTs) involving a total of 3139 men (including 18 double-blind trials) demonstrated that men treated with SP experienced decreased urinary tract symptom scores, less nocturia, better urinary tract symptom self-rating scores and peak urine flow improvements compared with men receiving placebo.[69] This analysis also showed that, matched up with men receiving the DHT inhibitor finasteride (Proscar), men treated with SP had similar improvements in urinary tract symptom scores and peak urine and sparked an increase in use in both clinical and research settings. A related review also reported that adverse effects due to SP were mild and infrequent with ED appearing more frequently with finasteride (4.9%) than with SP (1.1%).[76] However, the most recent update to this Cochrane review on the subject, which included studies comparing SP to either placebo or finasteride as well as studies using various doses of SP, demonstrated no significant benefit for treating any symptoms of BPH, including prostate size, nightly urination and peak urine flow among the high-quality studies. The large variability in patient population, severity of disease and extraction or source of SP, as demonstrated by a lack of heterogeneity between studies and wide confidence intervals for outcomes, highlights some of the challenges in herbal medicine research when applying research results to individuals. While this evidence of no effect cannot be ignored, one should note that clinical success in using SP for BPH is variable, and not considered the standard of care. If a decision is made to use SP as a part of a holistic treatment approach, clinicians should expect that improvement, if any, in men with mild to moderate symptoms receiving treatment within the first four to six weeks of onset.

Despite an efficacy profile similar to other single agents (finasteride) for mild to moderate severity, SP has a lower risk profile and is less expensive.[77] The most common side effect is gastrointestinal distress, and this is easily remedied by taking SP with food.

Cernilton, a proprietary combination of water-soluble and acetone-soluble extract of *Secale cereale*, has been used to treat prostatitis and BPH for years in Europe.[78,79] Several short clinical studies and one systematic review suggest it to be beneficial in the treatment of BPH,[80–86] with patients reporting moderate improvement. Patients who respond typically have reductions of nocturia and diurnal frequency of around 70%, as well as significant reductions in residual urine volume. The extract has been shown to exert some anti-inflammatory action and produce a contractile effect on the bladder while simultaneously relaxing the urethra.[87]

In one study the clinical efficacy of Cernilton in treating symptomatic BPH was examined over a one-year period.[79] Seventy-nine males of an average age of 68 years (range 62–89), with a mean baseline prostatic volume of 33.2 cm^2, were administered 63 mg of Cernilton pollen extract twice daily for 12 weeks. Average urine maximum flow rate increased from 5.1 to 6 mL/s. Average flow rate increased from 9.3 to 11 mL/s. Residual urine volume decreased from 54.2 mL to less than 30 mL. Urgency and discomfort improved by 76.9% with dysuria, incomplete emptying, intermittency, delayed or prolonged voiding all having 60–70% improvement. Nocturia improved by 56.8%. Overall, 85% of the test subjects experienced benefit, 11% reporting 'excellent', 39% reporting 'good', 35% reporting 'satisfactory' and 15% reporting 'poor' as a description of their outcome.

A systematic review conducted in 2000 compiling two placebo-controlled studies, two comparative trials (both lasting 12–24 weeks) and three double-blind studies of 444 men showed that, although Cernilton did not improve urinary flow rates, residual volume or prostate size compared with placebo or the comparative study agents, it did improve self-rated urinary symptom scores and reduced nocturia compared with placebo.[84] Again, this review highlights some of the variability in evidence for the use of this herbal extract with the chances of clinical success in using this as a stand-alone treatment remaining unclear.

Extracts from the bark of ***Pygeum africanum*** used in research studies are fat-soluble sterols and fatty acids. Virtually all of the research on pygeum has featured a *Pygeum africanum* extract standardised to contain 14% triterpenes including beta-sitosterol and 0.5% *n*-docosanol. The suggested therapeutic action has been suggested to be due, in part, to the inhibition of growth factors EGF, bFGF and IGF-1, which are responsible for the prostatic overgrowth.[88,89]

Very early evidence suggests a potential role for calcium–magnesium balance in cancerous prostatic tissue proliferation.[90] Although speculative, the herb *Corotn membranaceus* (ethanolic root extract 60 mg/day) was successfully used to correct this imbalance.

Clinical trials totalling more than 600 patients have demonstrated *Pygeum africanum* extract to be effective in reducing the symptoms and clinical signs of BPH, especially in early cases.[89,91] The research studies suggest *pygeum africanum* having a superiority in objective parameters, especially urine flow rate and residual urine content, over SP. However, as the two extracts have somewhat overlapping mechanisms of actions, they can be used in combination. Other proprietary herbal combinations (*Cucurbita pepo*, *Epilobium parviflorum*, lycopene, *Pygeum africanum* and SP) have been investigated and are suggestive of statistically significant benefit for the various symptoms of BPH, although these studies are small and bear repeating.[92]

Lepidium meyenii (**maca**) is a root belonging to the brassica family traditionally known for its aphrodisiac properties in both men and women.[93] A relatively recent randomised, double-blind placebo-controlled trial demonstrated a subjective improvement on the International Index of Erectile Function (IIEF-5) and Satisfaction Profile (SAT-P) using 2400 mg/day of dry extract of maca compared with placebo.[94] Although both groups improved significantly from baseline self-rated psychological performance scores, there was a statistically significant superiority in the maca group in physical and social performance. This represents a small but statistically significant clinical effect from using this dose of maca in men with mild ED. Two other randomised, placebo-controlled studies with limited information suggest that 1.5 and 3 g/day dose of maca can improve ED without altering testosterone levels in men with this disorder.[95,96] Further research is necessary to better determine the mechanism of action, the clinical relevance and optimal dose and constituents in maca for use in ED. No clinical evidence exists for the use of maca for treating BPH.

Extracts of **Urtica dioica** have also been shown to be effective in treating BPH, although less research evidence exists compared with other botanical medicines. A number of long-term, double-blind studies have shown it to be more effective than a placebo, with no adverse effects reported.[97,98] A randomised, multicentre, double-blind study in 431 patients using extracts of both SP and *Urtica dioica* found clinical benefit equal to that of finasteride,[99] with a larger, second study lasting 24 weeks confirming its benefit in reducing residual urine and improving peak flow.[97] A similar therapeutic action between *Urtica dioica* and SP extracts appears to exist in that each interact with binding of DHT to cytosolic and nuclear receptors.[100] Other in vitro studies also show that lignans found in *Urtica dioica* may modulate hormonal effects due to their affinity for sex hormone-binding globulin.[101]

In vitro studies of **Epilobium spp.** suggest steroid receptor and aromatase inhibition activity as well as potent cyclo-oxygenase-2 (COX-2) and antioxidant potential, so this herb could theoretically be used in BPH.[102,103] Other cell-line research supports this and elucidates the antihyperplastic and potential anticancer action of *Epilobium parviflorum* extract (oenothein B) as a potent inhibitor of DNA synthesis in a human prostate cell line. Aqueous extracts have also demonstrated plausible COX-2 action,[104] although ethanolic extracts appear to have the most potential inhibitory action on this enzyme linked to inflammatory pathways.[105] These results have yet to be duplicated in clinical trials.

Reduce inflammation

While limited, some studies suggest that the inflammatory process including the production of cytokines (interleukin 1 and 6, and tissue necrosis factor alpha) increases prostatic tissue proliferation.[67,78] Other research links the presence of platelet-derived growth factor (PDGF) (produced during the inflammatory processes) and androgens with the incidence of BPH and hyperproliferation of prostate cells.[106,107] In these studies, DHT failed to produce a mitogenic response in prostate cells without the presence of PDGF.

In a large, Italian, case-controlled study, **essential fatty acids** (**EFA**) consisting of linoleic, linolenic and arachidonic acids have resulted in significant improvement for many BPH patients.[108] All 19 subjects in an uncontrolled study showed diminution of residual urine, with 12 of the 19 having no residual urine by the end of several weeks of treatment. Prostatic and seminal lipid levels and ratios are often abnormal,[109] and supplementation may be addressing an underlying EFA deficiency. Cell-line research suggests differences in essential fatty acid composition in hyperplastic or cancerous prostate cells.[110,111] Because of concern regarding increased oxidation of unsaturated acids,[24] a basic antioxidant regimen should be employed when taking EFAs.

The role of tomatoes, tomato sauce and **lycopene** in BPH is not clear; however, epidemiological and population-based studies suggest that their consumption is linked to decreased incidence of BPH,[111] a reduction in PSA levels[112] and decreased progression of BPH to prostate cancer.[113,114] The therapeutic action of lycopene in this disorder may be due to its potent antioxidant properties.

The role of oxidative stress in relation to inflammation and the protective effects of antioxidants is a new area of exploration with respect to prevention and treatment of BPH. It may be prudent for clinicians to address the overall nutrition of the patient and look to support optimal antioxidant status, particularly relating to selenium and serum glutathione s-transferase α activity.[115]

Address sympathetic nervous system hyperactivity

Reduction of urethral stricture and relaxation of smooth muscles is aided by parasympathetic stimulation or parasympathetic mimetic agents.[116] Reduction in sympathetic nervous activity and/or parasympathetic stimulation may aid in LUTS relief, as evidenced by some studies suggesting that a combination of **glycine**, **alanine** and **glutamic acid** (in the form of two six-grain capsules administered three times daily for two weeks and one capsule three times daily thereafter) relieved many BPH symptoms. Nocturia was relieved or reduced in 95%, urgency reduced in 81%, frequency reduced in 73% and delayed micturition alleviated in 70% in one study,[117] with similar results reported in other controlled studies.[118] The mechanism of action is unknown. These amino acids may act as inhibitory neurotransmitters, providing symptom relief and reducing the feelings of a full bladder, or providing an overall nervine function that can positively affect urine flow in men suffering from BPH.[119]

While no clinical evidence supports the use of ***Humulus lupulus***, the antiproliferative effects of flavonoids on prostate cancer cell lines, as well as its nervine and parasympathetic action, may warrant further research as to clinical benefit.[72,120] Other **nervine and antispasmodic herbal medicines** may have a potential supportive role in managing BPH; examples are *Scutellaria lateriflora* and *Passiflora incarnata*. However, no studies have presently been conducted to assess this potential. See Table 29.1 for the evidence summary.

Enhance vascular functioning

Chronic ischaemia can result in thickening of the prostate and growth of tissue in response to an altered endothelial growth factor resulting from the diminished blood supply.[130] Atherosclerosis and diminished blood supply appear to be potential root causes in BPH and ED. Improving vascular function via herbal and nutrient interventions (discussed in the ED section later in this chapter), managing cholesterol and moderating alcohol consumption, in addition to dietary strategies to address cardiovascular risk, will possibly prove beneficial (see Chapters 11–13 on the cardiovascular system).

In addition to epidemiological studies suggesting a relationship between higher cholesterol levels and cardiovascular disease with higher incidence of BPH and ED, the breakdown products of cholesterol itself can also be cytotoxic and carcinogenic and have been shown to accumulate in hyperplastic or cancerous prostate tissue.[109]

Hypocholesterolaemic (statin) drugs have been shown to have a favourable influence on BPH, possibly by limiting subsequent formation of epoxycholesterols (metabolic by-products of cholesterol).[111] As discussed, the regulation of cardiovascular risk factors (such as elevated low-density lipoprotein (LDL) and total cholesterol) and decreased high-density lipoprotein (HDL) may help in the holistic prevention and treatment of BPH.

Although only beer has been associated with increasing prolactin levels, higher overall alcohol intake may be associated with BPH. In a large Hawaiian study involving 6581 men, an alcohol intake of at least 740 mL/month was directly correlated with the diagnosis of BPH,[35] with a stronger association for beer, wine and sake compared with distilled spirits. While this indicates a relationship in incidence, a smaller study suggested that men waiting for TURP surgery were more likely to avoid the surgical procedure (having remission of symptoms) with higher consumption of alcohol.[28] This study also described the correlation of higher rates of BPH in men with coronary disease. Although these studies are apparently contradictory in relationship to alcohol, it is possible that in men at higher risk for coronary artery disease due to higher levels of LDLs, alcohol may play an overall protective role by reducing these lipoproteins.

INTEGRATIVE MEDICAL CONSIDERATIONS

Overall, there is a distinct lack of evidence evaluating the safety and effectiveness of integrative therapy as a whole, though some studies exist supporting use of a combination of natural health product and a conventional pharmaceutical agent.

The nature of BPH suggests that a risk-based approach based on severity of symptoms may be appropriate in the selection of treatments, particularly for addressing modifiable risk factors for patients in the watchful waiting stage. Beyond that, severity of the symptoms will dictate whether surgery or catheterisation is necessary for acute urinary obstruction. **Counselling** may be necessary to address the psychological issues of sexual dysfunction. Progression of BPH to prostate cancer is of concern and should be monitored appropriately using regular digital rectal exams with possible PSA testing. **Acupuncture** and **moxibustion** can increase blood flow, and some studies have provided evidence that it may be considered as a viable adjunctive treatment,[125,131,132] particularly when combined with **hypnotherapy**.[133] Numerous studies on the effect of acupuncture on urinary frequency have been conducted; however, no studies exist on the use of acupuncture for BPH specifically, and many of these studies involve ageing women.[134–138] Other studies suggest trigger point release therapy and relaxation as being beneficial for addressing ED and BPH, particularly if chronic pelvic pain is involved.[139]

Counselling and psychiatry may be beneficial for addressing the psychological roots or manifestations of ED and the symptoms of BPH. Pelvic floor (Kegel) exercises have been shown to be beneficial in up to 35% of ED patients[140,141] with some potential shown for their ability to improve urinary function.[142]

CLINICAL SUMMARY

The initial case-taking process should assess both the clinical state of presenting symptoms as well as a thorough screening and diagnostic evaluation. This should include a complete patient history to identify the presence of comorbid conditions,

---

Erectile dysfunction

Overview

- ED is classified as organic (circulatory or a side effect of medication, particularly anti-depressant or neurogenic) or psychological.[143]
- Significant psychosomatic or mind/body connections affect this disorder.[144]
- Normal erectile function involves a balance between excitatory and inhibitory psychological, vascular and neural responses,[13,145] involves release of NO gas into the endothelial cells of the penis and causes the subsequent relaxation of smooth muscle cells lining the corpus cavernosum so there is increased blood to flow into the organ and retention of blood in the spongy erectile tissue.
- Parasympathetic nervous activity and conversion of guanosine triphosphate (GTP) into cyclic guanosine monophosphate (cGMP) by the enzyme guanylate cyclase.[8] An erection subsides when cGMP is hydrolysed by phosphodiesterase type 5 enzymes (PDE5), causing smooth muscle contraction and emptying of the corpus cavernosum.
- Screening and diagnostic evaluation should include a complete patient history to identify the presence of comorbid conditions, particularly diabetes, dyslipidaemia and hypertension[145] as well as assessment of any neurological or circulatory obstacles to proper innervation of the pelvic area.

Conventional treatments

Conventional treatments focus on providing symptomatic relief through pharmacological substances (phosphodiesterase type-5 (PDE-5) inhibitors such as sildenafil or tadalafil) as first-line therapy, removing causative agents (the side effects of beta-adrenergic blockers, antidepressants or spironolactone), and counselling.[14,146,147]

Nutrients

Three small, pilot, randomised, controlled studies provided relative support for the clinical effectiveness of L-arginine in doses ranging from 1500 mg–5 g/day used over a two- to six-week period for ED.[148–150] While the study[149] using 1500 mg/day for two weeks did not demonstrate a significant benefit over placebo, the other two studies demonstrated a 20–40% self-reported improvement in symptoms of ED. It is unclear whether foods rich in L-arginine such as legumes, whole grains and nuts consumed in moderate to large amounts would have a similar effect. Other studies using L-arginine in combination with other natural substances such as Pycnogenol[151] or yohimbine[152] generally supported the notion that L-arginine can have some positive effect on the symptoms of ED; however, further research is necessary.

Herbal medicines

As discussed earlier, double-blind RCTs involving *Lepidium meyenii* is effective in men with mild ED, providing a small but statistically significant clinical effect at doses between 1.5 g and 3 g.[87–89] *Panax ginseng* has the most promising evidence for safe and effective treatment of ED, with 900 mg/day for eight weeks showing clinical and physiological effectiveness in up to 60% of men with ED.[8,153] Yohimbine (5.4 mg t.i.d. for eight weeks) also shows promising results, although significant side effects associated with its therapeutic action as an alpha-2-adrenergic receptor make it a less desirable treatment option.[154] Based on vasodilatory actions, *Ginkgo biloba* may benefit some men where penile blood flow is impaired (however, the clinical evidence is mixed).[155,156] *Tribulus terrestris* may be a viable option to treat ED, via increasing the release of NO from the endothelium and nitrergic nerve endings in penile tissue (clinical studies are relatively limited in isolating safe and effective extracts or demonstrating clinically significant efficacy over placebo).[157–159]

---

particularly diabetes, dyslipidaemia, hypertension and chronic infection (bladder, urethral or other), an assessment of any neurological, structural (i.e. lumbar or sacral vertebral subluxations) or circulatory obstacles to proper innervation of the pelvic area, and investigations to detect the presence of any significant organic (circulatory or a side effects of medications, particularly antidepressant or neurogenic), psycho-somatic or mind–body connections that may affect these disorders. As detailed earlier, an evidence-based integrative prescriptive plan using a risk-based approach should be provided to comprehensively treat BPH and ED. Lifestyle factors should be addressed and incorporated as part of normal, healthy dietary and exercise patterns consistent with the patient's state, capabilities and overall goals. Motivational issues, their understanding of the disease and options, time restrictions, financial limitations, the perspective about the source of their difficulties and their treatment priorities may influence a patient's ability to make those changes. Adherence and engagement is increased by having ownership of the treatment plan and a sense of shared partnership in its development and planning. Due to this, all treatment strategies should be developed considering the above factors, and the management and treatment strategy should be individually tailored and offered in a stepwise manner, incorporating appropriate follow-up and monitoring of the disease state. General lifestyle advice should focus on encouraging a balance between -meaningful work, adequate rest and sleep, judicious exercise, positive social and sexual interactions and -pleasurable hobbies. If substance abuse, or other significant biopsychosocial challenges exist, these need to be discussed and incorporated as part of treatment or referral to other effective healthcare providers or existing services.

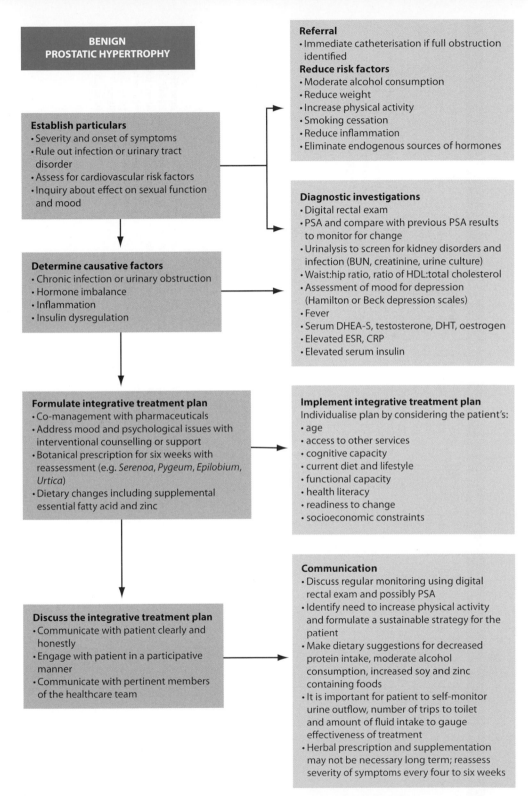

BENIGN PROSTATIC HYPERTROPHY

Establish particulars
• Severity and onset of symptoms
• Rule out infection or urinary tract disorder
• Assess for cardiovascular risk factors
• Inquiry about effect on sexual function and mood

Determine causative factors
• Chronic infection or urinary obstruction
• Hormone imbalance
• Inflammation
• Insulin dysregulation

Formulate integrative treatment plan
• Co-management with pharmaceuticals
• Address mood and psychological issues with interventional counselling or support
• Botanical prescription for six weeks with reassessment (e.g. *Serenoa, Pygeum, Epilobium, Urtica*)
• Dietary changes including supplemental essential fatty acid and zinc

Discuss the integrative treatment plan
• Communicate with patient clearly and honestly
• Engage with patient in a participative manner
• Communicate with pertinent members of the healthcare team

Referral
• Immediate catheterisation if full obstruction identified
Reduce risk factors
• Moderate alcohol consumption
• Reduce weight
• Increase physical activity
• Smoking cessation
• Reduce inflammation
• Eliminate endogenous sources of hormones

Diagnostic investigations
• Digital rectal exam
• PSA and compare with previous PSA results to monitor for change
• Urinalysis to screen for kidney disorders and infection (BUN, creatinine, urine culture)
• Waist:hip ratio, ratio of HDL:total cholesterol
• Assessment of mood for depression (Hamilton or Beck depression scales)
• Fever
• Serum DHEA-S, testosterone, DHT, oestrogen
• Elevated ESR, CRP
• Elevated serum insulin

Implement integrative treatment plan
Individualise plan by considering the patient's:
• age
• access to other services
• cognitive capacity
• current diet and lifestyle
• functional capacity
• health literacy
• readiness to change
• socioeconomic constraints

Communication
• Discuss regular monitoring using digital rectal exam and possibly PSA
• Identify need to increase physical activity and formulate a sustainable strategy for the patient
• Make dietary suggestions for decreased protein intake, moderate alcohol consumption, increased soy and zinc containing foods
• It is important for patient to self-monitor urine outflow, number of trips to toilet and amount of fluid intake to gauge effectiveness of treatment
• Herbal prescription and supplementation may not be necessary long term; reassess severity of symptoms every four to six weeks

Figure 29.3
Naturopathic treatment decision tree—benign prostatic hypertrophy

Table 29.1
Review of the major evidence

Intervention	Mechanisms of action	Key literature	Summary of results	Comment
Serenoa repens	Androgen receptor: inhibits cellular and nuclear receptor binding to increase metabolism and elimination of DHT Anti-inflammatory: inhibit cyclo-oxygenase and lipoxygenase and mast cell accumulation Antiproliferative: increase apoptosis of fibroblasts and epithelial cells from prostatic tissue Hormonal: inhibit 5-alpha-reductase activity on testosterone	Meta-analyses: Wilt et al. 2002[121] Tacklind et al. 2012[122] (update of Wilt 2002)	Initial review[121]: significant improvements in urinary symptoms compared with placebo or pharmaceutical treatment (21 trials) Updated review[122]: no statistically significant benefits for nocturia, peak urinary flow or prostate size Relative risk (RR) compared with tamsulosin: 0.91 (not significant superiority)	Significant heterogeneity among the RCTs in most recent analyses, particularly with respect to dose and extract of *Serenoa repens* as well as length of study (range 4–26 weeks) Serenoa does not appear to provide statistically significant benefit as a monotherapy; use as combination therapy is recommended.[123]
Beta-sitosterol	Cholesterol: interferes with intestinal absorption of cholesterol and increases bile acid secretion; inhibition of sterol (24)-reductase, an essential enzyme in the process of cholesterol biosynthesis	Systematic review: Wilt et al. 1999[62]	Four studies of varied extracts/doses over a four- to 26-week period: significant improvements in peak urine flow Two studies showing a 4.9 decrease in International Prostate Symptom Scores (IPSS) (95% CI = −6.3 to −3.5, $p < 0.05$), no observed reduction in prostate size on palpation	Longer term studies with sufficient reporting of safety are required, although among these studies only 8% of participants experienced any adverse reactions
Lepidium meyenii	Improvements in penile endothelial L-arginine–nitric-oxide	Systematic review: Shin 2010[124]	Systematic review for effects on sexual function concluded further research is necessary based on the small number of studies and limited sample sizes	Limited reporting of adverse events and small sample sizes of studies limit the clinical utility of the existing literature, though the mechanism of action and effect size suggests promise as a vasodilator Effect on BPH is not established

Table 29.1
Review of the major evidence (continued)

Intervention	Mechanisms of action	Key literature	Summary of results	Comment
Zinc	Anti-inflammatory: decreases C-reactive protein, lipid peroxidation and inflammatory cytokines and increasing anti-inflammatory proteins Cell proliferation: nutritional cofactor in multiple pathways relating to healthy cell production, regulation and oxidant Hormonal: Varied role in testosterone and prolactin regulation (5-alpha-reductase)	Preclinical models: Sinquin 1984[66] Fahim 1993[32]	Metabolites of testosterone produced via 5-alpha reductase were significantly increased in prostate cells with addition of zinc Significant ($p < 0.05$) reduction in prostate weight and 5-alpha reductase activity following intraprostatic zinc injections compared with sham and placebo in rat model	Mechanism of action for altering testosterone/androgen profile using zinc is established Based on this and epidemiological data on zinc in men with BPH, human clinical studies are warranted
Acupuncture	Circulatory: increased micro-circulatory vascular contractility to improve blood flow Neurological: possible mediation by release of beta-endorphins, changes in vagal tone	Systematic reviews: Lee et al. 2009[125] Cui et al. 2016[126]	Up to 63% responder rate from 4 to 10 weeks 1–2×/week of acupuncture or electro-acupuncture Not statistically superior to sham acupuncture RR: 2.73 (95% CI = 0.42–17.78, $p = 0.29$). Large heterogeneity between studies	A total of four studies evaluating acupuncture for ED were included for review; however, 25 case reports/series as well as studies combining acupuncture and herbs or moxibustion were also identified Studies suffered from small sample size and poor design, including control groups, randomisation and blinding Large response to sham acupuncture (43%) Further research is warranted

Table 29.1
Review of the major evidence (continued)

Intervention	Mechanisms of action	Key literature	Summary of results	Comment
Diet	Cholesterol: maintenance of healthy cholesterol levels and prevention of reduced circulation due to atherosclerosis
Hormonal: inhibition of 5-alpha reductase	Epidemiological studies:
Kristal et al. 2008[112]
Rohrmann et al. 2007[127]
Meyer et al. 2005[42]	Daily consumption of red meat (increased HR 1.38), high fat (HR 1.31), vegetables (> 3 servings/day) (decreased HR 0.68) and alcohol (> 2 servings/day) (HR 0.68)
Vegetable consumption (but not fruit) inversely associated with BPH (5th compared with 1st quintile OR 0.89; 95% CI = 0.80–0.99; $p = 0.03$)
Consumption of fruit and vegetables rich in beta-carotene ($p = 0.004$), lutein ($p = 0.0004$), or vitamin C ($p = 0.05$) was inversely related to BPH
Population-based study: no significant effect from supplements containing zinc, vitamin E, vitamin C, selenium and beta-carotene over eight-year period on PSA or IGF levels ($p > 0.05$)	With increasing vitamin C intake from foods, men were less likely to have BPH
Neither alpha- nor gamma-tocopherol intake from foods was associated with BPH
Supplementation with antioxidants did significantly reduce the hazard ratio of developing prostate cancer in men with normal PSA at baseline
Lifestyle	Circulatory: possibly mediated by endorphins, increased blood flow, prevention of atherosclerosis, metabolic syndrome and other comorbidities related to BPH and ED	Epidemiological studies:
Platz et al. 1998[128]
Rohrmann et al. 2005[127]
Shiels et al. 2009[129]
Platz 2003[160]	Physical activity inversely related with total BPH (extreme quintiles: OR 0.75, 95% CI = 0.67–0.85, $p < 0.001$), surgery for BPH (OR 0.76, 95% CI = 0.64–0.90, $p < 0.001$), and symptomatic BPH (OR 0.75, 95% CI = 0.64–0.87, p for trend < 0.001)
Former heavy smokers ($\geq$ 50 pack-years) had higher odds of LUTS than never smokers (OR 2.01, 95% CI = 1.04–3.89)
Daily alcohol use showed lower chance of LUTS than non-drinkers (OR 0.59, 95% CI = 0.37–0.95, $p = 0.07$). All levels of moderate and vigorous activity inversely associated with LUTS ($p = 0.06$), zero physical activity increased odds of LUTS (OR 2.06, 95% CI = 1.26–3.39)
Men currently smoking had higher serum testosterone, free testosterone and oestradiol levels ($p < 0.05$ for all measures)
A moderate increased risk of metastatic or fatal prostate cancer was found for extreme quintiles (RR 1.38 95% CI 0.96–1.98 $p = 0.07$), particularly pronounced in younger men	Walking, the most prevalent activity, was inversely related to BPH risk; men who walked two to three hours/week had a 25% lower risk of total BPH
Confirmation across multiple epidemiological studies among varied populations of men that smoking is linked to hormone levels and incidence of BPH and that physical activity is inversely associated with LUTS
High caloric intake may be associated with metabolic profiles that favour enhanced growth factor production and increase the risk of metastatic disease

KEY POINTS

- BPH shares many properties with cardiovascular, metabolic syndrome, ED, depression and urinary tract infection disorders.

- The holistic treatment approach should look beyond hormonal regulation and include therapies to reduce inflammation, reduce oxidative stress and improve NO production.

- BPH is predominantly an androgen-mediated disorder. Factors that decrease the production of dihydrotestosterone should be included in most treatment protocols.

- Counselling to address issues of ageing, mood and sexual health may be important in moderating quality of life and the mental/emotional aspects of these diseases.

FURTHER READING

Abrams DI. An integrative approach to prostate cancer. J Altern Complement Med 2018;24(9–10):872–80.

Espinosa G. Nutrition and benign prostatic hyperplasia. Curr Opin Urol 2013;23(1):38–41.

Malviya N, Malviya S, Jain S, et al. A review of the potential of medicinal plants in the management and treatment of male sexual dysfunction. Andrologia 2016;48(8):880–93.

Ooi SL, Pak SC. Serenoa repens for lower urinary tract symptoms/benign prostatic hyperplasia: current evidence and Its clinical implications in naturopathic medicine. J Altern Complement Med 2017;23(8):599–606.

Roehrborn CG. Benign prostatic hyperplasia and lower urinary tract symptom guidelines. Can Urol Assoc J 2012;6(5 Suppl. 2):S130–2.

REFERENCES

1. Edwards JL. Diagnosis and management of benign prostatic hyperplasia. Am Fam Physician 2008;77(10):1403–10.

2. Arrighi HM, et al. Natural history of benign prostatic hyperplasia and risk of prostatectomy. The Baltimore Longitudinal Study of Aging. Urology 1991;38(1 Suppl.):4–8.

3. Dull P, et al. Managing benign prostatic hyperplasia. Am Fam Physician 2002;66(1):77–84.

4. Feldman HA, et al. Impotence and its medical and psychosocial correlates: results of the Massachusetts Male Aging Study. J Urol 1994;151(1):54–61.

5. Goldstein I. Male sexual circuitry. Working Group for the Study of Central Mechanisms in Erectile Dysfunction. Sci Am 2000;283(2):70–5.

6. Shankar PR, Subish P. Disease mongering. Singapore Med J 2007;48(4):275–80.

7. Nehra A, Kulaksizoglu H. Global perspectives and controversies in the epidemiology of male erectile dysfunction. Curr Opin Urol 2002;12(6):493–6.

8. McKay D. Nutrients and botanicals for erectile dysfunction: examining the evidence. Altern Med Rev 2004;9(1):4–16.

9. Thomas JA. Diet, micronutrients, and the prostate gland. Nutr Rev 1999;57(4):95–103.

10. Comhaire F, Mahmoud A. Preventing diseases of the prostate in the elderly using hormones and nutriceuticals. Aging Male 2004;7(2):155–69.

11. Rakel D, editor. Integrative medicine. 2nd ed. Philadelphia: Saunders; 2007.

12. Zakaria L, et al. Common conditions of the aging male: erectile dysfunction, benign prostatic hyperplasia, cardiovascular disease and depression. Int Urol Nephrol 2001;33(2):283–92.

13. Sullivan ME, et al. Nitric oxide and penile erection: is erectile dysfunction another manifestation of vascular disease? Cardiovasc Res 1999;43(3):658–65.

14. Rosenberg MT. Diagnosis and management of erectile dysfunction in the primary care setting. Int J Clin Pract 2007;61(7):1198–208.

15. Jacobsen SJ. Risk factors for benign prostatic hyperplasia. Curr Urol Rep 2007;8(4):281–8.

16. Moyad MA. Lifestyle changes to prevent BPH: heart healthy = prostate healthy. Urol Nurs 2003;23(6):439–41.

17. Kwon H, et al. Relationship between predictors of the risk of clinical progression of benign prostatic hyperplasia and metabolic syndrome in men with moderate to severe lower urinary tract symptoms. Urology 2013;81(6):1325–9.

18. Roehrborn CG. Benign prostatic hyperplasia and lower urinary tract symptom guidelines. Can Urol Assoc J 2012;6(5 Suppl. 2):S130–2.

19. Engl T, et al. Uropharmacology: current and future strategies in the treatment of erectile dysfunction and benign prostate hyperplasia. Int J Clin Pharmacol Ther 2004;42(10):527–33.

20. Nickel JC, et al. 2010 Update: guidelines for the management of benign prostatic hyperplasia. Can Urol Assoc J 2010;4(5):310–16.

21. Roehrborn CG, et al. The effects of combination therapy with dutasteride and tamsulosin on clinical outcomes in men with symptomatic benign prostatic hyperplasia: 4-year results from the CombAT study. Eur Urol 2010;57(1):123–31.

22. Hoffman RM, et al. Microwave thermotherapy for benign prostatic hyperplasia. Cochrane Database Syst Rev 2012;(9):CD004135, doi:10.1002/14651858.CD004135.pub3.

23. Soygur T, et al. Effect of obesity on prostatic hyperplasia: its relation to sex steroid levels. Int Urol Nephrol 1996;28(1):55–9.

24. Suzuki S, et al. Intakes of energy and macronutrients and the risk of benign prostatic hyperplasia. Am J Clin Nutr 2002;75(4):689–97.

25. Wisard M. Erectile dysfunction: physical exercise, losing weight, stop smoking, reducing alcohol, relaxing, it could also work! Rev Med Suisse 2007;3(136):2773–4, 2776, 2778.

26. Morrison AS. Epidemiology and environmental factors in urologic cancer. Cancer 1987;60(3 Suppl.):632–4.

27. Lagiou P, et al. Diet and benign prostatic hyperplasia: a study in Greece. Urology 1999;54(2):284–90.

28. Gass R. Benign prostatic hyperplasia: the opposite effects of alcohol and coffee intake. BJU Int 2002;90(7):649–54.

29. Demark-Wahnefried W, et al. Pilot study to explore effects of low-fat, flaxseed-supplemented diet on proliferation of benign prostatic epithelium and prostate-specific antigen. Urology 2004;63(5):900–4.

30. Kappas A, et al. Nutrition-endocrine interactions: induction of reciprocal changes in the delta 4–5 alpha-reduction of testosterone and the cytochrome P-450-dependent oxidation of estradiol by dietary macronutrients in man. Proc Natl Acad Sci USA 1983; 80(24):7646–9.

31. Zhang SX, et al. Comparison of incidence of BPH and related factors between urban and rural inhabitants in district of Wannan. Zhonghua Nan Ke Xue 2003;9(1):45–7.

32. Fahim MS, et al. Zinc arginine, a 5 alpha-reductase inhibitor, reduces rat ventral prostate weight and DNA without affecting testicular function. Andrologia 1993;25(6):369–75.

33. Leake A. The effect of zinc on the 5 alpha-reduction of testosterone by the hyperplastic human prostate gland. J Steroid Biochem 1984;20(2):651–5.

34. Leake A. Subcellular distribution of zinc in the benign and malignant human prostate: evidence for a direct zinc androgen interaction. Acta Endocrinol (Copenh) 1984;105(2):281–8.

35. Chyou PH, et al. A prospective study of alcohol, diet, and other lifestyle factors in relation to obstructive uropathy. Prostate 1993;22(3):253–64.

36. Zaichick V, et al. Zinc in the human prostate gland: normal, hyperplastic and cancerous. Int Urol Nephrol 1997;29(5):565–74.

37. Leake A, et al. The effect of zinc on the 5 alpha-reduction of testosterone by the hyperplastic human prostate gland. J Steroid Biochem 1984;20(2):651–5.

38. Leake A, et al. Subcellular distribution of zinc in the benign and malignant human prostate: evidence for a direct zinc androgen interaction. Acta Endocrinol (Copenh) 1984;105(2):281–8.

39. Wallace AM, Grant JK. Effect of zinc on androgen metabolism in the human hyperplastic prostate. Biochem Soc Trans 1975;3(4):540–2.

40. Johnson AR, et al. High dose zinc increases hospital admissions due to genitourinary complications. J Urol 2007;177(2):639–43.

41. Silk R, LeFante C. Safety of zinc gluconate glycine (Cold-Eeze) in a geriatric population: a randomized, placebo-controlled, double-blind trial. Am J Ther 2005;12(6):612–17.

42. Meyer F, et al. Antioxidant vitamin and mineral supplementation and prostate cancer prevention in the SU.VI.MAX trial. Int J Cancer 2005;116(2):182–6.

43. Neuhouser ML, et al. Dietary supplement use in the Prostate Cancer Prevention Trial: implications for prevention trials. Nutr Cancer 2001;39(1):12–18.

44. Patterson RE, et al. Vitamin supplements and cancer risk: the epidemiologic evidence. Cancer Causes Control 1997;8(5):786–802.

45. Judd AM, et al. Zinc acutely, selectively and reversibly inhibits pituitary prolactin secretion. Brain Res 1984;294(1):190–2.

46. Login IS, et al. Zinc may have a physiological role in regulating pituitary prolactin secretion. Neuroendocrinology 1983;37(5):317–20.

47. Farnsworth WE, et al. Interaction of prolactin and testosterone in the human prostate. Urol Res 1981;9(2):79–88.

48. De Rosa G, et al. Prolactin secretion after beer. Lancet 1981;2(8252):934.

49. Corenblum B, Whitaker M. Inhibition of stress-induced hyperprolactinaemia. Br Med J 1977;2(6098):1328.

50. Farrar DJ, Osborne JL. The use of bromocriptine in the treatment of the unstable bladder. Br J Urol 1976;48(4):235–8.

51. Boyd A. Bromocriptine and psychosis: a literature review. Psychiatr Q 1995;66(1):87–95.

52. Miettinen TA, et al. Serum plant sterols and cholesterol precursors reflect cholesterol absorption and synthesis in volunteers of a randomly selected male population. Am J Epidemiol 1990;131(1):20–31.

53. Tilvis RS, Miettinen TA. Serum plant sterols and their relation to cholesterol absorption. Am J Clin Nutr 1986;43(1):92–7.

54. Berges RR, et al. Randomised, placebo-controlled, double-blind clinical trial of beta-sitosterol in patients with benign prostatic hyperplasia. Beta-sitosterol Study Group. Lancet 1995;345(8964):1529–32.

55. Denis L, et al. Diet and its preventive role in prostatic disease. Eur Urol 1999;35(5–6):377–87.

56. Engelhardt PF, Riedl CR. Effects of one-year treatment with isoflavone extract from red clover on prostate, liver function, sexual function, and quality of life in men with elevated PSA levels and negative prostate biopsy findings. Urology 2008;71(2):185–90, discussion 190.

57. Messina MJ. Emerging evidence on the role of soy in reducing prostate cancer risk. Nutr Rev 2003;61(4):117–31.

58. Jarred RA, et al. Anti-androgenic action by red clover-derived dietary isoflavones reduces non-malignant prostate enlargement in aromatase knockout (ArKo) mice. Prostate 2003;56(1):54–64.

59. Drewes SE, et al. Hypoxis hemerocallidea—not merely a cure for benign prostate hyperplasia. J Ethnopharmacol 2008;119(3):593–8.

60. Katz AE. Flavonoid and botanical approaches to prostate health. J Altern Complement Med 2002;8(6):813–21.

61. Wilt T, et al. Beta-sitosterols for benign prostatic hyperplasia. Cochrane Database Syst Rev 2000;(2):CD001043.

62. Wilt TJ, et al. Beta-sitosterol for the treatment of benign prostatic hyperplasia: a systematic review. BJU Int 1999;83(9):976–83.

63. Gerber GS. Phytotherapy for benign prostatic hyperplasia. Curr Urol Rep 2002;3(4):285–91.

64. Yamashita A, et al. Influence of diethylstilbestrol, Leuprorelin (a luteinizing hormone-releasing hormone analog), Finasteride (a 5 alpha-reductase inhibitor), and castration on the lobar subdivisions of the rat prostate. Prostate 1996;29(1):1–14.

65. Lahtonen R. Zinc and cadmium concentrations in whole tissue and in separated epithelium and stroma from human benign prostatic hypertrophic glands. Prostate 1985;6(2):177–83.

66. Sinquin G, et al. Testosterone metabolism by homogenates of human prostates with benign hyperplasia: effects of zinc, cadmium and other bivalent cations. J Steroid Biochem 1984;20(3):773–80.

67. Sivkov AV, et al. Morphological changes in prostatic tissue of patients with benign prostatic hyperplasia treated with permixon. Urologiia 2004;5:10–16.

68. Buck AC. Phytotherapy for the prostate. Br J Urol 1996;78(3):325–36.

69. Dedhia RC, et al. Impact of phytotherapy on utility scores for 5 benign prostatic hyperplasia/lower urinary tract symptoms health states. J Urol 2008;179(1):220–5.

70. Fleshner N, et al. Evidence for contamination of herbal erectile dysfunction products with phosphodiesterase type 5 inhibitors. J Urol 2005;174(2):636–41, discussion 641; quiz 801.

71. Gryniewicz CM, et al. Detection of undeclared erectile dysfunction drugs and analogues in dietary supplements by ion mobility spectrometry. J Pharm Biomed Anal 2009;49(3):601–6.

72. Buck AC. Is there a scientific basis for the therapeutic effects of serenoa repens in benign prostatic hyperplasia? Mechanisms of action. J Urol 2004;172(5 Pt 1):1792–9.

73. Magri V, et al. Activity of Serenoa repens, lycopene and selenium on prostatic disease: evidences and hypotheses. Arch Ital Urol Androl 2008;80(2):65–78.

74. Vela Navarrete R, et al. BPH and inflammation: pharmacological effects of Permixon on histological and molecular inflammatory markers. Results of a double blind pilot clinical assay. Eur Urol 2003;44(5):549–55.

75. Vela-Navarrete R, et al. Efficacy and safety of a hexanic extract of Serenoa repens (Permixon®) for the treatment of lower urinary tract symptoms associated with benign prostatic hyperplasia (LUTS/BPH): systematic review and meta-analysis of randomised controlled trials and observational studies. BJU Int 2018;122:1049–65. doi:10.1111/bju.14362.

76. Wilt TJ, et al. Phytotherapy for benign prostatic hyperplasia. Public Health Nutr 2000;3(4A):459–72.

77. Asakawa K, et al. Effects of cernitin pollen-extract (Cernilton) on inflammatory cytokines in sex-hormone-induced nonbacterial prostatitis rats. Hinyokika Kiyo 2001;47(7):459–65.

78. Yasumoto R, et al. Clinical evaluation of long-term treatment using Cernilton pollen extract in patients with benign prostatic hyperplasia. Clin Ther 1995;17(1):82–7.

79. Buck AC, et al. Treatment of outflow tract obstruction due to benign prostatic hyperplasia with the pollen extract, cernilton. A double-blind, placebo-controlled study. Br J Urol 1990;66(4):398–404.

80. Dutkiewicz S. Usefulness of Cernilton in the treatment of benign prostatic hyperplasia. Int Urol Nephrol 1996;28(1):49–53.

81. Hayashi J, et al. Clinical evaluation of Cernilton in benign prostatic hypertrophy. Hinyokika Kiyo 1986;32(1):135–41.

82. Horii A, et al. Clinical evaluation of Cernilton in the treatment of the benign prostatic hypertrophy. Hinyokika Kiyo 1985;31(4):739–46.

83. MacDonald R, et al. A systematic review of Cernilton for the treatment of benign prostatic hyperplasia. BJU Int 2000;85(7):836–41.

84. Maekawa M, et al. Clinical evaluation of Cernilton on benign prostatic hypertrophy—a multiple center double-blind study with Paraprost. Hinyokika Kiyo 1990;36(4):495–516.

85. Ueda K, et al. Clinical evaluation of Cernilton on benign prostatic hyperplasia. Hinyokika Kiyo 1985;31(1):187–91.

86. Habib FK, et al. Identification of a prostate inhibitory substance in a pollen extract. Prostate 1995;26(3):133–9.

87. Yablonsky F, et al. Antiproliferative effect of Pygeum africanum extract on rat prostatic fibroblasts. J Urol 1997;157(6):2381–7.

88. Boulbes D, et al. Pygeum africanum extract inhibits proliferation of human cultured prostatic fibroblasts and myofibroblasts. BJU Int 2006;98(5):1106–13.

89. Edgar AD, et al. A critical review of the pharmacology of the plant extract of Pygeum africanum in the treatment of LUTS. Neurourol Urodyn 2007;26(4):458–63, discussion 464.

90. Asare GA, Ngala RA, Afriyie D, et al. Calcium–magnesium imbalance implicated in benign prostatic hyperplasia and restoration by a phytotherapeutic drug—Croton membranaceus Müll.Arg. BMC Complement Altern Med 2017;17(1):152. doi:10.1186/s12906-017-1663-x.

91. Kamatenesi-Mugisha M, Oryem-Origa H. Traditional herbal remedies used in the management of sexual impotence and erectile dysfunction in western Uganda. Afr Health Sci 2005;5(1):40–9.

92. Coulson S, et al. A phase II randomised double-blind placebo-controlled clinical trial investigating the efficacy and safety of ProstateEZE Max: a herbal medicine preparation for the management of symptoms of benign prostatic hypertrophy. Complement Ther Med 2013;21(3):172–9.

93. Zenico T, et al. Subjective effects of Lepidium meyenii (maca) extract on well-being and sexual performances in patients with mild erectile dysfunction: a randomised, double-blind clinical trial. Andrologia 2009;41(2):95–9.

94. Gonzales GF, et al. Effect of Lepidium meyenii (maca), a root with aphrodisiac and fertility-enhancing properties, on serum reproductive hormone levels in adult healthy men. J Endocrinol 2003;176(1):163–8.

95. Gonzales GF, et al. Effect of Lepidium meyenii (maca) on sexual desire and its absent relationship with serum testosterone levels in adult healthy men. Andrologia 2002;34(6):367–72.

96. Lopatkin N, et al. Efficacy and safety of a combination of sabal and urtica extract in lower urinary tract symptoms—long-term follow-up of a placebo-controlled, double-blind, multicenter trial. Int Urol Nephrol 2007;39(4):1137–46.

97. Safarinejad MR. Urtica dioica for treatment of benign prostatic hyperplasia: a prospective, randomized, double-blind, placebo-controlled, crossover study. J Herb Pharmacother 2005;5(4):1–11.

98. Sokeland J. Combined sabal and urtica extract compared with finasteride in men with benign prostatic hyperplasia: analysis of prostate volume and therapeutic outcome. BJU Int 2000;86(4):439–42.

99. Wagner H, et al. Biologically active compounds from the aqueous extract of Urtica dioica]. Planta Med 1989;55(5):452–4.

100. Schottner M, et al. Lignans from the roots of Urtica dioica and their metabolites bind to human sex hormone binding globulin (SHBG). Planta Med 1997;63(6):529–32.

101. Ducrey B, et al. Inhibition of 5 alpha-reductase and aromatase by the ellagitannins oenothein A and oenothein B from Epilobium species. Planta Med 1997;63(2):111–14.

102. Hevesi Toth B, Kery A. Epilobium parviflorum—in vitro study of biological action. Acta Pharm Hung 2009;79(1):3–9.

103. Hevesi BT, et al. Antioxidant and antiinflammatory effect of Epilobium parviflorum Schreb. Phytother Res 2009;23(5):719–24.

104. Steenkamp V, et al. Studies on antibacterial, anti-inflammatory and antioxidant activity of herbal remedies used in the treatment of benign prostatic hyperplasia and prostatitis. J Ethnopharmacol 2006;103(1):71–5.

105. Vlahos CJ, et al. Platelet-derived growth factor induces proliferation of hyperplastic human prostatic stromal cells. J Cell Biochem 1993;52(4):404–13.

106. Gleason PE, et al. Platelet derived growth factor (PDGF), androgens and inflammation: possible etiologic factors in the development of prostatic hyperplasia. J Urol 1993;149(6):1586–92.

107. Bravi F, et al. Macronutrients, fatty acids, cholesterol, and risk of benign prostatic hyperplasia. Urology 2006;67(6):1205–11.

108. Boyd E, Berry N. Prostatic hypertrophy as part of generalized metabolic disease. J Urol 1939;41:406–11.

109. Chaudry AA, et al. Arachidonic acid metabolism in benign and malignant prostatic tissue in vitro: effects of fatty acids and cyclooxygenase inhibitors. Int J Cancer 1994;57(2):176–80.

110. Narayan P, Dahiya R. Alterations in sphingomyelin and fatty acids in human benign prostatic hyperplasia and prostatic cancer. Biomed Biochim Acta 1991;50(9):1099–108.

111. Kristal AR, et al. Dietary patterns, supplement use, and the risk of symptomatic benign prostatic hyperplasia: results from the prostate cancer prevention trial. Am J Epidemiol 2008;167(8):925–34.

112. Edinger MS, Koff WJ. Effect of the consumption of tomato paste on plasma prostate-specific antigen levels in patients with benign prostate hyperplasia. Braz J Med Biol Res 2006;39(8):1115–19.

113. Schwarz S, et al. Lycopene inhibits disease progression in patients with benign prostate hyperplasia. J Nutr 2008;138(1):49–53.

114. Bullock TL, Andriole Jnr GL. Emerging drug therapies for benign prostatic hyperplasia. Expert Opin Emerg Drugs 2006;11(1):111–23.

115. Eichholzer M, et al. Effects of selenium status, dietary glucosinolate intake and serum glutathione S-transferase α activity on the risk of benign prostatic hyperplasia. BJU Int 2012;110(11 Pt C):E879–85.

116. Damrau F. Benign prostatic hypertrophy: amino acid therapy for symptomatic relief. J Am Geriatr Soc 1962;10:426–30.

117. Feinblatt HM, Gant JC. Palliative treatment of benign prostatic hypertrophy; value of glycine-alanine-glutamic acid combination. J Maine Med Assoc 1958;49(3):99–101. passim.

118. Thor PJ, et al. The autonomic nervous system function in benign prostatic hyperplasia. Folia Med Cracov 2006;47(1–4):79–86.

119. Delmulle L, et al. Anti-proliferative properties of prenylated flavonoids from hops (Humulus lupulus L.) in human prostate cancer cell lines. Phytomedicine 2006;13(9–10):732–4.

120. Kozlowski R, et al. Chronic ischemia alters prostate structure and reactivity in rabbits. J Urol 2001;165(3):1019–26.

121. Wilt T, et al. Serenoa repens for benign prostatic hyperplasia. Cochrane Database Syst Rev 2002;(3):CD001423.

122. Tacklind J, et al. Serenoa repens for benign prostatic hyperplasia. Cochrane Database Syst Rev 2012;(12):CD001423, doi:10.1002/14651858. CD001423.pub3.

123. Ooi SL, Pak SC. Serenoa repens for lower urinary tract symptoms/benign prostatic hyperplasia: current evidence and its clinical implications in naturopathic medicine. J Altern Complement Med 2017;23(8):599–606.

124. Shin BC, et al. Maca (L. meyenii) for improving sexual function: a systematic review. BMC Complement Altern Med 2010;10(44):doi:10.1186/1472–6882–10–44.

125. Yang YK, et al. Effects of moxibustion on erectile function and NO-cGMP pathway in diabetic rats with erectile dysfunction. Zhongguo Zhen Jiu 2007;27(5):353–6.

126. Cui X, Zhou J, Qin Z, et al. Acupuncture for erectile dysfunction: a systematic review. Biomed Res Int 2016;2016:2171923.

127. Rohrmann S, et al. Association of cigarette smoking, alcohol consumption and physical activity with lower urinary tract symptoms in older American men: findings from the third National Health And Nutrition Examination Survey. BJU Int 2005;96(1):77–82.

128. Platz EA, et al. Physical activity and benign prostatic hyperplasia. Arch Intern Med 1998;158(21):2349–56.

129. Shiels MS, et al. Association of cigarette smoking, alcohol consumption, and physical activity with sex steroid hormone levels in US men. Cancer Causes Control 2009;20(6):877–86.

130. Hinman F, editor. Benign prostatic hypertrophy. New York: Springer-Verlag; 1983.

131. Zhao L. Clinical observation on the therapeutic effects of heavy moxibustion plus point-injection in treatment of impotence. J Tradit Chin Med 2004;24(2):126–7.

132. Rowland DL, Slob AK. Understanding and diagnosing sexual dysfunction: recent progress through psychophysiological and psychophysical methods. Neurosci Biobehav Rev 1995;19(2):201–9.

133. Kim JH, et al. Randomized control trial of hand acupuncture for female stress urinary incontinence. Acupunct Electrother Res 2008;33(3–4):179–92.

134. Tian FS, et al. Study on acupuncture treatment of diabetic neurogenic bladder. Zhongguo Zhen Jiu 2007;27(7):485–7.

135. Emmons SL, Otto L. Acupuncture for overactive bladder: a randomized controlled trial. Obstet Gynecol 2005;106(1):138–43.

136. Katz AR. Urinary tract infections and acupuncture. Am J Public Health 2003;93(5):702, author reply 702–703.

137. Alraek T, et al. Acupuncture treatment in the prevention of uncomplicated recurrent lower urinary tract infections in adult women. Am J Public Health 2002;92(10):1609–11.

138. Anderson RU, et al. Sexual dysfunction in men with chronic prostatitis/chronic pelvic pain syndrome: improvement after trigger point release and paradoxical relaxation training. J Urol 2006;176(4 Pt 1):1534–8, discussion 1538–1539.

139. Dorey G, et al. Pelvic floor exercises for treating post-micturition dribble in men with erectile dysfunction: a randomized controlled trial. Urol Nurs 2004;24(6):490–7.

140. Dorey G, et al. Pelvic floor exercises for erectile dysfunction. BJU Int 2005;96(4):595–7.

141. Vasconcelos M, et al. Voiding dysfunction in children. Pelvic-floor exercises or biofeedback therapy: a randomized study. Pediatr Nephrol 2006;21(12):1858–64.

142. Rohrmann S. Meat and dairy consumption and subsequent risk of prostate cancer in a US cohort study. Cancer Causes Control 2007;18(1):41–50.

143. Sachs BD. The false organic-psychogenic distinction and related problems in the classification of erectile dysfunction. Int J Impot Res 2003;15(1):72–8.

144. Price D, Hackett G. Management of erectile dysfunction in diabetes: an update for 2008. Curr Diab Rep 2008;8(6):437–43.

145. Mikhail N. Management of erectile dysfunction by the primary care physician. Cleve Clin J Med 2005;72(4):293–4, 296–297, 301–305. passim.

146. Chen J, et al. Effect of oral administration of high-dose nitric oxide donor L-arginine in men with organic erectile dysfunction: results of a double-blind, randomized, placebo-controlled study. BJU Int 1999;83(3):269–73.

147. Baldwin D. Sexual dysfunction associated with antidepressant drugs. Expert Opin Drug Saf 2004;3(5):457–70.

148. Klotz T, et al. Effectiveness of oral L-arginine in first-line treatment of erectile dysfunction in a controlled crossover study. Urol Int 1999;63(4):220–3.

149. Zorgniotti AW, Lizza EF. Effect of large doses of the nitric oxide precursor, L-arginine, on erectile dysfunction. Int J Impot Res 1994;6(1):33–5, discussion 36.

150. Stanislavov R, Nikolova V. Treatment of erectile dysfunction with pycnogenol and L-arginine. J Sex Marital Ther 2003;29(3):207–13.

151. Kernohan AF, et al. An oral yohimbine/L-arginine combination (NMI 861) for the treatment of male erectile dysfunction: a pharmacokinetic, pharmacodynamic and interaction study with intravenous nitroglycerine in healthy male subjects. Br J Clin Pharmacol 2005;59(1):85–93.

152. Rowland DL, Tai W. A review of plant-derived and herbal approaches to the treatment of sexual dysfunctions. J Sex Marital Ther 2003;29(3):185–205.

153. Ernst E, Pittler MH. Yohimbine for erectile dysfunction: a systematic review and meta-analysis of randomized clinical trials. J Urol 1998;159(2):433–6.

154. Wheatley D. Triple-blind placebo-controlled trial of Ginkgo biloba in sexual dysfunction due to antidepressant drugs. Hum Psychopharmacol 2004;19(8):545–8.

155. Cohen AJ, Bartlik B. Ginkgo biloba for antidepressant-induced sexual dysfunction. J Sex Marital Ther 1998;24(2):139–43.

156. Adimoelja A. Phytochemicals and the breakthrough of traditional herbs in the management of sexual dysfunctions. Int J Androl 2000;23(Suppl. 2):82–4.

157. Adaikan PG, et al. Proerectile pharmacological effects of Tribulus terrestris extract on the rabbit corpus cavernosum. Ann Acad Med Singapore 2000;29(1):22–6.

158. Lee MS, et al. Acupuncture for treating erectile dysfunction: a systematic review. BJU Int 2009;104(3):366–70.

159. GamalEl Din SF, Abdel Salam MA, Mohamed MS, et al. Tribulus terrestris versus placebo in the treatment of erectile dysfunction and lower urinary tract symptoms in patients with late-onset hypogonadism: a placebo-controlled study. Urol J 2018. https://doi.org/10.1177/0391560318802160.

160. Platz EA, et al. Interrelation of energy intake, body size, and physical activity with prostate cancer in a large prospective cohort study. Cancer Res 2003;63(23):8542–8.

CHAPTER **30**

Recurrent urinary tract infection

Michelle Boyd
ND, MHSc

OVERVIEW

A urinary tract infection (UTI) is by simplest definition an infection that affects any part of the urinary tract, including the kidneys, ureters, bladder and urethra. Most infections will involve the lower tract, which includes the urethra and the bladder. UTIs are most commonly caused by the organism *Escherichia coli*.[1] Infections typically develop when bacteria or viruses enter the urinary system through the urethra. Once inside the bladder, the bacteria begin multiplying until their numbers are large enough to cause infectious symptoms (usually more than 100 000 organisms per millilitre in a midstream urine sample). Infections may cause swelling of the urethra (urethritis), bladder (cystitis), epididymis (epididymitis) or one or both testicles (orchitis).[1] Females are far more likely to present with UTIs than males, as the female urethra is closer to the anus (and its bacterial load) than the male urethra. Most UTIs are classified as 'uncomplicated', being caused by a transient infection of a single strain of proliferative bacteria.[2] Other cases, however, are classed as 'complicated' and are caused by urinary tract dysfunction or disease, or via an overarching medical condition such as diabetes. In the latter case concern exists regarding potential renal damage; medical referral is advised.

Common symptoms associated with UTI include urgency to urinate, a burning sensation during micturition, haematuria, cloudy or foul (or otherwise abnormal) smelling urine and frequently passing small amounts of urine.[1,3] Symptoms suggestive of urethritis include a burning sensation during micturition and, in men, penile discharge. Symptoms suggestive of cystitis may include pelvic pressure, lower abdominal pain and painful and frequent urination.[1,3] Symptoms suggestive of epididymitis in men include: scrotal pain; tenderness in the testes and groin; painful intercourse, ejaculation and urination; and orchitis.[1,3]

Some populations are particularly prone to recurrent asymptomatic bacteriuria including those with indwelling catheters; pregnant and older women; people with diabetes; and those with spinal cord injury. Treating these individuals with antibiotics has not been shown to improve long-term outcomes. In addition, antimicrobial resistance is common (and especially in postmenopausal women) and therefore other interventions are more likely to be successful in the long run.[4,5] A number of factors are potentially involved in the increased rate of recurrent UTIs in older women and these include oestrogen deficiency and thinning of urethral mucosa, previous urogenital surgery, incontinence, cystocoele and incomplete bladder emptying and having had a previous history of more than six UTIs. Oestrogen normally maintains vaginal flora, which reduce risk of UTI.[6]

Screening of asymptomatic women has shown that approximately 5% will have some form of UTI, 11% will experience UTI in any given year and 50% will experience symptoms of cystitis at some stage in their life.[7,8] All males who present with a UTI should be referred for investigation to exclude any underlying abnormality such as prostatitis. The differential diagnoses of vaginitis or vulvovaginal infections (such as *Candida* spp.) are also often associated with vaginal discharge.[1]

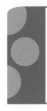

DIFFERENTIAL DIAGNOSIS

- Acute pyelonephritis
- Atrophic vaginitis
- Bladder cancer
- Cystitis
- Genital herpes
- Interstitial cystitis

Source: Kodner et al. 2010[9]

RISK FACTORS

Sexual intercourse frequency is the strongest risk factor for UTIs in younger populations.[1] Exposure to spermicide and new sexual partners are additive risk factors.[10] Diabetes is also a risk factor for UTIs, particularly for complicated UTIs, and women who require medical management for this condition will run roughly twice the risk of developing a UTI than non-diabetic women.[11] Low levels of oestrogen can -dramatically change the microflora from one dominated by *Lactobacillus* spp. to one dominated by *Escherichia coli*, therefore increasing the risk of UTI. (It should be noted that this may be of clinical relevance only in postmenopausal women.)[5,12]

CONVENTIONAL TREATMENT

Conventional treatment of UTIs relies on antibiotic therapy and most cases of uncomplicated infection can be managed easily, with antibiotic treatment expected to cure 80–90% of uncomplicated UTIs.[8] Optimal treatment also includes adjuvant recommendations such as increasing fluid intake, encouraging complete bladder emptying and urinary alkalinisation for severe dysuria.[8] Simple analgesics such as paracetamol are recommended for pain. Recurrent UTIs are usually defined as three or more UTIs in a 12-month period, and in these women a larger focus on preventive treatment is advised, even as far as prophylactic antibiotic use after sexual intercourse.[8]

KEY TREATMENT PROTOCOLS

The primary naturopathic treatment goals for UTIs are to initially combat the urinary pathogen and ameliorate symptoms such as pain and fever. Long-term treatment

Naturopathic Treatment Aims

- Educate the patient with lifestyle advice to aid in UTI prevention.
- Target a UTI with antimicrobials and bacterial antiadhesives, and increase water intake.
- Remove aggravating factors such as a highly acidic diet.
- Promote appropriate immune function.
- Restore urinary tract microflora balance.

protocols are to enhance the patient's immune function to appropriately remove and resist infection, remove possible irritants, restore urinary tract microflora, prevent bacteria from adhering to the mucosal wall of the bladder and promote preventive behaviours. Herbal medicine has a strong tradition of use in genitourinary conditions (Table 30.1), although many herbal medicines' mechanisms of action and clinical efficacy have yet to be validated.

Provide antimicrobial activity

Encouraging healthy bacterial balance may be achieved by preventing dysbiosis and promoting healthy gastrointestinal bacteria populations. As most infections are the result of *Escherichia coli* from the digestive tract, promoting a diet that favours healthy microflora ratios may be beneficial in reducing the incidence of UTI. A Finnish study, for example, found that women who consumed fermented dairy products containing probiotic strains had a reduced risk of developing UTI.[13] The consumption of fresh juices, particularly berry juices, was also associated with decreased risk of developing UTI. Clinical investigation of women who are predisposed to recurrent UTI has also uncovered reduced beneficial microflora populations, even during times of non-infection.[14,15]

Although it is known that pathogenic urogenital flora proliferate at the time of infection, attempts to restore balance with **probiotic supplements** to reduce UTI show mixed results.[6] Specific strains of probiotics can be beneficial for preventing recurrent UTIs in women and generally have a good safety profile. In a recent study, young women experiencing recurrent UTIs were randomised to insert either an intravaginal suppository containing *Lactobacillus crispatus* (Lactin-V) or a placebo daily for five days, then once weekly for 10 weeks. A reduction in UTI incidence was observed among the women using the probiotic.[16] *Lactobacillus rhamnosus* and *Lactobacillus reuteri* either intravaginally or orally are most effective, while *Lactobacillus casei* Shirota and *Lactobacillus crispatus* showed efficacy in some studies; *Lactobacillus rhamnosus* does not seem as effective.[17,18] Controversy still surrounds the use of probiotics for UTI prophylaxis due to limited and mixed evidence. As with all instances in using specific probiotic strains for specific therapeutic effects, care needs to be taken to identify the appropriate strain. (See Chapter 4 on irritable bowel syndrome for more discussion on suitable probiotic strains for specific conditions.)

The isoquinoline alkaloid **berberine** from **Hydrastis canadensis**, **Coptis chinensis** and **Berberis vulgaris** has a strong effect in treating UTIs due to bacteriostatic activity.[19] Its effects have been confirmed against a number of bacteria including *Staphylococcus* spp., *Escherichia coli* and *Streptococcus* spp.[20] **Arctostaphylos uva-ursi**, rich in the phenolic constituent arbutin, also provides strong antimicrobial activity and has preliminary clinical evidence.[21] Clinical studies using these botanicals are now required to confirm this activity in humans. The acetone and ethanol extracts from rhizome of **Drynaria quercifolia** shows promise in treating UTIs. It is used to treat various kinds of health problems including UTIs and has been shown to possess antibacterial effect on isolated bacterial pathogens of urinary tract such as *Streptococcus pyogenes*, *Enterococcus faecalis* and *Pseudomonas aeruginosa*.[22]

Inhibit bacteria adhering to bladder wall

A key protocol in treating UTIs is to reduce bacterial proliferation in the bladder and their adherence to the bladder wall. In addition to increasing diuresis and providing

Table 30.1
Traditional herbal actions in urinary tract infection*

Herb	Anti-adherent	Anti-inflammatory	Antilithic	Antiseptic (urinary)	Astringent	Bladder tonic	Diuretic	Demulcent (urinary)	Immune modulating	Spasmolytic
Androgriphis paniculata		✓							✓	
Agathosma betulina		✓		✓			✓	✓		
Zea mays		✓	✓				✓	✓		
Agropyron repens							✓	✓		
Viburnum opulus					✓					✓
Vaccinium macrocarpon	✓			✓						
Crataeva nurvala		✓	✓			✓				
Solidago virgaurea		✓		✓			✓			
Equisetum arvense					✓	✓	✓			
Hydrangea spp.		✓	✓				✓	✓		
Glycyrrhiza glabra		✓							✓	
Althaea officinalis		✓						✓		
Urtica dioica		✓					✓			
Petroselinum crispum		✓		✓			✓			✓
Arctostaphylos uva-ursi		✓		✓	✓					

*Adapted from Commission E and British Herbal Pharmacopoeia monographs[13,14]

603

an antimicrobial and bacteriostatic action, interventions that interfere with bacterial adherence will be of benefit. A key lifestyle measure in reducing bacterial colonisation and adherence on bladder tissue is complete urination after sexual intercourse. The main phytotherapy studied for this action is *Vaccinium macrocarpon* (**cranberry**) and as well as other plants in the *Vaccinium* genus including *Vaccinium myrtilus* and *Vaccinium vitis-idaea*. *Agropyron repens* and the stigmata of *Zea mays* have also been shown to decrease bacterial adhesion by interacting with outer membrane proteins of bacteria.[23] In vitro and animal studies have demonstrated that cranberry consumption inhibits the binding of bacterial strains such as *Escherichia coli* to uroepithelial cells.[19,21] It appears, that the proanthocyanidins (PACs), and particularly those with A-type linkages found in cranberry, are responsible for this activity. Further, these PACs have been shown to be important inhibitors of various (including antibiotic-resistant) strains of *Escherichia coli*.[24,25]

A previous 2008 Cochrane review and meta-analysis found that cranberry or cranberry and lingonberry significantly reduced people's chances of developing UTIs over a 12-month period and concluded that women rather than men or people with bladder infections due to catheterisation might preferentially benefit from cranberry juice or tablets.[26] In contrast, a 2012 Cochrane review concluded that cranberry was less effective than previously indicated. Although some of the small studies demonstrated limited benefit for women with recurrent UTIs, there were no statistically significant differences when the results of a much larger study were included. One point raised was the high numbers of dropouts/withdrawals from studies (mainly attributed to the acceptability of consuming cranberry products [particularly juice] over long periods). In addition, only five studies tried to describe the amount of PAC—the compound considered to be the active ingredient in cranberry juice. Even so, there was no correlation between the dose and/or individual products used and efficacious outcomes.[27] However, the French Agency for Food Health Safety (AFSSA) identifies the bacterial anti-adherence effects of cranberry juice and endorses daily use equivalent to 300 mL containing 36 mg PACs for decreasing the frequency of UTIs in adult women.[28]

Of the many reviews assessing cranberry, a key point raised is the need to use suitable medications that avoid long-term antibiotic prophylaxis and the risk of antibiotic resistance.[29,30] Older women with asymptomatic UTIs can develop malaise; anorexia and frequency of urine and are therefore possible candidates for cranberry therapy. A study assessing the benefits of cranberry capsules in female nursing home residents with bacteriuria found that cranberry PAC in various doses given over one month reduced numbers of bacteria in the urine, particularly *Escherichia coli* in a dose-dependent manner.[31] A botanical with traditional use in UTIs is *Juniperus* **spp.** This medicinal plant may provide an anti-UTI effect via bacteriostatic, diuretic and anti-adhesion effects, but to date no human clinical trials substantiate this.[21] It should be noted that a common misconception exists about *Juniperus* spp. and nephrotoxicity. Close evaluation of the literature reveals that a review of the evidence does not support this effect and that previous case studies may be based on adulteration of the juniper oil.[21] As mentioned previously, the isoquinoline alkaloid **berberine** has a potential effect in treating UTIs due to bacteriostatic action; this constituent also has demonstrated anti-adhesion activity against a number of bacteria including *Staphylococcus* spp., *Escherichia coli* and *Streptococcus* spp.[19,20] The nutrient **D-mannose** may also provide anti-adhesion activity against bacteria such as *Escherichia coli*. This simple sugar has been shown to bind to uroepithelial cells to which bacteria normally adhere, thereby interfering with colonisation.[19] While a promising intervention it should be noted that current evidence is based on in vitro and animal studies. See Table 30.4 for the evidence summary.

Enhance diuresis

The most obvious way to increase diuresis is by use of aquaretics: agents that increase water excretion via effects on glomerular filtration as opposed to affecting electrolyte control with diuretics.[21] Water and herbal teas related to treatment are the preferable methods of increasing liquid intake. Although most botanicals used for this effect are regarded as being aquaretic, there have been some studies on the diuretic effects of certain herbs that are noted to be potentially beneficial in conditions like oedema and hypertension.[21] Reference is particularly made in this instance to the herb *Taraxacum officinale* where the leaf especially has demonstrated diuretic effects due in part to potassium content.[32] An added benefit for use of *Taraxacum officinale* in diuresis is that potassium levels are compensated for the loss of this mineral in urine output.[33] The first human study to evaluate the diuretic effects of this herb showed promise for its use as a diuretic.[34] The pilot study used fresh leaf hydroethanolic extract of *Taraxacum officinale* (8 mL t.d.s.) in 17 participants to investigate whether an increased urinary frequency and volume would result (compared with pre-recorded baseline measurements). Results revealed a significant increase in the frequency of urination in the five-hour period after the first dose. There was also a significant increase in the excretion ratio in the five-hour period after the second dose of extract. The third dose, however, failed to significantly alter any of the measured parameters. For more detail on the use of *Taraxacum officinale* as a diuretic refer to Chapter 12 on hypertension.

Reduce inflammation and pain

Symptomatic relief of pain and inflammation is also important in treating UTIs. The use of **herbal anti-inflammatories** and **demulcents** are specifically indicated and are highly recommended (see the detailed lists in Tables 30.1 and 30.2). Further details on treating pain and inflammation may be found in Chapter 25 on osteoarthritis, Chapter 31 on autoimmunity and Chapter 40 on pain management.

Encourage preventative measures

Clinicians are advised to provide lifestyle advice to assist in UTI prevention (see box). A key consideration is to advise that the patient communicate to their sexual partner(s) about the potential influence their sexual hygiene may have on the genesis of a UTI. To effectively prevent UTIs, the sexual partner is advised to adopt the same lifestyle advice as the patient being treated (especially males) because they may be the prime source of recurrent infection. Although studies on fluid intake and susceptibility to UTI appear inconclusive, adequate hydration is important and may improve the results of interventional treatment.[35] Supporting healthy immune function is also an important preventive measure. One small trial found that 100 mg of **vitamin C** reduced the incidence of UTI in pregnant women.[36] A recent meta-analysis noted, however, that vitamin C may be of little use as an acidifying agent lowering urinary pH.[37] The preventive action for using vitamin C in the case of UTIs may be by way of its indirect rather than direct effects.

Lifestyle factors useful in the prevention of UTIs

Hydration and urination

- Drink at least eight glasses of water per day.
- Urinate often because retaining urine in the bladder may promote bacterial growth.
- Completely empty the bladder when urinating.

Urogenital area hygiene

- Good hygiene and urination should be observed (by both sexual partners) before and after sexual activity.
- Any potential irritants that are vaginally inserted should be avoided where possible in women with recurrent infections—these may include diaphragms or tampons that contain potentially irritating chemicals.
- Always cleanse the urogenital and anal areas from front to back.

Clothing

- Wear appropriate clothing—avoid tight-fitting underwear and wear breathable natural fibres like cotton for underwear and stockings.

Sensitivities and allergies

- Allergens and sensitivity by-products may cause irritation of the bladder wall so avoidance is recommended.
- UTIs after sexual activity may also result from latex or spermicidal allergies. Therefore reviewing birth control methods may be advised.

Sources: Kodner et al. 2010,[9] Jepson & Craig 2008[26] and Jepson et al. 2012[27]

Remove bladder irritants

Some substances may have an irritant effect on bladder epithelial tissue, predisposing patients to infection and delaying treatment effects. These are caffeine, refined sugars, dietary allergens, nicotine, alcohol and certain medications.

Source: Wyman 2009[38]

Medicinal teas

One potentially beneficial complementary and alternative medicine (CAM) intervention in the treatment of UTIs is **medicinal teas**, which, in addition to providing anti-microbial, anti-inflammatory, demulcent or diuretic activity, also increase the amount of water consumed. As Reinard Ludewig (1989)[39] espoused, 'persons who prefer their daily coffee, cocoa, or tea to caffeine tablets are unknowingly accepting and enjoying the pleasure of gentle-acting phytomedicines'. Traditional herbal pharmacopoeias advocate the use of medicinal herbal teas (infusions and decoctions) for treating UTIs, promoting diuresis, disinfecting the urine and preventing the formation of renal gravel and stones (Table 30.2).[39]

Writings in *The American Eclectic Materia Medica and Therapeutics* (1863) reflected the practice of the day, declaring without doubt that 'infusion and decoction are the most eligible forms of administering such vegetable remedies' as they 'yield either a part or all of their virtues to water infusion'. They reiterated that, although much 'tea' was laughed at, 'this practice has proven eminently successful' and the added advantage was 'that the patient will receive sufficient [liquid], a matter that is of the first importance in the treatment of many diseases'.[42]

Teas, as aqueous preparations, are efficient in extracting water-soluble plant chemicals, in particular essential oils, and the presence of saponins enhances the bioavailability of

Table 30.2
Teas commonly used in UTIs

	Herb details			Monograph indications					
Botanical name	Plant part	Dosage and administration	German commission E	World Health Organization	European Scientific Cooperative on Phytotherapy	German standard licence	British Herbal Compendium	British Herbal Pharmacopoeia
Agathosma betulina	Leaf	1–2 g by infusion t.d.s.					Mild UTI	Cystitis, urethritis Specific: acute catarrhal cystitis
Agropyron repens	Rhizome	4–8 g in decoction t.d.s.						Cystitis, urethritis, lithuria Specific: cystitis with irritation or inflammation of urinary tract
Althaea officinalis	Leaf	Leaf: 2–5 g by infusion t.d.s.						Leaf: cystitis, urethritis, urinary gravel or calculus
Arctostaphylos uva-ursi	Leaf	Steep 3 g in 150 mL boiled water 15 mins up to q.i.d.	Inflammatory disorders of efferent urinary tract		Uncomplicated UTIs, cystitis	Support therapy for bladder and kidney catarrh		Cystitis, urethritis, dysuria, pyelitis and lithuria Specific: acute catarrhal cystitis with dysuria and highly acid urine
Armoracia rusticana	Root	Steep 2 g in 150 mL boiled water for 5 mins	Supportive therapy for UTIs				Inflammation or mild infections of the genitourinary tract	
Echinacea spp.	Root	Steep 2 g in 150 mL boiled water for 5 mins		Supportive therapy for UTIs				

Table 30.2
Teas commonly used in UTIs (continued)

| Herb details | | | | Monograph indications | | | | | |
Botanical name	Plant part	Dosage and administration	German commission E	World Health Organization	European Scientific Cooperative on Phytotherapy	German standard licence	British Herbal Compendium	British Herbal Pharmacopoeia
Equisetum arvense	Green stems	Steep 2 g in 150 mL boiled water 10–15 mins t.d.s.	Lower UTIs and inflammation and renal gravel			Lower UTIs and inflammation and renal gravel		
Juniperus communis	Berry	Dried ripe fruits infusion 1:20 in boiling water dosed 100 mL t.d.s.						Acute or chronic cystitis Specific: cystitis, in absence of renal inflammation
Petroselinum crispum	Herb and root	Steep 2 g in 150 mL water t.d.s.	Diuresis and prevent and treat kidney gravel					
Solidago virgaurea	Aerial (above ground)	Steep 3 g in 150 mL boiled water for 10–15 mins, two to four times daily between meals	Diuresis for inflammatory lower UTIs, prevent and treat urinary calculi and kidney gravel		Diuresis for inflammatory urinary tract and renal gravel, adjuvant bacterial UTIs	Diuresis in inflammation of kidneys and bladder	Mild infections of UT	Cystitis
Urtica dioica	Leaf	Steep 2–5 g in 150 mL boiled water for 10–15 mins t.d.s.	Diuresis for inflammatory lower urinary tract, prevent and treat kidney gravel		Irrigation therapy in inflammatory conditions of lower urinary tract	Increase urine volume and treat urine associated complaints		
Zea mays	Styles and stigmas	4–8 g by infusion t.d.s.						Cystitis, urethritis and nocturnal enuresis Specific: acute or chronic inflammation of urinary system

Sources: Blumenthal et al. 2000[40] and British Herbal Medicine Association Scientific Committee 1983[41]

other, less-soluble compounds.[43] Furthermore, therapeutic infusions have added benefits not gleaned from herbal liquid extracts and solid dose forms. The ritual of preparing a herbal tea, savouring the aroma and slowly sipping to ultimately experience the soothing, warm sensation that, at some level, brings relaxation to an otherwise stressed individual has added therapeutic value.

There are important considerations in the selection of herbs to create a balanced blend that is both therapeutic and palatable. Weiss instructs that every formulation requires three components: the basic remedy (the *remedium cardinal*); an adjuvant to enhance or complement the action of the basic remedy; and a 'corrigent' to improve palatability and compliance.[44] Preparation instructions also need to be communicated well as the method used has the potential to impede or potentiate the therapeutic benefits of a herbal tea. Herbal parts containing volatile oils (e.g. in delicate leaves and seeds) should be gently infused in hot water in an enclosed vessel (teapot) so as not to damage or lose these therapeutic plant compounds. Chemical compounds contained in harder bark or root components may need to be 'drawn out' in boiling water for 10–15 minutes. Furthermore, dosage instructions will potentiate the curative properties attributed to both the preparation and the ingestion practices of taking tea. Unless otherwise indicated, one or two teaspoons of herb are used per cup (150 mL) of hot water, of which two to three cups are to be taken daily on an empty stomach to aid absorption, preferably drunk on rising, mid-afternoon and before bed.[44]

INTEGRATIVE MEDICAL CONSIDERATIONS

Warning
There are important medical implications associated with UTIs. UTIs elevate the risk of pyelonephritis and are associated with impaired renal function and end-stage renal disease.[1] It is therefore imperative that anyone presenting with a UTI with suspected kidney disease should be referred to a general practitioner for assessment with possible further referral to a urologist (see Table 30.3 for other common urinary conditions).[45]

Conventional treatment of UTIs with antibiotics along with a high recurrence rate of UTIs, especially among young women, has led to issues of antibiotic resistance. Various authors have reported on antibiotic resistance and its implications for the long-term use of antibiotics for the effective management of urinary tract and kidney infections.[47–50] One case-control study concluded that exposure to antibiotics is a strong risk factor for a resistant *Escherichia coli* UTI.[51] An integrative approach using various herbal and nutritional therapeutics to support and resolve UTIs may provide promise. A Norwegian study found that acupuncture reduced the UTI rate by around half in women who had a history of recurrent UTIs.[52] However, treatment needs to be individualised based on the diagnosis and prescription of trained practitioners. Acupuncture also seems to result in improved quality of life of women with recurrent UTIs.[53]

Dietary and lifestyle advice

Recommendations are made to further reduce susceptibility to and incidence of UTIs and to promote general wellbeing and healthy immune function. Dietary advice may include reducing or eliminating intake of refined sugar and alcohol, and increase pre- and probiotic foods (mucopolysaccharides and cultured yoghurts). Calcium

Table 30.3
Treatment of other urogenital conditions

Urogenital disorder	Treatment protocol	CAM interventions	Comment
Kidney stones	Reduce inflammation Assist breakdown of urinary gravel Increase diuresis Provide analgesia	Low-oxalate diet Low-purine diet Increase water intake Antilithic, anti-inflammatory botanicals Vitamin B6, magnesium	Monitor closely for referral for medical help if condition worsens, such as increased pain or blood in urine Address pain with analgesic medicines Evidence of antilithic activity is currently based only on traditional evidence Ultrasound may assist
Pyelonephritis/ kidney infection	Refer immediately for medical help (antibiotics are usually prescribed) Support adjuvantly Reduce inflammation Provide analgesia Tonify kidneys (traditional protocol)	Antimicrobial, anti-inflammatory, demulcent, diuretic botanicals More water (with adequate electrolytes) Urogenital hygiene Low renal-irritant diet	Chronic recurring kidney infections and nephritis may be unresponsive to repeated antibiotics Antimicrobial herbs, such as *Arctostaphylos uva-ursi, Hydrastis canadensis, Echinacea* spp. may assist in this case
Vaginal thrush	Antifungal action Recolonise tissue with appropriate microflora Reduce itching Support immune and nervous systems	Antifungal/microbial pessary or douche containing tea tree oil, *Hydrastis canadensis*, probiotics Low-yeast diet Immune tonics Nervines	Screen for trigger, such as stress, diet change or antibiotic use Considered in traditional Chinese medicine as a 'damp' condition—avoid 'damp' diets and exposure to wet environments

Sources: Kumar & Clark 2002,[3] Reid 2001,[17] Barrons & Tassone 2008,[19] Beetz 2003[35] and Manz & Wentz 2005[46]

supplementation (not from fermented dairy products) may be associated with increased risk of UTI (calcium ions increase bacterial adherence to uroepithelial cells) as has the consumption of non-organic retail chicken (four to six days per week) and pork (one to three days per week) due to antimicrobial resistant UTI-causing *Escherichia coli* found in these foods and possibly being transferred via faeces to urogenital area.[54,55] Increased fluid intake, using fresh vegetable juices (e.g. a blend of celery, carrot, lemon and ginger), herbal teas and pure water, is also advised. Urogenital hygiene practices— pre- and postcoital hygiene and increased urination—are also recommended.

CLINICAL SUMMARY

UTIs are common, especially in young women, and recurrence rate is high. UTIs elevate the risk of pyelonephritis and are associated with impaired renal function and end-stage renal disease, so UTIs should be treated assertively and comprehensively. Conventional treatment of UTIs with antibiotics may lead to patterns of antibiotic resistance, so judicious use is advised. Various CAM therapeutics (herbal and nutritional) have value in the treatment and prevention of UTIs and can be considered as stand-alone interventions or adjuvants with antibiotics. Regardless, medical referral is needed if the UTI is serious or is not responding to CAM. Implementation of dietary and lifestyle advice (e.g. sexual hygiene) is still, however, advised to help prevent recurrence (see decision tree at Figure 30.1).

It would be expected that within a few days of starting a naturopathic prescription (potentially after the first day) there would be relief of symptoms. Reduced UTI recurrence can be promoted by increasing immune resistance and improved balance of bowel and urogenital flora. Furthermore, a reduced UTI recurrence rate may be affected if diet and lifestyle advice is adhered to. Herbal prescription should be continued a couple of days after the symptoms have resolved to completely address the pathogen. Preventive measures should be continued. A prophylactic prescription can be provided to enhance immune function, maintain bowel and urogenital flora, improve mucous membrane integrity and urinary tract function, and to address any contributing factors such as stress. The use of the herbal teas and cranberry tablets/capsules can be continued long term and is advised in people with chronic recurrent UTIs.

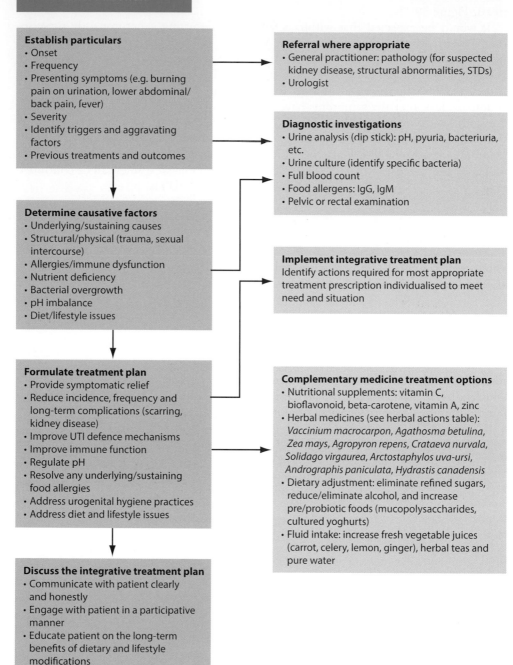

Figure 30.1
Naturopathic treatment decision tree—urinary tract infection

Table 30.4
Review of the major evidence

Intervention	Mechanisms of action	Key literature	Summary of results	Comment
Probiotics: *Lactobaccilus* **spp.**	Restoration of vaginal flora as treatment and prophylaxis of bacterial urogenital infections	Review: Barrons & Tassone 2008[17]	Use of lactobacilli for prophylaxis of UTI remains inconclusive due to small sample sizes and invalidated dosing strategies. Of four RCTs: One (12 months, 55 subjects) study reported 73% reduction of recurrent UTI compared with previous year ($p = 0.001$); one study (12 months, 149 subjects) showed no reduction in recurrent UTI compared with placebo or cranberry-lingonberry juice (CLJ) – CLJ group reduced recurrence of UTI vs control ($p = 0.023$); and two remaining studies (26 and 36 weeks, 47 and 41 subjects respectively) showed no effect on recurrence	Authors raised concerns about lack of detail provided for probiotic product stability and strain-specificity
***Vaccinium macrocarpon* (cranberry)**	Prevent bacteria from sticking on walls of bladder to help prevent bladder infection and other UTIs	Cochrane review: Jepson & Williams 2012[27]	24 RCTs (14 studies added to this update) involving 4473 participants showed: cranberry juice has no significant benefit in prevention of UTIs and long-term use may be unacceptable; cranberry tablets or capsules were also shown to be ineffective, however, they were as effective as antibiotics—lack of effectiveness may be due to lack of potency of 'active ingredient'	Cranberry less effective than previous (2008) Cochrane review indicated. Although some small studies demonstrated limited benefit for women with recurrent UTIs, there were no statistically significant differences when results of larger study were included. Only five studies provided active (PAC) ingredient details; most others didn't and may not have had enough potency to be effective. Large number of dropouts/withdrawals mainly due to acceptability of consuming cranberry juice over long periods of time

KEY POINTS

- UTIs are common, especially in young women, and recurrence rate is high.
- UTIs elevate the risk of pyelonephritis and are associated with impaired renal function and end-stage renal disease, so UTIs should be treated assertively and comprehensively.
- Conventional treatment of UTIs with antibiotics may lead to patterns of antibiotic resistance, so judicious use is advised.
- Various CAM therapeutics (herbal and nutritional) have value in the treatment and prevention of UTIs and can be considered as stand-alone interventions or adjuvants with antibiotics.
- Implementation of lifestyle advice (e.g. sexual hygiene) is advised to help prevent recurrence.

FURTHER READING

Barrons R, Tassone D. Use of Lactobacillus probiotics for bacterial genitourinary infections in women: a review. Clin Ther 2008;30:453–68.

Fu Z, Liska D, Talan D, et al. Cranberry reduces the risk of urinary tract infection recurrence in otherwise healthy women: a systematic review and meta-analysis. J Nutr 2017;147(12):2282–8. doi:10.3945/jn.117.254961. Epub 2017 Oct 18.

Grigoryan L, Trautner BW, Gupta K. Diagnosis and management of urinary tract infections in the outpatient setting: a review. JAMA 2014;312(16):1677–84. doi:10.1001/jama.2014.12842. Review.

Raditic DM. Complementary and integrative therapies for lower urinary tract diseases. Vet Clin North Am Small Anim Pract 2015;45(4):857–78. doi:10.1016/j.cvsm.2015.02.009. Epub 2015 Mar 31.

REFERENCES

1. Wein AJ, et al. Campbell-Walsh urology. 11th ed. Philadelphia: Saunders Elsevier; 2015.
2. Boon NA, et al. Davidson's principles and practice of medicine, 23rd edn. Edinburgh: Churchill Livingstone; 2018.
3. Kumar P, Clark M. Clinical medicine. 9th ed. London: W.B. Saunders; 2016.
4. Miotla P, et al. Antimicrobial resistance patterns in women with positive urine culture: does menopausal status make a significant difference? BioMed Res Int 2017;1–6. https://doi.org/10.1155/2017/4192908.
5. Concia E, et al. Clinical evaluation of guidelines and therapeutic approaches in multi drug-resistant urinary tract infections. J Chemother 2017;29(sup1):19–28.
6. Muhleisen AL, Herbst-Kralovetz MM. Menopause and the vaginal microbiome. Maturitas 2016;91:42–50.
7. Foxman B, et al. Urinary tract infection: self reported incidence and associated costs. Ann Epidemiol 2000;10:509–15.
8. Murtagh J. General practice. 6th ed. Sydney: McGraw-Hill; 2015.
9. Kodner CM, Thomas Gupton EK. Recurrent urinary tract infections in women: diagnosis and management. Am Fam Physician 2010;82(6):638–43.
10. Scholes D, et al. Risk factors for recurrent urinary tract infection in young women. J Infect Dis 2000;182:1177–82.
11. Boyko E, et al. Diabetes and the risk of acute urinary tract infection among postmenopausal women. Diabetes Care 2002;25:1778–83.
12. Wang C, et al. Estrogenic modulation of uropathogenic Escherichia coli infection pathogenesis in a murine menopause model. Infect Immun 2013;81(3):733–9.
13. Kontiokari T, et al. Dietary factors protecting women from urinary tract infection. Am J Clin Nutr 2003;77:600–4.
14. Gupta K, et al. Inverse association of H2O2-producing lactobacilli and vaginal Escherichia coli colonization in women with recurrent urinary tract infections. J Infect Dis 1998;178:446–50.
15. Kirjavainen P, et al. Abnormal immunological profile and vaginal microbiota in women prone to urinary tract infections. Clin Vaccine Immunol 2009;16:29–36.
16. Stapleton AE, et al. Randomized, placebo-controlled phase 2 trial of a Lactobacillus crispatus probiotic given intravaginally for prevention of recurrent urinary tract infection. CID 2011;52:1212–17.
17. Barrons R, Tassone D. Use of Lactobacillus probiotics for bacterial genitourinary infections in women: a review. Clin Ther 2008;30:453–68.
18. Reid G. Probiotic lactobacilli for urogenital health in women. J Clin Gastroenterol 2008;42:S234–6.
19. Head K. Natural approaches to prevention and treatment of infections of the lower urinary tract. Altern Med Rev 2008;13:227–44.
20. Scazzocchio F, et al. Antibacterial activity of Hydrastis canadensis extract and its major isolated alkaloids. Planta Med 2001;67:561–4.
21. Yarnell E. Botanical medicines for the urinary tract. World J Urol 2002;20:285–93.
22. Mithraja MJ, et al. Antibacterial efficacy of Drynaria quercifolia (L.) J. Smith (Polypodiaceae) against clinically isolated urinary tract pathogens. Asian Pac J Trop Biomed 2012;(Suppl. 1):S131–5.
23. Rafsanjany N, et al. Antiadhesion as a functional concept for protection against uropathogenic Escherichia coli: in vitro studies with traditionally used plants with

antiadhesive activity against uropathogenic Escherichia coli. J Ethnopharmacol 2013;145:591–7.

24. Howell AB, et al. Dosage effect on uropathogenic Escherichia coli anti-adhesion activity in urine following consumption of cranberry powder standardized for proanthocyanidin content: a multicentric randomized double blind study. BMC Infect Dis 2010;10:94.

25. Lavigne JP, et al. In-vitro and in-vivo evidence of dose-dependent decrease of uropathogenic Escherichia coli virulence after consumption of commercial Vaccinium macrocarpon (cranberry) capsules. Clin Microbiol Infect 2008;14(4):350–5.

26. Jepson RG, Craig JC. Cranberries for preventing urinary tract infections (Review). Cochrane Database Syst Rev 2008;(1):CD001321.

27. Jepson RG, et al. Cranberries for preventing urinary tract infections (Review). Cochrane Database Syst Rev 2012;(10):CD001321.

28. Haesaerts G. The quantitation of cranberry proanthocyanidins (PAC) in food supplements: challenges and latest developments. Phytotherapy 2010;8:218–23.

29. Hisano M, et al. Cranberries and lower urinary tract infection prevention. Clinics 2012;67(6):661–7.

30. Wang C-H, et al. Cranberry-containing products for prevention of urinary tract infections in susceptible populations. Arch Intern Med 2012;172(13):988–96.

31. Bianco L, et al. Pilot randomized controlled dosing study of cranberry capsules for reduction of bacteriuria plus pyuria in female nursing home residents. JAGS 2012;60(6):1180–1.

32. Hook I, et al. Evaluation of dandelion for diuretic activity and variation of potassium content. Int J Pharmacog 1993;31(1):29–34.

33. Schütz K, et al. Taraxacum—a review on its phytochemical and pharmacological profile. J Ethnopharmacol 2006;107:313–23.

34. Clare BA, et al. The diuretic effect in human subjects of an extract of Taraxacum officinale folium over a single day. J Altern Complement Med 2009;15(8):929–34.

35. Beetz R. Mild dehydration: a risk factor of urinary tract infection. Eur J Clin Nutr 2003;57:S52–8.

36. Ochoa-Brust G, et al. Daily intake of 100 mg ascorbic acid as urinary tract infection prophylactic agent during pregnancy. Acta Obstet Gynecol Scand 2007;86:783–7.

37. Masson P, et al. Meta-analyses in prevention and treatment of urinary tract infections. Infect Dis Clin North Am 2009;23:355–85.

38. Wyman JF, et al. Practical aspects of lifestyle modifications and behavioural interventions in the treatment of overactive bladder and urgency urinary incontinence. Int J Clin Pract 2009;63(8):1177–91.

39. Schulz V, et al. Rational phytotherapy: a physicians' guide to herbal medicine. Berlin: Springer; 2001.

40. Blumenthal M, et al. Herbal medicine expanded Commission E monographs. Newton: Integrative Medicine Communications; 2000.

41. British Herbal Medicine Association Scientific Committee. British herbal pharmacopoeia. Bournemouth: British Herbal Medicine Association; 1983.

42. Bergner P. Tinctures vs teas. Med Herb 2001;10(4):3.

43. Bone K, Mills S. Principles and practice of phytotherapy. Edinburgh: Churchill Livingstone; 2013.

44. Weiss R. Herbal medicine. Gothenburg: Ab Arcanum and Beaconsfield. Beaconsfield Publishers; 1985.

45. Foxman B. Epidemiology of urinary tract infections: incidence, morbidity, and economic costs. Dis Mon 2003;49:53–70.

46. Manz F, Wentz A. The importance of good hydration for the prevention of chronic diseases. Nutr Rev 2005;63(6):S2–5.

47. Foxman B, et al. Antibiotic resistance and pyelonephritis. Clin Infect Dis 2007;45:281–3.

48. Karlowsky JA, et al. Fluoroquinolone-resistant urinary isolate of Escherichia coli from outpatients are frequently multidrug resistant: results from the North American Urinary Tract Infection Collaborative Alliance-Quinolone Resistance Study. Antimicrob Agents Chemother 2006;50(6):2251–4.

49. McNulty CAM, et al. Clinical relevance of laboratory-reported antibiotic resistance in acute uncomplicated urinary tract infection in primary care. J Antimicrob Chemother 2006;58:1000–8.

50. Mazzulli T. Resistance trends in urinary tract pathogens and impact on management. J Urol 2002;168:1720–2.

51. Hillier S, et al. Prior antibiotics and risk of antibiotic-resistant community-acquired urinary tract infection: a case-control study. J Antimicrob Chemother 2007;60:92–9.

52. Alraek T, et al. Acupuncture treatment in the prevention of uncomplicated recurrent lower urinary tract infections in adult women. Am J Public Health 2002;92:1609–11.

53. Alraek T, Baerheim A. An empty and happy feeling in the bladder … : health changes experienced by women after acupuncture for recurrent cystitis. Complement Ther Med 2001;9:219–23.

54. Kontiokari T, et al. Dietary factors affecting susceptibility to urinary tract infection. Pediatr Nephrol 2004;19:378–83.

55. Manges AR, et al. Retail meat consumption and the acquisition of antimicrobial resistant Escherichia coli causing urinary tract infections: a case-control study. Foodborne Pathog Dis 2007;4(4):419–31.

CHAPTER 31

Autoimmune disease

Neville Hartley
ND, MPhil

OVERVIEW

Autoimmune diseases are chronic inflammatory conditions in which the immune system causes organ or systemic damage to the host.[1] Autoimmune diseases refer to a large and heterogeneous group of diseases that affects 7–9% of the population, with women affected disproportionately more than men.[2] Apart from adult-onset diabetes, which affects males more than females, and childhood diseases, which are proportionate across the sexes, the prevalence for autoimmune diseases in females is generally much higher—more than 85% in thyroiditis, systemic sclerosis, systemic lupus erythematosus (SLE) and Sjögren's syndrome patients and up to 60–75% in multiple sclerosis and rheumatoid arthritis (RA).[3] Autoimmune diseases are one of the 10 leading causes of death in women aged under 65 years in the United States.[4]

Although different systems may be involved in different autoimmune diseases, they are generally characterised by chronic inflammation with a loss of tolerance to self-(auto) antigens. The causes for the loss of tolerance—the shift from normal immune function to autoimmune pathology—are poorly understood but are generally agreed to be multifactorial, involving a combination of genetic, environmental, hormonal and immune factors.[5,6] Key mechanisms include abnormal cytokine biology and the direct activation of larger than normal levels of autoreactive (self-reactive) CD4 positive (CD4+) T-cells.

Autoimmunity is a normal event, while autoimmune diseases result from an aberration of this normal phenomenon.[6]

Many theories and hypotheses have been postulated to explain the pathogenesis of autoimmune disease. Perhaps the most dominant is that it occurs in genetically susceptible individuals and is triggered after exposure to certain environmental factors. The order of events seems to be genetic susceptibility, environmental trigger, active autoimmune processes, metabolic alterations and clinical symptoms.

Some specific environmental factors have been identified but many remain to be proven. The most potent environmental factors are viral and bacterial infections. The search for mechanisms for how infections and other environmental factors influence genetic function has led to focused attention on epigenetic regulation—how gene expression is altered without changing DNA sequencing. The most influential points for epigenetic regulation appear to be at the level of DNA methylation and histone modification. Environmental factors that interact with these pathways are of particular interest as they may influence the course of autoimmunity.

Recently, a new theory for understanding chronic inflammatory and autoimmune diseases has been proposed. This theory builds upon the recent discovery of the extent of the human microbiome, various communities of microbial organisms and their genomes known to colonise humans. One of the most striking discoveries of the Human Genome Project (HGP) was that the human genome is not the only genome present in modern humans but there are many more genomes of microbial origin present inside human tissue, outweighing human genomes by an order of magnitude. Further, these microbial organisms are metabolically active, using similar metabolic processes to humans, perhaps with the potential to profoundly affect human metabolism and physiology through gene–gene interactions between microbe and human genes. Based on the findings from the HGP, Marshall et al. propose that host microbes play a critical role in human chronic inflammatory diseases, particularly autoimmune diseases.[7,8] There are significant research projects currently underway to elucidate the role of human microbiota in health and chronic diseases. The next few years of findings will be an exciting time for health research and may hold some breakthroughs in our understanding of the underlying causes and drivers of chronic inflammatory diseases.

Conventionally, autoimmune disorders were diagnosed and treated by clinicians specialising in the particular system involved, as shown in Table 31.1. This was followed by a move to group the wide spectrum of autoimmune diseases by their common

Table 31.1
Major autoimmune diseases

Autoimmune disease	System(s)	Main organs affected
SLE	Systemic	Skin, joints, kidneys, lungs, heart, brain and blood cells
RA	Systemic; muscular skeletal	Connective tissue in joints
Dermatitis herpetiformis	Integumentary	Skin, particularly elbows, knees, back and back of neck
Multiple sclerosis	Nervous	Myelin sheath in neurons of brain and spinal chord
Myasthenia gravis	Nervous; neuromuscular junction	Muscles, particularly the muscles around the eyes
Pernicious anaemia	Blood (haematological); gastrointestinal	Parietal cells in stomach
Goodpasture's syndrome	Renal; respiratory	Kidney and lungs
Graves' disease (hyperthyroidism)	Endocrine	Thyroid gland
Hashimoto's thyroiditis	Endocrine	Thyroid gland
Type 1 diabetes mellitus	Endocrine	Pancreatic beta cells
Coeliac disease	Gastrointestinal	Villi in small intestine
Ulcerative colitis (inflammatory bowel disease)	Gastrointestinal	Mucosa of colon, particularly large colon
Crohn's disease	Gastrointestinal	Can affect entire colon wall, most commonly the lower ileum

underlying mechanisms—chronic inflammation driven by abnormal cytokine biology and the direct activation of larger than normal levels of autoreactive CD4+ T-cells.[9] Future research should continue to provide further insights into autoimmune disease processes, perhaps by shifting our understanding to include genetic relationships with microbiological genomes living within humans in symbiotic homoeostasis, disturbances to which may lead to and drive chronic diseases. Working clinically with people with autoimmune diseases involves taking a holistic approach to the person and also taking account of these multiple approaches (conventional systems-based approach, underlying inflammatory imbalance and genetic and epigenetic factors, including potential interactions with microbial and environmental factors).

Genetic factors

In the immune system, cell surface protein molecules called human leucocyte antigens (HLA) recognise self from non-self. HLA antigens are unique for each individual and are encoded by a group of genes called the major histocompatibility complex (MHC). Certain MHC class II genotypes have been associated with increased susceptibility to autoimmune diseases. In practice, most autoimmune diseases involve multiple mutations. Critically, not everyone who is positive for a genetic mutation associated with an autoimmune disease clinically manifests the disease. Of those who do, there is a wide variation in the progression and severity of the disease. This implies there are other factors, genetic and non-genetic, controlling and regulating genes in the pathogenesis of autoimmune disease and providing the potential for lifestyle and clinical interventions.[10]

As a result of the complete coding of the human genome and subsequent work on haplotype maps, there are currently 68 known genetic mutations associated with autoimmune diseases. Many are clustered across multiple autoimmune diseases, suggesting common underlying pathologies.[11] Specific gene-environment interactions are increasingly being discovered. For researchers, it is challenging to understand precisely which genetic contexts are vulnerable to which environmental factors and by which mechanisms. This research will take time, but this knowledge will be critical for future prevention strategies. For instance, a nutrient–genetic interaction has been identified that increases the risk of multiple sclerosis (MS). Individuals with a certain mutated allele in the MHC class II genes have a threefold increase in the risk of developing MS. In addition, this mutant allele is sensitive to vitamin D, and the risk of MS in those with the mutation is significantly increased by the deficiency of vitamin D.[12] Children of parents with MS are therefore advised to supplement with **vitamin D** as a precautionary measure.

Epigenetics

Epigenetics are the changes to the genetic function that do not structurally change the genetic DNA sequence. Epigenetic changes occur through marks that appear on the genome, which permanently alters genetic expression and cell function. While the genetic traits determine the genotype, the epigenetic traits largely determine the phenotype. Unlike genetic traits, which remain stable over the life span, epigenetic traits are readily influenced by environmental factors. Epigenetic marks are heritable from generation to generation. The main types of epigenetic marks observed in autoimmune disease involve changes to DNA methylation and/or histone modifications. Defects in DNA methylation are associated with autoimmune diseases, including SLE, RA, systemic sclerosis, dermatomyositis and insulin-dependent (type 1) diabetes.

Dietary micronutrients, such as genistein and polyphenols, can modify epigenetic marks, particularly those pertaining to DNA methylation and histone modification.[13] For instance, DNA methylation is readily influenced by the availability of methyl donors, such as folate, or the cofactors required by the enzymes that are involved in methylation, vitamin B6, vitamin B12, choline and methionine. A deficiency or excess in any of these micronutrients could directly alter the production of *S*-adenosylmethionine (SAMe), which is required for the methylation of DNA. Other nutrients required for DNA methylation include selenium, genistein and green tea polyphenols. Nutritional factors can influence histone modification by altering the functioning of histone-modifying enzymes or altering the concentration of their substrates. Copper, dietary and green tea polyphenols and butyrate (a short-chain fatty acid produced in the colon by bacterial fermentation of carbohydrates) have all been shown to suppress various histone-modifying enzymes.[13]

Environmental factors

Of all the environmental factors known to induce active autoimmunity in susceptible individuals, infections are the most significant. In addition to ordinary infections, there has recently been the emergence of superantigens that are able to short circuit the inflammatory response and initiate a cytokine storm. Other known environmental factors include certain chemicals, such as cigarette smoke and crystalline silica, reproductive hormones and mechanical injury.[10,14,15]

Infections may be viral, bacterial and other infectious microorganisms. Infections can trigger autoimmunity via molecular mimicry and promote autoimmune pathology via bystander activation (see Delogu et al.[16] for a comprehensive review on these processes). Bystander activation refers to the spontaneous activation of local autoreactive CD4 cells as part of a coordinated inflammatory response, which may occur as a result of any threat to homoeostasis, such as infection.[17] Molecular mimicry is the term given to the process of activation of autoreactive helper CD4 cells or cytotoxic CD8 cells through cross-reactivity between foreign antigens and autoantigens. The foreign antigen may so closely resemble an autoantigen that the immune system, having reacted successfully to this foreign antigen, starts reacting to the autoantigen as well.[18] In humans molecular mimicry is implicated in the progression of gastric disease to pancreatic autoimmune disease via *Helicobacter pylori* infection.[19]

A group of bacteria called superantigens (SAs), which includes *Staphylococcus aureus* and *Streptococcus pyogenes*, are the most potent naturally occurring biological activators of T helper lymphocytes. SAs seem to short-cut the usual immune mechanisms of presentation to MHC II complexes on the cell surface and directly trigger both CD4 and CD8 cells to launch the full inflammatory response. The result is a sudden and enormous release of pro-inflammatory cytokines from T-cells, especially tumour necrosis factor alpha (TNF-α) and interleukin-2 beta IL-2. This is known as systemic inflammatory response syndrome and has been associated with serious infections, pneumonia, sepsis and toxic shock syndrome. Chronic, low-level exposure to SAs is thought to contribute to autoimmune pathology, and that such exposure may occur naturally in carriers of SAs. Roughly 20–30% of the population are asymptomatic permanent or intermittent carriers of *Staphylococcus aureus*, particularly in the skin or upper airways. Under favourable conditions, these colonies also produce one or more SAs, which can be readily absorbed through the skin or respiratory mucosa and bind to antigen-presenting cells. Whether full immune response is activated, launching active autoimmunity, depends on many factors including the strain of the SAs, the cells that bind them, the presence of autoreactive antigens and the co-stimulation signals by nearby cytokines.

While environmental factors are an important trigger, the progression from exposure to disease is mediated and regulated by cytokines.[20] Cytokine biology therefore provides a useful intervention point for lifestyle and clinical interventions.[15]

Inflammatory mechanisms

For the past two decades the field of immunology has embraced a Th1–Th2 hypothesis paradigm,[21] which depicted many disease states to be characterised by the functional relationship between T helper type 1 (Th1) cells and T helper type 2 (Th2) cells. Th1 cells augment a predominately cellular immune response and a dominance of Th1 differentiation mediates a potent inflammatory response and an ongoing predominance of Th1 cytokines, such as IL-1 and TNF-α.[9] Th2 cells activate and coordinate a predominately humoral immune response.[22] It was generally believed that Th1 dominant responses evolved to aid host clearance of intracellular pathogens and Th2 dominant responses evolved to defend primarily against parasitic helminth.[23] Within this Th1–Th2 paradigm, most autoimmune diseases had been viewed as Th1-driven disorders.[22]

The discovery of T helper 17 cells demonstrated that CD4 subsets were much more diverse than had previously been appreciated. It is believed that Th17 cells have evolved as a specific response to extracellular bacteria, fungi and microbes that were not particularly well handled by either the Th1 or the Th2 dominated responses.[23] Increased levels of Th17 cells have been found to be associated with both animal and human autoimmune diseases.[24] Many cytokines, such as IL-1, IL-6, IL-21, TNF-α, IL-23 and TGF-β, are known to stimulate IL-17 production from naive CD4 cells in the presence of inflammatory stimuli such as toll-like receptors (TLRs).[24] TLRs are pattern recognition receptors that have evolved to recognise specific bacteria and are found on many antigen-presenting cells, such as dendritic cells, in the innate immune system. When activated TLRs induce inflammation via activation of inflammatory transcription factors such as nuclear factor kappa B (NF-κB), which up-regulates the production of pro-inflammatory cytokines such as IL-17 from Th17 cells and IFG-γ from Th1 cells. Th17 cells are now recognised as representing a new arm of adaptive immunity, specific for chronic inflammatory and autoimmune states.

In summary, there are four established subsets of Th differentiation; Th1, Th2, Th17 and T_{reg} (Figure 31.1); Th17 and T_{reg} have the most relevance to autoimmunity. These subsets are not static but have demonstrated placidity; for instance, Th17 and T_{reg} cells can convert from one to another.[25] T_{reg} is an area offering new potential for clinical interventions in preventing and treating autoimmune pathology. Infusion and injection with iT_{reg} cells have shown clinical benefit in animal studies; more simple, natural interventions are also being demonstrated. For instance, a dietary intervention was shown to enhance iT_{reg} cell functioning in mice. Lupus-prone mice were fasted to induce a reduction in circulating levels of a pro-inflammatory cytokine secreted from adipose cells called leptin.[26] During fasting there was a significant reduction in blood leptin levels. When leptin was introduced back into the diet, the enhancement of T_{reg} cells was reversed. It was therefore concluded that leptin has a suppressive effect on T_{reg} cell function. There may be other dietary and/or lifestyle interventions that may enhance T_{reg} cell function via leptin or other mechanisms. This is an area of significant potential for future research and clinical development.

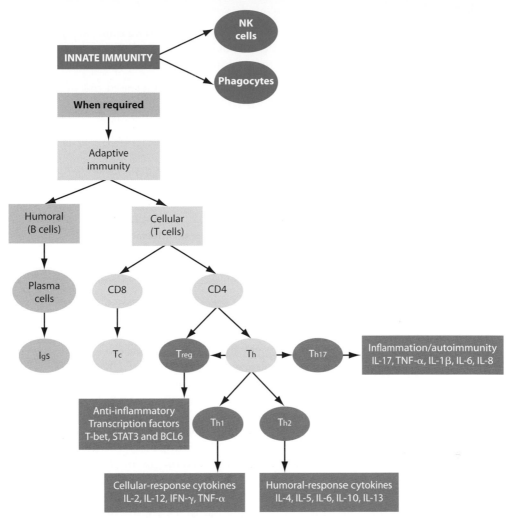

Figure 31.1
Structural overview of immune function*

*Simplified model

DIFFERENTIAL DIAGNOSIS

Due to the multifaceted expression of autoimmune disease affecting a range of bodily systems, the myriad differential diagnoses are not outlined. The diagnosis of an autoimmune disease must be made by a medical practitioner and in many cases a specialist. However, a measure of the professionalism of allied and complementary primary healthcare practitioners is being able to recognise when to refer on for a medical diagnosis. The clinical features provide the biggest clues for doctors and should also red flag allied and complementary practitioners as to when to refer. Medical tests such as blood tests, histology, diagnostic imaging and aspirations generally confirm the diagnosis for medical specialists made on the basis of the clinical history. The clinical features of some specific autoimmune conditions are discussed at the end of this chapter.

RISK FACTORS

The relative importance of genetic and environmental factors to autoimmune pathogenesis and progression remain unclear after decades of intense research. For a comprehensive review of the environmental risk factors in autoimmunity see Dooley et al.[27]

- *Infections.* There is strong epidemiological evidence of an increased risk of SLE with a history of shingles and frequent cold sores (i.e. more than one per year). While infection is a well-known trigger for many autoimmune diseases, the processes involved are at the molecular level and remain subclinical for substantial periods of time. The infection may have been cleared from the system by the time that clinical symptoms arise, making it difficult to gather evidence linking particular pathogens to autoimmune disease.[27]

- *Smoking.* There is strong evidence for an effect of smoking on RA but not SLE. Smoking was a significant risk factor for RA in men and women in a Swedish case control study of 422 cases and 859 controls.[28] In men there was a significant dose-dependent relationship between smoking and RA.

- *Hair dyes.* Weak evidence exists for an effect of the chemicals in permanent hair dye on SLE and connective tissue diseases in a case control study of 265 SLE patients and 355 community controls.[29] There was a 50% increased risk of developing SLE by using permanent hair dyes for all users compared with non-users, but this risk increased with longer term use.

- *Reproductive hormones.* The link between hormones and autoimmune disease has not been well established, despite the prevalence rates being much higher for women. In SLE, 85% of cases are women, yet a case control study of women with the disease ($n = 240$) compared with female controls without the disease ($n = 321$) found little difference in oestrogen or prolactin. In fact, increased exposure to these hormones seemed to offer some protection from SLE. In women who had breastfed, there was a reduced risk of SLE. In women who had early menopause, reducing subsequent exposure to oestrogen by three years or more increased the risk of SLE compared with controls.[27]

- *Occupational exposures.* Silica dust has a strong association with RA, lupus, scleroderma and glomerulonephritis.[30] A meta-analysis of 13 studies of organic solvents in multiple sclerosis found an increased risk after occupational exposure, such as shoe and leather workers and the chemical industry.[31] Solvent exposure has also been found weakly associated with other autoimmune disease risk, including scleroderma and connective tissue disease, and farming and pesticide exposure have also been weakly associated with RA.

- *Psychological stress.* Psychological stress has been shown to increase the risk of autoimmunity in children. In a study of 4400 one-year-old children in the United States,[32] parental stress at birth was associated with increased autoimmune activity at one year. A modern theory is that early trauma influences epigenetic markings, which in turn regulate post-transcriptional expression, increasing pro-inflammatory mediators and/or reducing stress regulatory hormones.[33] In a case-controlled study[34] 22 patients (cases) with autoimmune liver disease and 11 case controls in long-term remission were studied to identify factors associated with relapse. Cases experienced significantly higher psychological stress than controls, while controls identified more coping strategies than cases. Helping people identify resources to facilitate psychological resilience may be an area of clinical importance.

CONVENTIONAL TREATMENT

The goals of conventional treatment include treating the symptoms, controlling the pathology and helping the body's resistance to disease. Specific treatment will depend on the type and severity of the autoimmune disease present. Many people suffer from more than one autoimmune disease. In the first line of defence, simple over-the-counter analgesics and anti-inflammatories are given for symptomatic relief from inflammation.[35] Further medication is determined on a case-by-case basis but is generally anti-inflammatory and/or immunosuppressive in nature.

Anti-inflammatories can be categorised as steroidal or nonsteroidal. Steroidal anti-inflammatories include corticosteroid drugs, such as cortisone, hydrocortisone, prednisone and prednisolone. They work by binding to cortisol receptors. High doses may be given for short periods of time, with the goal of reduction to the minimum effective dose. Long-term use is not advisable but may not be avoidable for some people, and serious side effects should be discussed with patients including the risk of adrenal insufficiency, osteoporosis and cataracts. Nonsteroidal anti-inflammatory drugs (NSAIDs) inhibit the enzyme cyclooxygenase (COX), which is a key mediator of pro-inflammatory prostaglandins. Commonly used NSAIDs include ibuprofen, aspirin and naproxen. These drugs are also associated with serious side effects and long-term use is not recommended.

Immunosuppressive medication works by preventing the immune system from reacting to or reducing the efficacy of immune responses. An undesirable side effect is that this approach leaves the body vulnerable to opportunistic infections. Cortisone was first discovered in 1950. It is a steroid hormone that is administered by injection; the side effects may include pain around the injection site, weight gain and thinning of skin. Azathioprine was identified in the late 1950s. It suppresses immune cell function by inhibiting purine synthesis that is required for the proliferation of cells. It is listed as a potential carcinogen. Cyclosporine was the third immunosuppressant identified in the 1970s, initially from a fungus. It is a peptide that inhibits intracellular calcium activity of T-cells, thereby preventing the secretion of pro-inflammatory cytokines. Cyclosporine interacts with a wide variety of other drugs and substances. It is associated with a number of serious side effects including hyperplasia, convulsions, peptic ulcers, fever and vomiting.

Disease-modifying drugs are the next tier of autoimmune medications. They aim to improve symptoms by slowing disease progression. Methotrexate inhibits an enzyme required for folate metabolism, curbing cell proliferation. Although it was designed as a high-dosage anticancer drug, in low doses it appears to have anti-inflammatory effects by inhibiting the production of pro-inflammatory cytokines. It is used widely in RA, as it seems to be effective for some people (rapid onset of four to six weeks in responders) and well tolerated. Side effects may include stomatitis, mouth ulcers and digestive disturbances. Etanercept is a biopharmaceutical (uses recombinant DNA) that binds TNF-α (both in the circulation and locally) and reduces its activity. It is administered by subcutaneous injection. Side effects include susceptibility to opportunistic infection. Abatacept inhibits the activation of T-cells by its actions as a selective co-stimulation modifier, thereby delaying progression to structural damage in autoimmunity. It can be administered intravenously or subcutaneously. Side effects may include back pain, wheezy chest, dizziness and headache and susceptibility to opportunistic infection. Future research is continuing to provide new directions for clinical interventions, perhaps the most promising with IL17 and iT_{regs}.

KEY TREATMENT PROTOCOLS

An overarching naturopathic approach to any autoimmune condition aims to correct the underlying imbalance in cytokine biology in order to reduce the impact of chronic inflammation and associated tissue damage. Factors that are known to influence cytokine biology should be explored in those with autoimmune conditions on a case-by-case basis. In organ-specific conditions, the affected organ should also be supported according to the details given in the relevant chapters in this book. In systemic autoimmune conditions, the affected tissues and organs should also be supported as outlined in other relevant chapters. See Table 31.4 for a general summary of evidence.

Lifestyle and nutraceutical interventions to reduce inflammation

Anti-inflammatory dietary modifications

Two major nutritional factors known to influence cytokine biology beneficially are omega-3 fatty acids and antioxidants. The

> **Naturopathic treatment aims**
>
> - Regulation of cytokine biology:
>   - reduce production of pro-inflammatory cytokines
>   - increase production of regulatory cytokines.
> - Reduce oxidative stress.
> - Reduce and prevent exposure to chronic infection.
> - Support the affected organ/tissue (see relevant chapters).
> - Reduce low-grade systemic metabolic acidosis.
> - Support hypothalamic–pituitary–adrenal (HPA) axis resiliency (see Chapter 18 on stress and fatigue).
> - Reduce and manage psychological, emotional and physical stress and increase psychological coping/resiliency (see Chapters 14–17 on the nervous system).
> - Increase capacity of cellular detoxification pathways.
> - Instigate a program of moderate physical exercise if required.

Western diet is losing the protective antioxidants and omega-3 fatty acids, as they have been gradually processed out of the food supply over time. The loss of these protective factors together with a gain of dietary precursors to inflammatory and pro-oxidant mediators has led to a chronic imbalance in our diet and physiology. The Western diet has effectively become a pro-inflammatory diet.

It is essential that the imbalances of the background diet be fully understood and corrected as a priority in dealing with chronic inflammation. Correcting dietary imbalances has been shown to augment medical interventions, and may reduce reliance upon them.[36,37] **Dietary modifications** that favour balanced immune function should, for the most part, be sustained throughout life. **Lifestyle factors** must also be explored thoroughly for potential pro-inflammatory and protective influences. Pro-inflammatory influences need to be identified and minimised. Psychological stress induces an inflammatory state in the immune system by generating the production of pro-inflammatory cytokines.[38] The impact of stress on pro-inflammatory mediators can be buffered by coping mechanisms.[39]

In broader evolutionary terms the last century or two is an incredibly short period of time. While human protein-coding genes have not significantly changed, there has been a significant and dramatic change in our diet, which corresponds with the rise of 'lifestyle' diseases such as chronic stress, heart disease, cancer, obesity, diabetes, depression and autoimmune diseases. Chronic inflammatory processes form an underlying component of all these diseases. Evidence is mounting that the modern Western diet is a pro-inflammatory diet characterised by high caloric intake made up of a high intake of carbohydrates, saturated, *trans*-fats and an imbalance in essential fatty acids (EFAs).

EFA intakes have the potential to create balance or imbalance in immune function. An imbalance has been related to many modern-day diseases, from mental health problems to chronic inflammation and autoimmune disease. According to Simopoulos[40] the **Palaeolithic diet** consisted of an equal ratio of the two families of EFAs—omega-6 and omega-3 fatty acids. This ratio is currently estimated to be highly unbalanced at 10–15:1 in Australia and even more so in the United States at 20–30:1. Correction of the imbalance between the EFAs has major clinical implications for inflammatory diseases. For example, inflammation was reduced in patients with RA by reducing the ratio of omega-6 to omega-3 fatty acids to 2–3:1.[40]

Carbohydrate intake in the Western diet is much higher than that of most traditional diets and there is a compelling argument that the modern high-carbohydrate diet is associated with negative health outcomes including increased risk of various autoimmune diseases.[41] Grains may contain antinutrients, such as lectins, that reduce absorption of micronutrients in the small intestine and also have been shown to induce intestinal secretion of inflammatory cytokines and up-regulate MHC class II expression in enterocytes, exacerbating inflammation in coeliac disease.[42] The grain protein gliadin was also shown to up-regulate MHC class II presentation in the presence of cytokines in inflammatory bowel disease.[43] Several gliadins are suspected of molecular mimicry.[41]

Early work in nutritional immunology showed that protein- and **calorie-restricted diets** were associated with dramatic alterations in immune function, which were readily demonstrated in several animal models of autoimmune diseases.[44] In animal studies, low-protein diets delayed the onset of autoimmunity and blunted the clinical progression of autoimmune disease. Further, caloric restriction has more than doubled life span.[45] Based on such findings, a 25–40% caloric reduction has been recommended as a safe and effective preventative strategy and treatment for autoimmune diseases in humans. This is, however, a huge undertaking for most people and requires an extraordinary commitment over a very long period of time.

Omega-3 fatty acids

Dietary **omega-3 fatty acids** influence the production of inflammatory metabolites from the omega-6 polyunsaturated fatty acids, arachidonic acid. Recently, the long-chain omega-3 fatty acids, eicosapentaenoic acid (EPA) and docosahexaenoic acid (DHA), have been shown to directly activate gene transcription factors responsible for the regulation of gene expression and activity of cytokines, such as NF-κB and peroxisome proliferator activated receptors (PPARs). DHA has also recently been identified as a substrate for a family of proactive anti-inflammatory mediators called resolvins and protectins.[46]

As a general rule omega-6 fatty acids promote while omega-3 fatty acids inhibit the expression, production, secretion and target cell responsiveness of pro-inflammatory cytokines.[47] Omega-3 and omega-6 fatty acids share the same enzyme system, as illustrated in Figure 31.2. When high levels of omega-6 fatty acids are present, the enzyme shifts its preference to favour omega-6 fatty acids acid metabolism.[48] This means that diets rich in omega-6 fatty acids reduce EFA metabolism and promote the production of arachidonic acid-derived eicosanoids.[49] That is, through competitive inhibition, diets low in omega-3 fatty acids may promote inflammation.

Notes on the images: Sunflower oil and most vegetable oils are rich in linoleic acid, while evening primrose oil capsules are rich in gamma-linolenic acid (GLA), which is quickly metabolised into dihomo-gamma-linolenic acid (dGLA), a precursor for the anti-inflammatory PGE_1 eicosanoids.

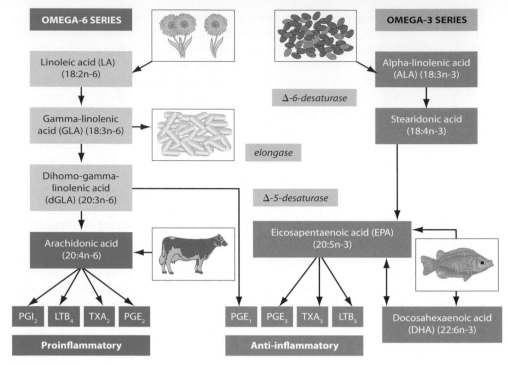

Figure 31.2
The metabolic pathways of essential fatty acids*

*Diagram shows the enzymatic competition for the desaturases and elongases and common food sources.

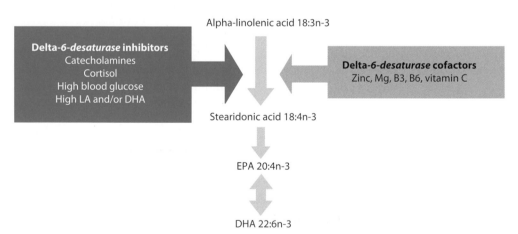

Figure 31.3
Enzyme modifiers of fatty acid conversion

Vegetarians and vegans rely heavily on the activity of liver enzymes for the production of the long-chain omega-3 fatty acids, as they do not consume them in their diet. Figure 31.3 illustrates some of the known influences on delta-6-desaturase. Essential cofactors include **zinc**, **magnesium**, **niacin (B3)**, **pyridoxine (B6)** and **vitamin C**. The stress hormones adrenaline, noradrenaline and cortisol inhibit the enzyme as does high blood sugar levels and high levels of linoleic acid as in the modern Western diet. DHA, as in those taking fish oil supplements, also inhibits these enzymes, hampering the production of arachidonic-derived inflammatory mediators such as prostaglandins and leukotrienes.

The enzyme delta-6-desaturase is the rate-limiting step in eicosanoid synthesis. The stress hormones cortisol and the catecholamines (adrenaline and noradrenaline) inhibit the enzyme. Dietary cofactors, such as zinc, magnesium, vitamins B3 and B6 and vitamin C are also required for optimal enzyme functioning.

Plant sources of omega-3 fatty acids contain **alpha-linolenic acid (ALA)** and are perhaps the predominant source of fatty acids in Western diets. However, the enzymatic conversions from ALA to the longer chain EPA and DHA molecules are not efficient, and are influenced by many factors including the amount of fat in the diet. A rough conversion rate has been proposed at 10–15% from ALA to EPA, and less through to DHA. Fish oil sources such as EPA and DHA predominate in traditional diets such as of the Inuit. Good natural sources of EPA and DHA are directly obtained from oily fresh fish such as sardines, herrings, mackerel, salmon, tuna and other seafood including seaweeds. The box below shows the Australian Government's recommendations for the intake of omega-3 fatty acids. For the prevention of chronic disease, the recommendation is to eat around two oily fish meals per week.

Australian Government recommendations for the intake of omega-3 fatty acids—NHMRC* recommendations

Adequate intake

ALA: 1.3 g/day for men; 0.8 g/day for women

EPA + DHA: 160 mg/day for men; 90 mg/day for women

Strategic daily intake (prevention of chronic disease)

EPA + DHA: 610 mg/day for men; 430 mg/day for women

*National Health and Medical Research Council

Dietary considerations to reduce pro-inflammatory cytokines

- Limit red meat to maximum of three meals per week.
- Cut down all junk food, pre-packaged food, take-away meals and all foods containing 'vegetable oil' such as corn chips, mayonnaise and biscuits.
- Eat at least three fish meals per week, preferably oily fish.
- Reduce consumption of grains.
- Use dairy sparingly.
- Limit simple sugars.
- Reduce salt intake; choose no-added-salt products, such as tinned tomatoes.
- Snack on dried fruits and nuts.
- Drink fresh vegetable juices weekly.
- Limit coffee and caffeinated beverages.
- Drink green tea and herbal teas daily.
- Use olive oil for all cooking; use vegetable oils sparingly or not at all.
- Eat plenty of brightly coloured vegetables.

Antioxidants

One mechanism by which the production of pro-inflammatory cytokines may be reduced is via suppression of NF-κB. Within minutes of activation it up-regulates the expression of the genes for many pro-inflammatory cytokines. Activators of NF-κB include reactive oxygen species (ROS), pro-inflammatory cytokines, bacteria and viruses, ultraviolet radiation, hypoxia and growth factors. Activation of NF-κB is involved in the pathogenesis of autoimmune diseases such as RA. Thus, agents that can block NF-κB activation, such as the glucocorticoids, may be effective interventions in autoimmune diseases.[50] The major polyphenol in **green tea**, epigallocatechin-3-gallate (EGCG), has been shown to block the activation of NF-κB, coinciding with reduced activation of autoantigen-specific T-cells in humans with MS.[51,52] DHA[53] has also been shown to be an effective inhibitor of NF-κB through multiple mechanisms.

High levels of the amino acids **arginine** and **glutamine** were shown to inhibit NF-κB. In 10 patients with Crohn's disease, colonic biopsies were cultured with low or high amounts of arginine and glutamine, respectively. The formula with the pharmacological levels of both amino acids significantly reduced the production of the pro-inflammatory gene transcription factor NF-κB and the cytokines TNF-α, IL-1β, IL-6 and IL-8 in the culture medium.[54] The **citrus bioflavonoids** luteolin,[55] quercetin[56] and 3'-hydroxy-flavone have been shown to block activation of NF-κB.[57] These studies indicate that there may be many nutritional factors that influence this important early stage of inflammation.

Alpha-lipoic acid is a potent antioxidant that appears to work in a multitude of ways. It is a free radical scavenger, it regenerates other antioxidants such as vitamin C and E, raises intracellular glutathione (GTS), crosses the blood–brain barrier and has important anti-inflammatory properties. It prevented the onset of autoimmune disease in the mouse model of MS and also reduced the severity of symptoms in established disease.[58] A pilot randomised clinical trial in people with MS who took the study medication before meals for two weeks[59] found that alpha-lipoic acid suppressed markers of leucocyte trafficking in a dose-dependent manner. High doses of alpha-lipoic acid reduced leucocyte trafficking into the brain of people with MS.[58]

Genistein is an isoflavone with anti-inflammatory, antioxidant and apoptotic properties. Genistein binds to human oestrogen receptors on immune cells.[60] Genistein reduced inflammatory and increased anti-inflammatory mediators during autoimmune pathology in animals.[60] This corresponded with significant improvements in clinical signs of disease progression for the genistein-treated group, evident in less weight loss and lower total clinical score, reduced leucocyte trafficking and less endothelial adherence in the brain. Such animal studies suggest that genistein may offer effective protection at the blood–brain barrier by regulating cytokine profiles. **Quercetin** is a phyto–oestrogenic flavanol with anti-inflammatory properties.[61] Quercetin reduced the severity and duration of paralysis as well as effecting reductions of central nervous system demyelination and inflammation in animal models of MS.[62]

Resveratrol is a polyphenol compound found in red wine with oestrogenic, antioxidant and anti-inflammatory properties.[63] Its mechanisms of action include inhibition of the production of pro-inflammatory cytokines and COX-2 via inhibition of NF-κB.[64] Resveratrol significantly delayed the onset of autoimmune pathology and halved the clinical symptoms in a dose-dependent manner in animal models. The reduction in the clinical scores corresponded with less inflammatory-related damage in the central nervous system. Serum IL-17 was significantly reduced in the resveratrol group as compared with placebos. Resveratrol also increased IL-6 as compared with controls. Resveratrol was also found to induce cell death in activated autoreactive T-cells.[63]

In summary, promising research into the mechanisms for dietary anti-inflammatory agents in autoimmune disease continues. Clinical trials are required to determine the optimal amount of these compounds required for effective interventions. However, it is likely that a diet rich in these and other anti-inflammatory compounds may have a cumulative, possibly synergistic, effect, all helping to keep oxidative stress levels low and preventing the unnecessary activation of NF-κB, thereby helping to regulate pro-inflammatory cytokine expression and activity.

Herbs with anti-inflammatory properties

Boswellia serrata (BS) was traditionally used for treating a range of conditions, including inflammation. The anti-inflammatory agents in BS resin are the boswellic acids, which have been shown to act as nonsteroidal anti-inflammatory agents, inhibiting 5-lipoxygenase activity and thereby suppressing leukotriene production.[65–67] A systematic review of all randomised controlled trials (RCTs) of *Boswellia serrata* in inflammatory disease states concluded that there was 'encouraging but not compelling' evidence for the use of BS for inflammatory conditions. Although the study of RA patients did not find any significant differences between groups, the BS group cut their NSAID use more than did the placebo group.[68]

Boswellia caution

Boswellia serrata has been shown to inhibit in vitro all the major human drug detoxification enzymes, cytochrome P450 1A2/2C8/2C9/2C19/2D6 and 3A4 enzymes.[69] This has implications for herb–drug interactions, as these enzymes are involved in the metabolism of 95% of pharmaceutical drugs.[70] By inhibiting the metabolism of pharmaceuticals, *Boswellia serrata* may potentiate an overdose of other drugs. Until further research can clarify the clinical relevance of these interactions for therapeutic doses of *Boswellia serrata*, it may be best to avoid this herb in patients taking other medications.

Harpagophytum procumbens has been used traditionally for centuries to treat arthritic conditions, pain and a range of other conditions.[71] The extract from the roots is now a licensed medicine in Germany.[72] A systematic review found there is good evidence for the use of *Harpagophytum procumbens* in degenerative joint diseases and other chronic inflammatory diseases.[71] The main active is harpagoside, which was shown to inhibit COX-2 expression comparable with ibuprofen but harpagide, another active compound found in the extract, was shown to significantly stimulate COX-2 activity by twofold.[72] Therefore, anti-inflammatory activity will be most effective in solutions with high harpagosides and low harpagides. The mechanism of action is not clear, but it was shown to inhibit the secretion of the pro-inflammatory cytokines, COX-2, iNOS and other inflammatory mediators.[73]

Uncaria **spp.** has been used for centuries in Peru to support immune function.[74] It is widely used as an anti-inflammatory herb and has been shown to significantly inhibit the activation of NF-κB,[75] and pro-inflammatory cytokines by 65–85%.[76] There are two species, *Uncaria tomentosa* and *Uncaria guianensis,* which are used interchangeably in South America, but most Western preparations contain *Uncaria tomentosa* due to its ease of standardisation.[77] In a study comparing the antioxidant and anti-inflammatory activity of the two species, it was found that *Uncaria guianensis* was the better antioxidant and stronger anti-inflammatory.

Curcumin, the active constituent of **Curcuma longa**, has demonstrated therapeutic effects in a wide range of autoimmune diseases.[78] Curcumin was found to be twice as potent as the NSAID phenylbutazone during acute inflammation but only half as powerful during chronic inflammation.[79] Curcumin was shown to inhibit the ex vivo stimulated production of pro-inflammatory cytokines.[80]

A study of 54 traditional Mexican Indian herbs found that only three were able to inhibit NF-κB. All belong to the *Asteraceae* family and are rich in sesquiterpene lactones (SL).[81] **Tanacetum parthenium** contains high levels of the SL parthenolide, which has been shown to be anti-inflammatory by inhibiting the activation of NF-κB.[82,83] **Urtica dioica** has also been shown to be a potent inhibitor of NF-κB. A standardised extract used in Germany as a commercial drug preparation (IDS23, Rheuma-Hek) was shown to be effective at the inhibition of ex vivo NF-κB activation in human cells.[84] After oral administration of IDS23 for 7 and 21 days in 20 healthy volunteers, there was an inhibition in the ex vivo lipopolysaccharide (LPS) stimulated TNF-α release of 14.6% and 24.0%, respectively, while IL-1β was inhibited by 19.2% and 39.3%, respectively.[85]

Hemidesmus indicus was shown to inhibit the ex vivo production of the pro-inflammatory cytokines.[80] Anethole, a constituent of **Foeniculum vulgare**, has been shown to block NF-κB activation.[86] In 14 renal patients with increased blood levels of TNF-α and reduced levels of IL-10, glomerular dysfunction and proteinuria, 900–1125 mg/day **Ganoderma lucidum** was shown to reduce TNF-α and increase IL-10 and correct renal dysfunction, including suppressing proteinuria.[87]

Essential oils have been used since antiquity for religious and medicinal purposes. In the ancient world Egyptians consumed vast quantities of *Boswellia papyrifera* and *Commiphora erythraea* in their religious cults and in later times the French discovered that essential oils possess strong antimicrobial activity.[88] Recently the ingestion of essential oils has shown promise in various animal studies for reducing inflammation (Table 31.2) and modulating the immune response (Table 31.3), suggesting a potential role in treating autoimmune disorders.

Lifestyle modifications with potential anti-inflammatory effects

Lifestyle factors, such as diet, physical exercise, mental stress and resilience, all have profound effects on the body physiology. Indeed, even **body posture** has been shown to have an effect on body physiology concerning the stress hormone cortisol. When people express power through open, expansive postures it increases testosterone and reduces cortisol.[96]

All relevant lifestyle factors should be identified and managed on a case-by-case basis with people with autoimmune disease seeking treatment. As information on epigenetics becomes available in future, individual tailoring of lifestyle advice will become much more individualised.

Maintain adequate physical activity

There appears to be many mechanisms by which physical exercise mediates beneficial effects on the immune system (see Chapter 3 on wellness, Chapter 25 on osteoarthritis and Chapter 26 on fibromyalgia).[97] Perhaps the most interesting is that skeletal muscle acts as a storehouse of the branched-chain amino acids, which supply nitrogen for the synthesis of glutamine by skeletal muscle. Skeletal glutamine supplies the rest of the body with glutamine as a precursor for the antioxidant glutathione.

Table 31.2
Anti-inflammatory essential oils

Intervention	Key findings	Comment
Eucalyptus citriodora, Eucalyptus tereticornis and *Eucalyptus globulus*[89]	Subcutaneous administration of essential oil extracts from three eucalyptus species inhibited carrageenan-induced rat paw oedema and neutrophil migration into rat peritoneal cavities, and vascular permeability induced by carrageenan and histamine	These findings suggest that essential oil extracts from three eucalyptus species possess neutrophil-dependent and independent anti-inflammatory activities
Aloe barbadensis[90]	Aloe vera oil inhibited lipoxygenase activity by 96% at a concentration of 0.5 µg/mL in vitro using the lipoxygenase inhibitor-screening assay	Aloe vera oil exhibited very strong anti-inflammatory activity
Thymus vulgaris[90]	Thyme oil inhibited lipoxygenase activity by 86% at a concentration of 0.5 µg/mL in vitro using the lipoxygenase inhibitor-screening assay	Thyme oil exhibited strong anti-inflammatory activity
Citrus bergamia[90]	Bergamot oil inhibited lipoxygenase activity by 85% at a concentration of 0.5 µg/mL in vitro using the lipoxygenase inhibitor-screening assay	Bergamot exhibited strong anti-inflammatory activity
Anthemis nobilis[90]	Chamomile oil showed slight lipoxygenase inhibitory activity at 0.5 µg/mL but strong lipoxygenase inducing activity at 5 µg/mL (−123%) in vitro using the lipoxygenase inhibitor-screening assay	Chamomile oil exhibited weak anti-inflammatory activity in low doses and inflammatory activity in higher doses
Melaleuca alternifolia[91]	Tea tree oil inhibited pro-inflammatory cytokine IL-2 from human peripheral blood mononuclear cells (PBMC) and increased anti-inflammatory cytokines IL-4 (at 0.1% concentration) and IL-10 (at 0.01% concentration) in vitro. Tea tree oil reduced ROS production throughout the kinetic study	Tea tree oil is an anti-inflammatory mediator due to its antioxidant activity and by reducing the proliferation of inflammatory cells without affecting their capacity to secrete anti-inflammatory cytokines

Cells that rapidly proliferate—such as immune cells, especially during inflammation—are highly dependent on skeletal glutamine release via muscle contractions during physical exercise. This has particular implications for autoimmune diabetes, as pancreatic beta cells have reduced expression and activity of glutathione and rely heavily on a systemic supply. Skeletal muscles release glutamine into the blood stream after physical

Table 31.3
Immunomodulating essential oils

Intervention	Key findings	Comment
Syzygium aromaticum (clove)[92]	Clove essential oil administered orally to immunised mice for one week increased total white blood cell (WBC) count, and enhanced the delayed-type hypersensitivity (DTH) response Cellular and humoral immune responses were restored in cyclophosphamide-immunosuppressed mice in a dose-dependent manner	Clove essential oil improved cell-mediated and humoral immune response mechanisms, demonstrating immunomodulatory activity Clove essential oil exerted immunomodulatory/ anti-inflammatory effects by inhibiting LPS action
Syzygium aromaticum[93]	Clove essential oil inhibited the production of pro-inflammatory cytokines IL-6 and IL-1β from LPS-stimulated peritoneal macrophages	
Zingiber officinale (ginger)[92]	Ginger essential oil administered orally to immunised mice for one week restored the humoral immune response in cyclophosphamide-immunosuppressed mice No significant effect on total WBC or DTH response	Ginger essential oil recovered the humoral immune response in immunosuppressed mice
Rosmarinus officinalis (rosemary)[94]	Rosemary essential oil administered orally to rats reduced the number of leucocytes that rolled, adhered and migrated to the scrotal chamber after carrageenan injection (in vivo) All doses of rosemary essential oil tested significantly inhibited leucocyte chemotaxis induced by casein (in vitro)	The effects of rosemary essential oil on leucocyte migration highlight an important mechanism of the anti-inflammatory action of rosemary
Petroselinum crispum (parsley)[95]	Parsley essential oil suppressed phytohaemagglutinin (PHA) and LPS-stimulated splenocyte proliferation and nitric oxide production in LPS-stimulated macrophages	Parsley essential oil demonstrated immunomodulatory activity on cellular and humoral immune responses

exercise at a very high rate.[98] Muscle contractions during physical exercise may therefore offset pancreatic beta cell glutamine depletion, and subsequent increase in GHS levels and antioxidant protective mechanisms.

Physical exercise elicits a cytokine response in the body. The type of physical exercise is a determinant of the particular cytokine response. **Moderate physical exercise** has been shown to induce anti-inflammatory cytokines (IL-1 receptor antagonist and IL-10), which offers protection against inflammation and autoimmune diseases.[99] Therefore, physical exercise affects immune function in a number of different ways including increasing regulatory cytokines and increasing antioxidants.

Enhance psychological resilience

Potential stressors need to be identified and reduced and available coping resources need to be increased (see nervous [Chapters 14–16] and endocrine [Chapters 18–20] system sections for further detail). This may include access to resources that help to increase psychological resilience. This may include referral for **psychological counselling**, **yoga**, **meditation** or **relaxation training**, **relationship counselling**, financial advice or other stress and mood management interventions. Protective lifestyle factors need to be instigated and sustained throughout life in all individuals interested in balancing immune function, and especially those with chronic inflammation.

Research into the newly established field of psychoneuroimmunology (PNI) (see box) has greatly advanced our understanding of the psychological and emotional factors that influence immune function. We know that negative and stressful emotions directly stimulate the production of pro-inflammatory cytokines that mediate and intensify disease.[100] The idea that emotions affect health outcomes is not new and can be dated as far back as Hippocrates. What is new is that, through PNI, science is providing evidence to support the 'mind–body' link.[101] **Laughter**,[102] **meditation**,[103,104] **spiritual beliefs**,[105] **positive thinking**[106] and even **choir singing and listening**[107] have all been shown to beneficially influence immune parameters.

Psychoneuroimmunology

Psychoneuroimmunology (PNI) is the interaction between psychological processes and the nervous and the immune systems. The relationship between the nervous and the immune systems is bidirectional, with cytokines playing a pivotal role in this relationship. For instance, negative emotions directly stimulate the production of pro-inflammatory cytokines that intensify disease and, accordingly, disease produces cytokines that have substantial effects on the nervous system, including production and enhancement of negative moods, a range of sickness behaviours from shivering to loss of appetite and physical symptoms including fatigue and lethargy.[108]

Stress is one of the most well-studied and well-known psychological processes that have been shown to affect the immune system. Chronic stress most often appears to be associated with suppressed immune function. In vivo studies have shown that chronic stress reduces natural killer cell activity, T lymphocyte proliferation in response to a mitogen, T helper cells and antibody levels.[109–111] Furthermore, chronic stress increases the susceptibility to infection and is associated with the onset, duration and recovery from illness.[112,113]

The link between emotions and illness is well known, with negative emotions such as anxiety, depression and hostility being shown to contribute to disease and verifiable health outcomes.[114] Anxiety, depression and hostility have been associated with increased risk of heart disease and coronary related death. In the normative ageing study higher levels of anxiety were associated with almost double the risk of fatal coronary heart disease.[115] In a 13-year prospective study individuals with major depression had 4.5 times greater risk of heart attack compared with those with no history of depression.[116] A nine-year population study including 2125 male subjects aged 42–60 years found that men with high hostility had more than twice the risk of all-cause and cardiovascular mortality compared with men low in hostility.[117,118]

In a study the effects of interpersonal stress on disease activity were examined for married women with RA who had differing qualities of spousal relationships. Women with better spousal relationships did not show increases in disease activity following an episode of interpersonal stress, suggesting that women with stronger marital relationships were less vulnerable to interpersonal stress.[119]

INTEGRATIVE MEDICAL CONSIDERATIONS

Psychological counselling and cognitive behaviour therapy

Strong emotions usually accompany autoimmune disease diagnoses but must be managed, particularly as chronic stress and depression can lead to increased inflammation and the potential for flares.[120] Refer these patients for counselling to help work through any stress and distress about the disease and other life stress. Education about how to manage the disease, the medications and the role of emotions can help to cope with the diagnosis.[121] Accessing supportive resources such as professional counselling in the community is measure of reliance.

A brief pain and stress management program incorporating biofeedback and cognitive behaviour therapy was shown to be significantly more effective than symptom monitoring (placebo) or usual care (no intervention controls) at reducing pain and physical symptoms in 92 people with SLE in a randomised placebo-controlled trial.[122] Psychological functioning was improved in the active intervention group compared with placebo, while the usual care group (controls) actually deteriorated over time.

Homeopathy

Many people with autoimmune diseases believe that homeopathy may be helpful, though whether this is due to specific homeopathic activity or placebo response is contested.[123] In a survey of 413 people with IBD, 52% had tried complementary and alternative medicine (CAM), and homeopathy was the most frequent CAM reported (55% of CAM users).[124] A survey of people with MS showed a similar trend.[125] Part of the reasons for the common use of homeopathy seems to be dissatisfaction with conventional treatment and its side effects, and the fact that homeopathy can be used alongside conventional medicine.[126]

In a randomised placebo-controlled trial of 112 patients using homeopathy in RA, there were significant improvements in pain (18%) and articular index (24%) for both the placebo and active group. There was a huge dropout rate in the six-month study, which caused some methodological issues. Most of the homeopathic prescriptions were for sulfur 30C and *Rhus toxicodendron* 6C and 30C.[127] In an earlier RCT using homeopathy or placebo in RA patients who were also using their own medication, those in the homeopathy group had significant improvement in pain, articular index, stiffness and grip compared with the placebo group.[128]

This body of research is promising and provides some preliminary evidence for an effect for homeopathy. There is obviously a need for much more research into the efficacy of homeopathy in autoimmune conditions. These conditions are complex and require multifaceted approaches. Perhaps there is a role for homeopathy, which may one day be validated with much stronger evidence than we have today.

Traditional Chinese medicine

In a randomised, double-blinded controlled trial 53 patients with mild to moderate SLE disease activity took the Chinese medicine formula Dan-Chi-Liu-Wei (composed of 2.7 g Liu-Wei-Di-Huang Wan and 125 mg Dan-Chi San) three times per day for six months as an add-on therapy to steroid and disease-modifying antirheumatic drugs (DMARDs). These patients demonstrated a reduction in SLE disease activity index compared with control, but it was not possible to taper the dosage of steroid after six months of the clinical trial.[129]

Jianpi Qingchang decoction (JQD) is a Chinese formula consisting of nine medicinal herbs (*Astragalus membranaceus, Coptis chinensis, Codonopsis pilosula, Portulaca oleracea, Radix sanguisorbae, Panax notoginseng, Bletillae rhizome, Radix aucklandiae, Glycyrrhiza uralensis*) used to treat TCM 'spleen deficiency' and 'dampness-heat syndrome' ulcerative colitis (UC). For eight weeks, 120 active UC patients with spleen deficiency and dampness-heat syndrome were randomly treated with JQD 400 mL/day or first-line medical treatment (5-amino salicyclic acid). Both treatment groups significantly reduced the Sutherland Disease Activity Index, but no significance was found between the two groups. JQD significantly relieved bowel and systemic symptoms and improved bodily pain, physical function, vitality and mental health compared to first-line medical treatment. Thus, JQD can improve the quality of life in active UC patients with spleen deficiency and dampness-heat syndrome. Although JQD showed promising results, a multicentered clinical trial with a larger sample population is required to validate this study.[130]

Tripterygium wilfordii Hook F (TwHF) is a traditional Chinese herb with therapeutic effect in inflammatory and autoimmune conditions such as RA and CD, and is widely used in China to treat CD. In a randomised, controlled, open-labelled trial, 2 mg/kg/day of TwHF significantly lowered CD Activity Index scores and Simple Endoscopic Scores for CD (SESCD) compared to mesalazine and a lower dose TwHF (1.5 mg/kg/day) in 198 patients with mild-moderate CD after 52 weeks. Clinical recurrence was significantly lower in patients receiving the high-dose TwHF compared to patients taking mesalazine or the lower dose TwHF. The overall findings of the study suggest TwHF as an effective maintenance treatment for CD; however, further research blinding the participants and the researchers would increase the validity of the study.[131]

Acupuncture

Pain and fatigue are common complaints in autoimmune diseases, particularly SLE. A double-blinded pilot RCT evaluated the effects of acupuncture as an adjunct to usual medical care on pain and fatigue in 24 patients over five weeks (two sessions per week). Forty per cent of patients who received acupuncture or minimal needling had 30% or more improvement on standard measures of pain, but no improvement in pain was demonstrated in those who received usual medical treatment without needling. Clinical improvement in fatigue was less striking, with 13% and 25% of acupuncture and minimal needling reporting greater vitality, whereas no usual-care participants met the improvement standard.[132]

Acupuncture was investigated for its effects on pain in RA patients in a systematic review. Eight RCTs were included in the review, which consisted of acupuncture with or without moxibustion. The findings provided no convincing evidence that acupuncture with or without moxibustion was beneficial for treating RA.[133] In another systematic review conducted in the same year acupuncture was shown in six out of eight studies included in the review to decrease pain in RA patients compared with controls; however, conflicting evidence existed in placebo-controlled trials concerning the efficacy of acupuncture for RA.[134] In a prospective, randomised, controlled, single-blind clinical trial 51 patients with mild to moderate active Crohn's disease were treated with acupuncture and moxibustion over a period of four weeks (10 sessions) and followed up for 12 weeks. The results showed a statistically significant change in the Crohn's activity index (CDAI) in the traditional Chinese medicine group versus the control group, which correlated with improved general wellbeing in the traditional Chinese medicine group compared with the control.[135]

SPECIFIC AUTOIMMUNE DISORDERS

Rheumatoid arthritis

RA is a common chronic inflammatory joint disease affecting 1–1.5% of the population worldwide, with a female preponderance of 3:1 and a peak onset in the fifth decade of life.[136,137] The main presenting symptoms are pain, stiffness and swelling of synovial joints typically in a symmetrical fashion and, as the disease progresses, cartilage destruction, bone erosion and joint deformities are evident.[138] RA is associated with systemic disturbance and a range of extra-articular features (see box) and the presence of auto-antibodies (anticyclic citrullinated peptide antibody [ACPA] and rheumatoid factor [RF]).[139] The classification criteria for early and established RA are shown in the box below.

Genetic factors account for 50–60% of the risk of developing RA, with the HLA-DRB1 and PTPN22 genes being strongly associated with developing RA. RA patients who carry these genes are likely to produce ACPA.[140] ACPA predates the clinical onset of RA and is associated with a higher rate of joint destruction and it predicts a more severe and erosive natural history.[141] The main environmental factors implicated in the development of RA are infections, smoking, pollutants and dietary factors.[140] Smoking is by the far the most studied and well-accepted environmental risk factor. Smoking increases the risk of developing seropositive RA (RF and/or ACPA) and may account for up to a third of seropositive cases. Furthermore, tobacco smoking may be associated with the development of a more aggressive disease, greater joint damage and a worse response to antirheumatic therapy.[142]

Conventional treatment consists of patient education, physical/occupational therapy and medications. Medications are generally administered in a three-pronged approach: NSAIDs and low-dose oral or intra-articular corticosteroids; DMARDs; and consideration of biologicals.[143] The earlier RA is diagnosed and treated the better its long-term outcome. The disease seems to be more responsive to treatment in its earlier stages during which therapeutic intervention has the potential to alter the disease course.[144]

Extra-articular features of RA

- Nodules
- Pulmonary
- Pulmonary nodules
- Pleural effusion
- Fibrosing alveolitis
- Ocular
- Keratoconjunctivitis sicca
- Episcleritis
- Scleritis
- Vasculitis
- Nail fold
- Systemic
- Cardiac
- Pericarditis

- Pericardial effusion
- Valvular heart disease
- Conduction defects
- Neurological
- Nerve entrapment
- Cervical myelopathy
- Peripheral neuropathy
- Mononeuritis multiplex
- Cutaneous
- Palmar erythema
- Pyoderma gangrenosum
- Vasculitic rashes
- Leg ulceration
- Amyloidosis

Source: Scott et al. 2010[139]

ACR/EULAR criteria

Joint involvement (0–5)

- One medium-to-large joint (0)
- Two to 10 medium-to-large joints (1)
- One to three small joints (large joints not counted) (2)
- Four to 10 small joints (large joints not counted) (3)
- More than 10 joints (at least one small joint) (5)

Serology (0–3)

- Negative RF *and* negative ACPA (0)
- Low positive RF *or* low positive ACPA (2)
- High positive RF *or* high positive ACPA (3)

Acute-phase reactants (0–1)

- Normal CRP *and* normal ESR (0)
- Abnormal CRP *or* abnormal ESR (1)

Duration of symptoms (0–1)

- Less than six weeks (0)
- Six weeks or more (1)

Points are shown in parentheses. Threshold for RA is six points or more. Patients can also be classified as having RA if they have typical erosions and longstanding disease previously satisfying the classification criteria.

ACR = American College of Rheumatology; EULAR = European League Against Rheumatism; RF = rheumatoid factor; ACPA = antibodies against citrullinated peptide antigens; CRP = C-reactive protein; ESR = erythrocyte sedimentation rate

2010 ACR/EULAR criteria are intended to classify both early and established disease.

Source: Scott et al. 2010[139]

Key treatment protocols

The goal of treating RA naturopathically is twofold: reduce the inflammatory burden placed on the system and remove the toxic debris accumulated in the tissues. Inflammation in the joints causes much of the pain, stiffness and swelling in the joints. The pro-inflammatory cytokines IL-1, IL-6 and TNF-α are present at high levels in arthritic joints, and their blood concentration correlates with the severity of RA.[145] Diet, lifestyle and herbal medicines can be used in a holistic approach to help to reduce both joint and systemic inflammation by increasing intracellular antioxidants, inhibiting inflammatory cytokines and also by encouraging the removal of wastes thereby preserving the joints and preventing further joint destruction.

Naturopathic Treatment Aims

- Reduce inflammation by balancing cytokine biology.
- Improve detoxification pathways.
- Reduce oxidative stress.
- Improve coping strategies to stressors.
- Modulate immune response.
- Improve digestive function.
- Alleviate pain.
- Address incorrect dietary habits and food allergies.

Reduce joint inflammation

Paeonia lactiflora is a traditional Chinese medicine for inflammation and pain. The major active is paeoniflorin and has been used to treat RA. Numerous in vitro and in vivo studies have demonstrated total glycosides of paeony (TGP)/paeoniflorin to exert anti-inflammatory effects in RA models by suppressing the production of pro-inflammatory, prostaglandin E_2, leukotriene B_4, nitric oxide and reactive oxygen species.[146] A meta-analysis found that the TGP combined with methotrexate (MTX) was more effective than the MTX treatment alone and the combined therapy significantly reduced adverse drug effects, such as the incidence rate of impaired liver function in RA.[147] Another meta-analysis found that TGP combined with an immunosuppressant might be more effective than the immunosuppressant alone for RA in the early stage of treatment.[148] The results from both meta-analyses demonstrate that combination therapies may be more effective than single therapies; however, high-quality and large-scale RCTs are needed to further confirm the results because of the limited quality of the included studies.[149]

In a randomised pilot clinical study 45 people with active RA received 1 g/day **curcumin** (*Curcuma longa*) or 100 mg/day diclofenac sodium or a combination of both over eight weeks. Curcumin was more effective in alleviating pain compared with diclofenac, had fewer adverse events and had the highest percentage of improvement in reducing tenderness and swelling of joints.[150] A small randomised double-blinded study compared a highly bioavailable curcumin at 250 or 500 mg twice daily over 90 days in active RA patients. Curcumin at both doses improved symptoms and diagnostic indicators in RA patients compared to placebo. These findings suggest curcumin acts as an anti-inflammatory and analgesic agent in the management of RA.[151] An open study in people with rheumatic conditions in the United Kingdom assessed the safety and efficacy of 960 mg (480 mg twice daily) of ***Harpagophytum procumbens*** in 259 patients over eight weeks. They reported significant improvements in global pain, stiffness and function; 66% of patients had reduced or stopped their pain medication by week 8.[152] The treatment was considered safe and well tolerated, with no serious adverse events (see Chapters 24–26 on musculoskeletal system and Chapter 40 on pain for more anti-inflammatory interventions). **Vitamin D** is a valuable nutrient known to exert anti-inflammatory and immunomodulatory properties. A recent meta-analysis involving 24 studies and 3489 patients revealed that RA patients had lower vitamin D levels than controls which correlated with an increased disease activity score in 28 joints.[153]

Support the removal of metabolic waste

An old naturopathic interpretation of unresolved inflammation was that it may be a sign of persisting toxicity or damage in the affected tissues.[154] RA is a chronic inflammatory condition considered to be of toxic nature where there is an accumulation of cellular waste products and ingested toxins, which may cause significant changes in tissue function.[155] From this perspective, then, a treatment strategy for RA is to remove such toxins in a gentle manner by employing **depurative herbs**. 'Depuratives' non-specifically cleanse the tissues and blood stream and have traditionally been used to treat chronic conditions including autoimmune diseases, cancer and inflamed skin conditions.[100]

There are a number of herbs that have been traditionally used as depuratives, including *Arctium lappa*, *Berberis* spp., *Echinacea* spp. (root), *Galium aparine*, *Hydrastis canadensis*, *Iris versicolor*, *Rumex crispus*, *Smilax* spp., *Trifolium pratense* and *Urtica dioica*.[156] Unfortunately there have been few scientific studies to support their traditional use as depuratives.[155] However, the alkaloid berberine from *Berberis* spp. and *Hydrastis canadensis* has been shown to up-regulate the expression and function of P-glycoprotein therefore increasing the ability of the cell to remove toxins and unwanted material, providing a potential scientific mode of action.[155]

Inflammatory bowel disease

Crohn's disease and ulcerative colitis (UC) represent the two main types of inflammatory bowel disease (IBD). Both diseases are idiopathic, have periodic flare-ups and frequently present with abdominal pain, fever, weight loss and clinical signs of bowel obstruction or diarrhoea with passage of blood or mucus, or both.[157,158] Crohn's can affect any part of the gastrointestinal tract (GIT) and is characterised by a patchy distribution throughout the GIT with inflammation extending the entire thickness of the intestinal wall, whereas UC affects the lining of the large intestinal wall and rectum, sparing the deeper layers of the intestinal wall.[157,158] The highest incidence rates and prevalence of Crohn's and UC have been reported in North America, northern Europe and the United Kingdom, where the rates are beginning to stabilise. Rates continue to rise in low-incidence areas including Asia, southern Europe and most developing countries.[159]

Although the pathogenesis of IBD remains unknown, there is now a body of evidence to suggest that genetic, immunological and environmental factors initiate the autoimmune process.[160] It is thought that IBD results from normal luminal flora inappropriately and continually activating the mucosal immune system. This aberrant response is probably facilitated by defects in the barrier function of the intestinal epithelium and the mucosal immune system.[161]

Conventional medical treatment for IBD consists of a variety of anti-inflammatory, immunosuppressive and biological agents to induce and/or maintain remission in IBDs.[158] However, clinical efficacy is limited as only 60% of IBD patients respond to a particular IBD therapy currently on the market and the majority of current IBD therapies are associated with severe side effects, sometimes rendering the treatment more deleterious than the disease itself.[162] Due to the limitations of conventional medicine there has been increased use of natural and complementary medicine in those with Crohn's and UC, with significantly more UC patients than Crohn's patients reporting its use.[163]

Key treatment protocols

The key goal of treating IBD naturopathically is to reduce intestinal inflammation and correct alterations in intestinal microflora (dysbiosis). Specific herbal medicines can be employed to dampen the inflammatory assault on the GIT and probiotics can be administered to beneficially alter intestinal microflora.

> **Naturopathic Treatment Aims**
>
> - Restore GIT microflora
> - Decrease intestinal inflammation.
> - Improve digestive function.
> - Manage GIT symptoms.
> - Improve coping strategies to stressors.
> - Modulate immune response.
> - Address incorrect dietary habits and food allergies.
> - Address nutritional deficiencies.

Reduce intestinal inflammation

Curcuma longa has been used for centuries in Asia for infections, inflammation and digestive disorders.[164] Numerous in vivo and in vitro studies have shown **curcumin** to be beneficial in chemically induced colitis by improving colonic morphology and survival, dampening local cytokine and chemokine production and reducing mucosal neutrophil infiltration.[164] Curcumin was recently evaluated for its effect on interferon-gamma, a pro-inflammatory cytokine that profoundly affects the intestinal epithelium by disrupting the epithelial barrier function, preventing epithelial cell migration and wound healing. Curcumin was shown to inhibit interferon-gamma signalling in colonocytes.[165] In a randomised placebo-controlled double-blind clinical trial of curcumin compared with placebo in 89 patients with quiescent UC, 2 g/d curcumin was significantly better than placebo at preventing remissions, and improving the clinical activity index and endoscopic index.[37] A systematic review and meta-analysis of RCTs investigated curcumin treatment in mild to moderate ulcerative colitis. Three studies (*n* = 184) met the inclusion criteria and were included in the analysis. Daily administration of curcumin for 4–8 weeks taken either orally (2–3 gm) or via rectal enema (140 mg) plus mesalamine (aminosalicylate anti-inflammatory drug) (1600–4000 mg daily) was superior to placebo plus mesalamine in achieving endoscopic improvement.[166]

Boswellia serrata has beneficial effects in intestinal inflammatory disease, thought to be via inhibition of 5-lipoxygenase.[167] *Boswellia serrata* gum resin extract (BSE) was shown to prevent diarrhoea and normalise intestinal motility in chemically induced colitis in rodents.[168] In a small clinical study of 30 patients with UC, 900 mg/day BSE taken for six weeks was shown to be more effective and have fewer side effects than sulfasalazine.[169] However, one should be cautious translating these results into clinical practice as the study was not randomised and had no control. See the box for cautions with using *Boswellia*. In an open-label observational study of 43 patients with UC in the remission phase, 250 mg/day of standardized BSE in a lecithin-based delivery system (Casperome®) taken for four weeks was shown to attenuate symptoms associated with mild UC compared to placebo.[170]

Aloe vera has been used traditionally in Ayurvedic and Thai medicine for peptic ulcers and locally for burns, wounds, mouth ulcers and inflamed areas.[156] A randomised, double-blinded, placebo-controlled trial examined the efficacy and safety of *Aloe vera* gel for treating mildly to moderately active UC. Thirty patients took 100 mL of oral *Aloe vera* gel and 14 patients had 100 mL of a placebo twice daily for four weeks. *Aloe vera* demonstrated a significant decrease in Simple Clinical Colitis Activity Index and histological scores were compared with placebo and appeared to be safe.[171] The exact mechanism of action of *Aloe vera* remains unknown. In vitro studies on human colonic mucosa have shown *Aloe vera* gel to inhibit prostaglandin E_2 and IL-8 secretion, suggesting a role in antimicrobial and anti-inflammatory responses.[172]

Triticum aestivum (**wheat grass**) juice has been used for treating various gastro-intestinal conditions but little information is known of its clinical effectiveness. In a randomised, double-blind, placebo-controlled trial 23 patients diagnosed clinically and sigmoidoscopically with active distal UC received either 100 mL of wheat grass juice, or a matching placebo, daily for one month. Treatment with *Triticum aestivum* juice was associated with significant reductions in the overall disease activity index and in the severity of rectal bleeding compared with placebo.[173] Thus, *Triticum aestivum* juice appeared effective and safe as a single or adjuvant treatment of active distal UC.

Punica granatum (**pomegranate**) is a fruit that has been traditionally and medically used for treating infections, diarrhea, ulcers and inflammation. A randomised, double-blinded, placebo-controlled trial examined the efficacy of *P. granatum* peel extract for symptomatic management in UC. Seventy-eight patients took 8 mL of an aqueous extract syrup containing 6 g of *P. granatum* peel daily or equivalent placebo complementary to standard medications for four weeks. *P granatum* was associated with significant clinical improvement in faecal incontinence and need for antidiarrhoeal medication compared to placebo.[174] **Silymarin** (an extract from *Silybum marianum* [milk thistle] seeds) is known for its hepatoprotective effects; however, in recent years it has been reported to reduce bowel inflammatory cytokines and control immune-based murine colitis. In a randomised, double-blinded placebo-controlled trial with 80 UC patients in remission, 140 mg Siymarin taken daily for six months along with standard medical treatment showed a significant improvement in disease activity index, hemoglobin levels and erythrocyte sedimentation rate.[175] **Resveratrol** is a polyphenolic compound found in grapes and berries and has antioxidant and anti-inflammatory properties.

The anti-inflammatory effects of resveratrol were investigated in 50 UC patients in a randomised, double-blinded, placebo-controlled pilot study. Resveratrol taken 500 mg/day over six weeks demonstrated a significant improvement in the inflammatory bowel disease questionnaire, a significant reduction in plasma hs-CRP, TNF-α levels, NF-kB activity in peripheral blood mononuclear cells, and the clinical colitis activity index compared to placebo. Thus, resveratrol reduced inflammation and improved the quality of life and disease activity in UC patients.[176] A prospective physician-blinded study investigated whether serum **vitamin D** status in currently remitted UC patients is associated with clinical relapse. The study was conducted over 12 months in 70 UC patients in clinical remission and the findings showed an increased risk of UC relapse when serum vitamin D levels are 35 ng/mL or lower during the remission phase of UC.[177]

Correcting alterations in gut microbial flora (dysbiosis)

Intestinal microbial flora (microbiota) has been implicated in inducing and maintaining intestinal inflammation through a complex interplay with the gut immune system.[178] Any alteration in the intestinal microbial flora (i.e. dysbiosis) that involves an alteration in the balance between 'protective' and 'harmful' intestinal bacteria[179] may play a key role in IBD. In faecal culture studies, mucosal analysis in IBD has found decreased concentrations of beneficial *Bifidobacteria* species and increased concentrations of anaerobes and *Escherichia coli*.[179] Certain antibiotics, including metronidazole and ciprofloxacin, have been used successfully to treat IBD; however, long-term antibiotic use is inadvisable due to systemic side effects.[178] Probiotics provide a safer therapeutic option. Probiotics beneficially affect the host by improving the intestinal microbial balance, blocking adhesion sites on the colonocytes thus enhancing gut barrier function and improving local immune response.[180]

Saccharomyces boulardii (SB) is a non-pathogenic **yeast** probiotic with beneficial effects on the human intestine. SB was evaluated for its clinical efficacy in maintenance and remission in 32 Crohn's patients in clinical remission. The results found that 1 g daily of SB taken for six months, when added to mesalazine (a salicylates-based anti-inflammatory medication) was more effective than mesalazine alone in maintaining remission of inactive Crohn's disease.[181] Another study evaluated the influence of SB on the intestinal permeability in Crohn's as measured by the lactulose/mannitol ratio. Thirty-four patients currently taking medications (mesalazine, azathioprine, prednisone, metronidazole and/or thalidomide) were randomly assigned to receive either SB or placebo. The results demonstrated SB reduced the lactulose:mannitol ratio in Crohn's patients in remission in comparison to placebo indicating an improvement in intestinal barrier function and thus intestinal permeability compared with placebo.[182] In a pilot study 25 patients with mild to moderate clinical flare-up of UC, 250 mg of SB taken three times a day for four weeks during maintenance treatment with mesalazine resulted in clinical remission, which was endoscopically confirmed.[183] Despite the promising preliminary results a recent prospective study of 165 patients showed no beneficial effects of taking 1 g/day of SB for 52 weeks in patients with Crohn's in remission following steroid or salicylate therapies.[184]

In a randomised, double-blind, placebo-controlled trial in 144 patients with mild to moderate active UC, **high-potency probiotic VSL#3** (consisting of a fixed ratio of three *Lactonbacillus* strains, three *Biofidobacterium* strains and one strain of *Streptococcus thermophilus*) had a significantly greater decrease in Ulcerative Colitis Disease Activity Index (UCDAI) scores and individual symptoms at weeks 6 and 12, compared with placebo.

Thus, VSL#3 is safe and effective in achieving clinical responses and remissions in patients with mild-to-moderately active UC.[185] A placebo-controlled, double-blind study in children with active UC demonstrated, at six months, 12 months or at time of relapse, endoscopic and histological scores significantly lower in the VSL#3 group than in the placebo, confirming VSL#3's efficacy and role in maintenance of remission in paediatric active UC.[180] In an open-labelled study 34 ambulatory patients with active UC received VSL#3, 3600 billion bacteria daily in two divided doses for six weeks. The results demonstrated a combined induction of remission/response rate of 77% with no adverse events.[186]

Systemic lupus erythematous

SLE is a chronic autoimmune connective tissue disease characterised by multiorgan involvement and variable clinical presentation.[187] Some patients may present with skin rash and joint pain, show spontaneous remissions and require little medication, whereas others demonstrate severe and progressive kidney involvement (glomerulonephritis) that requires therapy with high doses of steroids and cytotoxic drugs such as cyclophosphamide.[188] Women outnumber men almost 10-fold and the typical lupus patient is a young woman during her reproductive years, although men and woman of all age groups can be affected.[189] The incidence of the disease is four to five times higher among African Americans and Hispanics.[187] Although the aetiology of SLE is not fully understood, current understanding suggests that environmental factors, including microbial antigens, ultraviolet light, drugs and hormones act on genetically susceptible individuals causing loss of self-tolerance and the development of auto-reactivity.[187,190] The hallmark of the disorder is an elevated number of serum antinuclear antibodies (ANA).[188] Conventional treatment consists of immunosuppressive therapy with high doses of steroids remaining the first line of treatment for many manifestations of SLE.[187]

Naturopathic treatment protocols

SLE is a complex disorder affecting many systems of the body, therefore naturopathic treatment needs to address these systems and the underlying immune dysregulation and inflammation. The main goal of treating SLE is to modulate immune function and reduce systemic inflammation with herbal and nutritional medicines.

> **Naturopathic Treatment Aims**
>
> - Modulate immune response—inhibit excess apoptosis.
> - Reduce inflammation by balancing cytokine biology.
> - Reduce oxidative stress.
> - Improve coping strategies to stressors.
> - Improve digestive function.
> - Alleviate pain.
> - Encourage lifestyle changes.

Modulate immune function

Widespread inflammation characterises SLE and may affect multiple organs and systems simultaneously. Reducing systemic inflammation is central to controlling disease progression and flare-ups.

Astragalus membranaceus is a Western herb originating in traditional Chinese medicine, where it was believed to modulate Qi, blood and spleen.[156] It is used in Western medicine as an immune-modulating herb.[191] In a randomised trial involving 80 SLE patients, an injection of *Astragalus membranaceus* as an adjunct to conventional treatment was evaluated for its effect on apoptosis of lymphocytes and immune function. *Astragalus membranaceus* injection regulated the ratio and function of T-cell subsets to normal range.[114] In another study 43 patients diagnosed with SLE complicated by kidney damage and 'Qi-deficiency syndrome', a high-dose *Astragalus membranaceus* injection

Warning signs and symptoms of a lupus flare-up	
• Increased fatigue	• Mouth ulcers
• Increased pain in joints	• Headache
• Skin rash	• Dizziness
• Sensitivity to the sun	• Abdominal discomfort
• High temperature	

used together with cyclophosphamide was more effective than cyclophosphamide alone at improving immune function and reducing infection rate and urine protein.[192]

Bupleurum falcatum has been used traditionally in Chinese medicine for fever management and regulating and restoring gastrointestinal and liver function.[156] The active saikosaponins are anti-inflammatory, immunomodulatory and antibacterial.[193] In an in vivo study saikosaponin A inhibited T-cell activation and proliferation by cell arrest and induction of apoptosis. Additionally, it potently suppressed concanavalin A (Con A)-stimulated production of pro-inflammatory cytokines.

Glutathione is a tripeptide composed of cysteine, glutamic acid and glycine, and is a major endogenous antioxidant produced by cells. In a randomised, double-blinded placebo-controlled trial 36 SLE patients received daily placebo or 1.2 g, 2.4 g or 4.8 g of **N-acetylcysteine** (NAC) (a precursor to glutathione) for three months. The results demonstrated that 2.4 g/day and 4.8 g/day of NAC reduced SLE disease activity by blocking mammalian target of rapamycin (mTOR) (an enzyme that regulates cell growth, proliferation and death) in T-cells. Reversible nausea was experienced in 33% of patients taking 4.8 g/day of NAC and 2.4 g/day of NAC was safe and tolerated by all patients.[194]

In clinical trials, **fish oil** supplements have shown beneficial outcomes in SLE. For instance, in a randomised placebo-controlled, double-blind study of fish oil in SLE, 59 subjects were allocated into one of four groups. Subjects were given 3×1 g MaxEPA (180 g EPA + 120 mg DHA) per day or 3 mg of copper (as copper di-glycinate amino acid complex) per day or both copper and fish oil or placebo (olive oil). The primary outcome was scored on the revised Systemic Lupus Activity Measure (SLAM-R), a routinely used reliable and validated measure of disease activity. After 24 weeks of supplementation, participants in the fish oil groups significantly reduced scores on the SLAM-R.[195] This study demonstrated that six months of high doses of fish oil could improve clinical symptoms in SLE. **Vitamin D** is a steroid hormone that regulates endothelial function. Vascular tone and inflammation are regulated by the endothelium and SLE patients have deficits in these endothelial functions. A double-blind, randomised pilot study found that 5000 IU/day of vitamin D in vitamin D-deficient SLE patients after 16 weeks improved endothelial function as measured by flow-mediated dilation. Thus, repletion of vitamin D improves endothelial function in SLE patients.[196]

Reducing fatigue and stress

Fatigue is a particularly prevalent and debilitating symptom among SLE patients.[197] In a recent study, the relationship between oxidative stress and fatigue was investigated in SLE. The findings revealed that fatigue in SLE patients with low disease activity is associated with increased plasma levels of F_2-isoprostane, a biomarker for oxidative stress.[197] During chronic stress high levels of ROS, a marker of oxidative stress, have been observed in mice.[198] Inhalation of a novel aroma, **Praescent**, a mixture of plant-derived chemicals cis-3-hexen-1-ol, trans-2-hexenal and alpha-pinene, was shown to significantly reduce levels of ROS in chronically stressed immunised mice compared with controls.[198] Further studies are required to determine whether the reduction in oxidative stress correlated with clinical outputs, such as reduced fatigue. For more details, refer to Chapter 18 on stress and fatigue. A randomised, single-blind, placebo-controlled trial evaluated the impact **fish oil** has on fatigue, quality of life and disease activity in SLE patients. Fifty patients received six capsules per day of fish oil (2.25 g EPA and 2.25 g DHA) or six capsules per day of olive oil (placebo) for six months. Fish oil supplementation significantly improved the Physician Global Assessment (PGA) score, significantly reduced plasma ESR levels, and improved the quality of life in SLE patients in comparison to placebo. However, the Fatigue Severity Scale and SLE Disease Activity Index showed no clear difference between fish oil supplementation and placebo.[199]

CLINICAL SUMMARY

Autoimmune diseases are serious, chronic, degenerative conditions. As such, if there is any doubt that you are in the presence of undiagnosed autoimmune disease, refer immediately to a medical practitioner and cite this referral in your clinical notes. If the condition has been diagnosed by a medical specialist, you should advise the person to discuss with their specialist that they are seeing you and to inform him or her of any nutritional/herbal supplements that you may prescribe, and make a citation to this effect in your clinical notes.

These procedures should be conducted routinely by allied and complementary primary care practitioners in any serious, chronic disease as ethical and legal consider-ations to protect your client and yourself from inadvertent harm. For instance, should your client suddenly find themselves in surgery, their doctor should know what herbs/ supplements they were taking in the lead-up to surgery, as some herbs/nutrients interact with pharmaceuticals. For example, large doses of fish oil may increase bleeding time, although probably not enough to be a sufficient harm but may interact with other medi-cations the person may also be taking such as warfarin. Making a medical referral (write a letter addressed to their doctor) and keeping a copy or writing notes to this effect also protects you from any potential harm from future litigation.

Once the ethical and legal implications of treating someone with a chronic disease have been considered, apply the most fundamental naturopathic principle: treat the whole person, not the disease. Work out whether the person is dealing with systemic or organ-specific disease, and ensure to support those organs most affected (Figure 31.4). Most autoimmune diseases present in clusters of autoimmune/inflammatory diseases, so check whether there is more than one organ affected.

Take the clinical history with due diligence to potential environmental triggers, such as stressors and other exposures that may stimulate inflammation. Investigate any medication interactions or side effects. Perhaps there are complementary medicines that may help alleviate some of the side effects or help to enable a reduction of medica-tions, under medical supervision. If the person is on a number of different medications you may consider referral for a polypharmacy review; many pharmacists conduct these reviews in the community.

Treatment of autoimmune diseases would ideally occur in an integrative healthcare model, with the person themselves encouraged to take on the role of their own case manager. Support empowerment and resilience-building through accessing resources that can help with the symptoms of disease and the distress of the diagnosis.

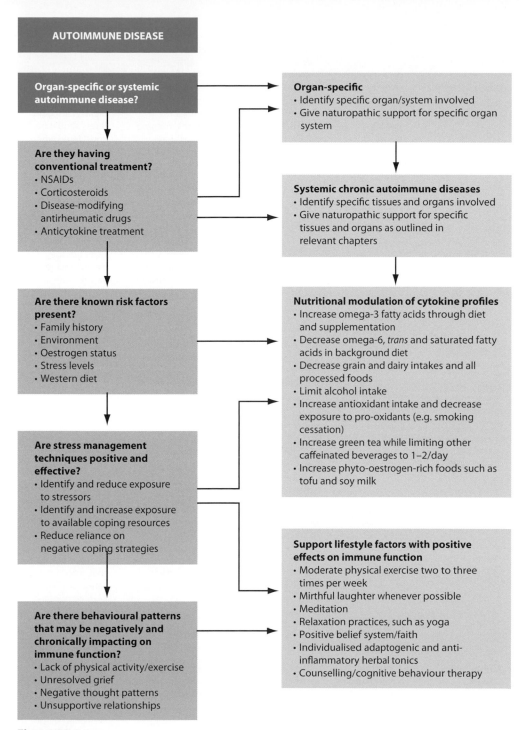

Figure 31.4
Naturopathic treatment decision tree—autoimmune disease

Table 31.4
Review of the major evidence

Intervention	Mechanisms of action	Key literature	Summary of results	Comments
Omega-3 fatty acids	Suppresses production of omega-6 eicosanoids and pro-inflammatory cytokines	Fortin et al. 1995[200] American meta-analysis on fish oil in RA in 368 patients	Three months' supplementation significantly reduces morning stiffness (rate difference (RD) [95% CI] = −25.9 [−44.3 to −7.5] [$p < 0.01$]) and tender joint count [RD] [95% CI] = −2.9 [−3.8 to −2.1] [$p = 0.001$] and as compared with heterogeneous dietary control oils	In clinical practice, background dietary omega-6 levels should be considered when recommending fish oil supplements or a high omega-3 diet Researchers conclude that fish oil is beneficial for symptomatic relief but they did not include withdrawals in the final analyses, therefore these results could be biased
		James & Cleland 1997[36] Australian review of 12 RCTs of fish oil in RA	Found good evidence for modest beneficial effects of fish oils in RA	
		Duffy et al. 2004[195] double-blind RCT using 3×1 g MaxEPA (180 mg EPA + 120 mg DHA) in 52 patients with SLE for six months	Significant improvement in disease activity compared with controls SLAM-R score of 6.12 to 4.69 ($p < 0.05$)	
Curcumin	Down-regulates inflammatory cytokines Strong antioxidant effects	Hanai et al. 2006[37] Double-blind RCT involving 89 patients with quiescent UC, 2 g/d curcumin or placebo alongside usual medications (sulfasalazine or mesalazine) for six months	Prevents remissions and improves both the clinical activity index and endoscopic index compared with placebo ($p < 0.05$)	This was a rigorous study as it used intention to treat analysis, demonstrating that curcumin is a safe and effective complementary therapy in the prevention of relapse in people with UC
Alpha-lipoic acid (MS)	Reduced two immunological markers of MS activity that are indirectly associated with T-cell migration into the central nervous system	Yadav et al. 2005[59] American pilot double-blind RCT of 37 patients with MS taking various amounts of lipoic acid ranging from 600 mg/d to 2400 mg/d for two weeks	1200 mg/d lipoic acid for 24 weeks significantly reduced clinical features on the SLAM-R between groups from 6.12 to 4.69 ($p < 0.05$)	Although a pilot study, these results provide good preliminary evidence for the safety and efficacy of lipoic acid as an intervention in people with MS

Table 31.4
Review of the major evidence (continued)

Intervention	Mechanisms of action	Key literature	Summary of results	Comments
Selenium	Antioxidant and anti-inflammatory effects and is involved in the production of active thyroid hormone	Rayman 2012[201] review on the impact of selenium on immune function and other parameters of health	80 μg or 200 μg per day as sodium selenite or selenomethionine is effective in Hashimoto's thyroiditis Was also effective in Graves' disease, improving quality of life, less eye involvement and slower deterioration of disease	Selenium has a U curve of effects on health and the immune system, with supplementation beneficial to those with inadequate selenium but there may be an increased risk of type 2 diabetes in those who have adequate selenium
Borage oil and other CAMs	Not known/discussed	Systematic review of efficacy in rheumatism[202]	No conclusive efficacy for CAM in rheumatism Positive results from two RCTs of borage oil demonstrated positive effects on reducing pain and swelling of rheumatism	1.4 g/d and 2.4 g/d respectively for six months resulted in significant reduction in borage seed oil intervention group compared with controls
Boswellia serrata resin extract	Boswellic acids have anti-inflammatory effect via modulation of leukotrienes	Sander et al. 2006[68] Double blind pilot study in outpatients with RA	Reduced use of NSAIDs in *Boswellia* group compared with controls 5.8% (*Boswellia*) and 3.1% (placebo)	The pilot study did not have the statistical power to find a significant effect Abstract only available in English so cannot study methodology
Harpagophytum procumbens	Anti-inflammatory activity and analgesic effects from the active constituent harpagoside	Warnock et al. 2007[152] British open study of 960 mg (480 mg twice daily) in 259 patients with rheumatic disease over eight weeks Brien et al. 2006[203] systematic review	Improvements in global pain, stiffness and function ($p < 0.0001$) and 66% of patients had reduced or stopped their pain medication by week 8	Poor-quality studies do not allow for any firm conclusions

KEY POINTS

- Balance the dietary fatty acids to modulate inflammatory pathways.
- Consider the impact of the gut flora (microbiota) on autoimmune conditions.
- Reduce the impact of oxidative stress by including plenty of antioxidants in the diet.
- Decrease low-grade metabolic acidosis.
- Consider adjustment towards the Palaeolithic diet.
- Minimise intake of salt, grains and dairy.
- Increase physical exercise to release endorphins, antioxidant precursors and anti-inflammatory cytokines, at least 30 minutes three times per week.
- Advise to practise relaxation techniques or meditation every day.

FURTHER READING

Michalsen A. The role of complementary and alternative medicine (CAM) in rheumatology—it's time for integrative medicine. J Rheumatol 2013;40(5):547–9. doi:10.3899/jrheum.130107.

Proal AD, Albert PJ, Marshall T. Autoimmune disease in the era of the metagenome. Autoimmun Rev 2009;8(8):677–81.

Vliet Vlieland TP, Vliet Vlieland TPM. Non-drug care for RA—is the era of evidence-based practice approaching? Rheumatology 2007;46(9):1397–404.

Vojdani A, Lambert J, Kellermann G. The role of Th17 in neuroimmune disorders: a target for CAM therapy. part III. Evid Based Complement Alternat Med 2011;2011:548086. doi:10.1093/ecam/nep064.

Acknowledgment: The author would like to acknowledge Joanne Bradbury, who authored this chapter in previous editions.

REFERENCES

1. Kumar P, Clark M. Clinical medicine. Edinburgh: W. B. Saunders; 1998.
2. Cooper GS, Bynum ML, Somers EC. Recent insights in the epidemiology of autoimmune diseases: improved prevalence estimates and understanding of clustering of diseases. J Autoimmun 2009;33(3–4):197–207.
3. Cooper GS, Stroehla BC. The epidemiology of autoimmune diseases. Autoimmun Rev 2003;2(3):119–25.
4. Walsh SJ, Rau LM. Autoimmune diseases: a leading cause of death among young and middle-aged women in the United States. Am J Public Health 2000;90(9):1463–6.
5. Shoenfeld Y, Zandman-Goddard G, Stojanovich L, et al. The mosaic of autoimmunity: hormonal and environmental factors involved in autoimmune diseases—2008. Isr Med Assoc J 2008;10(1):8–12.
6. Brickman CM, Shoenfeld Y. The mosaic of autoimmunity. Scand J Clin Lab Invest 2001;61(7):3–15.
7. Proal AD, Albert PJ, Marshall T. Autoimmune disease in the era of the metagenome. Autoimmun Rev 2009;8(8):677–81.
8. Marshall TG, Lee RE, Marshall FE. Common angiotensin receptor blockers may directly modulate the immune system via VDR, PPAR and CCR2b. Theor Biol Med Model 2006;3:1.
9. Kuek A, Hazleman BL, Ostor AJK. Immune-mediated inflammatory diseases (IMIDs) and biologic therapy: a medical revolution. Postgrad Med J 2007;83(978):251–60.
10. Davidson A, Diamond B. Autoimmune diseases. N Engl J Med 2001;345(5):340–50.
11. Lettre G, Rioux JD. Autoimmune diseases: insights from genome-wide association studies. Hum Mol Genet 2008;17(R2):R116–21.
12. Ramagopalan SV, Maugeri NJ, Handunnetthi L, et al. Expression of the multiple sclerosis-associated MHC Class II Allele HLA-DRB1*1501 is Regulated by Vitamin D. PLoS Genet 2009;5(2):e1000369.
13. McKay JA, Mathers JC. Diet-induced epigenetic changes and their implications for health. Acta Physiol (Oxf) 2011;202(2):103–18.
14. Mackay IR. Science, medicine, and the future: tolerance and autoimmunity. BMJ 2000;321(7253):93–6.
15. Hill N, Sarvetnick N. Cytokines: promoters and dampeners of autoimmunity. Curr Opin Immunol 2002;14(6):791–7.
16. Delogu LG, Deidda S, Delitala G, et al. Infectious diseases and autoimmunity. J Infect Dev Ctries 2011;5(10):679–87.
17. Sospedra M, Martin R. Immunology of multiple sclerosis. Annu Rev Immunol 2005;23(1):683–747.
18. Porth CM. Pathophysiology: concepts of altered health states. 4th ed. Philadelphia: J.B. Lippincott Company; 1994.
19. Kountouras J, Zavos C, Gavalas E, et al. Challenge in the pathogenesis of autoimmune pancreatitis: potential role of helicobacter pylori infection via molecular mimicry. Gastroenterology 2007;133(1):368–9.
20. Falcone M, Sarvetnick N. Cytokines that regulate autoimmune responses. Curr Opin Immunol 1999;11(6):670–6.

21. Coffman RL. Origins of the T(H)1-T(H)2 model: a personal perspective. Nat Immunol 2006;7(6):539–41.

22. Elenkov IJ, Lessoni DG, Daly A, et al. Cytokine dysregulation, inflammation and well-being. Neuroimmunomodulation 2005;12: 255–69.

23. Weaver CT, Hatton RD, Mangan PR, et al. IL-17 Family cytokines and the expanding diversity of effector T-cell lineages. Annu Rev Immunol 2007;25(1):821–52.

24. Mills KHG. Induction, function and regulation of IL-17-producing T cells. Eur J Immunol 2008;38(10): 2636–49.

25. Kong N, Lan Q, Chen M, et al. Antigen-specific transforming growth factor -induced Treg cells, but not natural Treg cells, ameliorate autoimmune arthritis in mice by shifting the Th17/Treg cell balance from Th17 predominance to Treg cell predominance. Arthritis Rheum 2012;64(8):2548–58.

26. Liu Y, Yu Y, Matarese G, et al. Cutting edge: fasting-induced hypoleptinemia expands functional regulatory T cells in systemic lupus erythematosus. J Immunol 2012;188(5):2070–3.

27. Dooley MA, Hogan SL. Environmental epidemiology and risk factors for autoimmune disease. Curr Opin Rheumatol 2003;15(2):99–103.

28. Reckner Olsson A, Skogh T, Wingren G. Comorbidity and lifestyle, reproductive factors, and environmental exposures associated with rheumatoid arthritis. Ann Rheum Dis 2001;60(10):934–9. Erratum appears in Ann Rheum Dis 2001 Dec;60(12):1161.

29. Cooper GS, Dooley MA, Treadwell EL, et al. Smoking and use of hair treatments in relation to risk of developing systemic lupus erythematosus. J Rheumatol 2001;28(12):2653–6.

30. Cooper GS, Miller FW, Germolec DR. Occupational exposures and autoimmune diseases. Int Immunopharmacol 2002;2(2–3):303–13.

31. Landtblom AM, Flodin U, Soderfeldt B, et al. Organic solvents and multiple sclerosis: a synthesis of the current evidence. Epidemiology 1996;7(4):429–33.

32. Sepa A, Wahlberg J, Vaarala O, et al. Psychological stress may induce diabetes-related autoimmunity in infancy. Diabetes Care 2005;28(2):290–5.

33. Miller GE, Chen E, Parker KJ. Psychological stress in childhood and susceptibility to the chronic diseases of aging: moving toward a model of behavioral and biological mechanisms. Psychol Bull 2011;137(6):959–97.

34. Srivastava S, Boyer JL. Psychological stress is associated with relapse in type 1 autoimmune hepatitis. Liver Int 2010;30(10):1439–47.

35. Brooks PM, Day RO. COX-2 inhibitors. Med J Aust 2000;173(8):433–6.

36. James MJ, Cleland LG. Dietary n-3 fatty acids and therapy for rheumatoid arthritis. Semin Arthritis Rheum 1997;27(2):85–97.

37. Hanai H, Iida T, Takeuchi K, et al. Curcumin maintenance therapy for ulcerative colitis: randomized, multicenter, double-blind, placebo-controlled trial. Clin Gastroenterol Hepatol 2006;4(12):1502–6.

38. Maes M, Song C, Lin A, et al. The effects of psychological stress on humans: increased production of pro-inflammatory cytokines and a Th1-like response in stress-induced anxiety. Cytokine 1998;10(4):313–18.

39. Bradbury J. Modelling stress constructs with biomarkers: the importance of the measurement model. Clin Exp Med Sci 2013;1(3):197–216.

40. Simopoulos AP. Omega-3 fatty acids in inflammation and autoimmune diseases. J Am Coll Nutr 2002;21(6):495–505.

41. Cordain L. Cereal grains: humanity's double-edged sword. In: evolutionary aspects of nutrition and health: diet, exercise, genetics and chronic disease. World Rev Nutr Diet 1999;84:19–73.

42. Lowes JR, Radwan P, Priddle JD, et al. Characterisation and quantification of mucosal cytokine that induces epithelial histocompatibility locus antigen-DR expression in inflammatory bowel disease. Gut 1992;33(3):315–19.

43. Mothes T, Bendix U, Pfannschmidt C, et al. Effect of gliadin and other food peptides on expression of MHC class II molecules by HT-29 cells. Gut 1995;36(4):548–52.

44. Fernandes G, Fernandes G. Progress in nutritional immunology. Immunol Res 2008;40(3):244–61.

45. Good RA, Fernandes G, Yunis EJ, et al. Nutritional deficiency, immunologic function, and disease. Am J Pathol 1976;84(3):599–614.

46. Kohli P, Levy BD, Kohli P, et al. Resolvins and protectins: mediating solutions to inflammation. Br J Pharmacol 2009;158(4):960–71.

47. Endres S, von Schacky C. n-3 polyunsaturated fatty acids and human cytokine synthesis. Curr Opin Lipidol 1996;7(1):48–52.

48. Huang YS, Nassar BA. Modulation of tissue fatty acid composition, prostaglandin production and cholesterol levels by dietary manipulation of n-3 and n-6 essential fatty acid metabolites. In: Horrobin D, editor. Omega 6 essential fatty acids: pathophysiology and roles in clinical medicine. USA: Wiley-Liss; 1990. p. 127–44.

49. Brenner R. Nutritional and hormonal factors influencing desaturation of essential fatty acids. Prog Lipid Res 1981;20:41–7.

50. Baldwin AS. The NF-kB and kB Proteins: new discoveries and insights. Annu Rev Immunol 1996;14(1): 649–81.

51. Aktas O, Prozorovski T, Smorodchenko A, et al. Green tea epigallocatechin-3-Gallate Mediates T cellular NF-{kappa} B inhibition and exerts neuroprotection in autoimmune encephalomyelitis. J Immunol 2004;173(9):5794–800.

52. Wheeler DS, Catravas JD, Odoms K, et al. Epigallocatechin-3-gallate, a green tea-derived Polyphenol, inhibits IL-1{beta}-dependent proinflammatory signal transduction in cultured respiratory epithelial cells. J Nutr 2004;134(5):1039–44.

53. Komatsu W, Ishihara K, Murata M, et al. Docosahexaenoic acid suppresses nitric oxide production and inducible nitric oxide synthase expression in interferon-[gamma] plus lipopolysaccharide-stimulated murine macrophages by inhibiting the oxidative stress. Free Radic Biol Med 2003;34(8):1006–16.

54. Schreiber S, Nikolaus S, Hampe J. Activation of nuclear factor kappa B in inflammatory bowel disease. Gut 1998;42(4):477–84.

55. Kim SH, Shin KJ, Kim D, et al. Luteolin inhibits the nuclear factor-kappa B transcriptional activity in Rat-1 fibroblasts. Biochem Pharmacol 2003;66(6):955–63.

56. Ruiz PA, Braune A, Holzlwimmer G, et al. Quercetin inhibits TNF-induced NF-{kappa}B transcription factor recruitment to proinflammatory gene promoters in murine intestinal epithelial cells. J Nutr 2007;137(5):1208–15.

57. Ruiz PA, Haller D. Functional diversity of flavonoids in the inhibition of the proinflammatory NF-{kappa}B, IRF, and Akt signaling pathways in murine intestinal epithelial cells. J Nutr 2006;136(3):664–71.

58. Marracci GH, Jones RE, McKeon GP, et al. Alpha lipoic acid inhibits T-cell migration into the spinal cord and suppresses and treats experimental autoimmune encephalomyelitis. J Neuroimmunol 2002;131(1–2):104–14.

59. Yadav V, Marracci G, Lovera J, et al. Lipoic acid in multiple sclerosis: a pilot study. Mult Scler 2005;11(2):159–65.

60. De Paula ML, Rodrigues DH, Teixeira HC, et al. Genistein down-modulates pro-inflammatory cytokines and reverses clinical signs of experimental autoimmune encephalomyelitis. Int Immunopharmacol 2008;8(9):1291–7.

61. Miodini P, Fioravanti L, Fronzo GD, et al. The two phyto-oestrogens genistein and quercetin exert different effects on oestrogen receptor function. Br J Cancer 1999;80(8):1150–5.

62. Muthian G, Bright JJ, Muthian G, et al. Quercetin, a flavonoid phytoestrogen, ameliorates experimental allergic encephalomyelitis by blocking IL-12 signaling through JAK-STAT1 pathway in T lymphocyte. J Clin Immunol 2004;24(5):542–52.

63. Singh NP, Hegde VL, Hofseth LJ, et al. Resveratrol (trans-3,5,4'-trihydroxystilbene) ameliorates experimental allergic encephalomyelitis, primarily via induction of apoptosis in T-cells involving activation of aryl hydrocarbon receptor and estrogen Receptor. Mol Pharmacol 2007;72(6):1508–21.

64. de la Lastra CA, Villegas I. Resveratrol as an anti-inflammatory and anti-aging agent: mechanisms and clinical implications. Mol Nutr Food Res 2005;49(5):405–30.

65. Safayhi H, Sailer ER, Ammon HP. Mechanism of 5-lipoxygenase inhibition by acetyl-11-keto-beta-boswellic acid. Mol Pharmacol 1995;47(6):1212–16.

66. Ammon HP, Mack T, Singh GB, et al. Inhibition of leukotriene B4 formation in rat peritoneal neutrophils by an ethanolic extract of the gum resin exudate of Boswellia serrata. Planta Med 1991;57(3):203–7.

67. Singh GB, Atal CK. Pharmacology of an extract of salai guggal ex-Boswellia serrata, a new non-steroidal anti-inflammatory agent. Inflamm Res 1986;18(3):407–12.

68. Sander O, Herborn G, Rau R. Is H15 (resin extract of Boswellia serrata, 'incense') a useful supplement to established drug therapy of chronic polyarthritis? Results of a double-blind pilot study. Z Rheumatol 1998;57(1):11–16.

69. Frank A, Unger M. Analysis of frankincense from various Boswellia species with inhibitory activity on human drug metabolising cytochrome P450 enzymes using liquid chromatography mass spectrometry after automated on-line extraction. J Chromatogr A 2006;1112(1–2):255–62.

70. Guengerich FP. Cytochromes P450, drugs, and diseases. Mol Interv 2003;3(4):194–204.

71. Brendler T, Gruenwald J, Ulbricht C, et al. Devil's Claw (Harpagophytum procumbens DC): an evidence-based systematic review by the Natural Standard Research Collaboration. J Herb Pharmacother 2006;6(1):89–126.

72. Abdelouahab N, Heard C. Effect of the major glycosides of Harpagophytum procumbens (Devil's Claw) on epidermal cyclooxygenase-2 (COX-2) in vitro. J Nat Prod 2008;71(5):746–9.

73. Grant L, McBean DE, Fyfe L, et al. A review of the biological and potential therapeutic actions of Harpagophytum procumbens. Phytother Res 2007;21(3):199–209.

74. National Institutes of Health. National Centre for Complementary and Alternative Medicine; Cat's claw; 2008. Available from: http://nccam.nih.gov/health/catclaw/. [Accessed 15 April 2009].

75. Sandoval-Chacon M, Thompson JH, Zhang XJ, et al. Antiinflammatory actions of cat's claw: the role of NF-kappaB. Aliment Pharmacol Ther 1998;12(12):1279–89.

76. Sandoval M, Charbonnet RM, Okuhama NN, et al. Cat's claw inhibits TNFalpha production and scavenges free radicals: role in cytoprotection. Free Radic Biol Med 2000;29(1):71–8.

77. Hardin SR, Hardin SR. Cat's claw: an Amazonian vine decreases inflammation in osteoarthritis. Complement Ther Clin Pract 2007;13(1):25–8.

78. Jagetia GC, Aggarwal BB, Jagetia GC, et al. 'Spicing up' of the immune system by curcumin. J Clin Immunol 2007;27(1):19–35.

79. Srimal RC, Dhawan BN. Pharmacology of diferuloyl methane (curcumin), a non-steroidal anti-inflammatory agent. J Pharm Pharmacol 1973;25(6):447–52.

80. Jain A, Basal E. Inhibition of Propionibacterium acnes-induced mediators of inflammation by Indian herbs. Phytomedicine 2003;10(1):34–8.

81. Bork PM, Schmitz ML, Kuhnt M, et al. Sesquiterpene lactone containing Mexican Indian medicinal plants and pure sesquiterpene lactones as potent inhibitors of transcription factor NF-[kappa]B. FEBS Lett 1997;402(1):85–90.

82. Hehner SP, Hofmann TG, Droge W, et al. The antiinflammatory sesquiterpene lactone parthenolide inhibits NF-{kappa}B by targeting the I{kappa}B kinase complex. J Immunol 1999;163(10):5617–23.

83. Kwok BH, Koh B, Ndubuisi MI, et al. The anti-inflammatory natural product parthenolide from the medicinal herb feverfew directly binds to and inhibits IkappaB kinase. Chem Biol 2001;8(8):759–66.

84. Riehemann K, Behnke B, Schulze-Osthoff K. Plant extracts from stinging nettle (Urtica dioica), an antirheumatic remedy, inhibit the proinflammatory transcription factor NF-kappaB. FEBS Lett 1999;442(1):89–94.

85. Teucher T, Obertreis B, Ruttkowski T, et al. Cytokine secretion in whole blood of healthy volunteers after oral ingestion of an Urtica dioica L. leaf extract. Zytokin-Sekretion im Vollblut gesunder Probanden nach oraler Einnahme eines Urtica dioica L-Blattextraktes. Arzneimittelforschung 1996;46(9):906–10.

86. Chainy GB, Manna SK, Chaturvedi MM, et al. Anethole blocks both early and late cellular responses transduced by tumor necrosis factor: effect on NF-kappaB, AP-1, JNK, MAPKK and apoptosis. Oncogene 2000;19(25):2943–50.

87. Futrakul N, Panichakul T, Butthep P, et al. Ganoderma lucidum suppresses endothelial cell cytotoxicity and proteinuria in persistent proteinuric focal segmental glomerulosclerosis (FSGS) nephrosis. Clin Hemorheol Microcirc 2004;31(4):267–72.

88. Battaglia S. The complete guide to aromatherapy. 2nd ed. Brisbane: The International Centre of Holistic Aromatherapy; 2003.

89. Silva J, Abebe W, Sousa SM, et al. Analgesic and anti-inflammatory effects of essential oils of Eucalyptus. J Ethnopharmacol 2003;89(2–3):277–83.

90. Wei A, Shibamoto T. Antioxidant/lipoxygenase inhibitory activities and chemical compositions of selected essential oils. J Agric Food Chem 2010;58(12):7218–25.

91. Caldefie-Chezet F, Fusillier C, Jarde T, et al. Potential anti-inflammatory effects of Melaleuca alternifolia essential oil on human peripheral blood leukocytes. Phytother Res 2006;20(5):364–70.

92. Carrasco FR, Schmidt G, Romero AL, et al. Immunomodulatory activity of Zingiber officinale Roscoe, Salvia officinalis L. and Syzygium aromaticum L. essential oils: evidence for humor- and cell-mediated responses. J Pharm Pharmacol 2009;61(7):961–7.

93. Bachiega TF, de Sousa JP, Bastos JK, et al. Clove and eugenol in noncytotoxic concentrations exert immunomodulatory/anti-inflammatory action on cytokine production by murine macrophages. J Pharm Pharmacol 2012;64(4):610–16.

94. Nogueira de Melo GA, Grespan R, Fonseca JP, et al. Rosmarinus officinalis L. essential oil inhibits in vivo and in vitro leukocyte migration. J Med Food 2011; 14(9):944–6.

95. Yousofi A, Daneshmandi S, Soleimani N, et al. Immunomodulatory effect of Parsley (Petroselinum crispum) essential oil on immune cells: mitogen-activated splenocytes and peritoneal macrophages. Immunopharmacol Immunotoxicol 2012;34(2):303–8.

96. Cuddy A. Your body language shapes who you are. YouTube; 2012 [updated 1 Oct 2012]. Available from: https://http://www.youtube.com/watch?v=Ks-_Mh1QhMc. [Accessed 14 May 2013].

97. Pedersen BK, Toft AD. Effects of exercise on lymphocytes and cytokines. Br J Sports Med 2000;34(4):246–51.

98. Costa Rosa LFBP. Exercise as a time-conditioning effector in chronic disease: a complementary treatment strategy. Evid Based Complement Alternat Med 2004;1(1): 63–70.

99. da Silva Krause M, de Bittencourt PIH Jr. Type 1 diabetes: can exercise impair the autoimmune event? The L-arginine/glutamine coupling hypothesis. Cell Biochem Funct 2008;26(4):406–33.

100. Kiecolt-Glaser JK, McGuire L, Robles TF, et al. Emotions, morbidity, and mortality: new perspectives from psychoneuroimmunology. Annu Rev Psychol 2002;53:83–107.

101. Salovey P, Rothman AJ, Detweiler JB, et al. Emotional states and physical health. Am Psychol 2000;55(1): 110–21.

102. Yoshino S, Fujimori J, Kohda M. Effects of mirthful laughter on neuroendocrine and immune systems in patients with rheumatoid arthritis. J Rheumatol 1996;23(4):793–4.

103. Davidson RJ, Kabat-Zinn J, Schumacher J, et al. Alterations in brain and immune function produced by mindfulness meditation [see comment]. Psychosom Med 2003;65(4):564–70.

104. Solberg EE, Halvorsen R, Sundgot-Borgen J, et al. Meditation: a modulator of the immune response to physical stress? A brief report. Br J Sports Med 1995;29(4):255–7.

105. Seeman TE, Dubin LF, Seeman M, et al. Religiosity/spirituality and health. A critical review of the evidence for biological pathways. Am Psychol 2003;58(1):53–63.

106. Prather AA, Marsland AL, Muldoon MF, et al. Positive affective style covaries with stimulated IL-6 and IL-10 production in a middle-aged community sample. Brain Behav Immun 2007;21(8):1033–7.

107. Kreutz G, Bongard S, Rohrmann S, et al. Effects of choir singing or listening on secretory immunoglobulin A, cortisol, and emotional state. J Behav Med 2004;27(6):623–35.

108. Kiecolt-Glaser JK, McGuire L, Robles TF, et al. Emotions, morbidity, and mortality: new perspectives from psychoneuroimmunology. Annu Rev Psychol 2002;53:83–107.

109. Glaser R, Rice J, Speicher CE, et al. Stress depresses interferon production by leukocytes concomitant with a decrease in natural killer cell activity. Behav Neurosci 1986;100(5):675–8.

110. Silberman DM, Wald MR, Genaro AM. Acute and chronic stress exert opposing effects on antibody responses associated with changes in stress hormone regulation of T-lymphocyte reactivity. J Neuroimmunol 2003;144(1–2):53–60.

111. Frick LR, Arcos ML, Rapanelli M, et al. Chronic restraint stress impairs T-cell immunity and promotes tumor progression in mice. Stress 2009;12(2):134–43.

112. Glaser R, Rice J, Sheridan J, et al. Stress-related immune suppression: health implications. Brain Behav Immun 1987;1(1):7–20.

113. Kiank C, Holtfreter B, Starke A, et al. Stress susceptibility predicts the severity of immune depression and the failure to combat bacterial infections in chronically stressed mice. Brain Behav Immun 2006;20(4):359–68.

114. Cai XY, Xu YL, Lin XJ. Effects of radix Astragali injection on apoptosis of lymphocytes and immune function in patients with systemic lupus erythematosus. Zhongguo Zhong Xi Yi Jie He Za Zhi 2006;26(5):443–5.

115. Kawachi I, Sparrow D, Vokonas PS, et al. Symptoms of anxiety and risk of coronary heart disease. The normative aging study. Circulation 1994;90(5):2225–9.

116. Pratt LA, Ford DE, Crum RM, et al. Depression, psychotropic medication, and risk of myocardial infarction. Prospective data from the Baltimore ECA follow-up. Circulation 1996;94(12):3123–9.

117. Everson SA, Kauhanen J, Kaplan GA, et al. Hostility and increased risk of mortality and acute myocardial infarction: the mediating role of behavioral risk factors. Am J Epidemiol 1997;146(2):142–52.

118. Sharma JN, Srivastava KC, Gan EK. Suppressive effects of eugenol and ginger oil on arthritic rats. Pharmacology 1994;49(5):314–18.

119. Zautra AJ, Hoffman JM, Matt KS, et al. An examination of individual differences in the relationship between interpersonal stress and disease activity among women with rheumatoid arthritis. Arthritis Rheum 1998;11(4):271–9.

120. Frieri M, Frieri M. Neuroimmunology and inflammation: implications for therapy of allergic and autoimmune diseases. Ann Allergy Asthma Immunol 2003;90(6 Suppl. 3):34–40.

121. Halverson PB, Holmes SB. Systemic lupus erythematosus: medical and nursing treatments. Orthop Nurs 1992;11(6):17–24.

122. Greco CM, Rudy TE, Manzi S. Effects of a stress-reduction program on psychological function, pain, and physical function of systemic lupus erythematosus patients: a randomized controlled trial. Arthritis Rheum 2004;51(4):625–34.

123. Linde K, Clausius N, Ramirez G, et al. Are the clinical effects of homoeopathy placebo effects? A meta-analysis of placebo-controlled trials. Lancet 1997;350(9081): 834–43.

124. Joos S, Rosemann T, Szecsenyi J, et al. Use of complementary and alternative medicine in Germany—a survey of patients with inflammatory bowel disease. BMC Complement Altern Med 2006;6:19.

125. Schwarz S, Knorr C, Geiger H, et al. Complementary and alternative medicine for multiple sclerosis. Mult Scler 2008;14(8):1113–19.

126. Quattropani C, Ausfeld B, Straumann A, et al. Complementary alternative medicine in patients with inflammatory bowel disease: use and attitudes. Scand J Gastroenterol 2003;38(3):277–82.

127. Fisher P, Scott DL. A randomized controlled trial of homeopathy in rheumatoid arthritis. Rheumatology 2001;40(9):1052–5.

128. Gibson RG, Gibson SLM, Macneill AD, et al. Homeopathic therapy in rheumatoid arthritis: evaluation by double blind clinical therapeutic trial. Br J Clin Pharmacol 1980;9(5):453–9.

129. Liao YN, Liu CS, Tsai TR, et al. Preliminary study of a traditional Chinese medicine formula in systemic lupus erythematosus patients to taper steroid dose and prevent disease flare-up. Kaohsiung J Med Sci 2011;27(7):251–7.

130. Dai YC, Zheng L, Zhang YL, et al. Effects of Jianpi Qingchang decoction on the quality of life of patients with

ulcerative colitis: a randomized controlled trial. Medicine 2017;96(16):e6651.

131. Sun J, Shen X, Dong J, et al. Tripterygium wilfordii Hook F as maintenance treatment for Crohn's disease. Am J Med Sci 2015;350(5):345–51.

132. Greco CM, Kao AH, Maksimowicz-McKinnon K, et al. Acupuncture for systemic lupus erythematosus: a pilot RCT feasibility and safety study. Lupus 2008;17(12):1108–16.

133. Lee MS, Shin BC, Ernst E. Acupuncture for rheumatoid arthritis: a systematic review. Rheumatology (Oxford) 2008;47(12):1747–53.

134. Clement-Kruzel S, Hwang SA, Kruzel MC, et al. Immune modulation of macrophage pro-inflammatory response by goldenseal and Astragalus extracts. J Med Food 2008;11(3):493–8.

135. Joos S, Brinkhaus B, Maluche C, et al. Acupuncture and moxibustion in the treatment of active Crohn's disease: a randomized controlled study. Digestion 2004;69(3):131–9.

136. Khurana R, Berney SM. Clinical aspects of rheumatoid arthritis. Pathophysiology 2005;12(3):153–65.

137. Alamanos Y, Drosos AA. Epidemiology of adult rheumatoid arthritis. Autoimmun Rev 2005;4(3):130–6.

138. Fishman P, Bar-Yehuda S. Rheumatoid arthritis: history, molecular mechanisms and therapeutic applications. In: Borea PA, editor. A3 adenosine receptors from cell biology to pharmacology and therapeutics. New York: Springer; 2010. p. 291–8.

139. Scott DL, Wolfe F, Huizinga TW. Rheumatoid arthritis. Lancet 2010;376(9746):1094–108.

140. Tobon GJ, Youinou P, Saraux A. The environment, geo-epidemiology, and autoimmune disease: rheumatoid arthritis. Autoimmun Rev 2010;9(5):A288–92.

141. Pratt AG, Isaacs JD, Mattey DL. Current concepts in the pathogenesis of early rheumatoid arthritis. Best Pract Res Clin Rheumatol 2009;23(1):37–48.

142. Ruiz-Esquide V, Sanmarti R. Tobacco and other environmental risk factors in rheumatoid arthritis. Reumatologia Clinica 2012;8(6):342–50.

143. Majithia V, Geraci SA. Rheumatoid arthritis: diagnosis and management. Am J Med 2007;120(11):936–9.

144. Bonciani D, Verdelli A, Bonciolini V, et al. Dermatitis herpetiformis: from the genetics to the development of skin lesions. Clin Dev Immunol 2012;2012:239691.

145. Badolato R, Oppenheim JJ. Role of cytokines, acute-phase proteins, and chemokines in the progression of rheumatoid arthritis. Semin Arthritis Rheum 1996;26(2):526–38.

146. Zhang W, Dai SM. Mechanisms involved in the therapeutic effects of Paeonia lactiflora Pallas in rheumatoid arthritis. Int Immunopharmacol 2012;14(1):27–31.

147. Shang W, Guo J, Cai H. Meta-analysis of total glucosides of paeony combined with methotrexate for treatment of rheumatoid arthritis. Mod J Integr Tradit Chin West Med 2010;19:653–6.

148. Zhong X, Su N, Zhou SH, et al. Meta-analysis of the efficacy and safety of total glucosides of paeony combined with immunosuppressant in the treatment of rheumatoid arthritis. China Pharm 2010;21:3731–4.

149. Zhang C, Jiang M, Lu AP. Evidence-based Chinese medicine for rheumatoid arthritis. J Tradit Chin Med 2011;31(2):152–7.

150. Chandran B, Goel A. A randomized, pilot study to assess the efficacy and safety of curcumin in patients with active rheumatoid arthritis. Phytother Res 2012;26(11):1719–25.

151. Amalraj A, Varma K, Jacob J, et al. A novel highly bioavailable curcumin formulation improves symptoms and diagnostic indicators in rheumatoid arthritis patients: a randomized, double-blind, placebo-controlled,

two-dose, three-arm, and parallel-group study. J Med Food 2017;20(10):1022–30.

152. Warnock M, McBean D, Suter A, et al. Effectiveness and safety of Devil's Claw tablets in patients with general rheumatic disorders. Phytother Res 2007;21(12):1228–33.

153. Lin J, Liu J, Davies ML, et al. Serum vitamin D level and rheumatoid arthritis disease activity: review and meta-analysis. PLoS ONE 2016;11(1):e0146351. https://doi.org/10.1371/journal.pone.0146351.

154. Mills S. The essential book of herbal medicine. London: Penguin Books; 1991.

155. Glastonbury S. Scientific evaluation of the use of traditional herbal depuratives via modulation of ABC transporters. Aust J Med Herbalism 2003;15(2):34–8.

156. Bone K. A clinical guide to blending liquid herbs. Missouri: Churchill Livingstone; 2003.

157. Baumgart DC, Sandborn WJ. Crohn's disease. Lancet 2012;380(9853):1590–605.

158. Fatahzadeh M. Inflammatory bowel disease. Oral Surg Oral Med Oral Pathol Oral Radiol Endod 2009;108(5):e1–10.

159. Loftus EV Jr. Clinical epidemiology of inflammatory bowel disease: incidence, prevalence, and environmental influences. Gastroenterology 2004;126(6):1504–17.

160. Fasano A, Shea-Donohue T. Mechanisms of disease: the role of intestinal barrier function in the pathogenesis of gastrointestinal autoimmune diseases. Nat Clin Pract Gastroenterol Hepatol 2005;2(9):416–22.

161. Podolsky DK. Inflammatory bowel disease. N Engl J Med 2002;347(6):417–29.

162. Li R, Alex P, Ye M, et al. An old herbal medicine with a potentially new therapeutic application in inflammatory bowel disease. Int J Clin Exp Med 2011;4(4):309–19.

163. Opheim R, Bernklev T, Fagermoen MS, et al. Use of complementary and alternative medicine in patients with inflammatory bowel disease: results of a cross-sectional study in Norway. Scand J Gastroenterol 2012;47(12):1436–47.

164. Ali T, Shakir F, Morton J. Curcumin and inflammatory bowel disease: biological mechanisms and clinical implication. Digestion 2012;85(4):249–55.

165. Midura-Kiela MT, Radhakrishnan VM, Larmonier CB, et al. Curcumin inhibits interferon-gamma signaling in colonic epithelial cells. Am J Physiol Gastrointest Liver Physiol 2012;302(1):G85–96.

166. Moole H, Yerasi C, Moole V, et al. A systematic review and meta-analysis of randomized controlled trials: improvement in endoscopic disease activity of ulcerative colitis with curcumin treatment. Gastrointest Endosc 2016;83(5):AB294.

167. Ammon HP. Salai Guggal—Boswellia serrata: from a herbal medicine to a non-redox inhibitor of leukotriene biosynthesis. Eur J Med Res 1996;1(8):369–70.

168. Borrelli F, Capasso F, Capasso R, et al. Effect of Boswellia serrata on intestinal motility in rodents: inhibition of diarrhoea without constipation. Br J Pharmacol 2006;148:553–60.

169. Gupta I, Parihar A, Malhotra P, et al. Effects of gum resin of Boswellia serrata in patients with chronic colitis. Planta Med 2001;67(5):391–5.

170. Pellegrini L, Milano E, Franceschi F, et al. Managing ulcerative colitis in remission phase: usefulness of Casperome®, an innovative lecithin-based delivery system of Boswellia serrata extract. Eur Rev Med Pharmacol Sci 2016;20(12):2695–700.

171. Langmead L, Feakins RM, Goldthorpe S, et al. Randomized, double-blind, placebo-controlled trial of oral

aloe vera gel for active ulcerative colitis. Aliment Pharmacol Ther 2004;19(7):739–47.

172. Langmead L, Makins RJ, Rampton DS. Anti-inflammatory effects of aloe vera gel in human colorectal mucosa in vitro. Aliment Pharmacol Ther 2004;19(5):521–7.

173. Ben-Arye E, Goldin E, Wengrower D, et al. Wheat grass juice in the treatment of active distal ulcerative colitis: a randomized double-blind placebo-controlled trial. Scand J Gastroenterol 2002;37(4):444–9.

174. Kamali M, Tavakoli H, Khodadoost M, et al. Efficacy of the Punica granatum peels aqueous extract for symptom management in ulcerative colitis patients. A randomized, placebo controlled, clinical trial. Complement Ther Clin Pract 2015;21(3):141–6.

175. Rastegarpanah M, Malekzadeh R, Vahedi H, et al. A randomized, double blinded, placebo-controlled clinical trial of silymarin in ulcerative colitis. Chin J Integr Med 2015;21(12):902–6.

176. Samsami-kor M, Daryani NE, Rezanejad P, et al. Anti-inflammatory effects of resveratrol in patients with ulcerative colitis: a randomized, double-blind, placebo-controlled pilot study. Arch Med Res 2015;46(4):280–5.

177. Gubatan J, Mitsuhashi S, Zenlea T, et al. Low serum vitamin D during remission increases risk of clinical relapse in patients with ulcerative colitis. Clin Gastroenterol Hepatol 2017;15(2):240–6.e1.

178. Guslandi M. A natural approach to treatment of inflammatory bowel disease. Br J Clin Pharmacol 2008;65(4):468–9.

179. Tamboli CP, Neut C, Desreumaux P, et al. Dysbiosis in inflammatory bowel disease. Gut 2004;53(1):1–4.

180. Miele E, Pascarella F, Giannetti E, et al. Effect of a probiotic preparation (VSL#3) on induction and maintenance of remission in children with ulcerative colitis. Am J Gastroenterol 2009;104(2):437–43.

181. Guslandi M, Mezzi G, Sorghi M, et al. Saccharomyces boulardii in maintenance treatment of Crohn's disease. Dig Dis Sci 2000;45(7):1462–4.

182. Garcia Vilela E, De Lourdes De Abreu Ferrari M, Oswaldo Da Gama Torres H, et al. Influence of Saccharomyces boulardii on the intestinal permeability of patients with Crohn's disease in remission. Scand J Gastroenterol 2008;43(7):842–8.

183. Guslandi M, Giollo P, Testoni PA. A pilot trial of Saccharomyces boulardii in ulcerative colitis. Eur J Gastroenterol Hepatol 2003;15(6):697–8.

184. Bourreille A, Cadiot G, Le Dreau G, et al. Saccharomyces boulardii does not prevent relapse of Crohn's disease. Clin Gastroenterol Hepatol 2013;11:982–7.

185. Sood A, Midha V, Makharia GK, et al. The probiotic preparation, VSL#3 induces remission in patients with mild-to-moderately active ulcerative colitis. Clin Gastroenterol Hepatol 2009;7(11):1202–9, 9 e1.

186. Bibiloni R, Fedorak RN, Tannock GW, et al. VSL#3 probiotic-mixture induces remission in patients with active ulcerative colitis. Am J Gastroenterol 2005;100(7):1539–46.

187. Franchin G, Peeva E, Diamond B. Pathogenesis of SLE: implications for rational therapy. Drug Discov Today 2004;1(3):303–8.

188. Kotzin BL. Systemic lupus erythematosus. Cell 1996;85(3):303–6.

189. Putterman C, Caricchio R, Davidson A, et al. Systemic lupus erythematosus. Clin Dev Immunol 2012;2012:437282.

190. Jönsen A, Bengtsson AA, Nived O, et al. Gene–environment interactions in the aetiology of systemic lupus erythematosus. Autoimmunity 2007;40(8):613–17.

191. Pan HF, Fang XH, Li WX, et al. Radix astragali: a promising new treatment option for systemic lupus erythematosus. Med Hypotheses 2008;71(2):311–12.

192. Su L, Mao JC, Gu JH. Effect of intravenous drip infusion of cyclophosphamide with high-dose Astragalus injection in treating lupus nephritis. Zhong Xi Yi Jie He Xue Bao 2007;5(3):272–5.

193. Sun Y, Cai TT, Zhou XB, et al. Saikosaponin a inhibits the proliferation and activation of T cells through cell cycle arrest and induction of apoptosis. Int Immunopharmacol 2009;9(7–8):978–83.

194. Lai ZW, Hanczko R, Bonilla E, et al. N-acetylcysteine reduces disease activity by blocking mammalian target of rapamycin in T cells from systemic lupus erythematosus patients: a randomized, double-blind, placebo-controlled trial. Arthritis Rheum 2012;64(9):2937–46.

195. Duffy EM, Meenagh GK, McMillan SA, et al. The clinical effect of dietary supplementation with omega-3 fish oils and/or copper in systemic lupus erythematosus. J Rheumatol 2004;31(8):1551–6.

196. Kamen DL, Oates JC. A pilot study to determine if vitamin D repletion improves endothelial function in lupus patients. Am J Med Sci 2015;350(4):302–7.

197. Segal BM, Thomas W, Zhu X, et al. Oxidative stress and fatigue in systemic lupus erythematosus. Lupus 2012;21(9):984–92.

198. Hartley N. The effect of chronic stress on cellular immunity: a possible alleviation by Praescent [MPhil]. St Lucia: University of Queensland; 2011.

199. Arriens C, Hynan LS, Lerman RH, et al. Placebo controlled randomized clinical trial of fish oil's impact on fatigue, quality of life, and disease activity in Systemic Lupus Erythematosus. Nutr J 2015;14:82.

200. Fortin PR, Lew RA, Liang MH, et al. Validation of a meta-analysis: the effects of fish oil in rheumatoid arthritis. J Clin Epidemiol 1995;48(11):1379–90.

201. Rayman MP. Selenium and human health. Lancet 2012;379(9822):1256–68.

202. Macfarlane GJ, El-Metwally A, De Silva V, et al. Evidence for the efficacy of complementary and alternative medicines in the management of rheumatoid arthritis: a systematic review. Rheumatology 2011;50(9):1672–83.

203. Brien S, Lewith GT, McGregor G. Devil's claw (Harpagophytum procumbens) as a treatment for osteoarthritis: a review of efficacy and safety. J Altern Complement Med 2006;12(10):981–93.

CHAPTER **32**

Cancer

Janet Schloss
ND, PhD

OVERVIEW

Cancer is a multifactorial disease characterised by uncontrollable cell growth. Many theories exist as to what may cause cancer with few cancers having definitive risk factors (e.g. cigarette smoking and lung cancer,[1] or human papilloma (HPV) and cervical cancer).[2] However, not everyone who smokes gets lung cancer and not everyone with HPV results in cervical cancer.

In Australia it is estimated that there will be 138 321 new cases of cancer diagnosed in 2018, with an estimated number of deaths being 48 586. The chances of survival for 5 years have now risen to over 68% for all cancers (2009–2013) which indicates more people are surviving diagnosis and treatment and living longer.[3–5] Worldwide, the World Health Organisation (WHO) states that cancer, cardiovascular disease, respiratory disease and diabetes are responsible for 80% of all deaths.[6]

The most common types of cancer in Australia are breast cancer in women and prostate cancer in men. Other common cancers diagnosed in Australia excluding non-melanoma skin cancers include colorectal, melanoma and lung cancer. It has been found that by 85 years of age, one in two Australian men and one in three Australian women will be diagnosed with some type of cancer.[3,4]

Cancer prevention

Cancer prevention is a broad topic with varied information on different types of cancer. To simplify, several areas of an individual's life can be taken into consideration to possibly prevent this disease. It should be noted that a person may encompass all of these aspects and could still be diagnosed with cancer. With such a multifactorial disease, people can only do the best they can to prevent its initiation and growth in their body. In saying this, it is estimated that a third of all cancers can be attributed to diet and lifestyle.[7]

A basic list of areas to consider in preventing cancer includes:

- diet—eat a balanced diet with lots of fresh fruit and vegetables (refer to the information on diet in Chapter 3) and ensure adequate nutrition[8]
- exercise and physical activity[8]
- maintenance of an optimal body weight[8,9]

- decrease negative stress[10]
- adequate sleep[11]
- having fun and enjoyment in life[12]
- reducing alcohol intake, reducing or stopping smoking and illicit drug use[13]
- having safe sex[14]
- spirituality or religion or some form of belief[12]
- moderation in everything.

Certain cancers have been linked with particular dietary and lifestyle choices (Table 32.1).

Table 32.1
Links between cancer and lifestyle

Causal factor	Implicated cancer
Smoking	Lung cancer[1] Cervical cancer in people with HPV[15] Vulvar squamous cell carcinoma (SCC)[15]
Alcohol	Total cancer risk[16] Liver cancer[16] Breast cancer—especially oestrogen-dependent cancers[17] Colon cancer[18]
Low fruit, vegetable and fibre intake; high intake of processed meats and nitrosamines; highly salted foods	Gastric cancer[19]
Obesity	Gastric cancer[20] Breast cancer—linked with leptin regulation[21]

RISK FACTORS

The types of risk factors vary depending on the type of cancer. These may include diet and lifestyle factors, viruses, genetics and environmental exposure. Other risk factors include lack of physical exercise,[22] high body mass index (BMI)/obesity,[22] exposure or lack of exposure to sun (due to low vitamin D),[23,24] nutrient deficiencies,[25] medication (in some cases medication can increase the risk of other cancers, such as tamoxifen causing endometrial carcinoma),[26] country/nationality,[27] stress,[28] gender (e.g. prostate cancer in males and ovarian cancer in females), age[29] and occupation.[30–32] The question of 'what causes cancer' has intrigued scientists and medical specialists for generations. There are a number of different theories with no one theory being totally correct.

Theorised cause factors for cancers are summarised in Table 32.2.

DIFFERENTIAL DIAGNOSIS

A differential diagnosis for cancer can be quite complex considering there are more than 200 different types of cancer and that cancer can cause almost any sign or symptom. Differential diagnosis for specific cancers should be sought.[54–57] However, there are 'red flag' signs and symptoms that may assist in identifying when a patient needs to be referred to a medical practitioner for further testing. These signs and symptoms can be due to the tumour pushing on organs, blood vessels, nerves or blocking ducts or passages such as a bile duct. Insomuch as some cancers can be found early, other cancers may not

Table 32.2
Theorised causative factors in cancer

Possible cause	Explanation
Genetics	Certain cancers, such as breast, prostate and colon cancer, have been found to have hereditary links. There are certain genetic markers that the medical fraternity can test for to check if someone has the genetic markers for that cancer, such as the BRCA gene for breast cancer.[33]
Viruses and infection	Viruses have been linked with the development of certain cancers. Examples of these include: HPV (cervical cancer)[2]; Epstein-Barr virus (non-Hodgkin's lymphoma)[34]; HIV (Kaposi's sarcoma, primary central nervous system lymphoma, invasive cervical cancer and non-Hodgkin's lymphoma)[35]; hepatitis B virus (hepatocellular carcinomas)[36]; retroviruses (adult T-cell leukaemia)[37]; *Helicobacter pylori* (gastric cancer in people with certain polymorphisms)[38]; and simian virus 40 (non-Hodgkin's lymphoma).[39]
Mitochondrial dysfunction	Cancer progression has been linked with mitochondrial dysfunction. This can be a result of mitochondrial DNA (mtDNA) mutations and/or depletion. These mutations or mitochondrial depletions have also been linked with an increase of drug resistance within cells. This mitochondrial dysfunction has been found in certain cancers such as prostate cancer.[40]
Environmental influences	Over time the prevalence of cancer in the Western world has increased.[41] Epidemiological studies have found an association between this increase and the exposure to environmental toxins such as organochlorides and synthetic pesticides.[42] Further research is being conducted, but it seems at this stage that fetuses, infants, children and young adults are most at risk.[42] There are specific cancers, such as mesothelioma, which have been directly linked with exposure to asbestos.[43]
Immune system	It has been postulated that a lowered immune system may increase the chance of cancer developing. The natural killer cells are the main surveillance system of the body, protecting against cancer formation and infection. These natural killer cells are a main part of the innate immune system and, if they are not functioning correctly, can allow tumours to develop through abnormal cell development.[44]
Cell cycle mitosis malfunction	In cell replication certain checkpoints and cellular activity maintain the health of the cell. If these checkpoints, such as p53, have mutations[45] or there are abnormal centrosomes in a cell, cancer cells may develop.[46] The elderly in particular are prone to malignant tumours that are related to the accumulation of damaged DNA from malfunctioning cell mitosis.[47]
Oxidative damage	There are several schools of thought that oxidative damage, especially to DNA and cellular components, can be attributed to developing cancer. Reactive species such as ROS (reactive oxygen species) and RNS (reactive nitrogen species) are a natural by-product of normal biochemical and physiological reactions in the body. These reactive species can cause damage to the DNA, cellular membrane and cellular organelles, and can interfere with cellular regulators.[48] The body is highly regulated and, normally, cell damage will result in cellular death. There are no human studies to support this theory, with in vitro studies not supporting normal physiological aspects of human cellular activity.
Mind–body connection	The pathogenesis of cancer may have a psychological aspect. There are theories on a connection between the mind and the development of certain cancers, but this has not been confirmed. However, there is good evidence that mind–body medicine should be taken into consideration when addressing cancer.[49]
Polymorphisms	There are numerous studies on polymorphisms and genetic mutations increasing the risk of nearly all cancers. As this is a relatively new area of research, more studies will emerge on new polymorphisms that can be linked with certain cancers, and testing procedures will become more accessible and less expensive.[29,50,51]

Table 32.2
Theorised causative factors in cancer (continued)

Possible cause	Explanation
Epigenetics	The increase of scientific knowledge on how chromatin organisation modulates gene transcriptions has highlighted how epigenetic mechanisms are involved in the initiation and progression of human cancer. These epigenetic changes have been found to affect nearly every step in tumour progression, especially the aberrant promoter hypermethylation that is associated with gene silencing.[52]
Exposure to carcinogens	The IARC designated 109 agents as group 1 carcinogens in 2012. Exposure to carcinogenic agents can be linked as theory that can cause cancer development. (www.iarc.fr)[53]

cause any signs or symptoms until they have grown quite large such as pancreas, kidney or ovarian. Other tumours can release cells into the blood stream and cause symptoms not normally associated with cancer such as blood clots in veins from pancreatic cancer or raised calcium levels from lung cancer.

Treatment for cancer is best if the cancer is diagnosed early, so all signs and symptoms that may indicate cancer development, no matter how small, should be investigated further. Sometimes people like to ignore signs or symptoms believing that nothing is wrong or they are frightened of what might be found. Some of these signs and symptoms can easily be from other causes and may seem unimportant but no signs or symptoms should be ignored or overlooked.

Cancer warning signs*

- Unexplained weight loss
- Development of a lump or thickening of an area
- Fever for an extended period of time
- Fatigue or lethargy that does not get better with rest
- Pain (e.g. headache that does not disappear, back ache)
- Skin changes such as darker looking skin, jaundice, reddened skin, itching, mole changes, excessive hair growth
- Change in bowel or urination habits
- Sores that do not heal
- White patches inside the mouth or on the tongue (leukoplakia)
- Unusual bleeding or discharge
- Indigestion or trouble swallowing
- Nagging cough or hoarseness

*General signs and symptoms to be aware of for potential cancer development[58]

CONVENTIONAL TREATMENT

Traditional treatment of cancer is based on four forms of treatment: surgery, chemotherapy, radiation and hormone therapy.[1] Any one or a combination of these treatments may be used, depending on the type of tumour, the location, the aggressiveness, the age of the patient and what has been found to be most effective by clinical trials.

The Cochrane database is an important source of information; there are a variety of Cochrane reviews on chemotherapy and radiation for different types of cancer and adjunct medications or complementary and alternative medicines (CAM) with cancer treatment. The information is extensive and beyond the scope of this chapter to list in detail. Entering 'chemotherapy' and 'radiation' separately into the Cochrane search engine will provide a broad overview of current effective treatments. Table 32.3 provides specific evidence pertaining to integrative cancer treatment only; see the relevant chapters in this book for generalised information, and Appendix 3 for a chemotherapeutic CAM interaction table.

Table 32.3
CAM treatment of common side effects of chemotherapy and radiation

Side effect	CAM therapy
Mouth ulcers	Calcium phosphate, honey, zinc sulfate,[59] *Aloe vera, Camellia sinensis, Acacia catechu, Matricaria recutita, Achillea millifolium*, Chinese herbs,[60] Glutamine[61]
Diarrhoea	Glutamine,[62] probiotics[63]
Constipation	*Senna alexandrina*[64]
Intestinal permeability	Glutamine[65]
Radiation enteritis or enteropathy	Hyperbaric oxygen chambers,[66] probiotics during radiation,[67] glutamine during radiation[68]
Neutrophilia	Vitamin E[69]
Anaemia	Iron[70]
Fibrosis	Lipoic acid[71]
Fatigue	L-carnitine,[72] coenzyme Q10[73]
Memory loss	Egg phosphocholine and low-dose vitamin B12[74]
Weight loss	Omega-3 fatty acids[75]
Weight gain	Dietary suggestions to keep BMI in range[76]
Stress/anxiety	L-theanine,[77] nervine herbs, B vitamins[78]
Peripheral neuropathy	Vitamin B1, B6, B12,[79] omega-3 fatty acids, lipoic acid, glutamine, vitamin E[80]
Cardiomyopathy	Coenzyme Q10[81]

Potential interactions

Potential interactions between orthodox and CAM therapies need to be considered when treating a patient with cancer. As there are a variety of drugs used for cancer, it is important for the CAM practitioner to address each drug and check for any possible interactions both beneficial and contradictory (Figure 32.1). More research is required on potential interactions of cancer drugs and complementary medicine as there is limited human data (most studies are animal or in vitro based).[82] A chart of potential interactions between naturopathic medicines and chemotherapeutics is in the appendices at the back of this book.

There are, however, ways in which the potential risk for interaction with chemotherapy can be moderated. Because many naturopathic medicines can protect and support not only the body from the deleterious effects of chemotherapy but the cancerous tissue as well, it may be prudent to apply a cautionary approach to CAM prescription.[83] In principle it takes five half-lives to reach a steady state and five half-lives to eliminate virtually all of a drug in the body. Knowing both the half-lives of naturopathic medicine and chemotherapy can allow for a dosing regimen that can reduce risk of possible interactions (see Table 32.4).

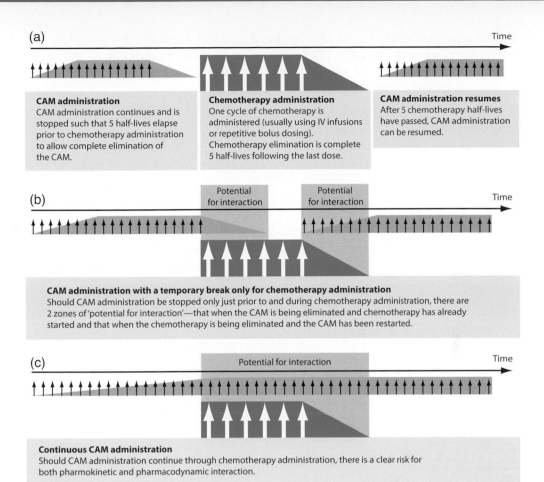

Figure 32.1
Risk of interactions associated with different CAM treatment protocols

Source: Seely et al. 2007[83]

Table 32.4
Selected natural products and their half-life

Naturopathic intervention	Half-life
Green tea	3.4 hours ± 0.3 hours
Curcumin	< 1 hour
Selenium	102–252 days
Vitamin C	30 minutes

Source: Seely et al. 2007[83]

Tumour markers

Certain types of cancers have been found to release specific molecules in the blood or tissues; these markers can be measured or identified. They can be used to aid diagnosis or in the clinical management of a patient. Blood tests are used to ascertain these markers.

Ideally, a positive result should only be found in a patient with a malignancy, and it should correlate with the stage of the cancer or the patient's response to treatment. Tumour markers can be used only as a guide as no tests meet all requirements.

Tumour markers have four purposes:

- screening of a healthy population or a high-risk population for the presence of cancer
- aid making a diagnosis of cancer or of a specific type of cancer
- determining the prognosis in a patient
- monitoring a patient in remission or while receiving surgery, radiation or chemotherapy.

Cell mitosis

The regulation of cell division is the most important part of cell mitosis (Figure 32.2). Without the cell regulators, abnormal cell development can occur. There are three main areas to consider in cell mitosis: oncogenes and tumour-suppressor genes; p53 and p21 checkpoints; and centrosomes. All three interact to allow abnormal cell development.

Common tumour markers

- **PSA**: prostate specific antigen. Range 0–4 µg/L
- **CEA**: carcinoembryonic antigen for colon cancer, but can also indicate pancreatic, gastric, lung or breast cancer. Range < 2.5 µ/L in non-smoker, < 5 µg/L in a smoker
- **CA 19-9**: mainly for pancreatic cancer, but can also be present in colon and gastric cancer
- **CA 125**: mainly ovarian cancer
- **AFP**: alpha-fetoprotein for hepatocellular carcinoma. Range < 10 µg/L
- **HCG**: human chorionic gonadotrophin, normally elevated in pregnancy, can also be found in gestational trophoblastic disease and germ cell tumours as well breast, lung and gastrointestinal tract (GIT) tumours
- **CA 15.3, CA 27–29**: mainly breast cancer
- **HMB**-45: melanoma
- **Thyroglobulin**: most thyroid cancer

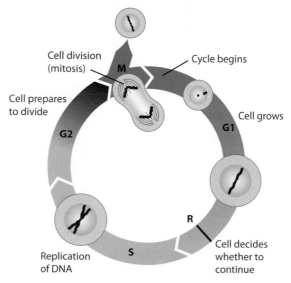

Figure 32.2
The cell cycle for normal cell division

KEY TREATMENT PROTOCOLS

Adjuvant use of nutraceuticals

Oncogenes and tumour-suppressor genes

Oncogenic processes have long been associated with cancer development and progression. These genes stimulate the process of cell mitosis and DNA replication and studies have shown that these genes are altered in cancer. The two main genes that are focused on are the proto-oncogenes and tumour-suppressor genes.[84]

Recent studies have identified a specific small class of RNA molecules called microRNAs (miRNAs). These miRNAs negatively regulate gene expression post-transcriptionally and aid the development of cell identity. These are important as they can affect cellular transformation, carcinogenesis and metastasis because they can act as an oncogene or tumour-suppressor gene.[85]

According to naturopathic treatment, keeping cellular oncogenes working efficiently and decreasing the development of cancer requires both dietary regulation and maintaining levels of particular nutrients within the body. Epidemiological and experimental data have found that Western diets that are high in fat and low in calcium and vitamin D may accelerate tumour growth by causing genetic manipulation.[86] Maintaining a **diet** low in detrimental fats and increasing calcium and vitamin D levels may therefore prevent gene alteration.

p53, p21

Abnormalities in the regulatory marker p53 have been found in most cancer cells. Cancer cells may have either mutations of the p53 gene or an accumulation of p53 proteins in the cells.[87,88] p21-activated kinases (PAKs) aid controlling G(2)/M transition and mitosis and are tumour-suppressor genes regulated by p53. Therefore they are necessary for cell proliferation, mitotic progression and other regulators.[89,90]

A number of different nutrients can play a role in the p53 and p21 genes, which can be of benefit for cell regulation. Low levels of **folate** and **vitamin B6** may influence p53, increasing the risk of colorectal cancer.[91] The mechanism of this deficiency involves the mutation of the p53 gene, therefore changing its expression. It is recommended that people consume more than 400 µg of folate a day to prevent this occurring.

Resveratrol has been found to modulate p53 to induce apoptosis (programmed cell death that is an integral part of normal biological processes to kill abnormal cell development) and decrease excessive p53, thereby expressing a beneficial effect in preventing abnormal cell division. Resveratrol has also been found to induce apoptosis via modulating other cellular molecules such as cyclin D1, p21, BCL2, BAX, Bcl XL, caspase 9 and p27.[92,93]

Green tea is another nutrient that has been found to modulate p53 and p21. Huang et al. found that green tea enhanced *Ziziphus jujuba*'s selective cytotoxic activity by causing cell death via up-regulation of p53 and p21 while decreasing cyclin E levels in HepG2 cells.[94] Green tea has also been found to inhibit tumour growth and angiogenesis as well as induce apoptosis.[95] **Genistein** has been found to influence p21 transcription by markedly inhibiting proliferative activity and inducing the expression of p21 plus oestrogen receptor beta (ERbeta).[96]

Vitamin D has been found to influence p53 and p21. Both p21 and p53 have vitamin D binding sites.[87] If a patient is deficient in vitamin D, both p53 and p21 may be affected, possibly influencing cell division. Flavonoids—such as **quercetin**—have also been found to influence p53 in relation to cancer. In 2008 Tanigawa found that quercetin helped to stabilise p53 at both the mRNA and the protein level to reactive p53-dependent cell cycle arrest and apoptosis.[97] This was achieved by quercetin inducing p53 phosphorylation and total p53 protein, but not up-regulating p53 miRNA at transcription. It also stimulates p21 expression and suppresses cyclin D1 to activate cell cycle arrest. Quercetin was also found to inhibit p53 mRNA degradation post transcriptionally.

Centrosomes

These microtubules aid cell mitosis by creating the polar rejection force that pushes the chromosomes away from the spindle poles by wobbling at high frequencies. A rise in intracellular **calcium** aids the regulation of the polar force at the onset of chromosomal splitting. If this is defective, chromosomal instability (characteristic of most cancers) can occur.[98] It has also been found that cells that have dysfunctional p53s have more centrosomes.[99]

Vitamin A plays a key role in centrosomes and chromosome replication through the retinoblastoma protein, which is a regulating protein of cyclins D and E, cdk 4 and 6, cdk inhibitors p16, p15 and p53.[100] A **vitamin B12** deficiency has been associated with enlarged, disrupted centrioles in monocytes and neutrophils.[101]

Proteasomes play an important role in a variety of cellular processes such as cell cycle progression, signal transduction and the immune response, and are important in maintaining rapid turnover of short-lived proteins. They also prevent accumulation of misfolded or damaged proteins. **Zinc** increases proteasome substrates such as p5 and p21, as well as decreasing the enzyme that degrades these substrates in centrosomes.[102]

Folate also plays a critical role in the prevention of chromosome breakage and hypomethylation of DNA. A folate deficiency can cause centromere defects that can induce abnormal distribution of replicated chromosomes during mitosis. It has also been found to be a risk factor for chromosomes 17 and 21 aneuploidy, which has been observed in breast cancer and leukaemia.[103]

Glycolysis and p53

A common theory sometimes postulated in the naturopathic treatment of cancer is that tumours or cancer feed on sugar. This theory is based on the idea that some cancer cells have different biochemical activity compared with 'normal cells'. Research has found that most solid cancer cells have higher rates of glycolysis than 'normal cells'.[88] It has also found that, after a loss of functional p53, there were mitochondrial changes, up-regulation of rate-limiting enzymes and proteins in glycolysis and intracellular pH regulation, hypoxia-induced switching to anaerobic metabolism leading to higher lactic acid levels and metabolic reprogramming.[88]

Extrapolation of these results has led to various diets being developed to 'starve' the cancer. This theory has not been proven. An epidemiological diet and health study conducted in 2012 investigated the association of total sugars, sucrose, fructose, added sugars, added sucrose and added fructose in the diet with the risk of 24 malignancies.[104] The authors found no association between dietary sugars and risk of colorectal or any other major cancer; however, they did observe a strong positive association between added sugars and the risk for oesophageal adenocarcinoma, a twofold increased risk of small intestine cancer and high fructose (especially added fructose) consumption and strong risk of pleural cancer with all investigated sugars.[104]

Other interesting findings from this study included a decreased risk of liver cancer, with high added fructose intake in women and a decrease risk of all cancers with added fructose in men. Men also had a decreased risk of oral cancer with both added sucrose and added fructose. Pancreatic cancer has been suggested to be associated with an increased sugar intake[105]; however, Tasevska's study found no association between added sugars and pancreatic risk but did find a mild association with high fructose intake.[104]

Overall, it is still recommended that people with cancer decrease their processed sugar intake and follow a low glycaemic index diet. It has been found that insulin-like growth factor 1 (IGF-1) and the synthesis of insulin by added sugars may enhance tumour development by promoting cell proliferation, inhibiting apoptosis, stimulating the synthesis of sex steroids or promoting the production of vascular endothelial growth factor (VEGF).[106–109]

The high usage of glycolysis by tumours is also why it is often recommended in traditional naturopathic theory to alkalise the body of a patient with cancer. It is hoped that the spread of cancer can be decreased by increasing buffers and trying to decrease the acidic environment. This theory has yet to be validated, though alkalising diets (higher fruit and vegetable intake, and lower meat intake) generally have positive effects in cancer.

Another theory (the Warburg effect) suggests 'oxygenating' the body, as cancer cells utilise anaerobic glycolysis more than normal cells, which prefer the aerobic system of the mitochondria.[110] This theory also has not been proven; however, increasing oxygen availability (e.g. through breathing exercises and circulatory stimulants) to cells may aid the normal cells rather than the cancer cells and potentially increase the removal of toxins and carcinogens.

Attenuation of inflammation

Inflammation has been linked with a variety of different cancers as inflammatory markers have been suggested to aid tumour progression, promotion and growth. It has been found that a cellular inflammatory microenvironment and an increased level of nitric oxide can stimulate or accelerate tumour development.[111] Cyclooxygenase enzymes such as prostaglandins and thromboxanes play an important role in cancer, particularly in gastrointestinal, oesophageal, gastric, liver, pancreatic and colorectal cancers.[112]

A key approach to cancer is to modulate the inflammatory cascade; this can have a positive effect on cancer initiation, promotion, progression and metastasis. Anti-inflammatory nutrients such as **curcumin**,[113] **bromelain**,[114] **quercetin**[114] and **EPA/DHA**[114] can decrease the progressive effect of the inflammation in cancer. Herbal medicines such as *Zingiber officinale*, *Curcuma longa*,[113] *Withania somnifera*[115] and *Boswellia serrata* may also be useful.[114]

Immunological factors

A functioning immune system appropriately monitors and attacks any foreign cells or pathogenic invaders. A dysregulated immune system may allow cancer cells to develop and spread.[116] States that can cause a dysregulated immune system affecting cancer include stress,[117,118] diabetes,[119] HIV (and other viruses)[120] and nutritional deficiencies.[121,122]

An important fact to consider is that once a tumour has developed the immune system cannot recognise it as a foreign object or 'non-self' due to the tumour coating.

The tumour can don a coat of the host's own protein on the cell's surface that is composed of fibrin and a polymeric form of human serum albumin (HAS), which is resistant to fibrinolytic degradation. The tumour cell than appears to the immune system as 'self' or a normal cell thus it is not detected by the immune system. This allows the tumour to be able to continue growing without the immune system attacking it.[123]

It has also been found that tumours can influence the immune system once formed. In many cancers, a malignant progression is accompanied by profound immune suppression that can interfere with the anti-tumour response and tumour elimination. The immune response to tumours resides in the recognition of tumour antigens and certain tumour aspects which has lead to the development of immunotherapy.[124] A randomised controlled trial (RCT) investigated the detection of immunoglobulin M (IgM) and immunoglobulin G (IgG) complexes in 979 patients with oesophagus, intestinal, lung, naropharyngeal, ovarian, breast, uterine, thyroid and hepatocellular carcinoma and Hodgkin's and non-Hodgkin's lymphoma compared with 401 healthy controls. This trial found that IgM and IgG, two-component-determined circulating immune complexes (TCIC), may play a significant role in immune regulation during the malignancy course. Patients with cancer were found to have a decreased IgM and IgG-TCIC accompanied by a diverse IgG/IgM-TCIC.[125] This allows scientists to have a better understanding of the immune system during malignancies and hopefully aid in the development of specific treatment regimens.

Although the immune system may not recognise some tumour cells, it is still considered important to support the immune system for the health benefits of the patient. Nutrients and herbs that support immune function can therefore be very important in assisting people with cancer. Those clinical **nutritional interventions** with particular benefit in cancer include vitamin D,[126] antioxidants,[127] vitamin C,[127] zinc[127] and **medicinal mushrooms** such as shiitake or reishi.[128,129] **Herbal medicines** that may be of benefit include *Astragalus membranaceus*,[130] *Uncaria tomentosa*,[131] *Eleutherococcus senticosus*,[132] *Rhodiola rosacea*,[132] *Schisandra chinensis*,[132] *Panax ginseng*[133] and *Echinacea* spp.[134]

Hormonal factors

Some specific cancers, including breast,[135] ovarian, endometrial,[136] cervical, prostate and testicular, are well known to have hormonal influences.[137] Other cancers, including both gastric and lung, may also have hormonal influences.[138,139]

Breast cancer can be stimulated by oestrogen and/or progesterone,[135] whereas ovarian, endometrial and cervical cancers may be oestrogen-stimulated via receptor sites on the cancer cells.[136] Testosterone is the key hormone related to prostate- or male genitalia-based cancers, whereas testicular cancer may be related to either oestrogen or androgens, and approximately 7–11% of males who get testicular cancer have also been found to have gynaecomastia.[137]

Oestrogen may have protective effects on gastric cancer. The prevalence of gastric cancer is higher in men while being lower in premenopausal women, women on hormone replacement and men undergoing oestrogen therapy.[138] The actual mechanism of protection is unclear, but it is thought that oestrogen may increase the expression of trefoil factor proteins, which have been found to protect mucous epithelia or inhibit the expression of c-erbB-2 oncogene.

Lung cancer has also been found to have an oestrogen connection. Adenocarcinoma is the most common type of lung cancer in non-smokers, and it has been suggested that there is a distinct pattern concerning oestrogen beta receptors.[139]

A number of nutrients and herbs can have a positive effect in the integrative treatment of hormonal tumours. For oestrogen- and progesterone-stimulated tumours, cruciferous indoles—particularly **indole-3-carbinol**—aids in a number of different ways: it aids the induction of apoptosis in breast and cervical cancer cells by inducing DNA breakage in the nucleus of the cells,[140] and it alters the metabolism of active oestrogen hormones indicated in urinary excretion (16-oestradiol to 2-oestradiol).[141]

Other nutrients that have been found to be of assistance include: **zinc** for testosterone via the enzyme 5 alpha-reductase[142]; **resveratrol** via inhibiting the cytochrome p450 19 enzymes (also called aromatase catalases, which are the rate-limiting step of oestrogen synthesis)[143] and **genistein**, which, although controversial and having mixed results, has shown positive results by inhibiting cell proliferation and inducing apoptosis in breast cancer cell lines.[144] However, it has also been shown to stimulate growth in oestrogen-dependent human tumour cells (MCF-7) and may negate the inhibitory effect of tamoxifen.[145]

Herbs that have shown to be of potential benefit include ***Serenoa repens*** for prostate cancer. *Serenoa repens* has been found to induce growth arrest of prostate cancer cells as well as increasing p21 and p53 in the prostate cells.[146] ***Actaea racemosa*** has been found to improve symptoms associated with breast cancer by alleviating vasomotor symptoms associated with the decrease of oestrogen.[147]

Trifolium pratense has also been found to be of benefit for oestrogen-based cancers. The isoflavone constituent biochanin A has been found to inhibit cytochrome p19 (aromatase) activity and gene expression, thereby decreasing the effect of active oestrogen.[148]

Mitochondrial function

Mitochondrial dysfunction has been linked with the increased risk of cancer.[149] Most of the mitochondrial influence is via its link to apoptosis (p53) and anaerobic glycolysis; however, there may be another area in which mitochondrial function plays an important role. Cancer cells may have impaired mitochondria and mitochondrial activity, which may support Warburg's theory as to why cancer cells use the anaerobic glycolysis pathway rather than the aerobic system.[150] Concentrating on mitochondrial reprogramming and support may therefore assist in addressing cancer. Nutrients that have been found to assist mitochondrial function include **coenzyme Q10**,[151] **lipoic acid**,[152] **carnitine**[153] and **B vitamins** such as niacin (NAD).[154]

Angiogenesis

The role of angiogenesis (a physiological process whereby new blood vessels develop from pre-existing vessels)[155] in tumours is well recognised.[149] Certain chemotherapeutics currently target this angiogenic process such as bevacizumab (Avastin)[156]; however, some naturopathic medicines have also been found to possess an antiangiogenic action. These include **intravenous nutraceuticals** such as vitamin C,[157] *Curcuma longa*,[158,159] *Artemisia annua, Viscum album, Scutellaria baicalensis,* resveratrol and proanthocyanidins, *Magnolia officinalis, Camellia sinensis, Ginkgo biloba,* quercetin, *Poria cocos, Zingiber officinale, Panax ginseng* and *Rabdosia rubescens hora*.[160] Using any number of these naturopathic medicines may help reduce angiogenesis by virtue of possibly having a positive effect on decreasing tumour initiation, promotion, progression and metastasis.

Diet and cancer

There have been a number of studies on diet and its effect on cancer. Certain dietary deficiencies have been associated with cancer development. Dietary factors account for approximately 30% of cancer cases in developed countries and 20% in developing nations, and are second only to tobacco as a preventable cause of cancer.[161] Other studies have been conducted on specific foods or beverages linked with cancer. There are also a multitude of diets that are promoted as 'anticancer diets', most of which have not been studied specifically and are based on broader empirical evidence.

The most common dietary link to cancer is the crude lack of fruit and vegetables.[162] Currently, the literature is showing that following a Mediterranean diet reduces the risk of overall cancer mortality, risk of different types of cancer and cancer mortality and aids in reducing recurrence in cancer survivors. The benefits from this diet are mainly driven by a higher intake of fruits, vegetables and wholegrains. In particular, breast cancer risk was found to decrease by 6% by pooling results from seven studies on a Mediterranean diet.[163] An increased intake of fruit and vegetables has been found to be protective against lung,[164] oesophageal[165] and colon cancer.[166] Fruit and vegetable intake has also been suggested to be protective from breast and ovarian cancer although results at this stage state that the lack of fruit and vegetables is not a risk factor for either.[167,168]

In addition to an increased consumption of fruit and vegetables, a low intake of meat and potatoes has been found to be protective against colorectal and oesophageal cancer.[165,166] High meat consumption—particularly through adolescence—has also been found to be a risk factor for premenopausal breast cancer.[169] Both high meat consumption and high sugar intake have also been linked as risk factors for pancreatic cancer.[170] High poultry intake and high-fat dairy intake are associated with an increased risk of gastric cancer.[165] Adherence to a Western-style diet and high alcohol intake are also associated with an increased risk of gastric cancer.[171] A high intake of alcohol has been associated with not only gastric cancer but also breast[172] and liver cancer.[17]

Fat intake is another area of concern in relation to cancer. High-fat diets have been linked with numerous cancers, including breast, prostate and colon cancers.[173,174] Studies have also found that high fat intake increases the oxidation of DNA and encourages damaged cell proliferation.[173] However, specific fats, such as **omega-3 fatty acids** as found in fish oil, have demonstrated protective effects for breast, prostate and colon cancer.[173,174] The current Western diet has a disproportionate ratio of omega-6 fatty acids to omega-3 fatty acids compared with more traditional diets; this may result in increased risk of cancer development.[174]

Iodine has been studied for a number of cancers, including thyroid cancer and breast cancer. Both a deficiency and an excessive amount of iodine have been associated with an increased risk of thyroid cancer.[175,176] For breast cancer, recent studies have suggested that iodine may play a protective role on breast tissue by inhibiting cancer development via the modulation of the oestrogen pathway.[176]

Green tea[177] has also been extensively studied for cancer with positive results, and **black tea**[178] and **coffee**[179] have also shown beneficial effects. Green tea and black tea have demonstrated benefit across a broad range of cancers; however, coffee seems to be mainly beneficial in protection against liver, kidney and, to a lesser extent, premenopausal breast cancer and colorectal carcinoma.[180] The protective effect of coffee seems to be related to the presence of a variety of biological compounds including caffeine, diterpenes, caffeic acid, polyphenols, volatile aroma and heterocyclic. Most studies indicate a moderate intake equivalent to one or two coffee drinks a day or less than 250 mg of caffeine intake a day although further study is required to ascertain the right serving size for protective benefits.[179]

Studies looking at vegetarian or plant-based diets have also achieved reasonable results, though nothing conclusive has been found at this stage. It seems that a vegetarian or plant-based diet or a macrobiotic diet may be of benefit, particularly for colorectal, prostate and breast cancer.[181,182] This may be related not merely to the vegetarian nature of the diet but also to the increased proportions of fibre and fruit and vegetable intakes often associated with these diets.

Although some studies focus on specific components or diets, the general consensus is that broad improvements in diet are extremely beneficial in the prevention and treatment of cancer. Increasing fruit and vegetable consumption has clear benefit. Patients should be encouraged to 'have a rainbow on their plate'—eating as many colours (often associated with specific phytochemical compounds) each day as they can. The less adventurous could be given the task of exploring a new fruit or vegetable each week. Increasing fibre and reducing the intake of simple carbohydrates also show great benefit, and these changes can be achieved by encouraging patients to experiment with lesser known grains such as buckwheat, quinoa, millet, brown rice and bulghur. Legumes can also be a beneficial addition in this respect. While these additions are clearly beneficial, they are in many cases large diversions from current eating habits, and patients may require practical support as well as suggestions if they are to implement these changes successfully.

INTEGRATIVE MEDICAL CONSIDERATIONS

Injection of nutraceuticals

Using intravenous or injecting particular vitamins and herbs is becoming more popular as science advances (see Chapter 38 on chronic fatigue for more detail on injecting nutraceuticals). **Intravenous Vitamin C** has been found to be widely used by CAM practitioners.[183] It has an illustrious past with initial observations and anecdotal clinical data from Cameron and Pauling indicating an increase in survival in some patients receiving 10 g of ascorbic acid daily compared with retrospective controls.[184,185] Two double-blind placebo-controlled trials were then conducted, showing no efficacy of ascorbic acid using the same dose. Vitamin C was therefore seen as ineffective and injectable ascorbate was dismissed.[186,187] Oral doses of vitamin C were then investigated, with a review in 2006 finding that oral doses of ascorbic acid demonstrated no benefit to cancer patients.[188]

Renewed interest in injectable ascorbic acid came after pharmacokinetics studies investigating oral intake versus intravenous ascorbic acid in healthy adults found that only intravenous ascorbic acid resulted in high ascorbic acid concentrations until renal excretion restored homeostasis.[189,190] A number of studies have now been conducted on intravenous vitamin C safety and efficacy with promising results.[191-195]

Intravenous vitamin C's mechanism of action is based on the high plasma concentrations of ascorbate, which increases production of hydrogen peroxide both inside and outside cells and tissues. Intravenous vitamin C therefore acts as a pro-drug delivering a significant influx of hydrogen peroxide to and around all cells including tumour cells. Normal cells have been found to rapidly and effectively remove excessive hydrogen peroxide but tumour cells do not. Therefore tumour cells go into apoptosis resulting in cell death.[196]

Other vitamins that have been investigated for cancer intravenously either by themselves, in conjunction with vitamin C or with chemotherapy include **vitamin D₃**,[197–199] **glutathione**,[200–204] **lipoic acid**[205,206] and **vitamin E**.[207]

The most widely used intravenous herb is ***Viscum album*** such as Iscador.[208] Iscador has been used as an adjunct treatment in patients with cancer, particularly in Germany and Switzerland.[209] The active components from mistletoe include cytotoxic glycoproteins (mistletoe lectins), which can stimulate effector cells of the innate and adaptive immune system. Its actions also include antitumoural properties, immune modulation, growth inhibition and cell death induction in tumour cells. As an adjunct to conventional medicine, it has been found to assist in patients' quality of life, reduce side effects such as nausea and fatigue and is associated with prolonged survival.[208,210] A current meta-analysis found that *Viscum album* is an effective adjuvant treatment; however, limitations particularly focused on study quality remain an issue and further well-constructed trials are suggested.[211]

Other herbs that have been investigated intravenously include ***Rosmarinus officinalis***, but more studies are required for confirmation of use.[197] A controversial injectable is that of laetrile or B17. A Cochrane review conducted in 2011[212] found more than 200 references; however, no studies were identified that met the inclusion criteria of an RCT or quasi-RCT. Laetrile is a semi-synthetic form of amygdalin, which is a compound isolated from the seeds of many fruits such as apricots, peaches and bitter almonds. Both laetrile and amygdalin contain similar chemical structures that contain cyanide.

The Therapeutic Goods Administration (TGA) and the American Food and Drug Agency (FDA) have both banned the use of laetrile or amygdalin due to its lack of effectiveness and risk of side effects from cyanide poisoning. Certain clinics and doctors promote infusion of laetrile or amygdalin or suggest oral ingestion, but cancer patients need to make an informed decision and acknowledge the high risk of developing serious adverse side effects. At this stage no reliable evidence for the alleged benefits of laetrile or amygdalin for curative effects in cancer have been found.

An injectable compound of toad venom has and is used in certain countries such as China and South America; however, in Australia this injectable is banned by the TGA. Current in vitro investigations into toad venom in 2013 have found beneficial results on selected components of toad venom for hepatocellular carcinoma[213] and leukaemia cells.[214] Both compounds indicated cytotoxic and antineoplastic mechanisms, although, being in vitro, no side effects were noted. A case report from Australia in 2009 highlighted a sudden death from an intravenous injection of toad extract.[215] Injections using CAM products should only be conducted in countries in which the product is approved and used legally by registered practitioners as unforeseen adverse events can occur such as the sudden death noted in the case report.

Melatonin

The natural endocrine hormone **melatonin** is present in the body and is released by the pineal gland to assist with sleep. Melatonin can also be given in pharmacological concentrations for a number of conditions including cancer as it has been found to have specific actions including decreasing cellular and secreted VEGF levels, inducing apoptosis, reducing adhesion and migratory abilities of tumour cells and suppressing proliferation.[216,217] Studies have found that melatonin can have an inhibitory effect on multiple malignant tumours including breast cancer,[218,219] brain tumours,[220] osteosarcoma cells[216] and liver cancer[217] to name a few. Melatonin has also been found to increase the efficacy of certain chemotherapy drugs and decrease side effects such as the doxorubicin-induced cardiotoxicity.[218–220]

Alteratives/depuratives and cancer—Essiac formula

A number of teas containing herbs that have alterative or depurative activity have been promoted for cancer. One of the best known teas suggested to people with cancer is the Essiac tea. It is a mixture of four herbs: *Arctium lappa*, *Rumex acetosella*, *Rheum officinale* and *Ulmus fulva*. It was originally a herbal formulation from the Ojibway Indians in Canada and was discovered in 1922 by Rene Caisse, who reports to have 'cured' hundreds of people with cancer with this formula.[221]

Rumex acetosella is reported in anecdotal references to destroy cancer cells while the other three herbs aid purifying the blood. A chiropractor, Gary Glum, stated that the burdock root also contains inulin, which is considered to be a powerful immune modulator.[221] Most of the information is anecdotal; however, there have been a few recent studies on the mechanism of action of Essiac using in vitro or cell analysis. Several studies found beneficial results; others found no real benefit and human studies are lacking.

The Department of Research and Clinical Epidemiology in the Canadian College of Naturopathic Medicine in Toronto conducted the first real investigation of Essiac in 2007.[222] This study came about as a response to the negative recommendations from the Task Force on Alternative Therapies of the Canadian Breast Cancer Research Initiative, as very little research had been conducted on this formula.[222]

The activity of Essiac was measured using assays to establish the antioxidant, fibrinolytic, antimicrobial, anti-inflammatory, immune-modulation and cell-specific cytotoxicity effects on cytochrome P450 enzymes. It was found that Essiac exhibited significant antioxidant activity and had immunomodulating effects through stimulation of granulocyte phagocytosis, increasing CD8+ cell activation and moderately inhibiting inflammatory pathways. It also exhibited significant cell-specific cytotoxicity towards ovarian epithelial carcinoma cells. In regard to cytochrome P450 enzymes, it inhibited CYP1A2 and CYP2C19. Clot fibrinolytic activity was dose-dependent.[222]

Two other in vitro studies found that Essiac had positive results, with one indicating inhibition of tumour growth in prostate cells.[223,224] However, one of the studies also showed that Essiac tea stimulated some pro-inflammatory molecules as well as nitric oxide.[225] This same study found that it had no anti-proliferative effect on leukaemic cell lines but that it inhibited 50% of MCF-7 breast cancer cell lines, as did Flor-Essence tea—a similar product containing *Arctium lappa*, *Rumex acetosella* and *Ulmus fulva*, but also containing *Nasturtium officinale*, *Rheum palmatum*, *Cnicus benedictus* and *Trifolium pratense*.[225] A more recent study conducted on prostate cells lines in mice also refuted the positive results initially found in prostate cancer cell lines. It found there was no significant difference between proliferation levels and markers in Essiac-treated or -untreated prostate cancer cells in mice.[225]

In another in vivo study conducted on mice the tea was administered orally, mimicking human intake. The result found that it did demonstrate a modest gastric protective effect by reducing ethanol-induced gastric ulceration. However, there was no demonstration of hepatoprotective, hypoglycaemic or immunomodulatory effects, not supporting the suggested actions of Essiac.[226]

There seems to be no toxicity associated with Essiac tea and in vitro studies seem to indicate potential positive anticancer properties. However, further studies on humans are required to scientifically support or discredit the use of Essiac tea in cancer treatment. At this stage there appears to be no or very little harm to patients with cancer if they consume Essiac tea as an adjuvant.

Cancer 'cures' and their potential risks/benefits

When people are diagnosed with cancer they are surrounded by a plethora of information given to them by doctors, hospitals, organisations, family and people in general. They may also look on the internet for potential 'cures' or information on CAM therapies. Not all of these therapies are approved or found to be 'safe' or 'effective' and in some cases are considered dangerous. Some examples of both approved and non-approved therapies can be found in Table 32.5.

Table 32.5
Examples of alternative interventions for cancer*

Product	Comments and research
Black salve or cansema	Black salve or 'cansema' is available as an ointment and a liquid herbal and is considered one of the 'top selling' products on many alternative medicine websites. It is a 'non-approved' corrosive topical irritant and banned in a lot of countries including Australia. The main ingredient is a bloodroot extract, in addition to galangal, red clover and sheep sorrel. It originally claimed to 'cure' skin cancers but is now touted to cure other cancers such as breast and osteosarcomas. Case studies published in peer-reviewed journals have discussed the physical disfigurement and pain associated with this treatment.[227–229] Use of this product can be dangerous and may result in extreme pain and severe skin damage and disfigurement. It does not guarantee that the cancer has been eradicated.
Laetrile or B17	Banned substance and is discussed under *Injectables*.
Zapper	One of the main pioneers of the zapper is Dr Hulda Clark, who wrote the book *Cure for all cancers*. The basis behind the zapper is that all diseases, especially cancer, are caused by parasites (including flukes) and that to cure cancer all you have to do is eliminate the parasites and flukes. The zapper is usually used in conjunction with anti-parasitic herbs. There is a lot of controversy regarding Clark's treatment protocol and Dr Clark herself died in 2009 of cancer (multiple myeloma). There are no peer review publications on this product or protocol.
Antineoplastons	These are peptides or amino acid compounds discovered by Stanislaw Burzynski in 1967. They are natural peptides found in the blood and urine of healthy people but not so much in cancer patients. Dr Burzynski developed a substances of these peptides called 'antineoplastons' and administered them to cancer patients. Burzynski has published some clinical trials using antineoplaston therapy as well as in vitro work,[230–237] but the veracity of these studies remains controversial, and Burzynski's work has had fierce opposition from the American Medical Association and the Food and Drug Administration.
Electronic therapies	This includes devices such as the Rife, Beck, Clark (mentioned above), radiowave therapy and electro-cancer treatment. *Rife machine*: This was developed by Royal Rife and are devices that transmit specific electronic signals to deactivate or destroy living pathogens, bacteria and cancers. Rife was banned in the United States and outlawed by the FDA. No scientific proof of the machine is documented. *Radiowave therapy*: These machines, such as the 'Holt' in Australia, are set to resonate with certain frequencies that can harm cancer cells. Several journal articles have been published on radiowave therapy and it is an approved therapy in certain countries.[238,239] *Electro-cancer treatment*: This was developed in Europe by Swedish professor Bjorn Nordenstrom and Austrian doctor Rudolf Pekar. This therapy uses galvanic electrical stimulations to treat tumours and skin cancers and is normally used in conjunction with other therapies such as chemotherapy agents.[240]
Graviola	This is an extract from the tropical tree *Annona muricata*, commonly known as graviola. The fruit from this tree is called 'soursop' and both graviola and soursop can be found as supplements. Graviola has been researched for both breast and pancreatic cancer, finding that it down-regulates epidermal growth factor receptor (EGFR) expression and inhibits multiple signalling pathways involving metabolism, cell cycle, survival and metastatic properties in pancreatic cells.[241,242] Graviola is only available in certain countries and banned in others. There are known side effects from this extract and, if administered, the patient needs regular monitoring.

Table 52.5
Examples of alternative interventions for cancer* (continued)

Product	Comments and research
Hydrazine sulfate	This is a common industrial chemical and was postulated for cancer treatment by Dr Joseph Gold. His theory was that a metabolic circuit existed in cancer patients that allows tumours to derive energy from normal metabolic pathways. A number of research trials have been conducted on hydrazine sulfate; however, results are not conclusive as an anticancer treatment and it is not approved by the FDA. It has also shown a number of side effects upon administration.[243-245]
Frankincense essential oil	Public support for the use of Frankincense oil internally and topically for cancer is growing. Currently, there are no human trials supporting the use of Frankincense essential oil although several in vitro studies on pancreatic cancer and breast cancer cell lines have shown potential benefit. Further human trials are required to confirm any benefit from topical application or ingestion of Frankincense essential oil.[246,247]

*Controversial treatments not scientifically supported and are not recommended for treatment. These summaries are provided solely to inform practitioners on major alternative treatments promoted publicly for cancer treatment that patients may identify in their own research.

Mind–body medicine

Many studies have shown beneficial effects of **acupuncture** for cancer, for a variety of different reasons. Studies using acupuncture to treat cancer pain,[248] vasomotor and fatigue symptoms of both breast and prostate cancer[249,250] show that it boosts the immune system and decrease tumour growth[251] and is beneficial for the treatment of nausea and other side effects.[252] Acupuncture has had documented success in improving nausea symptoms associated with chemotherapy.[253–255] Electro-acupuncture seems more effective than manual acupuncture for this purpose.

Meditation can be of assistance to people with cancer by reducing stress, improving mood and quality of life and aiding sleep problems.[256] Counselling has been found to assist with the anxiety, depression and life decisions that cancer patients experience.[257]

Yoga is another therapy that has growing support to assist with quality of life, sleep and mood. Other therapies that may be of assistance include creative therapies such as visual arts, painting, dance and music, which may help patients to express their feelings and help them cope with what they are experiencing.[256] A review of 50 studies found that Qi gong was mostly associated with positive outcomes in cancer patients.[258] It should be noted, however, that while interventions such as support groups can help cancer patients in numerous ways, evidence does not at this stage seem to suggest that this translates into prolonging their lives.[259]

Religious or spiritual beliefs have been found to be of benefit for cancer patients. The supportive environment and thought of an afterlife can be very important for cancer patients[260]; however, this should not translate to the encouragement of false hope.

Homeopathy

A Cochrane review on homeopathy and cancer treatment involving eight controlled trials and a total of 664 participants found preliminary data to support the efficacy of topical homeopathic calendula treatment for prophylaxis of acute dermatitis during radiotherapy. It also found the proprietary homeopathic Traumeel S mouthwash to be beneficial in treating chemotherapy-induced stomatitis.[261] They found no convincing evidence

> ## Treatment of people at different stages of cancer and levels of vitality
>
> It is important for naturopaths to fully consider a person's condition and level of vitality when recommending treatment modalities. For example, someone with a stage 4 cancer who has been told they have little time left to live or is in palliative care because there is nothing else that can be done medically may react several ways. They may be ready to pass away and just want assistance in managing pain and quality of life, or they may not accept the diagnosis and want to try other options to 'beat the cancer'. Either way, naturopaths need to acknowledge where the person is at emotionally and physically and support that person in their treatment decisions.
>
> Vitality at this stage is also important as some people who have been told they have a couple of months to live may actually have a lot of vitality and are able to take on a rigorous regimen to assist their health. Others may be very sick, so taking on a rigorous regimen is not appropriate because their body may not be able to withstand it. In most cases they won't have the energy or body function to allow it. An example of this is someone at end-stage cancer in extreme cachexia with or without the start of peripheral shutdown. This indicates that their body can take only very little stress and is very close to passing away. Normally they have no appetite, and have difficulty swallowing and performing normal bodily functions.
>
> Another example is radiation enteropathy where the person has severe vomiting, diarrhoea and inflammation along their entire GIT. They may go into severe cachexia quite rapidly and have problems consuming solids or liquids. It is nearly impossible to prescribe anything orally to assist, so other options need to be considered.
>
> For all these reasons, understanding the patient's level of vitality and emotional status is an essential aspect of treatment.

for the efficacy of homeopathic medicines for other adverse effects of cancer treatment. Pilot studies from British hospitals have demonstrated positive patient outcomes when homeopathy has been used in conjunction with conventional treatment.[262]

Massage

Massage has been found to give immediate beneficial effects for pain and improving mood for patients with cancer.[263] While positive outcomes have been found for stress and anxiety, adverse effects from massage therapy—including pathological fractures of metastatic bones and bruising in patients with coagulopathy—may be more likely in cancer patients.[264]

CLINICAL SUMMARY

As discussed, cancer is a multifactorial disease and, as such, is not a single condition. To date there are approximately 200 different types of cancer (plus subtypes) that can develop in any organ. Considering the human body has around 60 organs, each comprising different types of tissues, it's not surprising that different tumours can also be found in one organ. Each cancer has a different aetiology so there is no evidence based on 'just' cancer.

Naturopathic philosophy is based on treating the individual not the 'disease' and this also goes for people with cancer. In addition to treating the individual with cancer, it is also important to treat the stage they are at and not try to treat everything at once because that will overwhelm them. For example, treating a person with cancer going through chemotherapy will be different from what you suggest to them during radiation or in maintenance stage (Figure 32.2). If they are undergoing treatment, it is imperative that you know the drugs that they are being administered, the mechanism of action, the side effects and that each person reacts differently.

People who have been diagnosed with cancer go through a series of different mental states and acknowledging where they are at and what they want to achieve is very important. They must feel comfortable with you and as this is a high stress phase of their life, giving realistic hope is important, even if it's helping them to be more comfortable and have quality of life in palliative care. Moreover, a number of different modalities may be of assistance to that person, so working with a team of practitioners for best care of the patient is really important. Build a rapport with a variety of practitioners in various modalities to assist with referrals that you feel will be of assistance.

Overall, and most importantly, listen to the person and take one step at a time. Be very careful of overwhelming them as they will most likely be inundated with numerous hospital appointments, tests, scans and, in some cases, medication. Many people will want to give them advice. They may seek out information themselves online. This may or may not be appropriate and understanding what is out there and the evidence behind it is imperative. Always remember: First do no harm and guide and assist your patients as best you can.

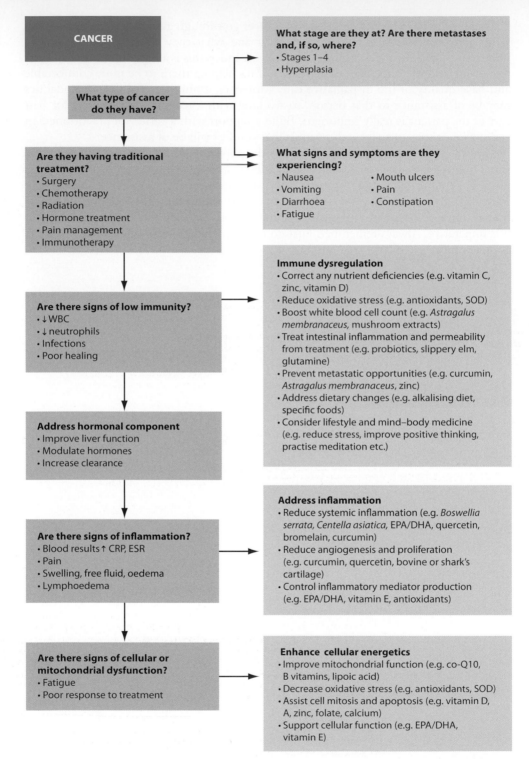

Figure 32.3
Naturopathic treatment decision tree—cancer

KEY POINTS

- Treat the person first, not the disease.

- Cancer is a complex condition with myriad different causes and interactions. It is important to address this multifactorial condition from many different aspects by addressing each stage rather than everything at once.

- Keep supplementation and diet simple, and don't overwhelm the patient with too many things to take, especially if they are also undergoing traditional treatment.

- Many nutritional and lifestyle factors can be involved with cancer and it is important to address the specific factors associated with the person as well as the type of cancer.

- Always address nutritional deficiencies and ensure a balanced body weight.

- Encourage a supportive environment and refer if required for psychological support.

FURTHER READING

Aucoin M, Cooley K, Knee C, et al. Fish-derived omega-3 fatty acids and prostate cancer: a systematic review. Integr Cancer Ther 2017;16(1):32–62. doi:10.1177/1534735416656052. Published online 2016 Jun 29.

Bahall M. Prevalence, patterns, and perceived value of complementary and alternative medicine among cancer patients: a cross-sectional, descriptive study. BMC Complement Altern Med 2017;17:345. doi:10.1186/s12906-017-1853-6. Published online 2017 Jun 30.

Davies NJ, Batehup L, Thomas R. The role of diet and physical activity in breast, colorectal, and prostate cancer survivorship: a review of the literature. Br J Cancer 2011;105(Suppl. 1):S52–73. doi:10.1038/bjc.2011.423. Published online 2011 Nov 3.

Fritz H, Seely D, Flower G, et al. Soy, red clover, and isoflavones and breast cancer: a systematic review. PLoS ONE 2013;8(11):e81968. doi:10.1371/journal.pone.0081968. Published online 2013 Nov 28.

Greenlee H, Balneaves LG, Carlson LE, et al.; for the Society for Integrative Oncology Guidelines Working Group. Clinical practice guidelines on the use of integrative therapies as supportive care in patients treated for breast cancer. J Natl Cancer Inst Monogr 2014;2014(50):346–58. doi:10.1093/jncimonographs/lgu041. Published 2015 May; 2015(51):98.

Potter J, Brown L, Williams RL, et al. Diet quality and cancer outcomes in adults: a systematic review of epidemiological studies. Int J Mol Sci 2016;17(7):1052. doi:10.3390/ijms17071052. Published online 2016 Jul 5.

Schloss J, Steel A. Thriving after cancer: the role of integrative medicine (IM) in cancer survivorship and wellbeing programs. Adv Integr Med 2015;2(3):123–4.

Weeks L, Balneaves LG, Paterson C, et al. Decision-making about complementary and alternative medicine by cancer patients: integrative literature review. Open Med 2014;8(2):e54–66. Published online 2014 Apr 15.

REFERENCES

1. Cancer Council NSW. Lung cancer: causes and symptoms. myDR. Canberra: Australian Government; 2002.

2. Krambeck WM, et al. HPV detection and genotyping as an earlier approach in cervical cancer screening of the female genital tract. Clin Exp Obstet Gynecol 2008;35(3):175–8.

3. Australian Institute of Health and Welfare & Australasian Association of Cancer Registries 2012. Cancer in Australia: an overview, 2012. Cancer series no. 74. Cat. no. CAN 70. Canberra: AIHW.

4. Australian Institute of Health and Welfare 2012. Cancer incidence projections: Australia, 2011 to 2020. Cancer Series no. 66. Cat. No. CAN 62. Canberra: AIHW.

5. Cancer Australia. Cancer in Australia Statistics. Australian Government; 2019. Available: https://canceraustralia.gov.au/affected-cancer/what-cancer/cancer-australia-statistics.

6. World Health Organization. Noncommunicable diseases. WHO. 219. Available: https://www.who.int/news-room/fact-sheets/detail/noncommunicable-diseases.

7. Parkin DM, Boyd L, Walker LC. The fraction of cancer attributable to lifestyle and environmental factors in the UK in 2010. Br J Cancer 2011;105:S77–81.

8. Amin AR, et al. Perspectives for cancer prevention with natural compounds. J Clin Oncol 2009;27(16):12–25.

9. Thomas CC, et al. Endometrial cancer risk among younger, overweight women. Obstet Gynecol 2009;114(1):22–7.

10. Andrykowski MA, et al. Psychological health in cancer survivors. Semin Oncol Nurs 2008;24(3):193–201.

11. Blask DE. Melatonin, sleep disturbance and cancer risk. Sleep Med Rev 2009;13(4):257–64.

12. Mystakidou K, et al. Exploring the relationships between depression, hopelessness, cognitive status, pain, and

spirituality in patients with advanced cancer. Arch Psychiatr Nurs 2007;21(3):150–61.

13. Frieden TR, et al. A public health approach to winning the war against cancer. Oncologist 2008;13(12):1306–13.

14. Stanley M. Prevention strategies against the human papillomavirus: the effectiveness of vaccination. Gynecol Oncol 2007;107(2 Suppl. 1):S19–23.

15. Hussain SK, et al. Cervical and vulvar cancer risk in relation to the joint effects of cigarette smoking and genetic variation in interleukin 2. Cancer Epidemiol Biomarkers Prev 2008;17(7):1790–9.

16. Gomaa AI, et al. Hepatocellular carcinoma: epidemiology, risk factors and pathogenesis. World J Gastroenterol 2008;14(27):4300–8.

17. Deandrea S, et al. Alcohol and breast cancer risk defined by estrogen and progesterone receptor status: a case-control study. Cancer Epidemiol Biomarkers Prev 2008;17(8):2025–8.

18. Mizoue T, et al. Alcohol drinking and colorectal cancer risk: an evaluation based on a systematic review of epidemiologic evidence among the Japanese population. Jpn J Clin Oncol 2006;36(9):582–97.

19. Liu C, Russell RM. Nutrition and gastric cancer risk: an update. Nutr Rev 2008;66(5):237–49.

20. Gravaghi C, et al. Obesity enhances gastrointestinal tumorigenesis in Apc-mutant mice. Int J Obes (Lond) 2008;32:1716–19.

21. Perera CN, et al. Leptin regulated gene expression in MCF-7 breast cancer cells: mechanistic insights into leptin regulated mammary tumor growth and progression. J Endocrinol 2008;199(2):221–33.

22. Moayyedi P. The epidemiology of obesity and gastrointestinal and other diseases: an overview. Dig Dis Sci 2008;53(9):2293–9.

23. Dobbinson S, et al. Prevalence and determinants of Australian adolescents' and adults' weekend sun protection and sunburn, summer 2003–2004. J Am Acad Dermatol 2008;59:602–14.

24. Bouillon R, et al. Vitamin D and human health: lessons from vitamin D receptor null mice. Endocr Rev 2008;16:200–57.

25. Ames BN. Low micronutrient intake may accelerate the degenerative diseases of aging through allocation of scarce micronutrients by triage. Proc Natl Acad Sci USA 2006;103(47):17589–94.

26. Bläuer M, et al. Effects of tamoxifen and raloxifene on normal human endometrial cells in an organotypic in vitro model. Eur J Pharmacol 2008;592(1–3):13–18.

27. Moore M, et al. Cancer registration literature update (2006–2008). Asian Pac J Cancer Prev 2008;9(2):165–85.

28. Chan C, et al. Stress-associated hormone, norepinephrine, increases proliferation and IL-6 levels of human pancreatic duct epithelial cells and can be inhibited by the dietary agent, sulforaphane. Int J Oncol 2008;33(2):415–19.

29. Mosor M, et al. Polymorphisms and haplotypes of the NBS1 gene in childhood acute leukaemia. Eur J Cancer 2008;44:627–30.

30. Lahti TA, et al. Night-time work predisposes to non-Hodgkin lymphoma. Int J Cancer 2008;123(9):2148–51.

31. Karunanayake CP, et al. Occupational exposures and non-Hodgkin's lymphoma: Canadian case-control study. Environ Health 2008;7(1):44.

32. Swiatkowska B, et al. Occupational risk factors for lung cancer—a case-control study, Lódź industrial center. Med Pr 2008;59(1):25–34.

33. Bourret P. BRCA patients and clinical collectives: new configurations of action in cancer genetics practices. Soc Stud Sci 2005;35(1):41–68.

34. Queiroga EM, et al. Viral studies in Burkitt lymphoma: association with Epstein-Barr virus but not HHV-8. Am J Clin Pathol 2008;130(2):186–92.

35. Nutankalva L, et al. Malignancies in HIV: pre- and post-highly active antiretroviral therapy. J Natl Med Assoc 2008;100(7):817–20.

36. Tao X, et al. The role of hepatitis B virus x gene in development of primary hepatocellular carcinoma. Sci China C Life Sci 2000;43(3):293–301.

37. Yoshida M. Identification of adult T-cell leukemia virus and its gene structure. Gan to Kagaku Ryoho 1983;10(2):680–9.

38. Zhou SZ, et al. Association of single nucleotide polymorphism at interleukin-10 gene 1082 nt with the risk of gastric cancer in Chinese population. Nan Fang Yi Ke Da Xue Xue Bao 2008;28(8):1335–8.

39. Amara K, et al. Presence of simian virus 40 DNA sequences in diffuse large B-cell lymphomas in Tunisia correlates with aberrant promoter hypermethylation of multiple tumor suppressor genes. Int J Cancer 2007;121(12):2693–702.

40. Moro L, et al. Mitochondrial DNA depletion reduces PARP-1 levels and promotes progression of the neoplastic phenotype in prostate carcinoma. Cell Oncol 2008;30(4):307–22.

41. Kamangar F, et al. Patterns of cancer incidence, mortality, and prevalence across five continents: defining priorities to reduce cancer disparities in different geographic regions of the world. J Clin Oncol 2006;24(14):2137–50.

42. Newby JA, Howard CV. Environmental influences in cancer aetiology. J Nutr Environ Med 2006;1–59.

43. Frost G, et al. Occupational exposure to asbestos and mortality among asbestos removal workers: a Poisson regression analysis. Br J Cancer 2008;99(5):822–9.

44. Schmitt C, et al. NK cells and surveillance in humans. Reprod Biomed Online 2008;16(2):192–201.

45. Bell HS, Ryan KM. Targeting the p53 family for cancer therapy: 'big brother' joins the fight. Cell Cycle 2007;6(16):1995–2000.

46. Pelletier L. Centrosomes: keeping tumors in check. Curr Biol 2008;18(16):R702–4.

47. Arai T, et al. Role of DNA repair systems in malignant tumor development in the elderly. Geriatr Gerontol Int 2008;8(2):65–72.

48. Hoye AT, et al. Targeting mitochondria. Acc Chem Res 2008;41(1):87–97.

49. Gordon JS. Mind–body medicine and cancer. Hematol Oncol Clin North Am 2008;22(4):683–708.

50. Ma Z, et al. Polymorphisms of fibroblast growth factor receptor 4 have association with the development of prostate cancer and benign prostatic hyperplasia and the progression of prostate cancer in a Japanese population. Int J Cancer 2008;123:2574–9.

51. Zhang Z, et al. Genetic variants in RUNX3 and risk of bladder cancer: a haplotype-based analysis. Carcinogenesis 2008;29(10):1973–8.

52. Jones PA, Baylin SB. The fundamental role of epigenetic events in cancer. Nat Rev Genet 2002;3:415–28.

53. International Agency for Research on Cancer. IARC Monographs on the Identification of Carcinogenic Hazards to Humans. IARC. Available at: http://monographs.iarc.fr/ENG/Classification/index.php.

54. Medscape. Breast cancer differential diagnosis. Online. Available: http://emedicine.medscape.com/article/1947145-differential 1 Nov 2013.

55. Medscape. Prostate cancer differential diagnosis. Online. Available: http://emedicine.medscape.com/article/1967731-differential 1 Nov 2013.

56. Medscape. Colon adenacarcinoma differential diagnosis. Online. Available: http://emedicine.medscape.com/article/277496-differential 1 Nov 2013.

57. El-Hashemy S. Naturopathic standards of primary care. Toronto: CCNM Press; 2007.

58. American Cancer Society. What are the signs and symptoms? Online. Available: http://www.cancer.org/cancer/cancerbasics/signs-and-symptoms-of-cancer 1 Nov 2013.

59. Worthington HV, et al. Interventions for preventing oral mucositis for patients with cancer receiving treatment. Cochrane Database Syst Rev 2007;(4):CD000978.

60. Baharvand M, Jafari S, Mortazavi H. Herbs in oral mucositis. J Clin Diagn Res 2017;11(3):ZE5–11. doi:10.7860/JCDR/2017/21703.9467. Published online 2017 Mar 1, PMCID: PMC5427456.

61. Tsujimoto T, Yamamoto Y, Wasa M, et al. L-glutamine decreases the severity of mucositis induced by chemoradiotherapy in patients with locally advanced head and neck cancer: a double-blind, randomized, placebo-controlled trial. Oncol Rep 2015;33(1):33–9. doi:10.3892/or.2014.3564. Published online 2014 Oct 23.

62. Daniele B, et al. Oral glutamine in the prevention of fluorouracil induced intestinal toxicity: a double blind, placebo controlled, randomized trial. Gut 2001;48(1):28–33.

63. Liu MM, Li ST, Shu Y, et al. Probiotics for prevention of radiation-induced diarrhea: a meta-analysis of randomized controlled trials. PLoS ONE 2017;12(6):e0178870. doi:10.1371/journal.pone.0178870. Published online 2017 Jun 2.

64. Thorpe DM. Management of opioid-induced constipation. Curr Pain Headache Rep 2001;5(3):237–40.

65. Li Y, et al. Oral glutamine ameliorates chemotherapy-induced changes of intestinal permeability and does not interfere with the antitumor effect of chemotherapy in patients with breast cancer: a prospective randomized trial. Tumori 2006;92(5):396–401.

66. Marshall GT, et al. Treatment of gastrointestinal radiation injury with hyperbaric oxygen. Undersea Hyperb Med 2007;34(1):35–42.

67. Demirer S, et al. Effects of probiotics on radiation-induced intestinal injury in rats. Nutrition 2006;22(2):179–86.

68. Erbil Y, et al. The effect of glutamine on radiation-induced organ damage. Life Sci 2005;78(4):376–82.

69. Branda RF, et al. Vitamin E but not St John's wort mitigates leukopenia caused by cancer chemotherapy in rats. Transl Res 2006;148(6):315–24.

70. Wojtukiewicz MZ, et al. The Polish Cancer Anemia Survey (POLCAS): a retrospective multicenter study of 999 cases. Int J Hematol 2009;89(3):276–84.

71. Liu R, et al. Therapeutic effects of alpha-lipoic acid on bleomycin-induced pulmonary fibrosis in rats. Int J Mol Med 2007;10(6):865–73.

72. Cruciani RA, et al. Safety, tolerability and symptom outcomes associated with L-carnitine supplementation in patients with cancer, fatigue, and carnitine deficiency: a phase I/II study. J Pain Symptom Manage 2006;32(6):551–9.

73. Nicolson GL, Conklin KA. Reversing mitochondrial dysfunction, fatigue and the adverse effects of chemotherapy of metastatic disease by molecular replacement therapy. Clin Exp Metastasis 2008;25(2):161–9.

74. Masuda Y, et al. EGG phosphatidylcholine combined with vitamin B12 improved memory impairment following lesioning of nucleus basalis in rats. Life Sci 1998;62(9):813–22.

75. MacDonald N. Cancer cachexia and targeting chronic inflammation: a unified approach to cancer treatment and palliative/supportive care. J Support Oncol 2007;5(4):157–62.

76. Campbell KL, et al. Resting energy expenditure and body mass changes in women during adjuvant chemotherapy for breast cancer. Cancer Nurs 2007;30(2):95–100.

77. Yamada T, et al. Effects of theanine, r-glutamylethylamide, on neurotransmitter release and its relationship with glutamic acid neurotransmission. Nutr Neurosci 2005;8(4):219–26.

78. Chandwani KD, Ryan JL, Peppone LJ, et al. Cancer-related stress and complementary and alternative medicine: a review. Evid Based Complement Alternat Med 2012;2012:979213. doi:10.1155/2012/979213. Published online 2012 Jul 15.

79. Caram-Salas NL, et al. Thiamine and cyanocobalamin relieve neuropathic pain in rats: synergy with dexamethasone. Pharmacology 2006;77(2):53–62.

80. Schloss J, Colosimo M, Vitetta L. New insights into potential prevention and management options for chemotherapy-induced peripheral neuropathy. Asia Pac J Oncol Nurs 2016;3(1):73–85. doi:10.4103/2347-5625.170977.

81. Conklin KA. Coenzyme q10 for prevention of anthracycline-induced cardiotoxicity. Integr Cancer Ther 2005;4(2):110–30.

82. Engdal S, et al. Identification and exploration of herb-drug combinations used by cancer patients. Integr Cancer Ther 2009;8(1):29–36.

83. Seely D, et al. A strategy for controlling potential interactions between natural health products and chemotherapy: a review in pediatric oncology. J Pediatr Hematol Oncol 2007;29(1):32–47.

84. Furney SJ, et al. Prioritization of candidate cancer genes—an aid to oncogenomic studies. Nucleic Acids Res 2008;36(18):e115.

85. Medina PP, Slack FJ. MicroRNAs and cancer: an overview. Cell Cycle 2008;7(16):2485–92.

86. Yang K, et al. Dietary components modify gene expression: implications for carcinogenesis. J Nutr 2005;35(11):2710–14.

87. Azarhoush R, et al. Relationship between p53 expression and gastric cancers in cardia and antrum. Arch Iran Med 2008;11(5):502–6.

88. Yeung SJ, et al. Roles of p53, MYC and HIF-1 in regulating glycolysis—the seventh hallmark of cancer. Cell Mol Life Sci 2008;65:3981–99.

89. Maroto B, et al. P21-activated kinase is required for mitotic progression and regulates P1k1. Oncogene 2008;27(36):4900–8.

90. Saramäki A, et al. Regulation of the human p21(waf1/cip1) gene promoter via multiple binding sites for p53 and the vitamin D3 receptor. Nucleic Acids Res 2006;34(2):543–54.

91. Schernhammer ES, et al. Folate and vitamin B6 intake and risk of colon cancer in relation to p53 expression. Gastroenterology 2008;135:770–80.

92. Cecconi D, et al. Induction of apoptosis in Jeko-1 mantle cell lymphoma cell line by resveratrol: a proteomic analysis. J Proteome Res 2008;7(7):2670–80.

93. Chan JY, et al. Resveratrol displays converse dose-related effects on 5-fluorouracil-evoked colon cancer cell apoptosis: the roles of caspase-6 and p53. Cancer Biol Ther 2008;7(8).

94. Huang X, et al. Green tea extract enhances the selective cytotoxic activity of Zizyphus jujuba extracts in HepG2 Cells. Am J Chin Med 2008;36(4):729–44.

95. Lee SC, et al. Effect of a prodrug of the green tea polyphenol (-)-epigallocatechin-3-gallate on the growth

of androgen-independent prostate cancer in vivo. Nutr Cancer 2008;60(4):483–91.

96. Matsumura K, et al. Involvement of the estrogen receptor beta in genistein-induced expression of p21(waf1/cip1) in PC-3 prostate cancer cells. Anticancer Res 2008;28(2A):709–14.

97. Tanigawa S, et al. Stabilization of p53 is involved in quercetin-induced cell cycle arrest and apoptosis in HepG2 cells. Biosci Biotechnol Biochem 2008;72(3):797–804.

98. Wells J. Do centrioles generate a polar ejection force? Riv Biol 2005;98(1):71–95.

99. Dutertre S, et al. The absence of p53 aggravates polyploidy and centrosome number abnormality induced by Aurora-C overexpression. Cell Cycle 2005;4(12):1783–7.

100. Krämer A, et al. Centrosome replication, genomic instability and cancer. Leukemia 2002;16(5):767–75.

101. Crist WM, et al. Dysgranulopoietic neutropenia and abnormal monocytes in childhood vitamin B12 deficiency. Am J Hematol 1980;9(1):89–107.

102. Kim I, et al. Pyrrolidine dithiocarbamate and zinc inhibit proteasome-dependent proteolysis. Exp Cell Res 2004;298(1):229–38.

103. Wang X, et al. Folate deficiency induces aneuploidy in human lymphocytes in vitro-evidence using cytokinesis-blocked cells and probes specific for chromosomes 17 and 21. Mutat Res 2004;551(1–2):167–80.

104. Tasevska N, Jiao L, Cross AJ, et al. Sugars in diet and risk of cancer in the NIH-AARP Diet and Health Study. Int J Cancer 2012;130(1):159–69.

105. Nothlings U, Murphy SP, Wilkens LR, et al. Dietary glycemic load, added sugars and carbohydrates as risk factors for pancreatic cancer: the Multiethnic Cohort Study. Am J Clin Nutr 2007;86:1495–501.

106. Kaaks R, Lukanova A. Energy balance and cancer: the role of insulin and insulin-like growth factor-1. Proc Nutr Soc 2001;60:91–106.

107. Bustin SA, Jenkins PJ. The growth hormone-insulin-like growth factor-1 axis and colorectal cancer. Trends Mol Med 2001;7:447–54.

108. Kuramoto H, et al. Immunohistochemical evaluation of insulin-like growth factor I receptor status in cervical cancer specimens. Acta Med Okayama 2008;62(4):251–9.

109. Haluska P, et al. HER receptor signaling confers resistance to the insulin-like growth factor-I receptor inhibitor, BMS-536924. Mol Cancer Ther 2008;7(9):2589–98.

110. Samudio I, et al. The Warburg effect in leukemia-stroma cocultures is mediated by mitochondrial uncoupling associated with uncoupling protein 2 activation. Cancer Res 2008;68(13):5198–205.

111. Hussain SP, et al. Nitric oxide is a key component in inflammation-accelerated tumorigenesis. Cancer Res 2008;68(17):7130–6.

112. Wang D, DuBois RN. Pro-inflammatory prostaglandins and progression of colorectal cancer. Cancer Lett 2008;267(2):197–203.

113. Aggarwal BB, Harikumar KB. Potential therapeutic effects of curcumin, the anti-inflammatory agent, against neurodegenerative, cardiovascular, pulmonary, metabolic, autoimmune and neoplastic diseases. Int J Biochem Cell Biol 2008;41:40–59.

114. Wallace JM. Nutritional and botanical modulation of the inflammatory cascade—eicosanoids, cyclooxygenases, and lipoxygenases—as an adjunct in cancer therapy. Integr Cancer Ther 2002;1(1):7–37.

115. Kaileh M, et al. Screening of indigenous Palestinian medicinal plants for potential anti-inflammatory and cytotoxic activity. J Ethnopharmacol 2007;113(3):510–16.

116. de Visser KE, et al. Paradoxical roles of the immune system during cancer development. Nat Rev Cancer 2006;6:24–37.

117. Caserta MT, et al. The associations between psychosocial stress and the frequency of illness, and innate and adaptive immune function in children. Brain Behav Immun 2008;22(6):933–40.

118. Littrell J. The mind–body connection: not just a theory anymore. Soc Work Health Care 2008;46(4):17–37.

119. Bartella V, et al. Insulin-dependent leptin expression in breast cancer cells. Cancer Res 2008;68(12):4919–27.

120. Silberstein J, et al. HIV and prostate cancer: a systematic review of the literature. Prostate Cancer Prostatic Dis 2008;12(1):6–12.

121. Pérez-López FR. Sunlight, the vitamin D endocrine system, and their relationships with gynaecologic cancer. Maturitas 2008;59(2):101–13.

122. Friedlander AH, et al. The relationship between measures of nutritional status and masticatory function in untreated patients with head and neck cancer. J Oral Maxillofac Surg 2008;66(1):85–92.

123. Lipinski B, Egyud G. Resistance of cancer cells to immune recognition and killing. Med Hypotheses 2000;54(3):456–60.

124. Finn OJ. Immuno-oncology: understanding the function and dysfunction of the immune system in cancer. Ann Oncol 2012;23(Suppl. 8):viii6–9. doi:10.1093/annonc/mds256.

125. Yang T, Li H, Huang G, et al. Detection of IgM and IgG complexes provides new insights into immune regulation of patients with malignancies: a randomized controlled trial. Int Immunopharmacol 2007;7:1433–41.

126. Fleet JC. Molecular actions of vitamin D contributing to cancer prevention. Mol Aspects Med 2008;29(6):388–96.

127. Maggini S, et al. Selected vitamins and trace elements support immune function by strengthening epithelial barriers and cellular and humoral immune responses. Br J Nutr 2007;98(Suppl. 1):S29–35.

128. Shen J, et al. Potentiation of intestinal immunity by micellary mushroom extracts. Biomed Res 2007;28(2):71–7.

129. Nozaki H, et al. Mushroom acidic glycosphingolipid induction of cytokine secretion from murine T cells and proliferation of NK1.1 alpha/beta TCR-double positive cells in vitro. Biochem Biophys Res Commun 2008;373(3):435–9.

130. Dong JC, Dong XH. Comparative study on effect of astragalus injection and interleukin-2 in enhancing anti-tumor metastasis action of dendritic cells. Zhongguo Zhong Xi Yi Jie He Za Zhi 2005;25(3):236–9.

131. Pilarski R, et al. Antiproliferative activity of various Uncaria tomentosa preparations on HL-60 promyelocytic leukemia cells. Pharmacol Rep 2007;59(5):565–72.

132. Kormosh N, et al. Effect of a combination of extract from several plants on cell-mediated and humoral immunity of patients with advanced ovarian cancer. Phytother Res 2006;20(5):424–5.

133. Choi KT. Botanical characteristics, pharmacological effects and medicinal components of Korean Panax ginseng C A Meyer. Acta Pharmacol Sin 2008;29(9):1109–18.

134. Zhai Z, et al. Enhancement of innate and adaptive immune functions by multiple Echinacea species. J Med Food 2007;10(3):423–34.

135. Ogba N, et al. HEXIM1 regulates 17beta-estradiol/estrogen receptor-alpha-mediated expression of cyclin D1 in mammary cells via modulation of P-TEFb. Cancer Res 2008;68(17):7015–24.

136. Tan DS, et al. ESR1 amplification in endometrial carcinomas: hope or hyperbole? J Pathol 2008;216:271–4.

137. Hassan HC, et al. Gynaecomastia: an endocrine manifestation of testicular cancer. Andrologia 2008;40(3):152–7.

138. Chandanos E, Lagergren J. Oestrogen and the enigmatic male predominance of gastric cancer. Eur J Cancer 2008;44(16):2397–403.

139. Alì G, et al. Different estrogen receptor beta expression in distinct histologic subtypes of lung adenocarcinoma. Hum Pathol 2008;39(10):1465–73.

140. Chen DZ, et al. Indole-3-carbinol and diindolylmethane induce apoptosis of human cervical cancer cells and in murine HPV16-transgenic preneoplastic cervical epithelium. J Nutr 2001;131(12):3294–302.

141. Higdon JV, et al. Cruciferous vegetables and human cancer risk: epidemiologic evidence and mechanistic basis. Pharmacol Res 2007;55(3):224–36.

142. Om AS, Chung KW. Dietary zinc deficiency alters 5 alpha-reduction and aromatization of testosterone and androgen and estrogen receptors in rat liver. J Nutr 1996;126(4):842–8.

143. Wang Y, et al. A positive feedback pathway of estrogen biosynthesis in breast cancer cells is contained by resveratrol. Toxicology 2008;248(2–3):130–5.

144. Li Z, et al. Genistein induces cell apoptosis in MDA-MB-231 breast cancer cells via the mitogen-activated protein kinase pathway. Toxicol In Vitro 2008;22:1749–53.

145. Ju YH, et al. Dietary genistein negates the inhibitory effect of letrozole on the growth of aromatase-expressing estrogen-dependent human breast cancer cells (MCF-7Ca) in vivo. Carcinogenesis 2008;29(11):2162–8.

146. Yang Y, et al. Saw palmetto induces growth arrest and apoptosis of androgen-dependent prostate cancer LNCaP cells via inactivation of STAT 3 and androgen receptor signaling. Int J Oncol 2007;31(3):593–600.

147. Kanadys WM, et al. Efficacy and safety of black cohosh (Actaea/Cimicifuga racemosa) in the treatment of vasomotor symptoms–review of clinical trials. Ginekol Pol 2008;79(4):287–96.

148. Wang Y, et al. The red clover (Trifolium pratense) isoflavone biochanin A inhibits aromatase activity and expression. Br J Nutr 2008;99(2):303–10.

149. Mumber M, editor. Integrative oncology: principles and practice. London: Taylor & Francis; 2005.

150. Ortega AD, et al. Glucose avidity of carcinomas. Cancer Lett 2008;276:125–35.

151. Littarru GP, Tiano L. Bioenergetic and antioxidant properties of coenzyme Q10: recent developments. Mol Biotechnol 2007;37(1):31–7.

152. McCarty MF, et al. The 'rejuvenatory' impact of lipoic acid on mitochondrial function in aging rats may reflect induction and activation of PPAR-gamma coactivator-1alpha. Med Hypotheses 2009;72(1):29–33.

153. Inazu M, Matsumiya T. Physiological functions of carnitine and carnitine transporters in the central nervous system. Nihon Shinkei Seishin Yakurigaku Zasshi 2008;28(3):113–20.

154. Ahn BH, et al. A role for the mitochondrial deacetylase Sirt3 in regulating energy homeostasis. Proc Natl Acad Sci USA 2008;105(38):14447–52.

155. Risau W, Flamme I. Vasculogenesis. Annu Rev Cell Dev Biol 1995;11:73–91.

156. Veytsman I, Aragon-Ching JB, Swain SM. Bevacizumab and Angiogenesis Inhibitors in the treatment of CNS metastases: the Road less Travelled. Curr Mol Pharmacol 2013;5(3):382–91.

157. Mikirova NA, et al. Anti-angiogenic effect of high doses of ascorbic acid. J Transl Med 2008;6(1):50.

158. Anand P, et al. Biological activities of curcumin and its analogues (Congeners) made by man and Mother Nature. Biochem Pharmacol 2008;76:1590–611.

159. Binion DG, et al. Curcumin inhibits VEGF mediated angiogenesis in human intestinal microvascular endothelial cells through COX-2 and MAPK inhibition. Gut 2008;57:1509–17.

160. Sagar SM, et al. Natural health products that inhibit angiogenesis: a potential source for investigational new agents to treat cancer-part 2. Curr Oncol 2006;13(3):99–107.

161. Lock K, et al. The global burden of disease attributable to low consumption of fruit and vegetables: implications for the global strategy on diet. Bull World Health Organ 2005;83(2):100–8.

162. Riboli E, Norat T. Epidemiologic evidence of the protective effect of fruit and vegetables on cancer risk. Am J Clin Nutr 2003;78(3 Suppl.):559S–69S.

163. Schwingshackl L, Schwedhelm C, Galbete C, et al. Adherence to Mediterranean diet and risk of cancer: an updated systematic review and meta-analysis. Nutrients 2017;9(10):1063. doi:10.3390/nu9101063. Published online 2017 Sep 26.

164. Wright ME, et al. Intakes of fruit, vegetables, and specific botanical groups in relation to lung cancer risk in the NIH-AARP Diet and Health Study. Am J Epidemiol 2008;168:1024–34.

165. Navarro Silvera SA, et al. Food group intake and risk of subtypes of esophageal and gastric cancer. Int J Cancer 2008;123(4):852–60.

166. Flood A, et al. Dietary patterns as identified by factor analysis and colorectal cancer among middle-aged Americans. Am J Clin Nutr 2008;88(1):176–84.

167. van Gils CH, et al. Consumption of vegetables and fruits and risk of breast cancer. JAMA 2005;293(2):183–93.

168. Koushik A, et al. Fruits and vegetables and ovarian cancer risk in a pooled analysis of 12 cohort studies. Cancer Epidemiol Biomarkers Prev 2005;14(9):2160–7.

169. Linos E, et al. Red meat consumption during adolescence among premenopausal women and risk of breast cancer. Cancer Epidemiol Biomarkers Prev 2008;17(8):2146–51.

170. Hart AR, et al. Pancreatic cancer: a review of the evidence on causation. Clin Gastroenterol Hepatol 2008;6(3):275–82.

171. Bahmanyar S, Ye W. Dietary patterns and risk of squamous-cell carcinoma and adenocarcinoma of the esophagus and adenocarcinoma of the gastric cardia: a population-based case-control study in Sweden. Nutr Cancer 2008;54(2):171–8.

172. Duffy CM, et al. Alcohol and folate intake and breast cancer risk in the WHI Observational Study. Breast Cancer Res Treat 2008;168(9):1024–34.

173. Bartsch H, et al. Dietary polyunsaturated fatty acids and cancers of the breast and colorectum: emerging evidence for their role as risk modifiers. Carcinogenesis 1999;20(12):2209–18.

174. Berquin IM, et al. Multi-targeted therapy of cancer by omega-3 fatty acids. Cancer Lett 2008;269(2):363–77.

175. Dal Maso L, et al. Risk factors for thyroid cancer: an epidemiological review focused on nutritional factors. Cancer Causes Control 2008;42(2–3):53–61.

176. Stoddard FR 2nd, et al. Iodine alters gene expression in the MCF7 breast cancer cell line: evidence for an anti-estrogen effect of iodine. Int J Med Sci 2008;5(4):189–96.

177. Ishii T, et al. Covalent modification of proteins by green tea polyphenol (–)–epigallocatechin-3-gallate through autoxidation. Free Radic Biol Med 2008;45:384–94.

178. Arts IC. A review of the epidemiological evidence on tea, flavonoids, and lung cancer. J Nutr 2008;138(8):1561S–6S.

179. Tao KS, et al. The multifaceted mechanisms for coffee's anti-tumorigenic effect on liver. Med Hypotheses 2008;71:730–6.

180. Nkondjock A. Coffee consumption and the risk of cancer: an overview. Cancer Lett 2009;277(2):121–5.

181. Young GP, Le Leu RK. Preventing cancer: dietary lifestyle or clinical intervention? Asia Pac J Clin Nutr 2002;11(Suppl. 3):S618–31.

182. Kushi LH, et al. The macrobiotic diet in cancer. J Nutr 2001;131(11 Suppl.):3056S–64S.

183. Padayatty SJ, Sun AY, Chen Q, et al. Vitamin C: intravenous use by complementary and alternative medicine practitioners and adverse effects. PLoS ONE 2010;5(7):e11414.

184. Cameron E, Pauling L. Supplemental ascorbate in the supportive treatment of cancer: prolongation of survival times in terminal human cancer. Proc Natl Acad Sci USA 1976;73(10):3685–9.

185. Cameron E, Pauling L. Supplemental ascorbate in the supportive treatment of cancer: reevaluation of prolongation of survival times in terminal human cancer. Proc Natl Acad Sci USA 1978;75(9):4538–42.

186. Creagan ET, Moertel CG, O'Fallon JR, et al. Failure of high-dose vitamin C (ascorbic acid) therapy to benefit patient with advanced cancer. A controlled trial. N Engl J Med 1979;301:687–90.

187. Moertel CG, Fleming TR, Creagan ET, et al. High-dose vitamin C versus placebo in the treatment of patients with advanced cancer who have had no prior chemotherapy. A randomized double-blind comparison. N Engl J Med 1985;312:137–41.

188. Coulter ID, Hardy ML, Morton SC, et al. Antioxidants vitamin C and vitamin E for the prevention and treatment of cancer. J Gen Intern Med 2006;21(7):735–44.

189. Padayatty SJ, Levine M. Reevaluation of ascorbate in cancer treatment: emerging evidence, open minds and serendipity. J Am Coll Nutr 2000;19(4):423–5.

190. Padayatty SJ, Sun H, Wang Y, et al. Vitamin C pharmacokinetics: implications for oral and intravenous use. Ann Intern Med 2004;140:533–7.

191. Monti DA, Mitchell E, Brazzan JA, et al. Phase I evaluation of intravenous ascorbic acid in combination with gemcitabine and erlotinib in patients with metastatic pancreatic cancer. PLoS ONE 2012;7(1):e29794.

192. Mikirova N, Casciari J, Rogers A, et al. Effect of high-dose intravenous vitamin C on inflammation in cancer patients. J Transl Med 2012;10:189.

193. Vollbracht C, Schneider B, Leendert V, et al. Intravenous vitamin C administration improves quality of life in breast cancer patients during chemo-/radiotherapy and aftercare: results of a retrospective, multicentre, epidemiological cohort study in Germany. In Vivo 2011;25(6):983–90.

194. Chen P, Yu J, Chalmers B, et al. Pharmacological ascorbate induces cytotoxicity in prostate cancer cells through ATP depletion and induction of autophagy. Anticancer Drugs 2012;23(4):437–44.

195. Takemura Y, Satoh M, Satoh K, et al. High dose of ascorbic acid induces cell death in mesothelioma cells. Biochem Biophys Res Commun 2010;394(2):249–53.

196. Du J, Cullen JJ, Beuttner GR. Ascorbic acid: chemistry, biology and the treatment of cancer. Biochim Biophys Acta 2012;1826(2):443–57.

197. Shabtay A, Sharabani H, Barvish Z, et al. Synergistic antileukemic activity of carnosic acid-rich rosemary extract and the 19-nor Gemini vitamin D analogue in a mouse model of systemic acute myeloid leukemia. Oncology 2008;75(3–4):203–14.

198. Petrioli R, Pascucci A, Francini E, et al. Weekly high-dose calcitriol and docetaxel in patients with metastatic hormone-refractory prostate cancer previously exposed to docetaxel. BJU Int 2007;100(4):775–9.

199. Chadha MK, Tian L, Mashtare T, et al. Phase 2 trial of weekly intravenous 1,25 dihydroxy cholecalciferol (calcitriol) in combination with dexamethasone for castration-resistant prostate cancer. Cancer 2010;116(9):2132–9.

200. Chen P, Stone J, Sullivan G, et al. Anti-cancer effect of pharmacologic ascorbate and its interaction with supplementary parenteral glutathione in preclinical cancer models. Free Radic Biol Med 2011;51(3):681–7.

201. Cascinu S, Cordella L, Del Ferro E, et al. Neuroprotective effect of reduced glutathione on cisplatin-based chemotherapy in advanced gastric cancer: a randomized double-blind placebo-controlled trial. J Clin Oncol 1995;13:26–32.

202. Cascinu S, Catalano V, Cordella L, et al. Neuroprotective effect of reduced glutathione on oxaliplatin-based chemotherapy in advanced colorectal cancer: a randomized, double-blind, placebo-controlled trial. J Clin Oncol 2002;20:3478–83.

203. Smyth JF, Bowman A, Perren T, et al. Glutathione reduces the toxicity and improves quality of life of women diagnosed with ovarian cancer treated with cisplatin: results of a double-blind, randomised trial. Ann Oncol 1997;8:569–73.

204. Bohm S, Oriana S, Spatti G, et al. Dose intensification of platinum compounds with glutathione protection as induction chemotherapy for advanced ovarian carcinoma. Oncology 1999;57:115–20.

205. Berkson BM, Rubin DM, Berkson AJ. Revisiting the ALA/N (alpha-lipoic acid/low-dose naltrexone) protocol for people with metastatic and nonmetastatic pancreatic cancer: a report of 3 new cases. Integr Cancer Ther 2009;8(4):416–22.

206. Berkson BM, Rubin DM, Berkson AJ. The long-term survival of a patient with pancreatic cancer with metastases to the liver after treatment with the intravenous alpha-lipoic acid/low-dose naltrexone protocol. Integr Cancer Ther 2006;5(1):83–9.

207. Dufès C. Delivery of the vitamin E compound tocotrienol to cancer cells. Ther Deliv 2011;2(11):1385–9.

208. Podlech O, Harter PN, Mittlebronn M, et al. Fermented mistletoe extract as a multimodal antitumoral agent in gliomas. Evid Based Complement Alternat Med 2012;2012:501796.

209. Bussing A. Overview on Viscum album L. products. In: Bussing A, editor. Mistletoe. The genus Viscum. Medicinal and aromatic plants—industrial profiles. Amsterdam: Harwood Academic Publishers; 2000. p. 209–21.

210. Bar-Sela G, Wollner M, Hammer L, et al. Mistletoe as complementary treatment in patients with advanced non-small-cell lung cancer treated with carboplatin-based combinations: a randomised phase II study. Eur J Cancer 2013;49(5):1058–64.

211. Ostermann T, Büssing A. Retrolective studies on the survival of cancer patients treated with mistletoe extracts: a meta-analysis. Explore (NY) 2012;8(5):277–81.

212. Milazzo S, Ernst E, Lejeune S, et al. Laetrile treatment for cancer (Review). Cochrane Database Syst Rev 2006;(2):CD005476.

213. Zhang DM, Lui JS, Deng LJ, et al. Arenobufagin, a natural bufadienolide from toad venom, induces apoptosis and autophagy in human hepatocellular carcinoma cells through inhibition of P13K/Akt/mTOR pathway. Carcinogenesis 2013;34(6):1331–42.

214. Ferreira PMP, Lima DJB, Debiasi BW, et al. Antiproliferative activity of Rhinella marina and Rhaebo guttatus venom extracts from Southern Amazon. Toxicon 2013;72:43–51.

215. Kostakis C, Byard RW. Sudden death associated with intravenous injection of toad extract. Forensic Sci Int 2009;V188:e1–5.

216. Cheng Y, Cai L, Jiang P, et al. SIRT1 inhibition by melatonin exerts antitumour activity in human osteosarcoma cells. Eur J Pharmacol 2013;715(1–3):219–29.

217. Carbajo-Pescador S, Ordoñez R, Benet M, et al. Inhibition of VEGF expression through blockade of Hif1α and STAT3 signalling mediates the anti-angiogenic effect of melatonin in HepG2 liver cancer cells. Br J Cancer 2013;109(1):83–91.

218. Zhang Y, Li L, Xiang C, et al. Protective effect of melatonin against Adriamycin-induced cardiotoxicity. Exp Ther Med 2013;5(5):1496–500.

219. Jung JH, Sohn EJ, Shin EA, et al. Melatonin suppresses the expression of 45S preribosomal RNA and upstream binding factor and enhances the antitumor activity of puromycin in MDA-MB-231 breast cancer cells. Evid Based Complement Alternat Med 2013;2013:879746.

220. Martín V, Sanchez-Sanchez AM, Herrera F, et al. Melatonin-induced methylation of the ABCG2/BCRP promoter as a novel mechanism to overcome multidrug resistance in brain tumour stem cells. Br J Cancer 2013;108(10):2005–12.

221. Majchrowicz MA. Essiac. Notes Undergr 1995;29:6–7.

222. Seely D, et al. In vitro analysis of the herbal compound Essiac. Anticancer Res 2007;27(6B):3875–82.

223. Ottenweller J, et al. Inhibition of prostate cancer-cell proliferation by Essiac. J Altern Complement Med 2004;10(4):687–91.

224. Cheung S, et al. Antioxidant and anti-inflammatory properties of ESSIAC and Flor-Essence. Oncol Rep 2005;14(5):1345–50.

225. Eberding A, et al. Evaluation of the antiproliferative effects of Essiac on in vitro and in vivo models of prostate cancer compared to Paclitaxel. Nutr Cancer 2007;58(2):188–96.

226. Leonard BJ, et al. An in vivo analysis of the herbal compound Essiac. Anticancer Res 2006;26(4B):3057–63.

227. Ma L, Dharamsi JW, Vandergriff T. Black salve as self-treatment for cutaneous squamous cell carcinoma. Dermatitis 2012;23(5):239–40.

228. Eastman KL, McFarland LV, Raugi GJ. Buyer beware: a black salve caution. J Am Acad Dermatol 2011;65(5):e154–5.

229. Cienki JJ, Zaret L. An Internet misadventure: bloodroot salve toxicity. J Altern Complement Med 2010;16(10):1125–7.

230. Burzynski SR, Janicki TJ, Weaver RA, et al. Targeted therapy with antineoplastons A10 and AS2–1 of high-grade, recurrent, and progressive brainstem glioma. Integr Cancer Ther 2006;5(1):40–7.

231. Burzynski SR, Weaver RA, Janicki T, et al. Long-term survival of high-risk pediatric patients with primitive neuroectodermal tumors treated with antineoplastons A10 and AS2–1. Integr Cancer Ther 2005;4(2):168–77.

232. Burzynski SR, Weaver RA, Lewy RI, et al. Phase II study of antineoplaston A10 and AS2–1 in children with recurrent and progressive multicentric glioma: a preliminary report. Drugs R D 2004;5(6):315–26.

233. Burzynski SR, Lewy RI, Weaver R, et al. Long-term survival and complete response of a patient with recurrent diffuse intrinsic brain stem glioblastoma multiforme. Integr Cancer Ther 2004;3(3):257–61.

234. Burzynski SR, Lewy RI, Weaver RA, et al. Phase II study of antineoplaston A10 and AS2–1 in patients with recurrent diffuse intrinsic brain stem glioma: a preliminary report. Drugs R D 2003;4(2):91–101.

235. Lee SS, Mohabbat MO, Burzynski SR. In vitro cancer growth inhibition and animal toxicity studies of antineoplaston A3. Drugs Exp Clin Res 1987;13(Suppl. 1):13–16.

236. Burzynski SR, Burzynski B, Mohabbat MO. Toxicology studies on antineoplaston AS2–1 injections in cancer patients. Drugs Exp Clin Res 1986;12(Suppl. 1): 25–35.

237. Burzynski SR. Antineoplastons: history of the research (I). Drugs Exp Clin Res 1986;12(Suppl. 1):1–9.

238. Nelson AJ, Holt JA. Combined microwave therapy. Med J Aust 1978;2(3):88–90.

239. Cardinal J, Klune JR, Chory E, et al. Noninvasive radiofrequency ablation of cancer targeted by gold nanoparticles. Surgery 2008;144(2):125–32. doi:10.1016/j.surg.2008.03.036.

240. Nordenström BE. Survey of mechanisms in electrochemical treatment (ECT) of cancer. Eur J Surg Suppl 1994;574:93–109.

241. Torres MP, Rachagani S, Purohit V, et al. Graviola: a novel promising natural-derived drug that inhibits tumorigenicity and metastasis of pancreatic cancer cells in vitro and in vivo through altering cell metabolism. Cancer Lett 2012;323(1):29–40. doi:10.1016/j.canlet.2012.03.031.

242. Dai Y, Hogan S, Schmelz EM, et al. Selective growth inhibition of human breast cancer cells by graviola fruit extract in vitro and in vivo involving downregulation of EGFR expression. Nutr Cancer 2011;63(5):795–801.

243. Gold J. Hydrazine sulfate in nonsmall-cell lung cancer. J Clin Oncol 1990;8(6):1117–18.

244. Gold J. Anabolic profiles in late-stage cancer patients responsive to hydrazine sulfate. Nutr Cancer 1981;3(1):13–19.

245. Gold J. Use of hydrazine sulfate in terminal and preterminal cancer patients: results of investigational new drug (IND) study in 84 evaluable patients. Oncology 1975;32(1):1–10.

246. Ni X, Suhail MM, Yang Q, et al. Frankincense essential oil prepared from hydrodistillation of Boswellia sacra gum resins induces human pancreatic cancer cell death in cultures and in a xenograft murine model. BMC Complement Altern Med 2012;12:253. doi:10.1186/1472-6882-12-253. Published online 2012 Dec 13.

247. Suhail MM, Wu A, Cao A, et al. Boswellia sacra essential oil induces tumor cell-specific apoptosis and suppresses tumor aggressiveness in cultured human breast cancer cells. BMC Complement Altern Med 2011;11:129. doi:10.1186/1472-6882-11-129. Published online 2011 Dec 15.

248. Robb K, et al. A Cochrane Systematic Review of transcutaneous electrical nerve stimulation for cancer pain. J Pain Symptom Manage 2009;37(4):746–53.

249. Harding C, et al. Auricular acupuncture: a novel treatment for vasomotor symptoms associated with luteinizing-hormone releasing hormone agonist treatment for prostate cancer. BJU Int 2008;103(2):186–90.

250. Johnston MF, et al. Acupuncture and fatigue: current basis for shared communication between breast cancer survivors and providers. J Cancer Surviv 2007;1(4):306–12.

251. Lai M, et al. Effects of electroacupuncture on tumor growth and immune function in the Walker-256 model rat. Zhongguo Zhen Jiu 2008;28(8):607–9.

252. Naeim A, et al. Evidence-based recommendations for cancer nausea and vomiting. J Clin Oncol 2008;26(23):3903–10.

253. Streitberger K, et al. Acupuncture for nausea and vomiting: an update of clinical and experimental studies. Auton Neurosci 2006;129:107–17.

254. Choo SP, et al. Electroacupuncture for refractory acute emesis caused by chemotherapy. J Altern Complement Med 2006;12:963–9.

255. Ezzo JM, et al. Acupuncture-point stimulation for chemotherapy-induced nausea or vomiting. Cochrane Database Syst Rev 2006;(2):CD002285.

256. Carlson L, Bultz B. Mind-body interventions in oncology. Curr Treat Options Oncol 2008;9(2–3):127–34.

257. Montazeri A. Health-related quality of life in breast cancer patients: a bibliographic review of the literature from 1974 to 2007. J Exp Clin Cancer Res 2008;27(1):32.

258. Chen K, Yeung R. Exploratory studies of Qigong therapy for cancer in China. Integr Cancer Ther 2002;1(4):345–70.

259. Smedslund G, Ringdal G. Meta-analysis of the effects of psychosocial interventions on survival time in cancer patients. J Psychosom Res 2004;57(2):123–31.

260. Breitbart W. Spirituality and meaning in supportive care: spirituality-and meaning-centered group psychotherapy interventions in advanced cancer. Support Care Cancer 2002;10(4):272–80.

261. Kassab S, et al. Homoeopathic medicines for adverse effects of cancer treatments. Cochrane Database Syst Rev 2009;(2):CD004845.

262. Thompson EA, et al. Towards standard setting for patient-reported outcomes in the NHS homoeopathic hospitals. Homeopathy 2008;97(3):114–21.

263. Kutner JS, et al. Massage therapy versus simple touch to improve pain and mood in patients with advanced cancer: a randomized trial. Ann Intern Med 2008;149(6):369–79.

264. Corbin L. Safety and efficacy of massage therapy for patients with cancer. Cancer Control 2005;12(3):158–64.

CHAPTER 33

Paediatrics

Diana Bowman
ND, MHSc

OVERVIEW

Working with children can be extremely rewarding, but it is markedly different from treating adults. Children often face very different medical conditions from adults and require specialised care. Practitioners need to be aware of children's special needs, the sensitivity and vitality of the child and the child's parents and siblings.

Most paediatric conditions are acute and self-limiting and recovery can be as sudden as the onset. However, while many childhood conditions can be treated in the family home, it is wise to seek the help of medical intervention, and often to do so as soon as possible, as children (especially babies) can become gravely ill quite quickly. It is also wise to constantly work with the diet and a positive healthy family lifestyle, to improve the vitality of the child. Additionally, as children are constantly developing physiologically, emotionally and mentally, protective and preventive factors are of paramount importance. Although medication and therapeutic interventions are important, focus should also be put on encouraging behaviours such as maternal breastfeeding, exercise and physical activity and appropriate diet and nutrition, which encourage healthy growth and development, and as such protection from many conditions.

Classification of the paediatric patient was defined at the International Conference on Harmonisation,[1] which defined the following categories: newborn (0–27 days); infants and toddlers (28 days to 23 months); children (2–11 years) and adolescents (12–16 or 18 years depending on region). According to the WHO paediatric age categories, a minor is defined as anyone under the age of 18.[2] Just as is observed in adult populations, there is an increase in the use of complementary medicines (CM) in paediatric patients.[3]

Paediatric medication considerations

Academic and clinical consensus recommends that children are not viewed as 'small adults'.[5] There are marked differences in pathology, physiology, pharmacokinetics and pharmacodynamics between paediatric and adult populations.[6-8] The efficacy of a medication in a paediatric patient depends on the practitioner selecting an appropriate preparation, calculating the correct dosage and motivating the family to ensure regular administration.[9]

Naturopathic paediatric ethical and legal considerations[4]

- A cautious yet balanced approach can help guide the paediatric naturopath towards clinical advice (including referral) that is clinically responsible, ethically appropriate and legally defensible. Employing an approach that embraces both clinical and legal concerns can help to protect the child's welfare.
- Employ judicious use of CM to prevent financial and emotional burdens to the family.
- Serious and life-threatening conditions must only be treated in conjunction with the child's primary doctors/paediatrician.
- Most research on CM therapies is being conducted on adults and may therefore not be directly applicable to paediatric populations.
- Older children or adolescents may have the cognitive and emotional capacity to fully participate in healthcare decisions. If so, the adolescent should be provided with the same information as would be given to an adult patient.
- Differences in cultural or religious beliefs may lead to conflict between patients, families and medical practitioners over treatment options. Healthcare practitioners need to remain sensitive to and maintain an attitude of respect for these differences. An obligation exists to provide effective treatment to the child.

There are some important considerations when deciding the dose of medications at different life stages. Drugs are metabolised very differently in neonates and children compared with adults, or even adolescents. Absorption is affected by differences in gastric acid secretion, bile salt formation, gastric emptying, intestinal motility and microflora.[5] These are mostly reduced in a neonate and may also be reduced—though sometimes raised—in an ill child. The distribution of the volume of drugs in children can change with age because of the differences in the body's composition of minerals, lipids, proteins and water (Figure 33.1); plasma protein binding capacity also changes with age. Drug elimination can be longer in babies than adults. So, when medicating babies and children younger than 12 years old, body weight and age should be considered.[6] (See Table 33.1 for formulas.)

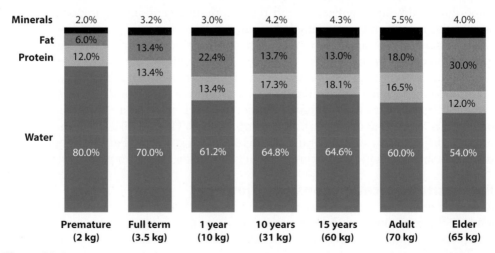

Figure 33.1
Changes in body proportions of body composition with growth and ageing
Adapted from Puig 1996[10]

Table 33.1
Calculating medication dosages

Rule	Formula
Fried's rule	$\dfrac{\text{Age in months}}{150} \times \text{adult dose} = \text{child's dose}$
Young's rule	$\dfrac{\text{Age in years}}{(\text{age} + 12)} \times \text{adult dose} = \text{child's dose}$
Dilling's rule	$\dfrac{\text{Age in months}}{20} \times \text{adult dose} = \text{child's dose}$
Clark's rule	$\dfrac{\text{Weight in kg}}{67} \times \text{adult dose} = \text{child's dose}$
Ausberger's rule	$1.5 \times \text{weight in kg} + 10 = \%$ of adult dose
Unless the teenager is of small stature, adult doses may be considered	

Sources: Mosby, Inc. 2013[11] and Dorland 2011[12]

Individual practitioners will have a preference for one dosage calculation formula over another when selecting a dose for children. Table 33.1 can be used to guide those in doubt when considering a herbal formula. Ausberger's rule and Clark's rule for calculations of paediatric doses of medications are based on weight as opposed to age and may be more suitable to allow for the faster metabolism of children at certain ages,[13] while Fried's rule, Dilling's rule and Young's rule are based on age alone. Adult doses may be considered for teenagers unless they are of small stature, in which case dosage may be calculated using either Clark's rule or Ausberger's rule.

Hepatic metabolism

Medications are metabolised by enzymatic and metabolic reactions in the body. Phase I activity for drug metabolism is reduced in neonates, increases progressively during the first six months of life, slows during adolescence and usually attains adult rates by late puberty.[6,7] Neonates metabolise medications much more slowly than adults do. By six months of age the immature reactions involving acetylation, glucuronidation and conjugation with amino acids have matured to adult levels.[7] The metabolic pathways for phase II reactions reach adult levels by 3–4 years of age.[7,12,14,15]

Digestive flora

Colonisation of the gastrointestinal tract (GIT) begins at birth and is usually established by week 1. The infant microbiota is varied in composition and less stable over time and progresses from sterility to dense colonisation similar to an adult by age one year.[16] The type of microorganism will depend on hygiene and diet. *Bifidobacterium* spp. are the most prolific organism in a breastfed baby.[16] After infancy, intestinal microbiota composition does not change significantly. Hence, older children and adults have less variable faecal flora composition which is not as dependent on diet.[10] Implications of this altered flora are discussed in the chapters on irritable bowel syndrome, atopic skin disorders and asthma, and it is known that functions of the microbiota include protection against pathogens, stimulation of angiogenesis, regulation of fat storage and the processing of nutrients.[16] Factors that underlie the development of microbiota include mode of delivery (birth), maternal vaginal microbiota, maturity/prematurity at birth, hospitalisation and method of feeding.[16]

Nutrition in children

The physiological differences in children when compared with adults also result in differing nutritional requirements for children. This reflects the population's unique needs for growth and development, as well as their differing maintenance requirements due to higher metabolisms. The estimated average requirements for the main nutrients are listed in Tables 33.2 and 33.3.[17–19]

Principles for a good diet include avoiding allergens, sugar, fried and processed foods and having varied fresh fruits and vegetables, nuts, seeds and whole grains (not for babies), yoghurt and bitter (usually well hidden) foods.[20] Following a course of antibiotics, if there is a suspicion of intestinal worms, consistent poor appetite, pica, diarrhoea or constipation, consult a naturopath.

Herbal medicine in children

The conditions encountered in paediatric practice may be different from those encountered in general practice (e.g. otitis media and colic). Therefore the herbal medicines most commonly used will also differ. Table 33.4 outlines common paediatric conditions and herbal medicines used to treat these conditions, according to traditional use.

Herbal medicine considerations in paediatric practice

- Keep herbal medicines in a locked cupboard.
- Consideration of metabolic rate, constitution and temperament is important.
- Start the dosage in the lower part of the therapeutic range for the herb or nutrient and increase if needed.
- The 'vitality' of the child needs to be taken into consideration.
- Be particularly careful of sweetened medications with young children, and do not use honey as a sweetener in babies under 12 months of age.

Common paediatric conditions

Generally, common paediatric conditions can be treated in a similar manner as it would in adult populations (as suggested in appropriate chapters), while also paying attention to certain paediatric-specific conditions as recommended in this chapter. The more common presentations in paediatric naturopathic practice include[11,21]:

- acne
- asthma
- allergies and food intolerances
- conjunctivitis
- constipation
- colic
- cough
- dermatitis
- diarrhoea
- ear infections

- enuresis
- fever and infectious diseases
- 'fussy eaters'
- obesity
- otitis media
- recurrent colds
- stomach upset food regurgitation and vomiting
- stress and adjustment issues
- tantrums and bad behaviour
- vaccination decisions and reactions.

Mental health in children

It can be a difficult for parents or carers to notice possible mental health problems in children. Children are rapidly changing and maturing physically, mentally and

Table 33.2
Vitamins

Age group and gender	Vitamin C (mg/day)	Thiamine (mg/day)	Ribo-flavin (mg/day)	Niacin (mg/day) niacin equivalents	Vitamin B6 (mg/day)	Vitamin B12 (µg/day)	Folate (µg/day) as dietary folate equivalents	Pantothenic acid (mg/day)	Biotin (µg/day)	Choline (µg/day)	Vitamin A (retinol equivalents ts) (µg/day)	Vitamin D (µg/day)	Vitamin E α-tocopherol equivalents (mg/day)	Vitamin K (µg/day)
Infants 0–6 months	25	0.2	0.3	2	0.1	0.4	65	1.7	5	125	250	5	4	2.0
7–12 months	30	0.3	0.4	4	0.3	0.5	80	2.2	6	150	430	5	5	2.5
Children 1–3 years	25	0.4	0.4	5	0.4	0.7	120	3.5	8	200	210	5	5	25.0
4–8 years	25	0.5	0.5	6	0.5	1.0	160	4.0	12	250	275	5	6	35.0
Boys 9–13 years	28	0.7	0.8	9	0.8	1.5	250	5.0	20	375	445	5	9	45.0
14–18 years	28	1.0	1.1	12	1.1	2.0	330	6.0	30	550	630	5	10	55.0
Girls 9–13 years	28	0.7	0.8	9	0.8	1.5	250	4.0	20	375	420	5	8	45.0
14–18 years	28	0.9	0.9	11	1.0	2.0	330	4.0	25	400	485	5	8	55.0

Table 33.3
Main minerals

Age group and gender	Calcium (mg/day)	Magnesium (mg/day)	Iron (mg/day)	Potassium (mg/day)	Selenium (μg/day)	Sodium (mg/day)	Zinc (mg/day)
Infants 0–6 months	210	30	0.2	400	12	120	2.0
7–12 months	270	75	7.0	700	15	170	2.5
Children 1–3 years	360	65	4.0	2000	20	200–400	2.5
4–8 years	520	110	4.0	2300	30	300–600	3.0
Boys 9–13 years	800–1050	200	6.0	3000	40	400–800	5.0
14–18 years	1050	340	8.0	3600	60	460–920	11.0
Girls 9–13 years	800–1050	200	6.0	2500	40	400–800	5.0
14–18 years	1050	300	8.0	2600	50	460–920	6.0

Table 33.4
Commonly used herbs in paediatrics according to herbal tradition

Main conditions	Main treatment actions	Common herbs
Infants and toddlers		
Colic	Carminative	*Mentha piperita, Foeniculum vulgare, Matricaria recutita, Melissa officinalis* Essential oils: *Matricaria recutita, Foeniculum vulgare* or *Anaethum graveolens*
Common cold	Immune system-enhancing Circulatory stimulant Antiseptic	*Echinacea* spp., *Andrographis paniculata, Astragalus membranaceus* (not in the acute phase) *Zingiber officinale* *Verbascum thapsis, Thymus vulgaris* *Glycyrrhiza glabra*
Constipation	Laxatives Demulcent Spasmolytic Hydrative	*Iris versicolor, Angelica polymorpha, Rumex crispus, Taraxacum officinale* (radix), *Glycyrrhiza glabra* *Ulmus fulva* *Matricaria recutita, Melissa officinalis, Mentha piperita*
Children		
Respiratory tract infections	Anticatarrhals Respiratory demulcents Expectorants Mucolytics Antitussives Antiseptic Mucous membrane trophorestorative	*Solidago virgaurea, Hydrastis canadensis* *Althea officinalis, Chondus crispus* *Pelargonium sidoides, Grindelia camporum, Inula helenium* *Allium sativum, Amoracia rusticana* *Prunus serotina, Glycyrrhiza glabra* *Thymus vulgaris, Allium sativum, Inula helenium, Pelargonium sidoides* *Hydrastis canadensis*
Fever	Diaphoretics Cooling bitters	*Mentha piperita, Achillea millefolium, Sambucus nigra* *Taraxacum officinale, Gentiana lutea*
Allergy	Antiallergy	*Albizia lebbeck, Scutellaria baicalensis*
Asthma	Bronchodilator Expectorant Bronchodilator Trophorestorative Anticatarrhal	*Adhatoda vasica* *Coleus forskohlii* *Hydrastis canadensis*
Adolescents		
Acne	Depurative Hypoglycaemic Immune modulating Anti-inflammatory	*Rumex crispus, Berberis aquifolium, Arctium lappa* *Galega officinalis, Gymnema sylvestre* *Echinacea* spp., *Andrographis paniculata* *Glycyrrhiza glabra, Bupleurum falcatum, Rehmannia glutinosa*
Warts	Antiviral Immunomodulating	*Thuja occidentalis* *Echinacea* spp.
Stress	Adrenal tonic Adaptogen Nervine	*Glycyrrhiza glabra* *Eleutherococcus senticosus, Withania somnifera* *Hypericum perforatum, Scutellaria lateriflora, Passiflora incarnata*

Sources: Hull 2013,[13] Mosby, Inc. 2013[11] and Dorland 2011[12]

spiritually. Some degree of poor behaviour or changeable mood is therefore normal in children, especially with changing hormones.

Though children can be affected by many different mental health problems (see Chapters 14–17 on the nervous system and Chapters 36 and 37 on bipolar disorder and ADHD). The three most common groups of disorders are:

- emotional disorders such as anxiety, depression and obsessions
- conduct disorders characterised by awkward, troublesome, aggressive and antisocial behaviours
- hyperactivity disorders involving inattention and overactivity.[22]

Warning signs that indicate a clinical problem include mood changes, intense feelings, behaviour changes, concentration difficulties, unexplained weight loss and physical harm to self or others.[23] In addition to more interventionist forms of treatment, exercise, yoga and meditation are excellent family activities and equip children with lifelong beneficial life skills.

COMPLIANCE ISSUES

Babies

Babies clearly communicate differently from other populations until they grow and develop speech. Parents can quickly learn the different types of crying their baby has for hunger, pain or discomfort (including being wet or soiled), fear and frustration or being too hot or cold. If a baby requires medication it may be possible to give the medicine in an adult dose to a breastfeeding mother; however, a drug/herb must reach the maternal serum in order to penetrate into milk.[24]

If a baby is breastfed or bottle-fed, using a dropper to the side, close to the back of the baby's mouth will help to keep the tongue from thrusting the medicine out and the swallow reflex will take effect.

If a baby has thrush, the appropriate probiotic can be put on the nipple before feeding for a breastfed baby, or on the teat for a formula-fed infant.

Children

Children of all ages need to be given positive feedback on their progress and positive attitudes. Realistic goals should be set to increase the likelihood of compliance; for example, in the case of planned weight loss, planning to lose one of 10 kg by the next follow-up consultation if on a weight-loss plan or having three different-coloured vegetables at least four times a week if diversifying their foods has been recommended.[6]

If changes to lifestyle such as dietary changes or physical activities and exercise have been recommended, the instructions given to the family should be simplified, and introduced incrementally where possible (an important exception to this would be the need to immediately remove a highly allergic food such as peanuts in children who have experienced an anaphylactic reaction to the peanuts or other dangerous or life-threatening situations).

Young children may find it difficult to swallow pills and may dislike the taste of tablets and liquids. A child disliking the taste of medication is a common problem and may result in most of the liquid herbal formula not being ingested by the time they return for the next consultation. By explaining ways of taking the medications or having a printed handout with suggestions the naturopath may minimise the noncompliance. Crushed supplements and liquid medications can be added to other palatable foods, or mixed with a little apple or pear concentrate. Alternatively, they can be frozen into little ice blocks with a pleasant-tasting juice or fruit concentrate, and then they can be chipped into smaller pieces and easily swallowed.

Adolescents

Adolescents are mostly healthy and physical complaints are commonly associated with psychosocial issues which, combined with risk-taking behaviour, feature prominently as causes of morbidity and mortality. Key areas of physical, cognitive and psychosocial development vary greatly in individual adolescents. Healthcare for this age group needs to acknowledge a growing autonomy combined with withdrawal of parental control in the areas of health and wellbeing. Gaining trust and empathy are imperative to treatment success, but practitioners must be vigilant of professional boundaries.[25]

Taking a psychosocial history is an important part of the adolescent consultation as physical, emotional and social wellbeing are closely interlinked. One approach is using a psychosocial screening tool such as the HEADSSS psychosocial assessment tool.[26]

Parent care

Treating children inevitably interfaces with the child's parents. It is important to consider that, while the child is certainly the patient, treatment must often extend to the parent as well. Health issues in children are clearly a stressful and emotional time for parents, and they need to be supported throughout the treatment in a rational and appropriate manner. Parents need to be included in the treatment process and educated appropriately.

Parents may not fully understand the instructions and rationale of the prescription— for example, the medications, dietary advice or physical therapy. Giving written instructions in a language they can understand is useful.

An early follow-up telephone call can be made to see if the family has any residual questions and can assist with adherence to a new regimen.[6] People under financial stress (a common occurrence when raising children) may have priorities other than paying for medicine. Ask the family to bring the medication bottles with them to each consultation and record the pill or liquid count or an estimation. Discrepancies could explain why expected results have not been achieved—many parents may simply not understand that under-dosing can reduce effectiveness. These considerations need to be taken into account when formulating a treatment plan.

Some parents may have beliefs or attitudes that deter or prevent them from giving children medications or other treatments.[6] These considerations also need to be taken into account, and potential problems can be resolved by actively engaging the parents in the treatment process. Concise but informative and easily understandable oral and written instructions should be given to the parents for each suggested medication or other treatment. The instruction should explain what the medication or treatment is for, how it will work and any possible side effects that might occur.[14]

There may be potential challenges working with the parents. For example, a parent may become defensive about a child's diet or activity level, and if the need for this is not explained in a gentle but educational manner there may be a loss of confidence in parenting skills, or a reduction in patient compliance.

EXAMPLES OF TREATMENT FOR COMMON PAEDIATRIC CONDITIONS

There is relatively little information or specific evidence for naturopathic treatment of conditions in paediatric medicine. In most instances practitioners will need to refer to adult or general population evidence, with modifications based on recommendations in this chapter. Some manifestations are, however, more common in children. Some of these do have specific evidence. For example, otitis media will be rarely observed in most adult populations, and studies have demonstrated olive oil infused with extracts of *Allium sativum*, *Verbascum thapsus*, *Calendula officinalis* and *Hypericum perforatum* is effective in reducing pain in children with otitis media.[27] Additionally, examination of most Cochrane reviews for complementary medicine in paediatric populations finds that they are inconclusive due to dearth of paediatric-specific studies, inappropriately small study populations or poor methodological quality,[28] and similar findings appear to occur in even the majority of most current complementary medicine research in paediatric populations.[29] The breadth of paediatric practice also makes it difficult to recommend specific therapies across the paediatric population. Therefore, when examining evidence for naturopathic treatment, practitioners need to critically assess both the paediatric and the general population literature for evidence of specific interventions in naturopathic paediatric practice. However, it is usually the approaches to treatment, rather than specific treatments themselves, where major differences occur between general and paediatric naturopathic practice. For these reasons examples of treatment approaches for common naturopathic paediatric presentations follow.

Digestive issues

Recurrent abdominal pain (three distinct episodes of pain over three or more months) occurs in 10% of school-aged children.[30] An organic cause will be found in 5–10% of cases.[31] Digestive issues also need to consider that infants, toddlers and young children can be erratic eaters, have erratic and variable bowel motions and protuberant abdomens that come and go. The key is to establish with the parents/caregivers that which is normal and abnormal for the child. Stressors and other psychological factors must be considered and appropriate individual treatments tailored for the child and sometimes the family. Networks of care are needed to improve the digestion and nutritional health of children.[32,33] Some examples of core clinical considerations in paediatric digestive issues are listed in Table 33.5.

Stress and adjustment issues

A range of stress and adjustment issues are common in paediatric populations.[31] Stress refers to an individual's immediate reactions to external pressures and to prolonged internal states that may have long-term deleterious effects.[34] Children cannot advocate for themselves,[35] and therefore look for protection from reliable and familiar adults. Long-term involvement with trustworthy adults is a strong protective factor in childhood, especially when the adults can control their own reactions to the child's stress and adjustment issues.[36–39]

Being aware of the multidirectional forces within a child, supporting the child itself, the child's nervous system, other systems affected as sequelae, and the family unit, are within the realms of the healthcare practitioner. Children may have to adjust to many and varied life stressors, which may include: divorce of parents; death of a parent, sibling,

Table 33.5
Examples of treatments options for common paediatric conditions

Common presentation	Naturopathic aims	Protocol	Examples of treatments for digestive upsets
Treatments for digestive presentations			
Stomach upset Loss of appetite Hunger and excitement Functional abdominal pain Colic Nausea and/or vomiting Constipation and/or diarrhoea	Determine and treat the cause(s) to provide relief to the child and family Calm the nervous system and support psychologically Support a healthy appetite and normal bowel motions	Exclude conditions needing medical intervention and organic conditions Correct lifestyle issues including diet and ensure healthy GIT flora Judicious and preferably short-term use of medications (herbs and supplements) Encourage the mechanics of eating Reassurance and explanation to parents Pacifying techniques for child	Refer to primary doctor/paediatrician (especially if there is weight loss, frequent vomiting, loss of energy, fever, growth retardation, constant abdominal pain, an abdominal mass or severe diarrhoea) Refer for counselling if the stress is prolonged or the behaviour changes remarkably Reduce stimulants and external stressors Avoid highly processed foods and sugar (a common cause of diarrhoea in children) Increase foods containing magnesium, B vitamins, folate and zinc Determine if tolerant of high-fibre diet Try frequent nutrient-dense foods rather than three large meals and encourage to chew food slowly and don't drink with meals Recolonise the GIT with good bacteria such as *Bifidobacterium* and *Lactobacillus* if they have had a sugary diet, an illness or a course of antibiotics Use of anxiolytic and nervine herbs such as *Piper methysticum* (not for children under 12 years old), *Passiflora incarnata*, *Scutellaria lateriflora*, *Withania somnifera* and *Matricaria recutita*. Judicious use of carminatives, antinausea/vomiting herbs, sedatives, spasmolytics, possibly use of appetite stimulants and demulcents such as *Mentha X piperita*, *Matricaria recutita*, *Melissa officinalis*, *Filipendula ulmaria*, *Foeniculum vulgare* and *Althaea officinalis*

Table 33.5
Examples of treatments options for common paediatric conditions (continued)

Common presentation	Naturopathic aims	Protocol	Examples of treatments
		Treatments for common stress/adjustment-related presentations	Examples of treatments for digestive upsets
Mood reactivity/easily upset or angry or withdrawing Tiredness and insomnia Anxiety Nightmares Poor concentration Worsening of any existing condition such as eczema, asthma Loss of appetite Abdominal aches and pains Constipation and/or diarrhoea Nail biting Nervousness and restlessness Secondary enuresis Headaches, worry, depression	Ensure child safety Determine the cause Exclude conditions needing medical treatment/organic conditions Calm the nervous system and support psychologically	Refer to essential services if the child needs protection Remove stressors Support the nervous system Support other systems suffering as sequelae Psychological counselling for the child/adolescent and consider family counselling	Use of anxiolytic and nervine herbal medicines such as *Piper methysticum* (not for children under 12), *Passiflora incarnata*, *Scutellaria lateriflora*, *Withania somnifera*, *Matricaria recutita* Supplement with calcium, magnesium, B vitamin complex, vitamin C and zinc Lifestyle advice such as encouraging the child to talk about their feelings, reducing stimulants and external stressor(s), moderating exercise but avoiding excitement and physical activities before bed, tailored relaxation techniques or massage. Bathing with lavender, marjoram, ylang ylang, chamomile and clary sage aromatherapy oils. Use a hops and lavender herbal pillow Dietary increase of magnesium, B vitamins, folate, zinc, calcium and magnesium and vitamin C-containing foods such as whole grains, leafy vegetables, lean protein. Include foods such as oats, millet, brown rice, asparagus, onion, garlic, potatoes, turnips, carrots, lentils and kidney beans, and the culinary herbs rosemary, nutmeg, marjoram and oregano Exclude food allergies, fluctuating blood glucose levels and intestinal parasites Enquire about bullying at school Referral for psychological treatment may also be helpful

Table 33.5
Examples of treatments options for common paediatric conditions (continued)

Common presentation	Naturopathic aims	Protocol	Examples of treatments for digestive upsets
		Treatments for common skin-related presentations	
Inherently dry irritable skin Itchy skin condition occurring in the last 12 months plus at least three of the following: – onset below two years of age (often by six months) – distribution varies with age (in young infants cheeks, forehead and scalp are the most common site) – history of flexural involvement, history of xerosis – history of other atopic conditions – visible flexural rash Predisposition to develop asthma and/or allergic rhinitis Indications of essential fatty acid deficiency Indications of micronutrient and antioxidant deficiency Indications of immune deficiency; raised IgE level Stroking the skin produces a flat white line instead of usual red line, flare and wheal	Alleviate the skin irritation Detect and eliminate allergens Reduce inflammatory cascade Detect and eliminate psychological stressors	Check for candidiasis Check for dietary/ environmental allergens/irritants Ensure an appropriate diet Consider emotional tensions (see section above)	Careful attention to hygiene to minimise *Staphylococcus aureus* For *Candidiasis*, recolonise the GIT with good bacteria such as *Bifidobacterium lactis*, *Lactobacillus* GG, *Lactobacillus rhamnosus* and *Lactobacillus reuteri* and give *Tabebuia* and zinc For dietary allergens—in particular investigate dairy products, eggs, peanuts, tomatoes, wheat, sugar, chocolate, yeast extracts, pork, beef, nightshades, nuts and food additives; consider a rotation diet Use non-irritant clothing, avoid heat and sweating, use mild non-irritant soaps for clothing and rinse clothing well Supplement with gamma-linolenic-acid, antioxidants and anti-inflammatories (vitamins A, C, E and zinc in particular) Look for and correct hypochlorhydria Behaviour modification/counselling for stress and scratching Herbal medicine—Consider using immunomodulating herbs, depuratives, digestives, adaptogens, antiallergy and antioxidant classes of herbs such as *Echinacea* spp., *Albizia lebbeck*, *Hemidesmus indicus*, *Rumex crispus* or *Curcuma longa* Topically—*Avena sativa* baths or poultices for the itch can give immediate relief, and *Glycyrrhiza glabra* and *Matricaria recutita* mixed into a gentle cream base such as vitamin E cream b.d. or t.d.s. can give great relief. Experience shows that if the lesions are particularly advanced, applying wet packs over the cream and lesion and wrapping them in a protective plastic can aid absorption

significant other person or pet; adoption; conflicted marriage; drug or alcohol abuse within the home; or moving home or school and away from peers. Therefore the development of coping strategies is an important part of child development. Naturopaths—like all health professionals—have a duty of care to report suspected child abuse. Refer to your state, provincial or territory authority for laws governing your jurisdiction.

There are many tools available to the general public and health professionals that assist with rating or scaling adjustment issues in children. Some are best completed by teachers, some by the caregiver and some by health professionals. Many are available online such as the ASCA (Adjustment Scales for Children and Adolescents) and the BBAS (Basic Behavioural Adjustment Scale). Many paediatric presentations, such as bed wetting (secondary enuresis), may in fact be a manifestation of stress and an adjustment issue (Table 33.5).

Skin conditions (atopic dermatitis / eczema)

The presentations of skin conditions are one of the major treatment areas in paediatric naturopathic practice, with atopic dermatitis and eczema being the most common. The principles are avoidance of triggers, restoration of barrier function, reduction of the inflammatory cascade and avoidance of irritants (Table 33.5). Further detail on specific treatments can be found in the inflammatory skin conditions chapter (Chapter 28). There is the possibility that atopic dermatitis may have a lifelong tendency. It is a multifactorial condition in which allergy and food intolerance are just two of many factors. Eliminating allergens may ameliorate and breastfeeding may be protective. The premature introduction of solid foods (before four months) may increase the risk of developing the condition. The family can be reassured that there is no permanent disfiguration, it is not contagious and the condition improves with time. There is complete resolution in 5% of cases and relapse by five years in one-third of cases.[40]

INTEGRATIVE MEDICAL CONSIDERATIONS

Exercise and physical activity

A recent clinical review on physical complementary therapies in adolescents found that improving **exercise and physical activity** had benefits on weight control and lipid profiles, as well as improved outcomes in asthma diabetes and depression.[41] **Yoga** was found to have improvements on ADHD and anxiety, and **Tai Chi** on ADHD and asthma. The potential underlying mechanism for the positive effects of these therapies is thought to be the stimulation of pressure receptors leading to increased vagal activity, decreased stress hormones and increased production of anti-pain and antidepressant neurotransmitters (such as serotonin).

Hypnotherapy

Children generally are receptive to hypnosis and make good subjects for guided imagery and may have good results for some conditions, particularly in procedure-related pain and enuresis, though studies are usually of varying quality or clinical relevance.[42] Culbert and Banez[43] report four classic studies where hypnosis had better outcomes for bladder control than other treatments including pharmaceuticals, especially long term after cessation of treatments. Teaching children self-hypnosis is empowering for the child as they can take control of their own conditions.

Acupuncture

Laser acupuncture may be a more gentle approach than needling when treating children. However, examination of acupuncture safety does demonstrate that while adverse events do exist, they are usually mild in nature, and acupuncture is safe when practised by an appropriately trained practitioner.[42] The literature published on the effectiveness of acupuncture is conflicting and studies are usually of varying quality, with pain relief, treatment of postoperative or chemotherapy-induced nausea and nocturnal enuresis demonstrating the most promise for acupuncture intervention.[44]

Massage

Massage may also demonstrate some benefit in paediatric populations. Two large Cochrane reviews have been published on massage in paediatric populations. A review of massage for promoting physical growth and mental health of infants aged younger than six months found significant improvement in sleep hours compared with control but no improvement in growth measures.[45] Another review examined massage intervention in promoting growth and development in preterm and/or low-birthweight infants.[46] Infants receiving massage had reduced hospital stays and also gained more weight than controls, though weight gain was thought to be of statistical, and not clinical, relevance.

CLINICAL SUMMARY

Children are not just 'little adults'. Naturopathic paediatric practice requires a complex and flexible approach to patient treatment that understands and acknowledges the stage of child development.[47] There is relatively little information or specific evidence for naturopathic treatment of conditions in paediatric medicine,[48] and in most instances practitioners will need to refer to adult or general population evidence, with modifications based on recommendations in this chapter. In many instances therapeutic interventions may not be required at all, and a focus on preventive and protective factors can assist in reducing the need for further attention. However, while most presentations will be self-limiting, naturopaths need to be aware that the condition of paediatric patients can deteriorate quite quickly, and need to have appropriate resources, including referral pathways, at hand to provide appropriate care in these instances.

Children require routines and need to know that they are loved, respected and are important enough to be involved in the treatment plan for their condition. They also need the appropriate amount of sleep for their age, appropriate diet, exercise, fluid intake and fun and play. These need to be incorporated into the treatment plan. Children and adolescents of all ages may resist treatment regimens that take them away from activities or classes or make them appear different from their friends. Engaging adolescents appropriately in the treatment process may reduce these compliance issues. Parents and guardians are also an important element in naturopathic paediatric practice, and where appropriate should be actively involved in any treatment plan. See decision tree (Figure 33.2) for specific treatment considerations.

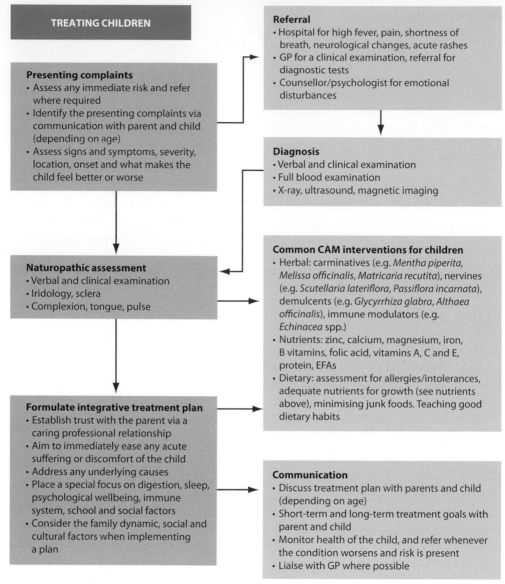

Figure 33.2
Naturopathic treatment decision tree—treating children

Note: Due to the extensive range of potential disorders, a *Review of the major evidence* table has not been formulated. Please see evidence throughout the chapter and consult other chapters for specific conditions.

KEY POINTS

- Children are not 'little adults' but have their own specific requirements.
- Children's symptoms can exacerbate quickly, so that they often need urgent and appropriate attention.
- Parents and siblings may also require some form of treatment or support.
- Education, explanation and motivation should form the basis of treatment.
- Children of all ages require positive feedback on their progress.
- Encourage healthy attitudes to digestion and elimination in the early years as this may assist in providing lifelong health.
- Identify and set achievable goals.

FURTHER READING

Garth M. Moonbeam meditations for children. North Blackburn: Collins Dove; 1993.

Glazner C, Evans J, Cheuk D. Complementary and miscellaneous interventions for nocturnal enuresis in children. Cochrane Database Syst Rev 2005;(2):CD005230.

Hunt K, Ernst E. The evidence-base for complementary medicine in children: a critical overview of systematic reviews. Arch Dis Child 2011;96(8):769–76.

Santich R, Bone K. Phytotherapy essentials: healthy children optimising children's health with herbs. Warwick: Phytotherapy Press; 2008.

United Nations. Conventions on the rights of the child. General Assembly resolution 44/25 of 20 November 1989. Geneva, Switzerland: Online. Available: http://www.unicef.org/crc.1989. [Accessed 1 November 2013].

Acknowledgments: The author would like to acknowledge Vicki Mortimer and Jon Wardle who co-authored this chapter in the previous edition and therefore contributed to the final version in this edition.

REFERENCES

1. International Conference on Harmonisation. Clinical investigation of medicinal products in the paediatric population E11. Online. Available: http://emea.europa.eu/htms/human/ich/ichefficacy.htm. [Accessed 1 November 2013].

2. United Nations. Conventions on the rights of the child. General Assembly resolution 44/25 of 20 November 1989. Geneva, Switzerland. Online. Available: www.unicef.org/crc. [Accessed 1 November 2013].

3. Surette S, Vohra S. Complementary, holistic, and integrative medicine: utilization surveys of the pediatric literature. Pediatr Rev 2014;35(3):114–27.

4. Kodish E, Weise K. Ethics in pediatric care. In: Kliegman RM, Behrman RE, Jenson HB, et al, editors. Nelson textbook of pediatrics. 19th ed. Philadelphia: Sanders; 2011.

5. Tillisch K. Complementary and alternative medicine for functional gastrointestinal disorders. Gut 2006;55:593–6.

6. Ethics Advisory Committee. Royal College of Paediatrics and Child Health: guidelines for the ethical conduct of medical research involving children. Arch Dis 2002;Ch82(2):177–82.

7. Beers MH, et al. Merck manual of diagnosis and therapy. Whitehouse Station: Merck Research Laboratories; 2006.

8. Suggs D. Pharmacokinetics in children: history, considerations, and applications. J Am Acad Nurse Pract 2000;12(6):236–9.

9. Jones B. Pharmacokinetics in children. MSD manual, professional version. Kenilworth: Merck Sharp & Dohme Corp; 2019. Available: https://www.msdmanuals.com/en-au/professional/pediatrics/principles-of-drug-treatment-in-children/pharmacokinetics-in-children#v1085281.

10. Winkler P, Ghadimi D, Schrezenmeir J, et al. Molecular and cellular basis of microflora-host interactions. The J Nutr 2007;137(3):756S–72S.

11. Mosby, Inc. Mosby's dictionary of medicine, nursing & health professions. Elsevier Health Sciences; 2013.

12. Dorland WA. Dorland's illustrated medical dictionary, 32nd edn. Elsevier Health Sciences; 2011.

13. Hull D, Johnston DI, editors. Essential paediatrics. 3rd ed. Edinburgh: Churchill Livingstone; 1993.

14. Zenk K. Challenges in providing pharmaceutical care for pediatric patients. Am J Hosp Pharm 1994;51:683–94.

15. Reed M. Principles of drug therapy. In: Nelson WE, Behrman RE, et al, editors. Textbook of pediatrics. 15th ed. Philadelphia: Sanders; 2011.

16. Thomas DW, Greer FR. Probiotics and prebiotics in pediatrics. Pediatrics 2010;126(6):1217–31.

17. Millard R, et al. Clinical efficacy and safety of tolterodine compared to placebo in detrusor overactivity. J Urol 1999;161:1551–5.

18. Braun L, Cohen M. Herbs and natural supplements, volume 2: an evidence-based guide. Elsevier Health Sciences; 2015.

19. Capra S. Nutrient reference values for Australia and New Zealand: including recommended dietary intakes. Commonwealth of Australia; 2006.

20. Buttriss JL. Eatwell Guide—the bare facts. Nutr Bull 2017;42:159–65. doi:10.1111/nbu.12265.

21. Pizzorno J, et al. The textbook of natural medicine. Philadelphia: Churchill Livingstone; 2008.

22. Green H, McGinnity Á, Meltzer H, et al. Mental health of children and young people in Great Britain. Palgrave Macmillan; 2004.

23. Mayo Health Clinic Online. Mental illness in children. Available: http://www.mayoclinic.com/health/ mental-illness-in-children/MY01915. [Accessed 18 August 2013].

24. Thomas J. Medications and breastfeeding: tips for giving accurate information to mothers. Am Acad Pediatr 2019; Available: https://www.aap.org/en-us/ advocacy-and-policy/aap-health-initiatives/Breastfeeding/ Pages/Medications-and-Breastfeeding.aspx.

25. Royal Children's Hospital Melbourne. Engaging with and assessing the adolescent patient. Clinical Practice Guidelines. Available: https://www.rch.org.au/clinicalguide/guideline_ index/Engaging_with_and_assessing_the_adolescent_ patient/.

26. Goldenring JM, Rosen D. Getting into adolescent heads: an essential update. Contemp Pediatr 2004;21:64–92.

27. Scott J, Barlow T. Herbs in the treatment of children. Missouri: Churchill Livingstone; 2003.

28. Meyer S, Gortner L, Larsen A, et al. Complementary and alternative medicine in paediatrics: a systematic overview/ synthesis of Cochran Collaboration reviews. Swiss Med Wkly 2013;143:w13794.

29. Snyder J, Brown P. Complementary and alternative medicine in children: an analysis of the recent literature. Curr Opin Pediatr 2012;24(4):539–46.

30. Bufler Ph, Gross M, Uhlig HH. Recurrent abdominal pain in childhood. Dtsch Arztebl Int 2011;108(17):295–304. doi:10.3238/arztebl.2011.0295.

31. Murtagh John E. Murtagh's general practice handbook. 4th ed. Sydney: McGraw Hill; 2007.

32. Voelker R. The world in medicine: diet and asthma. JAMA 2000;284(10):1235.

33. Laicouras C, Piccoli DA. Pediatric gastroenterology. St Louis: Mosby; 2007.

34. Sparrow J. Understanding stress in children. Pediatr Ann 2007;36(4):187–94.

35. Stanton B, Behrman R. Children cannot advocate for themselves. Nelson's textbook of pediatrics, 19th edn. Philadelphia: Sanders; 2011.

36. Garbarino J, Kosteilny K, Dubrow N. No place to be a child. San Francisco, CA: Jossey-Bass; 1991.

37. Osofsky JD. Young children and trauma: intervention and treatment. New York, NY: Guilford Press; 2004.

38. Lieberman A, Padron E, Van Horn P, et al. Angels in the nursery: the intergenerational transmission of benevolent parental influences. Infant Ment Health J 2005;26(6):504–20.

39. Anthony EJ, Cohler BJ, editors. The invulnerable child. New York, NY: Guilford Press; 1987.

40. Barnetson RSC, Rogers M. Childhood atopic eczema. BMJ 2002;324(7350):137.

41. Field T. Exercise research on children and adolescents. Complement Ther Clin Pract 2012;18(1):54–9.

42. Adams D, Cheng F, Jou H, et al. The safety of pediatric asthma: a systematic review. Pediatrics 2011;128(6):e1575–87.

43. Culbert T, Banez GA. Wetting the bed: integrative approaches to nocturnal enuresis. Explore (NY) 2008;4(3):215–20.

44. Lv ZT, Song W, Wu J, et al. Efficacy of acupuncture in children with nocturnal enuresis: a systematic review and meta-analysis of randomized controlled trials. Evidence-Based Complementary and Alternative Medicine, 2015.

45. Underdown A, Barlow J, Chung V, et al. Massage intervention for promoting mental and physical health in infants aged under 6 months. Cochrane Database Syst Rev 2006;(4):CD005038.

46. Vickers A, Ohlsson A, Lacy JB, et al. Massage for promoting growth and development of preterm and/or low birth-weight infants. Cochrane Database Syst Rev 2004;(2):CD000530.

47. Niederhauser V. Prescribing for children: issues in pediatric pharmacology. Nurse Pract 1997;22(3):16–30.

48. Hunt K, Ernst E. The evidence-base for complementary medicine in children: a critical overview of systematic reviews. Arch Dis Child 2011;96(8):769–76.

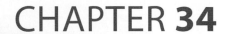

CHAPTER **34**

Fertility, preconception care and pregnancy

Amie Steel
ND, MPH, PhD

Karen Martin
ND, MDEd

OVERVIEW—PRECONCEPTION CARE

There is solid scientific evidence that infant health is inextricably linked to the health of the women who bear them, especially regarding preconception care.[1] Preconception care takes place prior to conception and focuses on the reduction of conception-related risk factors and increasing healthy behaviours. It can be said that preconception care epitomises the naturopathic principle to address the cause, not just the symptom, of illness. By ensuring health issues are addressed in both partners prior to conception, the aim is to improve the health of the infant at birth in a way that even early prenatal care cannot.[2] Ideally, preconception care involves both partners as some risk factors affect both males and females. Furthermore, involving both partners may help promote equal involvement in the preparation for a major life transition.[3] The nature of a preconception care plan will differ between couples. For ease of understanding, preconception care can be categorised into two broad categories: health promotion and disease attenuation. Health promotion preconception care describes couples who have not yet attempted conception and have no diagnosed illnesses, but would like to ensure optimum health before their baby is conceived. Disease attenuation preconception care, in contrast, applies to couples with current diagnosed health conditions, or who have already had unsuccessful attempts to conceive. There may be some crossover between these two categories and, once disease attenuation has been addressed, it is quite common to incorporate health promotion into the plan prior to conception (Figure 34.1). However, these are general guides only and the approach to the treatment plan should always be patient-centred, with the time and level of intervention required for each category determined based on couples' needs. As such, it is important to remind couples that, although many achieve conception soon after they commence attempting, for others patience is required.

Maximising fertility

Health promotion

Underlying conditions aside, preconception care benefits couples by promoting health. Many lifestyle factors dramatically affect fertility, birth success and infant

Disease attenuation
- Address any diagnosed health condition, e.g. diabetes, thyroid condition, depression.
- Safely reduce requirement of medication contraindicated in pregnant women, e.g. isotretinoids, antiepileptic drugs.

- Promote healthy body composition.
- Smoking and alcohol cessation.

Health promotion
- Address any general health imbalances.
- Investigate exposure to chemicals and other environmental toxins.
- Investigate family history of illness and enact prevention strategies.
- Encourage balanced dietary choices.
- Investigate intimate partner and sexual violence.

Figure 34.1
Approaches to preconception care

The World Health Organisation defines preconception care

Preconception care is the provision of biomedical, behavioural and social health interventions to women and couples before conception occurs, aimed at improving their health status, and reducing behaviours and individual and environmental factors that could contribute to poor maternal and child health outcomes. Its ultimate aim is improved maternal and child health outcomes, in both the long and short term.

At least three overlapping terms are used within this area of health care:

1. preconception care—provision of preventive, promotive or curative health and social interventions before conception occurs
2. periconception care—provision of these interventions in the period extending from three months before to three months after conception occurs
3. interconception care—provision of these interventions between two pregnancies.

Source: WHO 2012[4]

---

health.[5] Preconception care must address these factors in order to promote fertility, conception and healthy pregnancy outcome and if continued for at least two years this approach has been found to be highly successful for couples previously classified as infertile.[6]

Diet and nutritional status

Dietary change is an important intervention in any preconception plan and, although the focus is on a general healthy diet for couples, some specific dietary choices have been found to have direct benefits for fertility. Encouraging healthier eating habits more broadly improves fertility outcomes (see Appendix 4, 'Food sources of nutrients'). A range of dietary constituents have been linked with various aspects of subfertility including iron,[7,8] antioxidants,[9,10] selenium[11] and zinc.[12] Replacing animal protein with vegetable protein has been found to be beneficial in women seeking to get pregnant, particularly for those at increased risk of ovulatory infertility.[13] In contrast, a diet containing a large amount of dietary carbohydrates (particularly those with a high glycaemic load),[14] low-fat dairy products[15] and *trans*-unsaturated fats[15] have been associated with increased ovulatory infertility.

Developmental Onset of Health and Disease

The Developmental Onset of Health and Disease (DOHaD) hypothesis suggests that the offspring health status at birth contributes to the risk of non-communicable diseases (e.g. hypertension, insulin resistance) in adulthood. The hypothesis purports that intrauterine stresses such as nutrient deficiency during critical stages of development, effect changes in the genetic programming of the developing embryo and result in a variation in the offspring's phenotype. These *epigenetic* changes reflect modifications to the activation of the genetic code, rather than modification of the code itself. For example, otherwise dormant genes may be switched on or alternatively active genes may be switched off, thereby altering the offspring's metabolic processes and the risk of developing metabolic disease. A pictoral summary of the DOHaD hypothesis is seen in Figure 34.2.

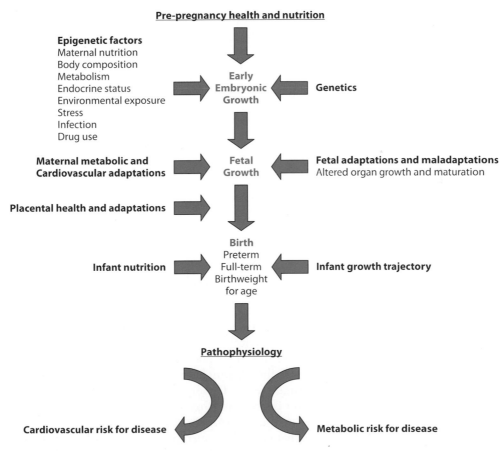

Figure 34.2
Fetal precursors to adult cardiovascular disease
Source: Adapted from Cota & Allen 2010[16]

Body composition

Overweight and obese women are less likely to conceive than those of normal weight.[17] These women also experience increased risk of pregnancy complications and adverse pregnancy outcomes in comparison with women who weigh less. Conversely, women who are very underweight may also experience problems conceiving.[17] Reproductive function can be affected by both obesity and low body weight due to hormone imbalances and ovulatory dysfunction.[18] Overall the relative risk of ovulatory infertility is increased for body mass index (BMI) below 20.0 kg/m^2 or above 24.0 kg/m^2.[19] There appears to be a 7% increase in the rate of fetal anomaly for each unit of BMI above 25.[18,20] Obesity affects fertility in ways that are complex and not well understood; however, the association with functional hyperandrogenism and hyperinsulinaemia is thought to play an important role.[21] Abdominal obesity in women with polycystic ovarian syndrome (PCOS) is considered to be co-responsible for the development of hyperandrogenism and chronic anovulation through mechanisms involving decreased concentrations of sex-hormone-binding globulin in the blood and insulin-mediated overstimulation of ovarian steroidogenesis.[21] Obesity may also contribute to reduced outcomes of in vitro fertilisation (IVF) or intracytoplasmic sperm injection (ICSI) procedures by promoting resistance to clomiphene and gonadotrophin-induced ovulation.[21] It has been demonstrated that weight loss in obese women can improve fertility through the recovery of spontaneous ovulation, and that others will have improved responses to ovarian stimulation in infertility treatment.[22]

Attenuating the hormonal imbalances resulting from high body fat can be achieved through both diet and exercise (as discussed in Chapter 23 on PCOS). Infertile overweight women commencing dietary and exercise intervention may experience favourable menstrual and metabolic outcomes conducive to conception in as little as 12 weeks.[23] In fact, lifestyle modification has proved more effective than fertility drugs in inducing ovulation in women with anovulatory disorders.[24] However, it is important to note that weight loss needs to be approached responsibly, as rapid weight loss is understood to lower progesterone levels, slow follicular growth and inhibit the luteinising hormone (LH) surge, disallowing ovulation.[25]

Lifestyle activity

Maintaining an active lifestyle is beneficial in promoting both male and female fertility; however, moderation is very important. While moderate exercise may improve the chances of conceiving spontaneously or through fertility treatment,[5,19] excessive physical exercise is associated with a spectrum of reproductive dysfunctions in both males and females. Female fertility issues associated with excessive exercise range from luteal phase defects to anovulation to infertility and finally to amenorrhoea.[19] Increase in vigorous activity (but not moderate activity) is associated with reduced relative risk of ovulatory infertility,[19] and has been linked to poor IVF outcomes.[26] This concern has also been found to affect male fertility, through subclinical changes in reproductive hormone profile and semen parameters.[27] For example, male endurance runners have been found to have a reduction in total and free testosterone, alterations in LH release and in pituitary responses to gonadotrophin-releasing hormone.[27] Furthermore, there has been evidence of a change in the semen parameters of some endurance athletes, such as low normal sperm count, decreased motility and various morphological changes.[27]

This apparent contradiction between the benefits and risks of exercise can be best explained by the role of exercise in preventing and managing conditions that detrimentally effect fertility, such as PCOS and obesity.[18] In contrast, any level of activity that induces metabolic stress will interfere with the hypothalamus–pituitary–gonadal (HPG) axis, and therefore affect fertility.[28] Overall, the focus when supporting couples prior to conception should be on moderate exercise that does not place undue stress on their systems.

Cigarette smoking

The practice of cigarette smoking adversely affects fertility in both males and females.[29–32] Smoking affects sperm production, motility, morphology and incidence of DNA damage in males.[5] This may be explained by increased reactive oxygen species, which has been linked with lowered sperm concentration, motility and morphology.[33] Cigarette smoking in females may affect the follicular microenvironment, and may cause alteration of hormone levels in the follicular phase.[5] Both active and passive smoking have been demonstrated to increase zona pellucida thickness, which may make it more difficult for sperm to penetrate.[34] In active smokers, the effect of delayed conception is increased with the number of cigarettes smoked.[35]

Caffeine

Higher levels of caffeine intake may also adversely affect fertility outcomes.[17] Some research has found that coffee and/or tea intake greater than six cups a day is associated with reduced fertility.[30] However, other researchers assert that coffee and tea consumption associated with reduced fertility rates in males and females is not dose related, and that constituents other than caffeine may also have an effect.[29]

Other drug use, such as recreational drugs and alcohol, may also contribute to certain subtypes of infertility.[17]

Window of fertility

Once baseline health issues have been addressed, the next priority when approaching preconception care and couples with fertility issues is to establish the window of fertility. The window of fertility is probably best defined as the period in the six days leading up to ovulation, when in theory the oocytes and sperm should have maximum viability and survivability.[36,37] However, in an individual clinical setting this can be more accurately garnered through analysis of intermenstrual intervals, cervical mucus and basal body temperature charts (see Chapter 23 on PCOS). Intercourse is most likely to result in pregnancy when it occurs within the three days prior to ovulation.

Although certainly not a prerequisite for pregnancy to occur, the probability of conception is highest when cervical mucus (vaginal secretions) is slippery and clear (Figure 34.3).[38–40] When combined with basal body temperature charts these simple and cheap analyses are able to predict peak fertility far better than menstrual charts alone. Cervical mucus analysis alone has been demonstrated to better predict peak fertility than either basal body temperature charts or biochemical ovulation detection kits based on LH.[41]

Monitoring cervical mucus may have other practical benefits as water-based vaginal lubricants can inhibit sperm motility by 60–100% in vitro.[43] Mineral oil, canola oil or hydroxyethylcellulose-based lubricants do not seem to have this effect.

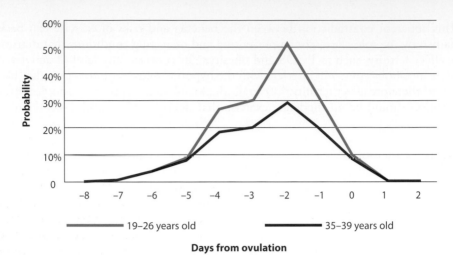

Figure 34.3
Probability of pregnancy by cycle day, involving recurrent intercourse, by age[42]

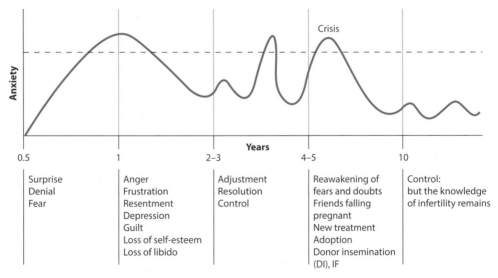

Figure 34.4
Emotional responses to infertility

Sources: Murtagh 2007[45] and Craig 1990[46]

Stress

The emotional journey of a subfertile couple is complex. Seemingly innocuous events such as friends falling pregnant, family events and birthdays may trigger underlying anxiety issues (Figure 34.4). Psychological stress is an added risk factor for reduced fertility in both females[20] and males.[44] Depression in males has been correlated with decrease in sperm concentration and poor coping mechanisms by male partners have been associated with increased occurrence of early miscarriage.[44]

The process of undergoing infertility treatment itself can also be stressful and exacerbate anxiety, depression and stress, often enough to negatively affect pregnancy outcomes.[47,48] This may be due to increased cortisol secretion, resulting from a normal stress response, down-regulating the HPG axis. It has been postulated that this may occur by inhibiting gonadotrophin-releasing hormone's (GnRH) release of follicle-stimulating hormone (FSH) and LH from the pituitary.[49]

Counselling or **psychological support**, particularly interventions that focus on stress management and coping-skills training, should be strongly recommended throughout this process,[50] particularly if time to conception becomes prolonged. It is equally as important for the infertile couple to build a support network. Both attending support sessions and using cognitive behavioural interventions are equally effective in reducing the emotional aspects of infertility and improving the chances of pregnancy.[51] Music therapy has also been associated with positive pregnancy outcomes.[52] Overall, couples should be encouraged to take part in stress reduction activities at all stages of preconception and pregnancy. Anecdotal stories of previously infertile couples conceiving after ceasing trying or while on holiday are not to be ignored.[53]

Environmental concerns

Exposure to herbicides, fungicides, pesticides and other chlorinated hydrocarbons has been associated with decreased fertility and a higher risk of spontaneous miscarriage.[54,55] Although more than 140 000 chemicals are in common use in today's society, evaluation of the effects on reproduction of common physical and chemical agents has occurred in only 5% of substances.[56] A substantial proportion of pregnant women have detectable levels of chemicals such as heavy metals (e.g. mercury, lead, cadmium), volatile organic compounds, perfluorinated compounds, polychlorinated biphenyls (PCBs), organo-chlorine pesticides, organophosphate insecticides, environmental phenols, phthalates and polycyclic aromatic hydrocarbons.[57] Not only are these linked with subfertility and miscarriage but exposure to these environmental toxins during pregnancy can increase the risk of a child developing attention deficit hyperactivity disorder (ADHD) and autism spectrum disorders.[57,58]

With this in mind, it is important to investigate potential exposure to environmental chemicals such as pesticides, herbicides, household chemicals, plastics and paint and paint thinners. Choosing organic whole food alongside avoidance of other environmental sources of toxins may be beneficial. Paradoxically many couples will subject themselves to high levels of environmental toxins during 'nesting' activities while trying to conceive or during pregnancy. While preparation for the child is certainly important, activities that include exposure to dust, paint or other chemicals and substances that release toxins, such as home renovations, may adversely affect pregnancy outcomes and should be considered carefully.

If exposure is identified, and particularly if it is occupational (e.g. factory workers, tradespeople, farmers and horticulturalists), then protective measures must be taken. Such measures include appropriate occupation health and safety interventions like wearing protective clothing and masks.[59] Beyond this, the preconception treatment plan needs to incorporate suitable detoxification protocols (see the box on liver detoxification in Chapter 22 on endometriosis).

Nutritional medicines

The primary conventional focus of nutrient supplementation in preconception care is on the role of **folic acid** in preventing neural tube defect.[60] The benefits attributed to folic acid in the prevention of this condition require maternal sufficiency in the first

28 days of gestation, before many women know they are pregnant.[60] It is this knowledge that has led to public health interventions such as folate fortification of bread flour and further supplementation of 400 µg/day for women of reproductive age.[60]

Folic acid is not the only nutrient required in preconception and the early stages of gestation. A recent longitudinal study[61] observed the effect of pregnancy on the micro-nutrient status of the mothers. It was noted that, while folate levels decreased slightly during pregnancy and remained decreased up to six weeks after delivery, **vitamin B12** progressively declined throughout gestation and reached marginal or deficient levels.[61] This is of particular concern, as vitamin B12 status has been associated with a threefold risk of neural tube defect.[62] This deviates from the previous approach to neural tube defect prevention, which has been firmly focused on folic acid supplementation and fortification of food. In fact, the focus on folic acid fortification of food, such as bread flour, may be contributing to a masking of vitamin B12 deficiency and an increased risk of neural tube defect[63] (see the box on vitamin B12 and folate). There is a growing body of evidence linking folate and other B-vitamin deficiencies and hyper-homocysteinaemia to altered spermatogenesis and impaired ovarian reserve.[64]

Various multivitamin and antioxidant nutritional supplements have improved pregnancy rates in those undergoing assisted reproduction[65] or lowered time to conception in couples seeking preconception care.[65,66] Preconception multivitamin use has also been associated with a higher incidence of multiple births for unknown reasons.[67] Folate needs to be taken at least three months prior to conception for optimal benefit in reducing neural tube defects or leukaemia development in the fetus. However, it is also associated with decreased incidence of ovulatory infertility more generally.[68] **Vitamin C** supplementation has also had improved fertility outcomes in women with luteal phase defects.[69] There is recent evidence that **vitamin D** also plays a role in modulating reproductive processes in both men and women.[70] In males vitamin D is positively associated with sperm motility and morphology, and with androgen levels.[70] In females with PCOS hypovitaminosis D may be involved in the pathogenesis of insulin resistance and metabolic syndrome.[70]

Vitamin B12 or folic acid?

Folic acid has been used for a number of years to prevent neural tube defect[60]; however, recent research has identified that vitamin B12 is also important in preventing this condition.[62] With this in mind, the most predictable course of action may be to incorporate vitamin B12 supplementation into standard preconception care approaches alongside folic acid. Unfortunately, just as some concerns regarding the risks of folic acid supplementation masking vitamin B12 deficiency have been raised,[63] excess vitamin B12 intake, resulting in potential cobalt toxicity,[71] may also be a concern. To avoid this, and to stay true to the naturopathic patient-centred approach, assessing the most appropriate nutrients required for supplementation and the relevant dosages are vital. Folic acid is found predominantly in legumes and green leafy vegetables, while vitamin B12 is found in its most bioavailable form in animal products.[72] As such, an assessment of a patient's diet will provide an initial indication as to whether supplementation of folic acid and/or vitamin B12 is required. In general, though, it is important to remember that the absorption of vitamin B12 is an incredibly complex process that relies on healthy gastric, pancreatic and intestinal function, and that dysfunction in any one of these organs can compromise B12 status.[72] A more thorough assessment of sufficiency of these nutrients can be gleaned through testing. The most accurate test to determine folic acid status is red blood cell folate, not the commonly used serum folate, which does not correlate with tissue stores.[73] Vitamin B12 status can be assessed using serum cobalamin, which is more specific and stable compared with serum folate; however, both pregnancy and folate deficiency can result in false low readings. A more accurate assessment, which is independent of both of these conditions, is that of methylmalonic acid. Unfortunately, this test is much more expensive and technically demanding.[74]

Herbal hormonal regulation

In general, due to the individual nature of preconception care, herbal treatment interventions used will vary significantly between couples. Common herbal medicines that may be useful when supporting couples during preconception care include ***Vitex agnus-castus*** and ***Tribulus terrestris***. *Vitex agnus-castus* is used traditionally in fertility disorders, particularly for women with progesterone deficiency or luteal phase defects. No large studies have explored this role, although preliminary data suggests women with secondary amenorrhoea and luteal insufficiency who use *Vitex agnus-castus* are twice as likely to achieve pregnancy.[75] *Tribulus terrestris* has also been associated with improving conception outcomes in women with endocrine sterility.[76]

The male partner

In 20% of infertile couples males are the sole cause of infertility and are an important contributing factor in a further 20–40% of infertile couples.[77] Although many infertile men may have physical or structural conditions that require surgical intervention, many may have reversible issues that can be corrected with non-invasive measures. Men also experience declining fertility as they age.[78]

A decline in male fertility has been reported over the past few decades in a number of countries, though this has been controversial.[79] It has been suggested that environmental and lifestyle factors such as increased occupational chemical and pesticide exposure are at least partly responsible for this decline.[80–82] Oestrogen-like products are thought to be partly responsible. The fact that organic farmers have higher sperm counts than regular farmers or other exposed occupational groups lends further credence to this theory.[83] Other environmental and lifestyle factors that may be affecting fertility include wearing tight-fitting clothing, using hot baths and spas and having occupations that require long periods of sitting down, as these behaviours all increase scrotal temperature.[84] Diet must also be considered as it may affect semen quality. Men consuming diets high in meat and dairy products[85] and soy protein[86] have compromised semen parameters, whereas diets high in fruits and vegetables show benefit.[85] The advantage in a fruit- and vegetable-rich diet may be attributed to an increased antioxidant intake.[87]

Beyond diet and lifestyle, some specific nutrients have been identified to improve fertility in men. For example, there is evidence that **coenzyme Q10** supplementation can improve semen parameters in men,[88,89] while **vitamin C**, **vitamin E**, **beta carotene**, **folate** and **zinc** are important for semen quality.[90] A similar trial that identified increased pregnancy rates in couples with severe male infertility when taking an antioxidant supplement containing ascorbic acid, zinc, vitamin E, folate, lycopene, garlic oil and selenium has been conducted.[91] In contrast, selenium has been demonstrated to improve sperm quality and motility in subfertile men but not those diagnosed with infertility,[92] or conversely with normal testicular selenium levels.[93] Similarly, **L-carnitine** has been associated with increased semen quality and sperm concentration, particularly in groups with lower baseline levels,[94] though one trial suggested that this may be true only in those with normal mitochondrial function.[95] ***Withania somnifera*** has been demonstrated to improve sperm count, sperm concentration, motility and hormonal profiles in normozoospermic, oligospermic and asthenozoospermic men compared pre- and post-treatment.[96]

INFERTILITY AND SUBFERTILITY

Impaired fertility affects approximately one in six couples.[97] In young, healthy couples, the probability of conception in one reproductive cycle is typically 20–25%, and in one year it is approximately 90%; however, this success rate can decline rapidly due to various age-related or health factors.[97]

Reproductive specialists use strict definitions of infertility.[90] Clinical infertility in a couple is defined as the inability to become pregnant after 12 months of unprotected intercourse. However, consensus is building that the diagnosis of clinical infertility should also be considered after six cycles of unprotected sex in women older than 35 years of age.[97] Clinical infertility may also be considered when the female is incapable of carrying a pregnancy to full term. At this time further investigation becomes warranted to establish whether there are physical conditions hindering conception and, if so, what intervention may be appropriate. Infertility is not necessarily analogous to subfertility, which is often caused by other underlying conditions such as endometriosis or PCOS.[98]

Causes of infertility and subfertility

Infertility can be considered to be primary or secondary. Couples with primary infertility have never been able to conceive, while secondary infertility is defined as difficulty conceiving after already having conceived (and either carried the pregnancy to term or had a miscarriage).[90]

Secondary infertility is not considered as a diagnosis if there has been a change of partners.[90]

Infertility may also be more broadly grouped into categories of sterility or relative infertility. Sterility can arise from various predominantly non-treatable underlying disorders involving:

- lack of oocytes (menopause, radiation damage or some autoimmune diseases)
- lack of sperm (infectious causes or immature sperm)
- fallopian tube obstruction (endometriosis, surgical or due to infection such as chlamydia), or
- hysterectomy.

In contrast, infertility may be caused by other factors (Table 34.1).

Table 34.1
Common causes of infertility in males and females

Male	Female
Low sperm count	Non-specific immune factors
Low percentage of progressively motile sperm	Irregular ovulation (e.g. PCOS)
Disorders of sperm morphology	Steroid–hormone imbalance (may be influenced by insulin, thyroid function, stress, adiposity or exposure to hormone-disrupting compounds)
High degree of abnormality on sperm	Hostile endometrial environment (may be influenced by hormonal imbalance, structural abnormalities, fibroids, infection or immunological factors)
Chromosome fragmentation	Genetic variations (e.g. MTHFR polymorphism)

Source: Adapted from Speroff and Fritz 2005[5]

RISK FACTORS

Like many conditions, factors that increase the risk of infertility can be both inherited and due to lifestyle. Lifestyle factors that contribute to infertility include common concerns such as cigarette smoking and alcohol misuse but also extend to the use of certain prescription medications.

Both maternal and paternal age have a bearing on the fertility level of a couple. Older women experience more difficulty achieving and maintaining pregnancy,[97] and are less likely to deliver a healthy infant than younger women.[99] In females spontaneous cumulative pregnancy rates begin to decline as early as 31–35 years of age.[97] One-third of women aged 35–39 years will experience difficulty achieving pregnancy, and half of women aged 40–44 years will have an impaired ability to reproduce.[97] Increasing maternal age results in a decreased number of oocytes, decreased oocyte quality, uterine age-related changes affecting endometrial receptivity and neuroendocrine system ageing.[97]

Another general risk factor to consider when approaching preconception care is the presence of underlying disease. Women with a chronic disease such as diabetes have an increased risk of congenital abnormalities in their offspring but are known to have improved birth outcomes when they plan their pregnancies and use preconception care.[100] Coeliac disease is another condition that is known to incur higher miscarriage rates, increased fetal growth restriction and lower birthweights.[101] Although not a disease, obesity may also affect fertility for both males[102] and females.[22] Sexually transmitted infections, particularly chlamydia and gonorrhoea, may lead to infertility.[17] Infection of any nature may be associated with reduced sperm motility.[103] Other conditions may affect fertility but, rather than the disease being detrimental, it is the medication used to manage the condition that is problematic. Several different types of medications, including hormones, antibiotics, antidepressants, pain-relieving agents and aspirin and ibuprofen, when taken in the middle of the cycle, have been reported to affect female fertility.[90] With this in mind, it is important to address any underlying health issues, resolving them where possible, to reduce reliance on medication. Alternatively, where the condition cannot be resolved, exploration of substitute medication may be necessary.

KEY TREATMENT PROTOCOLS

A key treatment approach when supporting couples with fertility issues (aside from treating any underlying pathology) is to optimise the general health of both partners. It is vital that the approach to the development of a treatment plan for such couples is patient-centred, and does not make assumptions about their individual needs without diligent exploration of their health history and current health complaints.

Address underlying pathology

Examination of the health requirements of couples with infertility or subfertility must extend beyond reproductive health, as a number of conditions not directly linked to the reproductive system, such as inflammatory bowel disease,[104] thyroid disease[105] and type 1 diabetes,[106] have been associated with infertility. Other conditions more directly associated with the reproduc-tive system that may need to be addressed include endo-metriosis[107] and PCOS.[108]

> **Naturopathic Treatment Aims**
>
> - Address lifestyle-related risk factors:
>   - smoking
>   - caffeine intake
>   - BMI
>   - stress
>   - diet.
> - Ensure sufficiency of key nutrients.
> - Address confounding and high-risk conditions:
>   - PCOS
>   - endometriosis
>   - hormone imbalances
>   - thyroid imbalances
>   - semen parameters.

Relationship issues

Preconception can be an exciting time for a couple, but it can also be challenging. Sometimes in the lead-up to starting a family relationship issues that may not have been apparent previously can surface. The process of becoming pregnant can consume time and substantial resources—emotional, physical and financial. If fertility problems become apparent and assisted fertility in the way of procedures such as IVF is required, this can further add to feelings such as loss of control, distance between the couple and feelings of guilt or blame. All of these issues can be a significant source of stress in the relationship. It is important that a couple remember that the reason they want to bring a baby into the world is that they are two people in love. Nurturing the relationship by continuing to do things as a couple is very important. Small suggestions like a candlelit dinner occasionally or a walk along the beach together should be as much a part of the preconception prescription as any naturopathic medications.

Let's talk about sex

Trying to conceive is a stressful time for any couple and this stress can creep into the bedroom. Some couples may have forgotten to have intercourse as often as required or have turned it into a chore. Others may have been trying for so long that they even forget to have intercourse at all—except for once a month according to the calendar. This places further stress on the couple and may be ultimately counterproductive. Couples should maintain intimacy and engage in sexual activity as they desire, not purely based on ovulatory cycles. A well-timed weekend away or regular date night may improve both the relationship and the chances of a couple falling pregnant.

Immune system

Immune system imbalances may adversely affect fertility outcomes through a number of ways, including high generalised inflammation and antibodies targeted to key tissues. High levels of inflammatory prostaglandins, for example, may reduce uterine receptivity to fertilised embryos,[110] possibly by affecting the regulation of genes necessary for human endometrial receptivity.[109] Chronic inflammation may also contribute to the development of anatomical abnormalities such as pelvic adhesions and occluded fallopian tubes, as well as premature ovarian failure.[109] Causes of inflammation in reproductive tissues vary and may include sexually transmitted infections such as *Chlamydia trachomatis*, endometriosis and autoimmune conditions.[109] Autoimmune conditions that can contribute to infertility may be non-specific, such as type 1 diabetes mellitus and Hashimoto's thyroiditis, or specific, such as antibodies that target FSH and LH and their receptors[111,112] and antibodies that target ovaries and sperm.[109] It is worth noting, however, that the inflammatory response is also an important mechanism within healthy, normal reproductive function (see the box on inflammation and healthy reproduction). With this in mind, various measures to reduce inflammation systemically and specifically can be found in other relevant chapters.

Inflammation and healthy reproduction

Inflammation is often approached as an undesirable adversary in the human body. In fact, inflammation is a mechanism necessary for the normal and healthy reproductive process. As the LH surge occurs prior to ovulation, LH stimulates granulosa cells to secrete inflammatory mediators (prostaglandins and cytokines) and progesterone. These compounds all trigger the secretion of matrix metalloproteinases, which break down the extracellular matrix, thereby allowing for follicular rupture and ovulation.[109] As such, indiscriminate use of anti-inflammatory interventions in preconception care should be avoided.

CONVENTIONAL TREATMENT

Conventional preconception care focuses on attenuating the impact of chronic diseases, infectious diseases, reproductive issues, genetic/inherited conditions, medications and medical treatment, and personal behaviours or exposures on the health of mother and future baby.[2] A number of these issues have established clinical practice guidelines. Folic acid supplementation is considered essential to reduce the incidence of neural tube defects in the fetus, and supplementation ideally begins three months prior to conception.[2] Prevention of congenital defects due to rubella infection is also recommended through rubella vaccination, and a similar approach is taken to hepatitis B due to the potential for vertical transmission to infants and resulting organ damage.[2] Management of chronic diseases such as diabetes and hypothyroidism is also considered important in pregnancy to reduce the effects on the developing fetus. Likewise, conditions managed with isotretinoids and anti-epileptic medication need to be approached with lower dosages or alternative medication as these drugs are teratogens and as such can cause birth defects.[2]

If a couple have been attempting to conceive for at least 12 months, then initial assessment of hormone levels, ovulation, weight/body composition and semen analysis is undertaken. In the longer term, gynaecological examination to check for physical factors interfering with conception (e.g. scarring from a previous sexually transmitted infection or endometriosis) is conducted.

Once the diagnosis of infertility has been made, the conventional treatment approach varies depending on the diagnosed reason for the infertility. If the diagnosis is male infertility, then the treatment will depend on the seminal analysis. If azoospermia (absence of sperm) is diagnosed, then conception relies upon donor insemination.[113] However, if there is severe oligospermia (fewer than five million sperm), then a single spermatozoon is recovered from the epididymis and microinjected in the ovum. This has a 30% success rate.[113] There have been some attempts to increase the sperm count of men with oligospermia using hormonal therapy (testosterone analogues and antioestrogens), with limited documented benefit.[108] Another alternative in this situation is IVF.[113]

Alternatively, infertility may be due to female reproductive pathophysiology. Anovulation is managed by encouraging the woman to aim for an appropriate body composition and use of an antioestrogen drug (clomifene), which has resulted in a 70% conception rate in amenorrhoeic women.[113] If tubal damage has been diagnosed, there are really only two options available: microsurgery to attempt to repair the fallopian tubes or IVF. With a diagnosis of cervical hostility, the traditional conventional approach is to encourage the couple to use condoms for six months in the hope that the antibodies attacking the sperm will be eliminated. Other, more invasive approaches include ingestion of oral corticoids by the male in the first 10 days of the woman's cycle, the use of washed sperm or IVF or gamete intrafallopian transfer techniques.[113]

Assisted reproductive technologies

Assisted reproductive technologies (ART) encompass a spectrum of methods and are valid options for infertile couples (Table 34.2). However, the usefulness of these therapies needs to be considered by any prospective couple in the context of the costs and risks. In 2005 a systematic review of studies measuring the prevalence of birth defects in infants conceived using ART found a 30–40% increased risk.[114] However, later studies that compared malformation risk for ART with subfertile couples conceiving naturally found no statistical difference with IVF,[115,116] although the increased risk with ICSI

Table 34.2
Types of assisted reproductive technologies

Type	Procedure	Pregnancy rate*
Assisted insemination with husband's sperm (AIH)	Sperm are transferred by catheter into uterus or fallopian tube	Up to 15% per cycle
IVF	Fertilised eggs are transferred in to the uterus or fallopian tube	10–25% per cycle; depends on maternal age
Gamete intrafallopian transfer (GIFT)	Unfertilised eggs and sperm are transferred into one or both fallopian tubes using laparoscopy or transvaginal ultrasound	Up to 30–40% per cycle
ICSI	Sperm is injected into the egg	More than 50% per cycle
Zygote intrafallopian transfer (ZIFT), tubal embryo stage transfer (TEST)	Zygote or early embryo is transferred into the fallopian tube using laparoscopy or transvaginal ultrasound the day after egg pick-up	Up to 30–40% per cycle

*Note that pregnancy rate is not the same as live birth rate. Naturopathic treatment of couples undergoing assisted reproductive techniques should not cease once these interventions have resulted in a successful pregnancy.
Adapted from Oats & Abraham 2005[7]

remained.[115] Furthermore, the average cost of IVF for Australian women is $32 903,[117] while the success rate is 10% for a single IVF procedure, and increases to 40% if the procedure is repeated five times.[113] Finally, the process of IVF requires constant emotional adjustment through each phase of the process,[118] and can be debilitating for the woman in particular. To support this, a questionnaire study[119] found that financial burden (23%), psychological stress (36%) and lack of success (23%) were the most predominant reasons couples discontinued IVF programs. In particular, a combination of lack of success and psychological stress was noted in 18% of participants.

Often this course of action is used as a symptomatic approach to infertility and does not have the added benefit of preparing the body for a healthy pregnancy or allowing for improved success of subsequent births. In one study 65% of couples who had previously undergone multiple IVF cycles were able to conceive within two years of a preconception program.[6] However, there will be instances where referral to this procedure will be appropriate.

Most patients attending assisted reproduction will be using some form of complementary therapy and are likely to be consulting a complementary therapist; they are perhaps using several options concurrently.[120] Therefore it may be prudent to identify the broad scope of treatment the patient is undertaking so as to reduce the risk of negative interactions. Non-ingestive therapies are better options during IVF cycles due to lower risk of negative interactions, and acupuncture performed on the day of IVF embryo transfer is demonstrated to have a beneficial effect on pregnancy rates and live births.[121]

OVERVIEW—PREGNANCY

Pregnancy is one area that lends itself to naturopathic treatment for a number of reasons. Although it is not a disease state (though it has certainly been managed and thought of as one in the past) it is a significant life transition that encompasses the mind, body and spirituality of the mother. It is also a time when the power of nature and the abilities of the body are apparent and there is a greater recognition of the immediate need and benefit of optimal health. Pregnancy care is also a time in which the accepted aim of treatments is to be as minimally invasive as possible. Therefore the aim of the naturopath is to avoid unnecessary treatment of any kind and instead support optimal health for the mother and child.

The management of the pregnant woman should be in conjunction with a qualified specialist practitioner—a midwife and/or obstetrician. Midwifery and naturopathy have traditionally had a supportive relationship due to their shared belief that pregnancy and birth are normal physiological processes that can be supported through adequate nutrition, psychological and physical support when required and avoidance of harmful substances.

Decision-making when supporting a pregnant woman requires careful thought. The potential for any therapy to do harm needs to be considered. This includes not only instances of possible direct harm to the fetus or mother (e.g. the use of potentially teratogenic herbs—see Safety in pregnancy later this chapter) but also the possibility of indirect harm. Indirect harm includes such things as potentially delaying a useful therapy (e.g. in the progression of pre-eclampsia to toxaemia) or financially exploiting the patient through the use of unnecessary or ineffective therapies. It can be easy to overcomplicate treatment in the pregnant woman, and a simple approach is often best.

Dietary requirements

Dietary requirements in pregnancy encompass nutrients that must be included and foods that should be avoided. Additional energy is needed in pregnancy and lactation to cover the needs of the growing fetus, the placenta and expanding maternal tissues, and additional maternal effort at rest and in physical activity, as well as the production of breast milk during lactation. Nothing additional over pre-pregnancy requirements is needed in the first trimester, though in the second trimester an extra 1.4 MJ/day and in the third trimester an extra 1.9 MJ/day over pre-pregnancy levels should be consumed.[123] **Protein** requirements also increase to 1.1 g/kg of body weight, as does the recommended daily intake of a number of nutrients including **folic acid**, **vitamin C**, **iron**, **zinc** and **calcium** (Table 34.3). Maternal vitamin D deficiency has been associated with increased risk for diabetes mellitus, pre-eclampsia and small-for-gestational-age birth.[70]

A number of dietary practices should be avoided or limited.[125] Higher levels of alcohol consumption during pregnancy are linked to a spectrum of disorders in the infant ranging from fetal alcohol syndrome through to alcohol-related birth defects or alcohol-related neurodevelopmental disorders.[125] While data is not conclusive, there is potentially no safe level of alcohol intake during pregnancy (see the box on ethanol-based herbal extracts and pregnancy). Fish consumption must also be approached with care in pregnancy due to the risks associated with fetal exposure to methylmercury. In general, this compound accumulates from industrial pollution (although it also occurs naturally) in some of the larger, longer lived fish, and those that consume other fish.[125] Examples include shark, swordfish, king mackerel and tuna.[125] In contrast, sardines and white fish have lower mercury levels and as much as 360 g can be safely consumed per week.[125] Another risk is food contamination with *Listeria monocytogenes* (listeriosis), which can cause spontaneous abortion, stillbirth and fetal infection.[125] To prevent this illness, pregnant women should avoid unpasteurised milk, undercooked or raw animal products, refrigerated smoked food, pâtés or meat spreads, soft cheeses and unwashed fruit

Table 34.3
Key nutrients in pregnancy*

Nutrient	Effect	Comment
DHA	Accumulates in the developing brain, and is important for prenatal and postnatal neurological development	Can be easily converted via desaturases from α-linolenic acid
Vitamin A	Important for the regulation of gene expression and for cell differentiation and proliferation	Direct studies of vitamin A status are lacking, but excess retinol is a known teratogen The threshold risk is still unclear, but the upper intake level is 3000 µg/day
Folate	Required for normal cell division, and methylation during nucleotide synthesis Associated with prevention of neural tube defect	Supplementation still needs to be approached judiciously as the upper limit is only 1000 µg/day and some women already have folate-rich diets
Vitamin B12	Supports methylation of nucleotides in conjunction with folate; also essential for neurological function Absorption decreases during pregnancy	Although vitamin B12 can be stored in adults long term, only newly absorbed vitamin B12 is readily transported across the placenta Vegan women will need to supplement
Biotin	Animal studies imply that deficiency is teratogenic	More evidence relating specifically to pregnant women is required to make confident clinical decisions
Calcium	Required for bones, teeth, vascular contraction, vasodilation, muscle contraction, nerve transmission and glandular secretion	Most fetal accretion occurs in the third trimester, and this is lower when maternal intake is low
Chromium	Potentates the action of insulin	Chromium is depleted throughout pregnancy and fetal tissue levels decline after birth, suggesting the need for deposition during pregnancy
Iodine	Required for thyroid hormones, and therefore associated with myelination of the central nervous system and general metabolism Most active in perinatal periods	Deficiency is damaging to the developing brain and includes mental retardation, hypothyroidism and goitre
Iron	Required for haem proteins and other iron-dependent enzymes	Deficiency in pregnancy is associated with increased perinatal maternal and infant mortality, premature delivery and low birthweight
Zinc	A cofactor to nearly 100 enzymes, with catalytic, structural and regulatory functions	Maternal zinc deficiency may lead to prolonged labour, intrauterine growth retardation, teratogenesis and embryonic or fetal death Lower dietary intakes can lead to a higher incidence of premature deliveries

Adapted from Turner 2006[124]
*Only key nutrients detailed (not an exhaustive list)

and vegetables.[125] Caffeine consumption must also be approached with caution during pregnancy, as it has been connected with fetal growth restriction and low-birthweight infants.[126] One of the concerns surrounding caffeine is that the enzyme responsible for caffeine clearance, CYP1A2, is not present in fetal tissue, although caffeine can easily pass through the fetoplacental barrier.[126] For this reason, it is important that if the pregnant woman is going to consume caffeine their own phase 1 detoxification pathway is functioning at its optimum. This should be addressed in preconception treatment, however, not during pregnancy. It has been recommended that women should not consume more than 200 mg/day of caffeine throughout gestation.[126]

Ethanol-based herbal extracts and pregnancy

It is recommended that all pregnant women minimise their alcohol consumption and abstain if possible.[126] But where does that leave the prescription of ethanol-based herbal extracts? If possible, other forms of herbal products should be prescribed to pregnant women to keep alcohol consumption to a minimum. This can include preformulated tablets, infusions, decoctions or glycetracts. However, the value in an individualised and extemporaneously dispensed formula of ethanol-based herbal extracts is well known to most practising naturopaths. If it is deemed that the best treatment for the individual is in the form of an ethanol-based herbal extract (with low-volatile oils), then a useful approach is the addition of hot water to the tincture prior to each dose. This encourages evaporation of the alcohol and, although it will only reduce the alcohol content modestly, it is a reduction nonetheless.

Ideally, people who smoke cigarettes will cease as part of their preconception health planning. If this has not occurred it is important to cease as soon as they are aware of conception. Maternal smoking during pregnancy has been linked to increased risk of wheezing in infants up to two years old[127] and reduced fetal brain development,[128] and may increase the infant's risk of adult development of diabetes, hypertension and metabolic syndrome.[31] Despite these statistics, more than 10% of pregnant women continue to smoke cigarettes.[99] Similarly, high alcohol consumption during pregnancy puts the developing fetus at risk of fetal alcohol syndrome.[129] Even lower level intake can potentially affect the neuroendocrine and behavioural functions of the offspring.[130]

Appropriate weight gain

There should be relatively little maternal weight gain until the second and third trimesters, with the bulk of the weight gain in the third trimester (Figure 34.5). Increased weight gain may lead to an increased risk of gestational diabetes, which has significant health implications for both mother and child.[90] High blood sugar levels are used as an energy source by the growing baby and will therefore lead to increased birthweight. Although there are several negative health consequences for the baby associated with high birthweight and gestational diabetes, one of the main concerns is the potential labour complications associated with giving birth to a larger baby. Patients should be made aware of these potentially alarming practical complications in addition to the negative health aspects.

Another potential cause of inappropriate weight gain is oedema, which may be linked to pre-eclampsia. Pre-eclampsia is a form of hypertension that occurs only in pregnancy, and is accompanied by proteinuria and excessive oedema.[126] Although obesity does increase the risk of developing pre-eclampsia,[126] it should not be assumed

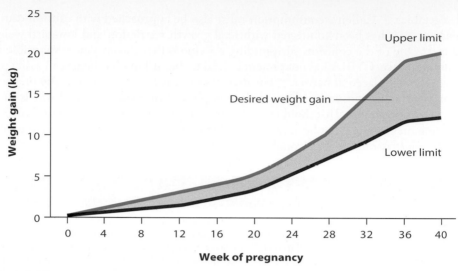

Figure 34.5
Appropriate weight gain in pregnancy

that weight gain is simply fat gain. Thorough dietary and physical assessment are needed to determine if fluid retention is an issue, or whether a high glycaemic, hypercaloric diet is the concern.

Anaemia

Maternal iron requirements increase in pregnancy because of the demands of the developing fetus, the formation of the placenta and the increasing maternal red cell mass.[123] Fetal iron requirements seem to come at the expense of maternal stores if there is insufficient intake. Even moderate iron deficiency is associated with a twofold risk of maternal death.[123] However, routine iron supplementation in women with normal haemoglobin is not associated with improved pregnancy outcomes. Furthermore, supplementation with high levels of iron increases the risk of oxidative stress, and should be approached with caution. With this in mind, one study[131] found that taking an iron supplement (60 mg **iron**, 200 μg **folic acid** and 1 μg **B12**) daily was no more beneficial than taking two tablets once per week. This may be an approach to reduce the risk of oxidative damage and still ensure iron sufficiency.

Safety in pregnancy

As the aim of pregnancy care is generally to move towards optimal health rather than treatment of particular disease states, herbal medicines and large doses of specific nutrients should generally be avoided during pregnancy (Table 34.4). Even seemingly innocuous herbal medicines with hormonal activity or uterine activity are best avoided during pregnancy. Although uterine tonics may have a role to play in preparation for labour, even they need to be avoided at early stages of pregnancy.

There is still a high use of many different herbal and nutritional medicines by pregnant women, and nearly three-quarters of these women do not discuss this use with their conventional doctor.[136,137] This may be due to the fact that specialist obstetricians generally have less favourable attitudes towards complementary medicines than women's non-obstetric doctors.[138]

Table 34.4
Herbs contraindicated during pregnancy*

Abrus precatorius	*Daphne mezereum*	*Podophyllum resin*
Achillea millefolium	*Datura* spp.	*Pteridium aquilinum*
Aconitum spp.	*Digitalis* spp.	***Pulsatilla vulgaris***
Acorus calamus	*Dryopteris filix-mas*	*Rauwolfia* spp.
Adhatoda vasica	*Duboisia* spp.	*Rhamnus frangula*
Adonis vernalis	*Echium vulgare*	*Ricinus communis*
Aloe vera	*Ephedra* spp.	*Robinia pseudoacacia*
Ammi visnaga	*Erysimum* spp.	***Salvia officinalis***
Angelica archangelica	*Euonymus europaeus*	*Sarpthamnus scoparius*
Angelica sinensis	*Galega officinais*	*Schoenocaulon officinale*
Apocynum spp.	*Galanthus* spp.	***Schisandra chinensis***
Aristolochia spp.	*Gelsemium* spp.	*Scopolia carniolica*
Arnica spp.	*Heliotropium* spp.	*Semecarpus anacardium*
***Artemisia* spp.**	*Helleborus* spp.	*Senecio* spp.
Arum maculatum	*Juglans cinerea*	*Solanum* spp.
Belladonna spp.	*Juniperus* spp.	*Sophora secundiflora*
Brugmansia spp.	*Hyoscyamus* spp.	*Spigelia marilandica*
Brunfelsia uniflora	*Lantana camara*	*Staphysagria* spp.
Calendula officinalis	*Larrea* spp.	*Strophanthus* spp.
Calotropis spp.	*Lathyrus sativus*	*Strychnos* spp.
Carbenia benedicta	*Lithospermum* spp.	*Symphytum* spp.
Caulophyllum thalictroides	*Lobelia* spp.	*Tamus communis* fruit and root
Catha edulis	*Mandragora* spp.	***Tanacetum* spp.**
Chenopodium ambrosioides	*Menispermum canadense*	*Teucrium* spp.
Cicuta virosa	*Mentha pulegium*	*Thevetia* spp.
Actaea racemosa	*Oleander* spp.	***Thuja occidentalis***
Cinchona spp.	*Opuntia cylindrica*	*Toxicodendron radicans*
Colchicum spp.	***Panax quinqefolium***	***Tribulus terrestris***
Convallaria spp.	***Panax notoginseng***	***Turnera diffusa***
Coronilla spp.	*Papaver somniferum*	*Tussilago farfara*
Corydalis ambigua	*Peganum harmala*	***Viscum album***
Crotalaria spp.	*Petasites* spp.	*Virola sebifera*
Croton spp.	*Peumus boldus*	*Yohimbine* spp.
Cynoglossum officinale	***Phytolacca* spp.**	

*Bold indicates common herbs more likely to be encountered regularly in clinical practice
Sources: Ensiyeh & Sakineh 2009,[132] Jewell & Young 2003,[133] Wergeland & Strand 1998[134] and Wolf et al. 2001[135]

To assist naturopaths to determine the safety of herbal medicines, a classification system[130] based on Therapeutic Goods Administration (Australia) and Food and Drug Administration (USA) categories for prescription medicines in pregnancy has been developed. Contraindicated herbs fit into categories D and X in this system (Table 34.5). However, it is recommended that most herbal medicines be avoided during pregnancy unless absolutely necessary.

Chronic miscarriage

Conservative estimates suggest that 10% of first trimester pregnancies end in spontaneous abortion or miscarriage.[90] ***Viburnum prunifolium*** was traditionally used by the eclectic physicians of North America to prevent miscarriage,[140] and was embraced by obstetricians in the late 1800s for the same purpose.[141–144] ***Dioscorea villosa*** and

Table 34.5
Examples of herbs classified for use in pregnancy

Category	Category definition	Relevant herbs
Category A	Drugs that have been taken by a large number of pregnant women and women of childbearing age without any proven increase in the frequency of malformations or other direct or indirect harmful effects on the fetus having been observed	*Rubus idaeus* *Zingiber officinale* *Echinacea* spp. *Matricaria recutita* *Panax ginseng* *Vaccinium myrtillus* *Curcuma longa*
Category B1	Drugs that have been taken by only a limited number of pregnant women and women of childbearing age, without an increase in the frequency of malformation or other direct or indirect harmful effects on the human fetus having been observed Studies in animals have not shown evidence of an increased occurrence of fetal damage	*Astragalus membranaceus* *Valeriana officinalis* *Ginkgo biloba* *Hypericum perforatum* *Bupleurum falcatum*
Category B2	Drugs that have been taken by only a limited number of pregnant women and women of childbearing age, without an increase in the frequency of malformation or other direct or indirect harmful effects on the human fetus having been observed Studies in animals are inadequate or may be lacking, but available data show no evidence of an increased occurrence of fetal damage	*Barosma betulina*
Category B3	Drugs that have been taken by only a limited number of pregnant women and women of childbearing age, without an increase in the frequency of malformation or other direct or indirect harmful effects on the human fetus having been observed Studies in animals have shown evidence of an increased occurrence of fetal damage, the significance of which is considered uncertain in humans	*Andrographis paniculata*
Category C	Drugs that, owing to their pharmacological effects, have caused or may be suspected of causing harmful effects on the human fetus or neonate without causing malformations; these effects may be reversible Accompanying texts should be consulted for further details	*Arctostaphylos uva-ursi* *Hydrastis canadensis* *Glycyrrhiza glabra* *Aesculus hippocastanum* *Salvia miltiorrhiza*
Category D	Drugs that have caused, are suspected to have caused or may be expected to cause an increased incidence of human fetal malformations or irreversible damage; these drugs may also have adverse pharmacological effects Accompanying texts should be consulted for further details	*Ruta graveolens* *Adhatoda* spp. *Tabebuia avellanedae* *Phytolacca* spp.
Category X	Drugs that have such a high risk of causing permanent damage to the fetus that they should not be used in pregnancy or when there is a possibility of pregnancy	*Aristolochia* spp. *Senecia* spp. *Peumus boldus*

Source: Mill & Bone 2005[139]

Chamaelirium luteum have also been traditionally used in threatened miscarriage.[145] Unfortunately, more recent research into the efficacy of these herbs has not been conducted; furthermore, concerns over the accurate identification of the herb used in earlier interventions have been raised.[146]

Other underlying factors may need to be considered and treated in cases of recurrent or threatened miscarriage. For example, an increased risk of miscarriage in both naturally conceived pregnancies and following fertility treatment has been associated with extremes of BMI,[147] and interventions that have addressed elevated BMI have been found to reduce the incidence of miscarriage in high-risk women.[148]

Nausea and vomiting

Up to 80% of all pregnant women experience some nausea and vomiting,[149] commonly referred to as 'morning sickness'. It has been noted, however, that one of the possible causes of nausea and vomiting in early pregnancy is elevated prostaglandin E_2 (PgE_2), stimulated by human chorionic gonadotrophin.[150] Due to the important functions PgE_2 performs in early stages of pregnancy, treatment of morning sickness in the first trimester needs to be tempered with respect for the natural process of gestation. In line with this, treatment for pregnancy nausea and vomiting should begin with the most minimal intervention.

Low blood sugar can play a role in pregnancy nausea, and simple interventions that address this such as a cup of tea and a biscuit before rising in the morning or nibbling on a small amount of carbohydrate-based food at regular intervals during the day can offer some relief.

The most common naturopathic treatment for nausea and vomiting in pregnancy is ***Zingiber officinale***. *Zingiber officinale* has been demonstrated to be an effective treatment for nausea and vomiting in early pregnancy.[151] Ginger tea and candied ginger are suitable therapeutic sources in pregnant patients. *Zingiber officinale* is also effective for postoperative nausea associated with childbirth.[152] Additional research has demonstrated **vitamin B6** to be an effective treatment for the nausea and vomiting of pregnancy.[132] The optimum dose for this is thought to be between 30 and 75 mg daily.[133]

Pre-eclampsia

Obesity and stress are both associated with increased risk of pre-eclampsia.[134,135] Exercise can help reduce the incidence of pre-eclampsia.[153] Insufficient protein, magnesium, calcium, iron, pyridoxine (B6), vitamin C, vitamin E, essential fatty acids and folic acid have all been directly indicated in the pathogenesis of pre-eclampsia.[154] Rather than focusing on one particular nutrient, consensus is moving towards nutritional education more generally as a preventive measure but these trends are contrasted with growing evidence of a profound relationship between specific nutrients such as calcium in the development of pre-eclampsia.[155]

Urinary tract infections

Women experience urinary tract infections (UTIs) more frequently during pregnancy. It is important to note that acute UTIs in pregnancy are a serious condition. Pregnant women are at increased risk of pyelonephritis, which is linked to low birthweight and preterm labour. ***Vaccinium macrocarpon***, which has a documented safety profile in pregnancy,[156,157] or the use of probiotics, either orally or as direct recolonisation of vaginal mucosal tissue,[158] offer effective prophylactic treatment options. However, all UTIs in pregnant women should be referred promptly for medical assessment.

Another potentially beneficial treatment option is the use of probiotics. The most direct route to increase the *Lactobacillus* spp. colony in vaginal mucosal tissue is through insertion of encapsulated probiotics, and should result in improved populations within three days.[158] If oral administration is preferred then 10×10^9 colony forming units are recommended, and will require 28–60 days to normalise vaginal colonies[158] (see Chapter 30 on recurrent UTIs).

Partus preparators

Rubus idaeus has long been traditionally used as a 'partus preparator'—preparing the uterus for delivery and to facilitate labour.[159] Animal studies have suggested that *Rubus idaeus* may modulate the frequency of uterine contractions.[160] Such an effect has not yet been identified in human research primarily due to limited research alongside poor-quality data and flawed research design from the few studies that have been conducted.[151]

Caulophyllum thalictroides is also a herb that has been traditionally used as a partus prepartor; however, recent low-level evidence has highlighted safety concerns with the use of this herb by pregnant and birthing women.[161] Case study reports of women using *Caulophyllum thalictroides* indicate a greater incidence of fetal complications such as cerebrovascular damage to the infant alongside other markers of fetal distress such as meconium-stained fluid and transient fetal tachycardia. Adverse effects such as nausea have also been reported for the mother. While in vitro research does confirm oxytocic effects of *Caulophyllum thalictroides*, teratogenicity and embryotoxicity have also been identified.[161] Overall, despite traditional evidence of its use, the current body of evidence indicates *Caulophyllum thalictroides* should not be used by pregnant and birthing women.

Childbirth

Childbirth is a culmination of between 37 and 42 weeks' gestation, and providing support to women at this important moment in time can prevent unnecessary interventions at later stages. Education and empowerment of women to trust their body and the birth process are paramount before labour begins.[162] This can be achieved successfully through group psychoeducation and support work to release fear surrounding the birth process.[163] It is also important that the woman feels supported by sensitive and nurturing birth companions at the time of birth.[161] Birth companions such as midwives[164–166] and doulas[167–170] have been associated with improved birth outcomes for women seeking low-intervention births.

Reducing interventions associated with birth not only benefits the birth experience of the woman if she desires a low-intervention birth but may also benefit the health of the infant. For example, an induced labour frequently results in a cascade of interventions such as the use of intravenous lines, enforced bed rest, continuous electronic fetal heart monitoring, amniotomy, increased pain and discomfort, epidural analgesia, operative (caesarean) delivery and prolonged hospital stay.[171] Postbirth health risks associated with induction and the potentially resulting caesarean delivery include maternal depression and neonatal respiratory illness,[172] as well as longer term risks to the infant of atopic diseases such as allergic rhinitis,[173] eczema and asthma[174] (see Chapter 28 on inflammatory skin disorders). Interventions such as induction and operative delivery may still be indicated in high-risk circumstances, but the importance lies not so much in avoiding the intervention as ensuring women are educated and empowered to feel in control of their birth process.[175]

Outside of the medical model, there are some low-intervention therapies that may benefit child birth. For example, **acupressure** has been used effectively to reduce pain or delivery time in labour.[176] A case report has also been published promoting the use of **homeopathic** *Caulophyllum* in conjunction with **nipple stimulation** to induce and augment labour,[177] and a small randomised-controlled trial (RCT) found that a combination of homeopathic *Arnica* and *Bellis perennis* resulted in an apparent reduction in postpartum blood loss.[178] Even less invasive models such as **muscle relaxation techniques**[179] and **lower back massage**[180] have been associated with reduced labour pain.

POSTNATAL SUPPORT

Lactation

The mammary glands develop during pregnancy, but the levels of progesterone and oestrogen secreted by the placenta prevent lactation occurring until 30–40 hours after birth.[181] Healthy and adequate lactation provides extensive health benefits to infants both at birth and later in life, and promoting efficient suckling and successful breastfeeding begins with timely skin-to-skin contact between mother and infant (father to child skin-to-skin contact is also recommended).[182] Furthermore, promotion of good health practices through preconception and pregnancy education reduces the risk of breastfeeding complications.[182] In contrast, delayed contact between mother and infant, washing the mother or infant prior to contact or the use of a pacifier ('dummy') before six weeks of age have all been shown to interfere with effective and successful breastfeeding.[182]

A number of **herbs** have been used traditionally to encourage lactation: *Trigonella foenum-graecum*, *Galega officinalis*, *Foeniculum vulgare*, *Pimpinella anisum*, *Cnicus benedictus*, *Silybum marianum*, *Asparagus racemosus* and *Urtica dioica*.[145,183] Of these, Trigonella *foenum-graecum* and *Silybum marianum* have been identified through preliminary clinical research to support improved breast milk supply for lactating women and *Asparagus racemosus*'s traditional Ayurvedic use as a galactagogue has also been confirmed in a clinical trial.[184]

Formula feeding

There is an undeniable weight of evidence that 'breast is best', although in some instances breastfeeding may not be an option. Formula supplementation may also be required in a nutritionally compromised mother.

Soy proteins have been used as an alternative protein source for infants with allergies or food intolerances, although there is little evidence to support their use. A Cochrane review of five studies found only one study comparing soy to cow's milk formula noted a reduction in childhood allergy, asthma and allergic rhinitis.[185] The other four studies that fit the inclusion criteria reported no significant benefit for any allergy or food intolerance. Many infants allergic to cow's milk may also be allergic to soy milk,[186] suggesting a deeper underlying immunological issue. Furthermore, intestinal permeability is higher in infants fed formula than those fed breast milk[187]; this may contribute to the risk of the development of atopic disease (see Chapter 28 on inflammatory skin disorders). In these circumstances, **colostrum** supplementation in the initial feeding of formula-fed infants may offer some protection.[188]

No formula will ever be able to replicate the comprehensive and complex nutritional profile of human breast milk. In addition, any nutritional deficiencies will be compounded by exclusive use of one formula. Therefore several specific formulas should be rotated regularly to ensure that the effects of possible deficiencies are minimised.

Postnatal depression

Some women develop a severe depression after childbirth. Sleep deprivation and general tiredness may worsen these symptoms.[189,190] Recent research has also acknowledged that in 50% of couples, if women are depressed, their partners are depressed also.[191] Unfortunately, current family health systems do not effectively balance the postnatal support to both members of the parenting team.[191] If either partner is experiencing fatigue, promoting adequate sleep is important and may simply require sleeping when the baby sleeps. If there is difficulty sleeping during these odd hours, sleeping aids may be considered (see Chapter 16 on insomnia). **Omega-3 essential fatty acids** are also indicated in general postnatal depression (see Chapter 15 on depression). Other underlying issues, particularly those associated with the development of menstrual disorders, should be investigated, as women with a history of postnatal depression are more likely to develop menstrual difficulties and perimenstrual symptoms when menstruation recommences.[192]

INTEGRATIVE MEDICAL CONSIDERATIONS

Traditional Chinese medicine

Acupuncture on the day of embryo transfer is demonstrated to have a beneficial effect on live births.[121] Acupuncture has been demonstrated to be a safe and effective treatment tool for pelvic and back pain associated with pregnancy.[193] Similarly, acupressure, a less invasive therapy similar to acupuncture, has been associated with reduced pain and shorter delivery time in labour.[176] Moxibustion is a method used in traditional Chinese medicine as a method for cephalic version of breech babies, which has also been associated with promising outcomes in clinical trials.[193]

Antenatal classes

Antenatal classes can provide appropriate supervision and advice on antenatal exercises, back care, labour pain relief, relaxation skills and posture. Women who attend antenatal classes have a much lower risk of caesarean section and are half as likely to bottle feed in hospital, as well as being more satisfied with the experience of childbirth.[194] Furthermore, group psychoeducation classes, which focus on releasing the fear surrounding the birth process, can improve a woman's pain tolerance and coping mechanisms in childbirth.[163] Similarly, fathers attending antenatal classes felt they were more prepared for the birth and for their role as a support person.[195]

Homeopathy

Individualised homeopathic treatment in subfertile men has been found through preliminary research to improve semen parameters (sperm count and motility in addition to general health parameters) equal to conventional treatment.[196] ***Caulophyllum thalictroides*** is a commonly used homeopathic remedy for third trimester cervical ripening and induction of labour. A Cochrane review[197] evaluating this remedy identified two trials involving 133 women, but the results of the review were inconclusive due to a lack of information about the methodology used in the studies. Although a lower level of evidence, a case report has also been published promoting the use of this remedy.[177]

Aromatherapy

A pilot randomised-controlled feasibility study that took an individualised approach to the prescription of aromatherapy oils in childbirth found that the intervention group rated a lower pain perception, and a higher proportion of the control group had their infants transferred to the neonatal intensive care unit.[198]

CLINICAL SUMMARY

Working with couples during this important time in their lives can be incredibly meaningful and rewarding. Providing preconception care to women and their partners not only increases the likelihood that the woman will have a healthy pregnancy and birth but that these benefits will also provide a strong foundation for lasting health for the infant into adulthood.

The journey to conception for couples having difficulty can be quite tumultuous and unpredictable. It is important to have a plan in mind and encourage couples to allow sufficient time for good foundations to be laid before conceiving. However, this also needs to be tempered with the often-present impatience expressed by couples who have 'tried everything' prior to their first naturopathic consultation. Furthermore, naturopaths also need to be flexible with their treatment plan and be prepared to cancel intended treatment protocols and compromise certain stages in preconception care if this does not fit in with the timeline of the couple, or alternatively if the couple unexpectedly fall pregnant outside of the intended plan. Either way, it is important that the naturopath value and appreciate the powerful role counselling and dietary and lifestyle changes can have on conception and pregnancy outcomes, rather than placing all of their focus on supplements and other such interventions.

Pregnancy and birth are normal physiological processes and the role of any health practitioner is to keep women's bodies following the best trajectory towards a healthy gestation and an easier birth. At times this requires substantial application of treatments and interventions while at others the most important function of the practitioner is to stand back and simply remind the woman of her innate capacity to grow and birth her baby.

Note: Due to the complexity of preconception care, pregnancy and childbirth (including multiple persons, treatment stages and approaches), no decision tree is provided in this chapter.

Table 34.6
Review of the major evidence

Intervention	Mechanisms of action	Key literature	Summary of results	Comment
Fertility and preconception care				
Multivitamins	Maternal nutrition has the most impact on placental and fetal growth during the periods of preimplantation and immediate postimplantation prior to pregnancy confirmation Teratogenesis of fetal organs are also most likely to occur in this early pregnancy period; for this reason, ensuring adequate maternal nutriture prior to conception is important[199]	Review: Zerfu & Ayele 2013[200] Cziezel et al. 2011[201] Cohort studies: Chavarro et al. 2008[68] Cziezel et al. 2006[202] Cziezel & Vargha 2004[67]	Increased prevalence of twin births (OR = 1.14 –2.0) Inverse dose-dependent association with ovulatory infertility (OR = 0.59–0.88) No effect on risk of multiple congenital abnormalities in following pregnancy Minor reductions in the incidence of neural tube defects in following pregnancy	The most significant barrier to a conclusive understanding of the effects of multivitamins in fertility and preconception care is the lack of consistency in formulas used Due to this, meta-analysis is not possible and current insights rely on cohort study data
Antioxidants	While small amounts of reactive oxygen species (ROS) are important to the capacitation of spermatozoa, excess amounts can be detrimental Lipid peroxidation can affect membrane fluidity, which is needed for sperm motility and fusion with oocytes ROS can also cause DNA damage, resulting in mutation and polymorphism, or apoptosis Antioxidants may help to prevent these effects by acting as free radical scavengers[203]	Systematic review/ meta-analysis: Showell et al. 2011[204] Youseff et al. 2015[205]	Male partner supplementation: Increased pregnancy rate (OR = 4.18) Increased live birth rate (OR = 4.85) No side effects reported Maternal supplementation: No difference in number of mature oocytes or pregnancy success rate in women with unexplained infertility	The studies included in this review compared any type or dose of antioxidant (single or combined) compared with either placebo, no treatment or another antioxidant These broad inclusion criteria may result in a lack of clarity around the effectiveness of discrete antioxidant supplements as some may be potentially more valuable than others

Table 34.6
Review of the major evidence (continued)

Intervention	Mechanisms of action	Key literature	Summary of results	Comment
N-acetylcysteine (NAC)	The exact mechanism by which NAC impacts on the effectiveness of ART is not clear NAC is, however, known to be the rate-limiting substrate for glutathione, which is an important endogenous antioxidant[72,206] As such, NAC may be acting as a free radical scavenger and thereby preventing DNA damage and the associated oocyte apoptosis NAC also has insulin-sensitising and androgen-reducing effects, which may be beneficial for anovulatory women with PCOS who are undergoing ART[207]	Systematic review/ meta-analysis: Thakker et al. 2015[208] RCT: Badawy et al. 2006[209] Badawy et al. 2007[210] Elgindy et al. 2010[211] Rizk et al. 2005[212] Salehpour et al. 2012[207]	Adjuvant for ICSI cycles: inconclusive Adjuvant with clomiphene: higher number of follicles and thicker endometrium Higher ovulation rate, improved oestrogen and progesterone levels for women with PCOS (including those resistant to clomiphene) but not those with unexplained fertility Higher odds of having a live birth (OR = 3.00), getting pregnant (OR = 3.58) and ovulation (OR = 5.46) as compared to placebo for women with PCOS but less likely to have pregnancy (OR = 0.40) or ovulation (OR = 0.13) as compared to metformin.	There was a particular focus for this intervention on women with PCOS For this reason, anovulatory women undergoing ovulation induction who do not have PCOS may not experience the same outcomes
Vitamin E	The role of vitamin E in facilitating ART has been hypothesised to be associated with its free radical scavenging activity as an antioxidant[213] Vitamin E also has an anticoagulant effect, which may facilitate blood flow to the endometrial lining or to the ovarian follicles and in doing so support endometrial thickening[213]	RCT: Cickek et al. 2012[213] Ghanem et al. 2010[214] ElSheikh et al. 2015[215]	Adjuvant with clomiphene: increase in sperm count and motility but no change to sperm morphology or semen volume Greater pregnancy success (OR = 3.76) Adjuvant to pentoxifylline: increase in endometrial thickness but no difference in implantation rates or pregnancy success	The research in this area is preliminary and the outcomes, while positive, are only indicating clinical relevance when used with males (i.e. greater pregnancy success)
L-arginine	Arginine is a substrate for the synthesis of nitric oxide (NO)[72] NO inactivates the superoxide free radicals, which effect lipid peroxidation in the membranes of spermatozoa[216]	RCT: Battaglia et al. 1999[122] Stanislavov et al. 2009[217] Kobori et al. 2015[218]	IVF response: inconclusive Combined with Pycnogenol®: increased semen volume, sperm count, motility and morphology compared with placebo	This was a small study with methodological flaws related to randomisation While the findings do indicate a possible benefit to poor responder IVF patients, the small sample size also limits the statistical power of the interpretation

Table 34.6
Review of the major evidence (continued)

Intervention	Mechanisms of action	Key literature	Summary of results	Comment
Folic acid	Folate is an important cofactor in the methylation pathway, which is responsible for DNA methylation—a process that is programmed during early embryogenesis Effective DNA methylation is important for embryonic development including proper neural tube closure[219]	Systematic review and meta-analysis: Blencowe et al. 2010[220]	Neural tube defects: 62% reduction in primary risk for NTD and 70% reduction in recurrence through supplementation Food fortification gives 46% reduction in neural tube defect (NTD) incidence	While food fortification still appears to prevent NTDs, supplementation is much more effective This is particularly the case for women who have had previous NTD births
Folic acid and zinc	Similar to embryogenesis, DNA methylation (for which folic acid is a necessary cofactor) is required for the maintenance and repair of DNA in spermatozoa[72] Zinc is also a cofactor for both zinc fingers, which stabilise DNA during replication and the endogenous antioxidant enzyme superoxide dismutase[72]	RCT: Wong et al. 2002[221]	Subfertile men: 74% increase in sperm count	While these results seem promising it is unclear whether the use of zinc and folate manifests with greater pregnancy success or live birth rate
Withania somnifera	*Withania somnifera* is used within Ayurvedic and Unani medicine traditions for stress, impotence, infertility, antiageing effects, aphrodisiac and geriatric tonic	PCRT: Ahmad et al. 2010[96] Ambiye et al. 2013[222]	Improvement in sperm concentration, sperm count, motility and hormone profiles compared with pretreatment ($p < 0.01$)	The focus of this trial was improvement of semen quality posttreatment in categorised infertile men (normozoospermic, oligozoospermic and asthenozoospermic) While these results show promise, outcomes of pregnancy success and live birth rate have yet to be examined

Table 34.6
Review of the major evidence (continued)

Intervention	Mechanisms of action	Key literature	Summary of results	Comment
Pregnancy				
Vitamin D	Due to the diverse conditions associated with vitamin D (Vit D) in pregnancy the mechanisms of action are quite broad Vit D is important in the regulation and homeostasis of calcium and as such all functions related to calcium are affected by Vit D status This means Vit D impacts on fetal skeletal development and general growth and may reduce risk of schizophrenia and other mental disorders Vit D also upregulates innate immunity and downregulates adaptive immunity[223]	Systematic review and meta-analysis: Christesen et al. 2012[224] Thorne-Lyman & Fawzi 2012[225]	Pre-eclampsia: protective dose-dependent effect Gestational diabetes mellitus: protective dose-dependent effect Low birthweight: protective effect (RR = 0.40) Preterm delivery: no effect Small for gestational age: inconclusive	The studies included in the meta-analysis were cohort studies Due to the observational nature of these studies causality cannot be assumed Also, these studies are identifying the effects of deficiency; this does not necessarily correspond to a positive effect on any of the identified conditions through supplementation of vitamin D
Zingiber officinale	The mechanism of action of *Zingiber officinale* for nausea and vomiting in pregnancy is currently unknown but has been hypothesised to be related to anti-inflammatory and antispasmodic activity[226]	Systematic review: Matthews et al. 2010[227] Viljoen et al. 2014[228] Cohort study: Heitmann et al. 2013[229] Sharifzadeh et al. 2018[230]	Compared with placebo: improvement in symptoms by day 6–9 (RR = 0.29–0.42) Compared with vitamin B6: no significant difference Compared with dimen-hydrinate: inconclusive Dosage: Lower daily dosage of <1500 mg ginger for nausea relief Safety: No increased risk for stillbirth/perinatal death, spontaneous abortion, preterm birth, low birthweight or low Apgar scores. No significant risk for the side-effects of heartburn or drowsiness	The most conclusive studies for this treatment compare it with placebo
Vitamin B6	The mechanism of action of vitamin B6 for nausea and vomiting in pregnancy is currently unknown	Systematic review: Matthews et al. 2010[227] Sharifzadeh et al. 2018[230]	Compared with placebo: improvement in nausea after day 3 No clear effect on vomiting	The small study size and heterogeneity between the two included studies limits the clinical confidence in the effectiveness of this treatment

Table 34.6
Review of the major evidence (continued)

Intervention	Mechanisms of action	Key literature	Summary of results	Comment
Multivitamins	The vast array of nutrients found in multivitamins may address maternal nutrient insufficiencies and thereby support healthy embryonic development as well as prevent maternal complications for the pregnancy and birth[231]	Meta-analysis: Goh et al. 2007[232] Goh et al. 2006[233] Ramakrishnan et al. 2012[234]	Paediatric cancer: protective against leukaemia (OR = 0.61), paediatric brain tumours (OR = 0.73) and neuroblastoma (OR = 0.53) Congenital abnormalities: protective against neural tube defect (OR = 0.52–0.67), cardiovascular defects (OR = 0.61–0.78), limb defects (OR = 0.48–0.57), cleft palate (OR = 0.42–0.76), urinary tract anomalies (OR = 0.48–0.68) No effects for Down syndrome, pyloric stenosis, undescended testis or hypospadias Low birthweight: protective effect (RR = 0.86) Small for gestational age: protective effect (RR = 0.83) Birthweight: higher compared with controls (+52.6 g) Neonatal death: higher risk compared with iron-folate supplement if started after first trimester (RR = 1.38)	The results from this meta-analysis were drawn from seven cohort studies There is still a lack of clarity whether it is the multivitamins more broadly or a specific micronutrient that conveys the protective effects
Calcium	The underlying mechanisms for the many effects of calcium deficiency in pregnancy have only been partially explored It is proposed that calcium deficiency may contribute to pre-eclampsia by stimulating parathyroid secretion, which increases intracellular calcium and smooth muscle contractility while also releasing renin from the kidney, which leads to vasoconstriction and retention of sodium and fluid The role of calcium in infant morbidities may be related to its skeletal function, which impacts on fetal growth and development[235]	Meta-analysis: Buppasiri et al. 2011[236] Hofmeyr et al. 2010[155] Imdad et al. 2011[237] Tang et al. 2015[238]	Preterm birth: no effect Low birthweight: no effect Gestational hypertension: protective effect (RR = 0.55–0.65) Pre-eclampsia: protective effect (RR = 0.36–0.62) Neonatal mortality: protective effect (RR = 0.70) Maternal death/serious morbidity: protective effect (RR = 0.80) Childhood hypertension: protective effect (RR = 0.59)	The meta-analyses were conducted on primarily cohort studies and as such causality between calcium and the reported conditions cannot be assumed Furthermore, as there was only one study examining childhood hypertension the effect reported here cannot be considered from meta-analysis data

Table 34.6
Review of the major evidence (continued)

Intervention	Mechanisms of action	Key literature	Summary of results	Comment
Omega-3 fatty acids	The mechanisms by which omega-3 impacts on these pregnancy-related health outcomes is not well known Explanatory mechanisms related to omega-3 in general depression may be also be applicable in antenatal depression; beyond this, further research is needed	Systematic review: Cohen et al. 2005[239] Gould et al. 2013[240] Saccone & Berghella 2015[241] RCT: Freeman et al. 2008[242] Su et al. 2008[243]	Preterm birth: no effect Birthweight: higher compared with controls (+71 g) Low birthweight: no effect Gestational age at delivery: higher compared with controls (+4.5 days) Antenatal depression: inconclusive Early childhood cognitive and visual development: inconclusive	Research in this area is still developing and, particularly for conditions such as antenatal depression, warrant further investigation However, given the potential value and safety of omega-3 this should be a priority area of maternity care research
Iodine	Iodine is required for the synthesis of maternal and fetal thyroid hormones[244]	Cross-sectional study: Rebagliato et al. 2010[244] Murcia et al. 2011[245]	Thyroid function: supplementation in iodine-sufficient or mildly deficient women may cause maternal thyroid dysfunction (RR = 2.5) Psychomotor development: iodine supplementation may contribute to reduced psychomotor development in the offspring	The level of evidence for this nutrient as it relates to maternal health is quite low for developed countries
Iron	Iron is an important component in haemoglobin and as such is necessary for red blood cell synthesis[72]	Meta-analysis: Peña-Rosas et al. 2012a[246] Peña-Rosas et al. 2012b[247] Haider et al. 2013[248]	Low birthweight: protective effect (daily use: RR = 0.81) Maternal anaemia: protective effect (daily use: RR = 0.30) Iron deficiency at term: protective effect (daily use: RR = 0.43) Side effects: more common (> 60 mg/day: RR = 2.36) Results from studies using intermittent iron supplementation was inconclusive	The importance of iron in maternity care is well established; however, the diversity of forms of iron and dosages given to women requires closer attention Daily iron supplementation may be found in multivitamins and as such may limit interpretation of the outcomes

FURTHER READING

Agarwal A, Durairajanayagam D, Du Plessis SS. Utility of antioxidants during assisted reproductive techniques: an evidence based review. Reprod Biol Endocrinol 2014;12(1):112.

Gleicher N, Barad D. Unexplained infertility: does it really exist? Hum Reprod 2006;21(8):1951–5.

Kotelchuck M, Lu M. Father's role in preconception health. Matern Child Health J 2017;21:2025–39.

McKerracher L, Moffat T, Barker M, et al. Translating the Developmental Origins of Health and Disease concept to improve the nutritional environment for our next generations: a call for a reflexive, positive, multi-level approach. J Dev Orig Health Dis 2018. Online. Available: https://doi.org/10.1017/S2040174418001034.

Pairman S, editor. Midwifery: preparation for practice. Sydney: Elsevier Churchill Livingstone; 2006.

Stephenson J, Heslehurst N, Hall J, et al. Before the beginning: nutrition and lifestyle in the preconception period and its importance for future health. Lancet 2018;391(10132):1830–41.

Acknowledgments: The authors would like to acknowledge Jon Wardle who co-authored this chapter in the previous edition and therefore contributed to the final version in this edition.

REFERENCES

1. Johnson K, Posner SF, Biermann J, et al. Recommendations to improve preconception health and health care—United States. MMWR Recomm Rep 2006;55:1–23. Online. Available: http://www.cdc.gov/mmwr/preview/mmwrhtml/rr5506a1.htm. 2 Dec 2013.

2. Atrash HK, Johnson K, Adams M, et al. Preconception care for improving perinatal outcomes: the time to act. Matern Child Health J 2006;10:3–11.

3. Hohmann-Marriott B. The couple context of pregnancy and its effects on prenatal care and birth outcomes. Matern Child Health J 2009;13:745–54.

4. WHO. Meeting to develop a global consensus on preconception care to reduce maternal and childhood mortality and morbidity. Meeting report. Geneva: World Health Organisation; 2012. p. 6.

5. Anderson K, Norman RJ, Middleton P. Preconception lifestyle advice for people with subfertility. Cochrane Database Syst Rev 2010;(4):CD008189.

6. Ward N. Preconceptual care questionnaire research project. J Nutr Environ Med 1995;5:205–8.

7. Chavarro JE, Rich-Edwards JW, Rosner BA, et al. Iron intake and risk of ovulatory infertility. Obstet Gynecol 2006;108:1145–52.

8. Physicians F. Iron supplements may reduce risk for ovulatory infertility CME/CE. Obstet Gynecol 2006;108:1145–52.

9. Ruder EH, Hartman TJ, Blumberg J, et al. Oxidative stress and antioxidants: exposure and impact on female fertility. Hum Reprod Update 2008;14:345.

10. Verit FF, Erel O, Kocyigit A. Association of increased total antioxidant capacity and anovulation in nonobese infertile patients with clomiphene citrate–resistant polycystic ovary syndrome. Fertil Steril 2007;88:418–24.

11. Boitani C, Puglisi R. Selenium, a key element in spermatogenesis and male fertility. Adv Exp Med Biol 2008;636:65–73.

12. Yuyan L, Junqing W, Wei Y, et al. Are serum zinc and copper levels related to semen quality? Fertil Steril 2008;89:1008–11.

13. Chavarro JE, Rich-Edwards JW, Rosner BA, et al. Protein intake and ovulatory infertility. Am J Obstet Gynecol 2008;198:210.e1–7.

14. Chavarro JE, Rich-Edwards JW, Rosner BA, et al. A prospective study of dietary carbohydrate quantity and quality in relation to risk of ovulatory infertility. Eur J Clin Nutr 2009;63(1):78–86.

15. Chavarro JE, Rich-Edwards JW, Rosner BA, et al. Dietary fatty acid intakes and the risk of ovulatory infertility. Am J Clin Nutr 2007;85:231–7.

16. Cota BM, Allen PJ. The developmental origins of health and disease hypothesis. Pediatr Nurs 2010;36(3):157–67.

17. Silva P, et al. Impact of lifestyle choices on female infertility. J Reprod Med 1999;44:288–96.

18. Nelson SM, Fleming RF. The preconceptual contraception paradigm: obesity and infertility. Hum Reprod 2007;22:912.

19. Rich-Edwards JW, et al. Physical activity, body mass index, and ovulatory disorder infertility. Epidemiology 2002;13(2):184–90.

20. Hjolland N, et al. Distress and reduced fertility: a follow up study of first-pregnancy planners. Fertil Steril 1999;72:47–53.

21. Pasquali R, et al. Obesity and reproductive disorders in women. Hum Reprod 2003;9:359–72.

22. Zain MM, Norman RJ. Impact of obesity on female fertility and fertility treatment. Womens Health (Lond) 2008;4:183–94.

23. Miller P, et al. Effect of short-term diet and exercise on hormone levels and menses in obese, infertile women. J Reprod Med 2008;53:315–19.

24. Karmizadeh M, Javedani M. An assessment of lifestyle modification versus medical treatment with clomiphene citrate, metformin, and clomiphene citrate-metformin in patients with polycystic ovary syndrome. Fertil Steril 2009;update.

25. Wynn M, Wynn A. Slimming and fertility. Mod Midwife 1994;4:17–20.

26. Morris SN, Missmer SA, Cramer DW, et al. Effects of lifetime exercise on the outcome of in vitro fertilization. Obstet Gynecol 2006;108:938–46.

27. Arce JC, De Souza MJ. Exercise and male factor infertility. Sports Med 1993;15:146.

28. Hill JW, Elmquist JK, Elias CF. Hypothalamic pathways linking energy balance and reproduction. Am J Physiol Endocrinol Metab 2008;294:E827.

29. Curtis K, et al. Effects of cigarette smoking, caffeine consumption and alcohol intake on fecundability. Am J Epidemiol 1997;146:32–41.

30. Hassan M, Killick S. Negative lifestyle is associated with a significant reduction in fecundity. Fertil Steril 2004;81:384–92.

31. Hunt KJ, Hansis-Diarte A, Shipman K, et al. Impact of parental smoking on diabetes, hypertension and the metabolic syndrome in adult men and women in the San Antonio Heart Study. Diabetologia 2006;49:2291–8.

32. Practice Committee of American Society for Reproductive Medicine. Smoking and infertility. Fertil Steril 2008;90:S254–94.

33. Agarwal A, Sharma RK, Nallella KP, et al. Reactive oxygen species as an independent marker of male factor infertility. Fertil Steril 2006;86:878–85.

34. Shiloh H, et al. The impact of cigarette smoking on zona pellucida thickness of oocytes and embryos prior to transfer into the uterine cavity. Hum Reprod 2004;19:157–9.

35. Hull M, et al. Delayed conception and active and passive smoking. Fertil Steril 2000;74:725–33.

36. Brosens I, et al. Managing infertility with fertility-awareness methods. Sex Reprod Menopause 2006;4:13–16.

37. Wilcox A, et al. Timing of sexual intercourse in relation to ovulation-effects on the probability of conception, survival of the pregnancy, and sex of the baby. N Engl J Med 1995;333:1517–21.

38. Scarpa B, et al. Cervical mucus secretions on the day of intercourse: an accurate marker of highly fertile days. Eur J Obstet Gynecol Reprod Biol 2006;125:72–8.

39. Stanford J, et al. Timing intercourse to achieve pregnancy: current evidence. Obstet Gynecol 2002;100:1333–41.

40. Stanford J, et al. Vulvar mucus observations and the probability of pregnancy. Obstet Gynecol 2003;101.

41. Bigelow J, et al. Mucus observations in the fertile window: a better predictor of conception than timing of intercourse. Hum Reprod 2004;19:889–92.

42. Stanford J, Dunson D. Effects of sexual intercourse patterns in time to pregnancy studies. Am J Epidemiol 2007;165:1088–95.

43. Kutteh W, et al. Vaginal lubricants for the infertile couple: effect on sperm activity. Int J Fertil Menopausal Stud 1996;41:400–4.

44. Zorn B, et al. Psychological factors in male partners of infertile couples: relationship with semen quality and early miscarriage. J Andrology 2007;31:55–264.

45. Murtagh J. General practice. Sydney: McGraw-Hill; 2007.

46. Craig S. A medical model for infertility counseling. Aust Fam Physician 1990;19:491–500.

47. Burns L. Psychiatric aspects of infertility and infertility treatments. Psychiatr Clin North Am 2007;30:689–716.

48. Champagne D. Should fertilization treatment start with reducing stress? Hum Reprod 2006;21:1651–8.

49. Damti OB, Sarid O, Sheiner E, et al. Stress and distress in infertility among women. Harefuah 2008;147:256.

50. Cousineau TM, Domar AD. Psychological impact of infertility. Best Pract Res Clin Obstet Gynaecol 2007;21:293–308.

51. Domar AD, et al. Impact of group psychological interventions on pregnancy rates in infertile women. Fertil Steril 2000;73:805–11.

52. Chang M, et al. Effects of music therapy on psychological health of women during pregnancy. J Clin Nurs 2008;17:2580–7.

53. Kotz D. Success at last. Couples fighting infertility might have more control than they think. US News World Rep 2007;142:62–4.

54. Greenlee A, et al. Risk factors for female infertility in an agricultural region. Epidemiology 2003;14:429–36.

55. Hruska K, et al. Environmental factors in infertility. Clin Obstet Gynecol 2000;43:821–9.

56. Gold E, et al. Reproductive hazards. Occup Med 1994;9:363–72.

57. Sutton P, Woodruff TJ, Perron J, et al. Toxic environmental chemicals: the role of reproductive health professionals in preventing harmful exposures. Am J Obstet Gynaecol 2012;September:164–73.

58. Sagiv T, et al. Prenatal exposure to mercury and fish consumption during pregnancy and attention-deficit/hyperactivity disorder-related behavior in children. Arch Pediatr Adolesc Med 2012;166:1123–31.

59. Claman P. Men at risk: occupation and male infertility. Sex Reprod Menopause 2004;2:19–26.

60. Johnston RB Jr. Folic acid: preventive nutrition for preconception, the fetus, and the newborn. NeoReviews 2009;10:e10.

61. Cikot R, Steegers-Theunissen RPM, Thomas CMG, et al. Longitudinal vitamin and homocysteine levels in normal pregnancy. Br J Nutr 2007;85:49–58.

62. Ray JG, Wyatt PR, Thompson MD, et al. Vitamin B12 and the risk of neural tube defects in a folic-acid-fortified population. Epidemiology 2007;18:362.

63. Ray JG, Goodman J, O'Mahoney PRA, et al. High rate of maternal vitamin B12 deficiency nearly a decade after Canadian folic acid flour fortification. QJM 2008;101(6):475–7.

64. Forges T, Monnier-Barbarino P, Alberto JM, et al. Impact of folate and homocysteine metabolism on human reproductive health. Hum Reprod Update 2007;13(3):225–38.

65. Westphal LM, et al. A nutritional supplement for improving fertility in women: a pilot study. J Reprod Med 2004;49:289–93.

66. Czeizel AE, et al. The effect of preconceptional multivitamin supplementation on fertility. Int J Vitam Nutr Res 1996;66:55–8.

67. Czeizel AE, Vargha P. Periconceptional folic acid/multivitamin supplementation and twin pregnancy. Am J Obstet Gynecol 2004;191:790–4.

68. Chavarro JE, Rich-Edwards JW, Rosner BA, et al. Use of multivitamins, intake of B vitamins, and risk of ovulatory infertility. Fertil Steril 2008;89:668–76.

69. Henmi H, et al. Effects of ascorbic acid supplementation on serum progesterone levels in patients with luteal phase defect. Fertil Steril 2003;80:459–61.

70. Lerchbaum E, Obermayer-Pietsch B. Vitamin D and fertility: a systematic review. Eur J Endocrinol 2012;166:765–78.

71. Karovic O, Tonazzini I, Rebola N, et al. Toxic effects of cobalt in primary cultures of mouse astrocytes: similarities with hypoxia and role of HIF-1. Biochem Pharmacol 2007;73:694–708.

72. Kohlmeier M. Nutrient metabolism. San Diego: Academic Press; 2003.

73. Carmel R. Folic acid. In: Shils ME, Shike M, Ross AC, et al., editors. Modern nutrition in health and disease. Philadelphia: Lippincott Williams & Wilkins; 2006.

74. Carmel R. Cobalamin (Vitamin B12). In: Shils ME, Shike M, Ross AC, et al., editors. Modern nutrition in health and disease. Philadelphia: Lippincott Williams & Wilkins; 2006.

75. Gerhard I, et al. Mastodynon(R) bei weiblicher Sterilität. Forsch Komplementarmed 1998;5:272–8.

76. Tabakova P, et al. Clinical study of Tribestan® in females with endocrine sterility. Sofia: Bulgarian Pharmacology Group; 2000.

77. Thonneau P, et al. Incidence and main causes of infertility in a resident population (1,850,000) of three French regions (1988–1989). Hum Reprod 1991;6:811–16.

78. Ford W, et al. Increasing paternal age is associated with delayed conception in a large population of fertile couples: evidence for declining fecundity in older men. The ALSPAC study team (Avon Longitudinal Study of Pregnancy and Childhood). Hum Reprod 2000;15:1703–8.

79. Jorgensen N, et al. Regional differences in semen quality in Europe. Hum Reprod 2001;16:1012–19.

80. Kumar S. Occupational exposure associated with reproductive dysfunction. J Occupational Health 2004;46:1–19.

81. Oliva A, et al. Contribution of environmental factors to the risk of male infertility. Hum Reprod 2001;16:1768–76.

82. Swan S, et al. Semen quality in relation to biomarkers of pesticide exposure. Environ Health Perspect 2003;111:1478–84.

83. Abell A, et al. High sperm density among members of Organic Farmers' Association. Lancet 1994;343:1498.

84. Wang C, et al. Effect of increased scrotal temperature on sperm production in normal men. Fertil Steril 1997;68:334–9.

85. Mendiola J, et al. Food intake and its relationship with semen quality: a case-control study. Fertil Steril 2009;91:812–18.

86. Chavarro JE, et al. Soy food and isoflavone intake in relation to semen quality parameters among men from an infertility clinic. Hum Reprod 2008;23:2584–90.

87. Eskanzi B, et al. Antioxidant intake is associated with semen quality in healthy men. Hum Reprod 2005;20:1006–12.

88. Balerica G, et al. Coenzyme Q(10) supplementation in infertile men with idiopathic asthenozoospermia: an open, uncontrolled pilot study. Fertil Steril 2004;81:93–8.

89. Lewin A, Lavon H. The effect of coenzyme Q10 on sperm motility and function. Mol Aspects Med 1997;18:S213–19.

90. Speroff L, Fritz M. Clinical gynecologic endocrinology and infertility. 7th ed. Philadelphia: Lippincott Williams & Wilkins; 2005.

91. Tremellen K. Antioxidant therapy for the enhancement of male reproductive health: a critical review of the literature. Male Infertility. New York: Springer; 2012.

92. Safarinejad MR, Safarinejad S. Efficacy of selenium and/or N-Acetyl-Cysteine for improving semen parameters in infertile men: a double-blind, placebo controlled, randomized study. J Urol 2009;181:741–51.

93. Hawkes W, Alkan Z, Wong K. Selenium supplementation does not affect testicular selenium status. J Androl 2009;30:525–33.

94. Lenzi A, et al. Use of carnitine therapy in selected cases of male factor infertility: a double-blind crossover trial. Fertil Steril 2003;79:292–300.

95. Garolla A, et al. Oral carnitine supplementation increases sperm motility in asthenozoospermic men with normal sperm phospholipid hydroperoxide glutathione peroxidase levels. Fertil Steril 2005;83:355–61.

96. Ahmad MK, Mahdi AA, Shukula KK, et al. Withania somnifera improves semen quality by regulating reproductive hormone levels and oxidative stress in seminal plasma of infertile males. Fertil Steril 2010;94(3):989–96.

97. Newman P, Morrell S, Black M, et al. Reproductive and sexual health in New South Wales and Australia: differentials, trends and assessment of data sources. eds. Sydney: Family Planning; 2011.

98. Gnoth C, et al. Definition and prevalence of subfertility and infertility. Hum Reprod 2005;20:1144–7.

99. Li Z, McNally L, Hilder L, et al., editors. Australia's mothers and babies 2009. Perinatal statistics series. Sydney: AIHW National Perinatal Epidemiology and Statistics Unit; 2011.

100. Ray JG, et al. Preconception care the risk of congenital anomalies in the offspring of women with diabetes mellitus: a meta-analysis. QJM 2001;94:435–44.

101. Eliakim R, Sherer DM. Celiac disease: fertility and pregnancy. Gynecol Obstet Invest 2001;51:3–7.

102. Sallmen M, Sandler DP, Hoppin JA, et al. Reduced fertility among overweight and obese men. Epidemiology 2006;17:520–3.

103. Diemer T, et al. Urogenital infection and sperm motility. Andrologia 2003;35:283–7.

104. Mahadevan U. Fertility and pregnancy in the patient with inflammatory bowel disease. BMJ 2006;55:1198.

105. Poppe K, Velkeniers B, Glinoer D. Thyroid disease and female reproduction. Clin Endocrinol (Oxf) 2007;66:309.

106. Jonasson JM, Brismar K, Sparén P, et al. Fertility in women with type 1 diabetes. Diabetes Care 2007;30:2271.

107. Kim HO, Yang KM, Kim JY, et al. Are IVF/ICSI outcomes of women with minimal to mild endometriosis associated infertility comparable to those with unexplained infertility? Fertil Steril 2007;88:S215.

108. Franks S. Polycystic ovary syndrome. N Engl J Med 1995;333:853–61.

109. Weiss G, Goldsmith LT, Taylor RN, et al. Inflammation in reproductive disorders. Reprod Sci 2009;16:216.

110. Simon C, et al. Cytokines and embryo implantation. J Reprod Immunol 1998;39:117–31.

111. Altuntas C, et al. Autoimmune targeted disruption of the pituitary-ovarian axis causes premature ovarian failure. J Immunol 2006;177:1988–96.

112. Tuohy V, Altuntas C. Autoimmunity and premature ovarian failure. Curr Opin Obstet Gynecol 2007;19: 366–9.

113. Oats J, Abraham S. Fundamentals of obstetrics and gynaecology. Philadelphia: Elsevier Mosby; 2005.

114. Hansen M, Bower C, Milne E, et al., editors. Assisted reproductive technologies and the risk of birth defects—a systematic review. Human Reproduction. ESHRE; 2005. p. 328–38.

115. Davies M, Moore VM, Willson KJ, et al. Reproductive technologies and the risk of birth defects. N Engl J Med 2012;366:1803–13.

116. Rimm AA, Katayama AC, Katayama KP. A meta-analysis of the impact of IVF and ICSI on major malformations after adjusting for the effect of subfertility. J Assist Reprod Genet 2011;28:699–705.

117. Chambers GM, Ho MT, Sullivan EA. Assisted reproductive technology treatment costs of a live birth: an age-stratified cost-outcome study of treatment in Australia. Med J Aust 2006;184:155.

118. Verhaak CM, Smeenk JMJ, Evers AWM, et al. Women's emotional adjustment to IVF: a systematic review of 25 years of research. Hum Reprod Update 2007;13:27.

119. Rajkhowa M, McConnell A, Thomas GE. Reasons for discontinuation of IVF treatment: a questionnaire study. Hum Reprod 2006;21:358–63.

120. Stankiewicz M, Smith C, Alvino H, et al. The use of complementary medicine and therapies by patients attending a reproductive medicine unit in South Australia: a prospective survey. Aust N Z J Obstet Gynaecol 2007;47:145–9.

121. Cheong Y, et al. Acupuncture and assisted conception. Cochrane Database Syst Rev 2008;(8):CD006920.

122. Battaglia C, Salvatori M, Maxia N, et al. Adjuvant L-arginine treatment for in-vitro fertilization in poor responder patients. Hum Reprod 1999;14:1690–7.

123. Food and Nutrition Board. Dietary reference intakes for energy, carbohydrate, fiber, fat, fatty acids, cholesterol, protein and amino acids (macronutrients). eds. Washington, DC: Institute of Medicine; 2002.

124. Turner RE. Nutrition during pregnancy. In: Shils ME, Shike M, Ross AC, et al., editors. Modern nutrition in health and disease. Philadelphia: Lippincott Williams & Wilkins; 2006. p. 71–83.

125. Moore MC. Nutritional assessment and care. Mosby's pocket guide series. Missouri: Elsevier Mosby; 2005.

126. Miles L, Foxen R. New guidelines on caffeine in pregnancy. Nutr Bull 2009;34:203.

127. Lannerö E, Wickman M, Pershagen G, et al. Maternal smoking during pregnancy increases the risk of recurrent wheezing during the first years of life (BAMSE). Respir Res 2006;7:3.

128. Roza SJ, Verburg BO, Jaddoe VWV, et al. Effects of maternal smoking in pregnancy on prenatal brain development. The Generation R Study. Eur J Neurosci 2007;25:611.

129. Guerri C, Bazinet A, Riley EP. Foetal alcohol spectrum disorders and alterations in brain and behaviour. Alcohol Alcohol 2009.

130. Weinberg J, Sliwowska JH, Lan N, et al. Prenatal alcohol exposure: foetal programming, the hypothalamic-pituitary-adrenal axis and sex differences in outcome. J Neuroendocrinol 2008;20:470.

131. Casanueva E, Viteri FE, Mares-Galindo M, et al. Weekly iron as a safe alternative to daily supplementation for nonanemic pregnant women. Arch Med Res 2006;37:674–82.

132. Ensiyeh J, Sakineh M-AC. Comparing ginger and vitamin B6 for the treatment of nausea and vomiting in pregnancy: a randomised controlled trial. Midwifery 2009;25:649–53.

133. Jewell D, Young G. Interventions for nausea and vomiting in early pregnancy. Cochrane Database Syst Rev 2003;(4):CD000145.

134. Wergeland E, Strand K. Work place control and pregnancy health in a population-based sample of employed women in Norway. Scand J Work Environ Health 1998;24:206–12.

135. Wolf M, et al. Obesity and preeclampsia: the potential role of inflammation. Obstet Gynecol 2001;98:757–62.

136. Adams J, Lui C-W, Sibbritt D, et al. Women's use of complementary and alternative medicine during pregnancy: a critical review of the literature. Birth 2009;36:237–45.

137. Steel A, Adams J, Sibbritt D, et al. Utilisation of complementary and alternative medicine (CAM) practitioners within maternity care provision: results from a nationally representative cohort study of 1,835 pregnant women. BMC Pregnancy Childbirth 2012;12:146.

138. Adams J, Lui C-W, Sibbritt D, et al. Attitudes and referral practices of maternity care professionals with regard to complementary and alternative medicine: an integrative review. J Adv Nurs 2011;67:472–83.

139. Mills S, Bone K. The essential guide to herbal safety. Missouri: Churchill Livingstone; 2005.

140. Felter HW, Lloyd JU. King's American dispensary. 18th ed. Portland: Eclectic Medical Publications; 1905. reprinted 1983.

141. Campbell WMF. Note on Viburnum prunifolium in abortion. BMJ 1886;1:391.

142. Chadwick CM. Embolus of the basilar artery. BMJ 1886;1:391.

143. Napier ADL. Viburnum prunifolium in abortion. BMJ 1886;1:489.

144. Wilson JH. Viburnum prunifolium, or black haw, in abortion and miscarriage. BMJ 1886;1:640.

145. Blumenthal M. British herbal pharmacopoeia. London: BHMA Publishing; 1996.

146. Bone K. A clinical guide to blending liquid herbs. Missouri: Churchill Livingstone; 2003.

147. Veleva Z, Tiitinen A, Vilska S, et al. High and low BMI increase the risk of miscarriage after IVF/ICSI and FET. Hum Reprod 2008;23:878.

148. Barclay L. Bariatric surgery before pregnancy may improve pregnancy outcomes in obese women CME. JAMA 2008;300:2286–96.

149. Gadsby R, Barnie-Adshead AM, Jagger C. A prospective study of nausea and vomiting during pregnancy. Br J Gen Pract 1993;43:245.

150. Gadsby R, Barnie-Adshead A, Grammatoppoulos D, et al. Nausea and vomiting in pregnancy: an association between symptoms and maternal prostaglandin E2. Gynecol Obstet Invest 2000;50(3):149–52.

151. Holst L, Wright D, Haavik S, et al. Safety and efficacy of herbal remedies in obstetrics—review and clinical implications. Midwifery 2011;27:80–6.

152. Chaiyakunaprak N, et al. The efficacy of ginger for the prevention of postoperative nausea and vomiting: a meta-analysis. Am J Obstet Gynecol 2006;194:95–9.

153. Weissberger T, et al. The role of regular physical activity in preeclampsia prevention. Med Sci Sports Exerc 2003;36:2024–31.

154. Roberts J, et al. Nutrient involvement in pre-eclampsia. J Nutr 2003;133:S1684–92.

155. Hofmeyr GJ, Lawrie TA, Atallah A, et al. Calcium supplementation during pregnancy for preventing hypertensive disorders and related problems. Cochrane Database Syst Rev 2010;(8):CD001059.

156. Dugoua J-J, et al. Safety and efficacy of cranberry (vaccinium macrocarpon) during pregnancy and lactation. Can J Clin Pharmacol 2008;15:80–6.

157. Jepson R, et al. Cranberries for preventing urinary tract infections. Cochrane Database Syst Rev 2004;(1):CD001321.

158. Barrons R, Tassone D. Use of Lactobacillus probiotics for bacterial genitourinary infections in women: a review. Clin Ther 2008;30:453–68.

159. Grieves M. A modern herbal. London: Penguin; 1980.

160. Zheng J, Pistilli MJ, Holloway AC, et al. The effects of commercial preparations of red raspberry leaf on the contractility of the rat's uterus in vitro. Reprod Sci 2010;17:494–501.

161. Dugoua J-J, Perri D, Seely D, et al. Safety and efficacy of blue cohosh (Caulophyllum thalictroides) during pregnancy and lactation. Can J Clin Pharmacol 2008;15:e66–73.

162. Thorpe J, Anderson J. Supporting women in labour and birth. In: Pairman S, Pincombe J, Thorogood C, et al., editors. Midwifery: preparation for practice. Sydney: Elsevier Churchill Livingstone; 2006.

163. Saisto T, Toivanen R, Salmela-Aro K, et al. Therapeutic group psychoeducation and relaxation in treating fear of childbirth. Acta Obstet Gynecol Scand 2006;85:1315–19.

164. Janssen PA, Ryan EM, Etches DJ, et al. Outcomes of planned hospital birth attended by midwives compared with physicians in British Columbia. Obstet Gynecol Surv 2007;62:701.

165. Morano S, Cerutti F, Mistrangelo E, et al. Outcomes of the first midwife-led birth centre in Italy: 5 years' experience. Arch Gynecol Obstet 2007;276:333–7.

166. Tan WM, Klein MC, Saxell LRM, et al. How do physicians and midwives manage the third stage of labor? Birth 2008;35:220.

167. Campbell DA, Lake MF, Falk M, et al. A randomized control trial of continuous support in labor by a lay doula. J Obstet Gynecol Neonatal Nurs 2006;35:456–64.

168. Mottl-Santiago J, Walker C, Ewan J, et al. A hospital-based doula program and childbirth outcomes in an urban, multicultural setting. Matern Child Health J 2008;12:372–7.

169. Nommsen-Rivers LA, Cullum A, Hansen RL, et al. Doula care improves birth and breastfeeding outcomes for low-income, primiparous mothers. APHA Annual Meeting, 28 Oct 2008.

170. Steel A, Diezel H, Johnstone K, et al. The value of care provided by student doulas: an examination of the perceptions of women in their care. J Perinat Educ 2013;22:39–48.

171. Thorogood C, Donaldson C. Disturbances in the rhythm of labour. In: Pairman S, Pincombe J, Thorogood C, et al., editors. Midwifery: preparation for practice. Sydney: Elsevier Churchill Livingstone; 2006.

172. Liston FA, Allen VM, O'Connell CM, et al. Neonatal outcomes with caesarean delivery at term. Arch Dis Child Fetal Neonatal Ed 2008;93:F176.

173. Pistiner M, Gold DR, Abdulkerim H, et al. Birth by cesarean section, allergic rhinitis, and allergic sensitization among children with a parental history of atopy. J Allergy Clin Immunol 2008;122:274–9.

174. Thavagnanam S, Fleming J, Bromley A, et al. A meta-analysis of the association between Caesarean section and childhood asthma. Clin Exp Allergy 2008;38:629–33.

175. Beebe KR, Lee KA, Carrieri-Kohlman V, et al. The effects of childbirth self-efficacy and anxiety during pregnancy on prehospitalization labor. J Obstet Gynecol Neonatal Nurs 2007;36:410–18.

176. Smith CA, Collins CT, Crowther CA, et al. Acupuncture or acupressure for pain management in labour. Cochrane Database Syst Rev 2011;(7):CD009232, doi:10.1002/14651858.CD009232.

177. Kistin SJ, Newman AD. Induction of labor with homeopathy: a case report. J Midwifery Womens Health 2007;52:303–7.

178. Oberbaum M, Galoyan N, Lerner-Geva L, et al. The effect of the homeopathic remedies Arnica montana and Bellis perennis on mild postpartum bleeding—A randomized, double-blind, placebo-controlled study—Preliminary results. Complement Ther Med 2005;13:87–90.

179. Smith CA, Levett KM, Collins CT, et al. Relaxation techniques for pain management in labour. Cochrane Database Syst Rev 2011;(12):CD009514, doi:10.1002/14651858.CD009514.

180. Smith CA, Levett KM, Collins CT, et al. Massage, reflexology and other manual methods for pain management in labour. Cochrane Database Syst Rev 2012;(2):CD009290.

181. Baddock S, Dixon L. Physiological changes in labour and the postnatal period. In: Pairman S, Pincombe J, Thorogood C, et al., editors. Midwifery: preparation for practice. Sydney: Elsevier Churchill Livingstone; 2006.

182. Henderson A, Scobbie M. Supporting the breastfeeding mother. In: Pairman S, Pincombe J, Thorogood C, et al., editors. Midwifery: preparation for practice. Sydney: Elsevier Churchill Livingstone; 2006.

183. Abascal K, Yarnell E. Botanical galactagogues. Altern Compliment Ther 2008;14:288–94.

184. Sharma S, et al. Randomized controlled trial of Asparagus racemosus (shatavari) as a lactogogue in lactational inadequacy. Indian Pediatr 1996;33:675–7.

185. Osborn DA, Sinn JKH. Probiotics in infants for prevention of allergic disease and food hypersensitivity. Cochrane Database Syst Rev 2009;(4):CD006475.

186. Allen L. Formulas and milks for infants and young children: making sense of it all. Mod Med 1999;42:24–30.

187. Taylor S, et al. Intestinal permeability in preterm infants by feeding type: mother's milk versus formula. Breastfeeding Med 2009;4:11–15.

188. Uruakpa FO, Ismond MAH, Akobundu ENT. Colostrum and its benefits: a review. Nutr Res 2002;22:755–67.

189. Hunter L, et al. A selective review of maternal sleep characteristics in the postpartum period. J Obstet Gynecol Neonatal Nurs 2009;38:60–8.

190. Ross L, et al. Sleep and perinatal mood disorders: a critical review. J Psychiatry Neurosci 2005;30:247–56.

191. Fletcher RJ, Matthey S, Marley CG. Addressing depression and anxiety among new fathers. Med J Aust 2006;185:461.

192. Steiner M. Female-specific mood disorders. Clin Obstet Gynecol 1992;35:599–611.

193. Smith CA, Cochrane S. Does acupuncture have a place as an adjunct treatment during pregnancy? A review of randomized controlled trials and systematic reviews. Birth 2009;36:246–53.

194. Spinelli A, Baglio G, Donati S, et al. Do antenatal classes benefit the mother and her baby? J Matern Fetal Neonatal Med 2003;13:94–101.

195. Fletcher R, Silberberg S, Galloway D. New fathers' postbirth views of antenatal classes: satisfaction, benefits, and knowledge of family services. J Perinat Educ 2004;13:18–26.

196. Gerhar I, Wallis E. Individualized homeopathic therapy for male infertility. Homeopathy 2002;91:133–4.

197. Smith CA. Homoeopathy for induction of labour. Cochrane Database Syst Rev 2003;(4):CD003399.

198. Burns E, Zobbi V, Panzeri D, et al. Aromatherapy in childbirth: a pilot randomised controlled trial. BJOG 2007;114:838–44.

199. Gardiner PM, Nelson L, Shellhaas CS, et al. The clinical content of preconception care: nutrition and dietary supplements. Am J Obstet Gynecol 2008;199:S345–56.

200. Zerfu TA, Ayele HT. Micronutrients and pregnancy; effect of supplementation on pregnancy and pregnancy outcomes: a systematic review. Nutr J 2013;12(1):20.

201. Czeizel AE, Dudás I, Paput L, et al. Prevention of neural-tube defects with periconceptional folic acid, methylfolate, or multivitamins? Ann Nutr Metab 2011;58:263–71.

202. Czeizel AE, Puhó EH, Bánhidy F. No association between periconceptional multivitamin supplementation and risk of multiple congenital abnormalities: a population-based case-control study. Am J Med Genet A 2006;140A:2469–77.

203. Choudhary R, Chawala V, Soni N, et al. Oxidative stress and role of antioxidants in male infertility. Pak J Physiol 2010;6.

204. Showell MG, Brown J, Yazdani A, et al. Antioxidants for male subfertility. Cochrane Database Syst Rev 2011;(1):CD007411.

205. Youssef MA, Abdelmoty HI, Elashmwi HA, et al. Oral antioxidants supplementation for women with unexplained infertility undergoing ICSI/IVF: randomized controlled trial. Hum Fertil 2015;18(1):38–42.

206. Gropper SS, Smith JL, Groff JL. Advanced nutrition and human metabolism. 5th ed. Belmont: Wadsworth; 2009.

207. Salehpour S, Akbari Sene A, Saharkhiz N, et al. N-acetylcysteine as an adjuvant to clomiphene citrate for successful induction of ovulation in infertile patients with polycystic ovary syndrome. J Obstet Gynaecol Res 2012;38:1182–6.

208. Thakker D, Raval A, Patel I, et al. N-acetylcysteine for polycystic ovary syndrome: a systematic review and meta-analysis of randomized controlled clinical trials. Obstet Gynecol Int 2015;2015.

209. Badawy A, Baker El Nashar A, El Totongy M. Clomiphene citrate plus N-acetyl cysteine versus clomiphene citrate for augmenting ovulation in the management of unexplained infertility: a randomized double-blind controlled trial. Fertil Steril 2006;86:647–50.

210. Badawy A, State O, Abdelgawad S. N-Acetyl cysteine and clomiphene citrate for induction of ovulation in polycystic ovary syndrome: a cross-over trial. Acta Obstet Gynecol Scand 2007;86:218–22.

211. Elgindy EA, El-Huseiny AM, Mostafa MI, et al. N-Acetyl cysteine: could it be an effective adjuvant therapy in ICSI cycles? A preliminary study. Reprod Biomed Online 2010;20:789–96.

212. Rizk AY, Bedaiwy MA, Al-Inany HG. N-acetyl-cysteine is a novel adjuvant to clomiphene citrate in clomiphene citrate–resistant patients with polycystic ovary syndrome. Fertil Steril 2005;83:367–70.

213. Cicek N, Eryilmaz O, Sarikaya E, et al. Vitamin E effect on controlled ovarian stimulation of unexplained infertile women. J Assist Reprod Genet 2012;29:325–8.

214. Ghanem H, Shaeer O, El-Segini A. Combination clomiphene citrate and antioxidant therapy for idiopathic male infertility: a randomized controlled trial. Fertil Steril 2010;93:2232–5.

215. ElSheikh MG, Hosny MB, Elshenoufy A, et al. Combination of vitamin E and clomiphene citrate in treating patients with idiopathic oligoasthenozoospermia: a prospective, randomized trial. Andrology 2015;3(5):864–7.

216. Srivastava S, Desai P, Coutinho D, et al. Mechanism of action of l-arginine on the vitality of spermatozoa is primarily through increased biosynthesis of nitric oxide. Biol Reprod 2006;74:954–8.

217. Stanislavov R, Nikolova V, Rohdewald P. Improvement of seminal parameters with Prelox®: a randomized, double-blind, placebo-controlled, cross-over trial. Phytother Res 2009;23(3):297–302.

218. Kobori Y, Suzuki K, Iwahata T, et al. Improvement of seminal quality and sexual function of men with oligoasthenoteratozoospermia syndrome following supplementation with L-arginine and Pycnogenol®. Arch Ital Urol Androl 2015;87(3):190–3.

219. Blom H, Smulders Y. Overview of homocysteine and folate metabolism. With special references to cardiovascular disease and neural tube defects. J Inherit Metab Dis 2011;34:75–81.

220. Blencowe H, Cousens S, Modell B, et al. Folic acid to reduce neonatal mortality from neural tube disorders. Int J Epidemiol 2010;39:i110–21.

221. Wong WY, Merkus HMWM, Thomas CMG, et al. Effects of folic acid and zinc sulfate on male factor subfertility: a double-blind, randomized, placebo-controlled trial. Fertil Steril 2002;77:491–8.

222. Ambiye VR, Langade D, Dongre S, et al. Clinical evaluation of the spermatogenic activity of the root extract of Ashwagandha (Withania somnifera) in oligospermic males: a pilot study. Evid Based Complement Alternat Med 2013;2013.

223. Wagner CL, Taylor SN, Dawodu A, et al. Vitamin D and its role during pregnancy in attaining optimal health of mother and fetus. Nutrients 2012;4:208–30.

224. Christesen HT, Falkenberg T, Lamont RF, et al. The impact of vitamin D on pregnancy: a systematic review. Acta Obstet Gynecol Scand 2012;91:1357–67.

225. Thorne-Lyman A, Fawzi WW. Vitamin D during pregnancy and maternal, neonatal and infant health outcomes: a systematic review and meta-analysis. Paediatr Perinat Epidemiol 2012;26:75–90.

226. Ryan JL, Heckler CE, Roscoe JA, et al. Ginger (Zingiber officinale) reduces acute chemotherapy-induced nausea: a URCC CCOP study of 576 patients. Support Care Cancer 2012;20:1479–89.

227. Matthews A, Dowswell T, Haas DM, et al. Interventions for nausea and vomiting in early pregnancy. Cochrane Database Syst Rev 2010;(9):CD007575.

228. Viljoen E, Visser J, Koen N, et al. A systematic review and meta-analysis of the effect and safety of ginger in the treatment of pregnancy-associated nausea and vomiting. Nutrition 2014;13(1):20.

229. Heitmann K, Nordeng H, Holst L. Safety of ginger use in pregnancy: results from a large population-based cohort study. Eur J Clin Pharmacol 2013;69:269–77.

230. Sharifzadeh F, Kashanian M, Koohpayehzadeh J, et al. A comparison between the effects of ginger, pyridoxine (vitamin B6) and placebo for the treatment of the first trimester nausea and vomiting of pregnancy (NVP). J Matern Fetal Neonatal Med 2018;31(19): 2509–14.

231. Ramakrishnan U. A review of the benefits of nutrient supplements during pregnancy: from iron-folic-acid to long-chain polyunsaturated fatty acids to probiotics. Annales Nestlé (English ed.) 2010;68:29–40.

232. Goh YI, Bollano E, Einarson TR, et al. Prenatal multivitamin supplementation and rates of pediatric cancers: a meta-analysis. Clin Pharmacol Ther 2007;81:685–91.

233. Goh Y, Bollano E, Einarson T, et al. Prenatal multivitamin supplementation and rates of congenital anomalies: a meta-analysis. J Obstet Gynaecol Can 2006;28:680.

234. Ramakrishnan U, Grant FK, Goldenberg T, et al. Effect of multiple micronutrient supplementation on pregnancy and infant outcomes: a systematic review. Paediatr Perinat Epidemiol 2012;26:153–67.

235. Hacker AN, Fung EB, King JC. Role of calcium during pregnancy: maternal and fetal needs. Nutr Rev 2012;70:397–409.

236. Buppasiri P, Lumbiganon P, Thinkhamrop J, et al. Calcium supplementation (other than for preventing or treating hypertension) for improving pregnancy and infant outcomes. Cochrane Database Syst Rev 2011;(10):CD007079.

237. Imdad A, Jabeen A, Bhutta ZA. Role of calcium supplementation in pregnancy in reducing risk of developing gestational hypertensive disorders: a meta-analysis of studies from developing countries. BMC Public Health 2011;11:S18.

238. Tang R, Tang IC, Henry A, et al. Limited evidence for calcium supplementation in preeclampsia prevention: a meta-analysis and systematic review. Hypertens Pregnancy 2015;34(2):181–203.

239. Cohen JT, Bellinger DC, Connor WE, et al. A quantitative analysis of prenatal intake of n-3 polyunsaturated fatty acids and cognitive development. Am J Prev Med 2005;29:366–366.e12.

240. Gould JF, Smithers LG, Makrides M. The effect of maternal omega-3 (n-3) LCPUFA supplementation during pregnancy on early childhood cognitive and visual development: a systematic review and meta-analysis

241. Saccone G, Berghella V. Omega-3 long chain polyunsaturated fatty acids to prevent preterm birth: a systematic review and meta-analysis. Obstet Gynecol 2015;125(3):663–72.

242. Freeman MP, Davis M, Sinha P, et al. Omega-3 fatty acids and supportive psychotherapy for perinatal depression: a randomized placebo-controlled study. J Affect Disord 2008;110:142–8.

243. Su K-P, Huang S-Y, Chiu T-H, et al. Omega-3 fatty acids for major depressive disorder during pregnancy: results from a randomized, double-blind, placebo-controlled trial. J Clin Psychiatry 2008;69:644.

244. Rebagliato M, Murcia M, Espada M, et al. Iodine intake and maternal thyroid function during pregnancy. Epidemiology 2010;21:62–9. doi:10.1097/EDE.0b013e3181c1592b.

245. Murcia M, Rebagliato M, Iniguez C, et al. Effect of iodine supplementation during pregnancy on infant neurodevelopment at 1 year of age. Am J Epidemiol 2011;173(7):804–12.

246. Peña-Rosas J, De-Regil L, Dowswell T, et al. Daily oral iron supplementation during pregnancy (Review). Cochrane Database Syst Rev 2012a;(12):CD004736.

247. Peña-Rosas JP, De-Regil LM, Dowswell T, et al. Intermittent oral iron supplementation during pregnancy. Cochrane Database Syst Rev 2012b;(7):CD009997.

248. Haider BA, Olofin I, Wang M, et al. Anaemia, prenatal iron use, and risk of adverse pregnancy outcomes: systematic review and meta-analysis. BMJ 2013;346: f3443.

of randomized controlled trials. Am J Clin Nutr 2013;97(3):531–44.

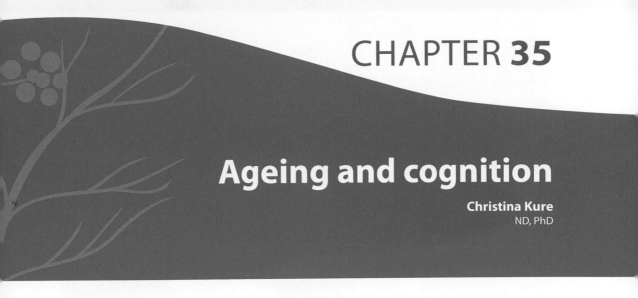

CHAPTER 35

Ageing and cognition

Christina Kure
ND, PhD

OVERVIEW

Ageing is a multidimensional process comprising physical, psychological and social factors that vary and interact over the lifespan.[1,2] Normal ageing is characterised by organ and system changes that vary among individuals depending on physical, emotional, psychological and social changes experienced during life.[3] These changes are influenced by such factors as genetics, physical and social environments, diet, health, stress and lifestyle choices. In the absence of disease, normal ageing involves changes and impairment of bodily systems leading to structural and functional changes, some of which are noticeable upon inspection of older patients.

In the recent decades, the elderly in developed countries have experienced a dramatic increase in life expectancy and a declining death rate, giving rise to a vastly older population. Consequently, public health systems have been burdened both logistically and financially by an increasing number of elderly individuals suffering from age-related diseases such as dementia,* cardiovascular disease and cancer, requiring ever higher rates of hospitalisation, surgery and visits to their clinician.[3] The holistic and preventative approach of naturopathic practices suggests a role for these disciplines in the promotion of healthy ageing and in meeting the health challenges of the future. A comprehensive naturopathic review provides a detailed account of systems that are most affected during the ageing process; given that the pattern of ageing is unique to each individual,[3] treatment needs to be tailored to individual needs.

Figure 35.1 indicates common diseases and illnesses in the elderly such as cardiovascular disease, arthritis, diabetes, infections, cancer and gastrointestinal disturbances. (Refer to the respective chapters in this book for details on how to address these conditions holistically.)

THERAPEUTIC CONSIDERATIONS IN THE ELDERLY

Age-related chronic diseases are often not successfully treated since conventional methods often fail to provide long-term relief and have adverse side effects. A survey among older Australian adults (50 year +) revealed that approximately 9% consulted a

---

*In the revised DSM-5 the term 'dementia' is classified as a 'major neurocognitive disorder'.[4]

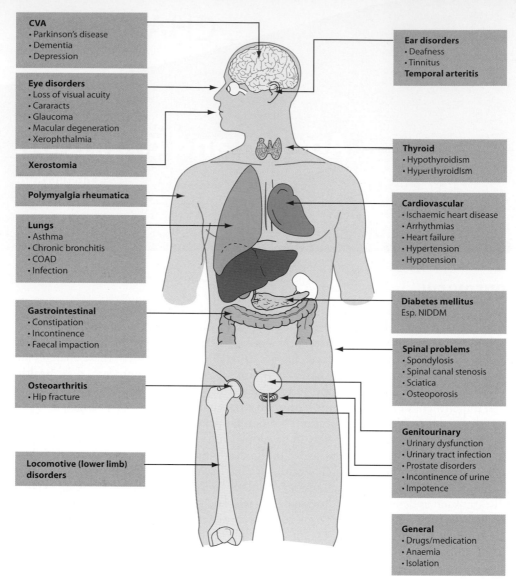

Figure 35.1
Common conditions seen in the elderly
Source: Adapted from Murtagh 2006[5]

complementary and alternative medicine (CAM) practitioner for a chronic condition in the previous three months (12% women and 4% men), with older adults (> 80 years) less likely to consult a CAM practitioner.[6]

A medical history will help determine the time of disease onset, and assessment using dementia screening tools, such as the Mini-Mental State Examination and measures of depression such as the geriatric depression scale,[7] are valuable. Additionally, full blood cell count tests for thyroid, kidney and liver function, and serum level of vitamin B12 are recommended. A naturopathic approach needs to consider the physical and mental stage the elderly individual is at in their ageing process. Each individual has been exposed to different factors in their lifetime that may either increase or decrease the risk of developing cognitive decline. A detailed account of the presenting case and patient history will help determine an appropriate treatment approach and aid in determining the risk factors that may have contributed to presenting cognitive complaints, and whether the presenting symptoms are due to normal or pathological ageing.

Wear and tear affects not only the brain and vascular system, but also other body parts. It is essential to consider these changes in elderly patients and treat other illnesses such as arthritis, hearing difficulties, diabetes or heart disease during naturopathic consultations. It is also essential to support changes to bodily systems, such as improving gastrointestinal function (with bitters, protease/amylases/lipase and gut bacteria), supporting the cardiovascular system (with circulatory stimulants and cardiac tonics), regulating cholesterol levels, treating infections (with immune system stimulants), encouraging exercise to improve bone mass and muscle tone, supporting the genitourinary system (with urinary tonics) and seeking regular hearing and vision tests.

Due to a number of changes in body composition, gastrointestinal and sensory function, older people are prone to dysfunction in the digestive system, and are thus at risk of malnutrition.[8] Oral health concerns (e.g. improperly fitted dentures, missing teeth), and reduced taste and olfactory sensations may result in reduced appetite and food intake.[8] In those with dentures, incorporating soft foods in the diet is recommended. Insufficient digestive enzyme production may lead to inadequate digestion and assimilation of micronutrients to vital tissues and organs, resulting in poor health, poor immunity and disability.[8] Therefore, it is vital to improve digestive functions (refer to the section on the digestive system in Chapters 4–6). The existence of multiple medical issues makes the elderly prone to polypharmacy; interactions with vitamins and herbs (see Appendix 1) need to be well thought out prior to prescribing a treatment regimen.

As it is imperative to use a holistic approach to treating seniors whereby diseases and illness in each bodily system needs to be addressed, this chapter focuses on ageing in general and age-related cognitive decline with particular reference to the dementias of the vascular and Alzheimer's types.

NORMAL BRAIN AGEING

Cognition encompasses a broad range of brain processes that are taken for granted until lost, or at least decline in functional capacity. There is no definition for cognitive health; however, the Critical Evaluation Study Committee defines cognitive health as 'the development and preservation of the multidimensional cognitive structure that allows the older adult to maintain social connectedness, a sense of purpose, and the ability to function independently, to permit functional recovery from illness or injury, and to cope with residual functional deficits'.[9]

Memory is a mental process where information is stored, processed and retrieved. Memory is divided into working memory (short-term memory) and episodic memory (long-term memory). Using focused attention, information in working memory is briefly stored over a period of seconds by means of manipulation through rehearsal.[10] Episodic memory, however, involves storing information over minutes, days and years that can subsequently be retrieved after a long period of time. The ability to store information in long-term memory requires focused activity.[11] Attention refers to an individual's ability to disengage, adjust their focus and to be responsive to surrounding stimuli.[11] Various functions defining attention include vigilance, which is the process

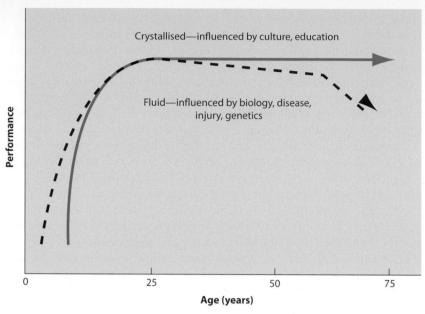

Figure 35.2
The change in fluid and crystallised abilities with age
Source: Anstey 2004[12]

of sustained attention, and information processing. Executive functions, on the other hand, are higher order cognitive processes involved in planning, attentional control and response inhibition.

Cognitive abilities can be classified as 'fluid' when they rely on short-term memory storage to process information, or 'crystallised' where knowledge and expertise accumulates and relies on long-term memory.[12] Fluid intelligence involves solving new problems, spatial manipulation, mental speed and identifying complex patterns. Fluid abilities peak in the mid 20s and then gradually decline until the age of 60 years, when the decline becomes more rapid.[12] In contrast, crystallised abilities increase during the life span through education, occupational and cultural experiences. Intellectual pursuits slow in late adulthood and may gradually decline from the age of 90 years (refer to Figure 35.2); they are affected by ageing and disease and often remain intact even in the early stages of dementia or after brain injury.[12]

Healthy ageing negatively affects general cognition, short-term memory, fine motor skills, processing speed and visuospatial ability, while long-term memories are well maintained.[12,13] It is important for the naturopathic practitioner to detect signs of early cognitive decline in older patients and, using a combination of herbal, nutritional and lifestyle interventions together with appropriate referrals to other medical practitioners, prepare older patients for making decisions about their future care before they have lost the ability to do so[14] (Table 35.1).

PATHOLOGICAL COGNITIVE DECLINE

Individuals who experience cognitive decline are at a greater risk of developing dementia, and researchers suggest that early detection and intervention may be effective strategies to slow the progress of dementia.[8] Alzheimer's disease (AD) is the most common of

Table 35.1
Common conditions seen in the elderly and naturopathic treatment approach*

Conditions commonly seen in the elderly	Naturopathic treatment approach
Osteoporosis	Calcium and vitamin D are important for improving bone mass and preventing bone fractures and falls; recommended dietary allowances for people aged 65 + years are[15]: • calcium 700–800 mg • vitamin D 400–800 IU (> 800 IU per day with calcium for preventing falls)[16] Increase dairy products (milk, yoghurts and cheese) and fish (sardines with bones)
Poor digestion[4,17]	This is the result of a decline in bifidobacteria and lactic acid bacteria (LAB) in the gut, leading to microbial infections Supplement with probiotics (bifidobacteria or lactobacilli) and address nutritional deficiencies Use herbal medicines with bitter or aromatic properties[18] Properly fitting dentures[4]
Urinary incontinence[19]	Seen in approximately 11.6% of 65+ year olds living in the community Encourage adequate hydration Avoid caffeine and alcohol Pelvic floor muscle therapy (Kegel exercises) Address nutritional deficiencies, especially Mg, Zn and B12
Sleep disorders	Effective treatments[20]: • melatonin for circadian disorders affecting sleep • valerian, Tai Chi, acupuncture, acupressure, yoga and meditation

*Except cardio/cerebrovascular disease and cancer (see Section 3 on the cardiovascular system and Chapter 32 on cancer).

the subtypes of the dementias[14] characterised by the presence of amyloid-beta-protein (AβP) and intraneural deposition of neurofibrillary tangles in the brain; although this pathology is also seen in non-demented individuals, it is the distribution of these plaques in the brain that differentiates normal and abnormal brain changes.[21] Mild cognitive impairment (MCI) is a condition presenting with memory deficits that are below the defined norms and in the absence of other cognitive dysfunctions, and although it is thought to be a preclinical state of dementia[22] approximately half of MCI individuals go on to develop AD.[23] This again furnishes a role for naturopaths to work in conjunction with other medical professionals qualified to diagnose and monitor the progression of cognitive decline and provide a complementary treatment approach to prescribing holistic remedies proven to slow the progression of cognitive decline in these individuals.

CEREBROVASCULAR CONDITIONS

Cerebrovascular disease (CVD) refers to brain lesions that are caused by: 1. vascular disorders including cerebral infarction or acute cessation of blood flow to a localised area of the brain; 2. brain haemorrhage caused by rupture in a vascular wall; and 3. vascular dementia (VaD),[†] caused by multiple small infarcts and subcortical Binswanger-like white-matter.[21] VaD is recognised as the second most prevalent type of dementia. Cerebrovascular health benefits from treatment of broader cardiovascular risk factors,[24] hence older patients presenting with the problems of cognitive decline should be assessed for vascular risk and treated more broadly.

[†]In the revised DMS-V vascular dementia is classified as vascular neurocognitive disorder.[7]

SCREENING TOOLS

When appropriate, naturopaths treating older patients are encouraged to arrange referrals to health professionals qualified to detect abnormal brain ageing. Although there is no universally accepted measure to detect preclinical signs of cognitive decline, psychologists, psychiatrists and neuropsychologists can administer screening tools which measure patients' subjective or objective cognitive decline. The patients' cognitive performance, which is compared with norms appropriate to the patient's age, education and cultural background, can help distinguish normal from abnormal brain ageing, and the progression or stabilisation of cognitive decline.[7,13] Such screening tools include the Mini-Mental State Examination (MMSE) and the Alzheimer's Disease Assessment Scale (ADAS-cog).

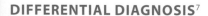

DIFFERENTIAL DIAGNOSIS[7]

- Neurocognitive disorder (NCD)—modest (mild NCD) or significant (major NCD) cognitive decline in one or more cognitive domains. Cognitive impairments do (major NCD) or do not (mild NCD) impede ability to carry out daily activities independently (e.g. paying bills, managing medicines).
- Neurocognitive disorder due to Alzheimer's disease—an 'insidious onset and gradual progression of cognitive impairment in one or more cognitive domains'.
- Vascular neurocognitive disorder—temporary cognitive impairment due to one or more cerebrovascular events. Cerebrovascular disease as the principal pathology related to cognitive impairments.
- Psychiatric disorders—schizophrenia, major depressive disorder.
- Delirium—decreased ability to maintain and shift attention appropriately; associated symptoms fluctuate whereas in dementia symptoms are usually stable.
- Major or mild neurocognitive disorder due to traumatic brain injury—post-traumatic amnesia with persistent memory impairment; behavioural symptoms (e.g. aphasia, attentional problems, irritability, anxiety, depression); can lead to risk-taking behaviours.
- Age-related cognitive decline—normal ageing process where cognitive dysfunction is within the normal range for the person's age; individuals may have difficulties remembering names and appointments or solving complex problems.
- Alterations in cognition from acute infections.
- Organic brain disease and central nervous system (CNS) disorders.

Source: American Psychiatric Association 2013[4]

RISK FACTORS

Several risk factors have been associated with the development of cognitive decline (e.g. VaD and AD) including[14,25–28]:

- cardiovascular disease
- hypertension
- central obesity
- diabetes
- excessive alcohol intake
- elevated homocysteine levels
- cigarette smoking
- inflammation
- a history of anxiety and depression.

Vascular risk factors (e.g. hypertension, diabetes, obesity and high cholesterol levels), especially when seen in young adulthood and midlife, may contribute to cognitive impairments seen in ageing.[29] Other vascular risk factors including heart disease (coronary heart disease, atrial fibrillation, heart failure) may be linked to cerebral hypoperfusion, hypoxia, emboli, or infarcts and neurodegenerative lesions such as ß amyloid deposition.[29] Elevated blood pressure has been found to influence cognitive ability: hypertension increases the risk of vascular and endothelial damage and disrupts the blood–brain barrier,[14] and it has been proposed that a reduction in high blood pressure may be a preventative measure against stroke and cognitive decline in elderly patients.[30] Increased central adipose tissue has been linked to vascular and metabolic factors that give rise to cognitive decline and dementia, and there is emerging evidence suggesting that metabolic syndrome is associated with an increased risk of dementia. A greater waist-to-hip ratio (WHR) and age are negatively correlated with hippocampal volumes, suggesting that a larger WHR may be related to neurodegenerative, vascular or metabolic processes that affect brain structures underlying cognitive decline and dementia.[26] Clinicians need to consider lifestyle interventions towards an early and effective cardiovascular risk-factor management to reduce the risk of cardiometabolic and the cognitive decline.[31] When exploring psychological factors, a history of nervous disorders such as anxiety and depression has also been linked to poor cognitive health later on in life.[8] Finally, researchers have recently theorised a possible link between age-related alterations in intestinal microbiomes and cognitive decline by promoting systemic- and neuro-inflammation, and peripheral insulin sensitivity.[32,33]

CONVENTIONAL TREATMENT

Pharmacological treatments such as cholinesterase inhibitors are available for the short-term symptoms of dementia, rather than modifying the disease as such.[34] The cholinergic system has a central role in regulating cognitive functioning, and a consistent deficit in the neurotransmitter acetylcholine (ACh) in the hippocampus is a key feature of AD.[35] Inhibition of acetylcholinesterase (AChE), the main enzyme involved in the breakdown of ACh, is the key strategy for the short-term relief of symptoms commonly seen in AD. These therapies include the medications donepezil, tacrine and galantamine, in addition to drugs such as rivastigmine and, although these treatments delay the symptomatic progression associated with AD by 6–12 months,[34] they can cause adverse effects including gastrointestinal disturbances, diarrhoea, muscle cramps, fatigue, nausea, rhinitis, vomiting, anorexia and insomnia.[36] Additionally, ACh inhibitors such as galantamine, huperzine A, physostigmine and its derivatives have been used to increase the levels of ACh to improve neural functioning.[37]

Since there is no cure for AD, preventative measures are very important and are commonly prescribed by medical practitioners. Some conventional medications, including non-steroidal anti-inflammatory, antidiabetic, hypertension and statin medications are thought to be effective in preventing the onset of dementia. Although there is insufficient evidence for the use of these drugs for the treatment of cognitive impairment,[38,39] the therapeutic action of these medications targets the brain systems that scientists think are impaired in dementia and other age-related diseases including CVD.[40]

KEY TREATMENT PROTOCOLS

The causes of age-related cognitive decline and pathologies such as AD are not known. The underlying mechanisms associated with normal ageing need to be understood in order to understand abnormal ageing associated with cognitive decline. It is thought that cognitive decline may be a multifactorial process; therefore, treatments simultaneously targeting these mechanisms may be the ideal preventative strategy.[38]

Attenuate oxidative stress

Oxidative stress is strongly implicated in the ageing process in addition to various disease states including cardiovascular conditions such as stroke, CVD and neurodegenerative diseases such as AD and dementia.[41,42] Antioxidant micronutrients such as vitamin C, vitamin E and carotenoids are important in combating the effects of oxidative stress; inadequate dietary intake of these is thought to increase the risk of degenerative diseases including AD and MCI.[42]

Rectifying deficiencies in these nutrients may be one aim of combating oxidative stress in the ageing individual. Vitamin C and vitamin E intake through vegetables and high-dose supplementation used chronically (average 4.3 years) have also been linked to lowering the risk of AD.[43,44]

Research examining the effects of multivitamin supplementation on cognitive function in older individuals has produced mixed results. Randomised trials have reported no effects of multivitamins on cognitive function or mood in healthy elderly following six months[45] or 12 months intervention.[46] However, when mixed with a herbal formula, multivitamins have shown positive effects on working memory in elderly women at risk of cognitive decline (16-week intervention),[47] and episodic memory in older male individuals (50–74 years; eight-week intervention).[48] Investigation of an integrated treatment approach on cognitive performance using antidepressants, cholinesterase inhibitors, and vitamins and supplements (multivitamins, vitamin E, alpha-lipoic acid, omega-3 and CoQ10) was found to delay cognitive decline for 24 months and also improve cognition, especially frontal lobe activity and memory in patients with mild dementia and depression.[49] Future studies need to explore whether positive effects of multivitamins are seen in older individuals with nutritional deficiencies.[46]

Polyphenols are antioxidants found in fruits, vegetables and plant extracts that have positive effects on cognitive function. The pine bark extract **Pycnogenol**, which is high in polyphenols, has significant beneficial effects on cognitive functioning (particularly memory) and oxidative stress following approximately three months administration (60–85 years; PYC 150 mg/day)[50,51] suggesting the potential benefit in improving cognition in the elderly. The polyphenolic compound **curcumin** has been shown to improve cognitive functioning in AD patients, possibly due to its cholesterol-lowering, antioxidant, anti-inflammatory and lipophilic actions, and inhibiting acetylcholinesterase and mediating the insulin signalling pathway.[52] An RCT in healthy older adults showed that acute doses (one and three hours post intervention) of a curcumin extract (400 mg Longvida®) significantly improved sustained attention and working memory compared to controls with a reduced range of effects seen chronically (four weeks post intervention).[53] A large epidemiological study showed that a diet rich in berries (blueberries and strawberries), anthocyanins and flavonoid-rich foods (e.g. apples, tea, oranges and onions) lowered the rate of cognitive decline by up to 2.5 years in older women.[54] Supporting this, a higher consumption of **Camellia sinensis** (green tea) in a Japanese population was associated with a lower prevalence of cognitive impairment,[55] possibly due to metal-chelating, antioxidant, anti-inflammatory and neuroprotectant properties.[56,57] Additionally, preliminary human and animal studies show promising effects of polyphenols found naturally in cocoa as a treatment to delay age-related cognitive decline.[58–61] In particular, a flavanol-rich cocoa drink (990 mg) has been shown to increase blood flow velocity in the middle cerebral artery, and decrease blood pressure, insulin resistance and lipid peroxidation in healthy older volunteers.[62] Finally, epidemiological studies have reported a link between **coffee** consumption and a reduced risk in developing cognitive impairments.[63] These effects may be attributed not only to caffeine but also chlorogenic acid, an active constituent in coffee that has only recently been explored.[64] Collectively, these studies suggest that flavanol-containing foods may be an effective treatment for delaying age-related cognitive deficits in normal ageing, and for cerebrovascular ischaemia syndromes including dementias and stroke by improving vascular health. Collectively, these studies suggest that flavanol-containing foods may be an effective treatment for delaying age-related cognitive deficits in normal ageing, and for cerebrovascular ischaemia syndromes including dementias and stroke by improving vascular health.

Reduce inflammatory markers

A number of molecules associated with inflammation are believed to be involved in the pathogenesis of AD. These include increases in inflammatory markers alpha 1-antichymotrypsin (ACT), interleukin-6 (IL-6), monocyte chemoattractant protein-1 (MCP-1) and oxidised low-density lipoprotein (oxLDL) in the plasma and cerebro-spinal fluid in patients with AD.[65] It has also been established that centenarians have a higher frequency of genetic markers associated with better control of inflammation; such control appears to exert a protective effect against the development of age-related pathologies that have a strong inflammatory pathogenetic component.[65]

Bacopa monnieri is an Ayurvedic herb used traditionally for memory decline. *B. monnieri* contains bacosides A and B (steroidal saponins) that are believed to be essential for the clinical efficacy of the product, and is an anti-inflammatory,[66] antioxidant[67] and removes β amyloid deposits.[68]

Studies have reported that in AD patients, *B. monnieri* (300 mg Bacognize® twice daily) improved attention, language, writing and comprehension following six months of intervention.[69] In older adults without dementia, compared to the placebo group, daily administration of *B. monnieri* reduced forgetting rates of newly acquired information, improved retention of new information (150 mg twice daily for three months),[70] improved working memory, attention, cognitive processing,[71] verbal learning, memory acquisition and delayed recall (300 mg/day for 12 weeks).[72,73] In addition to cognitive benefits, *B. monnieri* has been shown to improve mood (depression, trait anxiety) and reduce heart rate in healthy elderly participants (65+ years; 300 g/day for 12 weeks).[73] A nutraceutical combination comprising *B. monnieri* (320 mg), L-Theanine (100 mg), *Crocus sativus* (30 mg), vitamin B6 (9.5 mg), biotin (450 µg), folic acid (400 µg), vitamin B12 (33 µg), vitamin D (25 µg) and copper (2 mg) improved global cognition (MMSE scores) and stress following two months of administration.[74] Likewise, patients diagnosed with MCI demonstrated improvements in cognitive function following a 60-day intervention of another nutraceutical formula (Illumina®) which included extracts of *B. monnieri* and *Haematococcus pluvialis* (astaxanthin), soy-extracted phosphatidylserine, and vitamin E.[75]

A systematic review concluded that three months' *B. monnieri* supplementation improves learning and free recall of information in healthy individuals with doses ranging between 300–400 mg (KeenMind®) and 300–450 mg (BacoMind®).[76] Since shorter treatment duration of one month failed to find any significant effects of *B. monnieri* on cognitive function,[77] it is possible that longer periods of treatment are required to notice an effect. Most long-term studies have examined the effects of *B. monnieri* over three months; however, studies designed to investigate whether *B. monnieri* has positive effects on cognitive function over longer periods of time (e.g. 12 or 24 months) are necessary.[76] *B. monnieri* is well tolerated; however, gastrointestinal tract side effects including increased stool frequency, abdominal cramps and nausea have been reported.[72]

Enhance vascular system integrity and function

There is increasing evidence linking the role of vascular function to cognitive decline and dementia.[78] A review of the literature demonstrated that vascular factors resulting in brain ageing and cognitive decline include reduced cerebral blood flow, reduced cerebral blood volume, poor capillary elasticity and poor vasodilatory capacity.[79] Such factors may affect the uptake and use of glucose and oxygen in the brain[80] Therefore, interventions addressing these vascular mechanisms, before normal age-related cognitive decline accelerates to dementia, may be effective in preventing cognitive impairment.[79]

Ginkgo biloba is one of the most widely researched herbs for the treatment and prevention of cognitive decline and has yielded mixed results. In the Ginkgo Evaluation of Memory (GEM) study a longer administration period (median of 6.1 years) of *G. biloba* (120-mg/day) did not slow the rate of cognitive decline (e.g. memory, language, attention, psychomotor speed and executive function) in elderly individuals with normal cognition or MCI (aged 72–69 years).[81]

However, other studies have demonstrated opposing results. Short-term randomised, placebo-controlled trials showed improvements following six weeks' EGb 761 (180 mg/day) on certain neuropsychological and memory processes in cognitively intact older individuals ($n = 262$; > 60 years).[82] Also, a recently published 20-year longitudinal study showed that non-demented individuals taking the EGb 761 ginkgo extract had a lower reduction in global cognitive ability compared to those who did not take this herb.[83] In patients with MCI, a two-year EGb 761 (240 mg/day) supplementation improved cognitive performance (executive function, attention) and anxiety.[84]

Additionally, in patients with dementia (AD and VaD) compared to a placebo group, those taking *G. biloba* extract EGb 761 (240 mg/day) showed improvements in cognitive functioning (verbal fluency and memory), neuropsychiatric symptoms, quality of life and activities of daily living.[85,86] *G. biloba* has been shown to be as effective as cholinesterase inhibitors in delaying symptoms of AD and[87] delay the course of the dementia by six months,[88] and is more effective when used in combination with donepezil, suggesting a promising adjunctive treatment for dementia.[89] Overall, EGb 761 is safe, effective and well tolerated; however, adverse events have been reported including headaches, respiratory tract infections, increased blood pressure and dizziness.[85,86]

Centella asiatica has been used in traditional Ayurvedic medicine for centuries for its beneficial effects on the vascular system and in enhancing memory, and is listed as a treatment for dementia in the ancient Indian Ayurvedic medical text, *Caraka Susmita*.[90] Despite limited placebo-controlled trials, a recent study reported that two months' daily administration of a high *Centella asiatica* dose (750 mg) enhanced working memory and improved self-related mood (alertness and calmness) in healthy elderly participants (mean age = 65.05 ± 3.56 years; $n = 28$).[91]

Reduce heavy metal exposure

Levels of zinc, copper and iron are significantly altered in AD brain tissue, particularly in the hippocampus, amygdala and neocortex.[92] Recent findings suggest that metal complexing agents may have therapeutic benefits in AD.[93] Curcumin's anti-inflammatory actions are believed to be due in part to its metal-chelating effects; it also has the ability to bind to heavy metals—particularly copper and iron—and as a result prevent neurotoxicity caused by such metals.[94] *B. monnieri* is believed to modulate the cholinergic system and/or have antioxidant effects and remove β-amyloid deposits, in addition to acting as a metal chelator.[95]

Genetic factors

It has been suggested that genetic susceptibility is implicated in the cognitive impairment seen in ageing.[96] For example, apolipoprotein E (Apo E) and ACE genes have been associated with cognitive impairments seen in ageing and dementia. Individuals carrying the Apo E epsilon 4 allele exhibit lower memory performance on tests related to declarative (storing facts) and procedural (long-term) memory.[96] Furthermore, AD is an autosomal-dominant disease involving four specific genes located on chromosomes 1, 14, 19 and 21; these genes have been associated with the progression of AD. Further research, however, is required to understand the relationship between Apo E and cognition.

Enhance mental function with herbal cognitive enhancers

Chronic administration of *Panax ginseng* extracts has shown improvements in cognitive functioning and performance in older individuals and dementia. Compared to a placebo group, eight to nine weeks' administration of a standardised *P. ginseng* extract (400 mg/day) in healthy older participants (> 40 years) resulted in significant improvements in performance on cognitive tasks, specifically related to executive functioning.[97] Additionally, preliminary evidence revealed that treatment with a ginsenoside product (4.5 g/day) for 12 weeks' improved cognitive function in patients with moderately severe AD.[98] These cognitive effects were observed in patients even at a two-year follow-up assessment. A herbal combination formula consisting of *Panax ginseng*, *Ginkgo biloba* and *Crocus sativus* resulted in slight improvements in working memory; however, studies employing larger sample sizes are needed to confirm these findings.[99]

Salvia officinalis exhibits antioxidant, oestrogenic and anti-inflammatory properties, and both inhibits butyryl and acetyl-cholinesterase.[100] *S. officinalis* aroma improves mood, quality of memory and secondary memory.[101] When taken orally a different species, *Salvia lavandulaefolia* (50 μL of the essential oil), improved secondary memory and attention one hour post administration and reduced fatigue four hours post dose in healthy young participants.[102] Furthermore, a 16-week administration of *S. officinalis* significantly improved scores on the ADAS-cog in patients with mild to moderate dementia.[103] ***Melissa officinalis*** has cholinergic-binding properties in vitro and may ameliorate cognitive decline associated with AD. A randomised, placebo-controlled, double-blind, balanced crossover study[104] assessed the acute (1, 2.5, 4 and 6 hours post dosing) cognitive and mood effects of three single doses of *M. officinalis* (lemon balm 300 g, 600 g and 900 g) or matching placebo. Improvements were observed in accuracy of attention following 600 g of lemon balm and reductions in both secondary memory and working memory factors and self-rated 'calmness', as assessed by Bond-Lader mood scales, was elevated at the earliest time points by the lowest dose (lemon balm 300 mg). Interestingly, alertness was significantly reduced at all time points following the highest dose. Preliminary findings showed that compared to placebo a low dose of ***Rosmarinus officinalis*** (750 mg) improves speed of memory, which is the time it takes for someone to retrieve information from memory.[105] However, a high dose of *R. officinalis* (6000 mg) has negative effects with increased feelings of fatigue.

INTEGRATIVE MEDICAL CONSIDERATIONS

Cognitively stimulating activities and psychosocial factors

The 'use it' or 'lose it' theory of cognitive ageing proposes that a combination of intellectual, social and physical activities prevents cognitive decline in older age.[106] Numerous epidemiological studies observed that frequent participation in cognitively stimulating activities such as reading, playing mental games and doing crossword puzzles were associated with reduced dementia risk.[107,108] **Cognitive training** refers to non-pharmacological treatments (e.g. computer cognitive training, psychosocial interventions) aimed to improve cognitive functioning in individuals.[109] Studies have shown that cognitive training improved cognitive functioning in patients with AD[109] and in healthy older individuals with effects lasting up to five years.[110] Online computer cognitive training tools in particular improved simple and choice reaction times following two weeks[111] and overall cognitive function following six weeks.[112] Some possible limitations to consider with online computer-based cognitive tools is computer literacy, slow internet speed and individuals not willing to progress to more advanced levels.[112] Brain training mobile phone applications may also provide a convenient and user-friendly alternative to online computer games tools.

Social engagements and networks provide a setting for emotional support and together these psychosocial factors are known to prevent cognitive decline.[8] However, social isolation is common in the elderly and factors such as depression, income and loss of a loved one may prevent participation in **social activities**.[113] A systematic review found an association between social isolation in the elderly and cognitive decline, nutritional deficiencies, coronary heart disease and the common cold.[113] A health practitioner is in a position to identify social isolation by asking the patient questions about family, friends and daily activities and recommend volunteering and attending social events run by the local councils and communities. In addition to psychosocial factors, immobility and bodily pain may prevent elderly patients from taking part in social activities. Encourage regular exercises such as **Tai Chi** and **yoga** to develop muscle strength, improve balance, prevent falls and improve quality of life.[114,115]

The following is a summary of non-pharmacological factors to promote cognitive retention and healthy ageing[106–115]:

- reading
- playing mental games
- crossword puzzles
- social engagement
- preventing falls
- encourage exercise
- emotional support
- improve social networks
- computer-based cognitive training
- adequate nutrition.

Dietary and lifestyle advice

Human epidemiological studies provide convincing evidence that dietary patterns practised during adulthood are important contributors to age-related cognitive decline and dementia risk.[116] Diets high in fat, especially trans and saturated fats, adversely affect cognition, while those high in fruits, vegetables, cereals and fish are associated with better cognitive function and lower risk of dementia.

The **Mediterranean diet** is purported to be particularly useful for preventing the cognitive decline associated with ageing.[117] A Mediterranean diet intervention modified to target neuroprotective effects was shown in a large study to improve global cognitive scores over an average period of 4.7 years in an older population.[117] Fibre-rich foods and wheat germ oil are rich sources of tocopherols, which act as antioxidants and have anti-inflammatory actions, preventing the risk of AD.[17] A review paper outlined blueberries, grape seed, pomegranate, walnut, coffee and ginger as promising protective foods for AD, although evidence on these foods is scarce.[118] The Mediterranean herbs *Salvia officinalis* and *Rosmarinus officinalis* with memory effects[103,105] may be added to the diet.

There is increasing evidence suggesting that cognitive impairment and dementia in older subjects might be positively influenced by a diet including seafood. A large trial ($n = 2031$; 70–74 years) found that daily fish intake was associated with a lower prevalence of poor cognitive performance, and the association between total fish intake and cognition was dose-dependent with the greatest effect seen in those consuming 75 g of fish per day. The effects were more pronounced for non-processed lean fish and fatty fish.[119] Supporting this data from a cross-sectional population-based study ($n = 1613$; 45–70 years) indicated that marine omega-3 PUFA (EPA and DHA) and fatty fish consumption are inversely related to the risk of impaired overall cognitive function and speed.[120] However, contrary to these findings another study[121] failed to find that lean fish consumption had a protective effect against dementia.

Vitamin D deficiency is associated with reduced cognitive performance in older adults.[122] Vitamin D may protect the brain by reducing inflammation, regulating calcium and reducing oxidative stress,[123] and deficiencies are associated with cognitive decline. In a large prospective population-based study in elderly individuals, vitamin D deficiency (< 50 nmol/L) or insufficiency (< 50–70 nmol/L) predicted cognitive decline (reduced MMSE scores) over an average of 4.4 years.[122] Vitamin D deficiencies need to be rectified not only to possibly prevent cognitive decline but also other adverse events including falls. When combined with calcium, high doses of vitamin D (> 800 IU per day) reduces the risk of falls in elderly women and this may in turn prevent immobilisation and subsequent social isolation.[16]

A systematic review of the published literature reported that a variety of meditation techniques including transcendental meditation (TM), mindfulness, mental relaxation[124] (MR), Kirtan Kriya and Vipassana showed positive effects on attention, memory, executive function, processing speed and general cognition.[124] Meditation interventions varied from 12 minutes daily for eight weeks (Kirtan Kriya) to 20–30 minutes three times per week (TM and MR) and in more experienced meditators with > 10 years' experience (Vihangam yoga). Since adequate cognitive function is required for meditation, it might not be suitable for patients with AD.[124] Finally, a systematic review of 10 articles reported evidence that air pollution may be associated with cognitive decline; however, longitudinal studies are essential for strengthening this evidence.[125]

Physical activity

Regular **exercise** can be a protective factor for cognitive decline and dementia. Compared with no exercise, regular physical activity was associated with lower risks of cognitive impairment and dementia, particularly AD.[126] This suggests that regular physical activity may be an important protective factor for cognitive decline and dementia in the elderly. Exercise programs have positive effects on executive functioning in older adults[127] and in individuals with mild cognitive impairments.[128] Based on recent reviews of the literature, aerobic fitness training[129] and a six-week exercise regime consisting of at least three 60-minute sessions may have positive effects on cognitive functioning in older individuals.[130] Further, a two-year lifestyle-based intervention which included advice on a healthy diet, exercise (strength training 1–3 times a week and aerobic exercise 2–5 times a week), cognitive training, and monitoring vascular risk was shown to have positive effects on cognitive function (executive functioning and processing speed) and reduce risks for cognitive decline[38]

Homeopathy

Authors of a Cochrane review evaluating the safety and efficacy profile of homeopathic treatments in dementia failed to find any randomised trials with a sample size of more than 20; hence, the authors concluded that there was insufficient evidence to comment on the use of homeopathy in treating dementia.[131]

Compliance issues

Not complying with medical regimes can have detrimental effects on the health and quality of life of the elderly.[132] A recent systematic review noted common obstacles to medication non-compliance including poor health literacy, poor cognitive function, polypharmacy, adverse drug effects, lack of social support and the patient–health practitioner relationship.[132] Support of the patient in resolving or minimising these modifiable obstacles to increase treatment adherence is required to ensure naturopathic treatment protocols will be adhered to, especially when the patient is also taking conventional medicines.

To get an account of the patient's understanding of the treatment regimen and compliance, ask them to repeat the treatment regimen, address any possible challenges they might experience with incorporating the treatment regimen into their current lifestyle (such as cultural differences or lack of mobility) and ask the patient to return any surplus prescriptions at the next consultation. Ensure the patient's carer (family or nurse) understands the naturopathic treatment regimen and, if deemed appropriate, offer home and/or telephone consultations.

CLINICAL SUMMARY

When using evidence-based naturopathic remedies (Table 35.2), improvements in memory should be expected in patients following 4–6 weeks after commencing the treatment. When treating older individuals, refer them to their general practitioner for a full blood examination and address any nutritional deficiencies that may occur (see Figure 35.3; decision-making tree). Encourage patients to partake in social activities if socially isolated, in cognitive training and/or in online cognitive training tools. Encourage regular exercise, ideally three 60-minute sessions per week although consider possible physical limitations in patients who may be arthritic or physical pain.

Naturopathic treatments should be continued for 6–12 months and changes in cognitive function and mood, sleep and fatigue should be carefully monitored over time. Additionally, treat and monitor concomitant conditions and modify naturopathic treatment formulas accordingly. For example, change formulas based on improvements or exacerbations in sleep (hypnotics), anxiety (nervines, anxiolytics, magnesium), stress (adaptogens) and arthritic pain (anti-inflammatory, glucosamine sulfate, topical treatment such as warming liniments). Reassess the treatment protocol if deterioration is observed in cognitive functioning or mood and refer the patient to their general practitioner who may further refer on to a neuropsychologist. Be empathic to the elderly patient and ask open-ended questions to help ascertain whether they have appropriate support during life transitions. Also respect cultural differences.

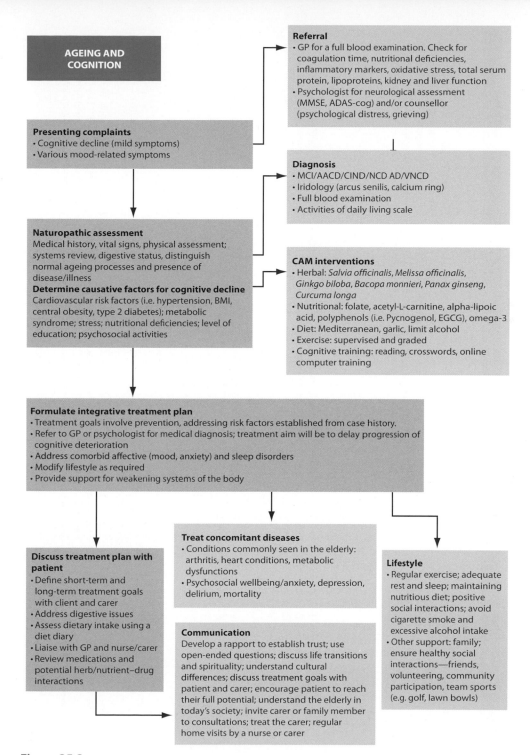

Figure 35.3
Naturopathic treatment decision tree

MCI = mild cognitive impairment, AACD = age-associated cognitive decline, CIND = cognitive impairment no dementia, NCD AD = neurocognitive disorder due to Alzheimer's disease, VNCD = vascular neurocognitive disorder.

Table 35.2
Review of the major evidence

Intervention	Mechanisms of action	Key studies	Summary of results	Comment
Ginkgo biloba	Platelet-activating factor (PAF) antagonist activity,[133] free radical scavenger activity, enhancing active choline uptake and improving cerebral blood flow[134–137]	Double-blind RCT: healthy sample Snitz et al. 2009[81] Amieva et al. 2013[83] Mix & Crews 2002[82] Double-blind RCT: Dementia Ihl et al. 2012[86] Herrschaft et al. 2012[85] Ihl 2012[89] Systematic review: Birks et al. 2009[138]	Improves cognitive functioning in AD and VaD Cognitive improvements following six weeks[82] Longitudinal studies not positive[81] Cognitive decline lower in elderly population reported using EGb 761[84]	Mixed evidence for use in dementia. In dementia, best used in combination with donepezil Mixed results for long-term effects on cognition in healthy elderly individuals without dementia
Bacopa monniera	Modulation of the cholinergic system and/or metal chelation,[67] removes β-amyloid deposits,[68] anti-inflammatory,[66] anxiolytic,[139] antidepressant,[140] adaptogenic properties[141] Suppress AChE activity[71] Modulates antioxidant enzyme activity[142]	Systematic review Pase et al., 2012[76] Double-blind RCT: Calabrese et al. 2008[73] Peth-Nui et al. 2012[71] Roodenrys et al. 2002[70] Barbhaiya et al. 2008[143] Morgan & Stevens 2010[72] Combination nutraceutical trials Cicero et al. 2016[74] Zanotta 2014[75] Open label, uncontrolled In AD patients[69]	Twelve-week supplementation in healthy older individuals • Improves learning and free recall of information[76] • Improves working memory, attention and cognitive processing in elderly[71] Effective dosages[76] KeenMind 300-400 mg; BacoMind 300-450 mg Improves attention, language writing and comprehension in AD[69] Nutraceutical combination comprising *Bacopa monnieri* improves cognition in MCI and the elderly	Chronic studies with positive effect have been on average 3 months long. One month treatment duration may not be sufficient to notice clinical effects. Clinical trials with longer administration periods are required Placebo-controlled, randomised trials using more comprehensive cognitive tools are required to assess effects in AD
Panax ginseng	Neuroprotection of ginsenoside Rg1 via attenuating cerebral amyloid beta, modulating amyloid precursor protein (APP)[144]	Double-blind RCT: Sørensen et al. 1996[97] Heo et al. 2012[98] Pilot combination study (RCT): Steiner et al. 2016[99]	Improvements seen in executive function after 8–9 weeks in older individuals[97] High-potency product improved cognitive function in AD after 12 and 24 weeks[98] *Panax ginseng*, *Ginkgo biloba* and *Crocus sativus* combination showed improvements in working memory	Acute (hours) and chronic studies show improvement in cognition, although studies on healthy older individuals and dementia are in their infancy

Table 35.2
Review of the major evidence (continued)

Intervention	Mechanisms of action	Key studies	Summary of results	Comment
Polyphenols: Berries	Antioxidant properties[54,145]	Epidemiological studies: Devore et al. 2012[54]	Diet rich in berries (blueberries and strawberries) and anthocyanidins and other flavonoid-rich foods (e.g. apples, tea, oranges and onions) lowered rate of cognitive decline in older women[54]	Large randomised controlled studies are required
Polyphenols Cocoa	Increase cerebral blood flow Decrease lipid peroxidation; decrease insulin resistance; decrease blood pressure[62]	RCTs: Sorond et al. 2008[60] Desideri et al. 2012[62] Sorond et al. 2008[60]	Two weeks flavanol-rich cocoa drink (FRC ~990 mg) increased blood flow velocity in middle cerebral artery in healthy older volunteers[60] Regular consumption of flavanol-rich cocoa drinks for eight weeks improves cognition	Regular cocoa flavanol consumption may have a promising role in the treatment of cerebrovascular ischaemic syndromes, including dementias and stroke Polyphenols found naturally in cocoa as a treatment to delay age-related cognitive decline[58–61]
Vitamins E and C	Vegetables, particularly those high in vitamins C and E, which have antioxidant properties, have also been linked to lowering the risk of AD[44]	Epidemiological studies: Morris MC et al. 1998[43] Morris MC et al. 2006[146]	High-dose vitamin E and vitamin C suplerdentation used chronically (average 4.3 years) may lower the risk of AD in elderly individuals aged 65 years and older[43] Older subjects with greater intakes of fruits and vegetables, and the corresponding nutrients vitamin C and folate, have been shown to perform better on cognitive tests[146]	Diets high in antioxidants including vitamins E and C and fruits and vegetables are encouraged
Omega-3	Ageing is associated with decreased levels of DHA and that a high intake of omega-3 polyunsaturated fatty acids may be protective against age-related cognitive decline and decrease the risk of AD[147]	Epidemiological studies: Nurk et al. 2007[119] Kalmijn et al. 2004[120] RCTs: Stough et al. 2012[148] Freund-Levi et al. 2006[149]	Daily fish intake associated with lower prevalence of poor cognitive performance, greatest effect with 75 g fish per day[119] Fatty fish consumption related to better cognitive function and speed[120] No improvements in cognition following three-month low-dose omega-3 (252 mg/day) intervention in healthy older individuals[148] No positive effects on patients with mild to moderate AD acid (1.7 g DHA and 0.6 g EPA)[149]	Daily fish intake is recommended for preventing cognitive decline No evidence to suggest fatty fish intake prevents dementia Omega-3 supplementation studies are not positive Positive effects on visual acuity after three months[148]

Table 35.2
Review of the major evidence (continued)

Intervention	Mechanisms of action	Key studies	Summary of results	Comment
Multivitamins and B vitamins	Involved in a range of critical neurological processes	RCTs: MacPherson et al. 2012[47] Harris et al. 2012[48] Cockle et al. 2000[45] McNeill et al. 2007[150] Cochrane review: Malouf & Evans 2008[151]	Multivitamin and herbal preparation improves working memory in women at risk of cognitive decline after 16 weeks[47] and episodic memory in males after eight-week intervention[48] No effects following 6 or 12 months[45,150] Folic acid (800 µg/day) improves global cognition, memory storage and information-processing speed in elderly individuals with high homocysteine levels[151]	Multivitamins are well tolerated[47] Folic acid is well tolerated with no adverse effects[151]
Centella asiatica	Neuroprotective Anti-inflammatory Antioxidant properties[152]	RCT: Wattanathorn et al. 2008[91] Review article: Seevaratnam et al. 2012[152]	Two-month intervention period 750 mg/ daily improves working memory, alertness and calmness in elderly (mean age 65 years)[91]	Limitec placebo-controlled studies
Salvia officinalis	Activities include: antioxidant, oestrogenic and anti-inflammatory properties, inhibits butyryl and acetylcholinesterase effects[100]	Double-blind RCTs: Moss et al. 2010[101] Akhondzadeh et al. 2003[103]	Improved mood, quality of memory and secondary memory.[101] Sixteen-week treatment improves cognitive function in patients with mild to moderate dementia[103]	Positive acute and chronic effects on cognitive function
Green tea	Metal-chelating, antioxidant, anti-inflammatory and neuroprotectant properties[56,153]	Cross-sectional study: Kuriyama et al. 2006[55]	Higher green tea consumption is associated with a lower prevalence of cognitive impairment in humans	Flavanol-containing foods may be an effective part of treatment for delaying age-related cognitive deficits in normal ageing and for dementia

FURTHER READING

Anstey KJ, Low L-F. Normal cognitive changes in aging. Aust Fam Physician 2004;33(10):783.

Kure C, Timmer J, Stough C. The immunomodulatory effects of plant extracts and plant secondary metabolites on chronic neuroinflammation and cognitive aging: a mechanistic and empirical review. Front Pharmacol 2017;8:117.

Masana MF, Koyanagi A, Haro JM, et al. n-3 Fatty acids, Mediterranean diet and cognitive function in normal aging: a systematic review. Exp Gerontol 2017;91:39–50.

Noble EE, Hsu TM, Kanoski SE. Gut to brain dysbiosis: mechanisms linking western diet consumption, the microbiome, and cognitive impairment. Front Behav Neurosci 2017;11:9.

Stough C, Pase MP. Improving cognition in the elderly with nutritional supplements. Curr Dir Psychol Sci 2015;24(3):177–83.

REFERENCES

1. Baltes MM, Carstensen LL. The process of successful ageing: selection, optimization, and compensation. In: Staudinger UM, Lindenberger U, editors. Understanding human development: dialogues with lifespan psychology. Boston, London: Kluwer Academic Publishers; 2003.
2. Kumar P, Clark M, editors. Clinical medicine. 5th ed. London: WB Saunders; 2002.
3. Eliopoulos C. Gerontological nursing. 6th ed. Philadelphia: Lippincott Williams & Wilkins; 2005.
4. American Psychiatric Association. Diagnostic and statistical manual of mental disorders: DSM-5. 5th ed. Washington, DC: American Psychiatric Association; 2013.
5. Murtagh J. General practice. 4th ed. Sydney: McGraw-Hill Australia; 2006.
6. Yen L, Jowsey T, McRae IS. Consultations with complementary and alternative medicine practitioners by older Australians: results from a national survey. BMC Complement Altern Med 2013;13(1):73.
7. Montorio I, Izal M. The geriatric depression scale: a review of its development and utility. Int Psychogeriatr 1996;8(1):103–12.
8. Brownie S. Why are elderly individuals at risk of nutritional deficiency? Int J Nurs Pract 2006;12(2):110–18.
9. Hendrie HC, Albert MS, Butters MA, et al. The NIH cognitive and emotional health project. Alzheimers Dement 2006;2(1):12–32.
10. Baddeley A. The episodic buffer: a new component of working memory? Trends Cogn Sci 2000;4(11):417–23.
11. Lezak MD. Neuropsychological assessment. 5th ed. New York: Oxford University Press; 2012.
12. Anstey KJ, Low LF. Normal cognitive changes in aging. Aust Fam Physician 2004;33(10):783–7.
13. Hoogendam YY, Hofman A, van der Geest JN, et al. Patterns of cognitive function in aging: the Rotterdam Study. Eur J Epidemiol 2014;29(2):133–40.
14. Qualls SH, Smyer MA. Changes in decision-making capacity in older adults: assessment and intervention. John Wiley & Sons; 2008.
15. Gennari C. Calcium and vitamin D nutrition and bone disease of the elderly. Public Health Nutr 2001;4(2b):547–59.
16. Murad MH, Elamin KB, Abu Elnour NO, et al. Clinical review: the effect of vitamin D on falls: a systematic review and meta-analysis. J Clin Endocrinol Metab 2011;96(10):2997–3006.
17. Remacle C. Functional foods, ageing and degenerative disease. Cambridge: Woodhead Publishing Limited; 2004.
18. Mills S, Bone K. Principles and Practice of Phytotherapy. 2nd ed. London: Churchill Livingston; 2013.
19. Campbell AJ, Reinken J, McCosh L. Incontinence in the elderly: prevalence and prognosis. Age Ageing 1985;14(2):65–70.
20. Gooneratne NS. Complementary and alternative medicine for sleep disturbances in older adults. Clin Geriatr Med 2008;24(1):121–38.
21. Thal DR, Del Tredici K, Braak H. Neurodegeneration in normal brain aging and disease. Sci Aging Knowledge Environ 2004;23:26.
22. Akhtar S, Moulin CJ, Bowie PC. Are people with mild cognitive impairment aware of the benefits of errorless learning? Neuropsychol Rehabil 2006;16(3):329–46.
23. Palmer K, Backman L, Winblad B, et al. Early symptoms and signs of cognitive deficits might not always be detectable in persons who develop Alzheimer's disease. Int Psychogeriatr 2008;20(2):252–8.
24. Flicker L. Vascular factors in geriatric psychiatry: time to take a serious look. Curr Opin Psychiatry 2008;21(6):551–4.
25. Whitmer RA, Gustafson DR, Barrett-Connor E, et al. Central obesity and increased risk of dementia more than three decades later. Neurology 2008;71(14):1057–64.

26. Jagust W, Harvey D, Mungas D, et al. Central obesity and the aging brain. Arch Neurol 2005;62(10):1545–8.

27. Xu G, Liu X, Yin Q, et al. Alcohol consumption and transition of mild cognitive impairment to dementia. Psychiatry Clin Neurosci 2009;63(1):43–9.

28. Whitmer RA. Type 2 diabetes and risk of cognitive impairment and dementia. Curr Neurol Neurosci Rep 2007;7(5):373–80.

29. Qiu C, Fratiglioni L. A major role for cardiovascular burden in age-related cognitive decline. Nat Rev Cardiol 2015;12(5):267.

30. Pedelty L, Gorelick PB. Management of Hypertension and Cerebrovascular Disease in the Elderly. Am J Med 2008;121(8):S23–31.

31. Milionis HJ, Florentin M, Giannopoulos S. Metabolic syndrome and Alzheimer's disease: a link to a vascular hypothesis? CNS Spectr 2008;13(7):606–13.

32. Caracciolo B, Xu W, Collins S, et al. Cognitive decline, dietary factors and gut–brain interactions. Mech Ageing Dev 2014;136–7:59–69.

33. Noble EE, Hsu TM, Kanoski SE. Gut to brain dysbiosis: mechanisms linking western diet consumption, the microbiome, and cognitive impairment. Front Behav Neurosci 2017;11:9.

34. Grutzendler J, Morris JC. Cholinesterase inhibitors for Alzheimer's disease. Drugs 2001;61(1):41–52.

35. Mukherjee PK, Kumar V, Mal M, et al. Acetylcholinesterase inhibitors from plants. Phytomedicine 2007;14:289–300.

36. Pratt RD, Perdomo CA, Surick IW, et al. Donepezil: tolerability and safety in Alzheimer's disease. Int J Clin Pract 2002;56(9):710–17.

37. Houghton PJ, Howes MJ. Natural products and derivatives affecting neurotransmission relevant to Alzheimer's and Parkinson's disease. Neurosignals 2005;14(1–2):6–22.

38. Ngandu T, Lehtisalo J, Solomon A, et al. A 2 year multidomain intervention of diet, exercise, cognitive training, and vascular risk monitoring versus control to prevent cognitive decline in at-risk elderly people (FINGER): a randomised controlled trial. Lancet 2015;385(9984):2255–63.

39. McGuinness B, O'Hare J, Craig D, et al. Cochrane review on 'Statins for the treatment of dementia'. Int J Geriatr Psychiatry 2013;28(2):119–26.

40. Desai AK, Grossberg GT. Diagnosis and treatment of Alzheimer's disease. Neurology 2005;64(12):S34–9.

41. Mariani E, Polidori MC, Cherubini A, et al. Oxidative stress in brain aging, neurodegenerative and vascular diseases: an overview. J Chromatogr B 2005;827(1):65–75.

42. Polidori MC. Antioxidant micronutrients in the prevention of age-related diseases. J Postgrad Med 2003;49(3):229–35.

43. Morris MC, Beckett LA, Scherr PA, et al. Vitamin E and vitamin C supplement use and risk of incident Alzheimer disease. Alzheimer Dis Assoc Disord 1998;12(3):121–6.

44. Engelhart M, Geerlings MI, Ruitenberg A, et al. Dietary intake of antioxidants and risk of Alzheimer disease. JAMA 2002;287(24):3223–9.

45. Cockle SM, Haller J, Kimber S, et al. The influence of multivitamins on cognitive function and mood in the elderly. Aging Ment Health 2000;4(4):339–53.

46. McNeill G, Avenell A, Campbell MK, et al. Effect of multivitamin and multimineral supplementation on cognitive function in men and women aged 65 years and over: a randomised controlled trial. Nutr J 2007;6(10):1–5.

47. Macpherson H, Ellis K, Sali A, et al. Memory improvements in elderly women following 16 weeks treatment with a combined multivitamin, mineral and herbal supplement. Psychopharmacology (Berl) 2012;220(2):351–65.

48. Harris E, MacPherson H, Vitetta L, et al. Effects of a multivitamin, mineral and herbal supplement on cognition and blood biomarkers in older men: a randomised, placebo-controlled trial. Hum Psychopharmacol 2012;27(4):370–7.

49. Bragin V, Chemodanova M, Dzhafarova N, et al. Integrated treatment approach improves cognitive function in demented and clinically depressed patients. Am J Alzheimers Dis Other Demen 2005;20(1):21–6.

50. Ryan J, Croft K, Mori T, et al. An examination of the effects of the antioxidant Pycnogenol® on cognitive performance, serum lipid profile, endocrinological and oxidative stress biomarkers in an elderly population. J Psychopharmacol 2008;22(5):553–62.

51. Belcaro G, Luzzi R, Dugall M, et al. Pycnogenol® improves cognitive function, attention, mental performance and specific professional skills in healthy professionals age 35–55. J Neurosurg Sci 2014;58(4):239–48.

52. Tang M, Taghibiglou C. The mechanisms of action of curcumin in Alzheimer's disease. J Alzheimers Dis 2017;58(4):1003–16.

53. Cox KHM, Pipingas A, Scholey AB. Investigation of the effects of solid lipid curcumin on cognition and mood in a healthy older population. J Psychopharmacol 2015;29(5):642–51.

54. Devore EE, Kang JH, Breteler MMB, et al. Dietary intakes of berries and flavonoids in relation to cognitive decline. Ann Neurol 2012;72(1):135–43.

55. Kuriyama S, Hozawa A, Ohmori K, et al. Green tea consumption and cognitive function: a cross-sectional study from the Tsurugaya Project 1. Am J Clin Nutr 2006;83(2):355–61.

56. Choi Y, Jung C, Lee S, et al. The green tea polyphenol (-)-epigallocatechin gallate attenuates beta-amyloid-induced neurotoxicity in cultured hippocampal neurons. Life Sci 2001;70(4):603–14.

57. Weinreb O, Amit T, Youdim MBH. The application of proteomics for studying the neurorescue activity of the polyphenol (-)-epigallocatechin-3-gallate. Arch Biochem Biophys 2008;476(2):152–60.

58. Bisson JF, Nejdi A, Rozan P, et al. Effects of long-term administration of a cocoa polyphenolic extract (Acticoa powder) on cognitive performances in aged rats. Br J Nutr 2008;100(1):94–101.

59. Faridi Z, Njike VY, Dutta S, et al. Acute dark chocolate and cocoa ingestion and endothelial function: a randomized controlled crossover trial. Am J Clin Nutr 2008;88(1):58–63.

60. Sorond FA, Lipsitz LA, Hollenberg NK, et al. Cerebral blood flow response to flavanol-rich cocoa in healthy elderly humans. Neuropsychiatr Dis Treat 2008;4(2):433–40.

61. Francis ST, Head K, Morris PG, et al. The effect of flavanol-rich cocoa on the fMRI response to a cognitive task in healthy young people. J Cardiovasc Pharmacol 2006;47:S215–20.

62. Desideri G, Kwik-Uribe C, Grassi D, et al. Benefits in cognitive function, blood pressure, and insulin resistance through cocoa flavanol consumption in elderly subjects with mild cognitive impairment: the cocoa, cognition, and aging (CoCoA) study. Hypertension 2012;60(3):794–801.

63. Nolidin K, Kure C, Scholey A, et al. Coffee and cognition: extending our understanding beyond caffeine. In: Bagchi D, Moriyama H, Swaroop A, editors. Green coffee bean extract in human health. CRC Press; 2016.

64. Camfield DA, Silber BY, Scholey AB, et al. A randomised placebo-controlled trial to differentiate the acute cognitive

and mood effects of chlorogenic acid from decaffeinated coffee. PLoS ONE 2013;8(12):e82897.

65. Sun YX, Minthon L, Wallmark A, et al. Inflammatory markers in matched plasma and cerebrospinal fluid from patients with Alzheimer's disease. Dement Geriatr Cogn Disord 2003;16(3):136–44.

66. Channa S, Dar A, Anjum S, et al. Anti-inflammatory activity of Bacopa monniera in rodents. J Ethnopharmacol 2006;104(1–2):286–9.

67. Stough C, Downey LA, Lloyd J, et al. Examining the nootropic effects of a special extract of Bacopa monniera on human cognitive functioning: 90 Day double-blind placebo-controlled randomized trial. Phytother Res 2008;22(12):1629–34.

68. Holcomb LA, Dhanasekaran M, Hitt AR, et al. Bacopa monniera extract reduces amyloid levels in PSAPP mice. J Alzheimers Dis 2006;9(3):243–51.

69. Goswami S, Saoji A, Kumar N, et al. Effect of Bacopa monniera on cognitive functions in Alzheimer's disease patients. Int J Collaborat Res Intern Med Public Health 2011;3(4):285–93.

70. Roodenrys S, Booth D, Bulzomi S. Chronic effects of Brahmi (Bacopa monnieri) on human memory. Neuropsychopharmacology 2002;27(2):279–81.

71. Peth-Nui T, Wattanathorn J, Muchimapura S, et al. Effects of 12-week bacopa monniera consumption on attention, cognitive processing, working memory, and functions of both cholinergic and monoaminergic systems in healthy elderly volunteers. Evid Based Complement Alternat Med 2012.

72. Morgan A, Stevens J. Does bacopa monnieri improve memory performance in older persons? Results of a randomized, placebo-controlled, double-blind trial. J Altern Complement Med 2010;16(7):753–9.

73. Calabrese C, Gregory WL, Leo M. Effects of standardized Bacopa monnieri extract on cognitive performance, anxiety, and depression in the elderly: a randomized, double-blind, placebo-controlled trial. J Altern Complement Med 2008;14(6):707–13.

74. Cicero A, Bove M, Colletti A, et al. Short-term impact of a combined nutraceutical on cognitive function, perceived stress and depression in young elderly with cognitive impairment: a pilot, double-blind, randomized clinical trial. J Prev Alzheimers Dis 2016;4:12–15.

75. Zanotta D, Puricelli S, Bonoldi G. Cognitive effects of a dietary supplement made from extract of Bacopa monnieri, astaxanthin, phosphatidylserine, and vitamin E in subjects with mild cognitive impairment: a noncomparative, exploratory clinical study. Neuropsychiatr Dis Treat 2014;10:225–30.

76. Pase MP, Kean J, Sarris J, et al. The cognitive-enhancing effects of bacopa monnieri: a systematic review of randomized, controlled human clinical trials. J Altern Complement Med 2012;18(7):647–52.

77. Stough C, Lloyd J, Clarke J, et al. The chronic effects of an extract of Bacopa monniera (Brahmi) on cognitive function in healthy human subjects. Psychopharmacology (Berl) 2001;156(4):481–4.

78. Alagiakrishnan K, McCracken P, Feldman H. Treating vascular risk factors and maintaining vascular health: is this the way towards successful cognitive ageing and preventing cognitive decline? Postgrad Med J 2006;82(964):101–5.

79. Reynolds NC Jr, Hellman RS, Tikofsky RS, et al. Single photon emission computerized tomography (SPECT) in detecting neurodegeneration in Huntington's disease. Nucl Med Commun 2002;23(1):13–18.

80. Reynolds J, Hamill R, Ellithorpe R, et al. Retarding Cognitive decline with science-based nutraceuticals. JANA 2008;11(1):23–31.

81. Snitz BE, O'Meara ES, Carlson MC, et al. Ginkgo biloba for preventing cognitive decline in older adults a randomized trial. JAMA 2009;302(24):2663–70.

82. Mix JA, Crews WD Jr. A double-blind, placebo-controlled, randomized trial of Ginkgo biloba extract EGb 761® in a sample of cognitively intact older adults: neuropsychological findings. Hum Psychopharmacol 2002;17(6):267–77.

83. Amieva H, Meillon C, Helmer C, et al. Ginkgo biloba extract and long-term cognitive decline: a 20-year follow-up population-based study. PLoS ONE 2013;8(1):e52755. doi:10.1371/journal.pone.0052755.

84. Gavrilova S, Preuss U, Wong J, et al. Efficacy and safety of Ginkgo biloba extract EGb 761® in mild cognitive impairment with neuropsychiatric symptoms: a randomized, placebo-controlled, double-blind, multi-center trial. Int J Geriatr Psychiatry 2014;29(10):1087–95.

85. Herrschaft H, Nacu A, Likhachev S, et al. Ginkgo biloba extract EGb 761® in dementia with neuropsychiatric features: a randomised, placebo-controlled trial to confirm the efficacy and safety of a daily dose of 240 mg. J Psychiatr Res 2012;46(6):716–23.

86. Ihl R, Tribanek M, Bachinskaya N. Efficacy and tolerability of a once daily formulation of Ginkgo biloba extract EGb 761® in Alzheimer's disease and vascular dementia: results from a randomised controlled trial. Pharmacopsychiatry 2012;45(2):41–6.

87. Wettstein A. Cholinesterase inhibitors and Gingko extracts-are they comparable in the treatment of dementia? Comparison of published placebo-controlled efficacy studies of at least six months' duration. Phytomedicine 2000;6(6):393–401.

88. Le Bars PL, Kieser M, Itil KZ. A 26-week analysis of a double-blind, placebo-controlled trial of the ginkgo biloba extract EGb 761 in dementia. Dement Geriatr Cogn Disord 2000;11(4):230–7.

89. Ihl R. Gingko biloba extract EGb 761®: clinical data in dementia. Int Psychogeriatr 2012;24(S1):S35–40.

90. Dhanasekaran M, Holcomb LA, Hitt AR, et al. Centella asiatica extract selectively decreases amyloid β levels in hippocampus of Alzheimer's disease animal model. Phytother Res 2009;23(1):14–19.

91. Wattanathorn J, Mator L, Muchimapura S, et al. Positive modulation of cognition and mood in the healthy elderly volunteer following the administration of Centella asiatica. J Ethnopharmacol 2008;116(2):325–32.

92. Atwood CS, Huang X, Moir RD, et al. Role of free radicals and metal ions in the pathogenesis of Alzheimer's disease. Met Ions Biol Syst 1999;36:309–64.

93. Cuajungco MP, Faget KY, Huang X, et al. Metal chelation as a potential therapy for Alzheimer's disease. Ann N Y Acad Sci 2000;920(1):292–304.

94. Hatcher H, Planalp R, Cho J, et al. Curcumin: from ancient medicine to current clinical trials. Cell Mol Life Sci 2008;65(11):1631–52.

95. Tripathi YB, Chaurasia S, Tripathi E, et al. Bacopa monniera Linn. as an antioxidant: mechanism of action. Indian J Exp Biol 1996;34(6):523–6.

96. Bartres-Faz D, Junque C, Lopez A, et al. Apo E influences declarative and procedural learning in age-associated memory impairment. Neuroreport 1999;10(14):2923–7.

97. Sørensen H, Sonne J. A double-masked study of the effects of ginseng on cognitive functions. Curr Ther Res Clin Exp 1996;57(12):959–68.

98. Heo JH, Lee ST, Chu K, et al. Heat-processed ginseng enhances the cognitive function in patients with moderately severe Alzheimer's disease. Nutr Neurosci 2012;15(6):278–82.

99. Steiner GZ, Yeung A, Liu JX, et al. The effect of Sailuotong (SLT) on neurocognitive and cardiovascular function in healthy adults: a randomised, doubleblind, placebo controlled crossover pilot trial. BMC Complement Altern Med 2016;16(1).

100. Kennedy DO, Scholey AB. The psychopharmacology of European herbs with cognition-enhancing properties. Curr Pharm Des 2006;12(35):4613–23.

101. Moss L, Rouse M, Wesnes KA, et al. Differential effects of the aromas of Salvia species on memory and mood. Hum Psychopharmacol 2010;25(5):388–96.

102. Kennedy DO, Dodd FL, Robertson BC, et al. Monoterpenoid extract of sage (Salvia lavandulaefolia) with cholinesterase inhibiting properties improves cognitive performance and mood in healthy adults. J Psychopharmacol 2011;25(8):1088–100.

103. Akhondzadeh S, Noroozian M, Mohammadi M, et al. Salvia officinalis extract in the treatment of patients with mild to moderate Alzheimer's disease: a double blind, randomized and placebo-controlled trial. J Clin Pharm Ther 2003;28(1):53–9.

104. Kennedy DO, Jackson PA, Haskell CF, et al. Modulation of cognitive performance following single doses of 120 mg Ginkgo biloba extract administered to healthy young volunteers. Hum Psychopharmacol 2007;22(8):559–66.

105. Pengelly A, Snow J, Mills SY, et al. Short-term study on the effects of rosemary on cognitive function in an elderly population. J Med Food 2012;15(1):10–17.

106. Salthouse TA. Theoretical perspectives on cognitive aging. Hillsdale, NJ: Erlbaum; 1991.

107. Wilson RS, Scherr PA, Schneider JA, et al. Relation of cognitive activity to risk of developing Alzheimer disease. Neurology 2007;69(20):1911–20.

108. Wilson RS, Mendes De Leon CF, Barnes LL, et al. Participation in cognitively stimulating activities and risk of incident Alzheimer disease. JAMA 2002;287(6):742–8.

109. Sitzer DI, Twamley EW, Jeste DV. Cognitive training in Alzheimer's disease: a meta-analysis of the literature. Acta Psychiatr Scand 2006;114(2):75–90.

110. Willis SL, Tennstedt SL, Marsiske M, et al. Long-term effects of cognitive training on everyday functional outcomes in older adults. JAMA 2006;296(23):2805–14.

111. Simpson T, Camfield D, Pipingas A, et al. Improved processing speed: online computer-based cognitive training in older adults. Educ Gerontol 2012;38(7):445–58.

112. Bozoki A, Radovanovic M, Winn B, et al. Effects of a computer-based cognitive exercise program on age-related cognitive decline. Arch Gerontol Geriatr 2013;57(1):1–7.

113. Nicholson NR. A review of social isolation: an important but underassessed condition in older adults. J Prim Prev 2012;33(2–3):137–52.

114. Patel NK, Newstead AH, Ferrer RL. The effects of yoga on physical functioning and health related quality of life in older adults: a systematic review and meta-analysis. J Altern Complement Med 2012;18(10):902–17.

115. Tsang HWH, Leung DPK, Chan CKL, et al. Tai chi as an intervention to improve balance and reduce falls in older adults: a systematic and meta-analytical review. Altern Ther Health Med 2011;17(1):40–8.

116. Parrott MD, Greenwood CE. Dietary influences on cognitive function with aging: from high-fat diets to healthful eating. Ann N Y Acad Sci 2007;1114(1):389–97.

117. Morris MC, Tangney CC, Wang Y, et al. MIND diet slows cognitive decline with aging. Alzheimers Dement 2015;11(9):1015–22.

118. Essa MM, Vijayan RK, Castellano-Gonzalez G, et al. Neuroprotective effect of natural products against Alzheimer's disease. Neurochem Res 2012;37(9):1829–42.

119. Nurk E, Drevon CA, Refsum H, et al. Cognitive performance among the elderly and dietary fish intake: the Hordaland Health Study. Am J Clin Nutr 2007;86(5):1470–8.

120. Kalmijn S, Van Boxtel MPJ, Ocké M, et al. Dietary intake of fatty acids and fish in relation to cognitive performance at middle age. Neurology 2004;62(2):275–80.

121. Huang TL, Zandi PP, Tucker KL, et al. Benefits of fatty fish on dementia risk are stronger for those without APOE epsilon4. Neurology 2005;65(9):1409–14.

122. Toffanello ED, Coin A, Perissinotto E, et al. Vitamin D deficiency predicts cognitive decline in older men and women The Pro. VA Study. Neurology 2014;83(24):2292–8.

123. Buell JS, Dawson-Hughes B. Vitamin D and neurocognitive dysfunction: preventing "D"ecline? Mol Aspects Med 2008;29(6):415–22.

124. Gard T, Hölzel BK, Lazar SW. The potential effects of meditation on age-related cognitive decline: a systematic review. Ann N Y Acad Sci 2014;1307(1):89–103.

125. Peters R, Peters J, Booth A, et al. Is air pollution associated with increased risk of cognitive decline? A systematic review. Age Ageing 2015;44(5):755–60.

126. Laurin D, Verreault R, Lindsay J, et al. Physical activity and risk of cognitive impairment and dementia in elderly persons. Arch Neurol 2001;58(3):498–504.

127. Colcombe S, Kramer AF. Fitness effects on the cognitive function of older adults: a meta-analytic study. Psychol Sci 2003;14(2):125–30.

128. Heyn PC, Johnson KE, Kramer AF. Endurance and strength training outcomes on cognitively impaired and cognitively intact older adults: a meta-analysis. J Nutr Health Aging 2008;12(6):401–9.

129. Hillman CH, Erickson KI, Kramer AF. Be smart, exercise your heart: exercise effects on brain and cognition. Nat Rev Neurosci 2008;9(1):58–65.

130. Tseng C-N, Gau B-S, Lou M-F. The effectiveness of exercise on improving cognitive function in older people: a systematic review. J Nurs Res 2011;19(2):119–31.

131. McCarney R, Warner J, Fisher P, et al. Homeopathy for dementia. Cochrane Database Syst Rev 2003;(1):CD003803.

132. Gellad WF, Grenard JL, Marcum ZA. A systematic review of barriers to medication adherence in the elderly: looking beyond cost and regimen complexity. Am J Geriatr Pharmacother 2011;9(1):11–23.

133. Smith PF, Maclennan K, Darlington CL. The neuroprotective properties of the Ginkgo biloba leaf: a review of the possible relationship to platelet-activating factor (PAF). J Ethnopharmacol 1996;50(3):131–9.

134. Krištofiková Z. In vitro effect of Ginkgo biloba extract (EGb 761) on the activity of presynaptic cholinergic nerve terminals in rat hippocampus. Dement Geriatr Cogn Disord 1997;8(1):43–8.

135. Nathan P. Can the cognitive enhancing effects of Ginkgo biloba be explained by its pharmacology? Med Hypotheses 2000;55(6):491–3.

136. Maitra I, Marcocci L, Droy-Lefaix MT, et al. Peroxyl radical scavenging activity of Ginkgo biloba extract EGb 761. Biochem Pharmacol 1995;49(11):1649–55.

137. Zhang SJ, Xue ZY. Effect of Western medicine therapy assisted by Ginkgo biloba tablet on vascular cognitive impairment of none dementia. Asian Pac J Trop Med 2012;5(8):661–4.

138. Birks J, Grimley Evans J. Ginkgo biloba for cognitive impairment and dementia. Cochrane Database Syst Rev 2009;(1):CD003120.

139. Bhattacharya SK, Ghosal S. Anxiolytic activity of a standardized extract of Bacopa monniera: an experimental study. Phytomedicine 1998;5(2):77–82.

140. Sairam K, Dorababu M, Goel RK, et al. Antidepressant activity of standardized extract of Bacopa monniera in experimental models of depression in rats. Phytomedicine 2002;9(3):207–11.

141. Rai D, Bhatia G, Palit G, et al. Adaptogenic effect of Bacopa monniera (Brahmi). Pharmacol Biochem Behav 2003;75(4):823–30.

142. Priyanka HP, Singh RV, Mishra M, et al. Diverse age-related effects of Bacopa monnieri and donepezil in vitro on cytokine production, antioxidant enzyme activities, and intracellular targets in splenocytes of F344 male rats. Int Immunopharmacol 2013;15(2):260–74.

143. Barbhaiya HC, Desai RP, Saxena VS, et al. Efficacy and tolerability of BacoMind® on memory improvement in elderly participants - A double blind placebo controlled study. J Pharmacol Toxicol 2008;3(6):425–34.

144. Fang F, Chen X, Huang T, et al. Multi-faced neuroprotective effects of Ginsenoside Rg1 in an Alzheimer mouse model. Biochim Biophys Acta 2012;1822(2):286–92.

145. Mishra S, Palanivelu K. The effect of curcumin (turmeric) on Alzheimer's disease: an overview. Ann Indian Acad Neurol 2008;11(1):13–19.

146. Morris MC, Evans DA, Tangney CC, et al. Associations of vegetable and fruit consumption with age-related cognitive change. Neurology 2006;67(8):1370–6.

147. Uauy R, Dangour AD. Nutrition in brain development and aging: role of essential fatty acids. Nutr Rev 2006;64(S2): S24–33.

148. Stough C, Downey L, Silber B, et al. The effects of 90-day supplementation with the Omega-3 essential fatty acid docosahexaenoic acid (DHA) on cognitive function and visual acuity in a healthy aging population. Neurobiol Aging 2012;33(4):824.e1–3.

149. Freund-Levi Y, Eriksdotter-Jönhagen M, Cederholm T, et al. Omega-3 fatty acid treatment in 174 patients with mild to moderate Alzheimer disease: OmegAD study—A randomized double-blind trial. Arch Neurol 2006;63(10):1402–8.

150. McNeill G, Avenell A, Campbell MK, et al. Effect of multivitamin and multimineral supplementation on cognitive function in men and women aged 65 years and over: a randomised controlled trial. Nutr J 2007;6(10):1–5.

151. Malouf R, Grimley Evans J. Folic acid with or without vitamin B12 for the prevention and treatment of healthy elderly and demented people. Cochrane Database Syst Rev 2008;(4):CD004514.

152. Seevaratnam V, Banumathi P, Premalatha MR, et al. Functional properties of Centella asiatica (L.): a review. Int J Pharm Pharm Sci 2012;4(S5):8–14.

153. Weinreb O, Amit T, Youdim MBH. A novel approach of proteomics and transcriptomics to study the mechanism of action of the antioxidant—iron chelator green tea polyphenol (-)-epigallocatechin-3-gallate. Free Radic Biol Med 2007;43(4):546–56.

CHAPTER 36

Bipolar disorder

James Lake
MD

OVERVIEW

Bipolar disorder is a heritable mental illness. Approximately 1% of American adults experience persisting mood swings and fulfil criteria for a diagnosis of bipolar disorder.[1] First-degree relatives of bipolar individuals are significantly more likely to develop the disorder than the population at large. Bipolar illness in one identical twin corresponds to a 70% risk that the other twin will also have the disorder and the concordance risk is estimated at 15% in non-identical twins.[2]

The aetiology of bipolar disorder is multifactorial and many genetic, neurobiological and immunological factors probably contribute to the risk of developing this disorder. Recent findings suggest that decreased expression of RNA coding may lead to mitochondrial dysfunction, resulting in dysregulation of brain energy metabolism and increased oxidative stress associated with increased risk of developing bipolar disorder.[3] Natural product therapies that address this problem are being investigated. Acute mania may be associated with abnormal immune activation indicated by elevated levels of cytokines such as TNF-α, inflammatory macromolecules, antibodies to infectious agents, food antigens and brain proteins.[4,5] Emerging understandings of complex relationships between immune function and bipolar disorder may lead to a new class of drugs aimed at both preventing and treating bipolar disorder by modulating the immune system.

Dysregulations in hypothalamic circuits involved in maintaining normal circadian rhythms probably cause the affective and behavioural symptoms described in Western psychiatric nosology as bipolar disorder I and bipolar disorder II. Findings from functional neuroimaging studies suggest that abnormal prefrontal modulation of amygdala activation may result in both phases of bipolar disorder.[6,7] Acutely manic patients frequently have abnormal electroencephalogram (EEG) activity, which may predict responsiveness to conventional pharmacological treatments.[8] Folate deficiency has also been observed in both phases of bipolar disorder; however, the role of folate in the pathogenesis of bipolar disorder has not yet been elucidated.[9]

According to conventional psychiatric nosology, mania is a complex symptom pattern that may encompass disparate affective, behavioural and cognitive symptoms, including pressured speech, racing thoughts, euphoric or irritable mood, agitation, inflated self-esteem, distractibility, excessive or inappropriate involvement in pleasurable activities, increased goal-directed activity, diminished need for sleep and, in severe cases, psychosis.[10] According to the *Diagnostic and Statistical Manual of Mental Disorders* (DSM-5) a manic episode is diagnosed when elevated or irritable mood persists for at least one week (or less if hospitalisation is necessary), is accompanied by at least three of the above symptoms (four if only irritable), is associated with severe social or occupational impairment and cannot be adequately explained by a pre-existing medical or psychiatric disorder or the effects of substance abuse. In contrast to frank mania, the diagnosis of a hypomanic episode requires: sustained irritable or euphoric mood lasting at least four days but does not cause severe impairment in social or occupational functioning; three or more of the above symptoms; and exclusion of medical or psychiatric disorders that may manifest as these symptoms. According to the DSM-5, bipolar I is diagnosed when an individual has experienced one or more manic episodes, while one or more hypomanic episodes are required for a diagnosis of bipolar II disorder. Bipolar I disorder can be diagnosed after only one manic episode; however, the typical bipolar I patient has had several manic episodes, and at least 80% of patients who experience mania will have recurring manic episodes.[11] According to the DSM-5 a history of depressive episodes is not required for a formal diagnosis of bipolar I disorder. In contrast, bipolar II disorder can be diagnosed only in cases when at least one hypomanic episode and at least one depressive episode have been documented. In both disorders moderate or severe depressive episodes typically alternate with manic symptoms; however, in 'mixed mania' symptoms of mania and depressed mood overlap. Another variant called rapid cycling is diagnosed when at least four complete cycles of depressed mood and mania occur during any 12-month period. A mild variant of bipolar disorder is called cyclothymic disorder. Cyclothymic disorder is diagnosed when several hypomanic and depressive episodes take place over a two-year period in the absence of severe manic, mixed or depressive episodes. It is estimated that individuals diagnosed with bipolar I disorder are symptomatic approximately 50% of the time. Bipolar patients experience depressive symptoms three times more often than mania, and five times more often than rapid cycling or mixed episodes.[12]

Distinguishing between transient episodes of mania and acute agitation caused by another psychiatric disorder or a primary medical disorder can pose diagnostical challenges. A careful history is needed to establish a persisting pattern of mood symptoms fluctuating between depression and mania or hypomania. Conventional laboratory tests and functional brain imaging studies are used to rule out the presence of neurological or other medical disorders that can mimic symptoms of depressed mood or mania including, for example, thyroid disease, strokes (especially in the right frontal area of the brain), multiple sclerosis (rarely), seizure disorders and other neurological

DIFFERENTIAL DIAGNOSIS

- Unipolar depression (for depressive phase)
- Organic disease or disorder (e.g. brain injury, tumour)
- Schizoaffective disorder
- Personality disorder
- Medication or recreational drug side effect

Source: Vieta & Phillips 2007[13]

disorders. Irritability or euphoria alternating with periods of depressed mood is often associated with chronic abuse of stimulants, marijuana or other drugs. It is often difficult to establish a primary diagnosis of bipolar disorder after ruling out pre-existing psychiatric or medical disorders because of the variety of symptoms that can take place during a manic episode. For example, symptoms of irritability, agitation and emotional lability are frequent concomitants of chronic drug or alcohol abuse, psychotic disorders and personality disorders. Furthermore acutely manic patients frequently experience psychotic symptoms including auditory hallucinations, delusions, paranoia and derailed thinking, making it difficult to distinguish bipolar mania from schizophrenia or other psychotic disorders, especially when there is limited information about a patient's history.

RISK FACTORS

Several risk factors contribute to the rate of relapse and response to treatment in patients diagnosed with bipolar disorder. A diagnosis of bipolar disorder is one of the largest risk factors for suicide.[14] Fewer than half of patients who take conventional maintenance treatments following an initial manic episode report sustained control of their symptoms.[15] Furthermore, as many as 40% of bipolar patients who adhere to pharmacological treatment experience recurring manic or depressive mood swings while taking medications at recommended doses.[15] As many as one-quarter of bipolar I patients attempt suicide, and many eventually succeed. Treatment of bipolar disorder should be maintained on a consistent, long-term basis to reduce the rate of re-hospitalisation and increase chances of full remission.[16] Failure to initiate effective treatment that is well tolerated in the early stages of illness significantly increases the risk of relapse associated increased risk of suicide.[17] In patients diagnosed with bipolar disorder, stressors, seasonal change, reduced sleep and stimulants or recreational drug use may provoke an episode of hypomania or mania (although sometimes the trigger may not appear to have a cause).[18] Regular exercise, good nutrition, a strong social support network and a predictable, low-stress environment help reduce relapse risk.[19,20]

Obesity, diabetes and cardiovascular disease commonly occur in bipolar patients and significantly increase morbidity and mortality in this population. Cardiovascular disease is the leading cause of death in bipolar disorder, resulting in an average life expectancy 10–25 years shorter than the population at large. Bipolar patients are diagnosed with cardiovascular disease 14 years earlier on average compared with people who do not have mood disorders. Furthermore, bipolar individuals with comorbid cardiovascular disease have more frequent and more severe mood symptoms compared with medically healthy bipolar patients.[21] The association between increased risk of cardiovascular disease and bipolar disorder has not been adequately explained and may be due to chronic unhealthy lifestyle choices, the psychological stress of dealing with bipolar mood swings or a variety of primary genetic and biological factors (above). Adverse effects of medications also contribute significantly to cardiovascular risk by causing weight gain. Approximately two-thirds of patients diagnosed with bipolar disorder are overweight and one-third are obese.[22] People diagnosed with bipolar disorder exercise less and are more sedentary compared with those who are not diagnosed with serious psychiatric disorders.[23] High rates of obesity, smoking and drug and alcohol use in bipolar patients lead to high prevalence rates of diabetes, hypertension and heart disease, resulting in increased mortality compared with the general population. Clinicians should be proactive in addressing diet, smoking and lifestyle when treating patients diagnosed with bipolar disorder.

There is an established relationship between abnormal sleep and increased risk of cardiovascular disease. Short sleep duration, long sleep duration and insomnia as predictors of cardiovascular morbidity and mortality[24] and sleep disturbance is associated with increased prevalence of obesity, hypertension and diabetes mellitus that are known risk factors for cardiovascular disease.[25] Disrupted sleep and circadian rhythm disturbances are associated with increased relapse risk and poor response in bipolar disorder.[26] Exercise is helpful for both improving the quality of sleep and reducing symptoms of anxiety or agitation that may interfere with sleep.[27]

CONVENTIONAL TREATMENT

Medication

The American Psychiatric Association endorses the use of different conventional pharmacological agents including mood stabilisers (e.g. lithium carbonate and valproate), antidepressants, antipsychotics and sedative-hypnotics to treat bipolar disorder.[28] Lithium is a first-line treatment for maintenance therapy of bipolar disorder, is safe in combination with other mood-stabilising agents and antipsychotics, has neuroprotective effects, and reduces the risk of recurrence of acute mania and suicide. A drawback of chronic lithium therapy is the requirement of regular monitoring of renal function and thyroid hormone levels.[29] Anti-psychotics are used to treat agitation and psychosis, which occur frequently in acute mania.

Antipsychotics, specifically newer second-generation antipsychotics (SGA), are regarded as treatments of first choice for bipolar mania with or without psychosis. However, the potential therapeutic benefits of all antipsychotic drugs are limited by frequent potentially serious adverse effects. While so-called 'first-generation' antipsychotics were problematic because of frequent neurological adverse effects, the newer SGAs cause weight gain and metabolic adverse effects. After decades of research there is still no consensus on which particular medication should be tried first.[30] Efforts to identify an optimal pharmacological strategy have been hampered by methodological problems in recent systematic reviews including use of non-representative patient samples, short trial durations and experimental design flaws that make it difficult to generalise findings.[31,32] In response to these concerns clinical pragmatic trials (also known as 'effectiveness trials') were recently introduced to examine the effectiveness and tolerability of antipsychotics in naturalistic settings and patient populations that more accurately reflect the complex biological causes and treatment issues in individuals diagnosed with bipolar disorder or schizophrenia.[33]

Uses of prescription drugs in both bipolar mania and schizophrenia are constrained by large variations in response and tolerance in people with the same diagnosis.[34] Because of the diverse genetic and neurobiological causes of both disorders treatment with the same drug may yield broad differences in response and adverse effect tolerance.[34] The mean weight gain seen in patients taking SGAs is a few kilograms; however, inter-individual metabolic differences can increase that amount 10- to 20-fold.[35] A recent systematic review and meta-analysis of drug trials in acute mania included 68 studies on all drug classes and over 16,000 patients.[36] All drugs were found to be moderately superior to placebo by standardised symptom rating scales. Overall antipsychotics were found to be more effective than other mood stabilisers. Haloperidol, olanzapine and risperidone had the highest efficacy compared with the other drugs and olanzapine and risperidone ranked highest in terms of adverse effect tolerance. In a meta-analysis of head-to-head trials of single SGAs versus mood stabilisers in acute mania SGAs were found to be superior to other mood stabilisers in terms of both efficacy and adverse effect tolerance.[37]

Sedative hypnotics are frequently prescribed for the severe insomnia that accompanies mania as well as for daytime management of agitation and anxiety.[38] A significant percentage of bipolar patients must rely on conventional antidepressants to control depressive mood swings. Repetitive transcranial magnetic stimulation (rTMS) is an emerging treatment of both the acute manic phase and the depressive phase of bipolar disorder and does not risk mania induction; however, findings of controlled trials to date are highly inconsistent.[39] Mania associated with psychosis is approached differently from a mixed episode that includes both manic and depressive symptoms. Conventional antipsychotics are appropriate first-line treatments of the auditory hallucinations that occur during an acute manic episode, while mixed episodes are often managed using a combination of two mood stabilisers or a mood stabiliser and antipsychotic.[18] Findings of a recent meta-analysis and systematic review suggest that non-steroidal anti-inflammatory drugs have both antidepressant and anti-manic effects; however, additional studies are needed to confirm these findings, determine optimal dosing strategies and clarify potential risks.[40]

Psychotherapy and psychosocial interventions

Psychotherapy and psychosocial interventions in stable bipolar patients may potentially reduce relapse risk by providing psychological support, enhancing medication adherence and helping patients address warning signs of recurring depressive or manic episodes before more serious symptoms emerge.[41] A review of randomised studies on adjunctive psychotherapy and psychosocial interventions in bipolar patients concluded that adjunctive psychotherapy reduces symptom severity and improves functioning.[41] Family therapy and interpersonal therapy were most effective in preventing relapse when started following an acute manic or depressive episode. Cognitive behaviour therapy and group psychoeducation were effective strategies for relapse prevention when initiated during stable periods. Psychotherapies and psychosocial interventions emphasising medication adherence and early recognition of mood symptoms were more effective in preventing recurrences of mania, and cognitive and interpersonal approaches had greater success in preventing depressive relapses. A specialised psychological intervention called 'enhanced relapse prevention' is aimed at recognising and managing the early warning signs of depressive or manic episodes by improving patients' understanding of bipolar disorder, enhancing therapist–patient relationships and optimising ongoing treatment. A study using qualitative interviews found that both therapists and their bipolar patients believe that enhanced relapse prevention increases awareness of early warning signs of recurring illness, leading to effective changes in medication management and fewer relapses.[42]

Clinical considerations

- When patients present with depressed mood, be aware that this may be a depressive phase of bipolar disorder.
- Always screen for the previous or current hypomanic or manic symptoms.
- If involved in the management of a patient with bipolar hypomania or mania, be aware that a depressive mood swing may occur after the 'high' has resolved.

INTEGRATIVE MEDICAL TREATMENT OPTIONS

A significant percentage of people diagnosed with bipolar disorder use non-pharmacological modalities together with prescription medications; however, at present there is little evidence for the safety and efficacy of most non-conventional modalities.[43,44] The most appropriate and effective integrative treatment approach is determined by the type and severity of symptoms (including psychotic symptoms), the presence of comorbid medical or psychiatric disorders, response to previous treatments, patient preferences and constraints on cost and availability of treatments. When prominent symptoms of anxiety, psychosis or agitation are present, effective integrative strategies should prioritise treatment of those symptoms. For example, reasonable integrative approaches when managing an acutely manic patient who is agitated and extremely anxious include an initial loading dose of valproic acid or another conventional mood stabiliser, high-potency benzodiazepines, an antipsychotic that is sedating at bedtime (preferably a newer SGA) and possibly adjunctive use of select amino acids known to have calming or sedating effects, such as L-tryptophan, 5-HTP or L-theanine.

While CAM interventions appear to have limited activity in treating the hypomanic or manic phase of bipolar disorder,[45] they may have benefit in treating bipolar disorder depression as monotherapies or as adjuvant treatments with synthetic antidepressants.[46]

Nutrition and nutraceuticals

There is emerging evidence that diet is an important modifiable factor in mental illness including depressed mood and bipolar disorder. Nutritional influences on mental health involve several mechanisms including changes in the gut microbiome, reductions in the body's oxidative stress level and induction of epigenetic changes that indirectly affect neurotransmitters. The Mediterranean diet and other healthy diets high in polyunsaturated fats as well as fruits and vegetables rich in anti-oxidant vitamins may be associated with overall improvement in mental health and reductions in the severity of depressed mood, anxiety and other symptoms.[47] Adjunctive natural product treatments may help alleviate residual symptoms of bipolar disorder including psychotic symptoms that occur during acute mania, thereby improving outcomes of conventional drug treatment. Recent reviews of clinical trials on nutritional supplements used alone or in combination with conventional drugs in the treatment of

> ### Integrative Medical Treatment Aims
>
> - Before making a diagnosis of bipolar disorder rule out comorbid psychiatric (e.g. severe personality disorders, substance abuse, schizoaffective disorder) or medical disorders (e.g. thyroid disease, multiple sclerosis, metabolic disturbances) that may confound a primary diagnosis of bipolar disorder or interfere with treatment response.
> - Document conventional, complementary and alternative medicine (CAM) and integrative therapies that have been previously tried and responses including adverse effects.
> - Identify core symptoms causing the greatest distress or dysfunction that will be the focus of clinical attention.
> - Stabilise the patient as rapidly as possible, starting with appropriate conventional or integrative treatment protocols.
> - Always start with the most validated conventional or integrative treatment protocols (see later discussion).
> - When more substantiated modalities are not effective, consider less validated modalities, with the patient's written informed consent.
> - After hypomania or mania has resolved continue appropriate maintenance treatment, carefully monitor for relapse into a depressive phase and treat accordingly.

bipolar disorder identified inconsistent but largely positive findings for omega-3 fatty acids and chromium and limited evidence for inositol in bipolar depressed mood, and limited evidence for magnesium, folate, choline and L-tryptophan in the treatment of residual symptoms of mania.[48,49]

Countries where there is high fish consumption have relatively lower prevalence rates of bipolar disorder.[50] A meta-analysis of controlled trials on **omega-3 fatty acids** in bipolar disorder that used rigorous inclusion criteria identified only one study in which omega-3s used adjunctively with a mood stabiliser showed a differential beneficial effect on depressive but not manic symptoms.[51] The reviewers cautioned that any conclusions about the efficacy of omega-3 fatty acids in bipolar disorder must await larger controlled studies of improved methodological quality. Large doses of omega-3 fatty acids may be more effective in the depressive phase of the illness.[52] Rare cases of increased bleeding times, but not increased risk of bleeding, have been reported in patients taking aspirin or anticoagulants together with omega-3s. Some studies suggest that the omega-3 essential fatty acid eicosapentaenoic acid (EPA) may have beneficial adjuvant effects when added to certain atypical antipsychotics[53,54]; however, one placebo-controlled trial did not confirm an adjuvant effect.[55] In contrast, the appropriate management of a severely depressed bipolar patient might include an integrative regimen that combines a mood stabiliser with an antidepressant and omega-3 fatty acids.

Adding **L-tryptophan** three times a day may have beneficial effects on anxiety associated with mania.[56,57] L-tryptophan can be safely added to mood stabilisers at bedtime and may improve sleep quality in agitated manic patients. Doses as high as 15 g may be required when insomnia is severe (although this should be closely monitored, and this dosage may be restricted in some countries).[58] When added to sedating antidepressants (such as trazodone) taken at bedtime L-tryptophan may accelerate anti-depressant response and improve sleep quality.[59] Rapid tryptophan depletion has been shown to induce transient depressive mood swings in stable patients diagnosed with major depressive disorder. In a seven-day double-blind placebo-controlled pilot study 23 acutely manic patients randomised to a daily tryptophan-free amino acid drink (100 mg/day) versus placebo showed greater improvements in mania compared with the placebo group by the Young Mania Rating Scale (YMRS) and Clinical Global Impressions (CGI); however, there was a high drop-out rate due to intolerance.[60] These preliminary findings suggest that rapid tryptophan depletion may have antimanic effects. Large placebo-controlled studies are needed to confirm this finding and determine optimal, safe dosing. Safety considerations may limit the potential therapeutic benefits of this approach. Patients taking an amino acid drink for brief periods are at little risk; however, prolonged depletion of L-tryptophan (or other essential amino acids) may result in protein depletion.[61] Serious adverse effects have not been reported using this protocol.

Magnesium may be an effective adjunctive therapy for treating acute mania or rapidly cycling bipolar disorder. In a small open trial, oral magnesium supplementation had comparable efficacy to lithium in rapid-cycling bipolar patients.[62] In a small case series intravenous magnesium sulfate used adjunctively with lithium, haloperidol and a benzodiazepine in bipolar patients with severe treatment-resistant mania resulted in significant improvement in global functioning and reduction in the severity of mania.[63] Many patients treated with intravenous magnesium sulfate remained stable on lower doses of conventional medications.

A proprietary 36-ingredient formula of vitamins and minerals **(EM Power Plus)** may significantly reduce symptoms of mania, depressed mood and psychosis in bipolar patients when taken alone or used adjunctively with conventional mood stabilisers.[64–66] Researchers believe the formula works by correcting inborn metabolic errors that result in bipolar-like symptoms in genetically predisposed individuals when certain micronutrients are deficient in the diet.[65] A retrospective review of clinical case reports included in a database representing 120 children and adolescents diagnosed with paediatric bipolar disorder (24% of whom were also diagnosed with attention deficit, hyperactivity disorder [ADHD]) and taking the proprietary nutrient formula found greater than 50% improvement from baseline symptoms of both bipolar disorder and ADHD following three to six months of treatment in almost half of the individuals taking the formula, and 74% reduction in the number of prescription medications being used.[67] Findings were similar for all ages and both genders. These findings are limited by methodological flaws including open study design, absence of placebo controls and self-selection bias. Gradually titrating stable bipolar patients on a proprietary nutrient formula (see Table 36.1 for review of the evidence) while continuing them on their conventional mood stabiliser may result in improved outcomes, reductions in therapeutic doses in some cases, lower adverse effect rates and improved treatment adherence. Large randomised placebo-controlled trials in bipolar disorder are needed to confirm efficacy and safety of the formula both as a monotherapy or adjunctive treatment, and to determine optimal dosing and duration of treatment for both disorders. Concerns have been raised over safety problems reported when the nutrient formula is taken together with a conventional mood stabiliser.[64]

Enhancing mitochondrial function

Emerging evidence suggests that dysregulation in the brain's ability to protect against oxidative damage caused by free radicals may result in abnormal functioning of neuronal mitochondria, contributing to the pathogenesis of bipolar disorder and other psychiatric disorders. Mitochondrial function is known to be abnormal in patients diagnosed with schizophrenia and mood disorders and therapeutic benefits of medications used to treat these disorders may be due in part to their modulatory effects on mitochondrial functioning.

In their 'mitochondrial psychiatry' model Gardner and Boles propose that genetic or acquired factors may result in moderate reduction in mitochondrial energy metabolism, predisposing certain people to develop bipolar disorder or other chronic psychiatric disorders.[84] Neutraceuticals being investigated for their roles as mitochondrial modulators that may alleviate symptoms of bipolar disorder include N-acetylcysteine (NAC), acetyl-L-carnitine, S-adenosylmethionine (SAMe), coenzyme Q10 (co-Q10), alpha-lipoic acid, creatine monohydrate, melatonin, or combinations of two or more of these used as a 'mitochondrial agents cocktail'.[85]

Glutathione is the brain's major free radical scavenger. Its immediate precursor **N-acetyl cysteine** (NAC) is known to replenish brain levels of this crucial molecule. In a two-month open-label phase of a randomised placebo-controlled study 149 moderately depressed people diagnosed with bipolar disorder were treated with NAC (1 g 2 × day).[86] By study end symptoms of depressed mood decreased significantly and indices of functioning and life quality improved. In a subsequent double-blind placebo-controlled study done by the same authors 149 stable bipolar patients randomised to NAC (2 g 2 × day) versus placebo while continuing on treatment as usual did not have significant differences in recurrence rates or outcome measures of functioning or quality of life.[87] At study end symptom scores remained low and there were minimal changes in outcome measures in the NAC and placebo groups. A large controlled trial of bipolar depression is currently being conducted to further characterise the potential role of NAC as a treatment of bipolar disorder.

Findings of two small randomised controlled trials (RCTs) suggest that certain **branch-chain amino acids** may rapidly improve acute mania by interfering with synthesis of noradrenaline and dopamine.[71,72] In one study 25 bipolar patients randomised to a special tyrosine-free amino acid drink (60 g/day) versus placebo experienced significant reductions in the severity of mania within six hours.[72] Improvements in mania were sustained with repeated administration of the amino acid drink. Restricting or excluding L-tryptophan from the diet may increase the susceptibility of bipolar patients to depressive mood swings; however, research findings to date are highly inconsistent.[88]

Choline is necessary for the biosynthesis of acetylcholine (ACh) and abnormal low brain levels of acetylcholine may cause some cases of mania.[73] Findings of a small RCT suggest that phosphatidylcholine (15–30 g/day) may reduce the severity of mania and depressed mood in bipolar patients.[74] Many case reports and case series suggest that choline (a B complex vitamin) reduces the severity of mania. It has been postulated that abnormal low brain levels of ACh are a primary cause of mania.[73] In a small case study of treatment-refractory, rapid-cycling bipolar patients who were taking lithium, four out of six people responded to the addition of 2000–7200 mg/day of free choline. It should be noted that two non-responders were also taking hypermetabolic doses of thyroid medication. Clinical improvement correlated with increased intensity of the basal ganglia choline signal as measured on proton magnetic resonance imaging (MRI). The effect of choline on depressive symptoms was variable.[74] Case reports, open trials and one small double-blind study suggest that supplementation with phosphatidylcholine 15–30 g/day reduces the severity of both mania and depressed mood in bipolar patients, and that symptoms recur when phosphatidylcholine is discontinued.[73,74] Findings of an RCT suggest that supplementation with **folic acid** 200 µg/day may enhance the beneficial effects of lithium carbonate in acutely manic patients.[9] Findings of a double-blind study suggest that folic acid 200 µg/day may enhance the beneficial effects of lithium carbonate in acutely manic patients.[9,89]

Findings of a small open study suggest that patients diagnosed with bipolar disorder who exhibit mania or depressed mood respond to low doses (50 µg with each meal) of a natural lithium preparation.[90] Post-treatment serum lithium levels were undetectable in patients who responded to **trace lithium supplementation**. Findings of a small pilot study suggest that magnesium supplementation of 40 mEq/day may be as effective as lithium in treating rapid-cycling bipolar patients.[62]

Findings from animal research and a small open study suggest that bipolar patients who take **potassium** 20 mEq twice daily with their conventional lithium therapy experience fewer side effects, including tremor, compared with patients who take lithium alone.[91] No changes in serum lithium levels were reported in patients taking potassium. Pending confirmation of these findings by a larger double-blind trial, potassium supplementation may provide a safe, cost-effective integrative approach for managing bipolar patients who are unable to tolerate therapeutic doses of lithium due to tremor and other adverse effects. Patients who have cardiac arrhythmias or are taking antiarrhythmic medications should consult with their clinicians before considering taking a potassium supplementation.

Herbal medicines

A meta-analysis of placebo-controlled trials comparing *Hypericum perforatum* to placebo or conventional antidepressants suggests that *Hypericum perforatum* and standard antidepressants have similar beneficial effects.[92] This herb may be beneficial in the depressive phase of bipolar disorder; however, no studies on this have currently been conducted. Several case reports of mania induction with *Hypericum perforatum*[93,94] and potential serious interactions with many drugs[95] have resulted in limited use of this herbal for the treatment of bipolar disorder. Findings of a large 12-week placebo-controlled trial suggest that a proprietary Chinese compound herbal formula consisting of at least 11 herbals **(Free and Easy Wanderer Plus)** may be a beneficial adjuvant of conventional mood stabilisers for treatment of the depressive phase of bipolar disorder.[96] Bipolar depressed (but not manic) patients randomised to the herbal formula plus a conventional mood stabiliser experienced significantly greater reductions in the severity of depressed mood compared with matched patients receiving a mood stabiliser only. These findings were replicated in a subsequent study, which confirmed that bipolar depressed patients treated with the herbal formula only improved more than patients treated with a placebo.[97] Early studies suggested that the Ayurvedic herbal *Rauwolfia serpentina* was an effective treatment of bipolar disorder that augmented the antimanic efficacy of lithium without risk of toxic interactions.[98,99] However, use of this herbal in Western countries is now very restricted because of safety concerns.

Mindfulness training

Stable patients with bipolar disorder frequently report residual mood symptoms that may increase the risk of recurrence of major mood episodes. Findings of a systematic review of studies on mindfulness for bipolar disorder found that symptomatic patients who participated in mindfulness-based cognitive therapy (MBCT) reported improvements in emotional regulation, reductions in symptoms of anxiety and depressed mood, and improvements in cognitive functioning. These gains were maintained at 12-month follow-up when patients engaged in MBCT at least three times per week. Euthymic bipolar patients with residual symptoms of mania or hypomania reported significant reductions in symptom severity with regular practice. The significance of findings was limited by small study size and the absence of control groups and the diversity of mindfulness protocols used in different studies.[100] Large prospective trials are needed to confirm these findings and determine the optimal type and frequency of MBCT for cognitive symptoms of bipolar disorder.

CLINICAL SUMMARY

Conventional pharmacological treatments of the depressive and manic phases of bipolar disorder have a mixed record of success; however, in most cases pharmaceutical treatment is a critical component of acute and/or ongoing treatment. It should, however, be noted that there are high rates of treatment discontinuation and limited efficacy when treatment is adhered to. Furthermore, less severe symptoms of mania are often unreported or misdiagnosed as anxiety disorders or sleep disorders, resulting in erroneous diagnoses of agitated depressed mood or other psychiatric disorders and, subsequently, inappropriate and ineffective treatment.[118] Fewer than half of patients who take conventional maintenance treatments following an initial manic episode report sustained control of their symptoms.[119] Furthermore, as many as 40% of bipolar patients who adhere to pharmacological treatment experience recurring manic or depressive mood swings while

Schizophrenia

Overview

Schizophrenia is a chronic progressive neuropsychiatric disorder characterised by a range of symptoms that interfere with social and occupational functioning and impair reality testing. The lifetime prevalence of schizophrenia in the global population is approximately 1%.[101] The causes of schizophrenia and other psychotic disorders have not been clearly established but many genetic, neurobiological, environmental and social factors probably contribute to the pathogenesis and development of these disorders.[102–104] Schizophrenia has a chronic relapsing-remitting course and is associated with significantly reduced life expectancy and an increased risk of serious medical disorders.[105] Core symptoms of schizophrenia include hallucinations, delusions, blunted affect, apathy, social withdrawal, disorganised thought and behaviour and abnormal motor functioning (e.g. catatonia).[102]

The new DSM-5 diagnostic criteria eliminate sub-types of schizophrenia and other psychotic disorders, grades the presentation according to first or multiple episodes and whether in remission and discusses psychotic syndromes in relationship to pervasive developmental disorders. Although biomedical psychiatry regards bipolar disorder and schizophrenia as distinct disorders many of their symptoms frequently overlap. For example, psychotic symptoms frequently occur during acute mania, and affective symptoms are commonly experienced in people diagnosed with schizophrenia.[106]

Conventional treatments

All currently available antipsychotics antagonise dopamine D_2 receptors resulting in central nervous system (CNS) changes that are believed to mediate their antihallucinatory and anti-delusional effects.[107] The D_2-blocking property of the first generation antipsychotics is associated with increased serum prolactin levels as well as serious neurological adverse effects including extrapyramidal syndrome (EPS), Parkinsonism, akathisia and tardive dyskinesias. Newer SGAs such as clozapine and risperidone antagonise both D_2 and serotonin 2A receptors. Anticonvulsants including valproate and carbamazepine are sometimes used to treat symptoms of aggression and behavioural dysregulation in people diagnosed with schizophrenia; however, little evidence supports their use.[108]

It is estimated that as many as 75% of people being treated for schizophrenia are poorly adherent to their medications resulting in frequent relapses and hospitalisation.[109] Meta-analyses of controlled studies on oral antipsychotics in people diagnosed with schizophrenia support that antipsychotics are moderately more effective than placebos.[110–112] A recent meta-analysis of studies examining both efficacy and tolerability of various antipsychotics suggests clozapine, olanzapine and risperidone have superior efficacy compared with other oral antipsychotics; however, clozapine and olanzapine are associated with the greatest incidence of adverse metabolic effects and weight gain.[113]

Adjunctive CAM

Omega-3 fatty acids alone or in combination with antipsychotics may improve auditory hallucinations, paranoia and confused thinking that frequently occur in acute mania and schizophrenia while possibly lessening adverse neurological effects of antipsychotics. In a 12-week placebo-controlled study 81 adolescents considered to be at extremely high risk for developing psychosis were randomised to omega-3s (1.2 g/day) versus placebo.[76] Outcome measures included rate of transition to psychotic disorders, changes in global functioning, and pre–post comparison of omega-6 to omega-3 ratios in red blood cells. Seventy-six asdolescents completed the intervention. At study end only 11 people (27.5%) in the placebo group had transitioned to a psychotic disorder versus only two (5%) people in the omega-3 group. Those receiving omega-3s has significantly fewer positive and negative psychotic symptoms and improved global functioning compared with the placebo group. A larger study confirming these findings is underway.

Vitamin E may slow the rate of deterioration of a severe permanent neurological disorder called tardive dyskinesia but vitamin E supplementation probably does not improve symptoms of antipsychotic-induced tardive dyskinesia once it is established.[114] *Ginkgo biloba* may be an effective adjuvant when taken with antipsychotics; however, more research is needed to confirm its beneficial effects and determine the most appropriate dose.[115] *Ginkgo biloba* may also reduce the risk of movement disorders and other adverse neurological effects associated with antipsychotics. Glycine (60 g/day) may be an effective adjuvant when combined with antipsychotics and may be especially effective for 'negative' symptoms such as apathy and social withdrawal.[116] Select mind–body approaches including music therapy, meditation and mindfulness techniques may lessen symptom severity and improve global functioning in people diagnosed with schizophrenia[117] (see Table 36.1 for more detail on adjunctive use of nutra-ceuticals in schizophrenia).

taking medications at recommended doses.[120] Only about half of all conventional medications used to treat bipolar disorder are supported by strong evidence.[121] As many as half of all bipolar patients who take mood stabilisers do not experience good control of their symptoms or refuse to take medications, and approximately 50% discontinue their medications because of serious adverse effects including tremor, weight gain, elevated liver enzymes and others.[122] Due to this, CAM therapies may have a potential role in improving quality of life, reducing side effects and improving compliance.

When approaching a patient with symptoms of mania and psychosis principal treatment goals are patient safety and rapid stabilisation, usually requiring psychiatric hospitalisation (see treatment decision tree at Figure 36.1). Atypical antipsychotics are probably the most effective and efficient conventional treatments of severe mania and accompanying psychosis, and generally result in stabilisation within hours or days. 'Loading' a manic patient with a conventional mood stabiliser (such as lithium or valproic acid) to rapidly achieve a therapeutic serum level is also an effective and safe strategy for managing acute mania. It is reasonable to use omega-3 fatty acids and NAC adjunctively both during the initial stages of treatment and for maintenance therapy. There is evidence that both natural products may permit lower effective doses of mood stabilisers, reduced incidence of treatment-emergent adverse effects and improved medication adherence over the long term. Residual symptoms of insomnia can be managed using melatonin, improved sleep hygiene and guided imagery.

Regular exercise and a mind–body practice provide a healthy preventative framework for people diagnosed with bipolar disorder. After stabilisation has been achieved with conventional medications it may be possible to gradually reduce doses of mood stabilisers, antipsychotics and other medications in patients diagnosed with bipolar disorder (or schizophrenia) who are responding to adjunctive natural products including omega-3 essential fatty acids and NAC. Clinical management decisions regarding the use of adjuvant natural product therapies should always be accompanied by careful monitoring for warning signs of recurring manic, depressive or psychotic episodes and treatment-emergent adverse effects or drug–natural product interactions. Ongoing psychoeducation about the importance of lifestyle and stress management, together with support groups and other psychosocial interventions, may enhance treatment adherence and help people diagnosed with bipolar disorder to recognise and respond to early warning signs of relapse.

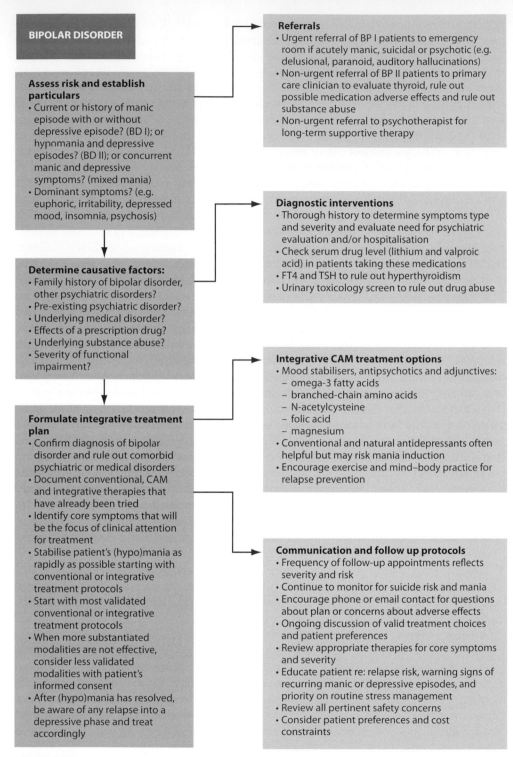

BIPOLAR DISORDER

Assess risk and establish particulars
- Current or history of manic episode with or without depressive episode? (BD I); or hypomania and depressive episodes? (BD II); or concurrent manic and depressive symptoms? (mixed mania)
- Dominant symptoms? (e.g. euphoric, irritability, depressed mood, insomnia, psychosis)

Referrals
- Urgent referral of BP I patients to emergency room if acutely manic, suicidal or psychotic (e.g. delusional, paranoid, auditory hallucinations)
- Non-urgent referral of BP II patients to primary care clinician to evaluate thyroid, rule out possible medication adverse effects and rule out substance abuse
- Non-urgent referral to psychotherapist for long-term supportive therapy

Determine causative factors:
- Family history of bipolar disorder, other psychiatric disorders?
- Pre-existing psychiatric disorder?
- Underlying medical disorder?
- Effects of a prescription drug?
- Underlying substance abuse?
- Severity of functional impairment?

Diagnostic interventions
- Thorough history to determine symptoms type and severity and evaluate need for psychiatric evaluation and/or hospitalisation
- Check serum drug level (lithium and valproic acid) in patients taking these medications
- FT4 and TSH to rule out hyperthyroidism
- Urinary toxicology screen to rule out drug abuse

Formulate integrative treatment plan
- Confirm diagnosis of bipolar disorder and rule out comorbid psychiatric or medical disorders
- Document conventional, CAM and integrative therapies that have already been tried
- Identify core symptoms that will be the focus of clinical attention for treatment
- Stabilise patient's (hypo)mania as rapidly as possible starting with conventional or integrative treatment protocols
- Start with most validated conventional or integrative treatment protocols
- When more substantiated modalities are not effective, consider less validated modalities with patient's informed consent
- After (hypo)mania has resolved, be aware of any relapse into a depressive phase and treat accordingly

Integrative CAM treatment options
- Mood stabilisers, antipsychotics and adjunctives:
  - omega-3 fatty acids
  - branched-chain amino acids
  - N-acetylcysteine
  - folic acid
  - magnesium
- Conventional and natural antidepressants often helpful but may risk mania induction
- Encourage exercise and mind–body practice for relapse prevention

Communication and follow up protocols
- Frequency of follow-up appointments reflects severity and risk
- Continue to monitor for suicide risk and mania
- Encourage phone or email contact for questions about plan or concerns about adverse effects
- Ongoing discussion of valid treatment choices and patient preferences
- Review appropriate therapies for core symptoms and severity
- Educate patient re: relapse risk, warning signs of recurring manic or depressive episodes, and priority on routine stress management
- Review all pertinent safety concerns
- Consider patient preferences and cost constraints

Figure 36.1
Integrative treatment decision tree—bipolar disorder

Table 36.1
Review of the major evidence

Intervention	Mechanisms of action	Key literature	Result	Comment
		Bipolar disorder		
Omega-3 fatty acids	Antidepressant and antipsychotic effects of omega-3s may be related to increased CNS serotonin activity[68] and suppression of pro-inflammatory cytokines[69]	Meta-analysis of RCTs using omega-3s in bipolar disorder (Sarris et al. 2011)[48]	Meta-analysis found a significant reduction of depressive symptoms ($p = 0.029$) for depressive but not manic symptoms ($p = 0.09$)	Possibly beneficial for BP depression No efficacy in BP mania. EPA more likely effective Uneven quality of studies Need larger controlled studies with improved quality
Magnesium	Currently an unknown mechanism of action Magnesium has been shown to be deficient in some psychiatric populations, and is involved with many neurotransmitter pathways	RCT using oral magnesium as an adjunctive to verapamil ($n = 20$, adults with mania)[70] Open trial magnesium versus lithium ($n = 9$, adults with rapid cycling)[62] Small case series intravenous magnesium sulfate with lithium, haloperidol and a benzodiazepine in bipolar patients with severe treatment-resistant mania[63]	Greater improvement with magnesium than placebo; verapamil + magnesium group improved more than verapamil + placebo Beneficial effects in seven patients Resulted in significant improvement in global functioning and reduction in the severity of mania[63]	Large prospective trials needed Oral magnesium and lithium had equivalent effects in over half of patients Many patients treated with intravenous magnesium sulfate remained stable on lower doses of conventional medications
Proprietary 36-ingredient nutrient formula	Select micronutrients may correct metabolic errors resulting in mood symptoms in genetically predisposed individuals[65]	Case series ($n = 11$, adults)[65] Case series ($n = 22$, children and adults)[64] Case series ($n = 19$, adults)[66]	Improvement in both depressive and manic symptoms; some patients stable on reduced doses of mood stabilisers Improvement in 19; 11 of 15 previously on medications remained stable without them Improvement in 16; 13 remained stable off conventional mood stabilisers	Large prospective trials needed Some subjects discontinue treatment due to recurring mania Adverse effects causing drop out include nausea and diarrhoea Safety problems reported when nutrient formula is taken with conventional mood stabiliser

Table 36.1
Review of the major evidence (continued)

Intervention	Mechanisms of action	Key literature	Result	Comment
Branched-chain amino acids	May rapidly improve acute mania by interfering with synthesis of noradrenaline and dopamine[71,72]	RCT (n = 25) special tyrosine-free amino acid drink (60 g/day) versus placebo[72]	Significant reductions in mania within six hours; sustained with continued use	Large prospective trials needed
Choline and phosphatidylcholine	ACh is abnormally low in acute mania. Choline supplementation increases ACh synthesis therefore reducing symptoms of mania[73]	Small RCT phosphatidylcholine (15–30 g/day)[74]	May reduce the severity of mania and depressed mood in bipolar patients	Large prospective trials needed
Folic acid	Folate is an essential cofactor in the synthesis of SAMe, which has antidepressant effects	RCT folic acid 200 μg/day + lithium versus lithium alone[9]	Differential improvement over lithium alone in acute mania	Large prospective trials needed
Schizophrenia				
Omega-3s	Omega-3 fatty acids reduce CNS oxidative stress and reduce inflammation, potentially correcting for neuropathological changes that eventually manifest as schizophrenia[75]	12-week placebo-controlled study of 81 individuals at extremely high risk for developing schizophrenia randomised to omega-3s (1.2 g/day) versus placebo (Amminger et al. 2010)[76] Meta-analysis of controlled studies in patients with chronic schizophrenia (Fusar-Poli et al. 2012)[77]	27.5% in placebo group transitioned to a psychotic disorder compared with 5% in the omega-3. Those taking omega-3s had significantly fewer positive and negative psychotic symptoms and improved global functioning compared with placebo group. No evidence for greater benefit of EPA augmentation over antipsychotic medications alone	EPA augmentation may be especially effective preventative strategy in individuals at high risk or early phase of illness but not as treatment of established chronic psychotic disorders (Fusar-Poli et al. 2007) Findings inconsistent; large controlled trials needed

Table 36.1
Review of the major evidence (continued)

Intervention	Mechanisms of action	Key literature	Result	Comment
Oestrogen	May antagonise the same neurotransmitter receptors targeted by atypical antipsychotics[78]	A Cochrane systematic review of studies on early studies on oestrogen augmentation in schizophrenia (Chua 2005)[79] More recent placebo-controlled augmentation studies in women and men (Kulkarni 2012)[80] diagnosed with schizophrenia	Systematic review of early studies found inconclusive evidence Recent studies reported significant improvement in positive and negative symptoms in both women and men	May be effective adjuvant when combined with antipsychotics permitting lower antipsychotic doses resulting in fewer adverse effects and improved adherence
DHEA	Affects several neurotransmitters reducing symptoms of schizophrenia and cognitive impairment	12-week placebo-controlled trial on DHEA (200 mg/day) in individuals diagnosed with schizophrenia continuing on antipsychotics (Ritsner 2010)[81]	DHEA group experienced greater improvement in cognitive functioning compared with the placebo group	More studies needed to confirm antipsychotic and cognitive enhancing benefits and determine safe and effective dosing *Caution:* men with prostate problems or prostate cancer should consult with their doctor before taking DHEA
Panax quinquefolium and Ginkgo biloba	The adjuvant use of both herbals may affect several neurotransmitters resulting in improved working memory and global cognitive functioning including in patients diagnosed with schizophrenia	A four-week placebo-controlled augmentation study on stable individuals diagnosed with schizophrenia randomised to a proprietary *Panax quinquefolium* extract versus placebo while remaining on treatment as usual (Chen & Hui 2012)[82] Augmentation study on *Ginkgo biloba* 360 mg/day in individuals diagnosed with schizophrenia while continuing haloperidol (Zhang 2001)[83]	Individuals in group taking ginkgo had significant improvements in visual working memory compared with placebo group Individuals in group taking ginkgo had significantly fewer neurological adverse effects compared with placebo group	Combining *Ginkgo biloba* or *Panax quinquefolium* with an antipsychotic may improve symptoms of schizophrenia more than taking an antipsychotic alone; however, more research is needed to confirm beneficial effects and determine optimal dosing strategies Ginkgo may reduce risk of movement disorders and other adverse neurological effects caused by antipsychotics

KEY POINTS

- Diverse genetic and metabolic factors potentially contribute to the pathogenesis of bipolar disorder.

- Available conventional pharmacological treatments of bipolar disorder have limited efficacy and significant safety issues, resulting in high rates of non-response, partial response and medication noncompliance. Emerging evidence suggests that omega-3 fatty acids and NAC are effective and safe adjuvants when combined with conventional medications, especially for the depressive phase of bipolar illness.

- Preliminary findings suggest that a proprietary nutrient formula may be an effective adjunctive therapy for bipolar disorder in combination with mood stabilisers; however, large RCTs are required to confirm efficacy claims and potentially serious safety issues need to be addressed before integrative regimens that include the formula can be generally recommended in bipolar disorder.

- Certain branched-chain amino acids (intravenous or oral), magnesium, choline and *Hypericum perforatum* may be beneficial in some cases of bipolar disorder. More studies are needed.

- Regular exercise, relaxation training, yoga or other mind–body practices may help reduce relapse risk in some cases of bipolar disorder.

FURTHER READING

Grande I, Berk M, Birmaher B, et al. Bipolar disorder. Lancet 2016;387(10027):156–72. doi:10.1016/S0140-6736(15)00241-X. [Epub 2015 Sep 18].

Lake J. An integrative paradigm for mental health care: ideas and methods shaping the future. Springer; 2019.

Qureshi NA, Al-Bedah AM. Mood disorders and complementary and alternative medicine: a literature review. Neuropsychiatr Dis Treat 2013;9:639–58.

Rakofsky JJ, Dunlop BW. Review of nutritional supplements for the treatment of bipolar depression. Depress Anxiety 2014;31(5):379–90. doi:10.1002/da.22220. [Epub 2013 Dec 18].

Sarris J, Lake J, Hoenders R. Bipolar disorder and complementary medicine: current evidence, safety issues, and clinical considerations. J Altern Complement Med 2011;17(10):881–90.

REFERENCES

1. Narrow WE, Rae DS, Robins LN, et al. Revised prevalence estimates of mental disorders in the United States: using a clinical significance criterion to reconcile 2 surveys' estimates. Arch Gen Psychiatry 2002;59(2):115–23.

2. Gurling H. Linkage findings in bipolar disorder. Nat Genet 1995;8–9:10.

3. Konradi C. Molecular evidence for mitochondrial dysfunction in bipolar disorder. Arch Gen Psychiatry 2004;61:300–8.

4. Kupfer DJ, Angst J, Berk M, et al. Advances in bipolar disorder: selected sessions from the 2011 International Conference on Bipolar Disorder. Ann N Y Acad Sci 2011;1242:1–25.

5. Anderson G, Maes M. Bipolar disorder: role of immune-inflammatory cytokines, oxidative and nitrosative stress and tryptophan cattabolites. Curr Psychiatry Rep 2015;17:8.

6. Altshuler L, Bookheimer S, Proenza MA, et al. Increased amygdala activation during mania: a functional magnetic resonance imaging study. Am J Psychiatry 2005;162:1211–13.

7. Foland LC, Altshuler LL, Bookheimer SY, et al. Evidence for deficient modulation of amygdala response by prefrontal cortex in bipolar mania. Psychiatry Res 2008;162(1):27–37.

8. Small JG. Topographic EEG studies of mania. Clin Electroencephalogr 1998;29(2):59–66.

9. Hasanah CI, et al. Reduced red-cell folate in mania. J Affect Disord 1997;46:95–9.

10. American Psychiatric Association: diagnostic and statistical manual of mental disorders. 4th ed. Arlington: American Psychiatric Association; 2000.

11. Winokur G. Manic depressive illness. St Louis: C.V. Mosby; 1969.

12. Judd L, et al. The long-term natural history of the weekly symptomatic status of bipolar I disorder. Arch Gen Psychiatry 2002;59(6):530–7.

13. Vieta E, Phillips ML. Deconstructing bipolar disorder: a critical review of its diagnostic validity and a proposal for DSM-V and ICD-11. Schizophr Bull 2007;33(4):886–92.

14. Ilgen MA. A collaborative therapeutic relationship and risk of suicidal ideation in patients with bipolar disorder. J Affect Disord 2008;115(1):246–51.

15. Culver JL. Bipolar disorder: improving diagnosis and optimizing integrated care. J Clin Psychol 2007;63(1):73–92.

16. Perlick DA. Symptoms predicting inpatient service use among patients with bipolar affective disorder. Psychiatr Serv 1999;50(6):806–12.

17. Altamura AC, Goikolea JM. Differential diagnoses and management strategies in patients with schizophrenia and bipolar disorder. Neuropsychiatr Dis Treat 2008;4(1):311–17.

18. Miklowitz DJ, Johnson SL. The psychopathology and treatment of bipolar disorder. Annu Rev Clin Psycholz 2006;2:199–235.

19. Benjamin AB. A unique consideration regarding medication compliance for bipolar affective disorder: exercise performance. Bipolar Disord 2007;9(8):928–9.

20. Lakhan SE, Vieira KF. Nutritional therapies for mental disorders. Nutr J 2008;21(7):2.

21. Goldstein BI, Fagiolini A, Houck P, et al. Cardiovascular disease and hypertension among adults with bipolar I disorder in the United States. Bipolar Disord 2009; 11(6):657–62.

22. Fagiolini A, Kupfer DJ, Houck PR, et al. Obesity as a correlate of outcome in patients with bipolar I disorder. Am J Psychiatry 2003;160:112–17.

23. Kilbourne AM, Rofey DL, McCarthy JF, et al. Nutrition and exercise behavior among patients with bipolar disorder. Bipolar Disord 2007;9:443–52.

24. Knutson KL. Sleep duration and cardiometabolic risk: a review of the epidemiologic evidence. Best Prac Res Clin Endocrinol Metab 2010;24:731–43.

25. Birkenaes AB, Opjordsmoen S, Brunborg C. The level of cardiovascular risk factors in bipolar disorder equals that of schizophrenia: a comparative study. J Clin Psychiatry 2007;68:917–23.

26. Harvey AG, Schmidt DA, Scarna A, et al. Sleep-related functioning in euthymic patients with bipolar disorder, patients with insomnia, and subjects without sleep problems. Am J Psychiatry 2005;162:50–7.

27. Dworak M, Wiater A, Alfer D, et al. Increased slow wave sleep and reduced stage 2 sleep in children depending on exercise intensity. Sleep Med 2008;9:266–72.

28. American Psychiatric Association. Practice guidelines: Treatment of patients with bipolar disorder. 7th edn. Online. Available: http://www.psychiatryonline.com/pracGuide/pracGuideTopic_8.aspx 2013.

29. Sani G, Perug G, Tondo L. Treatment of bipolar disorder in a lifetime perspective: is lithium still the best choice? Clin Drug Investig 2017;37:713–27.

30. Altamura A, Lietti L, Dobrea C, et al. Mood stabilizers for patients with bipolar disorder: the state of the art. Expert Rev Neurother 2011;11:85–99.

31. Leucht S, Heres S, Hamann J, et al. Methodological issues in current antipsychotic drug trials. Schizophr Bull 2008;34:275–85.

32. Stroup T, Alves W, Hamer R, et al. Clinical trials for antipsychotic drugs: design conventions, dilemmas and innovations. Nat Rev Drug Discov 2006;5:133–46.

33. Depp C, Lebowitz B. Clinical trials: bridging the gap between efficacy and effectiveness. Int Rev Psychiatry 2007;19:531–9.

34. Manschreck T, Boshes R. The CATIE schizophrenia trial: results, impact, controversy. Harv Rev Psychiatry 2007;15:245–58.

35. Arranz M, de Leon J. Pharmacogenetics and pharmacogenomics of schizophrenia: a review of last decade of research. Mol Psychiatry 2007;12:707–47.

36. Cipriani A, Barbui C, Salanti G, et al. Comparative efficacy and acceptability of antimanic drugs in acute mania: a multiple-treatments meta-analysis. Lancet 2011;378:1306–15.

37. Tarr G, Glue P, Herbison P. Comparative efficacy and acceptability of mood stabilizer and second generation antipsychotic monotherapy for acute mania—a systematic review and meta-analysis. J Affect Disord 2011;134:14–19.

38. Cousins DA, Young AH. The armamentarium of treatments for bipolar disorder: a review of the literature. Int J Neuropsychopharmacol 2007;10(3):411–13.

39. Rodriguez-Martin JL. Transcranial magnetic stimulation for treating depression. Cochrane Depression Anxiety and Eurosis Group. Cochrane Database Syst Rev 2001;(4):CD003493.

40. Husain M, Strawbridge R, Stokes P, et al. Anti-inflammatory treatments for mood disorders: systematic review and meta-analysis. J Psychopharmacol (Oxford) 2017;31(11):1137–48.

41. Miklowitz DJ. Adjunctive psychotherapy for bipolar disorder: state of the evidence. Am J Psychiatry 2008;165(11):1408–19.

42. Pontin E. Enhanced relapse prevention for bipolar disorder: a qualitative investigation of value perceived for service users and care coordinators. Implement Sci 2009;9(4):4.

43. Ernst E. Complementary medicine: where is the evidence? J Fam Pract 2003;52:630–4.

44. Dennehy E. Self-reported participation in nonpharmacologic treatments for bipolar disorder. J Clin Psychiatry 2004;65(2):278.

45. Sarris J, Lake J, Hoenders R. Bipolar disorder and complementary medicine: current evidence, safety issues, and clinical considerations. J Altern Complement Med 2011;17(10):881–90.

46. Sarris J, Kavanagh DJ, Byrne G. Adjuvant use of nutritional and herbal medicines with antidepressants, mood stabilizers and benzodiazepines. J Psychiatr Res 2010;44(1):32–41.

47. Marx W, Moseley G, Berk M, et al. Diet, nutrition and mental health and wellbeing. Plenary lecture: mental health as an emerging public health problem; Nutritional psychiatry: the present state of the evidence. P Nutr Soc 2017;76:427–36.

48. Sarris J, Mischoulon D, Schweitzer I. Adjunctive nutraceuticals with standard pharmacotherapies in bipolar disorder: a systematic review of clinical trials. Bipolar Disord 2011;13(5–6):454–65.

49. Sylvia LG, Peters AT, Deckersbach T, et al. Nutrient-based therapies for bipolar disorder: a systematic review. Psychother Psychosom 2013;82(1):10–19.

50. Hibbeln JR. Seafood consumption, the DHA content of mothers' milk and prevalence rates of postpartum depression: a cross-national, ecological analysis. J Affect Disord 2002;69:15–29.

51. Sarris J, Mischoulon D, Schweitzer I. Omega-3 for bipolar disorder: meta-analyses of use in mania and bipolar depression. J Clin Psychiatry 2012;73(1):81–6.

52. Chiu CC, et al. Omega-3 fatty acids are more beneficial in the depressive phase than in the manic phase in patients with bipolar I disorder. J Clin Psychiatry 2005;66:1613–14.

53. Emsley R. Randomized, placebo-controlled study of ethyl-eicosapentaenoic acid as supplemental treatment in schizophrenia. Am J Psychiatry 2002;1859:1596–8.

54. Peet M, Horrobin DF. E-E Multicentre Study Group). A dose-ranging exploratory study of the effects of ethyl-eicosapentaenoate in patients with persistent schizophrenic symptoms. J Psychiatr Res 2002;36(1): 7–18.

55. Fenton WS, et al. A placebo-controlled trial of omega-3 fatty acid (ethyl eicosapentaenoic acid) supplementation for residual symptoms and cognitive impairment in schizophrenia. Am J Psychiatry 2001;158(12):2071–3.

56. Soderpalm B, Engel JA. Serotonergic involvement in conflict behavior. Eur Neuropsychopharmacol 1990;1(1):7–13.

57. Kahn RS, et al. Effect of a serotonin precursor and uptake inhibitor in anxiety disorders; a double-blind comparison of 5-hydroxytryptophan, clomipramine, and placebo. Int Clin Psychopharmacol 1987;2(1):33–45.

58. Schneider-Helmert D, Spinweber CL. Evaluation of L-tryptophan for treatment of insomnia: a review. Psychopharmacology (Berl) 1986;89(1):1–7.

59. Levitan RD. Preliminary randomized double-blind placebo-controlled trial of tryptophan combined with fluoxetine to treat major depressive disorder: antidepressant and hypnotic effects. J Psychiatry Neurosci 2000;4:337–46.

60. Applebaum J, Bersudsky Y, Klein E. Rapid tryptophan depletion as a treatment for acute mania: a double-blind, pilot-controlled study. Bipolar Disord 2007;9(8):884–7.

61. Young SN. Rapid tryptophan depletion as a treatment for acute mania: safety and mechanism of the therapeutic effect. Bipolar Disord 2008;10(7):850–1.

62. Chouinard G. A pilot study of magnesium aspartate hydrochloride (Magnesiocard) as a mood stabilizer for rapid cycling bipolar affective disorder patients. Prog Neuropsychopharmacol Biol Psychiatry 1990;4:171–80.

63. Heiden A. Treatment of severe mania with intravenous magnesium sulphate as a supplementary therapy. Psychiatry Res 1999;89(3):239–46.

64. Popper C. Do vitamins or minerals (apart from lithium) have mood-stabilizing effects? J Clin Psychiatry 2001;62(12):933–5.

65. Kaplan BJ, et al. Effective mood stabilization with a chelated mineral supplement: an open-label trial in bipolar disorder. J Clin Psychiatry 2001;62:936–44.

66. Simmons M. Nutritional approach to bipolar disorder [Letter to the editor]. J Clin Psychiatry 2002;64:338.

67. Rucklidge JJ, Gately D, Kaplan BJ. Database analysis of children and adolescents with bipolar disorder consuming a micronutrient formula. BMC Psychiatry 2010;10:74.

68. Hibbeln JR. Fish consumption and major depression. Lancet 1998;351(9110):1213.

69. Maes M, Smith RS. Fatty acids, cytokines, and major depression. Biol Psychiatry 1998;43(5):313–14.

70. Giannini AJ, Nakoneczie AM, Melemis SM, et al. Magnesium oxide augmentation of verapamil maintenance therapy in mania. Psychiatry Res 2000;93(1):83–7.

71. Barrett S, Leyton M. Acute phenylalanine/tyrosine depletion: a new method to study the role of catecholamines in psychiatric disorders. Prim Psychiatry 2004;11(6):37–41.

72. Scarna A. Effects of a branched-chain amino acid drink in mania. Br J Psychiatry 2003;182:210–13.

73. Leiva D. The neurochemistry of mania: a hypothesis of etiology and rationale for treatment. Prog Neuropsychopharmacol Biol Psychiatry 1990;14(3):423–9.

74. Stoll AL. Choline in the treatment of rapid-cycling bipolar disorder: clinical and neurochemical findings in lithium-treated patients. Biol Psychiatry 1996;40:382–8.

75. Reddy R, Reddy R. Antioxidant therapeutics for schizophrenia. Antioxid Redox Signal 2011;15(7):2047–55.

76. Amminger GP, Schafer MR, Papageorgiou K, et al. Long-chain omega-3 fatty acids for indicated prevention of psychotic disorders: a randomized, placebo-controlled trial. Arch Gen Psychiatry 2010;67(2):146–54.

77. Fusar-Poli P, Berger G. Eicosapentaenoic acid interventions in schizophrenia: meta-analysis of randomized, placebo-controlled studies. J Clin Psychopharmacol 2012;32(2):179–85.

78. Hughes ZA, Liu F, Marquis K, et al. Estrogen receptor neurobiology and its potential for translation into broad spectrum therapeutics for CNS disorders. Curr Mol Pharmacol 2009;2(3):215–36.

79. Chua WL, De Izquierdo SA, Kulkarni J, et al. Estrogen for schizophrenia. Cochrane Database Syst Rev 2005;(4):CD004719.

80. Kulkarni J, Gavrilidis E, Worsley R, et al. Role of estrogen treatment in the management of schizophrenia. CNS Drugs 2012;26(7):549–57.

81. Ritsner MS, Strous RD. Neurocognitive deficits in schizophrenia are associated with alterations in blood levels of neurosteroids: a multiple regression analysis of findings from a double-blind, randomized, placebo-controlled, crossover trial with DHEA. J Psychiatr Res 2010;44(2):75–80.

82. Chen EY, Hui CL. HT1001, A proprietary North American ginseng extract, improves working memory in schizophrenia: a double-blind, placebo-controlled study. Phytother Res 2012;26(8):1166–72.

83. Zhang XY, Zhou DF, Zhang PY, et al. A double-blind, placebo-controlled trial of extract of Ginkgo biloba added to haloperidol in treatment-resistant patients with schizophrenia. J Clin Psychiatry 2001;62(11):878–83.

84. Gardner A, Boles RG. Beyond the serotonin hypothesis: mitochondria, inflammation and neurodegeneration in major depression and affective spectrum disorders. Prog Neuropsychopharmacol Biol Psychiatry 2011;35(3):730–43.

85. Nierenberg AA, Kansky C, Brennan BP, et al. Mitochondrial modulators for bipolar disorder: a pathophysiologically informed paradigm for new drug development. Aust N Z J Psychiatry 2013;47(1):26–42.

86. Berk M, Dean O, Cotton SM, et al. The efficacy of N-acetylcysteine as an adjunctive treatment in bipolar depression: an open label trial. J Affect Disord 2011;135(1–3):389–94.

87. Berk M, Dean OM, Cotton SM, et al. Maintenance N-acetyl cysteine treatment for bipolar disorder: a double-blind randomized placebo controlled trial. BMC Med 2012;10:91.

88. Hughes J. Effects of acute tryptophan depletion on cognitive function in euthymic bipolar patients. Eur Neuropsychopharmacol 2002;12(2):123–8.

89. Coppen A, et al. Folic acid enhances lithium prophylaxis. J Affect Disord 1986;10(1):9–13.

90. Fierro A. Natural low-dose lithium supplementation in manic-depressive disease. Nutr Perspectives 1988;1:10–11.

91. Tripuraneni B. Clin Psychiatry News. 1990;18(10):3, presented to the 143rd Annual Meeting of the American Psychiatric Association, 12–17 May 1990, abstracts NR 100 and NR 210.

92. Linde K. St John's wort for major depression. Cochrane Database Syst Rev 2008;(4):CD000448.

93. Moses EL, Mallinger AG. St. John's Wort: three cases of possible mania induction. J Clin Psychopharmacol 2000;20(1):115–17.

94. Fahmi M. A case of mania induced by hypericum. World J Biol Psychiatry 2002;3(1):58–9.

95. Izzo AA. Drug interactions with St. John's Wort (Hypericum perforatum): a review of the clinical evidence. Int J Clin Pharmacol Ther 2004;42(3):139–48.

96. Zhang ZJ, et al. Adjunctive herbal medicine with carbamazepine for bipolar disorders: a double-blind, randomized, placebo-controlled study. J Psychiatr Res 2007;41(3–4):360–9.

97. Zhang ZJ, et al. The beneficial effects of the herbal medicine Free and Easy Wanderer Plus (FEWP) for mood disorders: double-blind, placebo-controlled studies. J Psychiatr Res 2007;41:828–36.

98. Bacher NM, Lewis HA. Lithium plus reserpine in refractory manic patients. Am J Psychiatry 1979;136(6):811–14.

99. Berlant JL. Neuroleptics and reserpine in refractory psychoses. J Clin Psychopharmacol 1986;6(3):180–4.

100. Bojic S, Becerra R. Mindfulness-based treatment for bipolar disorder: a systematic review of the literature. Eur J Psychol 2017;13(3):573–98.

101. Kessler R, Petukhova M, Sampson N, et al. Twelve-month and lifetime prevalence and lifetime morbid risk of anxiety and mood disorders in the United States. Int J Methods Psychiatr Res 2012;21:169–84.

102. Tandon R, Nasrallah HA, Keshavan MS. Schizophrenia, 'just the facts' 4. Clinical features and conceptualization. Schizophr Res 2009;110:1–23.

103. Van Os J, Kenis G, Rutten BP. The environment and schizophrenia. Nature 2010;468:203–12.

104. Insel T, Cuthbert B, Garvey M, et al. Research domain criteria (RDoC): toward a new classification framework for research on mental disorders. Am J Psychiatry 2010;167:748–51.

105. De Hert M, Correll C, Bobes J, et al. Physical illness in patients with severe mental disorders. I. Prevalence, impact of medications and disparities in health care. World Psychiatry 2011;10:52–77.

106. Qian K, Di Lieto A, Corander J, et al. Re-analysis of bipolar disorder and schizophrenia gene expression complements the Kraepelinian dichotomy. Adv Exp Med Biol 2012;736:563–77.

107. Howes O, Kapur S. The dopamine hypothesis of schizophrenia: version III—the final common pathway. Schizophr Bull 2009;35:549–62.

108. Schwarz C, Volz A, Li C, et al. Valproate for schizophrenia. Cochrane Database Syst Rev 2008;(3):CD004028, Rev 11:CD006633.

109. Leucht S, Heres S. Epidemiology, clinical consequences, and psychosocial treatment of nonadherence in schizophrenia. J Clin Psychiatry 2006;67(Suppl. 5):3–8.

110. Leucht S, Arbter D, Engel R, et al. How effective are second-generation antipsychotic drugs? A meta-analysis of placebo-controlled trials. Mol Psychiatry 2009a;14:429–47.

111. Leucht S, Corves C, Arbter D, et al. Second-generation versus first-generation antipsychotic drugs for schizophrenia: a meta-analysis. Lancet 2009b;373:31–41.

112. Leucht S, Komossa K, Rummel-Kluge C, et al. A meta-analysis of head-to-head comparisons of second-generation antipsychotics in the treatment of schizophrenia. Am J Psychiatry 2009c;166:152–63.

113. Glick I, Correll C, Altamura A, et al. Mid-term and long-term efficacy and effectiveness of antipsychotic medications for schizophrenia: a data-driven, personalized clinical approach. J Clin Psychiatry 2011;72:1616–27.

114. Soares-Weiser K, Maayan N, McGrath J. Vitamin E for neuroleptic-induced tardive dyskinesia. Cochrane Database Syst Rev 2011;(2):CD000209.

115. Zhang XY, Zhou DF, Zhang PY, et al. A double-blind, placebo-controlled trial of extract of Ginkgo biloba added to haloperidol in treatment-resistant patients with schizophrenia. J Clin Psychiatry 2001;62:878–83.

116. Leiderman E, Zylberman I, Zukin S, et al. Preliminary investigation of high-dose oral glycine on serum levels and negative symptoms in schizophrenia: an open-label trial. Biol Psychiatry 1996;39:213–15.

117. Helgason C, Sarris J. Mind–body medicine for schizophrenia and psychotic disorders. Clin Schizophr Relat Psychoses 2013;1(1):1–29.

118. Benazzi F. Prevalence of bipolar II disorder in outpatient depression: a 203-case study in private practice. J Affect Disord 1997;43(2):163–6.

119. Tohen M. Outcome in mania: a 4-year prospective follow-up on 75 patients utilizing survival analysis. Arch Gen Psychiatry 1990;47:1106–11.

120. Strober M. Relapse following discontinuation of lithium maintenance therapy in adolescents with bipolar I illness: a naturalistic study. Am J Psychiatry 1990;147:457–61.

121. Boschert S. Evidence-based treatment largely ignored in bipolar disorder. Clinical Psychiatry News 1, June 2004.

122. Fleck DE, et al. Factors associated with medication adherence in African American and white patients with bipolar disorder. J Clin Psychiatry 2005;66: 646–52.

CHAPTER 37

Attention deficit and hyperactivity disorder

James Lake
MD

OVERVIEW

Attention deficit and hyperactivity disorder (ADHD) occurs in children and adults with roughly equal prevalence in all countries surveyed.[1] Recent surveys suggest that 7–8% of children[2] and 4–5% of adults[3] fulfil criteria for ADHD. The rate at which ADHD is diagnosed and treated in both children and adults has increased dramatically since the syndrome was first recognised as a specific disorder in the *Diagnostic and Statistical Manual of Mental Disorders* (DSM) in the 1970s. In the United States as many as 10% of males and 4% of females have been diagnosed with ADHD.[4] An objective epidemiological or scientific basis for the rapidly increasing prevalence of ADHD in general and the higher incidence of the syndrome in boys compared with girls is highly controversial and may reflect social issues and changes in diagnostic criteria more than actual changes in prevalence rates.[5]

The causes of ADHD are multifactorial. Data from twin studies show that ADHD is a highly heritable disorder[6] and the risk of developing this disorder is probably influenced by genes that affect central nervous system transport of dopamine and serotonin.[7] ADHD is also associated with premature birth, birth trauma, childhood illness and environmental toxins.[8] Increased risk of ADHD is associated with in utero exposure to alcohol, tobacco smoke and lead. As many as 20% of ADHD cases may be caused by brain injury around the time of birth. While certain food preservatives exacerbate the symptoms of ADHD, they are highly unlikely to *cause* the disorder.[6] Some cases of ADHD may be associated with delayed development of certain areas of the frontal and temporal lobes and relatively rapid maturation of motor areas of the brain.[9] Neuroimaging studies suggest that these brain regions may have relatively decreased activation in individuals diagnosed with ADHD. Children diagnosed with ADHD frequently experience disturbed sleep including restlessness, sleep walking, night terrors and restless leg syndrome; however, a causal relationship between sleep disorders and ADHD has not been clearly established.[10] Early childhood neglect or abuse may also increase the risk of developing ADHD. Most cases of ADHD probably result from multiple genetic, developmental, physiological, environmental and psychosocial factors.[11]

According to the DSM-5 a diagnosis of ADHD is considered to be a persistent pattern of inattention and/or hyperactivity-impulsivity that interferes with functioning or development.[12] An ADHD diagnosis requires the presence of at least six symptoms (five for ages > 17) of hyperactivity or inattention that begin before the age of 12, persist for at least six months, are maladaptive, are inconsistent with the child's development level, are present in two or more settings and are not better explained by a preexisting medical or psychiatric disorder. Specific symptoms of inattention may include careless mistakes in schoolwork, difficulty sustaining attention in school-related tasks or play, failure to follow through with instructions, difficulty organising tasks and activities, reluctance to engage in tasks requiring sustained attention and being distracted easily by extraneous stimuli. Specific symptoms of hyperactivity or impulsivity may include fidgeting with hands or feet or squirming while sitting, frequently getting up in a classroom or other situation in which remaining seated is expected, running or moving in inappropriate or disruptive ways or (in adults) subjective 'feelings of restlessness', difficulty engaging in quiet leisure activities and talking excessively.

DSM-5 ADHD subtypes
1. Predominantly inattentive type
2. Predominantly hyperactive type
3. Combined type (inattentive and hyperactive)

Symptoms of inattention, impulsivity or hyperactivity must cause clinically significant impairment in at least two spheres including social, academic or occupational functioning. Neuropsychological testing is frequently employed to assess inattention, processing speed and neurocognitive deficits. A diagnosis of ADHD should be made in childhood only after other childhood disorders, including pervasive developmental disorders, learning disorders and anxiety disorders, have been ruled out.[13]

DIFFERENTIAL DIAGNOSIS

- Bipolar disorder
- Hyperthyroidism
- Obsessive-compulsive disorder
- Chronic sleep deprivation
- Personality disorders

- Adjustment disorder
- Absence seizures
- Stimulatory effect from medications or illicit drugs

Source: Pearl et al. 2001[14]

RISK FACTORS

The hyperactivity of ADHD often resolves by late adolescence or adulthood; however, symptoms of distractibility may not lessen with age. It has been estimated that fewer than 20% of adults with ADHD have been correctly diagnosed and appropriately treated, resulting in significant social and occupational risk. ADHD is highly comorbid with oppositional defiant disorder (ODD) and learning disorders in children, and with major depressive disorder, anxiety disorders and substance abuse in adults.[15] It has been estimated that almost half of those diagnosed with ADHD never graduate from high school and fewer than 5% complete a four-year university degree program.[16] The high prevalence rate of ADHD significantly affects employment statistics. A large population survey of American adults found that a diagnosis of ADHD was associated with 35 days of lost work on average. Extrapolating these findings to the population suggests that US$19 billion in lost productivity and 120 million lost work days annually are attributable to ADHD.[17]

Psychostimulant abuse?

Stimulant abuse is an established risk factor in long-term prescription stimulant use among adults; however, a meta-analysis of six controlled trials found that when stimulants are used to treat childhood ADHD the risk of subsequent substance abuse actually *decreases*.[18] Although the American Academy of Pediatrics endorses the use of stimulants as safe and effective, considerable controversy surrounds their widespread use.

CONVENTIONAL TREATMENT

Stimulant medications are the standard Western treatment of ADHD; however, selective serotonin reuptake inhibitors (SSRIs) and other antidepressants are also used with varying degrees of success. Extended-release forms of stimulants are better tolerated and less often lead to abuse. Rates of stimulant abuse may be especially high in people with comorbid conduct disorder or substance abuse.[19] Stimulant use in these populations should be carefully monitored or avoided.[20] Long-acting stimulants are associated with relatively less abuse because they cross the blood–brain barrier more gradually than immediate release stimulants. The recently introduced long-acting stimulant lisdexamphetamine dimesylate is a pro-drug with comparable efficacy to existing long-acting stimulants but with less abuse potential as it must be metabolised in the gut before being converted into the active drug d-amphetamine.[21]

Approximately one-third of children and adolescents who take stimulants experience significant adverse effects, including abdominal pain, decreased appetite and insomnia, and 10% experience serious adverse effects.[22] Because stimulants are usually classified as scheduled or restricted medications (depending on the country), prescriptions are usually limited to a short supply; this can result in treatment interruptions and transient symptomatic worsening when refills are not obtained on time. One-third of all people who take stimulants for ADHD report significant adverse effects, including insomnia, decreased appetite and abdominal pain.[22] Sporadic cases of stimulant-induced psychosis have been reported.[23] Neurotoxic effects associated with long-term stimulant use have not been fully elucidated; however, chronic amphetamine use in childhood is associated with slowing in growth. Stimulants and other conventional treatments of adulthood ADHD may be only half as effective as they are in children.[15]

Only long-acting stimulants have been approved by the FDA for treatment of adult ADHD, while short-acting stimulants are the most prescribed conventional treatments in this population. Controlled-release stimulants, bupropion and the SSRI antidepressants are being increasingly used in the adult ADHD population; however, research findings suggest these medications may not be as efficacious as stimulants.[24] Atomoxetine, a serotonin noradrenaline reuptake inhibitor (SNRI), is the only non-stimulant drug that has been approved by the FDA for adults diagnosed with ADHD. Atomoxetine has less potential for abuse but may not be as efficacious as psychostimulants.[25] Atomoxetine is also FDA-approved for the treatment of childhood ADHD; however, there are growing concerns about its adverse effects, including hypertension, tachycardia, nausea and vomiting, liver toxicity and possibly increased suicide risk.[26,27] In Australia atomoxetine is registered for use by the Therapeutic Goods Administration. Other non-stimulant drugs recently approved by the FDA for treating childhood ADHD include modafinil,[28] reboxetine[29] and the α-2-adrenergic agonists clonidine and guanfacine.[30,31]

In addition to conventional prescription medications, behavioural modification is a widely used conventional treatment of ADHD in children. Psychotherapy and psycho-social support help reduce the anxiety and feelings of loss of control that frequently accompany ADHD. Some findings support that cognitive behaviour therapy (CBT) reduces symptom severity in adults diagnosed with ADHD.

Researchers are exploring the use of non-invasive brain stimulation techniques such as repetitive transcranial magnetic stimulation (rTMS) and transcranial direct current stimulation (tDCS) to treat ADHD. Both techniques work by modulating cortical excitability via transcranial electrical stimulation resulting in the amelioration of neuro-psychiatric symptoms. rTMS is being explored for its potential role in diagnosing ADHD, identifying medications that are more likely to be effective and to treat core symptoms of ADHD. Positive findings have been reported by a few small studies on rTMS in adult and paediatric populations diagnosed with ADHD.[32] Transcranial direct current stimulation (tDCS) has been demonstrated to enhance attention and working memory in healthy individuals and individuals diagnosed with psychiatric disorders such as major depressive disorder.[33,34] TDCS may increase functional brain connectivity in individuals diagnosed with ADHD (Cosmo 2015). In a pilot sham-controlled study ($n = 17$), adult patients diagnosed with ADHD were randomised to receive daily tDCS treatment consisting of 2 mA via electrodes placed over the right and left dorsolateral prefrontal cortex for 20 minutes versus sham over a five-day period. Individuals in the active treatment group reported greater reductions in symptoms of inattention compared to the sham group. Large sham-controlled studies are needed to confirm the benefits of rTMS and tDCS for ADHD.[35]

INTEGRATIVE MEDICAL TREATMENT OPTIONS

Overview

Many individuals diagnosed with ADHD use alternative therapies alone or adjunctively with conventional pharmacological treatments.[36] Growing concerns about inappropriate prescribing or over-prescribing by doctors of stimulant medications and incomplete understanding of risks associated with their long-term use have led to increasing acceptance of emerging non-conventional therapies.[37,38] Surveys suggest

---

Integrative Medical Treatment Aims*

- Take a complete history to determine possible relationships between diet, food allergies, etc. (including food colourings or additives) and ADHD symptoms.

- Document conventional and CAM treatments including doses, durations and brands of conventional medications and natural products that have been tried, including the patient's response and adverse effects.

- Develop an integrative treatment plan with the patient (or parent if the patient is younger than 18), including dietary changes if appropriate, behavioural therapy and psychosocial interventions, the use of select nutrients (such as essential fatty acids, or EFAs), trace elements, homeopathic remedies and electroencephalographic (EEG) biofeedback.

- Monitor symptoms using standardised symptom-rating scales and modify the treatment plan using conventional or CAM modalities until consistent improvement is achieved.

*Firstly confirm the diagnosis of ADHD, including symptoms starting in childhood, and rule out underlying primary psychiatric or medical causes.

that 12–68% of children diagnosed with ADHD use complementary and alternative medicine (CAM) therapies largely out of parental concerns over safety of conventional drugs.[39,40] Over half of parents of children diagnosed with ADHD treat their children's symptoms using one or more CAM therapies, including vitamins, dietary changes and expressive therapies, but few disclose this to their child's paediatrician.[41] Most CAM therapies for ADHD are supported by limited evidence; however, when any herbal or other naturopathic therapy is used to treat ADHD it is regarded as the primary treatment more than 80% of the time.[41]

A systematic review of clinical trials on **herbal and nutritional interventions** for ADHD found good support for zinc, iron, *Pinus marinus* and a Chinese herbal formula (Ningdong), and inconsistent findings for omega-3s and L-acetyl carnitine. Limited findings from clinical trials on *Bacopa monnieri* and *Piper methysticum* call for more research on these two herbals.[42] The most appropriate CAM and integrative treatment strategies for ADHD depend on the subtype of ADHD that is being addressed, symptom severity, previous treatment outcomes using conventional or CAM modalities, adverse effect issues, psychiatric or medical comorbidities, patient preferences, the availability of qualified CAM practitioners and access to reputable brands of specific supplements. Dietary modifications, including reduced sugar and caffeine intake and specialised restrictive diets, are reasonable first-line strategies in children diagnosed with the predominantly hyperactive subtype of ADHD.

Dietary modification

Early studies on a **restrictive diet** that eliminates all processed foods reported promising findings in children with ADHD,[43] although a review of controlled studies failed to support these findings.[44] Early studies suggested that artificial food colourings were associated with ADHD; however, a meta-analysis failed to confirm this.[45] The **oligoantigenic diet** (**OAD**) is a highly restrictive multiple elimination diet that excludes food colourings and additives, in addition to dairy products, sugar, wheat, corn, citrus, eggs, soy, yeast, nuts and chocolate. OADs permit a limited number of hypoallergenic foods, like lamb, chicken, potatoes, rice, banana, apple, cabbage, broccoli, brussels sprouts, carrots, peas, pears and cucumber, as well as salt, pepper, calcium and some vitamins. Studies involve several phases and require many weeks to complete. During phase I, which typically lasts four weeks, specific food items are withheld from the diet and the patient is monitored using standardised symptom rating scales. In cases where symptoms improve during the initial treatment phase, specific foods are gradually re-introduced in phase II. A third phase follows a placebo-controlled crossover design in which the patient is randomised to a food item that initially caused symptoms or an acceptable placebo for one week, followed by a washout period, and subsequently exposed to either placebo or a specific food item or additive for an additional week.

Several studies on the OAD regimen reported significant reductions in hyperactivity in children diagnosed with ADHD when specific food items were eliminated from the diet using the above protocol.[46–48] In all of these studies behavioural symptoms improved during the elimination and placebo phases and recurred when children were subsequently challenged with the eliminated food item following a blinded protocol. A meta-analysis of studies on restrictive diets in childhood ADHD including 14 open studies and six controlled trials concluded that roughly one-third of hyperactive children may benefit from some form of an elimination diet.[45] Although these results are promising they cannot be used to develop general ADHD treatment protocols because of study design flaws, including heterogeneity of patient populations, absence of standardised outcome measures, high dropout rates and, in some studies, non-blinded researchers.[49] A more recent systematic review of 14 meta-analyses of meta-analyses, six of which were confined to double-blind placebo-controlled trials evaluating the efficacy of diet interventions in children diagnosed with ADHD, found weak evidence for supplementation with polyunsaturated fatty acids (PUFA) and diets that eliminate artificial food colours, and substantial evidence for few-food diets that exclude specific food groups and additives.[50] The authors recommended that future studies should focus on the mechanism of action of dietary interventions at the level of the gut microbiota. In the face of these promising findings the American Academy of Pediatrics does not endorse elimination diets because of inconsistent findings of efficacy and concerns that highly restrictive diets do not provide balanced nutrition. Parents who are considering restrictive diets should consult with a nutritionist and highly restrictive diets should not be continued longer than two weeks in the absence of noticeable improvements in ADHD symptoms.[51]

The putative role of sugar in ADHD

Sugar is often regarded as a causative or exacerbating factor in ADHD, but research findings are inconsistent. In a nine-week randomised controlled trial (RCT), non-ADHD children randomised to high-sucrose diets versus aspartame or saccharin showed no differences in behaviour.[52]

This study failed to adequately control for fruits, juices or other high-glycaemic foods. Future studies are needed to investigate a possible link between high glycaemic index foods and hyperactivity.[53]

Parental expectations may bias perceptions of children's behaviour following consumption of large quantities of sugar. Mothers who believed their children had eaten sugar were more likely to label their child's behaviour as hyperactive.[54]

Large prospective studies on the therapeutic efficacy of dietary restrictions in ADHD are challenging because of difficulties controlling eating behaviour.[55]

Even though there is no causal link between dietary sugar and ADHD it is reasonable to limit dietary sugar during development because of the increasing prevalence of childhood obesity and associated risk of diabetes and other preventable weight-related medical problems.

EEG biofeedback

Many individuals diagnosed with ADHD have abnormal patterns of brain electrical activity, including 'under-arousal' in frontal and midline cortical regions and frontal 'hyper-arousal' that is more frequent in stimulant non-responders.[56] EEG biofeedback is aimed at normalising EEG activity in order to correct the brain's state of relative under-arousal and improve cognitive and behavioural functioning.[57] Two EEG biofeedback protocols have been extensively evaluated as treatments of ADHD. Sensorimotor rhythm (SMR) training reinforces EEG activity in the faster 'beta' frequency range (16–20 Hz) in the midline cortical regions, with the goal of reducing symptoms of impulsivity and hyperactivity. 'Theta suppression' reduces EEG activity in the slower 'theta' frequency range (4–8 Hz) and is primarily used to treat symptoms of inattention. An EEG biofeedback protocol directed at suppressing theta activity (4–8 Hz) over the midline regions is probably the most effective strategy when treating primarily symptoms of distractibility and inattention.

Controlled studies comparing EEG biofeedback with a stimulant medication versus a waitlist report positive clinical effects and EEG normalisation with select protocols have been conducted; however, it has not yet been established whether improved alertness is associated with increased or decreased alpha activity (12–18 Hz).[58,59] Neurofeedback sessions are typically 30–60 minutes in duration and are administered two to five times weekly for two to three months depending on symptom severity and response. A review of 14 randomised neurofeedback trials in children diagnosed with ADHD found consistent beneficial effects for all outcome measures.[60] The significance of neurofeedback research is limited by small study sizes, heterogeneous populations, absence of a control group, inconsistent outcome measures and limited or absent follow-up. The potential benefits of neurofeedback are limited by expensive treatments that are seldom covered by insurance. Further studies in which patients are randomly allocated to true versus sham biofeedback are needed to rule out positive group expectation effects. The use of sophisticated quantitative electroencephalography (QEEG) analysis with reference to a normative database may help future clinicians select the most efficacious treatment protocols for a particular ADHD symptom pattern.

Nutritional medicines

Children diagnosed with ADHD have lower plasma concentrations of certain **essential fatty acids** (EFAs) compared with the average population.[61] Findings to date on controlled trials of EFAs in ADHD are inconsistent. One study of EFAs as an adjunctive therapy to stimulants found no differential benefit of EFAs compared with stimulants plus a placebo.[62] Another adjunctive study found only modest improvements over placebo in disruptive behaviour and attention.[63] In a placebo-controlled trial on EFAs as a stand-alone treatment of ADHD, parents of children in the treatment group reported more improvement than parents of children receiving a palm oil placebo.[64] This study has been criticised because a high dropout rate biases findings in a positive direction.[53] The use of olive oil as a placebo may mask the beneficial clinical effects of EFAs because an active constituent of olive oil is converted into oleamide, which is known to affect brain function.[65] The short durations and low doses of EFAs used in most studies may not be adequate to result in the long-term changes in neuronal membrane structure required for clinical improvement.[62] The issue of dosing has been addressed by a small open-label study ($n = 9$) in which ADHD children were supplemented with high-dose eicosapentaenoic acid (EPA) or docosahexaenoic acid (DHA) concentrates (16.2 g/day) while continuing on stimulant medications. Most children were rated by a blinded psychiatrist as having significant improvements in both inattention and hyperactivity that correlated with reductions in the arachidonic acid (AA) to EPA ratio at the end of an eight-week treatment period.[66] A recent meta-analysis confirmed positive effects of adjunctive omega-3s in childhood ADHD; however, therapeutic benefits of this supplement were significantly less than for conventional pharmacological treatments.[67] A recent study comparing the efficacy of the omega-3 fatty acids DHA and EPA with the omega-6 fatty acid AA found improvement in a few specific areas of behaviour and cognition with increasing doses of omega-3s but no improvement in ADHD symptoms overall. Thirteen of 16 studies included in a systematic review of randomised controlled trials (total $n = 1514$) on essential fatty acids in ADHD children reported improvements in hyperactivity, impulsivity, attention, visual learning, word reading and short-term memory.[68] Four studies included in the review found that supplements containing a 9 : 3 : 1 ratio of eicosapentaenoic acid:docosahexaenoic acid:gamma linolenic acid increased red blood cell levels and were an effective adjunctive therapy in combination with stimulant medications. Pending confirmation by large controlled trials, supplementation with this ratio of fatty acids might permit lowering dosages of stimulant medications resulting in fewer adverse effects and improved compliance. Large prospective trials are needed to replicate these preliminary findings.[69]

Limited research findings suggest that **multivitamins** may improve concentration and attention in children[70]; however, large doses of single vitamins are ineffective in ADHD and may pose safety issues.[71] Some children diagnosed with ADHD may have abnormally low plasma zinc levels, which may interfere with optimal information processing and result in difficulties maintaining attention.[72,73] Findings of studies on **zinc** in ADHD are inconsistent. In a large 12-week prospective controlled randomised trial (PCRT) ($n = 400$), children and adolescents randomised to zinc (150 mg/day) experienced significant improvements in hyperactivity and impulsivity over placebo but not inattention.[74] A high dropout rate limits the significance of findings. In another study adding zinc to a stimulant resulted in greater improvement than stimulant alone.[75] In contrast to these findings a more recent placebo-controlled study failed to show efficacy.[76] Large prospective studies are needed to replicate these preliminary findings and confirm the optimum dosing of zinc sulfate.[77]

Abnormally low serum ferritin levels may be associated with hyperactivity in non-anaemic ADHD children but not with deficits in cognitive performance.[78] In an open trial non-iron-deficient children given oral **iron** for one month were perceived as less hyperactive and distractible by teachers but not by parents.[79] In a small 12-week PCRT non-anaemic ADHD children with abnormally low serum ferritin levels randomised to oral iron (ferrous sulfate 80 mg/day) showed progressive improvements in ADHD symptoms over placebo that were comparable to improvements obtained with stimulants.[80] A 2012 systematic review of studies on iron in children diagnosed with ADHD found mixed results in the relationship between serum iron levels and symptom severity, and inconsistent responses of ADHD symptoms to iron supplementation. Of note, two studies reviewed suggested that serum iron deficiency may reduce the effectiveness of stimulants.[81]

Acetyl-L-carnitine (ALC) is required for energy metabolism and synthesis of fatty acids. Findings of one small study suggested that L-carnitine significantly reduces the severity of ADHD symptoms; however, inconsistent findings and design flaws limit the significance of findings.[82] In a multi-site 16-week pilot study 112 ADHD children were randomised to placebo versus ALC (500 to 1500 mg b.i.d). Children in the ALC group with predominantly inattentive-type ADHD experienced greater improvement over placebo, but there was no differential benefit in children with combined-type ADHD. Significant adverse effects were not reported. In a six-week randomised placebo-controlled trial 40 children and adolescents (ages 7 to 13) diagnosed with ADHD were randomised to ALC (doses ranged from 500 to 1500 mg/day depending on weight) plus methylphenidate (20–30 mg/day) versus placebo plus methylphenidate. At the end of the study no differences were observed between the groups on Parent and Teacher Rating Scale scores.[83] Large prospective trials are needed to characterise the potential use of ALC as a stand-alone treatment or adjunctive treatment of childhood ADHD before this amino acid can be generally recommended.

Herbal medicines

In a four-week open study involving 36 children diagnosed with ADHD, a herbal preparation containing ***Ginkgo biloba*** and ***Panax quinquefolium*** was added to their existing ADHD medication.[84] Beneficial effects were observed in children taking the herbal combination after four weeks. It should be noted, however, that the absence of a placebo group (or a stimulant-only group) and the small size of the study limit the significance of findings. In a six-week double-blind randomised parallel group comparison 50 children with a diagnosis of ADHD treated with *Ginkgo biloba* showed significantly less improvement in symptom severity than matched children who received methylphenidate based on standardised parent and teacher ADHD rating scales.[85] Findings of open studies suggest that a standardised extract of *Pinus pinaster* (**Pycnogenol**) bark is beneficial in ADHD; however, only one PCRT has been published to date. Sixty-one children and adolescents randomised to Pycnogenol 1 mg/kg/day for one month experienced non-significant improvements in inattention, improved visual–motor coordination as evaluated by a psychologist but no improvements in symptoms of hyperactivity. Symptoms returned to pretreatment baseline levels after a one-month washout.[86] Only one case of mild gastric discomfort was reported. These findings should be regarded as preliminary pending replication by large prospective studies.

Bacopa monnieri is an Ayurvedic herbal used as a tonic and memory enhancer. In one RCT ($n = 85$) healthy men and women randomised to a extract containing *Ginkgo biloba* and *Bacopa monnieri* did not perform better than a placebo group in tests of short-term memory, working memory, executive processing, planning, problem-solving and information processing speed.[87] These findings cannot be generalised to ADHD, but they suggest that this herbal formula does not ameliorate the core symptoms of ADHD. A review of controlled trials investigating the effects of multi-herbal formulas containing *B. monnieri* on children and adolescents found modest evidence for improved cognition.[88] Findings were weakened by inconsistent statistical design and under-reporting of safety and tolerability data. Melatonin is sometimes used to treat ADHD in children, although a recent study failed to show clinical efficacy.[89]

In addition to single vitamins and herbals various proprietary herbal and nutrient formulas are sometimes used to treat ADHD; however, little research evidence supports their use. A four-month randomised double-blind placebo-controlled trial evaluated the efficacy of a patented herbal formula in 120 children diagnosed with ADHD. It evaluated the efficacy of a patented, compound herbal preparation (**Nurture and Clarity**) in improving attention, cognition and impulse control in children with ADHD.[90] Principle active ingredients included *Paeoniae alba*, *Withania somnifera*, *Centella asiatica*, *Spirulina platensis*, *Bacopa monnieri* and *Melissa officinalis*. At study end the group receiving the herbal formula showed statistically significant improvement in symptoms of inattention, impulse control and cognition in all four subscales of the test of variables of attention (TOVA) compared with no improvement in the control group. The herbal formula was well tolerated. Large prospective placebo-controlled studies are needed to confirm these preliminary findings.

Homeopathy

A systematic review of RCTs on homeopathic remedies in ADHD found no evidence of beneficial effects of homeopathy on symptom severity, core symptoms or the course of ADHD.[91] These findings have been criticised because conventional RCT study designs may not permit the demonstration of measurable clinical effects of individualised homeopathic remedies for ADHD. Long-term studies that include an initial open-label phase are needed to determine the 'optimal' homeopathic remedy for each unique patient over several months. In a subsequent placebo-controlled phase individuals could then be randomised to their 'optimum' remedy versus a randomly selected homeopathic preparation.[92]

These criticisms were addressed by a sequential case series comparing 20 children diagnosed with ADHD receiving homeopathic treatment with 10 ADHD children receiving usual care.[93] Eleven different homeopathic remedies were used and some children received concurrent treatment with prescription medications or other complementary therapies. Seventy-five per cent of children in the homeopathy treatment group reported experiencing cummulative improvements in core ADHD symptoms over the one-year study period.[93] The significance of findings is limited by small study size, non-random sample selection and the absence of outcome measures that could evaluate the effectiveness of different homeopathic remedies.

Acupuncture

A systematic review and meta-analysis of studies on acupuncture as a treatment for ADHD identified three studies that met inclusion criteria for methodological rigour and size.[94] Two sham-controlled studies reported improvement with electroacupuncture over sham electroacupuncture in children receiving concurrent behavioural therapy. A meta-analysis of two other studies using somatic acupuncture or auricular acupuncture combined with drug therapy showed significant differential effects of combined treatment. The authors of the systematic review regarded these findings as inconclusive due to small study size, the short duration of trials (less than one month), the absence of blinding in two studies resulting in a high risk of exaggerated treatment effects and the absence of an intention-to-treat analysis in all studies. The authors also noted that as all reviewed studies involved ethnic Chinese populations, findings cannot be generalised to other ethnic groups. Conclusive findings of acupuncture in the treatment of ADHD will emerge from studies of long duration that are large enough to permit rigorous statistical analysis of findings, and include blinded protocols for treatment allocation.

A different review summarised positive findings of studies on Chinese medicine treatments of ADHD including acupuncture, Chinese massage (tui na), tai chi chuan and Chinese herbal formulas.[95] The authors commented that methodological problems limit the significance of findings and recommended large high-quality studies. The same review included a meta-analysis and systematic review of unpublished data from 54 controlled trials conducted between 1999 and 2013 on Chinese herbal medicine alone or in combination with methylphenidate identified 39 compound herbal formulas containing a total of 94 herbals, with each formula containing 5 to 17 herbals. The two most frequently used herbals, Shichangpu (*Rhizoma acori tatarinowii*) and Yuanzhi (*Polygala tenuifolia*) readily cross the blood–brain barrier, are used to treat symptoms of psychosis, and (according to the same unpublished findings) improve memory and reduce hyperactivity. The unpublished findings reportedly show that many Chinese herbal formulas can be safely combined with methylphenidate, resulting in greater clinical improvement than with stimulants alone. The authors remarked on methodological problems and heterogeneity of studies including use of different herbal formulas and different dosages, and the absence of standardised diagnostic criteria and outcome measures.

Exercise

A systematic review of studies on clinical benefits of physical activity for individuals with ADHD found that regular moderate to intense physical activity reduces cognitive, behavioral and physical symptoms of ADHD.[96] Larger studies are needed to identify the ideal exercise prescription for ADHD.

Mind–body techniques

In a recent systematic review of studies on meditation and mind–body practices (e.g. yoga, Tai Chi, Qi gong) as treatments of ADHD only four studies including a total of 83 participants met inclusion criteria for methodological rigour and size.[97] Two studies evaluated **mantra meditation** and two studies compared **yoga** with conventional drugs, relaxation training, non-specific exercise or treatment as usual. The authors reported that study design problems resulted in a high risk of bias in all studies and identified only one study that met criteria for formal analysis. In that small study ($n = 15$) the teacher rating ADHD scale failed to show significant outcome differences between the meditation group and the drug therapy group. The review authors commented that small sample sizes of a few well-designed studies and high risk of bias render current findings on meditation and mind–body techniques in the treatment of ADHD inconclusive. Larger and better designed studies are needed.

Two more recent meta-analyses on studies of mindfulness-based therapies for ADHD reported conflicting findings. A meta-analysis of 10 studies on mindfulness-based therapies found significant reductions in symptoms of inattention, impulsivity and hyperactivity across age groups with a larger effect size for reduction of symptoms of inattention in adults.[98] Another review included a total of 16 studies on mindfulness interventions for ADHD identified no definitive findings because of a high risk of bias and generally poor methodological quality across studies.[99] The significance of findings of both reviews are limited by heterogeneity in study design, small study size and limited information on the nature of mindfulness interventions used in many studies. Well-designed studies are needed to confirm the benefits of mindfulness for ADHD before recommendations can be made for children or adults with this condition.

In a small pilot study ADHD children randomised to yoga experienced greater improvement over time compared with children who exercised. Children who continued on stimulants while practising yoga experienced the greatest improvements.[100] Two small controlled studies suggest that yoga and regular **massage therapy** may reduce the severity of ADHD symptoms.[101,102]

A retrospective cast study identified four adolescents diagnosed with ADHD who received chiropractic treatment. The authors reported improvements in ADHD symptoms following **spinal manipulative therapy**; however, these findings are inconclusive because of the small sample size, the absence of controls and the likelihood of reporting bias as all authors are chiropractors.[103]

It has been hypothesised that ADHD may be associated with poor working memory and memory training may result in functional improvements in children and adolescents diagnosed with ADHD. A proprietary **computer-based memory training program** available over the internet is being explored as a treatment of ADHD.[104] The five-week training program consists of 25 sessions lasting 30–45 minutes.[104] In a non-blinded study of 52 children diagnosed with ADHD non-blinded parent raters reported significant improvements in attention; however, teachers did not observe improvements in ADHD symptoms. An RCT demonstrated improved working memory in adolescents diagnosed with ADHD but no improvement in ADHD symptoms.[105]

Occupational therapy

It has been suggested that a form of occupational therapy called sensory integration—widely used to treat autism—may help lessen symptoms of hyperactivity; however, findings to date are limited by small study sizes and methodological problems.[106]

'Green' play environments
ADHD may result from 'attention fatigue' caused by limited contact with 'green spaces' during early childhood.
Findings of a large observational study suggest that ADHD children who spend more time playing outdoors in natural environments may experience fewer and less severe symptoms.[107]
These findings have been criticised because of design flaws, such as a heterogeneous population that included children with comorbid ODD and the absence of independent raters.[108]

CLINICAL SUMMARY

ADHD remains a highly controversial diagnosis among mental health professionals and parents because of many unresolved issues, and some claim that the disorder does not even exist.[109,110] In spite of considerable research there is still no strong evidence of a genetic or physiological basis for the disorder.[111] As noted above diagnostic criteria used to diagnose ADHD according to the DSM continue to evolve, suggesting that there is still no consensus on the symptoms that constitute ADHD. Although there is probably little abuse potential when stimulants are used to treat childhood ADHD, this remains a central concern among parents.[112]

In spite of their adverse effects and associated risk of substance abuse stimulants continue to be the most widely used conventional treatments of ADHD. When stimulants fail to result in significant reductions in symptom severity or when adverse effects, toxicities or comorbid substance abuse preclude their use, EEG biofeedback and select naturopathic treatments should be considered. Amelioration of ADHD symptoms usually requires several weeks of specialised EEG biofeedback training protocols, specifically SMR training or theta suppression (Figure 37.1). Restrictive diets are reasonable interventions in cases where impulsivity and distractibility may be related to sugar intake or food allergies. There are no contraindications to taking stimulant medications while following a restrictive diet; however, parents of ADHD children should first consult their child's paediatrician before initiating a strict dietary regimen, and ideally with a nutritionist who can provide them with expert guidance.

When therapeutic doses of stimulants cannot be achieved with acceptable tolerance the adjunctive use of EFAs, and select herbals (see evidence in Table 37.1), including *Ginkgo biloba*, *Panax quinquefolium*, *Pinus pinaster* and *Bacopa monnieri* may improve response. The adjunctive use of acetyl-L-carnitine, zinc and iron may be beneficial, although these treatments are not substantiated by strong research findings. Regular yoga and massage therapy may also help improve attention and hyperactivity in some cases. When a person diagnosed with ADHD fails to respond to established pharmacological and more substantiated alternative treatments it is prudent to rule out possibly confounding psychiatric disorders, including learning disorders, depressed mood and anxiety disorders, which are frequently comorbid with the syndrome and may interfere with treatment outcomes.

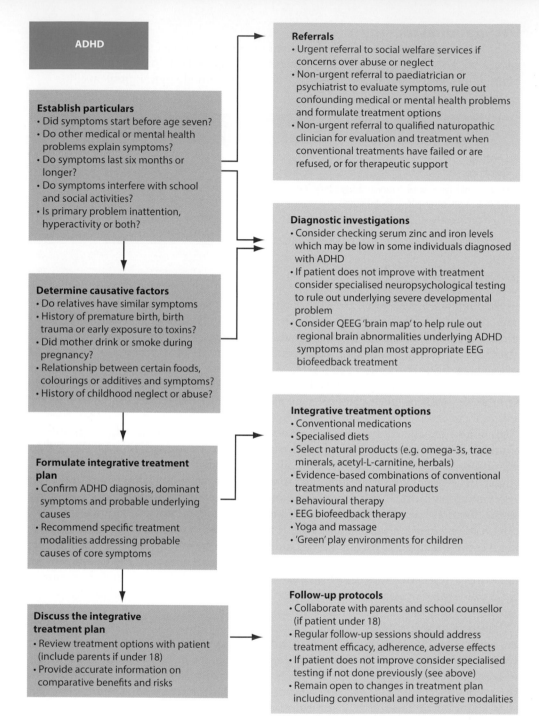

Figure 37.1
Integrative treatment decision tree—ADHD

Table 37.1
Review of the major evidence

Intervention	Mechanisms of action	Key literature	Summary of results	Comment
Dietary changes	A subset of children may be hypersensitive to certain foods or dietary additives resulting in symptoms of ADHD	Double-blind placebo-controlled challenge crossover trial ($n = 300$ ADHD children): phase I elimination, phase II challenge[113] Double-blind placebo-controlled challenge crossover trial ($n = 56$ children ages 4–12 years with behavioural problems): phase I open elimination followed by challenge[114]	75% improved with restricted diet but symptoms recurred when food colourings, additives re-introduced Improved behaviour and attention scores	No description of recruitment or eligibility of non-reactors in phase I More restrictive than Feingold but less restrictive than OAD protocol
EEG biofeedback	(EEG) biofeedback may normalise brain electrical activity, correcting the brain's state of relative under-arousal in ADHD and improving cognitive and behavioural functioning[57]	One-year clinical trial stimulants versus EEG biofeedback plus stimulants[57] ($n = 100$, ages 6–19 years) Twelve-week clinical trial EEG biofeedback SMR and beta rhythms three times a week versus stimulants ($n = 34$, boys aged 8–12 years)[115]	Symptoms improved on stimulants but only biofeedback group sustained improvement without stimulants at one-year follow-up TOVA and Conners' scores significantly improved in EEG biofeedback group	Group assignments based on parental preference; average of 43 sessions required for sustained improvement Group assignments based on parental preference
Herbal medicine	Herbals and other natural products may address ADHD through beneficial effects on different neurotransmitter systems	Four-week open study ($n = 34$): ADHD children randomised *Ginkgo biloba* + American ginseng added to ongoing stimulant medication[84] One-month RCT ($n = 61$): standardised extract of Pycnogenol (from *Pinus pinaster*) 1 mg/kg/day[74] RCT ($n = 85$ healthy men and women): extract of *Ginkgo biloba* and *Bacopa monnieri* versus placebo[80]	Improvements in ADHD symptoms were found after four weeks of treatment Significant improvements in hyperactivity, inattention and visual–motor coordination No improvements over placebo in short-term memory, working memory, executive processing, etc.	No comparison group treated with stimulants only Large studies needed to replicate findings Study population consisted of normal individuals Large prospective dose-finding trials on ADHD patients needed
Trace elements	Abnormally low plasma zinc levels in some children diagnosed with ADHD may interfere with optimal information processing and result in difficulties maintaining attention[72,73] Abnormally low serum ferritin levels may be associated with hyperactivity in some children[78]	Twelve-week RCT ($n = 400$ children and adolescents): high-dose zinc (150 mg/day) versus placebo[51] Twelve-week RCT: non-anaemic ADHD children with low serum ferritin treated with oral iron (80 mg/day) versus placebo[80]	Significant improvement in hyperactivity and impulsivity but *not* inattention Improvements with iron comparable to stimulants	High dropout rate limits significance Large prospective studies needed to confirm efficacy and determine optimal dosing

Table 37.1
Review of the major evidence (continued)

Intervention	Mechanisms of action	Key literature	Summary of results	Comment
Omega-3 fatty acids	Abnormal low plasma concentrations of certain EFAs needed for normal brain functioning may manifest as symptoms of ADHD[61]	Two-month double-blind placebo-controlled randomised trial (n = 40, ages 6–12); diet consisted of DHA-enriched foods versus olive-oil enriched foods[116] Eight-week open pilot study (n = 9): children given high dose EPA/DHA concentrates (16.2 g/day) then rated by blinded psychiatrist[66]	Short-term memory improved and commission errors decreased in control but not DHA group No differences in parent or teacher ratings of behavioural or cognitive symptoms Significant improvements in behaviour and inattention, correlating with reduced AA:EPA ratio and global severity of illness scores; no serious adverse effects were reported	Olive oil may not be inert (see text). Serum EFA levels were not measured Some subjects had comorbid Asperger's syndrome, conduct disorder, learning disorders and mood disorders No placebo group; some subjects had comorbid conduct disorder or ODD (which also improved during study) Dietary intake not recorded at baseline or during study; supplement intake not closely monitored
Acetyl-L-carnitine (ALC)	Taking ALC may lessen some symptoms of ADHD by increasing central nervous system energy production and fatty acid synthesis	A 16-week pilot study (n = 112 ADHD children) randomised to ALC (500–1500 mg b.i.d.) versus placebo[82]	ALC superior to placebo in inattentive-type children but not combined-type ADHD	A replication study is now needed
Yoga and massage	Yoga, massage and other mind–body approaches may reduce autonomic arousal enhancing baseline attention	In two small controlled studies ADHD children stable on medications were randomised to yoga or regular massage therapy[101,102]	Regular yoga and massage may reduce severity of ADHD symptoms	Possible group expectation effects Large prospective studies needed
Acupuncture	Acupuncture may address ADHD by correcting postulated 'energetic imbalances' that manifest as this disorder	Sham-controlled studies on electroacupuncture in children receiving concurrent behavioural therapy[72] ADHD children received somatic or auricular acupuncture combined with drug therapy	Children receiving electroacupuncture improved more than children receiving sham acupuncture Significant benefit of combined treatment over drugs alone	Longer, better designed studies needed to determine efficacy and optimal protocols Findings inconclusive due to small study size, methodological flaws and possible expectation bias
Exercise	Regular exercise may improve global brain functioning and assists in channelling excess or nervous energy	Open studies on exercise combined with drugs versus drugs only in children diagnosed with ADHD[117]	Exercise combined with drug therapy more beneficial for both cognitive and behavioural symptoms than drugs only	Findings limited by small sample size, methodological flaws and absence of documentation on ADHD subtype

KEY POINTS

- Take into account the unique causes of the syndrome in each patient, including genetic factors, perinatal insults or toxic exposure, food sensitivities and social factors.

- Stimulants and non-stimulant medications are beneficial and well-tolerated conventional treatments of ADHD for a significant percentage of children, adolescents and adults; however, there are legitimate concerns about safety and abuse potential whenever stimulants are used.

- Restricting food colourings, additives, sugar or specific foods may significantly reduce symptoms of hyperactivity in some cases.

- When stimulants are not effective, poorly tolerated or refused by the patient or parents, the use of validated EEG biofeedback protocols including SMR training for primarily hyperactive-type ADHD and theta suppression for primarily inattentive-type ADHD are appropriate first-line treatments.

- Zinc supplementation may be helpful when hyperactivity and impulsive behaviour do not respond to stimulants alone. Supplement with iron and ALC for the core symptoms of distractibility and inattention. More studies are needed.

- High doses of omega-3 EFAs (up to 16 g/day) may have therapeutic effects on symptoms of both inattention and hyperactivity. More studies are needed.

- *Ginkgo biloba*, *Panax quinquefolium*, *Pinus pinaster* and *Bacopa monnieri* may be beneficial in ADHD; however, conclusive findings from large prospective controlled trials are needed before any of these can be recommended as adjunctive or first-line treatments.

FURTHER READING

Katzman MA, Bilkey TS, Chokka PR, et al. Adult ADHD and comorbid disorders: clinical implications of a dimensional approach. BMC Psychiatry 2017;17(1):302. doi:10.1186/s12888-017-1463-3.

Lange KW, Hauser J, Lange KM, et al. The Role of Nutritional Supplements in the Treatment of ADHD: what the Evidence Says. Curr Psychiatry Rep 2017;19(2):8.

Sarris J, Kean J, Schweitzer I, et al. Complementary medicines (herbal and nutritional products) in the treatment of Attention Deficit Hyperactivity Disorder (ADHD): a systematic review of the evidence. Complement Ther Med 2011;19(4):216–27.

Thapar A, Cooper M. Attention deficit hyperactivity disorder. Lancet 2016;387(10024):1240–50.

REFERENCES

1. Polanczyk G, de Lima MS, Horta BL, et al. The worldwide prevalence of ADHD: a systematic review and metaregression analysis. Am J Psychiatry 2007;164(6):942–8.

2. Barbaresi WJ, Katusic SK, Colligan RC, et al. How common is attention-deficit/hyperactivity disorder? Incidence in a population-based birth cohort in Rochester, Minn. Arch Pediatr Adolesc Med 2002;156(3):217–24.

3. Kessler RC, Adler L, Barkley R, et al. The prevalence and correlates of adult ADHD in the United States: results from the National Comorbidity Survey Replication. Am J Psychiatry 2006;163(4):716–23.

4. Centers for Disease Control. National health interview survey. Atlanta: Centers for Disease Control; 2002. p. 2004.

5. Biederman J, Faraone SV. The Massachusetts General Hospital studies of gender influences on attention-deficit/hyperactivity disorder in youth and relatives. Psychiatr Clin North Am 2004;27(2):225–32.

6. Biederman J, Faraone SV. Attention-deficit hyperactivity disorder. Lancet 2005;366(9481):237–48.

7. Wallis D, et al. Review: genetics of attention deficit/hyperactivity disorder. J Pediatr Psychol 2008;33(10):1085–99.

8. Swanson JM, et al. Etiologic subtypes of attention-deficit/hyperactivity disorder: brain imaging, molecular genetic and environmental factors and the dopamine hypothesis. Neuropsychol Rev 2007;17(1):39–59.

9. Brennan AR, Arnsten AF. Neuronal mechanisms underlying attention deficit hyperactivity disorder: the influence of arousal on prefrontal cortical function. Ann N Y Acad Sci 2008;1129:236–45.

10. Silvestri R, et al. Sleep disorders in children with attention-deficit/hyperactivity disorder (ADHD) recorded overnight by video-polysomnography. Sleep Med 2009;10(10):1132–8.

11. Di Michele F, et al. The neurophysiology of attention-deficit hyperactivity disorder. Int J Psychophysiol 2005;58(1):81–93.

12. American Psychiatric Association. Diagnostic and Statistical Manual of Mental Disorders. 5th edn. Arlington: American Psychiatric Association; 2013.

13. American Psychiatric Association. Diagnostic and Statistical Manual of Mental Disorders. 4th edn. Arlington: American Psychiatric Association; 2000.

14. Pearl P, et al. Medical mimics of ADHD. In: Wasserstein J, editor. ADHD in adults: brain mechanisms and behavior. Ann NY Acad Sci; 2001. p. 99–111.

15. Newcorn JH, et al. The complexity of ADHD: diagnosis and treatment of the adult patient with comorbidities. CNS Spectr 2007;12(8 Suppl. 12):1–14.

16. Cimera R. Making ADHD a gift: teaching Superman how to fly. Lanham: Scarecrow Press, Inc; 2002. p. 16.

17. Kessler RC, et al. The prevalence and effects of adult attention deficit/hyperactivity disorder on work performance in a nationally representative sample of workers. J Occup Environ Med 2005;47(6):565–72.

18. Faraone SV, Wilens T. Does stimulant treatment lead to substance use disorders? J Clin Psychiatry 2003;64(Suppl. 11):9–13.

19. Rabiner DL, Anastopoulos AD, Costello EJ, et al. The misuse and diversion of prescribed ADHD medications by college students. J Atten Disord 2009;13(2):144–53.

20. Kollins SH. ADHD, substance use disorders, and psychostimulant treatment: current literature and treatment guidelines. J Atten Disord 2008;12(2):115–25.

21. Najib J. The efficacy and safety profile of lisdexamfetamine dimesylate, a prodrug of d-amphetamine, for the treatment of attention-deficit/hyperactivity disorder in children and adults. Clin Ther 2009;31(1):142–76.

22. Schachter HM, et al. How efficacious and safe is short-acting methylphenidate for the treatment of attention-deficit disorder in children and adolescents? CMAJ 2001;165(11):1475–88.

23. Berman SM, et al. Potential adverse effects of amphetamine treatment on brain and behavior: a review. Mol Psychiatry 2009;14(2):123–42.

24. Slatkoff J, Greenfield B. Pharmacological treatment of attention-deficit/hyperactivity disorder in adults. Expert Opin Investig Drugs 2006;15(6):649–67.

25. Findling RL. Evolution of the treatment of attention-deficit/hyperactivity disorder in children: a review. Clin Ther 2008;30(5):942–57.

26. Miller MC. What is the significance of the new warnings about suicide risk with Strattera? Harv Ment Health Lett 2005;22(6):8.

27. Nissen SE. ADHD drugs and cardiovascular risk. N Engl J Med 2006;354(14):1445–8.

28. Kahbazi M, Ghoreishi A, Rahiminejad F, et al. A randomized, double-blind and placebo-controlled trial of modafinil in children and adolescents with attention deficit and hyperactivity disorder. Psychiatry Res 2009;168(3):234–7.

29. Arabgol F, Panaghi L, Hebrani P. Reboxetine versus methylphenidate in treatment of children and adolescents with attention deficit-hyperactivity disorder. Eur Child Adolesc Psychiatry 2009;18(1):53–9.

30. Sallee FR, Lyne A, Wigal T, et al. Long-term safety and efficacy of guanfacine extended release in children and adolescents with attention-deficit/hyperactivity disorder. J Child Adolesc Psychopharmacol 2009;19(3):215–26.

31. Scahill L. Alpha-2 adrenergic agonists in children with inattention, hyperactivity and impulsiveness. CNS Drugs 2009;23(Suppl. 1):43–9.

32. Rubio B, Boes A, Laganiere S, et al. Noninvasive brain stimulation in pediatric ADHD: a review. J Child Neurol 2016;31(6):784–96.

33. Smith RC, Boules S, Mattiuz S, et al. Effects of transcranial direct current stimulation (tDCS) on cognition, symptoms, and smoking in schizophrenia: a randomized controlled study. Schizophr Res 2015;168(1–2):260–6.

34. Zaehle T, Sandmann P, Thorne JD, et al. Transcranial direct current stimulation of the prefrontal cortex modulates working memory performance: combined behavioural and electrophysiological evidence. BMC Neurosci 2011;12:2.

35. Cachoeiraa C, Leffab D, Mittelstadta L, et al. Positive effects of transcranial direct current stimulation in adult patients with attention-deficit/hyperactivity disorder—a pilot randomized controlled study. Psychiatry Res 2017;247:28–32.

36. Bussing R, et al. Use of complementary and alternative medicine for symptoms of attention-deficit hyperactivity disorder. Psychiatr Serv 2002;53(9):1096–102.

37. Stubberfield T, Parry T. Utilization of alternative therapies in attention-deficit hyperactivity disorder. J Paediatr Child Health 1999;35(5):450–3.

38. Anderson SL, Navalta CP. Altering the course of neurodevelopment: a framework for understanding the enduring effects of psychotropic drugs. Int J Dev Neurosci 2004;22(5–6):423–40.

39. Sinha D, Efron D. Complementary and alternative medicine use in children with attention deficit hyperactivity disorder. J Pediatr Child Health 2005;41:23–6.

40. Chan E, Rappaport LA, Kemper KJ. Complementary and alternative therapies in childhood attention and hyperactivity problems. J Dev Behav Pediatr 2003;24:4–8.

41. Chan E, et al. Complementary and alternative therapies in childhood attention and hyperactivity problems. J Dev Behav Pediatr 2003;24(1):4–8.

42. Sarris J, Kean J, Schweitzer I, et al. Complementary medicines (herbal and nutritional products) in the treatment of attention deficit hyperactivity disorder (ADHD): a systematic review of the evidence. Complement Ther Med 2011;19(4):216–27.

43. Feingold B. Why your child is hyperactive. New York: Random House; 1975.

44. Wender EH. The food additive-free diet in the treatment of behavior disorders: a review. J Dev Behav Pediatr 1986;7(1):35–42.

45. Nigg JT, Lewis K, Edinger T, et al. Meta-analysis of attention-deficit/hyperactivity disorder or attention-deficit/hyperactivity disorder symptoms, restriction diet, and synthetic food color additives. J Am Acad Child Adolesc Psychiatry 2012;51:86–97.

46. Egger J, et al. Controlled trial of hyposensitization in children with food-induced hyperkinetic syndrome. Lancet 1992;339:1150–3.

47. Carter CM, et al. Effects of a new food diet in attention-deficit disorder. Arch Dis Child 1993;69:564–8.

48. Schmidt MH, et al. Does oligoantigenic diet influence hyperactive/conduct-disordered children: a controlled trial. Eur Child Adolesc Psychiatry 1997;6:88–95.

49. Rojas NL, Chan E. Old and new controversies in the alternative treatment of attention-deficit hyperactivity disorder. Ment Retard Dev Disabil Res Rev 2005;11(2):116–30.

50. Pelsser LM, Frankena K, Toorman J, et al. Diet and ADHD, reviewing the evidence: a systematic review of meta-analyses of double-blind placebo-controlled trials evaluating the efficacy of diet interventions on the behavior of children with ADHD. PLoS ONE 2017;12(1):e0169277. doi:10.1371/journal.pone.0169277.

51. Arnold LE, Hurt E, Mayes T, et al. In: Evans SW, Hoza B, editors. Ingestible alternative and complementary treatments for treating attention deficit hyperactivity disorder: assessment and intervention in developmental context. Kingston: Civic Research Institute; 2010. p. 2–28.

52. Wolraich S, et al. Effects of diets high in sucrose or aspartame on the behavior and cognitive performance of children. N Engl J Med 1994;330(5):301–7.

53. Weber W, Newmark S. Complementary and alternative medical therapies for attention-deficit/hyperactivity disorder and autism. Pediatr Clin North Am 2007;54(6):983–1006, xii.

54. Hoover DW, Milich R. Effects of sugar ingestion expectancies on mother–child interactions. J Abnorm Child Psychol 1994;22(4):501–15.

55. Cormier E, Elder JH. Diet and child behavior problems: fact or fiction? Pediatr Nurs 2007;33(2):138–43.

56. Butnik SM. Neurofeedback in adolescents and adults with attention deficit hyperactivity disorder. J Clin Psychol 2005;61(5):621–5.

57. Monastra VJ, et al. The effects of stimulant therapy, EEG biofeedback, and parenting style on the primary symptoms of attention-deficit/hyperactivity disorder. Appl Psychophysiol Biofeedback 2002;27(4):231–49.

58. Monastra VJ, et al. Electroencephalographic biofeedback in the treatment of attention-deficit/hyperactivity disorder. Appl Psychophysiol Biofeedback 2005;30(2):95–114.

59. Ramirez P, et al. EEG biofeedback treatment of ADD: a viable alternative to traditional medical intervention? Ann NY Acad Sci. 2001;931:342–58.

60. Lofthouse N, Arnold LE, Hersch S, et al. A review of neurofeedback treatment for pediatric ADHD. J Atten Disord 2012;16:351–72.

61. Gedik Y, et al. Relationships between serum free fatty acids and zinc, and attention deficit hyperactivity disorder: a research note. J Child Psychol Psychiatry 1996;37:225–7.

62. Voigt RG, et al. A randomized, double-blind, placebo-controlled trial of docosahexaenoic acid supplementation in children with attention-deficit/hyperactivity disorder. J Pediatr 2001;139(2):189–96.

63. Stevens LJ, et al. Essential fatty acid metabolism in boys with attention-deficit hyperactivity disorder. Am J Clin Nutr 1995;62(4):761–8.

64. Sinn N, Bryan J. Effect of supplementation with polyunsaturated fatty acids and micronutrients on learning and behavior problems associated with child ADHD. J Dev Behav Pediatr 2007;28(2):82–91.

65. Richardson AJ, Puri BK. A randomized double-blind, placebo-controlled study of the effects of supplementation with highly unsaturated fatty acids on ADHD-related symptoms in children with specific learning difficulties. Prog Neuropsychopharmacol Biol Psychiatry 2002; 26:233–9.

66. Sorgi PJ, et al. Effects of an open-label pilot study with high-dose EPA/DHA concentrates on plasma phospholipids and behavior in children with attention deficit hyperactivity disorder. Nutr J 2007;6:16.

67. Bloch MH, Qawasmi A. Omega-3 fatty acid supplementation for the treatment of children with attention-deficit/hyperactivity disorder symptomatology: systematic review and meta-analysis. J Am Acad Child Adolesc Psychiatry 2011;50:991–1000.

68. Derbyshire E. Review article: do omega-3/6 fatty acids have a therapeutic role in children and young people with ADHD? J Lipids 2017;2017:Article ID 6285218.

69. Milte CM, Parletta N, Buckley JD, et al. Eicosapentaenoic and docosahexaenoic acids cognition and behavior in children with attention-deficit/hyperactivity disorder: a randomized controlled trial. Nutrition 2012;28:670–7.

70. Hurt E, Arnold LE, Lofthouse N. Dietary and nutritional treatments for attention-deficit/hyperactivity disorder: current research support and recommendations for practitioners. Curr Psychiatry Rep 2011;13:323–32.

71. Arnold LE, Hurt E, Mayes T, et al. Ingestible alternative and complementary treatments for treating attention deficit hyperactivity disorder: assessment and intervention in developmental context. In: Evans SW, Hoza B, editors. Treating attention deficit disorder. Kingston: Civic Research Institute; 2011. p. 15.1–12.

72. Yorbik O, et al. Potential effects of zinc on information processing in boys with attention deficit hyperactivity

disorder. Prog Neuropsychopharmacol Biol Psychiatry 2008;32(3):662–7.

73. Arnold LE, et al. Serum zinc correlates with parent- and teacher-rated inattention in children with attention-deficit/hyperactivity disorder. J Child Adolesc Psychopharmacol 2005;15(4):628–36.

74. Bilici M, et al. Double-blind, placebo-controlled study of zinc sulfate in the treatment of attention deficit hyperactivity disorder. Prog Neuropsychopharmacol Biol Psychiatry 2004;28(1):181–90.

75. Akhondzadeh S, et al. Zinc sulfate as an adjunct to methylphenidate for the treatment of attention deficit hyperactivity disorder in children: a double blind and randomized trial [ISRCTN64132371]. BMC Psychiatry 2004;4(1):9.

76. Arnold LE, DiSilvestro RA, Bozzolo D, et al. Zinc for attention-deficit/hyperactivity disorder: placebo-controlled double-blind pilot trial alone and combined with amphetamine. J Child Adolesc Psychopharmacol 2011;21(1):1–19.

77. Arnold LE, DiSilvestro RA. Zinc in attention-deficit/hyperactivity disorder. J Child Adolesc Psychopharmacol 2005;15(4):619–27.

78. Oner O, et al. Relation of ferritin levels with symptom ratings and cognitive performance in children with attention deficit-hyperactivity disorder. Pediatr Int 2008;50(1):40–4.

79. Sever Y, et al. Iron treatment in children with attention deficit hyperactivity disorder: a preliminary report. Neuropsychobiology 1997;35:178–80.

80. Konofal E, et al. Effects of iron supplementation on attention deficit hyperactivity disorder in children. Pediatr Neurol 2008;38(1):20–6.

81. Cortese S, Angriman M, Lecendreux M, et al. Iron and attention deficit/hyperactivity disorder: what is the empirical evidence so far? A systematic review of the literature. Expert Rev Neurother 2012;12(10):1227–40.

82. Van Oudheusden LJ, Scholte HR. Efficacy of carnitine in the treatment of children with attention-deficit hyperactivity disorder. Prostaglandins Leukot Essent Fatty Acids 2002;67(1):33–8.

83. Abbasi SH, Heidari S, Mohammadi MR, et al. Acetyl-L-carnitine as an adjunctive therapy in the treatment of attention-deficit/hyperactivity disorder in children and adolescents: a placebo-controlled trial. Child Psychiatry Hum Dev 2011;42(3):367–75.

84. Lyon MR, et al. Effect of the herbal extract combination Panax quinquefolium and Ginkgo biloba on attention-deficit hyperactivity disorder: a pilot study. J Psychiatry Neurosci 2001;26(3):221–8.

85. Salehi B, Imani R, Mohammadi MR, et al. Ginkgo biloba for attention-deficit/hyperactivity disorder in children and adolescents: a double blind, randomized controlled trial. Prog Neuropsychopharmacol Biol Psychiatry 2010;34(1):76–80.

86. Trebaticka J, et al. Treatment of ADHD with French maritime pine bark extract Pycnogenol™. Eur Child Adolesc Psychiatry 2006;6:329–35.

87. Nathan PJ, et al. Effects of a combined extract of Ginkgo biloba and Bacopa monnieri on cognitive function in healthy humans. Hum Psychopharmacol 2004;19(2):91–6.

88. Kean J, Downey L, Stough C. Review. Systematic overview of Bacopa monnieri (L.) Wettst. dominant poly-herbal formulas in children and adolescents. Medicine 2017;4:86. doi:10.3390/medicines4040086.

89. Hoebert M, van der Heijden KB, van Geijlswijk IM, et al. Long term follow-up of melatonin treatment in children with ADHD and chronic sleep onset insomnia. J Pineal Res 2009;4:1–7.

90. Katz M, Levine AA, Kol-Degani H, et al. A compound herbal preparation (CHP) in the treatment of children with ADHD: a randomized controlled trial. J Atten Disord 2010;14(3):281–91.

91. Coulter MK, Dean ME. Homoeopathy for attention deficit/hyperactivity disorder or hyperkinetic disorder. Cochrane Database Syst Rev 2007;(4):CD005648.

92. Frei H, et al. Randomised controlled trials of homoeopathy in hyperactive children: treatment procedure leads to an unconventional study design. Experience with open-label homoeopathic treatment preceding the Swiss ADHD placebo controlled, randomised, double-blind, cross-over trial. Homoeopathy 2007;96(1):35–41.

93. Fibert P, Relton C, Heirs M, et al. A comparative consecutive case series of 20 children with a diagnosis of ADHD receiving homeopathic treatment, compared with 10 children receiving treatment. Homeopathy 2016;105:194e201.

94. Lee MS, Choi TY, Kim JI, et al. Acupuncture for treating attention-deficit hyperactivity disorder: a systematic review and meta-analysis. Chin J Integr Med 2011;17(4):257–60.

95. Ni X, Zhang-James Y, Han X, et al. Traditional Chinese medicine in the treatment of ADHD: a review. Child Adolesc Psychiatr Clin N Am 2014;23:853–81.

96. Qin X, Hob C, Chanb H, et al. Managing childhood and adolescent attention-deficit/hyperactivity disorder (ADHD) with exercise: a systematic review. Complement Ther Med 2017;34:123–8.

97. Krisanaprakornkit T, Ngamjarus C, Witoonchart C, et al. Meditation therapies for attention deficit/hyperactivity disorder (ADHD). Cochrane Database Syst Rev 2010;(6):CD006507, 1–44.

98. Cairncross M, Miller C. The effectiveness of mindfulness-based therapies for ADHD: a meta-analytic review. J Atten Disord 2016;pii:.

99. Evans S, Ling M, Hill B, et al. Systematic review of meditation-based interventions for children with ADHD. Eur Child Adolesc Psychiatry 2017;doi:10.1007/s00787-017-1008-9. Epub.

100. Haffner J, et al. [The effectiveness of body-oriented methods of therapy in the treatment of attention-deficit hyperactivity disorder (ADHD): results of a controlled pilot study]. Z Kinder Jugendpsychiatr Psychother 2006;34(1):37–47.

101. Jensen PS, Kenny DT. The effects of yoga on the attention and behavior of boys with attention-deficit/hyperactivity disorder (ADHD). J Atten Disord 2004;7(4):205–16.

102. Khilnani S, et al. Massage therapy improves mood and behavior of students with attention-deficit/hyperactivity disorder. Adolescence 2003;38(152):623–38.

103. Alcantara J, Davis J. The chiropractic care of children with attention-deficit/hyperactivity disorder: a retrospective case series. Explore 2010;6:173–82.

104. 'CogMed Training Method'. CogMed. Pearson. Online. Available: http://http://www.cogmed.com/cogmed-training-method. 1 Nov 2013.

105. Gibson BS, Gondoli DM, Johnson AC, et al. Component analysis of verbal versus spatial working memory training in adolescents with ADHD: a randomized, controlled trial. Child Neuropsychol 2011;17:546–63.

106. American Academy of Pediatrics. Sensory integration therapies for children with developmental and behavioral disorders. Pediatrics 2012;129:1186–9.

107. Kuo FE, Taylor AF. A potential natural treatment for attention-deficit/hyperactivity disorder: evidence from a national study. Am J Public Health 2004;94(9):1580–6.

108. Canu W, Gordon M. Mother nature as treatment for ADHD: overstating the benefits of green. Am J Clin Nutr 2005;95:371.

109. Mayes R, et al. ADHD and the rise in stimulant use among children. Harv Rev Psychiatry 2008;16(3):151–66.

110. Foreman DM. Attention deficit hyperactivity disorder: legal and ethical aspects. Arch Dis Child 2006;91(2):192–4.

111. US Department of Health and Human Services. Treatment of attention-deficit/hyperactivity disorder. Washington DC: US Department of Health and Human Services; 1999.

112. Jadad AR, et al. The treatment of attention-deficit hyperactivity disorder: an annotated bibliography and critical appraisal of published systematic reviews and meta-analyses. Can J Psychiatry 1999;44(10):1025–35.

113. Rowe KS, Rowe KJ. Synthetic food coloring and behavior: a dose response effect in a double-blind, placebo-controlled, repeated-measures study. J Pediatr 1994;125(5 Pt 1):691–8.

114. Dengate S, Ruben A. Controlled trial of cumulative behavioural effects of a common bread preservative. J Paediatr Child Health 2002;38(4):373–6.

115. Fuchs T, et al. Neurofeedback treatment for attention-deficit/hyperactivity disorder in children: a comparison with methylphenidate. Appl Psychophysiol Biofeedback 2003;28(1):1–12.

116. Hirayama S, et al. Effect of docosahexaenoic acid-containing food administration on symptoms of attention-deficit/hyperactivity disorder—a placebo-controlled double-blind study. Eur J Clin Nutr 2004;58(3):467–73.

117. Gapin JI, Labban JD, Etnier JL. The effects of physical activity on attention deficit hyperactivity disorder symptoms: the evidence. Prev Med 2011;52:70–4.

CHAPTER 38

Chronic fatigue syndrome

Stephanie Gadsden
ND

Gary Deed
MBBS (Hons I)

OVERVIEW

Chronic fatigue syndrome (CFS) is a complex yet defined spectrum disorder. It is characterised by expert consensus to include persistent disabling fatigue lasting more than six months with other symptoms as listed in the box below. This definition is based upon the Centers for Disease Control and Prevention's (CDC) description of this illness.[1] Importantly there are medical conditions by their nature that may mimic CFS and need to be excluded prior to making an accurate diagnosis. These include untreated thyroid disease, sleep disorders such as sleep apnoea, alcohol abuse, major depressive disorders and schizophrenia. The presence of past and treated malignancy or unresolved infectious hepatitis is also considered exclusive of CFS.[1–4] However, the persistence of symptoms despite adequate treatment of the above conditions, including thyroid conditions or infections such as Lyme's disease, fibromyalgia and anxiety disorders, may possibly co-exist with a diagnosis of CFS.[2] CFS presents significant difficulties in diagnosis and assessment, as there is no single laboratory or clinically significant specific diagnostic test. Patients often appear clinically well, though express profound deterioration of social and occupational functioning and have significant physical and psychological distress.

CDC criteria for the diagnosis of CFS

- Patients have severe chronic fatigue of six months or longer duration with other known medical conditions excluded by clinical diagnosis.
- Patients concurrently have four or more of the following symptoms: substantial impairment in short-term memory or concentration; sore throat; tender lymph nodes; muscle pain; multi-joint pain without swelling or redness; headaches of a new type, pattern or severity; unrefreshing sleep; or postexertional malaise lasting more than 24 hours.
- The symptoms must have persisted or recurred during six or more consecutive months of illness and must not have predated the fatigue.
- The condition must also be defined by excluding other organic or psychiatric causes including that covered in the chapter on adrenal exhaustion.

Sources: CDC 2013,[1] CDC 2013,[2] Merck 2013[3] and CDC 2014[4]

Aetiology

Infectious agents

Clinically it is well known that many patients commence their illness after what appears to be an infectious episode. Certainly no single agent has been shown consistently to create all CFS cases; however, the CDC states 'the possibility remains that CFS may have multiple causes leading to a common endpoint, in which case some viruses or other infectious agents might have a contributory role for a subset of CFS cases, and infection with Epstein-Barr virus [EBV], Ross River virus and *Coxiella burnetii* will lead to a post-infective condition that meets the criteria for CFS in approximately 12% of cases'.[4]

Further research pointing to an infectious origin include:

- enterovirus in muscle biopsies of 20.8% of CFS patients, but not controls[5]
- *Mycoplasma* spp. (52%), *Chlamydia pneumoniae* (7.5%) and human herpesvirus 6 (HHV-6) (30.5%)[6]
- *Mycoplasma* infection[7]
- multiple active viral infections—HHV-7, parvovirus B19[8]
- tick-borne illnesses (e.g. Lyme's disease) and borreliosis[9]
- gram-negative enterobacteria causing increased intestinal permeability[10,11]; parasitic infestations such as giardia.[12]

Immunological abnormalities

CFS may potentially be the result of a complex interplay between an infectious insult and/or a disordered immune response in a susceptible individual. This complexity is revealed in research in the area of immunity and CFS; any one consistent abnormality (concerning interleukin abnormalities and altered cell-mediated immunity) has not been shown.[13,14] Recent studies are suggestive of defected Ca2+ dependent NK cell activity due to impaired TRPM3 receptors resulting in a dysfunctional response to potential pathogens, which could explain relapsing and remitting infections and flu-like symptoms experienced by the CFS patient.[15] There is also some speculation that the immune dysfunction in CFS patients could overlap with mast cell activation disorder but there is little current evidence to support this.

Neuroendocrine abnormalities

Hypoactivity of the hypothalamic–pituitary–adrenal (HPA) axis combined with hyper-activity of the serotonergic system has been postulated as a cause of CFS.[16,17] Other research suggests that up-regulation of hypothalamic serotonergic receptors may be the cause some of the HPA disorders—distinctly different from depression[18] and general fatigue. With respect to the HPA axis, lowered levels of dehydroepiandrosterone (DHEA, an adrenal steroidal hormone) have been assessed in CFS patients.[19] The interplay of dysfunctional immunity, cytokine imbalances leading to subtle neurotransmitter changes, is demonstrated in Figure 38.1. Importantly, as mentioned above, depression and its manifestations are distinctly different from CFS both in psychological distress and in physiological dysfunction.[20]

Genetic factors

Females are four times more likely to have CFS than males. Differential gene expression has been documented in patients suffering from CFS compared with healthy controls.[21,22] Certain genes effecting neurological, immunological and haematological processes have

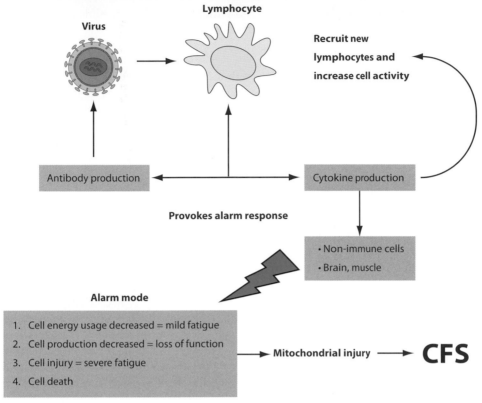

Figure 38.1
Cytokine-induced cell injury as the basis of CFS

been shown to be dysregulated in CFS patients.[21] Polymorphisms have been identified on genes affecting glutaminergic neurotransmission and circadian rhythms[21] and viral triggers such as EBV and enterovirus have thought to effect genes that play a role in immunological process.[22] Epigenetic changes have been identified in rDNA methylation in relation to glucocorticoid sensitivity, kinase activity, immune response and cellular metabolism; however, it is unclear if this changes are the result of CFS or predispose the condition.[23,24] Seven subtypes of CFS have been proposed due to the clustering of gene expression in relation to distinct clinical phenotypes associated with the severity of the disorder[22]; however, more research needs to be conducted into genetic variations in CFS patients to rely on this data for differential diagnosis.

Environmental factors

Exposure to certain environments and environmental pollutants may be linked to the development or sustained effects of the condition. It is common for disorders such as CFS, fibromyalgia and multiple chemical sensitivities (MCS) to co-occur[25,26]; however, whether there is a direct cause and effect relationship is unknown. Early childhood physical abuse in women was significantly associated with each of CFS, fibromyalgia, irritable bowel syndrome and MCS.[27] Sick building syndrome (SBS) shares characteristics with CFS including respiratory disturbance, neurological complaints and extreme fatigue.[28] It is important when treating CFS patients to look at possible environmental factors that could be contributing to or aggravating the condition.

Orthostatic intolerance

Patients with CFS have been shown to have abnormal autonomic responses to prolonged standing or sitting.[29] This 'orthostatic intolerance' (OI) manifests as fatigue plus elevated pulse rates, often associated with faintness when the above activities occur. In CFS patients, OI commonly is diagnosed as postural orthostatic tachycardia syndrome (POTS). The condition is diagnosable with a severe hypotensive and/or tachycardic response to 'tilt table' testing, where a patient is subjected to a head tilt when lying flat.[30] POTS is clinically defined as an increase in heart rate from the supine to upright position of more than 30 bpm or no more than 120 bpm with signs of OI.[31] Hypotheses have been made that POTS may contribute to postural cognitive loss due to a reduction in cerebral blood flow affecting vasomotor tone and neuronal activity.[32] There is also some speculation pointing to an infectious cause for POTS.

Nutrient deficiency

As the diagnosis is defined by the absence of other medical conditions, the fatigue that arises from iron deficiency, vitamin B and B12 deficiency is necessarily excluded as a cause. However, lowered levels of essential fatty acids L-carnitine, magnesium and coenzyme Q10 (co-Q10)[14] have been assessed in patients with CFS.[18] Interestingly, these nutrients give direct support to mitochondrial function—an essential pathway for the production of cellular energy.[33] Serum folic acid levels have been assayed in patients with CFS and 50% of 60 patients have been shown to have lowered levels.[34] Antioxidant nutrients such as vitamin E and zinc have been shown to be lowered, demonstrating that CFS patients may be more susceptible to oxidative damage.[14] However, many of these studies are of poor quality and no one consistent nutrient deficiency has been linked to clinical presentation.[35]

DIFFERENTIAL DIAGNOSIS
- General fatigue from over-exertion and/or lack of sleep
- Major depressive disorder
- Endocrine disorders including thyroid disease, hypogonadism and adrenal disease
- Sleep disorders
- Fibromyalgia
- Schizophrenia
- Iron deficiency or anaemia
- Alcohol abuse
- Hepatitis
- Malignancy

RISK FACTORS

No single risk factor has been strongly associated with CFS (Table 38.1). With a spectrum disorder with multiple aetiological factors it seems prudent to individually assess the clinical case as it presents. However, a study has commenced on what makes a person vulnerable to CFS, with the general consensus based upon observation that disordered immunity and infectious agents intervene in a susceptible individual.

Table 38.1
Factors contributing to CFS*

	Predisposing	Sustaining	Perpetuating
Physical	Infectious agents, nutrient deficiencies, neuroendocrine abnormalities, immune dysfunction, genetic factors	Nutrient deficiencies, immune dysfunction, orthostatic intolerance, decreased gut integrity	Postexertional fatigue
Mental	Posttraumatic stress disorder	Comorbidities of depression and/or anxiety, sleep abnormalities	Sleep abnormalities
Emotional	Trauma/abuse		
Environmental	MCS, food sensitivities	Food sensitivities	MCS, SBS, food sensitivities

*Systematic integrative approach to addressing these multifactorial issues

Predictive risks factors for developing CFS

- Older age
- Female > male (4:1)
- Low or middle rather than high educational level
- The presence of an anxiety disorder
- Mood disorder (pre-morbid or two months postinfection)
- Personality trait—emotional instability

- Musculoskeletal pain
- Low fitness two months postinfection
- Lower physical functioning at baseline assessment
- The presence of fatigue at time of viral illness
- Fatigue severity
- Other family members with symptoms of CFS

Source: Hempel et al. 2008[38]

Very recent research has revealed that childhood trauma—abuse of sexual or emotional type—may predispose an individual to developing CFS in the presence of other initiating factors.[36] Neuroendocrine dysfunction, as discussed in Chapter 18 on stress and fatigue, explains how the combination of these factors develop as a potential risk for CFS.[37]

CONVENTIONAL TREATMENT

There remains contention in some medical services about the existence of CFS, and its management. Fatigue is a common presentation to general practice; however, CFS is a unique and separate entity that requires understanding and knowledge of the condition itself and those things that may mimic it. Confusion arises because of the lack of a definitive laboratory test, plus uncertainty about management options available to patients.[18] Thus, much conventional therapy is directed to symptomatic control of distress, in the absence of single or definitive interventions.

Key interventions of conventional therapy include: sedating antidepressants such as tricyclic antidepressants; serotonergic reuptake inhibitors for sleep disorders[39–41]; and simple analgesia and nonsteroidal anti-inflammatory agents for ongoing pain management. Antiviral medications such as valganciclovir have been shown to help in a small population.[42] Serotonergic modulators such as fluoxetine or similar agents in this class are used for psychological support, especially for comorbid reactive mood disorders with or without anxiety. Serotonin-noradrenaline reuptake inhibitors (SNRIs), noradrenaline reuptake inhibitors (NRIs) or psychostimulants may also be potential treatment options. Hydrocortisone has also been shown to be mildly helpful in reducing fatigue and improving cognition as well as dexamphetamines.[43]

KEY TREATMENT PROTOCOLS

The primary clinical protocol is to be supportive and patient, and to address the individual needs of the person with CFS. Negotiation of a personalised plan recognising the patient's understanding of the nuances of their condition is also advised.

Treat the symptoms

Reduce pain and stiffness

Conventional therapies to reduce pain and suffering include regular doses of paracetamol and the use of a nocturnal dose of a tricyclic antidepressant such as amitryptyline—10–50 mg.[40,41] Integrative interventions favoured by people with CFS include massage and chiropractic therapies.[44] Recent research suggests that, in the presence of accompanying myofascial pain, **manual therapies** such as manipulation and myofascial trigger-point therapy may have some benefit.[45] **Acupuncture** may help to relieve pain or associated fibromyalgia (see Chapter 26). Nutritional interventions such as **magnesium** have also shown promise. Magnesium is a nutrient that is an essential cofactor in enzymes of energy metabolism; it acts on muscle tissue as a relaxant, and also is an essential cofactor in neurotransmitter regulation of pain.[46]

Vitamin D supplementation may be helpful as increased musculoskeletal pains were associated with a deficiency among select patient groups in rheumatology clinics.[47] Injection of either **magnesium sulfate** or oral chelates (such as citrate) at 500 mg two or three times a day has been shown to assist pain management.[48] A modified **intravenous Myers' cocktail** (Table 38.2) combination of water-soluble vitamins and minerals containing magnesium that is intravenously administered is widely used to treat symptoms of fibromyalgia and CFS by integrative practitioners in the United States, with reports of anecdotal success[49]; however, pilot data found the cocktail to be no more effective than placebo.[50] Herbal interventions may include combinations of *Curcuma longa*, *Boswellia serrata*, *Zingiber officinale* and *Apium graveolens*,[51] with an emphasis on management of pain and stiffness.

Integrative Medical Treatment Aims

- Individualisation of therapies allows a patient-centred approach. To assist this approach there are validated tools that assist assessment and goal setting for patients.
- Decrease symptoms:
  - reduce pain and stiffness
  - improve sleep.
- Improve immune dysfunction:
  - assess for infection, allergy and toxicity or deficiency
  - use nutrition and phytotherapy.
- Repair and restore gut functioning:
  - address any comorbid food and chemical sensitivities
  - address possible leaky gut and/or infection.
- Increase physical condition:
  - increase graded physical activity goals
  - use nutritional and herbal therapies for fatigue and weakness.
- Address psychological symptoms:
  - cognitive behaviour therapy (CBT)
  - nutrition and phytotherapy.

Table 38.2
Formulation of the modified Myers' cocktail

Magnesium chloride hexahydrate 20% (magnesium)	2–5 mL
Calcium gluconate 10% (calcium)	1–3 mL
Pyridoxine hydrochloride 100 mg/mL (B6)	1 mL
B complex 100 (B complex)	1 mL
Vitamin C 222 mg/mL (C)	4–20 mL
Dexpanthenol 250 mg/mL (B5)	1 mL

Note: Traditionally the Myers' cocktail also included hydroxocobalamin; this has been removed due to case reports of anaphylaxis[52,53]
Source: Kerr et al. 2008[54]

Improve sleep

Conventional therapies aimed at managing sleep include low-dose benzodiazepines or selective serotonin reuptake inhibitors (SSRIs), or **melatonin**, a naturally produced sleep hormone in the evening. Nutritional interventions include the use of **5-hydroxytryptophan**, which may increase serotonin production and melatonin production; however, clinicians need to be careful of nausea and also interactions with conventional antidepressants. Herbal interventions include *Withania somnifera*, which may promote sleep normalisation and may also provide antifatigue activity,[55] and *Valeriana officinalis*, which may assist in management of insomnia, irritability and restlessness.[56] Synergistic combinations of *Ziziphus jujuba* with *Valeriana officinalis* for nocturnal irritability and anxiety has also been shown to be helpful.[56] *Passiflora incarnata* also works synergistically with *Valeriana officinalis* to assist sleep and nervous agitation (see Chapter 16 on insomnia for further detail).[56]

Address any immune dysfunction

Assess first for infection, allergy and environmental toxicity (Table 38.3).[57–59] Dysfunctional immunity has been demonstrated in CFS[60,61]; this may manifest as sensitivity to environmental agents such as foods, pollens, dust mites and other agents. Assessment may range from skin prick/patch testing for inhalant allergens, foods and mites to immunoglobulin G (IgG) testing for food sensitivity.

Toxicity may involve allergy as mentioned above but also the possibility of immunological or metabolic injury from heavy metals and chemicals. The effects may range from displacement of energy cofactors such as copper antagonising zinc bioavailability, or mercury displacing selenium. Other effects may be from enzyme induction or inhibition by environmental or food chemicals (e.g. caffeine/nicotine), leading to altered metabolic clearance or altered production of physiological energy cofactors. An example of the latter is alteration of liver detoxification pathways (see Chapter 7 on liver dysfunction).

Nutritional interventions

As discussed, there is evidence to suggest that immunological and inflammatory pathways play a role in the pathophysiology of CFS. **Omega-3 fatty acids** may help to rebalance eicosanoid pathways.[62,63] Serum **zinc** levels have been correlated with severity of fatigue in patients with CFS; the higher the level of zinc the less fatigued the individual.[47,59]

Table 38.3
Tests for infection, allergy and environmental toxicity

Tests	Functional outcome	Management recommendation
Assess for infection	Detect any 'occult' or latent infections such as *Mycoplasma*, *Chlamydia*, *Rickettsia*, a virus or parasites	Requires specialised assessment and advice, but nutritional and herbal immune support can be used as a basis of management
Heavy metal assessment Tests to consider: hair analysis chelation challenge porphyrin assessment	Elevated heavy metals	Stabilise metal detoxification— improve digestion, antioxidants, replace displaced minerals— zinc, selenium etc. Specific chelation agents
Liver detoxification profile	Impaired phase I and/or phase II detoxification Uncoupled phase I to phase II	Enhance appropriate detoxification through nutritional support: phase I—vitamin B, phase II—amino acid support antioxidants
Food allergy assessment: skin/patch test IgG$_4$ blood test for food digestive stool analysis or faecal bacterial DNA assessment	Identification of possible triggers for persistent immune dysfunction	Elimination diet and challenge after exclusion Digestive support through probiotic supplementation and digestive enzymes

Sources: Regland et al. 2001[57] and Racciatti et al. 2001[58]

Zinc chelate at night may have direct effects on immune cell proliferation and function. **Glutamine** has been shown to modulate lymphocyte proliferation and assist immune outcomes.[64]

Injectable therapies

Intravenous vitamin C (IV-C) therapy[65] has been used in randomised blinded placebo-controlled trials with evidence of benefit in fatigued patients. IV-C has shown in active EBV to improve disease duration and decrease viral antibodies.[66] Also CFS and fatigue were seen to be the most common reason clinicians administered IV-C in 2006 in an American study (see section on injectable therapies later in this chapter).[67]

Herbal medicine

Due to the chronicity of CFS, adaptogenic herbal medicines may provide a potential beneficial therapeutic action; however, it is important to identify and remove any infection or insult before initiating a 'tonifying' phase. In the initial phase of treatment, antiviral, antimicrobial, anti-inflammatory herbal treatments and potentially the use of chelating agents are appropriate. Immunomodulatory herbs such as ***Echinacea* spp.** for its use in viral illness and immune disorders[68] can be beneficial (see Chapters 8–10 on the respiratory system). Where there is a viral infection with concomitant depressive symptoms ***Hypericum perforatum*** may be indicated due to its proposed action against encapsulated viruses such as EBV. In a randomised controlled trial (RCT), 39 patients treated with *Hypericum perforatum* showed significant improvement in symptoms after four weeks.[69] Other antiviral and antimicrobial herbs that may be appropriate include ***Andrographis paniculata*** and ***Thymus vulgaris***. ***Astragalus membranaceus*** is traditionally classified as a tonifying herb that contains polysaccharides and saponins, and is indicated for chronic immune enhancement (especially in cases of recurrent viral illness). A recent six-week study found that its effects on CFS involved its ability to balance abnormal cytokine levels.[51] For autoimmune presentations with chronic fatigue, **Hemidesmus indicus** may be indicated (see Chapter 31 on autoimmunity).

Increase physical conditioning

Graded physical activity

Negotiation of a balanced and achievable **exercise plan** with the patient (after a medical check-up) is advised.[70] This may involve a graded exercise program supervised by a qualified health professional such as an exercise physiologist or equivalent. Two reviews[71,72] of research show that after three months of exercise intervention, physical function improved and less fatigue was experienced by those who participated. However, improved responses were seen when education was combined with exercise therapy but not when antidepressants were also used in combination.[71] A large RCT[73] comparing GET, CBT and adaptive pacing showed significant improvement in fatigue scores and recovery rates; however, the results of this study are under review as the reliability of the data and methodology is questionable.[74] Due to an ongoing debate in the literature in relation to the effectiveness and safety of GET, it is important to make sure severity of symptoms and risk for rebound fatigue is assessed before implementing an exercise program. Recommendations suggest that managing daily activities should be prioritised over an exercise plan.[75,76]

Nutritional interventions

Acety-L-carnitine 500 mg three times a day has been shown to improve energy, especially mental fatigue.[77] Nutrients that have been specifically shown to improve energy metabolism in CFS patients are **magnesium citrate**,[48] **nicotinamide** (NADH) 10 mg a day[78] and oral **D-ribose** for mitochondrial support.[79] **Essential fatty acids** have been trialled, with reported benefit in relation to fatigue in patients treated with high-dose 1000 mg omega-3 marine oil four times a day.[57,62] Other interventions used with less evidence in CFS include **co-Q10**, with anecdotal evidence of improved exercise tolerance at 100 mg a day.[58]

Herbal interventions

Herbal adaptogens (improve adaptation to stress) are useful in this stage of treatment to improve physical conditioning and reduce fatigue. Herbal medicines to consider are **Eleutherococcus senticosus** for its ability to assist physical labour and mental tasks. An RCT study showed that moderately fatigued CFS patients who were prescribed *Eleutherococcus senticosus* had marked improvements in symptoms.[80] **Panax ginseng** is an adaptogen and tonic. Although never specifically studied in CFS, evidence for its ability to increase stamina and help normalise the HPA axis[81] would be beneficial in these patients. **Withania somnifera** is adaptogenic but a non-stimulant and has the added benefit of helping to normalise sleep[82]; however, there are no human trials to support its use in CFS. *Withania somnifera*'s traditional Ayurvedic indications can be applied to CFS patients for its use in assisting rejuvenation of the body in debilitating conditions and promoting mental and physical wellbeing.[51] **Rhodiola rosea**, also a herb with adaptogenic qualities,[83] may be helpful to improve cognitive performance, stamina and recall.

Consider orthostatic intolerance

Herbal medicines and sodium

Glycyrrhiza glabra contains glycyrrhizin and glycyrrhetinic acid, which have adrenal steroidal anti-inflammatory effects, plus elevation of blood pressure due to the promotion of sodium retention from the kidney.[33] (Exercise care with mineral imbalances in the presence of medication such as cardiovascular agents.) A herb that supports the adrenal gland and acts in a similar way to *Glycyrrhiza glabra* without the potential hypertensive effect is ***Rehmannia glutinosa***. It is traditionally used for fatigue in traditional Chinese medicine.[84,85] Venous tonics are another effective way to reduce symptoms of orthostatic intolerance. ***Ruscus aculeatus*** has been shown to help manage orthostatic hypotension.[63] It may be more effective when combined with ***Aesculus hippocastanum***. In orthostatic intolerance and neurally mediated hypotension, **increased intake of salt** (sodium chloride) 600 mg twice to three times a day with increased water intake may assist the control of this syndrome.[30]

Repair and restore gut function

Sufferers of CFS commonly complain of irritable bowel syndrome-type symptoms and often have many food sensitivities indicating possible dysbiosis. It has been shown that CFS patients have increased IgA and IgM, indicating an increased translocation of gram-negative enterobacteria and a weakening of the intestinal mucosal barrier allowing normally poorly invasive bacteria to cross the intestinal mucus.[11,86] This demonstrates a leaky gut pathology (see Chapters 4–6 on the gastrointestinal system).

Treatments to restore gut functioning and limit the effects of increased intestinal permeability involve using digestive enzymes to assist in the ability to digest protein and complex carbohydrates and **probiotics** if there are significant abnormalities on digestive bacterial analysis. However, a recent review found no clear evidence for any one strain of probitoic in improving symptoms in people with co-morbid CFS and IBS.[87] Oral glutamine powder not only has benefits on immune functioning but is also the main fuel for enterocytes and has been demonstrated along with whey protein to improve intestinal permeability measured by lactulose and mannitol excretion ratio in the urine.[25]

Address psychological symptoms

Psychological therapies

Short-term studies have shown that CBT is effective in reducing fatigue compared with other psychological therapies including relaxation, counselling and education/support.[88] This intervention has also shown benefit in randomised controlled studies in children and young adults. The long-term follow-up of CBT has shown benefits in fatigue, symptom reduction, physical functioning and school and work absences. It warrants further research.[38–40,88]

Nutritional and herbal interventions

Vitamin B12 replenishes central nervous system methylation imbalance and has improved cognitive function at doses of 1000 μg given intramuscularly, titrated to patient response (weekly to monthly).[79,89] Empirical research has shown that vitamin B12 injections may improve energy and cognitive ability and mood often with normal serum B12 levels.[38,78] **S-adenosylmethionine** may also be helpful.[33]

Hypericum perforatum improves depressive symptoms and has been postulated to have antiviral activity as well. It may be helpful for reactive depression; however, care should be taken with possible interactions with prescription antidepressants (see Chapter 15 on depression for more detail).[69,90]

INJECTABLE NUTRACEUTICALS

Injecting nutrients, herbs and homeopathic medicines is an area that is underresearched; however, more evidence is emerging to support the use of these types of treatment and validate numerous anecdotal claims of the benefits seen in acute and chronic disease states. A list of common injectable therapeutic interventions in CFS is provided in Table 38.4.

Examples where injectable herbal medicines have shown promising benefits include the use of **silymarin** for amatoxin poisoning from the *Amanita phalloides* mushroom[91] and viral hepatitis.[92] *Viscum album* as a chemotherapy agent and *Aesculus hippocastanum* have been used successfully intravenously to treat postoperative oedema[91] exudates. **Intramuscular B12** injections have shown some promise for CFS patients.[78]

Injecting nutrients and herbal medicines can have benefits over oral or topical routes. This can be seen in the example of silymarin and IV-C. The active constituent of silymarin, silybinin, has compromised bioavailability due to poor water solubility. Injection of silybinin along with a patent delivery system improves bioavailability, allowing for large amounts of the active ingredient to be administered and therefore is a successful treatment in acute, potentially fatal, hepatic toxicity. Vitamin C absorption via an oral route has limitations due to desaturation

Table 38.4
Injectable therapies used in the management of CFS

Substance	Administration	Benefits	Risks	Comments
Magnesium	Intramuscular (IM) injections / slow (IV)	Reduces muscle pain, cramps and fatigue[48]	Lowers blood pressure, cardiac rhythm changes and pain via intramuscular route	May be sufficient to use oral supplementation
Vitamin C	IV	Fatigue and immune function[65]	Needs careful infusion and care with renal disease and glucose-6-phosphate dehydrogenase deficiency	Training required for administration in sterile conditions Administration can be combined with other nutrients including magnesium and vitamin B
Vitamin B12	IM injections	Fatigue and neurocognitive or memory problems[38,78]	Care with site of injection	Usually supported by multivitamin B administration

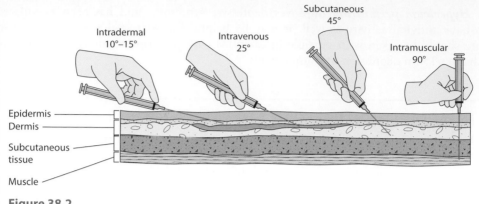

Figure 38.2
Site of injection

with doses greater than 2000 mg linked to gastric discomfort and diarrhoea. IV-C bypasses the gastrointestinal system leading to a higher concentration of ascorbic acid in the plasma. Benefits claimed of rapid pain relief with the use of mesotherapy including injection of saline solution and homeopathic medicines may occur due to the short time necessary for the active constituent to reach the targeted site[92]; however, evidence is lacking to support these methods (see also Chapter 26 on fibromyalgia).

There are many different methods of injectable therapies that can be incorporated into integrative practice (see below and Figure 38.2).

- **Intravenous nutrient therapy (IV)** is the process of injecting nutrients into the blood stream via accessing a vein with a small needle. Nutrients such as vitamin C, vitamin K3, glutathione, B vitamins, minerals, chelating agents and botanicals such as silymarin (from *Silybum marianum*) and *Viscum album* can be administered via IV (see Chapter 32 regarding use of IV nutraceuticals in cancer management).

- **Mesotherapy** is where multiple small injections are administered just below the skin's surface into the mesoderm.[92] These local minimally-invasive intradermal injections are commonly used for cosmetic purposes. Mesotherapy also involves the application of natural substances such as homeopathics, herbals and nutrients, injected locally for chronic pain relief and skin conditions; however, there is no conclusive evidence to support its effectiveness or safety.

- **Neural therapy**, developed in Germany by doctors Ferdinand and Walter Huneke, is the injection of local anaesthetic into specific sites.[93] Neural therapy although commonly used across Europe has not been shown to be effective through scientific evaluation.

- **Intramuscular (IM) injections** are commonly used to treat a deficiency because of its rapid systemic uptake (15–20 minutes) and prolonged action of the treatment.[94] Due to the increased absorption and large doses that can be administered via IM techniques safety concerns around possible allergic reactions are warranted.[94] IM vitamin D3 is commonly prescribed in some countries to treat deficiency; however, a recent RCT showed that patients who were given 300,000 IU of cholecalciferol orally in interval doses over a period of three months was marginally more effective than a single IM dose.[95] IM B12 is effective at correcting deficiency[96,97]; however, even without deficiency IM B12 has shown to improve fatigue and cognition in CFS patients.[78]

Safety considerations

Legal requirements for adequate training and patient care should be discussed with the practitioner's own training and accrediting association. Injection location and technique addressing safety around key anatomical structures is imperative.

Infection control is essential with use of all injectables (including safe disposal of any sharps) and is essential with any multiuse vials.

CLINICAL SUMMARY

CFS is a unique disorder with a spectrum of internationally recognised symptoms. Patients therefore require a variety of interventions to assist symptom reduction and address underlying individual pathology (Figure 38.3). Once a definitive diagnosis of CFS is reached by ruling out potential differentials including depression and adrenal fatigue, it is then time to develop an individualised treatment plan, agreed upon by the patient and addressing the physical, emotional and environmental causes.

Predisposing, sustaining and perpetuating factors need to be identified by taking a thorough case history. These could include past or present infection, nutrient deficiencies, diet quality, food sensitivities, history of trauma including physical abuse, exposure to environmental pollutants, autonomic nervous system dysregulation, sleep abnormalities, level of perceived stress and digestive functioning. Comorbidities such as fibromyalgia, depression, anxiety and irritable bowel syndrome can exist alongside CFS and it is essential that these are observed and addressed.

An integrative treatment plan using a range of modalities may benefit the treatment of CFS. Incorporating interventions such as psychological, herbal, nutritional, lifestyle therapies and pharmacotherapies often simultaneously is needed (see Table 38.1 for an evidence summary). Key integrative treatments should look to decrease symptoms of pain with the help of acupuncture and magnesium; sleep abnormalities can be addressed with botanicals such as *Valeriana officinalis*; and immune functioning can be enhanced with *Echinacea* spp., *Astragalus membranaceus*, zinc and omega-3 fatty acids. Herbal adaptogens such as *Eleutherococcus senticosus* are useful to improve physical conditioning along with graded exercise programs. Mitochondrial support can be given via interventions such as oral D-ribose, co-Q10 and NADH. Gut integrity needs to be assessed and food sensitivities avoided while optimising digestive function with probiotics, digestive enzymes and glutamine. Due to the chronicity of the disease plus potential history of emotional trauma in CFS patients, ongoing psychological care is essential and can be sought through avenues such as CBT co-administered with supportive botanicals such as *Hypericum perforatum*.

Integrative practitioners can also use interventions such as injectable therapies of vitamin C or B12 for symptomatic relief. It is essential that the treatment plan be communicated clearly, with realistic timeframes set. Practitioners need to encourage patients to employ a high level of self-management for their condition and to explain that patience is often required as CFS can be a condition that requires longer term management.

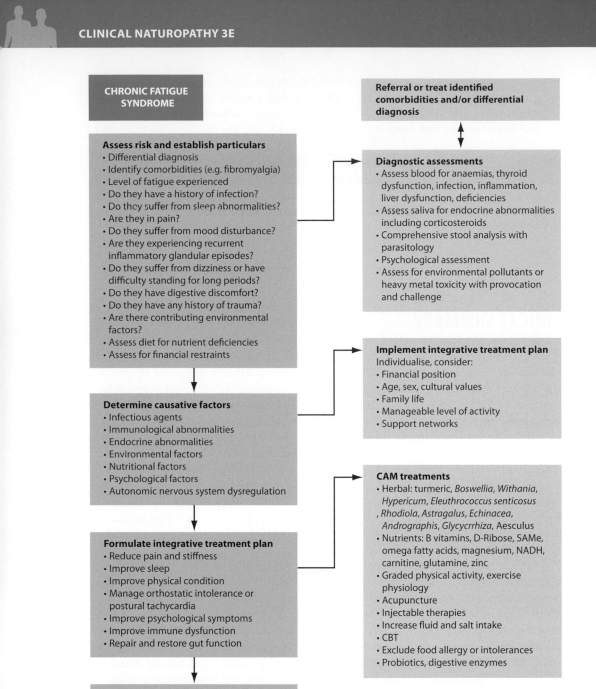

Figure 38.3
Integrative treatment decision tree—chronic fatigue syndrome

Table 38.5
Review of the major evidence

Intervention	Mechanisms of action	Key literature*	Summary of results	Comment
CBT	Identifying cognitive patterns to make changes to behaviour and thought processes and coping	Deale et al. 1997[98] (n = 60); five-year follow-up after 26-week intervention[98] Prins et al. 2001[99] (n = 278); 61-week follow-up after 35-week intervention[99] Sharpe et al. 1996[40] (n = 60); 52-week follow-up[40] Nijhof et al. 2012 (n = 135) six-month follow up[100]	All studies found significantly different positive effects for the intervention compared with controls The five-year follow-up study showed improvements remained for global improvements but not for physical functioning and fatigue scores	More participants withdrew from this intervention than in other trial interventions (19% versus 13% average) across most studies, possibly indicating that this therapy does not meet the needs of some patients with CFS
Graded exercise programs	Increases physical tolerance[71]	Fulcher & White 1997[101] (n = 66); follow-up 12 weeks[101] Powell et al. 2001[9] (n = 148); follow-up at 52 weeks after 26-week intervention[102] Wearden et al. 1998[103] (n = 136); follow-up at 26 weeks[103] White et al. 2011[104] (n = 641), GET arm n = 160; follow-up at 52 weeks	All trials showed significantly better results in overall benefit from this intervention Reliability of reporting is currently being contested in White et al. (2011)[104]	A combined RCT with an antidepressant (fluoxetine) showed no significant additional benefit
Magnesium	Essential cofactor for energy metabolism; muscle tissue relaxant, cofactor for neurotransmitter regulation of pain[46]	Cox et al. 1991[48] (n = 32); treated for six weeks; 15 patients with IMI magnesium sulfate and 17 with placebo[48]	Twelve of 15 treated patients experienced benefit versus three of the placebo arm Improvements were energy level, less pain and better emotional state	Study has been replicated without showing the same degree of benefit
Omega-3	Anti-inflammatory may help to rebalance eicosanoid pathways[62,63]	Behan et al. 1990[105] (n = 63); follow-up to 13 weeks[105] Warren et al. 1999[90] (n = 50); follow-up to 13 weeks[90]	The use of 4 g of marine-based omega fatty acids were given to active patients versus placebo	Appears to have potential benefit in CFS Larger studies are advised to validate these findings

Table 38.5
Review of the major evidence (continued)

Intervention	Mechanisms of action	Key literature*	Summary of results	Comment
Omega-3 (continued)			At one month 74% of active treated versus 23% placebo had benefit, with the three-month effect at 85% active versus 17% placebo ($p = 0.0001$)[105] Fifty participants were randomised to essential fatty acids = supplementation versus placebo showed some improvement of symptoms in treated group but did not reach significance[90]	The study[90] using the Beck's depression inventory and a physical function questionnaire may have adequate 'quality of life' data to assess a true effect of the intervention
Nutraceutical combination	Mitochondrial support	Menon et al. 2017[106]	Ten CFS patients were given an open-label trial of a nutraceutical combination (primary nutrients: Co Q10, Alpha lipoic acid, Acetyl-l-carnitine, N-acetyl cysteine, B vitamins, in addition to co-factors) over 16 weeks Significant improvement in fatigue symptoms across treatment period on the Chalder Fatigue Scale occurred. Specific improvements were found in tiredness, weakness, feeling sleepy or drowsy, as well as in sleep, and clinician-reported symptom improvement	While the open-label design prohibits a firm conclusion, the sample was largely treatment resistant, so the improvement is of note

Table 38.5
Review of the major evidence (continued)

Intervention	Mechanisms of action	Key literature*	Summary of results	Comment
Oral D-ribose	Mitochondrial support	Teitelbaum et al. 2012[14] (n = 203); follow-up baseline, week 1, 2 and 3	Patients were treated with 5 g of oral D-ribose for three weeks A visual analogue scale was used to measure outcomes of fatigue, sleep, cognitive function, pain and overall wellbeing Increase of 61.3% in energy, 37% in overall wellbeing	Authors acknowledged the need for a randomised control study; however, results look promising
Oral NADH	Mitochondrial support	Forsyth et al. 1999[107] (n = 26); follow-up to 12 weeks[107] Santaella et al. 2004[78] (n = 31); follow-up to 24 months[78] Castro-Marrero et al. 2015 (n = 80); follow-up in eight weeks[108]	Twenty-six active versus 26 placebos A four-week intervention with 10 mg NADH and then four weeks washout with a crossover treatment for four weeks; 31% versus 8% placebo had benefit[107] Eighty received 50 mg coq10 and 5 mg NADH or matching placebo BD. Significant reduction in fatigue and heart rate during cycle ergometer test[108] Twelve actively treated patients had initial three-month improvement versus placebo (p < 0.0001) on mean symptom scores of fatigue but this was not maintained at 24 months[78]	These are small studies that need replication The combination of CoQ10 and NADH showed no improvements in pain and sleep scores[108]
Homeopathy	Unknown action: Classical individualised homeopathy prescribing[109]	Weatherley-Jones et al. 2004[109] (n = 103); follow-up to 26 weeks	Forty-seven patients versus 42 placebo participants completed this triple-blinded RCT There was a weak but significant difference in effect	There appears to be some overall benefit from this intervention, but further trials may be needed to elucidate these outcomes

Table 38.5
Review of the major evidence (continued)

Intervention	Mechanisms of action	Key literature*	Summary of results	Comment
Massage therapy	Postulated that massage therapy may reduce inflammation[110] and improve parasympathetic nervous system conduction[111]	Field et al. 1997[112] (*n* = 20); follow-up to five weeks	This small RCT showed beneficial effect to five weeks	The study is considered flawed because comparisons were taken from within intervention groups rather than between them

*All studies are RCTs

KEY POINTS

- CFS is a complex disorder distinctive from depression and fatigue or other presentations including generalised fatigue.
- A spectrum of causes and symptom manifestations may require individualised management.
- Management should engage the patient through the use of a negotiated plan to address their physical and psychological needs while accepting that the patient is in charge of their health.
- Always observe and treat comorbid health conditions.
- An integrative approach using psychological, herbal, nutritional and lifestyle therapies should benefit the treatment of CFS, though pharmacotherapies may also be advised.

FURTHER READING

Joustra M, Minovic I, Janssens K, et al. Vitamin and mineral status in chronic fatigue syndrome and fibromyalgia syndrome: a systematic review and meta-analysis. PLoS ONE 2017;12(4):1–25.

Lorusso L, et al. Immunological aspects of chronic fatigue syndrome. Autoimmun Rev 2009;8(4):287–91.

Porter N, Jason L, Boulton A, et al. Alternative medical interventions used in the treatment and management of myalgic encephalomyelitis/chronic fatigue syndrome and fibromyalgia. J Altern Complement Med 2010;16(3):235–49.

Smith MB, Haney E, McDonagh M, et al. Treatment of myalgic encephalomyelitis/chronic fatigue syndrome: a systematic review for a National Institutes of Health Pathways to Prevention Workshop. Ann Intern Med 2015;162(12):841–50.

REFERENCES

1. Centers for Disease Control and Prevention. Diagnosis of chronic fatigue syndrome. Online. Available: http://www.cdc.gov/cfs. 1 Nov 2013.

2. Centers for Disease Control and Prevention. Definition of chronic fatigue syndrome. Online. Available: http://www.cdc.gov/cfs/cfsdefinition. 1 Nov 2013.

3. Merck & Co. The Merck manual for health care professionals. Chronic fatigue syndrome. Online. Available: http://www.merck.com. 1 Nov 2013.

4. Centers for Disease Control and Prevention. Causes of chronic fatigue syndrome. Online. Available: http://www.cdc.gov/CFS/cfscauses.htm. 1 Nov 2013.

5. Lane RJ, et al. Enterovirus related metabolic myopathy: a postviral fatigue syndrome. J Neurol Neurosurg Psychiatry 2003;74(10):1382–6.

6. Nicolson GL, et al. Multiple co-infections (Mycoplasma, Chlamydia, human herpes virus-6) in blood of chronic fatigue syndrome patients: association with signs and symptoms. APMIS 2003;111:557–66.

7. Endresen GK. Mycoplasma blood infection in chronic fatigue and fibromyalgia syndromes. Rheumatol Int 2003;23:211–15.

8. Koelle DM, et al. Markers of viral infection in monozygotic twins discordant for chronic fatigue syndrome. Clin Infect Dis 2002;35:518–25.

9. Gustaw K. Chronic fatigue syndrome following tick-borne diseases. Neurol Neurochir Pol 2003;37:1211–21.

10. Maes M, et al. Increased serum IgA and IgM against LPS of enterobacteria in chronic fatigue syndrome (CFS): indication for the involvement of gram-negative enterobacteria in the etiology of CFS and for the presence of an increased gut–intestinal permeability. J Affect Disord 2006;99(1):237–40.

11. Lloyd A, et al. Cell-mediated immunity in patients with chronic fatigue syndrome, healthy control subjects and patients with major depression. Clin Exp Immunol 1992;87(1):76–9.

12. Padayatty SJ, Sun AY, et al. Vitamin C: intravenous use by complementary and alternative medicine practitioners and adverse effects. PLoS ONE 2010;5(7):e11414.

13. Centers for Disease Control and Prevention. Chronic fatigue syndrome—causes. Online. Available: http://www.cdc.gov/cfs/causes/index.html. 1 Nov 2013.

14. Teitelbaum J, Jandrain J, McGrew R. Treatment of chronic fatigue syndrome and fibromyalgia with D-ribose: an open-label multicenter study. Open Pain J 2012;5:32–7.

15. Nguyen T, Johnston S, Clarke L, et al. Impaired calcium mobilization in natural killer cells from chronic fatigue syndrome/myalgic encephalomyelitis patients is associated with transient receptor potential melastatin 3 ion channels. Clin Exp Immunol 2017;2:284. Academic OneFile.

16. Smith AK, et al. Genetic evaluation of the serotonergic system in chronic fatigue syndrome. Psychoneuroendocrinology 2008;33(2):188–97.

17. Shephard RJ. Chronic fatigue syndrome: a brief review of functional disturbance and potential therapy. J Sports Med Phys Fitness 2005;45:381–92.

18. Griffith JP, Zarrouf AA. Systematic review of chronic fatigue syndrome: don't assume it's depression. Prim Care Companion J Clin Psychiatry 2008;10(2):120–8.

19. Kuratsune H, et al. Dehydroepiandrosterone sulfate deficiency in chronic fatigue syndrome. Int J Mol Med 1998;1(1):143–6.

20. Morriss RK, et al. The relation of sleep difficulties to fatigue, mood and disability in chronic fatigue syndrome. J Psychosom Res 1997;42(6):597–605.

21. Borody T, Nowak A, Finlayson S. The GI microbiome and its role in chronic fatigue syndrome: a summary of bacteriotherapy. Journal of the Australasian College of Nutritional and Environmental Medicine. Informit Health Collect 2012;31(3):3.

22. Senate Bill No. 1446, Chapter 333. An act to amend Sections 3640 and 3640.7 of, and to add Section 3640.8 to, the Business and Professions Code, relating to healing arts. Legislative Counsel's Digest SB 1446, Negrete McLeod. Online. Available: http://leginfo.legislature.ca.gov/faces/billNavClient.xhtml?bill_id=201120120SB1446. 22 Oct 2013.

23. de Vega W, Herrera S, Vernon S, et al. Epigenetic modifications and glucocorticoid sensitivity in myalgic encephalomyelitis/chronic fatigue syndrome (ME/CFS). BMC Med Genomics 2017;10:1–14.

24. de Vega W, Vernon S, McGowan P. DNA methylation modifications associated with chronic fatigue syndrome. PLoS ONE 2014.

25. Lavergne M, Cole D, Kerr K, et al. Functional impairment in chronic fatigue syndrome, fibromyalgia, and multiple chemical sensitivity. Can Fam Physician 2010;56(2):e57–65.

26. Brown M, Jason L. Functioning in individuals with chronic fatigue syndrome: increased impairment with co-occurring multiple chemical sensitivity and fibromyalgia. Dyn Med 2007;6:6.

27. Fuller-Thomson E, Sulman J, Brennenstuhl S, et al. Functional somatic syndromes and childhood physical abuse in women: data from a representative community-based sample. J Aggress Maltreat Trauma 2011;20(4):445–69.

28. Chester A, Levine P. Concurrent sick building syndrome and chronic fatigue syndrome: epidemic neuromyasthenia revisited. Clin Infect Dis 1994;18(Suppl. 1):S43–8.

29. Schondorf R, Freeman R. The importance of orthostatic intolerance in the chronic fatigue syndrome. Am J Med Sci 1999;317(2):117–23.

30. Rowe PC, Calkins H. Neurally mediated hypotension and chronic fatigue syndrome. Am J Med 1998;105(3a):15–21s.

31. Maes M, Twisk F, Kubera M, et al. Increased IgA responses to the LPS of commensal bacteria is associated with inflammation and activation of cell-mediated immunity in chronic fatigue syndrome. J Affect Disord 2012;136:3909–17.

32. Smith A, Fang H, Whistler T, et al. Convergent genomic studies identify association of GRIK2 and NPAS2 with chronic fatigue syndrome. Neuropsychobiology 2011;64(4):183–94.

33. Braun L, Cohen M. Herbs and natural supplements: an evidence based guide. 3rd ed. Sydney: Churchill Livingstone; 2010.

34. Jacobson W, et al. Serum folate and chronic fatigue syndrome. Neurology 1993;43(12):2645–7.

35. Joustra M, Minovic I, Janssens K, et al. Vitamin and mineral status in chronic fatigue syndrome and fibromyalgia syndrome: a systematic review and meta-analysis. PLoS ONE 2017;12(4):1–25.

36. Heim C, et al. Childhood trauma and risk for chronic fatigue syndrome: association with neuroendocrine dysfunction. Arch Gen Psychiatry 2009;66(1):72–80.

37. Nater UM, et al. Attenuated morning salivary cortisol concentrations in a population-based study of persons with chronic fatigue syndrome and well controls. Clin Endocrinol Metab 2008;93(3):703–9.

38. Hempel S, et al. Risk factors for chronic fatigue syndrome/myalgic encephalomyelitis: a systematic scoping review of multiple predictor studies. Psychol Med 2008;38:915–26.

39. Rimes KA, Calder T. Treatments for chronic fatigue syndrome. Occup Med 2005;55:32–9.

40. Sharpe M, et al. Cognitive behaviour therapy for the chronic fatigue syndrome: a randomised controlled trial. BMJ 1996;312:22–6.

41. Whiting P, et al. Interventions for the treatment and management of chronic fatigue syndrome: a systematic review. JAMA 2001;286(11):1360–401.

42. Montoya J, Kogelnik A, Bhangoo M, et al. Randomized clinical trial to evaluate the efficacy and safety of valganciclovir in a subset of patients with chronic fatigue syndrome. J Med Virol 2013;12:2101.

43. Collatz A, Johnston S, Staines D, et al. A systematic review of drug therapies for chronic fatigue syndrome/myalgic encephalomyelitis. Clin Ther 2016;38(6):1263–71.

44. Jones JF, et al. Complementary and alternative medical therapy utilization by people with chronic fatiguing illnesses in the United States. BMC Complement Altern Med 2007;7:12.

45. Vernon H, Schneider M. Chiropractic management of myofascial trigger points and myofascial pain syndrome: a systematic review of the literature. J Manipulative Physiol Ther 2009;32(1):14–24.

46. Murray ME. Brain and CSF magnesium concentrations during magnesium deficit in animals and humans. Magnes Res 1992;5:303–13.

47. Stewart J, Medow M, Messer Z, et al. Postural neurocognitive and neuronal activated cerebral blood flow deficits in young chronic fatigue syndrome patients with postural tachycardia syndrome. Am J Physiol Heart Circ Physiol 2012;302:H1185–94.

48. Cox IM, et al. Red blood cell magnesium and chronic fatigue syndrome. Lancet 1991;337:757–60.

49. Gaby AR. Intravenous nutrient therapy: the 'Myers' Cocktail'. Altern Med Rev 2002;7(5):389–403.

50. Jiaqiang L, Yongming L, Xiao Y, et al. Sodium β-aescin may be an effective therapeutic agent for Bell's palsy. Med Hypotheses 2008;71:762–4.

51. Bone K. Chronic fatigue syndrome and its herbal treatment. Townsend Letter for Doctors and Patients. 1 November 2001.

52. Mammucari M, Gatti A, Maggiori S, et al. Mesotherapy, definition, rationale and clinical role: a consensus report from the Italian Society of Mesotherapy. Eur Rev Med Pharmacol Sci 2011;15(6):682–94.

53. Benjamin J, Makharia G, Ahuja V, et al. Glutamine and whey protein improve intestinal permeability and morphology in patients with Crohn's disease: a randomized controlled trial. Dig Dis Sci 2012;57(4):1000–12.

54. Kerr JR, Petty R, Burke B, et al. Gene expression subtypes in patients with chronic fatigue syndrome/myalgic encephalomyelitis. J Infect Dis 2008;197(8):1171–84. doi:10.1086/533453.

55. Kulkarni SK, Dhira A. Withania somnifera Indian ginseng. Prog Neuropsychopharmacol Biol Psychiatry 2008;32(5):1093–105.

56. Burgoyne B. Herbal treatment of insomnia. Mod Phytotherapist 2002;7(1):12–21.

57. Regland B, et al. Nickel allergy is found in a majority of women with chronic fatigue syndrome and muscle pain—and may be triggered by cigarette smoke and dietary nickel intake. J Chronic Fatigue Syndrome 2001;8(1):57–65.

58. Racciatti D, et al. Chronic fatigue syndrome following a toxic exposure. Sci Total Environ 2001;270(1–3):27–31.

59. Graham B. Associations between zinc/copper, metabolic rate and disability scales in chronic fatigue syndrome. Unpublished data, 2005. Online. Available: http://www.nutritional-healing.com. 28 Sep 2013.

60. Tirelli U, et al. Immunological abnormalities in patients with chronic fatigue syndrome. Scand J Immunol 1994;40(6):601–8.

61. Racciatti D, et al. Study of immune alterations in patients with chronic fatigue syndrome with different etiologies. Int J Immunopathol Pharmacol 2004;17(2 Suppl.):57–62.

62. Behan PO, et al. Effect of high doses of essential fatty acids on the postviral fatigue syndrome. Acta Neurol Scand 1990;82:209–16.

63. Chen R, et al. Traditional Chinese medicine for chronic fatigue syndrome. eCAM, doi:10.1093/ecam/nen017.

64. Roth E. Immune and cell modulation by amino acids. Clin Nutr 2007;26(5):535–44.

65. Kumar A, Gopal H, et al. Vitamin D deficiency as the primary cause of musculoskeletal complaints in patients referred to rheumatology clinic: a clinical study. Indian J Rheumatol 2012;7(4):199–203.

66. Mikirova N, Hunninghake R. Effect of high dose vitamin C on Epstein-Barr viral infection. Med Sci Monit 2014;20:725–32.

67. Porter N, Jason L, Boulton A, et al. Alternative medical interventions used in the treatment and management of myalgic encephalomyelitis/chronic fatigue syndrome and fibromyalgia. J Altern Complement Med 2010;16(3):235–49.

68. Leigh E. Echinacea—Green paper 2001. Boulder: Herb Research Foundation, 2001; Leigh E. Ginseng—Green paper 1997–2001. Boulder: Herb Research Foundation. 2001.

69. Hübner WD, et al. Hypericum treatment of mild depressions with somatic symptoms. J Geriatr Psychiatry Neurol 1994;7(Suppl. 1):S12–14.

70. Larun L, Brurberg K, Odgaard-Jensen J, et al. Exercise therapy for chronic fatigue syndrome. Cochrane Database Syst Rev 2017;(4):CD003200, Science Citation Index.

71. Larun L, et al. Exercise therapy for chronic fatigue syndrome. Cochrane Database Syst Rev 2004;(3):CD003200.

72. Edmonds M, et al. Exercise therapy for chronic fatigue syndrome. Cochrane Database Syst Rev 2004;(3):CD003200.

73. White PD, Goldsmith KA, Johnson AL, et al. PACE trial management group. Comparison of adaptive pacing therapy, cognitive behaviour therapy, graded exercise therapy, and specialist medical care for chronic fatigue syndrome (PACE): a randomised trial. Lancet 2011;377(9768):823–36.

74. Wilshire CE, et al. Rethinking the treatment of chronic fatigue syndrome—a reanalysis and evaluation of findings from a recent major trial of graded exercise and CBT. BMC Psychology 2018;(1):1. doi: 10.1186/s40359-018-0218-3.

75. Rowe P, Underhill R, Friedman K, et al. Myalgic encephalomyelitis/chronic fatigue syndrome diagnosis and management in young people: a primer. Front Pediatr 2017;5:121.

76. Wilshire C, Kindlon T, Matthees A, et al. Can patients with chronic fatigue syndrome really recover after graded exercise or cognitive behavioural therapy? A critical commentary and preliminary re-analysis of the PACE trial. Fatigue 2017;5(1):43.

77. Ruud C, et al. Exploratory open label, randomized study of acetyl- and propionylcarnitine in chronic fatigue syndrome. Psychosom Med 2004;66:276–82.

78. Santaella ML, et al. Comparison of oral nicotinamide adenine dinucleotide (NADH) versus conventional therapy for chronic fatigue syndrome. P R Health Sci J 2004;23(2):89–93.

79. Pall ML. Cobalamin used in chronic fatigue syndrome therapy is a nitric oxide scavenger. J CFS 2001;8(2):39–44.

80. Hart AJ, et al. Randomised controlled trial of Siberian ginseng for chronic fatigue. Psychol Med 2004;34:51–61.

81. Morgan M, Bone K. Herbs to enhance energy and performance, A phytotherapist's perspective. Queensland: Mediherb; 2008. p. 124.

82. Mishra LC, et al. Scientific basis for the therapeutic use of Withania somnifera (ashwagandha): a review. Altern Med Rev 2000;5(4):334–46.

83. Rhodiola rosea. Monograph. Altern Med Rev 2002;7(5):421–3.

84. Redman D. Rusculus aculeatus (butcher's broom) as a potential treatment for orthostatic hypotension with a case report. J Altern Complement Med 2000;6(6):539–49.

85. PDRhealth. Online. Available: http://www.pdrhealth.com. 18 Oct 2013.

86. Kulkarni K, Ashish D. Review article: Withania somnifera: an Indian ginseng. Prog Neuropsychopharmacol Biol Psychiatry 2008;32:1093–105.

87. Corbitt M, Campagnolo N, Staines D, et al. A systematic review of probiotic interventions for gastrointestinal symptoms and irritable bowel syndrome in chronic fatigue syndrome/myalgic encephalomyelitis (CFS/ME). Probiotics Antimicrob Proteins 2018;10(3):466–77.

88. Price JR, et al. Cognitive behaviour therapy for chronic fatigue syndrome in adults. Cochrane Database Syst Rev 2008;(3):CD001027.

89. Lapp C. Using vitamin B12 for the management of CFS. CFIDS Chron 1999;Nov/Dec:14–16.

90. Warren G, et al. The role of essential fatty acids in chronic fatigue syndrome: a case controlled study of red-cell membrane essential fatty acids (EFA) and a placebo-controlled treatment study with high dose of EFA. Acta Neurol Scand 1999;99:112–16.

91. Ganzert M, Felgenhauer N, Schuster T, et al. Amanita poisoning—comparison of silibinin with a combination of silibinin and penicillin. Dtsch Med Wochenschr 2008;133(44):2261–7.

92. Frenci P, Scherzer T, Kerschner H, et al. Silibinin is a potent antiviral agent in patients with chronic hepatitis C not responding to pegylated interferon/ribaririn therapy. Gastroenterology 2008;135:1561–7.

93. Castelli M, Friedman K, Sherry J, et al. Comparing the efficacy and tolerability of a new daily oral vitamin B-12 formulation and intermittent intramuscular vitamin B-12 in normalizing low cobalamin levels: a randomized, open-label, parallel-group study. Clin Ther 2011;33(3):358–71. Science Citation Index.

94. Dosch P, Dosch J, Dosch M. Manual of neural therapy according to Huneke. Stuttgart: Thieme; 2007.

95. Hunter J. Intramuscular injection techniques. Nurs Stand 2008;22(24):35–40.

96. Zabihiyeganeh M, Jahed A, Nojomi M. Treatment of hypovitaminosis D with pharmacologic doses of cholecalciferol, oral vs intramuscular: an open labeled RCT. Clin Endocrinol (Oxf) 2013;78(2):210–16. Global Health.

97. Djuric V, Bogic M, Popadic A, et al. Anaphylactic reaction to hydroxycobalamin with tolerance to cyanocobalamin. Ann Allergy Asthma Immunol 2012;108(3):207–8.

98. Deale A, et al. Cognitive behavior therapy for chronic fatigue syndrome: a randomized controlled trial. Am J Psychiatry 1997;154:408–14.

99. Prins J, et al. Cognitive behaviour therapy for chronic fatigue syndrome: a multicentre randomised controlled trial. Lancet 2001;357:841–7.

100. Nijhof S, Bleijenberg G, Uiterwaal C, et al. Effectiveness of internet-based cognitive behavioural treatment for adolescents with chronic fatigue syndrome (FITNET): a randomised controlled trial. Lancet 2012;9824:1412.

101. Fulcher KY, White PD. Randomised controlled trial of graded exercise in patients with the chronic fatigue syndrome. BMJ 1997;314:1647–52.

102. Powell P, et al. Randomised controlled trial of patient education to encourage graded exercise in chronic fatigue syndrome. BMJ 2001;322:387–92.

103. Wearden AJ, et al. Randomised, double-blind, placebo-controlled treatment trial of fluoxetine and graded exercise for chronic fatigue syndrome. Br J Psychiatry 1998;172:485–92.

104. White PD, Goldsmith KA, Johnson AL, et al. PACE trial management group. Comparison of adaptive pacing therapy, cognitive behaviour therapy, graded exercise therapy, and specialist medical care for chronic fatigue syndrome (PACE): a randomised trial. Lancet 2011;377(9768):823–36.

105. Behan WM, Horrobin D. Effect of high doses of essential fatty acids on the postviral fatigue syndrome. Acta Neurol Scand 1990;82:209–16.

106. Menon R, Cribb L, Murphy J, et al. Mitochondrial modifying nutrients in treating chronic fatigue syndrome: a 12-week open-label pilot study. AIMED 2017;4(3):109–14. doi:10.1016/j.aimed.2017.11.001.

107. Forsyth LM, et al. Therapeutic effects of oral NADH on the symptoms of patients with chronic fatigue syndrome. Ann Allergy Asthma Immunol 1999;82:185–91.

108. Castro-Marrero J, Saez-Francas N, Segundo M, et al. Effect of coenzyme Q10 plus nicotinamide adenine dinucleotide supplementation on maximum heart rate after exercise testing in chronic fatigue syndrome—a randomized, controlled, double-blind trial. Clin Nutr 2016;35(4):826–34.

109. Weatherley-Jones E, et al. A randomised, controlled, triple-blind trial of the efficacy of homeopathic treatment for chronic fatigue syndrome. J Psychosom Res 2004;56(2):189–97.

110. Crane J, et al. Massage therapy attenuates inflammatory signaling after exercise-induced muscle damage. Sci Transl Med 2012;4(119):119ra13.

111. Diego M, Field T. Moderate pressure massage elicits a parasympathetic nervous system response. Int J Neurosci 2009;119:630–8.

112. Field TM, et al. Massage therapy effects on depression and somatic symptoms in chronic fatigue syndrome. J Chronic Fatigue Syndr 1997;3:43–51.

CHAPTER **39**

Human immunodeficiency virus

David Casteleijn
ND, MHSc

OVERVIEW

The human immunodeficiency virus (HIV) only contains ribonucleic acid (RNA) in conjunction with an enzyme (reverse transcriptase) which can convert RNA to deoxy-ribonucleic acid (DNA). This process is activated when the virus comes in contact with the host cell and proceeds to make viral DNA, utilising the host cell's capacity for cell metabolism and synthesis.[1] Antiretroviral therapy (ART) has revolutionised HIV care (including 'one daily' treatment options),[2] resulting in increasing numbers of people living with (well controlled) HIV (PLHIV), although adherence to antiretroviral therapy remains less than ideal with various factors involved.[2] However, assuming viral load is suppressed and CD4 levels are maintained, we are no longer treating an immune deficiency and our treatment focus needs to shift to managing comorbidities[3] and ensuring good quality of life. This also means encouraging early diagnosis, and medical treatment needs to become part of naturopathic care of PLHIV and at-risk populations.

RISK FACTORS AND PREVALENCE

Activities that increase exposure risk to HIV include any activity in which blood, semen, pre-seminal fluid, fluids from the vagina and rectum, and breast milk may be exchanged. It is possible for HIV to be passed to the fetus during pregnancy, birth or while breast-feeding.[4] The risk of transmission with oral sex is extremely low,[5] while urine, sweat, vomit and saliva are not considered infectious.[6] Since the beginning of the epidemic, more than 70 million people have been infected and about 35 million people have died. Globally, an estimated 36.7 million people were living with HIV at the end of 2016, although the burden of the epidemic continues to vary considerably among countries and regions. Sub-Saharan Africa remains most severely affected, with nearly 1 in every 25 adults (4.2%) living with HIV and accounting for nearly two-thirds of the people living with HIV worldwide.

Mitigating the risks

Traditionally, 'safe' or 'protected sex' has been equated with the use of condoms. Condoms continue to be the cheapest, most readily accessible, safe and practical way to prevent sexual transmission of HIV and some other sexually transmitted infections

(STIs). The adoption of condoms in high-risk groups, such as men who have sex with men and sex workers, in response to HIV has been one of the most effective strategies in minimising the transmission of HIV.[7]

Following a breakthrough study published in 2011,[8] the evidence continues to strengthen for the non-transmissibility of HIV from a virally suppressed HIV-positive person to their serodiscordant sexual partner,[8–11] leading to a 2017 statement that 'people living with HIV who take HIV medicine as prescribed and get and keep an undetectable viral load have effectively no risk of transmitting HIV to their HIV-negative sexual partners'[12] referred to as treatment as prevention (TasP).

Post-exposure prophylaxis (PEP), first recommended in 1996[13] with protocols regularly updated since, is a course of three (or more) antiretroviral drugs taken for four weeks within 72 hours of a high-risk exposure to HIV.[14,15]

Pre-exposure prophylaxis (PrEP) allows HIV-negative people to prevent HIV infection by taking one pill (usually Truvada®) containing two pharmaceuticals (tenofovir and emtricitabine also used in combination to treat HIV) every day[16]; when taken consistently prior to potential HIV exposure, PrEP can reduce the risk of HIV infection in people who are at high risk by up to 99%.[17] PrEP is also recommended for high-risk pregnant and breastfeeding mothers,[18] with very low concentrations secreted into breast milk,[19] and should not be discontinued during pregnancy if substantial risk of HIV continues.[20]

Both the Center for Disease Control in the United States[21] and the Australian Federation of AIDS Organisations[7] have extended the definition of the term 'protected sex' to refer to more than sex with condoms: people with HIV who take treatments and have an undetectable viral load are now considered to be practicing safe sex (TasP), as are people who are HIV negative taking antiretroviral drugs as PrEP. It is no longer accurate to equate condom-less sex with unprotected sex if TasP or PrEP are used.

Significant acronyms
PLHIV: people living with HIV
TasP: treatment as prevention
PEP: post-exposure prophylaxis
PrEP: pre-exposure prophylaxis
cART: combined anti-retroviral therapy
HAART: highly active anti-retroviral therapy
PIs: protease inhibitors
NNRTIs: non-nucleoside reverse transcriptase inhibitors
NRTIs: nucleoside/nucleotide reverse transcriptase inhibitors

CONVENTIONAL TREATMENT—AIMING FOR ZERO

With the advances in ART, HIV infection has been transformed into a chronic medical condition.[3] Treatment focus has moved on to a TasP approach, where newly diagnosed people are encouraged to commence treatment immediately to maintain an 'undetectable' viral load, improving health outcomes as well as dramatically reducing the risk (to zero) of transmission to sexual partners.[22]

PrEP allows HIV-negative people to prevent HIV infection by taking one pill containing two pharmaceuticals every day. When taken consistently, PrEP can reduce the risk of HIV infection in people who are at high risk by up to 99%.[17] PrEP consists of a combination of two reverse transcriptase inhibitors: tenofovir disoproxil fumarate (TDF) and emtricitabine with the trade name Truvada® when in combination. Development in this area continues, with the possibility of a once-a-week tablet or slow-release implanted device on the way.

Supporting medication compliance supports the patient

A critical aspect of the effectiveness of aiming for zero is taking medication regularly. This is one area in which naturopathy can offer significant benefit, improving medication compliance via reducing potential medication side effects and supporting quality of life during the patient's treatment.

Treatments are constantly evolving, and the prescribed drugs change often. The aim of primary therapy is to achieve an undetectable viral load using a combination of medications to target specific sites critical to viral replication, referred to as either highly active anti-retroviral therapy (HAART) or more recently combined anti-retroviral therapy (cART). The most common medications include nucleoside/nucleotide reverse transcriptase inhibitors (NRTIs), which insert faulty messages into the reverse transcriptase process; non-nucleoside reverse transcriptase inhibitors (NNRTIs), which bind to reverse transcriptase and halt the production of viral DNA; protease inhibitors (PIs), which are responsible for targeting the construction of new HIV; and fusion inhibitors, which block binding of the virus to the cell.

HAART and naturopathy

HAART medication should never be withdrawn in favour of naturopathic interventions.

Naturopathy offers a beneficial role in supporting medical treatment by improving the patient's wellbeing and quality of life and ameliorating the side effects of medications.

KEY TREATMENT PROTOCOLS (HIV POSITIVE AND ON TREATMENT)

With the drugs successfully managing HIV, the naturopathic focus moves away from the virus itself. Previously, as naturopaths, the focus was on herbs/nutrients which might be antiviral, or supportive of the immune system. However, immune deficiency is no longer an issue for someone on treatment and the focus needs to shift towards addressing chronic immune activation and inflammation, along with other age-related cardio-metabolic comorbidities, including cardiovascular disease, diabetes, obesity and frailty.[3] Our role will depend on what combination of ART the person is taking, whether HIV is undetectable, CD4 counts, comorbidities, risk factors, current state of health and anything else going on (treating the whole person).

Common side effects of HIV and HIV medications can include a spectrum of gastro-intestinal (GI) disorders, including diarrhoea, nutrient malabsorption, abdominal pain,

GI bleeding and hepatomegaly.[23] Supporting the gut in optimal function and promoting nutrient absorption can greatly improve an individual's ability to cope with the stresses of HIV.[24] Nutrients which support the gastric and intestinal mucosa include **L-glutamine**, **probiotics** and **prebiotics/dietary fibre**.[25] Probiotics have shown decreases in microbial translocation, inflammation markers and immune activation.[26–28] Herbs which support the gastric and intestinal mucosa include *Hydrastis canadensis*,[29] *Zingiber officinalis*[29] and *Althea officinalis*.[30]

KEY TREATMENT PROTOCOLS (HIV NEGATIVE AND ON PrEP)

We also need to consider the management of a person who is HIV negative and taking PrEP for an extended period. Overall, PrEP appears to have a good safety profile within the average period of three years studied. When starting PrEP there can be short-term side effects, including nausea, abdominal cramping, vomiting, dizziness, headache and fatigue,[31–34] typically arising in the first week or two but usually disappearing in the following few weeks. Useful support in this time is focused on mitigating the side effects with general gastrointestinal and liver support with *Hydrastis canadensis*,[29] *Zingiber officinalis*,[29] *Althaea officinalis*[30] and *Silybum marianum*[29] or *Cynara scolymus*.[29] People who elect to take PrEP will be doing so for many years and so the long-term side effects also need considering. Some PrEP trials have shown some creatinine elevations,[31–33,35] with variable findings for spontaneous reversal.[36–39] Some studies found an increased risk of osteoporotic fracture,[40] while others found no greater fracture risk despite decreasing bone mineral density.[41–44] It is regularly mentioned that liver irregularities are associated with TDF; however, this appears to be an extrapolation from studies in HIV-positive people with TDF as part of their cART,[45] with no reports of TDF-based PrEP involving serious hepatic complications.[46] Nevertheless, regular (quarterly) monitoring of liver enzymes in PrEP users is recommended and naturopathic support of general liver function is a logical preventative inclusion, particularly herbs like *Silybum marianum*.[29]

Optimise gut function

At six months after initial HIV infection, changes in mucosal integrity begin to occur,[47] due to a loss of CD4 T-cells resident in the gut mucosa.[48] As infection becomes chronic, alteration of the epithelium and changes in the composition and function of microbiota occur, creating an environment for translocation of pathogenic bacteria and systemic immune activation and inflammation[47] associated with impaired barrier function activation of pro-inflammatory cytokines and reduced IgA levels.[49] Commencing cART may not be enough to halt these alterations once they occur within the gastrointestinal tract.[47] A significant reason naturopaths would recommend early testing and treatment is to prevent this damage. Probiotics have

> ### Integrative Medical Treatment Aims
>
> - Treat underlying deficiencies that may lead to opportunistic infection.
> - Optimise GI mucosal integrity.
> - Optimise nutrition that will negate mitochondrial damage and oxidation.
> - Regulate digestion and support liver function, especially if on medications.
> - Work with prescribing physician to address the side effects of the HIV medications.
> - Focus on normalising blood lipids in order to decrease long-term cardiovascular damage.
> - Support the immune system in order to maintain high CD4 counts and low viral load.
> - Boost perceived quality of life and encourage mental health support.

shown decreases in microbial translocation and inflammation marker activation,[26–28] while prebiotics significantly improved microbiota composition decreasing a range of pathogenic microbes while concurrently improving bifidobacteria and decreasing CD4+ T-cell activation.[50] Herbs which support the gastric and intestinal mucosa include *Hydrastis canadensis*,[40] *Zingiber officinalis*,[40] *Althaea officinalis*[30] or *Cynara scolymus*.[40]

Reducing mitochondrial toxicity

Mitochondrial toxicity is a problematic side effect regularly observed with NRTI therapy.[51] Lipodystrophy (LD) is a disorder of metabolism that causes fat deposition in atypical sites, causing fat loss in the limbs and face, and excess fat deposits on the trunk, and can be responsible for the intense fatigue present in some HIV patients. Mitochondrial toxicity combined with the effects of increased cellular oxidation accelerates ageing and increases the risk of age-related comorbidities,[52] lactic acidosis, pancreatitis and peripheral neuropathy.[53] Treatment can slow the progression of adverse events and greatly improve quality of life on cART. Supplements which can reduce mitochondrial toxicity include **coenzyme Q10, riboflavin, thiamine**,[54,55] **N-acetyl cysteine, L-glutamine, L-carnitine and alpha-lipoic acid**.[56]

Coenzyme Q10 is lower in individuals with advanced HIV, and supplementation improves biochemical markers of health.[57] By acting as a sulfur donor, N-acetyl cysteine normalises lymphocyte glutathione production and thereby decreases the number of free radicals produced by the cell, leading to improved CD4 levels.[58,59] Glutamine deficiency is prevalent in HIV infection. It serves as the preferred fuel for lymphocytes, macrophages and enterocytes and, as it is primarily stored in muscle tissue, a deficiency exhibits as muscle wasting and overall weight loss.[60] Oral supplementation with glutamine or cysteine increases levels of glutathione in the body, decreasing tissue oxidation.[61] Supplementation at 40 g daily can reverse muscle wasting in HIV and increase weight gain in patients suffering from wasting syndrome.[62] L-carnitine acts as an antioxidant and aids the production of energy by supporting the mitochondria and decreasing oxidation. Studies show that L-carnitine has an analgesic effect in the treatment of HIV peripheral neuropathy and can also improve peripheral nerve function by supporting several mechanisms, including nerve regeneration.[63] Alpha-lipoic acid supports glutathione levels and decreases free radical activity generated by HIV infection, with 300 mg three times a day normalising blood glutathione and increasing lymphocyte reactivity to T-cell mitogens.[64] In addition, alpha-lipoic acid has been used with success to treat the peripheral neuropathy of HIV by decreasing oxidative stress and inflammation of the involved nerves.[65]

Emerging research points to the potential of herbs, nutrients and dietary phytochemicals to improve antioxidant status through activation or upregulation of the 'master regulator' of cellular antioxidant mechanisms (Nrf2 or nuclear factor [erythroid-derived 2] like 2). Nrf2 is a ubiquitous protein which regulates the gene expression of cytoprotective proteins including antioxidant, anti-inflammatory and detoxification enzymes.[66] In vitro and in vivo studies demonstrating upregulation of Nrf2 by *Ginkgo biloba*,[67] *Andrographis paniculata*,[66] *Rosmarinus officinalis*,[68] *Schisandra chinensis*[69] and *Withania somnifera*,[70] for example, suggest a potentially significant role in optimising cellular protection and maintaining cellular redox homeostasis, clearly highly desirable in supporting a HIV-positive patient.

Address nutrient deficiencies

Elevated oxidation in HIV infection, side effects of cART and the increased stress in general lead to accelerated use of nutrients and subsequent potential deficiencies. Staying ahead of nutritional deficiencies is an integral part of supporting individuals with HIV. Activities such as smoking,[71] excessive exercise and drinking excessive alcohol[72] can deplete glutathione, so reducing these activities, along with supplementation, may lead to improved intracellular glutathione levels. Enhanced glutathione levels can lead to significant improvement in physical and quality-of-life markers.[73] Gastrointestinal issues common in HIV may also exacerbate nutrient deficiencies via malabsorption. Vitamin B12, vitamin A, beta-carotene, zinc, selenium and folate may all be affected by decreased transit time, dysbiosis and gut inflammation due to HIV or cART.[71] **Antioxidants** are also metabolised at an increased rate in HIV, leading to the depletion of vitamin A, vitamin E and vitamin C.[72] Supplementing these nutrients can improve lymphocyte proliferation and apoptosis.[73] Herbs and nutrients to stimulate Nrf2 compounds should also be part of HIV patient care. Minerals are also depleted through various mechanisms involved in HIV pathogenesis. Supplementation with **minerals** such as zinc,[74] selenium,[75] magnesium and copper[76] have been shown to improve health outcomes and aid other nutrients in antioxidant functions.

Manage medication side effects

Combination ART is a life-saving intervention, prolonging life by controlling viral load.[77] Unfortunately, these benefits often come with systemic unwanted effects[78] (see Table 39.1 and Figure 39.1). From liver toxicity and chronic diarrhoea, to insomnia and lipodystrophy, the symptoms are varied and can be so severe that people will stop taking the medications just to avoid the side effects. The primary target of naturopathic therapy is helping PLHIV be more comfortable while they maintain treatment; stabilising their digestion, mood, sleep and cardiovascular health can have a profound influence on quality of life and ultimately survival.

Consider cardiovascular risk

HIV not only affects the immune system, but it also has a considerable effect on metabolism and in turn the cardiovascular system, and has been found to contribute to arteriosclerosis in infected individuals.[80] Protease inhibitors, NNRTIs or both are also contributing factors in developing cardiovascular pathologies. Dyslipidaemia, blood sugar abnormalities, inflammation and decreased fibrinolysis may all increase the occurrence of adverse cardiovascular events.[81,82] Fortunately, interventions that include **dietary and lifestyle changes** along with exercise can have a positive effect on lipid

Table 39.1
Common side effects of HIV medications[79]

Medication	Common side effects
NRTIs and NNRTIs	Lactic acidosis, hepatitis, pancreatitis, anaemia, lipoatrophy
PIs	Increased cholesterol and triglycerides, diabetes, lipodystrophy and lipoatrophy, osteoporosis and osteonecrosis
FIs	Pain at injection site, rashes, bad taste in mouth, increased occurrence of pneumonia

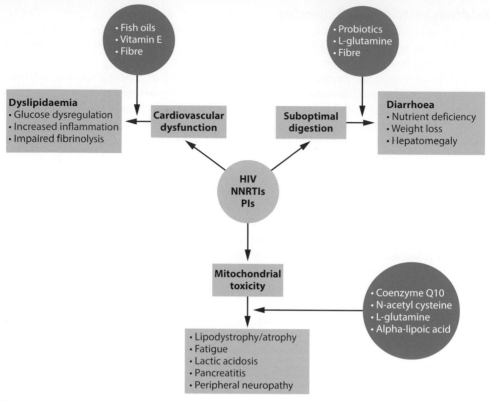

Figure 39.1
HIV/HAART side effects and nutritional interventions

levels and cardiovascular markers.[83] It has also been found that the use of **omega-3 fish oils** in combination with exercise can lead to a reduction in triglyceride levels, and would therefore be an important addition to any treatment protocol.[84] Another intervention demonstrated to change HIV-mediated cardiovascular markers is **vitamin E**.[85] Acting as an antioxidant, vitamin E reduces lipoprotein peroxidation, thus decreasing the potential for damage due to elevated blood lipids. Vitamin E also acts to decrease platelet aggregation, reducing the likelihood of vessel blockage and subsequent cardiovascular events.[86] The cardioprotective effects of **magnesium** might also be attributable to its effect on Nrf2.[87]

Maintaining wellbeing

One of the greatest challenges of treating HIV is that of maintaining general health and perceived wellbeing. Dealing with the mental and emotional stresses, along with the physical effects of the disease, can drain an individual and decrease their ability to cope with change. Patients can get extremely overwhelmed by the volume of new information that comes with a diagnosis of HIV, and with the continued therapies involved in their care. Health maintenance becomes the main goal, keeping physical as well as mental health balanced. Adaptogenic therapies can be extremely useful as an adjunct to other more aggressive medicines. The focus of adaptogenic medicines needs to be not only on supporting the adrenal glands, but also targeting the immune system.[88] Herbs such as *Withania somnifera*,[89] *Eleutherococcus senticosus, Panax ginseng, Ganoderma lucidum* and *Glycyrrhiza glabra* can all support the immune system while increasing tolerance to stress. **Withania somnifera**, in one study, was prescribed as an extract at 6 mL twice daily for four days, with a result of stimulating an increase in the expression of CD4 and natural killer cells, demonstrating its stimulatory effect on the immune system.[90] **Eleutherococcus senticosus** extracts have been found to increase CD4 counts and lymphocyte populations when used in healthy subjects.[91] Studies have also shown that *Eleutherococcus senticosus* aids in adrenal function through decreasing adrenal hypertrophy and increasing adrenal vitamin C levels.[92] **Panax ginseng** is a popular botanical used in traditional Chinese medicine and has demonstrated a broad range of effects on the immune system by enhancing both B- and T-cell mediated responses while acting as an antimicrobial against *Helicobacter pylori* and *Staphylococcus aureus*,[93] which can lead to infection in HIV-positive individuals. In addition, one animal study found it to increase CD4 cell function against the challenge of an induced systemic candida infection,[94] which is one of the main opportunistic infections found in HIV/AIDS.

Ganoderma lucidum, a fungus traditionally used in traditional Chinese medicine, has been proven to reduce physical and mental fatigue, while improving the function of the immune system.[95] Prescribing a botanical medicine based not only on its adaptogenic properties but also on its antimicrobial and immunosupportive qualities can help HIV-positive patients to maintain a high quality of life and improve their overall health.

Other **lifestyle interventions**, such as moderate exercise,[96] alternating hot and cold showers[97] and a daily meditation practice[98,99] also round out a treatment protocol for enhancing energy and boosting perceived quality of life.

Acupuncture is a very popular and effective method of treating the symptoms of HIV and the side effects of HAART. Due to the low probability of interaction between acupuncture and medical therapies and the cost-effective nature of this modality, it is a widely used tool in the treatment of HIV. One study recognised the value of acupuncture during structured treatment interruptions, where the group receiving the intervention during the interruption exhibited the suppression of viral load rebounds and the maintenance of immune function.[100] Many models exist to capture the effect that HIV has on the energetic balance of the body. Regardless of the specifics of how the retrovirus presents in the greater population, treating a person for their symptoms while also addressing the root of the imbalance can lead to a greater quality of life and a decrease in physical discomfort.[101] Evidence exists to support the use of acupuncture for a variety of complaints associated with HIV/AIDS, including insomnia, diarrhoea, fatigue, malaise and neuropathic pain associated with HIV peripheral neuropathy.[102] As with all patients, it is important to follow universal precautions when dealing with body fluids and employ sterile technique during acupuncture sessions.

Mental health support

Supporting the body includes supporting the mind as well. A diagnosis of HIV can be a devastating occurrence and often triggers acute anxiety and depression. What was once a death sentence has become a manageable ongoing illness, presenting new challenges in the treatment of mental health along the way. Long-term treatment fatigue can also take its toll as the constant reminder of illness counteracts attempts to live a meaningful and productive life.[103] Creating support networks of friends, healthcare providers and others living with HIV can validate and empower people to optimise their own health and that of the community.[104] It is important to recognise the symptoms of clinical depression and to treat or refer accordingly. Community support groups for people with HIV are particularly helpful in providing long-term coping strategies and creating a support network specific to HIV issues.

Drug–CAM interactions

It is important to recognise that there is a potential for interaction between the medications used for HAART and the botanical and nutraceutical supplements which naturopaths use on a daily basis. The literature recognises that botanicals that interact with CYP3A4 or P-glycoprotein can negatively affect the circulating levels of drugs in the system. One such interaction was considered to occur between *Hypericum perforatum* and PIs and NNRTIs, reducing their concentration in the body potentially leading to therapeutic failure.[105] However, more recent investigation of potential interactions with *Hypericum perforatum* identify hyperforin as the constituent largely responsible for these interactions and recommend using a product delivering less than 1 mg per day of hyperforin to minimise this risk.[106] It should also be noted that the pharmaceuticals used in PrEP are not from either of these classes and no interaction is expected.[107] A negative interaction may also occur between large amounts of garlic (*Allium sativum*) and ritonavir.[108] Criticism lies in that most of the studies involve the supplements in combination with a single drug, a situation rarely seen in current HIV therapy, and therefore may not be an accurate reflection of the interactions occurring in patients using drugs and CAM.[109]

> **No interaction expected between PrEP and *Hypericum perforatum***
>
> *Hypericum perforatum* is often avoided in patients taking medication with a narrow therapeutic range for fear of interaction. However, no known herb–drug interactions exist between PrEP and *Hypericum perforatum* and as such this useful herb can be safely employed in patients taking PrEP.

CLINICAL SUMMARY

Combination ART prescribing guidelines have been updated, recommending commencement as soon as possible after diagnosis with HIV. Previously, ART was delayed until CD4 levels were below a certain level or symptomatic HIV disease evident. This change should be embraced and supported by naturopaths, as early cART may prevent or at least delay the changes in mucosal integrity which begin to occur in the first six months after seroconversion,[47] from loss of CD4 T-cells resident in the gut mucosa.[48] Once these changes have occurred, cART does not appear to be able to completely correct the abnormalities which occur with ongoing untreated infection[47] and as such, naturopaths should no longer expect a window prior to antiviral medication being commenced. Rather, our focus needs to be on encouraging early diagnosis and treatment commencement followed by co-treatment. Naturopaths need to work as part of a team of people supporting someone living with HIV.

Assuming viral load is suppressed and CD4 levels are maintained, there is not an immune deficiency. A number of specific changes have been identified as occurring, due to chronic immune activation, inflammation (secondary to microbial translocation and increased gut permeability) and drug toxicity. Similarly, the focus of healthcare for PLHIV has moved away from the wasting, infections and cancers that were seen in AIDS, now focusing on healthy ageing and preventing and/or treating comorbidities.

While people may no longer be dying from AIDS-related illness, they continue to experience significant adverse health outcomes and naturopaths have numerous options to assist.

Optimising overall health exhibits significant improvement in many determinants of quality of life. Once on a protocol of antioxidants and adaptogens, with a good plan for proper nutrition and stress reduction, regular visits are often structured around acute complaints related to the medications or other aspects of the person's life. Patients seen in a naturopathic clinical practice should be expected to have commenced cART; and the real strength of naturopathic medicine lies in reducing side effects, improving vitality and empowering the patients to become part of the healing process.

Additionally, it is imperative practitioners working in this area are familiar with the current preventative options and encourage rather than oppose their use by their clients. PEP significantly reduces the risk of seroconversion post a risky exposure and PrEP provides an important additional layer of protection for people in high-risk groups. TasP is a significant additional mechanism in the ongoing work to eliminate new HIV infections.

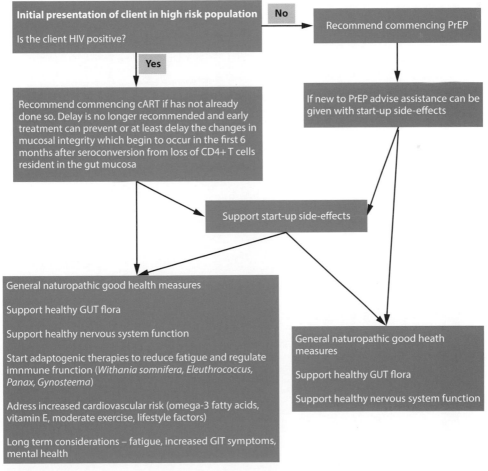

Figure 39.2
Naturopathic treatment decision tree

Table 39.2
Review of the major evidence

Intervention	Mechanisms of action	Key studies	Summary of results	Comment
Probiotics, soluble fibre and L-glutamine Supplementing cART with probiotics in HIV-positive individuals	Lactobacillus expresses CD4 receptor and can decrease HIV-1 binding, blocking HIV infection[110] • Soluble fibre acts as a prebiotic supporting increased probiotic population in gut • L-glutamine enhances glutathione stores, increases lean body mass in HIV, and also serves as the primary fuel for enterocytes[111]	Probiotics Reduce Inflammation in Antiretroviral Treated, HIV-Infected Individuals: Results of the 'Probio-HIV' Clinical Trial[26]	Inflammation and markers of microbial translocation were significantly reduced with probiotic supplementation. A clear and statistically significant reduction in the levels of immune activation on CD4 T-lymphocytes, for both markers CD38 and HLA-DR and their simultaneous expression, LBP and hsCRP plasma levels. A significant reduction of hsCRP after probiotics intake related to significant reduction of the cardiovascular diseases risk	Have shown decreases in microbial translocation, inflammation markers, immune activation
Antioxidant therapy	HIV precipitates altered metabolism and induces nutrient deficiencies including antioxidants Increased oxidative damage leads to an accelerated progression of the disease[112]	Dose comparison study: Batterham 2001[113]	Antioxidant supplementation significantly improved markers of oxidative defence. No difference in effectiveness noted between high and low doses	A significant difference in baseline antioxidant status was present between the two groups of participants. Future studies may account for this difference by grouping similar antioxidant baseline levels together for comparison of treatments
Omega-3 fatty acids	Omega-3 fatty acids reduce plaque inflammation, modulate very low-density lipoprotein (VLDL) and chylomicron metabolism and decrease hepatic secretion of VLDL[114]	RCTs: Carter 2006[115] DeTruchis 2007[116] Gerber 2008[117]	Significant reduction in the levels of triglycerides were found in each clinical trial, with 9 g of fish oil taken daily, 2 g of fish oil three times a day and 3 g of fish oil twice a day prescribed as the studied intervention	These studies included individuals receiving statin therapy and other lipid-lowering agents, providing a realistic representation of a HAART-prescribed population. Even factoring in the actions of these agents, omega-3 fatty acid supplementation in the form of fish oil still provided a statistically significant lipid-lowering effect which is very beneficial in people taking HAART

KEY POINTS

- Educate patients with potential risk of HIV infection.
- Support early testing and treatment (TasP) to limit gastrointestinal tract mucosal damage.
- Support PrEP commencement and adherence.
- No interaction between PrEP and St John's wort.
- Support body/mind with herbal tonics, adaptogens and nervines, and prescribe nutrients in cases of deficiency.
- Support optimal digestion and nutrition with a healthy diet and whole foods.
- Be sensitive to cultural beliefs and potential socioeconomic barriers.
- Stay alert to elevated cardiovascular risk, gastrointestinal symptoms and mental health challenges.
- Assist in establishing a network of care resources and make sure that psychological support is provided to the patient.

FURTHER READING

AIDS InfoNet. What is antiretroviral therapy (ART)? Fact Sheet 403. Online. Updated 23 July 2014. Available: http://www.aidsinfonet.org/fact_sheets/view/403.

Australian Federation of AIDS Organisations (AFAO) Living with HIV https://www.afao.org.au/about-hiv/living-with-hiv/.

Australian Federation of AIDS Organisations (AFAO). Online. Available: https://www.afao.org.au/.

Acknowledgments: The author would like to acknowledge Trent Wrightson and Fiona McCormick for their assistance. The author would also like to acknowledge Jennifer Hillier, who authored this chapter in previous editions.

REFERENCES

1. VanMeter KC, Hubert RJ. Pathophysiology for the health professions—e- book. St Louis: Elsevier; 2013.
2. Iacob SA, Iacob DG, Jugulete G. Improving the adherence to antiretroviral therapy, a difficult but essential task for a successful HIV treatment-clinical points of view and practical considerations. Front Pharmacol 2017;8:831. doi:10.3389/fphar.2017.00831.
3. Willig AL, Overton ET. Metabolic consequences of HIV: pathogenic insights. Curr HIV/AIDS Rep 2014;11(1):35–44. doi:10.1007/s11904-013-0191-7.
4. WHO. HIV/AIDS Online Q&A. 2009. Available: http://www.who.int/features/qa/71/en/24.
5. CDC. Oral Sex and HIV Risk. Centers for Disease Control and Prevention; 2016b. Available: https://www.cdc.gov/hiv/risk/oralsex.html.
6. AFAO. Low/No Risk Sexual Practices. 2018b.
7. AFAO. HIV Prevention. 2018a.
8. Cohen M, Chen YQ, McCauley M, et al. Prevention of HIV-1 infection with early antiretroviral therapy. N Engl J Med 2011;365(6):493–505.
9. Cohen M, Chen Y, McCauley M, et al. Antiretroviral therapy for the prevention of HIV-1 transmission. N Engl J Med 2016;375(9):830–9.
10. Grulich A, Bavinton B, Jin F, et al (2015). HIV transmission in male serodiscordant couples in Australia, Thailand and Brazil. Paper presented at the Seattle, Washington: 22nd Conference on Retroviruses and Opportunistic Infections.
11. Rodger A, Cambiano V, Bruun T, et al. Sexual activity without condoms and risk of HIV transmission in serodifferent couples when the HIV-positive partner is using suppressive antiretroviral therapy. JAMA 2016;316(2):171–81.
12. CDC. Evidence of HIV Treatment and Viral Suppression in Preventing the Sexual Transmission of HIV. 2017a. Available: https://www.cdc.gov/hiv/pdf/risk/art/cdc-hiv-art-viral-suppression.pdf.
13. CDC. Update: provisional Public Health Service recommendations for chemoprophylaxis after occupational exposure to HIV. MMWR Morb Mortal Wkly Rep 1996;45(22):468.
14. Kuhar D, Henderson D, Struble K, et al; Group, U. P. H. S. W. Updated US public health service guidelines for the management of occupational exposures to human immunodeficiency virus and recommendations for postexposure prophylaxis. Infect Control Hosp Epidemiol 2013;34(9):875–92.
15. McAllister J, Group., a. t. N. P. G. E. R. Literature review for the National Guidelines for Post-Exposure Prophylaxis after Non-Occupational and Occupational Exposure to HIV (Revised). Sydney: Australasian Society for HIV, Viral Hepatitis and Sexual Health Medicine (ASHM). 2016. Available: https://www.ashm.org.au/resources/PEP_Literature_Review_2016.PDF.
16. CDC. Pre-Exposure Prophylaxis (PrEP). 2017c. Available: https://www.cdc.gov/hiv/risk/art/index.html.
17. VAC. Pre Exposure Prophylaxis (PrEP). 2017. Available: http://vac.org.au/hiv-aids/pre-exposure-prophylaxis-prep.
18. WHO. WHO TECHNICAL BRIEF: preventing HIV during pregnancy and breastfeeding in the context of PrEP. Switzerland: World Health Organization; 2017.

19. Mugwanya K, Hendrix C, Mugo N, et al. Pre-exposure prophylaxis use by breastfeeding HIV-uninfected women: a prospective short-term study of antiretroviral excretion in breast milk and infant absorption. PLoS Med 2016;13(9):e1002132.

20. Mofenson L, Baggaley R, Mameletzis I. Tenofovir disoproxil fumarate safety for women and their infants during pregnancy and breastfeeding. AIDS 2017;31(2):213–32.

21. CDC. Anal Sex and HIV Risk. Centers for Disease Control and Prevention. 2016a. Available: https://www.cdc.gov/hiv/risk/oralsex.html.

22. CDC. HIV Treatment as Prevention. 2017b. Available: https://www.cdc.gov/hiv/risk/art/index.html.

23. Wilcox CM. Gastrointestinal consequences of infection with human immunodeficiency virus. In: Feldman M, Friedman LS, Brandt LJ, editors. Sleisenger and Fordtran's gastrointestinal and liver disease. 8th ed. Philadelphia: WB Saunders; 2006.

24. Fields-Gardner C. A review of mechanisms of wasting in HIV disease. Nutr Clin Pract 1995;10(5):167–76.

25. Heiser CR, et al. Probiotics, soluble fiber, and L-glutamine (GLN) reduce nelfinavir (NFV)-or lopinavir/ritonavir (LPV/r)-related diarrhea. J Int Assoc Physicians AIDS Care 2004;3(4):121–9.

26. d'Ettorre G, Ceccarelli G, Giustini N, et al. Probiotics reduce inflammation in antiretroviral treated, HIV-infected individuals: results of the 'Probio-HIV' clinical trial. PLoS ONE 2015;10(9):e0137200.

27. Stiksrud B, Nowak P, Nwosu FC, et al. Reduced levels of D-dimer and changes in gut microbiota composition after probiotic intervention in HIV-infected individuals on stable ART. J Acquir Immune Defic Syndr 2015;70(4):329–37.

28. Villar-García J, Hernández JJ, Güerri-Fernández R, et al. Effect of probiotics (Saccharomyces boulardii) on microbial translocation and inflammation in HIV-treated patients: a double-blind, randomized, placebo-controlled trial. J Acquir Immune Defic Syndr 2015;68(3):256–63.

29. Bone K, Mills S. Principles and practice of phytotherapy: modern herbal medicine. 2nd ed. Toronto: Churchill Livingston; 2013.

30. Schmidgall J, Schnetz E, Hensel A. Evidence for bioadhesive effects of polysaccharides and polysaccharide-containing herbs in an ex vivo bioadhesion assay on buccal membranes. Planta Med 2000;66(1):48–53. doi:10.1055/s-2000-11118.

31. Baeten JM, Donnell D, Ndase P, et al. Antiretroviral prophylaxis for HIV prevention in heterosexual men and women. N Engl J Med 2012;367(5):399–410.

32. Grant R, Lama J, Anderson P, et al. Preexposure chemoprophylaxis for HIV prevention in men who have sex with men. N Engl J Med 2010;363(27):2587–99.

33. Thigpen MC, Kebaabetswe PM, Paxton LA, et al. Antiretroviral preexposure prophylaxis for heterosexual HIV transmission in Botswana. N Engl J Med 2012;367(5):423–34.

34. Van Damme L, Corneli A, Ahmed K, et al. Preexposure prophylaxis for HIV infection among African women. N Engl J Med 2012;367(5):411–22.

35. Peterson L, Taylor D, Roddy R, et al. Tenofovir disoproxil fumarate for prevention of HIV infection in women: a phase 2, double-blind, randomized, placebo-controlled trial. PLoS Clin Trials 2007;2(5):e27.

36. Bonjoch A, Echeverría P, Perez-Alvarez N, et al. High rate of reversibility of renal damage in a cohort of HIV-infected patients receiving tenofovir-containing antiretroviral therapy. Antiviral Res 2012;96(1):65–9.

37. Dauchy F-A, Lawson-Ayayi S, de La Faille R, et al. Increased risk of abnormal proximal renal tubular function with HIV infection and antiretroviral therapy. Kidney Int 2011;80(3):302–9.

38. Liu AY, Vittinghoff E, Sellmeyer DE, et al. Bone mineral density in HIV-negative men participating in a tenofovir pre-exposure prophylaxis randomized clinical trial in San Francisco. PLoS ONE 2011;6(8):e23688.

39. Scherzer R, Estrella M, Yongmei L, et al. Association of tenofovir exposure with kidney disease risk in HIV infection. AIDS 2012;26(7):867.

40. Bedimo R, Maalouf NM, Zhang S, et al. Osteoporotic fracture risk associated with cumulative exposure to tenofovir and other antiretroviral agents. AIDS 2012;26(7):825–31.

41. Arribas JR, Pozniak AL, Gallant JE, et al. Tenofovir disoproxil fumarate, emtricitabine, and efavirenz compared with zidovudine/lamivudine and efavirenz in treatment-naive patients: 144-week analysis. J Acquir Immune Defic Syndr 2008;47(1):74–8.

42. Gallant JE, Staszewski S, Pozniak AL, et al. Efficacy and safety of tenofovir DF vs stavudine in combination therapy in antiretroviral-naive patients: a 3-year randomized trial. JAMA 2004;292(2):191–201.

43. Jacobson DL, Spiegelman D, Knox TK, et al. Evolution and predictors of change in total bone mineral density over time in HIV-infected men and women in the nutrition for healthy living study. J Acquir Immune Defic Syndr 2008;49(3):298–308.

44. McComsey GA, Kitch D, Daar ES, et al. Bone mineral density and fractures in antiretroviral-naive persons randomized to receive abacavir-lamivudine or tenofovir disoproxil fumarate-emtricitabine along with efavirenz or atazanavir-ritonavir: Aids Clinical Trials Group A5224s, a substudy of ACTG A5202. J Infect Dis 2011;203(12):1791–801.

45. Ryom L, Lundgren JD, De Wit S, et al. Use of antiretroviral therapy and risk of end-stage liver disease and hepatocellular carcinoma in HIV-positive persons. AIDS 2016;30(11):1731–43. doi:10.1097/qad.0000000000001018.

46. Tetteh RA, Yankey BA, Nartey ET, et al. Pre-exposure prophylaxis for HIV prevention: safety concerns. Drug Saf 2017;40(4):273–83. doi:10.1007/s40264-017-0505-6.

47. Tincati C, Douek DC, Marchetti G. Gut barrier structure, mucosal immunity and intestinal microbiota in the pathogenesis and treatment of HIV infection. AIDS Res Ther 2016;13:19. doi:10.1186/s12981-016-0103-1.

48. Nasi M, Pinti M, De Biasi S, et al. Aging with HIV infection: a journey to the center of inflammAIDS, immunosenescence and neuroHIV. Immunol Lett 2014;162(1):329–33.

49. Zilberman-Schapira G, Zmora N, Itav S, et al. The gut microbiome in human immunodeficiency virus infection. BMC Med 2016;14:83. doi:10.1186/s12916-016-0625-3.

50. Gori A, Rizzardini G, Van't Land B, et al. Specific prebiotics modulate gut microbiota and immune activation in HAART-naive HIV-infected adults: results of the 'COPA' pilot randomized trial. Mucosal Immunol 2011;4(5):554–63. doi:10.1038/mi.2011.15.

51. Caron M, et al. Contribution of mitochondrial dysfunction and oxidative stress to cellular premature senescence induced by antiretroviral thymidine analogues. Antivir Ther 2008;13(1):27–38.

52. Mallewa JE, et al. HIV-associated lipodystrophy: a review of underlying mechanisms and therapeutic options. J Antimicrob Chemother 2008;62(4):648–60.

53. Fitch KV, et al. Effects of a lifestyle modification program in HIV-infected patients with the metabolic syndrome. AIDS 2006;20(14):1843–50.

54. Bowers JM, Bert-Moreno A. Treatment of HAART-induced lactic acidosis with B vitamin supplements. Nutr Clin Pract 2004;19(4):375–8.

55. Khanh LVQ, Nguyen LTH. The role of thiamine in HIV infection, Review Article International Journal of Infectious Diseases, In Press, Corrected Proof, Available online 27 December 2012.

56. Patrick L. Nutrients and HIV: N-acetylcysteine, alpha-lipoic acid, L-glutamine, and L-carnitine. Altern Med Rev 2002;225:60.

57. Folkers K, et al. Biochemical deficiencies of coenzyme Q10 in HIV-infection and exploratory treatment. Biochem Biophys Res Commun 1988;153(2):888–96.

58. De Rosa SC, et al. N-acetylcysteine replenishes glutathione in HIV infection. Eur J Clin Invest 2000;30(10):915–29.

59. Droge W, Breitkreutz R. Glutathione and immune function. Proc Nutr Soc 2000;59:595–600.

60. Shabert JK, et al. Glutamine-antioxidant supplementation increases body cell mass in AIDS patients with weight loss: a randomized, double-blind controlled trial. Nutrition 1999;15(11–12):860–4.

61. Borges-Santos MD, et al. Plasma glutathione of HIV+ patients responded positively and differently to dietary supplementation with cysteine or glutamine. Nutrition 2012;28(7–8):753–6.

62. Wu G, et al. Glutathione metabolism and its implications for health. J Nutr 2004;134(3):489–92.

63. Chiechio S, et al. Acetyl-L-carnitine in neuropathic pain: experimental data. CNS Drugs 2007;21:31–8.

64. Curi R, et al. Molecular Mechanisms of glutamine action. J Cell Physiol 2005;204:392–401.

65. Jariwalla RJ, et al. Restoration of blood total glutathione status and lymphocyte function following alpha-lipoic acid supplementation in patients with HIV infection. J Altern Complement Med 2008;14(2):139–46.

66. Chen H-W, Huang Y-J, Yao H-T, et al. Induction of Nrf2-dependent antioxidation and protection against carbon tetrachloride-induced liver damage by Andrographis herba (穿心蓮 chuān xīn lián) ethanolic extract. J Tradit Complement Med 2012;2(3):211–19.

67. Liu X, Goldring C, Copple I, et al. Extract of Ginkgo biloba induces phase 2 genes through Keap1-Nrf2-ARE signaling pathway. Life Sci 2007;80(17):1586–91.

68. Lin C-Y, Wu C-R, Chang S-W, et al. Induction of the pi class of glutathione S-transferase by carnosic acid in rat Clone 9 cells via the p38/Nrf2 pathway. Food Funct 2015;6(6):1936–43.

69. He J-L, Zhou Z-W, Yin J-J, et al. Schisandra chinensis regulates drug metabolizing enzymes and drug transporters via activation of Nrf2-mediated signaling pathway. Drug Des Devel Ther 2015;9:127.

70. Sun GY, Li R, Cui J, et al. Withania somnifera and its withanolides attenuate oxidative and inflammatory responses and up-regulate antioxidant responses in BV-2 microglial cells. Neuromolecular Med 2016;18(3):241–52.

71. Cole SB, et al. Oxidative stress and antioxidant capacity in smoking and nonsmoking men with HIV/acquired immunodeficiency syndrome. Nutr Clin Pract 2005;20(6):662–7.

72. Colell A, et al. Selective glutathione depletion of mitochondria by ethanol sensitizes hepatocytes to tumor necrosis factor. Gastroenterology 1998;115(6):1541–51.

73. Namulema E, et al. When the nutritional supplements stop: evidence from a double-blinded, HIV clinical trial at Mengo Hospital, Kampala, Uganda. J Orthomol Med 2008;23(3):130–2.

74. Bobat R, et al. Safety and efficacy of zinc supplementation for children with HIV-1 infection in South Africa: a randomised double-blind placebo-controlled trial. Lancet 2005;366(9500):1862–9.

75. Ferencík M, Ebringer L. Modulatory effects of selenium and zinc on the immune system. Folia Microbiol (Praha) 2003;48(3):417–26.

76. Evans P, Halliwell B. Micronutrients: oxidant/antioxidant status. Br J Nutr 2001;85(Suppl. 2):S67–74.

77. Street E, Curtis H, Sabin CA, et al. British HIV Association (BHIVA) national cohort outcomes audit of patients commencing antiretrovirals from naïve. HIV Med 2009;10(6):337–42.

78. Gil L, et al. Altered oxidative stress indexes related to disease progression marker in human immunodeficiency virus infected patients with antiretroviral therapy. Biomed Pharmacother 2011;1(1):8–15.

79. Oelklaus MW, et al. Managing long-term side of effects of HIV therapy, Test Positive Aware Network, 2007. Online. Available from: http://www.thebody.com/content/treat/art40471.html March.

80. Schillaci G, et al. Aortic stiffness in untreated adult patients with human immunodeficiency virus infection. Hypertension 2008;52(2):308–13.

81. Grinspoon S, Carr A. Cardiovascular risk and body-fat abnormalities in HIV-infected adults. N Engl J Med 2005;352(1):48–62.

82. Dubé MP, Cadden JJ. Lipid metabolism in treated HIV infection. Best Pract Res Clin Endocrinol Metab 2011;25(3):429–42.

83. Triant VA, et al. Increased acute myocardial infarction rates and cardiovascular risk factors among patients with human immunodeficiency virus disease. J Clin Endocrinol Metab 2007;92(7):2506–12.

84. Wohl DA, et al. Randomized study of the safety and efficacy of fish oil (omega-3 fatty acid) supplementation with dietary and exercise counseling for the treatment of antiretroviral therapy — associated hypertriglyceridemia. Clin Infect Dis 2005;41(10):1498–504.

85. Gavrila A, et al. Exercise and vitamin E intake are independently associated with metabolic abnormalities in human immunodeficiency virus-positive subjects: a cross-sectional study. Clin Infect Dis 2003;36(12):1593–601.

86. Clarke MW, et al. Vitamin E in human health and disease. Crit Rev Clin Lab Sci 2008;45(5):417–50.

87. Mak IT, Kramer JH, Elzohary L, et al. Combination antiretroviral therapy (cART) altered redox/nitrosative genes, enhanced systemic stress and cardiac dysfunction in HIV-1 transgenic (HIV-Tg) rats: effects of magnesium supplementation (Mg-supp). Free Radic Biol Med 2017;112:117.

88. Jayakumar P, et al. Lipodystrophy and adrenal insufficiency: potential mediators of peripheral neuropathy in HIV infection? Med Hypotheses 2012;78(3):373–6.

89. Rege NN, et al. Adaptogenic properties of six rasayanan herbs used in Ayurvedic medicine. Phytother Res 1999;14(4):275–91.

90. Mikolai J, et al. In vivo effects of ashwagandha (Withania somnifera) extract on the activation of lymphocytes. J Altern Complement Med 2009;15(4):423–30.

91. Bohn B, et al. Flow-cytometric studies with eleutherococcus senticosus extract as an immunomodulatory agent. Arzneimittelforschung 1987;37(10):1193–6.

92. Eleutherococcus. Altern Med Rev 2006;11(2):151–5.

93. Tan BK, Vanitha J. Immunomodulatory and antimicrobial effects of some traditional Chinese medicinal herbs: a review. Curr Med Chem 2004;11(11):1423–30.

94. Lee JH, Han Y. Ginsenoside Rg1 helps mice resist to disseminated candidiasis by Th1 type differentiation of CD4+ T cell. Int Immunopharmacol 2006;6(9):1424–30.

95. Bone K. Phytotherapy review and commentary. Townsend Letter 2007;289/290:69–71.

96. Hand GA, et al. Moderate intensity exercise training reverses functional aerobic impairment in HIV-infected individuals. AIDS Care 2008;20(9):1066–74.

97. Goedsche K, et al. Repeated cold water stimulations (hydrotherapy according to Kneipp) in patients with COPD. Forsch Komplementmed 2007;14(3):158–66.

98. Creswell JD, et al. Mindfulness meditation training effects on CD4+ T lymphocytes in HIV-1 infected adults: a small randomized controlled trial. Brain Behav Immun 2009;23(2):184–8.

99. Fitzpatrick AL, et al. Survival in HIV-1 positive adults practicing psychological or spiritual activities for one year. Altern Ther Health Med 2007;13(5):18–20.

100. Zhao HX, et al. Effects of traditional Chinese medicine on CD4+ T cell counts and HIV viral loads during structured treatment interruption in highly active antiretroviral therapy. Zhongguo Yi Xue Ke Xue Yuan Xue Bao 2006;28(5):658–61.

101. Acupuncture Research Resource Centre. Briefing Paper No 6: HIV infection and traditional Chinese medicine, the evidence for effectiveness, February 2000. Online. Available: http://www.acupuncture.org.uk/content/Library/doc/hiv_bp6.pdf.

102. Burke A. The essential role of acupuncture, herbs and related therapies in HIV care, American Acupuncturist 41:26–28, 2007.

103. Reisner SL, et al. A review of HIV antiretroviral adherence and intervention studies among HIV-infected youth. Top HIV Med 2009;17(1):14–25.

104. Mosack KE, et al. Influence of coping, social support, and depression on subjective health status among HIV-positive adults with different sexual identities. Behav Med 2009;34(4):133–44.

105. Lee LS, et al. Interactions between natural health products and antiretroviral drugs: pharmacokinetic and pharmacodynamic effects. Clin Infect Dis 2006;43(8):1052–9.

106. Chrubasik-Hausmann S, Vlachojannis J, McLachlan AJ. Understanding drug interactions with St John's wort (Hypericum perforatum L.): impact of hyperforin content. J Pharm Pharmacol 2018.

107. MIMS. eMIMS. 2018. http://www.emims.com.au/Australia/interaction/advancedsearch?start=new.

108. Patel J, et al. In vitro interaction of the HIV protease inhibitor ritonavir with herbal constituents: changes in P-gp and CYP3A4 activity. Am J Ther 2004;11(4):262–77.

109. Mills E, et al. Natural health product–HIV drug interactions: a systematic review. Int J STD AIDS 2005;16(3):181–6.

110. Sua Y, Zhanga B, Sub L. CD4 detected from Lactobacillus helps understand the interaction between Lactobacillus and HIV. Microbiol Res 2013;168(5):273–7.

111. Patrick L. Nutrients and HIV: part three N-acetylcysteine, alpha-lipoic acid, L-Lglutamine, and L-carnitine. Altern Med Rev 2000;4:290–305.

112. Filteau S, Manno D. Nutrition and HIV/AIDS. Encyclopedia of Human Nutrition. 3rd ed. 2013. p. 303–308.

113. Batterham M, et al. Preliminary open label dose comparison using an antioxidant regimen to determine the effect on viral load and oxidative stress in men with HIV/AIDS. Eur J Clin Nutr 2001;55(2):107–14.

114. Weitz D, Weintraub H, Fisher E, et al. Fish oil for the treatment of cardiovascular disease. Cardiol Rev 2010;18(5):258–63.

115. Carter VM, et al. A randomised controlled trial of omega-3 fatty acid supplementation for the treatment of hypertriglyceridemia in HIV-infected males on highly active antiretroviral therapy. Sex Health 2006;3:287–90.

116. De Truchis P, et al. Reduction in triglyceride level with N-3 polyunsaturated fatty acids in HIV-infected patients taking potent antiretroviral therapy: a randomized prospective study. J Acquir Immune Defic Syndr 2007;44:278–85.

117. Gerber JG, et al. Fish oil and fenofibrate for the treatment of hypertriglyceridemia in HIV-infected subjects on antiretroviral therapy: results of ACTG A5186. J Acquir Immune Defic Syndr 2008;47(4):459–66.

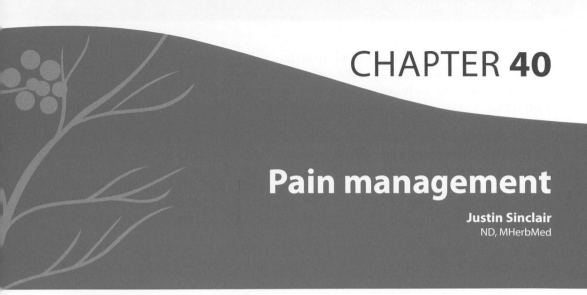

CHAPTER **40**

Pain management

Justin Sinclair
ND, MHerbMed

OVERVIEW

Pain is a disagreeable subjective physiological and psychosocial experience that often serves a biological purpose (warning of injury).[1-3] It incorporates both the perception of a painful stimulus and the response to the aforementioned perception.[4] It has been posited that the severity of pain does not necessarily correlate with the degree of tissue damage, and that a patient's individual expression and experience of pain is both complex and unique.[5] Being highly subjective, pain is therefore difficult to quantify. The most widely used scales for evaluating the experience of pain in patients are the visual analogue scale (VAS) and the numeric rating scale (NRS),[6] with behavioural rating scales also showing efficacy in estimating whether patients with cognitive impairment are in pain.[5]

Behavioural signs of pain
• Frowning or grimacing
• Crying/moaning or gritting teeth
• Irritability, anxiety, restlessness, hostility or anorexia
• Clenched fists or increased muscle tension
• Guarding or clutching the affected area/fetal position

Prevalence of pain, specifically chronic pain, varies greatly and is dependent on many factors.[7] A study conducted by the World Health Organization (WHO)[8] suggests that 22% of primary care patients reported pain that was persistent. Conversely, a review of 13 studies between 1991 and 2002 suggested a prevalence of chronic pain ranging from 10% to 55%,[9] with further studies suggesting a prevalence of chronic pain in the elderly of 23.7–50.2%.[10,11] In 2007, 3.1 million Australians were estimated to experience chronic pain, with a total cost impact on productivity valued at $11.7 billion.[12] Chronic pain has been found to affect more respondents than other chronic conditions such as diabetes, hypertension or asthma.[7]

Pain can be classified into being of either somatogenic (organic) or psychogenic (non-organic) origin.[13] Somatogenic pain occurs as a result of a direct physiological mechanism or insult (such as osteoarthritis or trauma) and can be further divided into nociceptive pain (e.g. ongoing activation of visceral nociceptors) or neuropathic pain (e.g. neurological dysfunction). Pain can further be explained by duration of effect, being either acute (lasting less than four weeks) or chronic (pain lasting longer than 12 weeks).[13] Acute pain is characterised by hyperactivity of the sympathetic nervous system and may present with anxiety, tachycardia, tachypnoea, hypertension and diaphoresis.[13] Conversely, chronic pain typically expresses vegetative signs such as lassitude, insomnia, anorexia, low libido, constipation and depression.[13] Due to the likelihood that most people with acute pain will seek out acute orthodox medical care, this chapter has focused more on chronic pain.

The aetiology of pain in its various presentations is complex and diverse. Nociceptive pain refers to conditions whereby pain is assumed to be predominantly driven by the activation of peripheral nociceptive sensory fibres,[14] with common examples including physical trauma in the form of burns, fractures or wounds (e.g. lacerations or contusions). These examples are seen as a response of primary afferent neurons (A-delta and C-fibres) to thermal, mechanical or inflammatory (chemical) stimulus.[15–17] Another definition of nociceptive pain promulgates that the noxious stimulus is delivered to an intact nervous system, which provides a point of differentiation to neuropathic pain.[18] Conditions such as cancer can exist within this nociceptive category, with two-thirds of patients experiencing moderate to severe pain; however, cancer pain can be of varied aetiology and 50% of cancer pain may be attributed to the neuropathic class.[5]

Figure 40.1 shows the dermatomes of the skin, which are each predominately supplied by a single spinal nerve.

Neuropathic pain is defined as 'pain initiated or caused by a primary lesion or dysfunction in the nervous system'.[19,20] Characterised by pain in the peripheral or central nervous systems caused by disease, surgical damage or trauma,[5,13] it is a clinical description and not an actual diagnosis. Neuropathic pain is distressing, chronic[21] and includes conditions such as nerve compression, neuroma formation, postamputation pain, post-stroke central pain, diabetic peripheral neuropathy and postherpetic and trigeminal neuralgia.[13,21,22] From a clinical standpoint, neuropathic pain presents as a constant burning, stabbing or pulsing pain with sharp exacerbations, allodynia, dysaesthesia or hyperalgesia[5,18] and causes considerable impact on quality of life.[21,23–26] As such, it is considered the most challenging type of pain to treat and manage,[27,28] with neuropathic pain patients having higher pain scores, lower health-related quality of life, requiring more medications and getting less pain relief from treatment.[28–30] Epidemiologically, chronic pain of a neuropathic origin has an estimated prevalence of 7–8% of the general population in various groups,[31–33] but exact figures of affliction worldwide are currently unavailable.[27]

Neuropathic pain definitions

- Allodynia: pain in response to non-harmful stimulus
- Dysaesthesias: unpleasant and abnormal sensations
- Hyperalgesia: increased pain in response to painful stimulus

Source: Colledge et al. 2010[5]

Psychogenic pain cannot be explained by a well-defined pathophysiological perspective and is considered to be of psychological origin.[34] As such, it poses a considerable challenge both clinically (i.e. diagnostics and treatment) and economically.[35,36] By the aforementioned definition, psychogenic pain can include functional somatic syndromes (e.g. irritable bowel syndrome [IBS], chronic fatigue syndrome [CFS], fibromyalgia, temporomandibular joint disorder [TMJ], globus syndrome, chronic low back pain and tension headache),[37] somatisation disorder[36] and even hypochondriasis.[13] Studies have shown that effective treatment

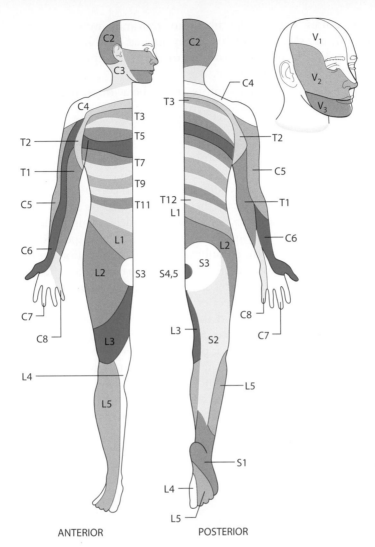

Figure 40.1
Dermatomal distribution

Source: Kumar & Clark 2012[1]

for disorders such as IBS and CFS is rarely supplied,[37,38] and leads to increasing rates of medical care.[39] There is currently little evidence on psychogenic pain prevalence.

The pathophysiology of pain is multifarious and generally in accordance with a suspected aetiology. The perception of nociceptive pain is physiologically mediated mainly by myelinated A-delta fibre and unmyelinated C-fibre terminal nerve endings, in combination with the neurotransmitter glutamate,[1] and follows the outline below.

1. In response to mechanical stimuli and subsequent chemical release at the site of injury, these nerve endings increase firing rates and cause pain by either direct stimulation or sensitising nerve endings.[1]
2. Both A-delta and C-fibres transmit electrical impulses from the peripheral nervous supply through the dorsal root and into the dorsal horn of the spinal cord.[40]

3. Myelination causes the A-delta fibres to transmit impulses extremely quickly compared with the slower travelling unmyelinated C-fibres. Acute and sharp pain travels via the A-delta fibres in contrast to the more chronic, dull pain generally associated with C-fibre transmission.[1]

4. Other fibres, such as silent nociceptors and A-beta fibres, occur in joints and the periosteum, and can also augment the pain response.[41]

Neuropathic pain pathophysiology is largely based on the causative aetiology in many instances; however, it is heavily characterised by dysfunction of pain fibres of the central nervous system.[42]

A multitude of biological and psychological models theorising the causes of pain have been posited over the years. Specificity theory (formulated by Schiff and Frey in 1858 theorised that pain is a specific sensation of its own, independent of touch and requiring its own sensory apparatus),[43] the intensive-summation theory (posited by Goldsheider, suggesting that the intensity of the stimulus and central summation are the major determinants of pain)[43] and the Aristotelian concept that pain was an affective quality were all competing for acceptance in the medical and scientific communities by the end of the 19th century.[43] Other notable theories included the fourth theory of pain,[43] which postulated the perception of pain and the reaction to it, and the sensory interaction theory, which promulgates the now accepted mechanism of the slow unmyelinated and small myelinated afferent fibre system for pain transmission.[44,45] It was not until the 1950s that observations such as referred pain, neuropathic pain, neurogenic inflammation and chemical mediators such as histamine and substance P were noted,[46] which has led to the more recent hypotheses of the 'gate control' theory of pain,[47] the discovery of the endogenous opioid system[48] and mechanisms for nociceptive pain plasticity.[43,49] Currently, no one unified and expansive theory of pain exists, but rather the foundation was laid with gate control and has been expanded on since then with new research into the concepts of interoception[50] and hyperalgesic priming.[51] All of these theories together form a cohesive working model of pain that will continue to evolve as new research comes to light.

Pain management prioritisation

- Classify/assess the pain: Using VAS, behavioural or numerical scales, identify pain intensity, location, type and duration. Physical assessment as required on a case-by-case basis.
- Identify cause: If a diagnosis has not been previously obtained, investigative tests or specialist referral may be required.
- Pain amelioration: Whether acute or chronic, pain needs to be reduced as a matter of urgency to improve patient wellbeing and mental health, comfort, improve quality of life and encourage healing.
- Address the underlying cause: Should be of top priority along with minimising any predisposing or sustaining causes.
- Enhance mental resilience: Cognitive behaviour therapy (CBT), mindfulness and meditation are all of use to assist in pain management. Referral for specific psychological counselling or group pain programs is also advised.
- Lifestyle modifications: Examples include loss of weight if obesity is increasing pain in the knees of an osteoarthritis (OA) patient or increasing social activities in a patient with depression.
- Close patient monitoring: This is to ensure correct analgesia and patient comfort but also for assessing potential side effects of treatment or drug dependence/tolerance; regular follow-ups are suggested.
- Social factors: These include lack of employment or financial concerns and can be referred to appropriate government or non-government agencies or *pro re nata* with severely impaired patients potentially needing full-time carers assigned (Figure 40.2).

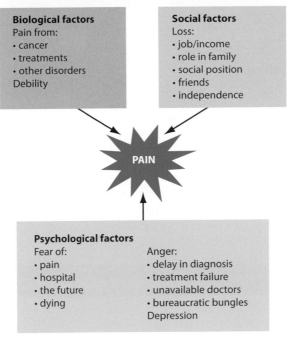

Figure 40.2
Contributing factors to pain

Source: Oxenham 2010[46]

DIFFERENTIAL DIAGNOSIS*

- Physiological (e.g. nociceptive acute trauma including either visceral, superficial or deep somatic pain)
- Chronic musculoskeletal (e.g. osteoarthritis, lumbago)
- Headaches (e.g. migraines, tension and cluster headaches)
- Nerve pain (e.g. herpes zoster, postherpetic neuralgia)
- Cancer (pain can be due to either the disease itself (i.e. the tumour affecting surrounding tissues) or potential treatment such as surgery or radiotherapy)
- Phantom pain (a form of neuropathic pain)
- Psychosomatic pain (i.e. psychogenic cause)

*Common conditions manifesting pain

RISK FACTORS

Further compounding the deleterious physiological effects of pain are social, emotional and psychological ramifications, which are especially prevalent in chronic pain, causing debilitating sequelae such as comorbid anxiety and/or depression.[13] Pain sufferers are often impaired in their ability to initiate or maintain fundamental daily activities such as eating, shopping and cleaning,[52,53] further isolating the patient and increasing morbidity scales (decreasing quality of life). Blyth and colleagues have found consistent evidence of the associations between chronic pain and the social determinants listed below:

- older age
- female gender

- low socioeconomic status
- poor education
- poor health
- employment disadvantage
- psychological distress.[7]

CONVENTIONAL TREATMENT

Modern medical treatment of pain, whether acute or chronic, is largely dependent on causation as this drives and directs treatment protocols. What follows is a basic overview of various analgesic drug classes and other orthodox therapies; for more detailed information, specific orthodox pain management texts or specialists should be consulted.

Treatment for acute pain conditions that are mild to moderate in presentation may be addressed by non-opioid analgesics such as acetaminophen and certain nonsteroidal anti-inflammatory drugs (NSAIDs).

Non-opioid analgesic examples*	
• Indoles (e.g. indomethacin, tolmetin) • Para-aminophenol derivatives (e.g. acetaminophen) • Propionic acids (e.g. ibuprofen, naproxen, ketoprofen, fenoprofen)	• Salicylates (e.g. aspirin, diflunisal) • Oxicams (e.g. piroxicam) • Fenamates (e.g. mefenamic acid) • Pyrazole (e.g. phenylbutazone)

*This list is not exhaustive.
Source: Beers & Berkow 1999[13]

More severe acute pain may require stronger medications in the form of opioid agonists such as codeine, morphine, oxycodone, hydromorphone or oxymorphone.[13] Co-administration of various types of analgesia may be necessary depending on the presenting condition, an example being acute urolithiasis where opioid analgesia and NSAIDs (ketorolac) administered together have shown superior analgesic performance than either alone.[54,55] In the most severe cases, or non-responders, various forms of anaesthesia or nerve blocks (such as an epidural in labour) may be considered by a specialist clinician, along with assorted other medications that may assist in treating the cause and, by doing so, reduce the pain.

Other drug classes used in pain management	
• Antibiotics (e.g. reducing bacterial infection) • Anticonvulsants • Antidepressants (e.g. comorbid depression) • Antispasmodics (e.g. colic)	• Muscle relaxants (e.g. cases of muscular spasticity) • Steroids (e.g. inflammatory conditions or arthropathies) • Tricyclics

Source: Kumar & Clark 2012[1]

Chronic, intractable pain generally entails multiple drug classes to help manage analgesia and other existing comorbidities. Of particular importance are mental health issues such as depression and anxiety (see Chapters 14 and 15 on depression and anxiety for further information). Other useful forms of therapy are ice and heat applications, transcutaneous electrical nerve stimulation (TENS) (which can be individualised to the patient based on pulse frequency and pulse pattern),[56] high-frequency spinal cord stimulation,[57,58] nerve blocks (somatic or sympathetic) and more specialised neurosurgeries (e.g. cordotomy, dorsal rhizotomy).[1] This last area is still considered controversial.

KEY TREATMENT PROTOCOLS

From a clinical perspective, the priority of treatment is focused upon pain amelioration as carefully and hastily as possible; however, no one model exists for treating all acute or chronic presentations of pain (see pain management prioritisation box earlier and the integrative decision tree in Figure 40.3 later in the chapter), so a degree of individual adaptability is required based on the presenting case.

> **Integrative Medical Treatment Aims**
>
> - Address the underlying causes of the pain.
> - Assist in the chronic management of pain.
> - Provide psychological support.
> - Address comorbidities such as depression, anxiety and insomnia.
> - Refer where appropriate.

Tying in with this need for adaptability is the ability for the clinician to prescribe extemporaneously from a herbal and nutritional perspective. Instead of relying upon pre-packaged mixtures of set pharmaceuticals at predefined doses, the modern naturopath and herbalist can manufacture individual holistic preparations that can take into account areas of therapeutic concern to the patient, comorbid conditions and bypass potential herb–drug–nutrient interactions (HDNIs), which have an increased likelihood in polypharmacy cases (see Chapter 41 on interactions for more information).

Ameliorate pain and reduce suffering

Herbal medicines work upon many different neuroreceptors, can modulate the central nervous system and have a complex phytochemistry, which makes them useful as analgesics, albeit they often fail to reach the strength or speed of onset that previously mentioned synthetic pharmaceuticals achieve.

Alkaloid-containing plants such as ***Eschscholzia californica*** have been shown to have gamma-aminobutyric acid (GABA) receptor binding affinity and anxiolytic activity,[59] with in-vitro evidence suggesting the extract can inhibit catecholamine degradation, synthesis of adrenaline and bind to opiate and benzodiazepine receptors.[60] ***Corydalis ambigua*** contains more than 20 different alkaloids including tetrahydropalmatine. This constituent imparts a sedative and analgesic action (1–10% that of opium but shares a naloxone-resistant analgesic action), with studies showing it is a dopamine receptor antagonist and is non-addictive, but tolerance can still be developed from administration.[61] Another alkaloid-containing plant is ***Passiflora incarnata***; however, it is the chrysin (flavone)[62] component that is currently considered the most biologically active constituent. While the herb itself does not convey notable analgesic action, it does possess significant anxiolytic, hypnotic and mild sedative action that can be of secondary clinical benefit.[60] Earlier studies, however, have shown the possibility of non-chrysin analgesic flavones within passion flower as having the ability to raise nociceptive thresholds.[63,64]

Piper methysticum has known anxiolytic, hypnotic, sedative, skeletal muscle relaxant, spasmolytic and mild analgesic actions.[60] While human clinical studies suggest positive outcomes in anxiety and insomnia, experimental models have shown that the *Piper methysticum* lactones may act as useful analgesics. The lactones dihydrokavain (DHK) and dihydromethysticin (DHM) have shown an analgesic effect via non-opiate pathways.[65]

Harpagophytum procumbens contains iridoid glycosides (primarily harpagoside) and has excellent anti-inflammatory and analgesic evidence for arthritis.[65,66] Proposed mechanisms of action for the herbal extract or isolated harpagoside include in-vitro evidence of suppression of lipopolysaccharide-induced inducible nitric oxide synthase (iNOS) and COX-2 expression through inhibition of nuclear factor kappaB (NF-κB) activation,[67,68] a reduction in COX-1[69] activity while also inhibiting the production of various inflammatory cytokines.[70]

Salix alba has a long history of use for pain management. First documented scientifically as an analgesic between 1763 and 1803,[65] the addition of an acetyl group to salicylic acid led to the development of the first NSAID, aspirin, in 1897. Unlike *Harpagophytum procumbens*, *Salix alba* demonstrates poor inhibitory activity against COX-1 and COX-2, albeit it has been posited that hyaluronidase and lipoxygenase inhibition alongside free radical scavenging activity contribute to its anti-inflammatory and analgesic action.[65]

Traditional analgesic evidence exists for *Piscidia erythrina*[71] and should not be discounted as it has shown central analgesic activity in preliminary studies.[72] Clinical evidence from randomised trials were not found in the literature.

A lesser known Brazilian vine *Dioclea grandiflora* (Mucanã) has shown central antinociceptive effects based upon a hydroalcoholic extract of the seeds in a rodent model.[73] The constituent dioflorin was isolated and shown to be a potent analgesic in mice, an activity that was reversed by naloxone suggestive of potential interaction with opioid receptors.[74,75]

While *Cannabis spp.* is considered an illegal substance in many countries due to United Nations Conventions,[76] this paradigm is currently changing with medical cannabis programs operating throughout Canada, Israel, the Netherlands and many states in the USA. More recently, Australia adopted a nationwide medicinal cannabis program in 2016 through amendments to the Narcotic Drugs Act 1967,[77] and utilises existing Special Access Scheme (Category B) and Authorised Prescriber pathways for patient access. New Zealand has recently followed suit, in 2018 voting in a bill for use in palliative care via the Misuse of Drugs (Medicinal Cannabis) Amendment Bill. It should be noted that in most of these international models, medical practitioners are the prescribers of medicinal cannabis products and that Australian and New Zealand naturopaths and herbalists cannot prescribe under the current systems. This being said, it is still of great clinical importance for naturopaths and herbalists to educate themselves about the endocannabinoid[78–81] system, the therapeutic benefits, adverse events and the interactions associated with cannabis as it is likely they will encounter this in clinical practice.

Cannabinoids from numerous cannabis cultivars show positive clinical evidence of reducing pain, with the Australian government writing a guidance document for cannabis use in chronic non-cancer pain in 2017[82] and a large academic review showing substantial and conclusive evidence for cannabis and cannabinoids in chronic pain in adults.[83] Delta-9-tetrahydrocannabinol (THC), a non-nitrogenous lipophilic compound, has been shown to be effective in both phasic and tonic pain[63] and interacts with cannabinoid G-protein coupled receptors.[75] Several other cannabinoids express analgesic action at the spinal cord level (e.g. 11-hydroxy-delta-9-THC, delta 9-THC, delta 8-THC).[63,84] THC has also shown benefit in the pain management of cancer, with one study showing that 10 mg of THC was roughly approximate to 60 mg of codeine.[63,85] Combination THC and cannabidiol (CBD) therapy has also shown significant effects on cancer pain.[86,87]

Interestingly, statistics now show that the majority of opioid deaths in Australia are attributed to pharmaceutical opioids,[88] and with many governments internationally now trying to curb this high incidence, evidence regarding cannabis is worthy of further investigation. A review in 2014 posits that medicinal cannabis laws in the USA are associated with significantly lower state-level opioid overdose mortality rates[89] and that there is a growing evidence base supporting the medical use of cannabis as an adjunct or substitute for opioid therapy.[90]

Acupuncture has been used as a treatment for more than 3000 years[91] and shows encouraging evidence for use in an array of different pain presentations including, but not limited to, chronic shoulder pain,[92] neck pain,[93,94] lumbar pain,[95,96] OA[97] and migraine.[91] WHO released a report in 2003 stating that acupuncture may be clinically useful in dental pain, tennis elbow, sciatica, rheumatoid arthritis, headache, trigeminal and intercostal neuralgia and peripheral neuropathy.[91,98] Of particular clinical interest is the successful use of acupuncture in certain neuropathic pain conditions that are notoriously difficult to ameliorate effectively. An electroacupuncture case report showed promising results in postherpetic neuralgia (PHN),[99] with a further acupuncture study documenting success in acute nerve pain from herpes zoster.[100] **Cupping**, another modality within the traditional Chinese medicine paradigm, may assist in reducing pain in conditions such as herpes zoster but not specifically PHN.[101]

Reduce local and systemic inflammation

Topical anaesthetics
Capsicum frutescens
• The alkaloid capsaicin, originally isolated from chilli, has been found to deplete neuronal stores of neuropeptides and substance P and is believed to target TRPV1 receptors.[102,103]
• This alkaloidal extract from chilli has modest evidence suggesting it can be of use in painful conditions such as postherpetic neuralgia (PHN) as a cream[104,105] and a patch[106–108] while also providing relief in conditions such as OA (see Chapters 25–26 on the musculoskeletal system).
Piper methysticum
• The local anaesthetic action of the kava pyrones was originally first observed by Lewin in 1886.[109,110]
• Kava lactones from *Piper methysticum* have shown local anaesthetic activity similar to that of procaine and cocaine.[65,111]
Gaultheria procumbens (wintergreen oil)
• Used topically as a counter-irritant for musculoskeletal and neuropathic pain[112]
Syzygium aromaticum (cloves)
• Clove oil has a long history of use as a dental anaesthetic and analgesic.
• Eugenol has been found to reverse mechanical allodynia after peripheral nerve injury by inhibiting hyperpolarisation activated cyclic nucleotide gated channels.[113]
• Further evidence for eugenol demonstrates inhibition of voltage-gated calcium and sodium channels in dental afferent neurons.[114–116] A similar action with sodium channels has also been demonstrated with *Erythroxylum coca* (containing the cocaine alkaloid), making it useful as a local anaesthetic,[75,117] although being a substance of addiction, it is illegal in most countries.

Inflammation represents a key requirement in managing many aspects of pain. Inflammation is a non-specific defence mechanism within the body and reflects an immune response focused on eliminating foreign substances either in response to invasion by pathogenic organisms or as a response to substances produced by damaged cells such as is observed in tissue injury.[118,119] Inflammation is a complex interaction between many inflammatory mediators such as histamine, kinins, prostaglandins and leukotrienes and has been implicated in the pathogenesis of various diseases, from cancer and arthritis to cardiovascular and neurodegenerative disease.[120] Of interest in regard to many herbal medicines and certain nutritional supplements are the eicosanoids, particularly arachidonic acid (AA), and its subsequent breakdown by either the cyclooxygenase or lipoxygenase (LOX) enzyme systems.[120]

Zingiber officinale has been shown in vitro to be a dual inhibitor of COX and LOX enzymes,[65,121,122] making it a valuable tool in stopping the leukotriene and prostaglandin pathways. A similar dual inhibitory activity has been noted in vitro for:

- liposterolic extracts of *Serenoa repens* on COX and 5-LOX pathways[123]
- *Curcuma longa* with the constituent curcumin down regulating COX-2, LOX and inducible nitric oxide synthase (it also inhibits NF-κB activation,[65,124] an action shared by withaferin A from *Withania somnifera*)[125]
- *Glycyrrhiza glabra* root and glabridin exhibit COX and 5-LOX inhibition, with glabridin showing inhibitory activity against reactive oxygen species[126,127]
- *Harpagophytum procumbens* (discussed previously).

Further evidence of herbs with anti-inflammatory activity is highlighted below but should not be considered exhaustive. Specific research should be conducted based on specific disease states. For more comprehensive information about anti-inflammatory herbs, consultation of an evidence-based compendium or *Materia Medica* is advised.

- *Boswellia serrata* has shown in-vitro evidence for inhibition of 5-LOX but not COX through its boswellic acids.[65]
- *Matricaria recutita* has shown evidence of inhibition of COX and 5-LOX formation.[65]
- *Arnica montana* extract and the isolated constituent helenalin demonstrate inhibition of NF-κB.[128]
- *Andrographis paniculata* shows in-vivo and in-vitro evidence of anti-inflammatory activity. The andrographolides may achieve this via increasing adrenocortical function via promotion of ACTH.[65]
- *Salix alba* (discussed previously).

Nutrients exhibiting anti-inflammatory action exist within the scientific literature. Omega-3 fish oil has been shown to decrease production of AA mediators by a partial replacement of AA by eicosapentaenoic acid (EPA) in cell membranes.[129] Competition for COX and LOX enzymes, reduced expression of COX-2 and 5-LOX, suppression of pro-inflammatory cytokines and modulation of adhesion molecule expression have all been implicated in the anti-inflammatory activity of fish oil.[129,130]

Vitamins play an important direct and indirect role in inflammation. Vitamin A, through its requirements for proper hormone synthesis (corticosteroids in the adrenal gland),[131] should be monitored for deficiency. Ascorbic acid and its role as an anti-oxidant is of clinical importance as higher **vitamin C** levels have been associated with lower C-reactive protein (CRP) levels.[132] **Vitamin E**, specifically alpha tocopherol, has also been shown to reduce CRP and pro-inflammatory cytokines, inhibits COX-2 and protein kinase C activity and is also a well-researched antioxidant.[133,134] All three of these vitamins are crucial in their role as antioxidants, which assist in the neutralising of free radicals and their subsequent pro-inflammatory effects. Other antioxidant sources include examples such as **selenium**, **alpha-lipoic acid** and **coenzyme Q10**. B-group vitamin supplementation may also be required in those patients with poor diet. A low level of **vitamin D** has been associated with various inflammatory diseases including the inflammatory bowel diseases in both adults and children.[135,136]

For specific examples of the use of anti-inflammatory herbal and nutritional substances in inflammatory disease states, refer to specific disease-focused chapters throughout this text.

Support the immune system (if applicable)

While not a typical presentation for most pain cases, dysfunction of the immune system can impact on the way many autoimmune or infectious diseases affect the human organism. Immunosuppressive herbs (e.g. *Hemidesmus indicus*, *Tylophora indica*) may play a role in the treatment of painful conditions such as systemic lupus erythematosus (SLE), Sjögren's syndrome or rheumatoid arthritis. Conversely, those suffering from painful chronic inflammation caused by an infectious source may benefit from immunostimulating/modulating herbs. Immune compromise is also a risk factor for the development of conditions such as herpes zoster; therefore, **herbs** such as *Echinacea spp.*, *Uncaria tomentosa*, *Andrographis paniculata* and *Astragalus membranaceus* all have evidence supporting this chosen action.[71,137–140] Immune modulating **medicinal fungi** such as *Ganoderma lucidum*, *Lentinula edodes*, *Trametes versicolor* and *Grifola frondosa* may also be of use. See Chapter 31 on autoimmune disease for further information.

Support the nervous system

Consideration of the nervous system in addressing pain is not solely focused upon supporting the psychological consequences of exposure to pain (such as depression, anxiety and insomnia) but should also concentrate upon those specific painful disease states that can affect the nervous system specifically such as trigeminal neuralgia, herpes zoster, PHN or postamputation pain.

The adaptogens form a herbal class of medicines that play an important supportive role in chronic pain and nervous system support, although this action is still not accepted in the current orthodox medical vernacular. **Adaptogens** have been shown to reduce stress reactions in the alarm phase and slow or prevent the exhaustion phase in accordance with the general adaptation syndrome theory posited by Selye, and therefore convey protection against exposure to long-term stress (see Chapter 18 on stress and fatigue).[141] *Eleutherococcus senticosus*,[142] *Withania somnifera*,[143] *Bacopa monnieri*,[144] *Panax quinquefolium*, *Panax ginseng*,[145,146] *Cordyceps*[147] *spp.*, *Rhodiola rosea*[148,149] and *Schisandra chinensis*[150] have all shown marked adaptogenic action, with many also exhibiting immune modulation, cognitive improvement and increased vigilance, all of which are important in chronic pain management. **Nervine tonics** are also a useful class in chronic pain as they are safe to take long term and convey a tonifying effect on the system. Representative examples of this class include *Scutellaria lateriflora*, *Hypericum perforatum*, *Verbena officinalis*, *Avena sativa*, *Bacopa monnieri* and *Centella asiatica*.[60]

Chronic and acute pain can also adversely affect sleep patterns, with statistics suggesting that sleep disturbance is one of the most prevalent complaints in patients with chronic pain,[151,152] with 50–70% of chronic pain patients complaining of sleep disturbance and considering it a significant quality-of-life issue.[153] It has been hypothesised that sleep deprivation or the disturbance of the sleep cycle enhances pain sensitivity and changes pain perception,[152,154,155] as well as causing fatigue, which flows on to potentially cause emotional lability. As such, effective analgesia to stop the patient from being awoken from sleep forms an integral approach to treatment. Supporting this action, herbs from the sedative and hypnotic classes may be required. Herbs such as ***Valeriana officinalis*** and ***Humulus lupulus*** show clinical evidence of being useful in assisting sleep. More traditional relaxants and hypnotics include ***Lavandula officinalis***, ***Ziziphus spinosa*** and ***Melissa officinalis***. For more detailed information about naturopathic treatment of sleep disorders, please refer to Chapter 16 on insomnia.

Address the psychological components of pain management

Long-term exposure to pain increases the likelihood of various psychological presentations, including depression, anxiety disorders and possible substance abuse. Pain and depression have been found to be two of the most prevalent and treatable cancer-related symptoms, present in 20–30% of oncology patients.[156] Depression as a comorbid condition has prevalence statistics of 50–87% in patients in chronic pain.[157] Comorbid anxiety in patients with chronic pain is also possible and usually includes presentations of panic disorder, posttraumatic stress disorder, substance use disorder or generalised anxiety disorder.[158]

Cognitive behaviour therapy (CBT) is a form of psychotherapy that focuses on assisting people to change unhelpful or negative thought patterns, feelings or behaviours. Evidence on CBT and pain intervention is growing; however, it is also the treatment of comorbid psychological factors that provides a valid foundation for treatment in chronic pain. CBT interventions have been shown to positively impact sleep quality,[154] fatigue, anxiety[159] and depression[160,161] so is of great importance in indirectly reducing pain. Further evidence that CBT can also increase relaxation, reduce pain catastrophising, identify patient pain beliefs and institute pain-coping mechanisms make it a worthwhile addition to patients.[162]

Mindfulness-based cognitive therapy (MBCT) can be defined as 'the practice of broad, present-focused and behaviourally neutral awareness'.[163] It is posited that sufferers of chronic pain become overly negative about their situation, focus on their pain and engage in recurrent thought patterns of struggling with pain that impacts daily functioning.[163] It has also been found that MBCT is of use in depression,[164] with a recent meta-analysis showing that MBCT as an adjunct to usual therapy for depression was significantly better in outcome than standard therapy alone.[165] Mindfulness-based interventions for chronic pain have been found to have a paucity of evidence in a recent systematic review, with the authors stating the topic requires better designed studies of larger power.[166]

Herbal medicines provide a useful clinical tool for the amelioration of mild to moderate depression and anxiety. *Hypericum perforatum* shows encouraging clinical evidence for use in depression, as do *Crocus sativus*, *Lavandula officinalis*, *Panax ginseng* and *Rhodiola rosea*.[59] Furthermore, herbs with anxiolytic activity include *Matricaria chamomilla*, *Ginkgo biloba*, *Bacopa monnieri*, *Withania somnifera*, *Scutellaria lateriflora* and *Passiflora incarnata*.[59] The reader should direct their attention to Chapters 14 and 15 on depression and anxiety for further information on naturopathic treatment of these conditions.

Nutraceuticals such as *S*-adenosylmethionine (SAMe),[167] folic acid (vitamin B9),[168] vitamin B12,[168] tryptophan, tyrosine and phenylalanine[169] may all play a part in assisting in managing depressive episodes. Omega-3 fatty acids have been found to be lower in people with unipolar and postpartum depression.[170] Similarly, tryptophan may be useful in clinical anxiety.[169]

Gamus and colleagues posit that acupuncture therapy may be effective in changing the patient's pain perception and enhance 'their sense of personal and treatment control over their pain', demonstrating that acupuncture can alter not only the physical aspects of pain but also the psychological as well.[171]

The referral of pain patients to specialist pain centres and pain support groups is an important aspect of the integrated treatment philosophy, the latter allowing patients to exchange stories and gain coping strategies from other patients that may be of great therapeutic value.

Monitor for herb–drug–nutrient interactions

The risk of herb–drug–nutrient interactions (HDNIs) is greatest in a population that is relying heavily on multiple medications (polypharmacy) or is of a greater age (due to age-related change to organ function). Chronic pain patients represent a particular clinical challenge when it comes to identifying and monitoring for HDNIs. Thorough research on the medications before the prescribing of herbal or nutritional therapies is of chief importance, as is open communication with clinicians and other members of the patient's pain management team. See Chapter 41 on managing interactions for further details.

INTEGRATIVE MEDICAL CONSIDERATIONS

It is rare that chronic pain conditions can be managed exclusively by CAM therapies, but rather would take on a more adjunctive or supportive role in approach to treatment. Further CAM therapies have been outlined below together with supportive evidence.

Manual therapies

Promising evidence exists for the use of **massage therapy** for reducing pain and improving mood status in conditions such as low back pain,[172] metastatic bone pain[173] and labour.[174] Other painful conditions such as fibromyalgia,[175] rheumatoid arthritis[176] and neck pain[177] also show benefit from massage treatment. **Chiropractic**[177] and **osteopathic services** would also be considered of clinical benefit in patients with musculoskeletal conditions causing pain, or pain caused by nerve compression (see the musculoskeletal section [Chapters 25 and 26] for more specific details).

Dietary modification

The need to ensure the patient is being supplied with a wide variety of healthful foods that can supply adequate vitamin and mineral requirements is paramount. Foods rich in B-complex vitamins, serine, taurine, biotin, lipoic acid and copper may be of value in pain associated with nerve involvement, so too foods rich in zinc, vitamin C and bioflavonoids to support healthy immune function.[169] A **polyamine-deficient diet** has been suggested as being useful in relieving abnormal and chronic pain due to the idea that polyamines modulate and excite glutamate/N-methyl-D-aspartate receptors (NMDA-R), which may be associated with central pain sensitisation,[178,179] although human clinical data on this is required.

Lifestyle advice and exercise

Strengthening and more dynamic exercises have been shown in the literature to be of benefit in low back pain[180,181] but also comorbidities such as depression[182] and anxiety.[183] Similarly, the holistic physical and spiritual practices of both **yoga** and **Tai Chi** exhibit promising clinical evidence for pain management of varying aetiology. Yoga has shown positive evidence for chronic low back pain, neck pain,[177] migraine without aura and pain associated with carpal tunnel syndrome[184] while also providing relief from comorbid psychological distress. Tai Chi has been recommended to patients with pain from OA, rheumatoid arthritis and fibromyalgia[185] and, like yoga, has also shown benefit in dealing with comorbid depression and anxiety[186] of varying cause.

As discussed earlier, mindfulness meditation should also be considered for chronic pain patients after an outpatient program showed positive outcomes.[187] Not surprisingly, deep breathing exercises have also shown benefit in pain management, particularly postoperatively.[188]

CLINICAL SUMMARY

The prognosis of patients with painful pathophysiological conditions obviously depends heavily upon the original diagnosis and available treatments. It is crucial where possible that an accurate diagnosis is found to direct appropriate treatment protocols, although this should not stop or delay symptomatic relief of the pain in the interim. Clinical measurement of pain, whether via visual or numerical scaling systems, is important to establish baseline statistics and gauge ongoing treatment success.

Patients with intractable cases of chronic pain are likely to explore CAM therapies as alternatives if orthodox management is failing to manage their condition, so working within a multidisciplinary team for individual patient outcomes is a likely outcome in such instances, driving the need for open communication channels between clinicians to minimise adverse effects and HDNIs while maximising pain amelioration and managing comorbidities.

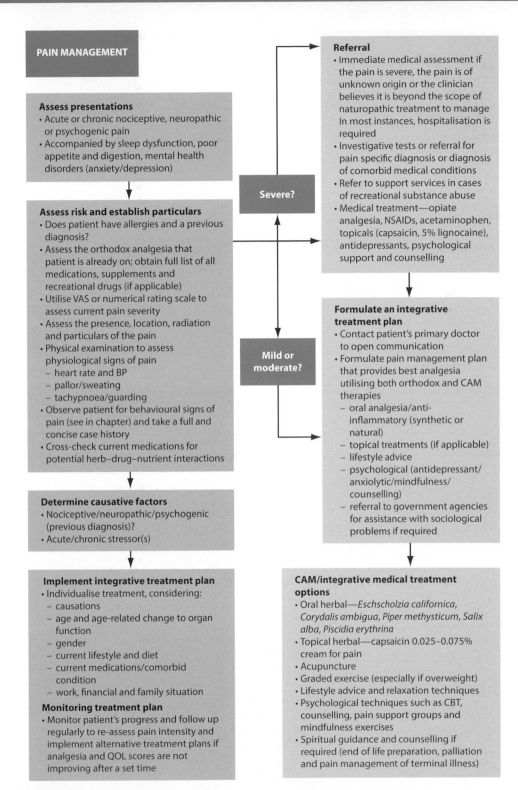

Figure 40.3
Integrative treatment decision tree—pain management*

*As pain manifests from various conditions, no evidence table is provided. Please refer to other chapters for specific information.

KEY POINTS

- Chronic pain management is one of the more complex clinical conditions to manage. As such, it is encouraged to include multiple disciplines in an integrative approach to improving patient outcomes.

- Polypharmacy and potential substance abuse is a likely event in chronic pain management; therefore, increasing the potential possibility of HDNIs. Close communication with the patient's primary clinician and other health professionals is of utmost importance, as is close patient monitoring and testing of organ function.

- Comorbid presentations of a psychological nature, including depression and anxiety, should be addressed swiftly as these can impact on the perception of pain experienced by the patient and have long-reaching consequences affecting patient quality of life.

FURTHER READING

Carli G. Historical perspective and modern views on pain physiology: from psychogenic pain to hyperalgesic priming. Arch Ital Biol 2011;149(Suppl.):175–86.

McCurdy CR, Scully SS. Analgesic substances derived from natural products (natureceuticals). Life Sci 2005;78(5):476–84.

McDermott AM, Toelle TR, Rowbotham DJ, et al. The burden of neuropathic pain: results from a cross-sectional survey. Eur J Pain 2006;10(2):127–35.

Mechoulam R, Parker LA. The endocannabinoid system and the brain. Annu Rev Psychol 2013;64:21–47.

National Academies of Sciences, Engineering and Medicine. The health effects of cannabis and cannabinoids: the current State of evidence and recommendations for research. Washington DC: The National Academies Press; 2017.

Vicker AJ, Linde K. Acupuncture for chronic pain. JAMA 2014;311(9):955–6.

REFERENCES

1. Kumar P, Clark M, editors. Clinical medicine. 8th ed. Edinburgh: Elsevier Saunders; 2012.
2. Fauci AS, Braunwald E, Kasper DL, et al, editors. Harrison's principles of internal medicine. 17th ed. New York: McGraw-Hill Medical; 2008.
3. Tortora GJ, Derrickson B, editors. Principles of anatomy and physiology. New York: John Wiley & Sons, Inc.; 2009.
4. Thomas CL. Pain. In: Thomas CL, Taber CW, editors. Taber's cyclopedic medical dictionary. Philadelphia: FA Davis Company; 1993.
5. Colledge NR, Walker BR, Ralston SH, editors. Davidson's principles and practice of medicine. 21st ed. Edinburgh: Churchill Livingstone Elsevier; 2010.
6. Ruyssen-Witrand A, Tubach F, Ravaud P. Systematic review reveals heterogeneity in definition of a clinically relevant difference in pain. J Clin Epidemiol 2011;64(5): 463–70.
7. Blyth FM, March LM, Brnabic AJ, et al. Chronic pain in Australia: a prevalence study. Pain 2001;89(2–3):127–34.
8. Gureje O, Von Korff M, Simon GE, et al. Persistent pain and well-being: a World Health Organization study in primary care. JAMA 1998;280(2):147–51.
9. Harstall C. How prevalent is chronic pain? Pain clinical updates IASP 2003;XI(2):1–4.
10. Brochet P, Michel P, et al. Population-based study of pain in elderly people: a descriptive survey. Age Ageing 1998;27:279–84.
11. Manchikanti L, Boswell MV, Raj PP, et al. Evolution of interventional pain management. Pain Physician 2003;6(4):485–94.
12. NPSI. National Pain Strategy: Pain management for all Australians. Pain Australia, 2007.
13. Beers MH, Berkow R, editors. The Merck manual of diagnosis and therapy. 17th ed. Whitehouse Station New York: Merck Research Laboratories; 1999.
14. Scholz J, Woolf CJ. Can we conquer pain? Nat Neurosci 2002;5(Suppl.):1062–7.
15. Julius D, McCleskey EW. Cellular and molecular properties of primary afferent neurons. In: McMahon S, Koltzenburg M, editors. Textbook of pain. 5th ed. Churchill Livingstone: : Elsevier; 2006.
16. Smart KM, Blake C, Staines A, et al. Mechanisms-based classifications of musculoskeletal pain: part 3 of 3: symptoms and signs of nociceptive pain in patients with low back (+/− leg) pain. Man Ther 2012;17(4):352–7.
17. Smart KM, Blake C, Staines A, et al. Clinical indicators of 'nociceptive', 'peripheral neuropathic' and 'central' mechanisms of musculoskeletal pain. A Delphi survey of expert clinicians. Man Ther 2010;15(1):80–7.
18. Chakravarty A, Sen A. Migraine, neuropathic pain and nociceptive pain: towards a unifying concept. Med Hypotheses 2010;74(2):225–31.
19. Dworkin RH. An overview of neuropathic pain: syndromes, symptoms, signs, and several mechanisms. Clin J Pain 2002;18(6):343–9.
20. Merskey H, Bogduck N. Classification of chronic pain. Seattle: Internation Association for the Study of Pain; 1994.
21. McDermott AM, Toelle TR, Rowbotham DJ, et al. The burden of neuropathic pain: results from a cross-sectional survey. Eur J Pain 2006;10(2):127–35.

22. Rasmussen PV, Sindrup SH, Jensen TS, et al. Symptoms and signs in patients with suspected neuropathic pain. Pain 2004;110(1–2):461–9.

23. Dieleman JP, Kerklaan J, Huygen FJ, et al. Incidence rates and treatment of neuropathic pain conditions in the general population. Pain 2008;137(3):681–8.

24. Cocito D, Paolasso I, Pazzaglia C, et al. Pain affects the quality of life of neuropathic patients. Neurol Sci 2006;27(3):155–60.

25. Galvez R, Marsal C, Vidal J, et al. Cross-sectional evaluation of patient functioning and health-related quality of life in patients with neuropathic pain under standard care conditions. Eur J Pain 2007;11(3):244–55.

26. Marchettini P. The burning case of neuropathic pain wording. Pain 2005;114(3):313–14.

27. Dworkin RH, O'Connor AB, Backonja M, et al. Pharmacologic management of neuropathic pain: evidence-based recommendations. Pain 2007;132(3):237–51.

28. O'Connor AB, Dworkin RH. Treatment of neuropathic pain: an overview of recent guidelines. Am J Med 2009;122(10 Suppl.):S22–32.

29. Torrance N, Smith BH, Watson MC, et al. Medication and treatment use in primary care patients with chronic pain of predominantly neuropathic origin. Fam Pract 2007;24(5):481–5.

30. Smith BH, Torrance N, Bennett MI, et al. Health and quality of life associated with chronic pain of predominantly neuropathic origin in the community. Clin J Pain 2007;23(2):143–9.

31. Torrance N, Smith BH, Bennett MI, et al. The epidemiology of chronic pain of predominantly neuropathic origin. Results from a general population survey. J Pain 2006;7(4):281–9.

32. Torrance N, et al. Neuropathic pain in the community: more under-treated than refractory? Pain 2013;154(5):690–9.

33. Bouhassira D, Lanteri-Minet M, Attal N, et al. Prevalence of chronic pain with neuropathic characteristics in the general population. Pain 2008;136(3):380–7.

34. Valdes M, Garcia L, Treserra J, et al. Psychogenic pain and depressive disorders: an empirical study. J Affect Disord 1989;16(1):21–5.

35. Pilowsky I, Barrow CG. A controlled study of psychotherapy and amitriptyline used individually and in combination in the treatment of chronic intractable, 'psychogenic' pain. Pain 1990;40(1):3–19.

36. Fjorback LO, Carstensen T, Arendt M, et al. Mindfulness therapy for somatization disorder and functional somatic syndromes: analysis of economic consequences alongside a randomized trial. J Psychosom Res 2013;74(1):41–8.

37. Henningsen P, Zipfel S, Herzog W. Management of functional somatic syndromes. Lancet 2007;369(9565):946–55.

38. Fink P, Rosendal M. Recent developments in the understanding and management of functional somatic symptoms in primary care. Curr Opin Psychiatry 2008;21(2):182–8.

39. Barsky AJ, Orav EJ, Bates DW. Somatization increases medical utilization and costs independent of psychiatric and medical comorbidity. Arch Gen Psychiatry 2005;62(8):903–10.

40. Hunter DJ, McDougall JJ, Keefe FJ. The symptoms of osteoarthritis and the genesis of pain. Med Clin North Am 2008;93(1):83–100.

41. Schaible H, Schmelz M, Tegeder I. Pathophysiology and treatment of pain in joint disease. Adv Drug Deliv Rev 2006;58(2):323–42.

42. Hanlon KE, Herman DS, Agnes RS, et al. Novel peptide ligands with dual acting pharmacophores designed for the pathophysiology of neuropathic pain. Brain Res 2011;1395:1–11.

43. Carli G. Historical perspective and modern views on pain physiology: from psychogenic pain to hyperalgesic priming. Arch Ital Biol 2011;149(Suppl.):175–86.

44. Hardy J, Wolff HD. Pain sensations and reactions. Baltimore: Williams and Wilkins; 1952.

45. Noordenbos W. Pain. Amsterdam: Elsevier; 1959.

46. Oxenham D. Davidson's principles and practice of medicine. 21st ed. Edinburgh: Churchill Livingstone Elsevier; 2010. p. 279–88.

47. Melzack R, Wall PD. Pain mechanisms: a new theory. Science 1965;150(3699):971–9.

48. Reynolds DV. Surgery in the rat during electrical analgesia induced by focal brain stimulation. Science 1969;164(3878):444–5.

49. Woolf CJ. Evidence for a central component of post-injury pain hypersensitivity. Nature 1983;306(5944):686–8.

50. Craig AD. How do you feel? Interoception: the sense of the physiological condition of the body. Nat Rev Neurosci 2002;3(8):655–66.

51. Reichling DB, Levine JD. Critical role of nociceptor plasticity in chronic pain. Trends Neurosci 2009;32(12):611–18.

52. Katz PP. The impact of rheumatoid arthritis on life activities. Arthritis Care Res 1995;8:272–8.

53. Keefe FJ, Smith SJ, Buffington ALH, et al. Recent advances and future directions in the biopsychosocial assessment and treatment of arthritis. J Consult Clin Psychol 2002;70(3):640–55.

54. Graham A, Luber S, Wolfson AB. Urolithiasis in the emergency department. Emerg Med Clin North Am 2011;29(3):519–38.

55. Safdar B, Degutis LC, Landry K, et al. Intravenous morphine plus ketorolac is superior to either drug alone for treatment of acute renal colic. Ann Emerg Med 2006;48(2):173–81, 181e1.

56. Johnson MI, Ashton CH, Thompson JW. The consistency of pulse frequencies and pulse patterns of transcutaneous electrical nerve stimulation (TENS) used by chronic pain patients. Pain 1991;44(3):231–4.

57. Vallejo R. High-frequency spinal cord stimulation: an emerging treatment option for patients with chronic pain. Tech Reg Anesth Pain Manag 2012;16(2):106–12.

58. Falowski S, Celii A, Sharan A. Spinal cord stimulation: an update. Neurotherapeutics 2008;5(1):86–99.

59. Sarris J, Panossian A, Schweitzer I, et al. Herbal medicine for depression, anxiety and insomnia: a review of psychopharmacology and clinical evidence. Eur Neuropsychopharmacol 2011;21(12):841–60.

60. Bone K. A clinical guide to blending liquid herbs: herbal formulations for the individual patient. St Louis: Churchill Livingstone; 2003.

61. Bone K. Clinical applications of Ayurvedic and Chinese herbs: monographs for the Western herbal practitioner. Warwick: Phytotherapy Press; 1996.

62. Dhawan K, Dhawan S, Sharma A. Passiflora: a review update. J Ethnopharmacol 2004;94(1):1–23.

63. Spinella M. The psychopharmacology of herbal medicine: plant drugs that alter mind, brain and behavior. Cambridge Massachusetts: Massachusetts Institute of Technology.; 2001.

64. Speroni E, Minghetti A. Neuropharmacological activity of extracts from Passiflora incarnata. Planta Med 1988;54(6):488–91.

65. Bone K, Mills S. Principles and practice of phytotherapy. 2nd ed. St Louis: Churchill Livingstone: Elsevier; 2013.

66. Chrubasik J, Roufogalis BD, Chrubasik S. Evidence of effectiveness of herbal antiinflammatory drugs in the treatment of painful osteoarthritis and chronic low back pain. Phytother Res 2007;21:675–83.

67. Huang TH, Tran VH, Duke RK, et al. Harpagoside suppresses lipopolysaccharide-induced iNOS and COX-2 expression through inhibition of NF-kappa B activation. J Ethnopharmacol 2006;104(1–2):149–55.

68. Kaszkin M, Beck KF, Koch E, et al. Down-regulation of iNOS expression in rat mesangial cells by special extracts of Harpagophytum procumbens derives from harpagoside-dependent and independent effects. Phytomedicine 2004;11(7–8):585–95.

69. Anauate MC, Torres LM, de Mello SB. Effect of isolated fractions of Harpagophytum procumbens DC (devil's claw) on COX-1, COX-2 activity and nitric oxide production on whole-blood assay. Phytother Res 2010;24(9):1365–9.

70. Inaba K, Murata K, Naruto S, et al. Inhibitory effects of devil's claw (secondary root of Harpagophytum procumbens) extract and harpagoside on cytokine production in mouse macrophages. J Nat Med 2010;64(2):219–22.

71. Scientific Committee of the BHMA British Herbal Medicine Association. British herbal pharmacopoeia. London: Scientific Committee of the BHMA British Herbal Medicine Association; 1983.

72. Almeida RN, Navarro DS, Barbosa-Filho JM. Plants with central analgesic activity. Phytomedicine 2001;8(4):310–22.

73. Almeida ER, Almeida RN, Navarro DS, et al. Central antinociceptive effect of a hydroalcoholic extract of Dioclea grandiflora seeds in rodents. J Ethnopharmacol 2003;88(1):1–4.

74. Bhattacharyya J, Majetich G, Jenkins TM, et al. Dioflorin, a minor flavonoid from Dioclea grandiflora. J Nat Prod 1998;61(3):413–14.

75. McCurdy CR, Scully SS. Analgesic substances derived from natural products (natureceuticals). Life Sci 2005;78(5):476–84.

76. Single Convention on Narcotic Drugs. United Nations. New York: NY. 1961.

77. Narcotic Drugs Amendment Act 2016. Australian Government. No. 12, pp. 1–153. Available: https://www.legislation.gov.au/Details/C2016A00012.

78. Battista N, Di Tommaso M, Bari M, et al. The endocannabinoid system: an overview. Front Behav Neurosci 2012;6:9.

79. Centonze D, Finazzi-Agro A, Bernardi G, et al. The endocannabinoid system in targeting inflammatory neurodegenerative diseases. Trends Pharmacol Sci 2007;28(4):180–7.

80. Di Marzo V, Bifulco M, De Petrocellis L. The Endocannabinoid System and its therapeutic exploitation. Nat Rev Drug Discov 2004;3(September):771–84.

81. Mechoulam R, Parker LA. The endocannabinoid system and the brain. Annu Rev Psychol 2013;64: 21–47.

82. Guidance for the use of medicinal cannabis and cannabinoids in the treatment of chronic non-cancer pain; 2017. Version 1. Australian Government: Department of Health. Therapeutic Goods Administration pp. 1-31.

83. National Academies of Sciences, Engineering and Medicine. The health effects of cannabis and cannabinoids: the current State of evidence and recommendations for research. Washington DC: The National Academies Press.; 2017.

84. Welch SP, Stevens DL. Antinociceptive activity of intrathecally administered cannabinoids alone, and in combination with morphine, in mice. J Pharmacol Exp Ther 1992;262(1):10–18.

85. Noyes R Jr, Brunk SF, Avery DA, et al. The analgesic properties of delta-9-tetrahydrocannabinol and codeine. Clin Pharmacol Ther 1975;18(1):84–9.

86. Johnson JR, Lossignol D, Burnell-Nugent M, et al. An open-label extension study to investigate the long-term safety and tolerability of THC/CBD oromucosal spray and oromucosal THC spray in patients with terminal cancer-related pain refractory to strong opioid analgesics. J Pain Symptom Manage 2013;46(2):207–18.

87. Johnson JR, Burnell-Nugent M, Lossignol D, et al. Multicenter, double-blind, randomized, placebo-controlled, parallel-group study of the efficacy, safety, and tolerability of THC:CBD extract and THC extract in patients with intractable cancer-related pain. J Pain Symptom Manage 2010;39(2):167–79.

88. Downey M Majority of overdose deaths in Australia are related to pharmaceutical opioids. National Drug & Alcohol Research Centre. 20 August 2018. https://ndarc.med.unsw.edu.au/news/majority-opioid-overdose-deaths-australia-are-related-pharmaceutical-opioids.

89. Bachhuber MA, Saloner B, Cunningham CO, et al. Medical cannabis laws and opioid analgesic overdose mortality in the United States, 1999-2010. JAMA Intern Med 2014;174(10):1668–73.

90. Lucas P. Rationale for cannabis-based interventions in the opioid overdose crisis. Harm Reduct J 2017;14(1):58.

91. Dorsher PT. Acupuncture for chronic pain. Tech Reg Anesth Pain Manag 2011;15(2):55–63.

92. Itoh K, et al. Randomized trial of trigger point acupuncture treatment for chronic shoulder pain: a preliminary study. J Acupunct Meridian Stud 2014;7(2):59–64.

93. Witt CM, Jena S, Brinkhaus B, et al. Acupuncture for patients with chronic neck pain. Pain 2006;125(1–2): 98–106.

94. Trinh K, Graham N, Gross A, et al. Acupuncture for neck disorders. Spine 2007;32(2):236–43.

95. Haake M, Muller HH, Schade-Brittinger C, et al. German Acupuncture Trials (GERAC) for chronic low back pain: randomized, multicenter, blinded, parallel-group trial with 3 groups. Arch Intern Med 2007;167(17): 1892–8.

96. Manheimer E, White A, Berman B, et al. Meta-analysis: acupuncture for low back pain. Ann Intern Med 2005;142(8):651–63.

97. Berman BM, Lao L, Langenberg P, et al. Effectiveness of acupuncture as adjunctive therapy in osteoarthritis of the knee: a randomized, controlled trial. Ann Intern Med 2004;141(12):901–10.

98. World Health Organization. Acupuncture: review and analysis of reports on controlled clinical trials. Geneva: WHO; 2003.

99. Carla G, et al. Electroacupuncture in post-herpetic neuralgia: a case report. Eur J Integr Med 2012;4(1): 139–40.

100. Ursini T, Tontodonati M, Manzoli L, et al. Acupuncture for the treatment of severe acute pain in herpes zoster: results of a nested, open-label, randomized trial in the VZV Pain Study. BMC Complement Altern Med 2011; 11:46.

101. Cao H, Han M, Li X, et al. Clinical research evidence of cupping therapy in China: a systematic literature review. BMC Complement Altern Med 2010;10:70.

102. Whitley RJ, Volpi A, McKendrick M, et al. Management of herpes zoster and post-herpetic neuralgia now and in the future. J Clin Virol 2010;48(Suppl. 1):S20–8.

103. Caterina MJ, Schumacher MA, Tominaga M, et al. The capsaicin receptor: a heat-activated ion channel in the pain pathway. Nature 1997;389(6653):816–24.

104. Bernstein JE, Korman NJ, Bickers DR, et al. Topical capsaicin treatment of chronic postherpetic neuralgia. J Am Acad Dermatol 1989;21(2 Pt 1):265–70.

105. Watson CP, Evans RJ, Watt VR. Post-herpetic neuralgia and topical capsaicin. Pain 1988;33(3):333–40.

106. Gawecka E, Oddbjorn V. Postherpetic neuralgia: new hopes in prevention with adult vaccination and in treatment with a concentrated capsaicin patch. Scand J Pain 2012;3:220–8.

107. Webster LR, Malan TP, Tuchman MM, et al. A multicenter, randomized, double-blind, controlled dose finding study of NGX-4010, a high-concentration capsaicin patch, for the treatment of postherpetic neuralgia. J Pain 2010;11(10):972–82.

108. Backonja M, Wallace MS, Blonsky ER, et al. NGX-4010, a high-concentration capsaicin patch, for the treatment of postherpetic neuralgia: a randomised, double-blind study. Lancet Neurol 2008;7(12):1106–12.

109. Lewin L. Uber piper methysticum (Kawa). Berlin: Hirschwald, A; 1886.

110. Singh YN. Kava: an overview. J Ethnopharmacol 1992;37(1):13–45.

111. Meyer HJ, May HU. [Local anesthetic properties of natural kava pyrones]. Klin Wochenschr 1964;42:407, Lokalanaesthetische eigenschaften natuerlicher kawa-pyrone.

112. Skidmore-Roth L. Mosby's handbook of herbs and natural supplements. 2nd ed. St Louis: Mosby; 2004.

113. Yeon KY, Chung G, Kim YH, et al. Eugenol reverses mechanical allodynia after peripheral nerve injury by inhibiting hyperpolarization-activated cyclic nucleotide-gated (HCN) channels. Pain 2011;152(9):2108–16.

114. Chung G, Rhee JN, Jung SJ, et al. Modulation of CaV2.3 calcium channel currents by eugenol. J Dent Res 2008;87(2):137–41.

115. Lee MH, Yeon KY, Park CK, et al. Eugenol inhibits calcium currents in dental afferent neurons. J Dent Res 2005;84(9):848–51.

116. Park CK, Li HY, Yeon KY, et al. Eugenol inhibits sodium currents in dental afferent neurons. J Dent Res 2006;85(10):900–4.

117. Matthews JC, Collins A. Interactions of cocaine and cocaine congeners with sodium channels. Biochem Pharmacol 1983;32(3):455–60.

118. Hechtman L, Harris K, Bridgeman K. The immune system. In: Hechtman L, editor. Clinical naturopathic medicine. Sydney Australia: Churchill Livingstone: Elsevier; 2011. p. 283.

119. Kanterman J, Sade-Feldman M, Baniyash M. New insights into chronic inflammation-induced immunosuppression. Semin Cancer Biol 2012;22(4):307–18.

120. Ricciotti E, FitzGerald GA. Prostaglandins and inflammation. Arterioscler Thromb Vasc Biol 2011;31(5):986–1000.

121. Flynn DL, Rafferty MF, Boctor AM. Inhibition of human neutrophil 5-lipoxygenase activity by gingerdione, shogaol, capsaicin and related pungent compounds. Prostaglandins Leukot Med 1986;24(2–3):195–8.

122. Mascolo N, Jain R, Jain SC, et al. Ethnopharmacologic investigation of ginger (Zingiber officinale). J Ethnopharmacol 1989;27(1–2):129–40.

123. Breu W, et al. Anti-inflammatory activity of sabal fruit extracts prepared with supercritical carbon dioxide. In vitro antagonists of cyclooxygenase and 5-lipoxygenase metabolism. Arzneimittelforschung 1992;42(4):547–51.

124. Jurenka JS. Anti-inflammatory properties of curcumin, a major constituent of Curcuma longa: a review of preclinical and clinical research. Altern Med Rev 2009;14(2):141–53.

125. Maitra R, Porter MA, Huang S, et al. Inhibition of NFkappaB by the natural product Withaferin A in cellular models of cystic fibrosis inflammation. J Inflamm (Lond) 2009;6:15.

126. Chandrasekaran CV, Deepak HB, Thiyagarajan P, et al. Dual inhibitory effect of Glycyrrhiza glabra (GutGard) on COX and LOX products. Phytomedicine 2011;18(4):278–84.

127. Kang JS, Yoon YD, Cho IJ, et al. Glabridin, an isoflavan from licorice root, inhibits inducible nitric-oxide synthase expression and improves survival of mice in experimental model of septic shock. J Pharmacol Exp Ther 2005;312(3):1187–94.

128. Klaas CA, Wagner G, Laufer S, et al. Studies on the anti-inflammatory activity of phytopharmaceuticals prepared from Arnica flowers. Planta Med 2002;68(5):385–91.

129. Calder PC. N-3 polyunsaturated fatty acids and inflammation: from molecular biology to the clinic. Lipids 2003;38(4):343–52.

130. Kim YJ, Kim HJ, No JK, et al. Anti-inflammatory action of dietary fish oil and calorie restriction. Life Sci 2006;78(21):2523–32.

131. Zimmermann M. Burgerstein's handbook of nutrition: micronutrients in the prevention and therapy of disease. Stuttgart Germany: Thieme; 2000.

132. Ford ES, Liu S, Mannino DM, et al. C-reactive protein concentration and concentrations of blood vitamins, carotenoids, and selenium among United States adults. Eur J Clin Nutr 2003;57(9):1157–63.

133. Calder PC, Albers R, Antoine JM, et al. Inflammatory disease processes and interactions with nutrition. Br J Nutr 2009;101(Suppl. 1):S1–45.

134. Singh U, Devaraj S, Jialal I. Vitamin E, oxidative stress, and inflammation. Annu Rev Nutr 2005;25:151–74.

135. Pappa HM, Gordon CM, Saslowsky TM, et al. Vitamin D status in children and young adults with inflammatory bowel disease. Pediatrics 2006;118(5):1950–61.

136. Gilman J, Shanahan F, Cashman KD. Determinants of vitamin D status in adult Crohn's disease patients, with particular emphasis on supplemental vitamin D use. Eur J Clin Nutr 2006;60(7):889–96.

137. Mills S, Bone K. Principles and practice of phytotherapy. London UK: Churchill Livingstone; 2000.

138. Braun L, Cohen M. Herbs and natural supplements: an evidence-based guide. 2nd ed. Marrickville: Elsevier.; 2007.

139. Gruenwald J, Brendler T, Jaenicke C, editors. Physicians desk reference for herbal medicines. 3rd ed. Montvale New Jersey: Thomson PDR; 2004.

140. Frawley D, Lad V. The Yoga of Herbs: an Ayurvedic guide to herbal medicine. Twin Lakes Wisconsin USA: Lotus Press; 1986.

141. Wagner H, Norr H, Winterhoff H. Plant adaptogens. Phytomedicine 1994;1(1):63–76.

142. Davydov M, Krikorian AD. Eleutherococcus senticosus (Rupr. & Maxim.) Maxim. (Araliaceae) as an adaptogen: a closer look. J Ethnopharmacol 2000;72(3):345–93.

143. Bhattacharya SK, Muruganandam AV. Adaptogenic activity of Withania somnifera: an experimental study using a rat model of chronic stress. Pharmacol Biochem Behav 2003;75(3):547–55.

144. Rai D, Bhatia G, Palit G, et al. Adaptogenic effect of Bacopa monniera (Brahmi). Pharmacol Biochem Behav 2003;75(4):823–30.

145. Nocerino E, Amato M, Izzo AA. The aphrodisiac and adaptogenic properties of ginseng. Fitoterapia 2000;71(Suppl. 1):S1–5.

146. Braz AS, Morais LC, Paula AP, et al. Effects of Panax ginseng extract in patients with fibromyalgia: a 12-week, randomized, double-blind, placebo-controlled trial. Rev Bras Psiquiatr 2013;35(1):21–8.

147. Cordyceps as an herbal Drug. Chapter 5: herbal medicine: biomolecular and clinical aspects. 2nd ed. Boca Raton: FL CRC Press/Taylor & Francis; 2011.

148. Spasov AA, Wikman GK, Mandrikov VB, et al. A double-blind, placebo-controlled pilot study of the stimulating and adaptogenic effect of Rhodiola rosea SHR-5 extract on the fatigue of students caused by stress during an examination period with a repeated low-dose regimen. Phytomedicine 2000;7(2):85–9.

149. Panossian A, Wikman G, Sarris J. Rosenroot (Rhodiola rosea): traditional use, chemical composition, pharmacology and clinical efficacy. Phytomedicine 2010;17(7):481–93.

150. Panossian A, Wikman G. Pharmacology of Schisandra chinensis Bail.: an overview of Russian research and uses in medicine. J Ethnopharmacol 2008;118(2):183–212.

151. Smith MT, Haythornthwaite JA. How do sleep disturbance and chronic pain inter-relate? Insights from the longitudinal and cognitive-behavioral clinical trials literature. Sleep Med Rev 2004;8(2):119–32.

152. Lautenbacher S, Kundermann B, Krieg JC. Sleep deprivation and pain perception. Sleep Med Rev 2006;10(5):357–69.

153. Casarett D, Karlawish J, Sankar P, et al. Designing pain research from the patient's perspective: what trial end points are important to patients with chronic pain? Pain Med 2001;2(4):309–16.

154. Pigeon WR, Moynihan J, Matteson-Rusby S, et al. Comparative effectiveness of CBT interventions for co-morbid chronic pain and insomnia: a pilot study. Behav Res Ther 2012;50(11):685–9.

155. Allen KD, Renner JB, Devellis B, et al. Osteoarthritis and sleep: the Johnston County Osteoarthritis Project. J Rheumatol 2008;35(6):1102–7.

156. Kroenke K, Theobald D, Wu J, et al. The association of depression and pain with health-related quality of life, disability, and health care use in cancer patients. J Pain Symptom Manage 2010;40(3):327–41.

157. Gallagher RM, Verma S. Managing pain and comorbid depression: a public health challenge. Semin Clin Neuropsychiatry 1999;4(3):203–20.

158. Erickson B. Depression, anxiety, and substance use disorder in chronic pain. Tech Reg Anesth Pain Manag 2005;9(4):200–3.

159. Covin R, Ouimet AJ, Seeds PM, et al. A meta-analysis of CBT for pathological worry among clients with GAD. J Anxiety Disord 2008;22(1):108–16.

160. Sudak DM. Cognitive behavioral therapy for depression. Psychiatr Clin North Am 2012;35(1):99–110.

161. Butler AC, Chapman JE, Forman EM, et al. The empirical status of cognitive-behavioral therapy: a review of meta-analyses. Clin Psychol Rev 2006;26(1):17–31.

162. Morley S, Keefe FJ. Getting a handle on process and change in CBT for chronic pain. Pain 2007;127(3):197–8.

163. McCracken LM, Gauntlett-Gilbert J, Vowles KE. The role of mindfulness in a contextual cognitive-behavioral analysis of chronic pain-related suffering and disability. Pain 2007;131(1–2):63–9.

164. Kuyken W, Watkins E, Holden E, et al. How does mindfulness-based cognitive therapy work? Behav Res Ther 2010;48(11):1105–12.

165. Chiesa A, Serretti A. Mindfulness based cognitive therapy for psychiatric disorders: a systematic review and meta-analysis. Psychiatry Res 2011;187(3):441–53.

166. Chiesa A, et al. Mindfulness-based interventions for chronic pain: a systematic review of evidence. J Altern Complement Med 2011;17(1):83–93.

167. Vahora SA, Malek-Ahmadi P. S-adenosylmethionine in the treatment of depression. Neurosci Biobehav Rev 1988;12(2):139–41.

168. Bottiglieri T. Folate, vitamin B(1)(2), and S-adenosylmethionine. Psychiatr Clin North Am 2013;36(1):1–13.

169. Osiecki H. The nutrient bible. 8th ed. Eagle Farm: Bio Concepts Publishing; 2010.

170. Sontrop J, Campbell MK. Omega-3 polyunsaturated fatty acids and depression: a review of the evidence and a methodological critique. Prev Med 2006;42(1):4–13.

171. Gamus D, Meshulam-Atzmon V, Pintov S, et al. The effect of acupuncture therapy on pain perception and coping strategies: a preliminary report. J Acupunct Meridian Stud. 2008;1(1):51–3.

172. Ernst E. Massage therapy for low back pain: a systematic review. J Pain Symptom Manage 1999;17(1):65–9.

173. Jane SW, Chen SL, Wilkie DJ, et al. Effects of massage on pain, mood status, relaxation, and sleep in Taiwanese patients with metastatic bone pain: a randomized clinical trial. Pain 2011;152(10):2432–42.

174. Gallo R, Santana LS, Ferreira CHJ, et al. Massage reduced severity of pain during labour: a randomised trial. J Physiother 2013;59(2):109–16.

175. Field T, Delage J, Hernandez-Reif M. Movement and massage therapy reduce fibromyalgia pain. J Bodyw Mov Ther 2003;7(1):49–52.

176. Field T, Diego M, Delgado J, et al. Rheumatoid arthritis in upper limbs benefits from moderate pressure massage therapy. Complement Ther Clin Pract 2013;19(2):101–3.

177. Plastaras CT, Schran S, Kim N, et al. Complementary and alternative treatment for neck pain: chiropractic, acupuncture, TENS, massage, yoga, Tai Chi, and Feldenkrais. Phys Med Rehabil Clin N Am 2011;22(3):521–37, ix.

178. Simonnet G, Laboureyras E, Sergheraert L. Polyamine deficient diet: a nutritional therapy for relieving abnormal and chronic pain. Pharma Nutr 2013.

179. Rivat C, Richebe P, Laboureyras E, et al. Polyamine deficient diet to relieve pain hypersensitivity. Pain 2008;137(1):125–37.

180. Vuori IM. Dose-response of physical activity and low back pain, osteoarthritis, and osteoporosis. Med Sci Sports Exerc 2001;33(6 Suppl.):S551–86, discussion 609–10.

181. Manniche C, Lundberg E, Christensen I, et al. Intensive dynamic back exercises for chronic low back pain: a clinical trial. Pain 1991;47(1):53–63.

182. Stanton R, Reaburn P. Exercise and the treatment of depression: a review of the exercise program variables. J Sci Med Sport 2013.

183. Herring M, Jacob ML, Suveg C, et al. Effects of short-term exercise training on signs and symptoms of generalised anxiety disorder. Ment Health Phys Act 2011;4(2):71–7.

184. Posadzki P, Ernst E, Terry R, et al. Is yoga effective for pain? A systematic review of randomized clinical trials. Complement Ther Med 2011;19(5):281–7.

185. Wang C. Tai chi and rheumatic diseases. Rheum Dis Clin North Am 2011;37(1):19–32.

186. Wang C, Bannuru R, Ramel J, et al. Tai Chi on psychological well-being: systematic review and meta-analysis. BMC Complement Altern Med 2010; 10:23.

187. Kabat-Zinn J. An outpatient program in behavioral medicine for chronic pain patients based on the practice of mindfulness meditation: theoretical considerations and preliminary results. Gen Hosp Psychiatry 1982;4(1):33–47.

188. Miller KM. Deep breathing relaxation. A pain management technique. AORN J 1987;45(2):484–8.

CHAPTER 41

Polypharmacy and drug–nutraceutical interactions

Justin Sinclair
ND, MHerbMed

OVERVIEW

Herbal, nutritional and other complementary medicines are continuing to experience a renewed interest and popularity in developed nations worldwide.[1–3] This increased trend in usage suggests that adverse herb–drug–nutrient interactions (HDNIs) may be of significant public health consequence[4] and highlights the importance of sustained pharmacovigilance and evidence-based appraisal with the concurrent use of herbs, nutrients and drugs in a clinical setting.[5,6]

STATISTICS

The Adverse Drug Reactions Advisory Committee (ADRAC) of the Australian Therapeutic Goods Administration started documenting adverse drug reactions in 1972,[7] and received its first report of an adverse drug reaction from a complementary medicine in 1979.[8] Since this time, some 4779 reports of suspected adverse drug reactions to 'other therapeutic products' (i.e. non-pharmaceuticals) have been voluntarily submitted in Australia, with herbal medicines accounting for 2350 reports.[7] As of 22 June 2018, there have been 356 460 reported adverse drug reactions to all forms of medicine.[8] While reported statistics on documented herbal and nutritional adverse drug reactions can be viewed as being comparatively low in contrast to orthodox medications, this may be a reflection of both the relative safety of complementary medicines and the under-reporting of potential HDNIs to regulatory agencies.[9,10] It is important that complementary medicine practitioners remain assiduous in identifying and reporting suspected adverse drug reactions to the regulatory authorities.

INTERACTION MECHANISMS

Given the multifarious array of substances currently used as medicines, it is not surprising that this correlates with multiple complex factors that can modify drug responses. Natural products, unlike those of the pharmaceutical/allopathic model, contain a complex mixture of bioactive entities, which greatly increases the likelihood of interactions due to many of these products being incompletely chemically characterised[11] and therefore they remain largely an unknown therapeutic entity until specific studies reveal phytochemical profiles and mechanisms of action. Current pharmacological opinion suggests that three heterogeneous interaction mechanisms exist, namely pharmacokinetic, pharmacodynamic and physicochemical models[9,12] (Figure 41.1).

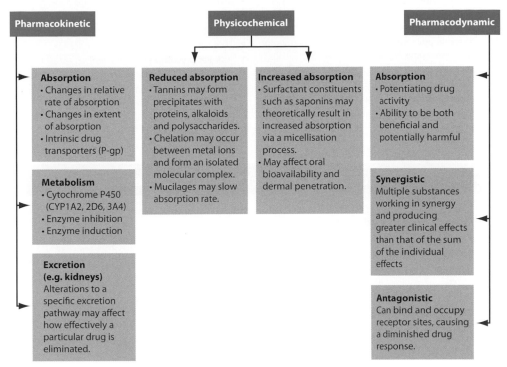

Figure 41.1
Interaction mechanisms

Adapted from Braun & Cohen 2010[9]

PHARMACOKINETIC INTERACTIONS

'Pharmacokinetics' is defined as the quantitative study of the absorption, distribution, metabolism and excretion of a medicine by the body (i.e. the effects the body has on the medicine).[13] Pharmacokinetic interactions occur when there is a modification to any of the four aforementioned processes, resulting in a change in the concentration of the drug in the target tissues or at the receptor sites.[9] A significant increase or decrease to bioavailability or clearance mechanisms has a higher potential to be clinically relevant.[6] Herbal and nutritional medicines, along with food, have the ability to modify the pharmacokinetic profile of a drug by either increasing or reducing its availability within the body and therefore modifying biochemical and physiological responses. Representative examples of pharmacokinetic interactions include the inhibition/induction of certain isoenzymes of the hepatic cytochrome P450 (CYP) system (particularly 1A2, 2D6 and 3A4), or the inhibition/induction of the drug transporter P-glycoprotein (P-gp). As interactions of this model are largely unpredictable[11,14] they are of far greater clinical concern in patients taking pharmaceutical medicines, especially those with a narrow therapeutic index.[11]

Other factors such as age-related organ changes in the elderly or very young (see box on the next page), interindividual variability and genetics, patient constitution,

Common narrow therapeutic index drugs

- Antiarrhythmics (e.g. quinidine and disopyramide)
- Hypoglycaemics (e.g. insulin)
- Antiepileptics/anticonvulsants (e.g. phenytoin, carbamazepine and valproic acid)
- Immunosuppressants (e.g. cyclosporine)
- Mood-altering drugs (e.g. lithium carbonate)
- Anti-HIV drugs (e.g. saquinavir)
- Monoamine oxidase inhibitors

- Antineoplastics (e.g. methotrexate)
- Opioid analgesics
- Barbiturates
- Theophylline
- Cardiac glycosides (e.g. digoxin)
- Tricyclic antidepressants
- Levothyroxine sodium

Factors that can affect paediatric patients

Paediatric patients require special consideration when it comes to pharmacokinetic and pharmacodynamic interactions in contrast to adults, due largely to:

- altered receptor sensitivity
- increased intramuscular absorption
- enhanced permeability of the blood–brain barrier
- underdeveloped hepatic enzymes
- higher gastric pH (generally > 4)

- immature renal function
- larger liver to body weight ratio
- reduced fat mass
- limited protein-binding capacity
- slower gastrointestinal absorption
- increased gastric emptying time.[15]

As such, special care needs to be taken.

gender, body composition, microbiome dysfunction, pregnancy and comorbid disease / sub-optimal organ function can also affect drug response,[12,16–19] and should be carefully considered when assessing potential HDNIs.[20]

Absorption

Absorption is a complicated and multifaceted phase in pharmacokinetic studies and is considered of prime importance in determining the clinical outcomes of drug therapy.[21] Individual factors affecting absorption are discussed in brief detail below.

Changes in gastric acid output or pH

The pH of the stomach plays a significant role in the absorption of drugs. Medications that increase gastric pH levels such as antacids, H_2 receptor antagonists and proton pump inhibitors can impact on other medications that may be best absorbed in a more acidic environment, such as ketoconazole.[22–24] Also worthy of note is that prolonged use of proton pump inhibitors can lead to B12 malabsorption.[25,26] Furthermore, in recent studies it has been shown that chronic proton pump inhibitor use has been associated with other micronutrient malabsorption (e.g. Fe),[27] interference with gastric bacteriocidal function and may predispose to enteric infections such as *Clostridium difficile*, *Campylobacter* and *Salmonella* gastroenteritis.[28,29] Conversely, agents such as herbal bitters (e.g. *Gentiana lutea*, *Andrographis paniculata*) that can increase hydrochloric acid output may work against agents that absorb better in a higher pH environment. Considerations should also be made for infants and toddlers as gastric acid secretion is reduced in this age bracket and does not reach adult pH levels until three to seven years of age.[15,30]

Reduction in bile acid concentration

Bile is required for the emulsification and subsequent absorption of fat-soluble compounds. Low bile concentration can result from increased drug binding and excretion or decreased production within the liver. An example of this is neomycin, which binds to bile acids and reduces their intraluminal concentration and increases excretion. This therefore has flow-on effects of reducing the absorption of fat-soluble vitamins (A, D, E and K).

Gastrointestinal microflora dysfunction

Certain drugs are predisposed to bacterial metabolism or, in some instances, drug cleavage by intestinal microorganisms, which is a required step in absorption/therapeutic effect. As such, any changes to the levels of the microflora within the intestines could detrimentally affect drug bioavailability or the availability of nutrients produced by the gut flora.

Changes in gastrointestinal motility

Certain medications can reduce gastrointestinal motility and therefore impact on gastric emptying by delaying the emptying of the stomach and increasing transit time (Table 41.1). Obesity is also of importance as increased abdominal fat can increase intra-abdominal pressure and impact gastric emptying (Table 41.1), especially in children.[15] High dietary fat has also been found to retard gastric emptying to a greater degree than either protein or carbohydrate.

Table 41.1
Drugs that can affect gastric emptying rate

Increase in gastric emptying rate	Decrease in gastric emptying rate
Morphine	Atropine
Phenytoin	Amitriptyline
Levodopa	Imipramine
Isoniazid	Anticholinergics

Source: Hirschberg 2012

Intrinsic transporters

Intestinal transport molecules are required for the absorption of certain herbs, drugs and nutrients through the intestinal epithelium and into systemic circulation.[15,31,32] One such example is P-glycoprotein (P-gp), a multidrug efflux transporter and the most studied adenosine 5'-triphosphate (ATP)-binding cassette transporter responsible for acting as a biological barrier by extruding toxic substances and xenobiotics out of cells.[33–37] The intracellular localisation of P-gp is tissue specific and exists on the apical surface of enterocytes, epithelial cells of the kidney and placenta but also in the brain, vessels and hepatocytes, which is indicative of its important role in absorption and subsequent assimilation, metabolism and excretion of substances within the body.[33,38,39] P-gp acts much like a gatekeeper as it can also operate in a counter-transport capacity, thereby expelling medicines from the blood back into the gastrointestinal lumen, reducing bioavailability.[9]

P-gp expression can be altered by a variety of substances such as drugs, herbal medicines, foods and nutraceuticals, causing either an inhibitory effect or one of induction. Induction implies that there would be a decrease in absorption and subsequent distribution of any P-gp substrates, whereas inhibition of substrates causes an increase in absorption and distribution. Depending on the substrate, especially those of narrow therapeutic index, this could have serious clinical implications.

The ability for foodstuffs, herbal and nutritional medicines to induce or inhibit P-gp is well documented in the literature; however, rarely is there more than in-vitro evidence. Clinical studies supporting the induction of P-gp by *Hypericum perforatum* exist,[40] along with in-vitro evidence for possible induction of genistein and diadzein.[9] Most evidence, however, is for P-gp inhibition, with grapefruit and orange (Seville) juice having supportive clinical evidence,[41] with an abundance of substances with in-vitro evidence such as polyphenols from *Camellia sinensis*,[42] *Rosmarinus officinalis*,[43] resveratrol,[42] curcumin (*Curcuma longa*),[44] quercetin[45] and *Silybum marianum*.[9,45] While the use of in-vitro data to form a basis for the cautionary use of many of the inhibitors of P-gp is wise, it is of unknown clinical significance until further evidence is obtained from more sophisticated models.

Important P-gp substrates

Substrates for the human multidrug resistance (MDR1) gene

- **Anticancer:** vincristine, vinblastine, tamoxifen, Taxol, doxorubicin, daunorubicin, colchicines, etoposide
- **Anti-emetics:** domperidone, ondansetron
- **Antimicrobials:** erythromycin, rifampicin, quinolones, ivermectin
- **Immunosuppressants:** cyclosporine, tacrolimus
- **Cardiac prescription:** digoxin, propafenone, quinidine, amiodarone, propranolol, verapamil, lovastatin, atorvastatin, diltiazem, timolol
- **Central nervous system prescription:** phenytoin, phenoxazine, fluphenazine
- **HIV protease inhibitors:** indinavir, ritonavir, saquinavir, nelfinavir
- **Morphins:** morphine, loperamide
- **Rheumatologicals:** quinine, methotrexate
- **Steroids:** hydrocortisone, dexamethasone

Sources: Braun & Cohen 2010,[9] Shapiro & Shear 2002,[46] Brinkmann & Eichelbaum 2001,[46] Brinkmann et al. 2001[47]

Local blood flow

When drugs are administered subcutaneously or intramuscularly, local blood flow in the surrounding tissue can impact upon absorption rates. An example of this is when local anaesthetics are administered in conjunction with a vasoconstrictor to provide a prolonged duration of action.[48]

Presence of food

The presence of food in the gastrointestinal tract can impact on drug absorption by altering gastric pH, gastric secretions, transit time and motility which can ultimately cause a change in the rate and extent of drug absorption.[49] Drugs like griseofulvin are lipid soluble and so enhanced absorption is obtained from a high-fat meal; so too is coenzyme Q10. Conversely, some drugs like isoniazid and acetaminophen should be taken on an empty stomach.[49] Dietary proteins can also impact on absorption. Drugs such as propranolol, metoprolol and lignocaine, which undergo extensive first-pass effect, have been shown in studies to have enhanced bioavailability after a high-protein meal.[15] This is attributed to the enhanced hepatic blood flow.

Since food can clearly affect absorption it is always best to ensure prescriptions are followed appropriately, or pharmacists consulted if the patient is unsure of when to take their medications.

Distribution

The distribution of medications depends on a variety of factors, including total body water concentration, extracellular fluid, adipose tissue percentage and capacity to bind to plasma proteins.[50] Most interactions that occur at this level are drug–drug, and for an interaction to occur the drugs involved need to be highly protein bound (> 95%) (or of narrow therapeutic index) and thus they compete for binding sites.[22,50] One such example is phenytoin, which is both a narrow therapeutic index drug and 89–93% protein bound, and is also involved in several metabolic interactions of the CYPs.[50]

Drugs that are highly protein bound	
• Amitriptyline	• Oxazepam
• Diazepam	• Phenytoin
• Indomethacin	• Thyroxine
• Ketoconazole	• Valproic acid
• Naproxen	• Warfarin
• Nifedipine	
Source: Manzi & Shannon 2005[50]	

Metabolism

For the great majority of pharmaceutical medications, the liver is the primary site for metabolism and is largely mediated by the CYP enzymes, and by this reasoning is of growing clinical and pharmacological interest.[51]

Cytochrome P450

While the highest concentration of these enzymes is found in hepatocytes,[52] they are also found in the intestines in both crypt cells and the tip of the villi of enterocytes,[22] and in smaller concentrations in the kidneys, skin and lungs.[9] The CYPs make up the major enzyme family capable of performing oxidative biotransformation of most drugs[53,54] (Table 41.2), a process that is divided into two categories comprised of phase I and phase II transformation reactions.[22,50] Phase I biotransformation reactions include intramolecular changes such as oxidation, reduction, hydroxylation and dealkylation, which can make the drug more polar.[9,22] During this process drugs are usually converted into inactive, less active or more active substances and can also render inactive pro-drugs biologically active.[9] Phase II biotransformation reactions are conjugation reactions (glucuronidation, sulfation, methylation and acetylation reactions) that allow for the drug conjugate to be easily eliminated from the body.[22,56]

Table 41.2
Examples of drugs metabolised by various CYP enzymes

CYP1A2	CYP2C9	CYP2D6	CYP3A4
Antidepressants Amitriptyline, imipramine, clomipramine	**Antidepressants** Amitriptyline, fluoxetine	**Antidepressants** Amitriptyline, clomipramine, fluoxetine	**Antiarrhythmics** Amiodarone, digoxin, quinidine
Antipsychotics Clozapine, olanzapine, haloperidol	**Antidiabetics** Nateglinide, glimepiride, rosiglitazone	**Antipsychotics** Haloperidol, risperidone, thioridazine	**Antidepressants** Amitriptyline, sertraline, imipramine
Miscellaneous Naproxen, paracetamol, propranolol, verapamil, warfarin, melatonin, oestradiol, theophylline	**NSAIDs** Celecoxib, diclofenac, naproxen, ibuprofen, suprofen	**Antiarrhythmics** Sparteine, flecainide, encainide	**Antibacterials** Erythromycin, rifampicin
	Miscellaneous Warfarin, tamoxifen, ketamine, fluvastatin, phenytoin	**Beta-blockers** Alprenolol, metoprolol, propranolol **Miscellaneous** Opioids Codeine, dextromethorphan, tramadol	**Benzodiazepines** Alprazolam, diazepam, midazolam, triazolam
			Calcium channel blockers Felodipine, amlodipine, nifedipine
			Chemotherapeutics Paclitaxel, vinblastine, vincristine, etoposide, docetaxel, cyclophosphamide, busulfan
			Immunosuppressive Corticosteroids, cyclosporine, dapsone, tacrolimus
			Miscellaneous Warfarin, theophylline, omeprazole, codeine, acetaminophen

Sources: Braun & Cohen 2010,[9] Shapiro & Shear 2002,[22] Manzi & Shannon 2005,[50] Jobst et al. 2003[55]

The five major P450 enzymes involved in the biotransformation of drugs are CYP1A2, 2C9, 2C19, 2D6 and 3A4, with the 1A2, 2D6 and 3A4 isoenzymes being involved in the metabolism of more than 50% of most pharmaceuticals.[57–59] Similar to P-gp, the CYP enzymes can be induced or inhibited, which can have a detrimental impact on circulating levels of drug.

Inhibition of specific enzymes can cause increased circulating levels of substrates due to reduced clearance/metabolism, causing increased drug response and toxic effects, which can obviously have catastrophic consequences in the case of narrow therapeutic index (NTI) medications.[22] Conversely, when enzymes are induced they cause the rapid metabolism of substrate from the body, which can cause reduced circulating levels of the drug and subtherapeutic outcomes or even treatment failure, again of particular importance for NTI medications. A well-known herbal medicine that has been shown to cause induction of CYP enzymes, especially 3A4, is *Hypericum perforatum*, due mainly to its hyperforin content.[60–63] Food has also been shown to be an inducer of various enzymes, especially cruciferous vegetables like broccoli, cabbage and brussels sprouts, red wine, ethanol and charcoal grilled beef.[64]

Genetic polymorphisms

The individual enzymes and their concentration within the different body environs is under genetic control.[55] This individual variability, known as genetic polymorphism, means that individuals may have different levels of activity of the various CYP isoforms—some may have a functional isoenzyme (such as CYP2D6), whereas others may not; the former would be classified as being 'extensive metabolisers' while the latter 'poor metabolisers'.[22,57] There also exists a class known as 'ultra-rapid metabolisers' due to the fact they may contain multiple copies of individual enzymes. The clinical ramifications of such genetic polymorphism is evident when drugs are administered to these groups; poor metabolisers are at higher risk of toxic effects with drugs that are metabolised by the enzymes that they lack, whereas ultra-rapid metabolisers may in most instances hypermetabolise the drug and therefore have treatment failure due to subtherapeutic plasma concentrations[22] (see Chapter 2 on diagnostic techniques for more information).

Excretion

The major organ of excretion are the kidneys; however, substances can still be excreted from the body in faeces (bile), saliva, sweat, tears, hair, breast milk and expired air (volatile substances).[50,65] Renal excretion requires that the substances being excreted are water-soluble, not too large and also not bound to proteins in the blood, and involves three major mechanisms in the form of glomerular filtration, tubular secretion and tubular reabsorption.[65] Anything that can impact on these processes, such as certain medications, being elderly or concurrent illness such as acute or chronic renal failure, is of significance.[50] Urine acidity is also clinically relevant and can affect the rate at which certain substances can be eliminated from the kidneys. Nutritional and herbal substances can directly impact on this parameter.

PHARMACODYNAMIC INTERACTIONS

Pharmacodynamics is concerned with the biochemical and physiological effect the drug has on the body and includes the relationship between drug concentration and the magnitude of drug effect. Pharmacodynamic interactions transpire when one drug alters the sensitivity or responsiveness of tissues to another drug via receptor-binding affinity and intrinsic activity, resulting in potential additive (agonistic), synergistic or antagonistic drug effects.[9] These drug effects have both positive and negative clinical repercussions, with synergistic and additive interactions frequently being utilised to improve patient outcomes.[9] There currently exists a paucity of clinical data in this area, making this class of interactions based largely on theoretical considerations rather than experimental data. As such, pharmacodynamic interactions may be theoretically predictable and can be identified by analysing the therapeutic profiles and mechanisms of action of the drugs, nutrients or herbal medicines used. Examples of pharmacodynamic interactions are listed below.

Antagonistic effects

When two substances that are receptor agonist and antagonist interact it is classed as an opposing or antagonistic interaction.[66]

- **Drugs:** Certain antagonistic interactions can be beneficial, such as naloxone reversal of opioid overdose or flumazenil reversal of benzodiazepine-induced sedation.[66]

When opposing actions interact they can also reduce the efficacy of one or both drugs, such as propranolol (beta-blocker) counteracting the way a beta-adrenergic stimulant such as albuterol works.

- **Herbs:** *Piper methysticum* has shown dopamine receptor antagonism activity and therefore poses a problem for dopamine agonists like L-dopa.[9,67,68] Similarly, stimulating herbs such as *Paullinia cupana, Camelia sinensis (Green tea), Coffea arabica/canephora (Coffee)*, high-grade *Theobroma cacao (Cacao)* and *Ilex paraguariensis* could work against the sedative effects of *Valeriana officinalis* or *Humulus lupulus*.
- **Nutrients:** Vitamin K reduces the international normalised ratio (INR) of patients on warfarin through inhibition of the anticoagulant effect.

Additive effects

Additive or synergistic interactions can occur when two substances with similar pharmacological properties are given together, therefore increasing therapeutic potency and physiological effect.

- **Drugs:** Mixing ethanol with other sedative drugs such as benzodiazepine anxiolytics or histamine H_1-receptor antagonists can produce an additive sedative effect.[66] Combinations of monoamine oxidase inhibitors with tricyclic or selective serotonin reuptake inhibitor (SSRI) antidepressants can have an additive effect by overstimulation of 5-HT[1] receptors causing serotonin syndrome.[66]
- **Foods:** In vivo[69] and case study[70] evidence suggests alcohol, when taken with *Piper methysticum*, can potentiate sedation, intoxication and impairment of cognition.
- **Herbs:** *Hypericum perforatum* could theoretically have an additive effect with SSRI medication and contribute to serotonin syndrome.[61,71–73] *Crataegus monogyna* may act synergistically with hypotensive medications and digitalis glycosides, therefore increasing its effect.[71]
- **Nutrients:** Vitamin E has been found to increase the response of warfarin and therefore increase bleeding risk.

PHYSICOCHEMICAL INTERACTIONS

The physicochemical model, also known as the pharmaceutical model, represents the interaction of substances that have conflicting physical or chemical properties.[9] This mechanism relates to the physicochemical properties of the drug and herb/nutrient not just on a molecular level, but also within the context of the environment in which they interact together (e.g. the lumen of the gastrointestinal system, in a closed vessel of manufacture or dispensation or a delivery device such as an enteral feeding tube).[6,74] This interaction will typically occur during the processes of digestion and absorption so is therefore most commonly localised to the stomach and small intestine.

Physicochemical interactions can have either a positive or a negative impact on the absorption of one or both substances and their subsequent assimilation and bioavailability within the body.[6] Examples of this type of interaction extend to herbal substances high in tannins, polyphenols, mucilages and saponins, and also metal ions via the process of chelation. Decreases or increases in absorption based on these substances is of particular importance when NTI drugs and alkaloid-based herbs or medications are being used.

Chelation

The process of chelation describes a process whereby drugs and other substances can bind metal ions (e.g. Mg^{2+}, Ca^{2+}, Fe^{2+}, Al^{3+}, Zn^{2+}). As such, decreased absorption or bioavailability is generally the result of chelation leading to poor treatment outcomes. Some examples of interactions that involve chelation are listed below.

- **Drugs:** Tetracycline and quinolone antibiotics form an insoluble complex with metals. Fluoroquinolones can interact with multivalent cation containing products such as antacids (aluminium or magnesium based) or products containing calcium, zinc or iron, which can trigger a marked decrease in oral absorption.[75]
- **Food:** Ciprofloxacin can have reduced bioavailability due to chelation with enteric nutrition formulation in nasogastric feeding tubes.[76] Food sources rich in oxalic and phytic acid have also been found to form insoluble complexes with calcium, reducing absorption.[9] Tetracycline has been found to chelate with calcium ions from concurrent milk consumption.[77]

Increased absorption

- **Saponins:** These have a long history of use for their detergent qualities.[78] Saponins largely occur as glycosides with a triterpenoid or steroidal aglycone, which gives them the 'ability to lower surface tension, producing the characteristic detergent like effect on mucous membranes and skin'.[79] Saponins can also irritate the gastric mucosa, increasing blood flow to the epithelium, which may theoretically enhance absorption. Some authors posit it could increase absorption through a micellisation process; more research is required and therefore such theories are still largely speculative.[9]

Decreased absorption

- **Tannins:** These are high molecular weight compounds that contain significant amounts of phenolic hydroxyl groups to permit the formation of stable cross-links with proteins.[79] They are astringent, work locally on tissues and can complex with metal ions.[13,78,80] Tannins can easily form precipitates with alkaloids and polysaccharides,[79] as well as reduce the absorption of certain minerals[81] and dietary protein. As such, experienced herbalists take care not to extemporaneously dispense herbs with high tannin content with these previously mentioned phytochemicals.
- **Mucilages and gums:** These are polysaccharides that combine with water to form a slimy mass[79] and can be found in plant seed coats (linseed and psyllium), barks (*Ulmus fulva*) and roots (*Althea officinalis*).[78] Having demulcent, emollient, antidiarrhoeal and bulk laxative actions, they are a highly useful class of phytochemicals (Table 41.3) for the gastrointestinal tract. This latter action can increase peristalsis, impacting on transit time and reducing drug absorption apart from potentially binding small drug fractions to it due to the large molecular size of the molecule. In-vitro studies have also highlighted the ability for non-starch polysaccharides[82] to bind to calcium, iron and zinc.
- **Food:** High-fibre diets and bulk-forming compounds have been found to interfere with the absorption of various medicines.[83] The narrow therapeutic index drug digoxin has shown reduced bioavailability when co-administered with a fibre-rich meal, with results showing almost half of the dose was sequestered or bound to the fibre.[15] Other drugs with similar reduced absorption on high-fibre diets include lithium salts, lovastatin[84] and tricyclic antidepressants.[85]

Table 41.3
Examples of specific phytochemically rich plants

Tannin-rich plants	Saponin-rich plants	Mucilage-rich plants
Agrimonia eupatoria	*Astragalus membranaceus*	*Chondrus crispus*
Arctostaphylos uva-ursi	*Withania somnifera*	*Althaea officinalis* (root)
Camellia sinensis	*Aesculus hippocastanum*	*Ulmus fulva*
Geranium maculatum	*Panax ginseng*	*Drosera rotundifolia*
Hamamelis virginicus	*Bupleurum falcatum*	*Aloe vera*
Potentilla tormentilla	*Glycyrrhiza glabra*	*Salvia hispanica*
Rubus idaeus	*Phytolacca americana*	*Plantago psyllium*

Sources: Braun & Cohen 2010,[9] Pengelly 2004[79]

Examples of alkaloid-containing plants	
Berberis vulgaris	*Passiflora incarnata (harmane type)*
Chelidonium majus	*Paullinia cupana*
Corydalis ambigua	*Piper nigrum or Piper longum*
Eschscholzia californica	*Stephania tetrandra*
Hydrastis canadensis	*Symphytum officinale*
Justicia adhatoda	*Tylophora indica*
Mahonia aquifolium	*Withania somnifera*

Sources: Pengelly 2004[79] and Bone 1996[86]

Challenges

The evidence available to guide practitioners in the decision-making process for assessing HDNIs is multifaceted and incorporates a variety of resources including human clinical trials, in-vivo studies and adverse drug reaction (ADR) database entries (see Table 41.4).

Clinical adverse events that have been ascribed to HDNIs are further complicated by such realities as botanical substitution (i.e. either intentional or accidental)[87] of a different plant species and contamination of the herb with pharmaceutically derived medications or other non-herbal substances, which should be taken into consideration before jumping to conclusions. This helps separate what Coxeter and colleagues[4] aptly term true 'interaction from overreaction'.

With conclusive evidence to substantiate HDNIs often lacking, it is usually the clinician that is left to speculate on a potential interaction between a herb, nutrient and drug. Current academics in the field of herbal pharmacology suggest that much greater research and funding to assess the clinical significance of HDNIs is required, and that until such a database exists, it is wise to closely monitor patients who are elderly, taking multiple medications, taking NTI drugs or suffering from serious diseases/conditions/disorders.

Table 41.4
Comparison of the evidence from studies of herb–drug interactions

Study design	Advantages	Disadvantages
Controlled clinical trial in patients	• High internal validity and generalisability to patients of interest	• Controlled trial may not reflect clinical reality • Difficult to implement (logistics, cost, ethics) • Increased sample size may be required to account for expected variability
Controlled clinical trial in healthy subjects	• High internal validity • Allows a full and rigorous assessment of herb–drug interaction mechanisms	• As above • May not predict significance of interaction in patients with diseases, organ dysfunction and/or other medications
Open label clinical trial	• Controlled patient group for comparison	• As above • Confounded by subjective endpoints
Case reports of series	• Informative and realistic information obtained in the patient group of interest • Generates hypotheses	• Uncontrolled observational study which may overestimate significance given the many possible confounders • May lead to over-reporting of cases with no insight into the clinical significance
Animal studies	• Allows a rigorous investigation of integrated pharmacological effects	• Some interspecies differences in drug response and metabolism may confound • Not possible to assess clinical significance
In-vitro studies in animal or human tissues	• Provides mechanistic information and allows fundamental understanding of interaction cause	• Isolated tissues may not reflect in vivo response • Concentrations of constituents may not reflect concentration or metabolites in vivo
Adverse event database entries	• Provides immediate reporting of potentially dangerous interactions • Provides an international perspective on the incidence of serious but rare interactions • Hypothesis generating	• Often cannot be evaluated due to non-existent or inaccessible extraneous data for critical interpretation

Source: Coxeter et al. 2004[4]

Overview of how to approach patients on medications

Dealing with patients taking medications is one of the most challenging areas of naturopathic practice, especially where polypharmacy is concerned.[9] A methodical and systematic approach (the INQUIRE method) to prescribing complementary medicines to people taking pharmaceutical medications is proposed as being best practice.

The INQUIRE method was designed specifically for students of herbal and naturopathic medicine to reduce the potential for oversight and implement foundational skills that can be honed while under supervision. The INQUIRE mnemonic stands for:

Investigate
Note
Qualify
Understand
Identify
Remember
Educate

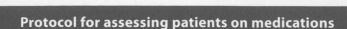

> ## Protocol for assessing patients on medications
>
> **I: Investigate** all aspects of the current medications the patient is taking (mechanisms of action, safety, adverse reactions, cautions, contraindications and interactions).
>
> **N: Note** the posology of the medications taken by the patient (dosage, when taken and duration of administration).
>
> **Q: Qualify** and rationalise the strengths and limitations of complementary medicines in being able to efficaciously assist in the management of the presenting conditions/disorders of the patient.
>
> **U: Understand.** Armed with the information obtained from research of the medications and case history, the naturopath can develop a treatment protocol/regimen specific to the patient.
>
> **I: Identify** any potential interactions with the intended treatment using reputable evidence-based texts and resources.
>
> **R: Remember** to contact the GP or medical practitioner (with patient consent) to outline the treatment plan if required.
>
> **E: Educate** the patient. Part of the strength of complementary medicine therapies lies in empowering and educating the patient to take an active role in their own health.

Investigate

All medications must be suitably researched and investigated to provide a rational foundation to identify potential interactions using appropriate pharmacological resources (e.g. MIMS). This should be done at the start of the consultation if possible so students can differentiate the signs and symptoms associated with disease from potential ADRs. This allows the practitioner to be cognisant of particularly problematic medications and therefore assists in selecting appropriate CAM therapies. Should the student still be uncertain or need clarification, contact a local pharmacist for expert opinion. Potential questions pertinent to this section include:

1. What types of medication are being taken? Are they prescription only (Schedule 4), controlled substances (S8) or pharmacy only (S3)?
2. Is there potential for interaction based on available pharmacodynamics/ pharmacokinetic information for the drug?
3. What are the cautions, side effects and contraindications of the drug?
4. Is the drug known to be of narrow therapeutic index? If so, use caution in your treatment strategy.

Note

Understanding the medication is only one part of this process, as posology is equally important. Significant questions relevant to this section include:

1. What is the dosage of the drug?
2. What is the frequency of dosing? Is it b.i.d., t.d.s. or other?
3. When is the drug taken? Is it taken before meals or after? Is the patient following the prescribed times for dosing?
4. How long have they been taking the medication?
5. Are they taking any other supplements? Many patients do not think of natural supplements as medicines. Many practitioners ask the patients to bring all of their current medications and supplements with them to the consult.

Qualify

There are many conditions and diseases that benefit from CAM treatment. Conversely, there are also those conditions that are considered too serious and beyond the scope of CAM practice.

1. Is there adequate evidence to support the use of CAMs in the patient's presenting case?
2. Should CAMs be applied as adjunct (supportive) rather than primary therapy?

Understand

Armed with a thorough understanding of the case and the patient's medication, and taking into account the constitution, general health and age of the patient, a treatment outline can be developed. Potentially beneficial pharmacodynamic interactions (synergistic or additive effects) can be explored further.

Identify

Once the treatment outline has been determined, it is now time to utilise CAM-specific evidence-based texts and other resources to identify any known HDNIs (see HDNI charts in appendices 1 and 2). In many cases, this can be done concurrently with the development of the treatment outline. At the conclusion of this, a prescription can be written.

Remember

If your patient is taking prescription-only drugs, or is being managed for a condition by a medical practitioner, it is wise to contact them before initiating treatment out of professional courtesy. This is paramount if your patient desires to reduce their prescription medications. It also establishes an open channel of communication between the medical practitioner and yourself and reduces the likelihood of you being unaware of a medication or management plan alteration, thus increasing patient safety due to the decreased chance of a potential HDNI or ADR. Remember to obtain patient consent before initiating contact due to confidentiality issues.

Educate

One of the major differences between naturopathic and orthodox medicine is the role the naturopath has in educating the patient and getting them actively involved in their own health. Key points of importance here are factors such as:

- foods/supplements/herbs to avoid or include
- potential interactions that could occur
- the importance of compliance
- the time it will take before noticeable effects are experienced
- empowering the patient and utilising positive reinforcement.

FURTHER READING

Braun L, Cohen M. Herbs & natural supplements: an evidence-based guide. 4th ed. Marrickville: Elsevier; 2015.
Boullata JI, Armenti VT. Handbook of drug-nutrient interactions. 2nd ed. Humana Press; 2010.
Caballero B, Allen LH, Prentice A. Encyclopaedia of human nutrition. 3rd ed. Academic Press; 2013.

ESCOP Monographs. 2nd ed. European Scientific Cooperative on Phytotherapy. Exeter. 2003.

ESCOP Monographs. 2nd ed Supplement. European Scientific Cooperative on Phytotherapy. Exeter. 2009.

Goey AKL, Beijnen JH, Schellens JHM. Herb-drug interaction in oncology. Clin Pharmacol Ther 2014;95(4):354–5.

Mechling KA. Nutrient-drug interactions. Florida: CRC Press; 2007.

Mills S, Bone K. The essential guide to herbal safety. St Louis: Churchill Livingstone; 2005.

Stargrove MB, et al. Herb, nutrient and drug interactions: clinical implications and therapeutic strategies. Missouri: Mosby Elsevier; 2008.

Williamson E, Driver S, Baxter K, editors. Stockley's herbal medicine interactions: a guide to the interactions of herbal medicines. 2nd ed. London: Pharmaceutical Press; 2013.

REFERENCES

1. MacLennan AH, Wilson DH, Taylor AW. The escalating cost and prevalence of alternative medicine. Prev Med 2002;35(2):166–73.

2. Thomas K, Nicholl JP, Coleman P. Use and expenditure on complementary medicine in England: a population based survey. Complement Ther Med 2001;9:2–11.

3. Eisenberg D, Davis RB, Ettner SL, et al. Trends in alternative medicine use in the United States, 1990–1997: results of a follow-up national survey. JAMA 1998;280(18):1569–75.

4. Coxeter PD, McLachlan AJ, Duke CC, et al. Herb-drug interactions: an evidence based approach. Curr Med Chem 2004;11(11):1513–25.

5. Patel J, Gohil KJ. Herb-drug interactions: a review and study based on assessment of clinical case reports in literature. Indian J Pharmacol 2007;39(3):129–39.

6. Boullata JI, Hudson LM. Drug–nutrient interactions: a broad view with implications for practice. J Acad Nutr Diet 2012;112(4):506–17.

7. Personal communication. Canberra: Office of Product Review: Therapeutic Goods Administration; 2018.

8. Personal communication. Canberra: Pharmacovigilance and Special Access Branch; 2018.

9. Braun L, Cohen M. Herbs and natural supplements: an evidence-based guide. 3rd ed. Sydney: Elsevier; 2010.

10. Farnsworth N. Relative safety of herbal medicines. HerbalGram 1993;29:36A–H.

11. Chavez ML, Jordan MA, Chavez PI. Evidence-based drug–herbal interactions. Life Sci 2006;78(18):2146–57.

12. Bryant B, Knights K, Salerno E. Pharmacology for health professionals. Marrickville NSW Australia: Elsevier; 2003.

13. Mills S, Bone K. Principles and practice of phytotherapy. 2nd ed. London UK: Churchill Livingstone; 2013.

14. Mills S, Bone K. The essential guide to herbal safety. St Louis: Churchill Livingstone; 2005.

15. Gura KM, Chan L-N. Drug therapy and Role of Nutrition. In: Duggan C, editor. Nutrition in paediatrics. 4th ed. Hamilton, Canada: Decker Inc; 2008. p. 191–208.

16. Schmucker D. Liver function and phase I drug metabolism in the elderly: a paradox. Drugs Aging 2001;18(11):837–51.

17. Bressler R, Bahl JJ. Principles of drug therapy for the elderly patient. Mayo Clin Proc 2003;78(12):1564–77.

18. Klotz U. Effect of age on pharmacokinetics and pharmacodynamics in man. Int J Clin Pharmacol Ther 1998;36(11):581–5.

19. Turnheim K. When drug therapy gets old: pharmacokinetics and pharmacodynamics in the elderly. Exp Gerontol 2003;38(8):843–53.

20. Mallet L, Spinewine A, Huang A. Prescribing in elderly people: the challenge of managing drug interactions in elderly people. Lancet 2007;370(9582):185–91.

21. Colalto C. Herbal interactions on absorption of drugs: mechanisms of action and clinical risk assessment. Pharmacol Res 2010;62(3):207–27.

22. Shapiro LE, Shear NH. Drug interactions: proteins, pumps, and P-450s. J Am Acad Dermatol 2002;47(4):467–84, quiz 485–8.

23. Bodey GP. Azole antifungal agents. Clin Infect Dis 1992;14 Suppl 1:S161–9.

24. Won CS, Oberlies NH, Paine MF. Mechanisms underlying food-drug interactions: inhibition of intestinal metabolism and transport. Pharmacol Ther 2012;136(2):186–201.

25. Conner KG. Drug–nutrient interactions. In: Caballero B, editor. Encyclopedia of human nutrition. Amsterdam: Elsevier; 2013. p. 90–8.

26. Jung SB, Nagaraja V, Kapur A, et al. Association between vitamin B12 deficiency and long-term use of acid-lowering agents: a systematic review and meta-analysis. Intern Med J 2015;45(4):409–16.

27. Lam JR, Schneider JL, Quesenberry CP, et al. Proton pump inhibitor and histamine-2 receptor antagonist use and iron deficiency. Gastroenterology 2017;152(4): 821–9, e1.

28. Yadlapati R, Kahrilas PJ. The 'dangers' of chronic proton pump inhibitor use. J Allergy Clin Immunol 2018;141(1):79–81.

29. Freedberg DE, Kim LS, Yang YX. The risks and benefits of long-term use of proton pump inhibitors: expert review and best practice advice from the American Gastroenterological Association. Gastroenterology 2017;152(4):706–15.

30. Stewart CF, Hampton EM. Effect of maturation on drug disposition in pediatric patients. Clin Pharm 1987;6(7):548–64.

31. Reuss L. One-hundred years of inquiry: the mechanism of glucose absorption in the intestine. Annu Rev Physiol 2000;62:939–46.

32. Balayssac D, et al. Does inhibition of P-glycoprotein lead to drug-drug interactions. Toxicol Lett 2005;156(3): 319–29.

33. Lin JH. Drug-drug interaction mediated by inhibition and induction of P-glycoprotein. Adv Drug Deliv Rev 2003;55(1):53–81.

34. Melchior DL, Sharom FJ, Evers R, et al. Determining P-glycoprotein-drug interactions: evaluation of reconstituted P-glycoprotein in a liposomal system and LLC-MDR1 polarized cell monolayers. J Pharmacol Toxicol Methods 2012;65(2):64–74.

35. Mizutani T, Nakamura T, Morikawa R, et al. Real-time analysis of P-glycoprotein-mediated drug transport across primary intestinal epithelium three-dimensionally cultured in vitro. Biochem Biophys Res Commun 2012;419(2):238–43.

36. Pal D, Kwatra D, Minocha M, et al. Efflux transporters- and cytochrome P-450-mediated interactions between drugs of abuse and antiretrovirals. Life Sci 2011;88(21–22):959–71.

37. Hennessy M, Spiers JP. A primer on the mechanics of P-glycoprotein the multidrug transporter. Pharmacol Res 2007;55(1):1–15.

38. Brewer L, Williams D. Drug interactions that matter. Medicine (Baltimore) 2012;40(7):371–5.

39. Loo TW, Clarke DM. Do drug substrates enter the common drug-binding pocket of P-glycoprotein through 'gates'? Biochem Biophys Res Commun 2005;329(2):419–22.

40. Hennessy M, Kelleher D, Spiers JP, et al. St Johns wort increases expression of P-glycoprotein: implications for drug interactions. Br J Clin Pharmacol 2002;53(1):75–82.

41. Di Marco M, et al. The effect of grapefruit juice and Seville orange juice on the pharmacokinetics of dextromethorphan: the role of gut CYP3A and P-glycoprotein. Life Sci 2002;71(10):1149–60.

42. Jodoin J, Demeule M, Beliveau R. Inhibition of the multidrug resistance P-glycoprotein activity by green tea polyphenols. Biochim Biophys Acta 2002;1542(1–3):149–59.

43. Plouzek CA, Ciolino HP, Clarke R, et al. Inhibition of P-glycoprotein activity and reversal of multidrug resistance in vitro by rosemary extract. Eur J Cancer 1999;35(10):1541–5.

44. Anuchapreeda S, Leechanachai P, Smith MM, et al. Modulation of P-glycoprotein expression and function by curcumin in multidrug-resistant human KB cells. Biochem Pharmacol 2002;64(4):573–82.

45. Chung SY, Sung MK, Kim NH, et al. Inhibition of P-glycoprotein by natural products in human breast cancer cells. Arch Pharm Res 2005;28(7):823–8.

46. Brinkmann U, Eichelbaum M. Polymorphisms in the ABC drug transporter gene MDR1. Pharmacogenomics J 2001;1(1):59–64.

47. Brinkmann U, Roots I, Eichelbaum M. Pharmacogenetics of the human drug-transporter gene MDR1: impact of polymorphisms on pharmacotherapy. Drug Discov Today 2001;6(16):835–9.

48. Corrie K, Hardman JG. Mechanisms of Drug Interactions: pharmacodynamics and pharmacokinetics. Anaesth Intensive Care Med 2011;12(4):156–9.

49. Ismail M. Drug–food interactions and role of pharmacist. Asian J Pharm Clin Res 2009;2(4):1–10.

50. Manzi SF, Shannon M. Drug interactions: a review. Clin Pediatr Emerg Med 2005;6:93–102.

51. Grime KH, Bird J, Ferguson D, et al. Mechanism-based inhibition of cytochrome P450 enzymes: an evaluation of early decision making in vitro approaches and drug-drug interaction prediction methods. Eur J Pharm Sci 2009;36(2–3):175–91.

52. Watkins PB. Drug metabolism by cytochromes P450 in the liver and small bowel. Gastroenterol Clin North Am 1992;21(3):511–26.

53. Zanger UM, Schwab M. Cytochrome P450 enzymes in drug metabolism: regulation of gene expression, enzyme activities, and impact of genetic variation. Pharmacol Ther 2013;138(1):103–41.

54. Guengerich FP. Cytochrome p450 and chemical toxicology. Chem Res Toxicol 2008;21(1):70–83.

55. Pirmohamed M, Park BK. Cytochrome P450 enzyme polymorphisms and adverse drug reactions. Toxicology 2003;192(1):23–32.

56. Venkataramanan R, Komoroski B, Strom S. In vitro and in vivo assessment of herb drug interactions. Life Sci 2006;78(18):2105–15.

57. Guengerich FP. Cytochrome P450 enzymes. In: McQueen CA, editor. Comprehensive toxicology. Elsevier; 2010. p. 41–76.

58. Blower P, de Wit R, Goodin S, et al. Drug-drug interactions in oncology: why are they important and can they be minimized? Crit Rev Oncol Hematol 2005;55(2):117–42.

59. Shimada T, Yamazaki H, Mimura M, et al. Interindividual variations in human liver cytochrome P-450 enzymes involved in the oxidation of drugs, carcinogens and toxic chemicals: studies with liver microsomes of 30 Japanese and 30 Caucasians. J Pharmacol Exp Ther 1994;270(1):414–23.

60. Dostalek M, Pistovcakova J, Jurica J, et al. Effect of St John's wort (Hypericum perforatum) on cytochrome P-450 activity in perfused rat liver. Life Sci 2005;78(3):239–44.

61. Hammerness P, Basch E, Ulbricht C, et al. St John's wort: a systematic review of adverse effects and drug interactions for the consultation psychiatrist. Psychosomatics 2003;44(4):271–82.

62. Roby CA, Anderson GD, Kantor E, et al. St John's Wort: effect on CYP3A4 activity. Clin Pharmacol Ther 2000;67(5):451–7.

63. Moore LB, Goodwin B, Jones SA, et al. St John's wort induces hepatic drug metabolism through activation of the pregnane X receptor. Proc Natl Acad Sci USA 2000;97(13):7500–2.

64. Jobst KA, McIntyre M, St George D, et al. Safety of St John's wort (Hypericum perforatum). Lancet 2000;355(9203):575.

65. Chillistone S, Hardman JG. Modes of drug elimination and bioactive metabolites. Anaesth Intensive Care Med 2011;12(8):371–4.

66. Pleuvry BJ. Pharmacodynamic and pharmacokinetic drug interactions. Anaesth Intensive Care Med 2005;6(4):129–33.

67. Schelosky L, Raffauf C, Jendroska K, et al. Kava and dopamine antagonism. J Neurol Neurosurg Psychiatry 1995;58(5):639–40.

68. Meseguer E, Taboada R, Sanchez V, et al. Life-threatening parkinsonism induced by kava-kava. Mov Disord 2002;17(1):195–6.

69. Jamieson DD, Duffield PH. Positive interaction of ethanol and kava resin in mice. Clin Exp Pharmacol Physiol 1990;17(7):509–14.

70. Foo H, Lemon J. Acute effects of kava, alone or in combination with alcohol, on subjective measures of impairment and intoxication and on cognitive performance. Drug Alcohol Rev 1997;16(?):147–55.

71. Bone K. A clinical guide to blending liquid herbs: herbal formulations for the individual patient. St Louis: Churchill Livingstone; 2003.

72. Barnes J, et al. Herbal medicines. 2nd ed. London: Pharmaceutical Press; 2002.

73. European Scientific Cooperative on Phytotherapy Monographs. Exeter: Thieme; 2003.

74. Lourenco R. Enteral feeding: drug/nutrient interaction. Clin Nutr 2001;20(2):187–93.

75. Fish DN. Fluoroquinolone adverse effects and drug interactions. Pharmacotherapy 2001;21(10 Pt 2): 253S–272S.

76. Mimoz O, Binter V, Jacolot A, et al. Pharmacokinetics and absolute bioavailability of ciprofloxacin administered through a nasogastric tube with continuous enteral feeding to critically ill patients. Intensive Care Med 1998;24(10):1047–51.

77. van Zyl M. The effects of drugs on Nutrition. South Afr J Clin Nutr 2011;24(3):S38–41.

78. Evans WC. Trease and Evans pharmacognosy. 15th ed. Philadelphia: Saunders; 2002.

79. Pengelly A. The constituents of medicinal plants: an introduction to the chemistry and therapeutics of herbal

medicine. 2nd ed. Crows Nest NSW: Allen and Unwin; 2004.

80. Heinrich M, et al. Fundamentals of Pharmacognosy and Phytotherapy. Philadelphia: Churchill Livingstone; 2004.

81. Brune M, Rossander L, Hallberg L. Iron absorption and phenolic compounds: importance of different phenolic structures. Eur J Clin Nutr 1989;43(8):547–57.

82. Stephane J, et al. In vitro binding of calcium, iron and zinc by non-starch polysaccharides. Food Chem 2001;73(4):401–10.

83. D'Arcy PF. Nutrient-drug interactions. Adverse Drug React Toxicol Rev 1995;14(4):233–54.

84. Richter WO, Jacob BG, Schwandt P. Interaction between fibre and lovastatin. Lancet 1991;338(8768):706.

85. Stewart DE. High-fiber diet and serum tricyclic antidepressant levels. J Clin Psychopharmacol 1992;12(6):438–40.

86. Bone K. Clinical applications of Ayurvedic and Chinese herbs: monographs for the Western herbal practitioner. Warwick Qld: Phytotherapy Press; 1996.

87. Saw JT, Bahari MB, Ang HH, et al. Potential drug–herb interaction with antiplatelet/anticoagulant drugs. Complement Ther Clin Pract 2006;12(4):236–41.

APPENDIX **1**

Drug–herb interaction chart

Justin Sinclair
ND, MHerbMed

Christy Sinclair
ND, MHSc

This chart is designed as a quick reference only. Further investigation may be required before making a clinical decision. This chart has been compiled using evidence-based texts, journal articles and monographs to give a current summary of known drug–herb interactions. Where applicable, supportive evidence has been referenced to allow for further investigation. The chart has been designed using a colour-coded system to highlight the different levels of supportive evidence and clinical significance. The table uses drug classes as major headings for ease of information retrieval and provides a summary of important or clinically relevant information at the end of each heading.

The authors acknowledge Jason Rainforest for designing the chart template.

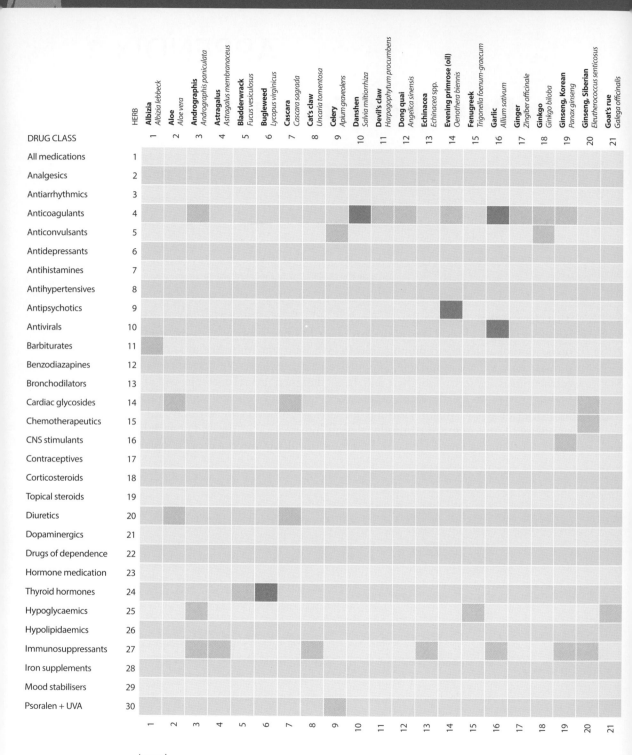

DRUG CLASS		Albizia *Albizia lebbeck* 1	Aloe *Aloe vera* 2	Andrographis *Andrographis paniculata* 3	Astragalus *Astragalus membranaceus* 4	Bladderwrack *Fucus vesiculosus* 5	Bugleweed *Lycopus virginicus* 6	Cascara *Cascara sagrada* 7	Cat's claw *Uncaria tomentosa* 8	Celery *Apium graveolens* 9	Danshen *Salvia miltiorrhiza* 10	Devil's claw *Harpagophytum procumbens* 11	Dong quai *Angelica sinensis* 12	Echinacea *Echinacea spp.* 13	Evening primrose (oil) *Oenothera biennis* 14	Fenugreek *Trigonella foenum-graecum* 15	Garlic *Allium sativum* 16	Ginger *Zingiber officinale* 17	Ginkgo *Ginkgo biloba* 18	Ginseng, Korean *Panax ginseng* 19	Ginseng, Siberian *Eleutherococcus senticosus* 20	Goat's rue *Galega officinalis* 21
All medications	1																					
Analgesics	2																					
Antiarrhythmics	3																					
Anticoagulants	4																					
Anticonvulsants	5																					
Antidepressants	6																					
Antihistamines	7																					
Antihypertensives	8																					
Antipsychotics	9																					
Antivirals	10																					
Barbiturates	11																					
Benzodiazapines	12																					
Bronchodilators	13																					
Cardiac glycosides	14																					
Chemotherapeutics	15																					
CNS stimulants	16																					
Contraceptives	17																					
Corticosteroids	18																					
Topical steroids	19																					
Diuretics	20																					
Dopaminergics	21																					
Drugs of dependence	22																					
Hormone medication	23																					
Thyroid hormones	24																					
Hypoglycaemics	25																					
Hypolipidaemics	26																					
Immunosuppressants	27																					
Iron supplements	28																					
Mood stabilisers	29																					
Psoralen + UVA	30																					

Legend

■ Implies a serious interaction with known potential to cause harm or changes in drug effectiveness. Avoid concurrent use.

▢ Use caution. Interactions have some supportive evidence. Concurrent medical supervision or avoidance is advised.

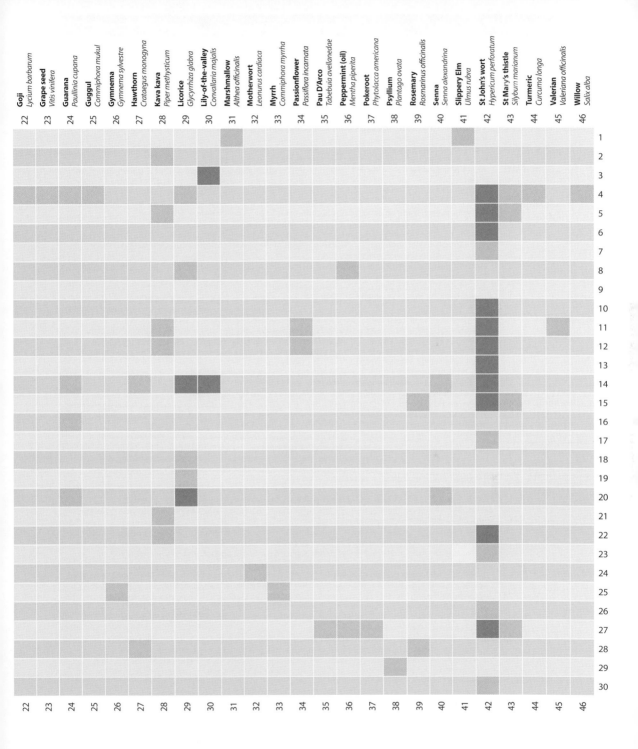

| | Goji
Lycium barbarum
22 | Grape seed
Vitis vinifera
23 | Guarana
Paullinia cupana
24 | Guggul
Commiphora mukul
25 | Gymnema
Gymnema sylvestre
26 | Hawthorn
Crataegus monogyna
27 | Kava kava
Piper methysticum
28 | Licorice
Glycyrrhiza glabra
29 | Lily-of-the-valley
Convallaria majalis
30 | Marshmallow
Althea officinalis
31 | Motherwort
Leonurus cardiaca
32 | Myrrh
Commiphora myrrha
33 | Passionflower
Passiflora incarnata
34 | Pau D'Arco
Tabebuia avellanedae
35 | Peppermint (oil)
Mentha piperita
36 | Pokeroot
Phytolacca americana
37 | Psyllium
Plantago ovata
38 | Rosemary
Rosmarinus officinalis
39 | Senna
Senna alexandrina
40 | Slippery Elm
Ulmus rubra
41 | St John's wort
Hypericum perforatum
42 | St Mary's thistle
Silybum marianum
43 | Turmeric
Curcuma longa
44 | Valerian
Valeriana officinalis
45 | Willow
Salix alba
46 | |

Drug	Herb	Drug–herb interaction
1	31	Mucilages in marshmallow may reduce the absorption of pharmaceutical medications. This is of particular importance in NTI drugs. Separate doses by a minimum of two hours.
1	41	Mucilages in slippery elm may reduce the absorption of pharmaceutical medications. This is of particular importance in NTI drugs. Separate doses by a minimum of two hours.
2	28	Kava may theoretically increase the central nervous system depressant activity of codeine and morphine. Close patient monitoring is advised.
3	30	Concurrent administration of quinidine and *Convallaria* may enhance both drug effects and side effects. Lily-of-the-valley is currently a scheduled (Schedule 4) medicine. Avoid concurrent use.
4	3	Andrographis has shown ex vivo antiplatelet activity. Andrographolide has been shown to inhibit PAF-induced platelet aggregation.[5]
4	10	Case reports suggest danshen can increase INR and prolong PTT.[5] In vitro studies have shown danshen to possess anticoagulant and fibrinolytic activity.[5] Avoid concurrent use.
4	11	A case of purpura was reported in a patient taking concurrent devil's claw and warfarin.[5] Due to lack of other medications, doses and duration of use in this case report the clinical significance is questionable. Monitor closely.
4	12	Concurrent use may increase risk of bleeding as dong quai may potentiate effects of warfarin.[5] Intravenous administration of dong quai caused prothrombin time to be significantly longer. Uncertain clinical significance for oral dosage forms of this herb.[5,7] Monitor closely.
4	14	Evening primrose oil contains gamma-linolenic acid, which can affect prostaglandin synthesis leading to inhibition of platelet aggregation.[1] Avoid high doses of the oil with concurrent use. Interaction is theoretical and of uncertain clinical significance.
4	16	Case reports have suggested that garlic may increase INR in patients on warfarin.[2] Poses a potential risk for postoperative bleeding. Caution should be exercised with patients taking any anticoagulant medication.[9] Avoid high doses of the herb (> 4 g/day equivalent fresh).
4	17	Ginger has been shown to inhibit platelet aggregation in high dose. Daily doses of 2 g/day of ginger should not be exceeded in pregnancy.[8] Avoid high dose (> 10 g/day) unless under medical supervision,[1] whereas Mills and Bone suggests > 4 g/day dried ginger requires supervision.[5] Monitor closely or avoid concurrent use.
4	18	Isolated case reports have reported increased bleeding tendency for both warfarin and aspirin.[5] Recent clinical studies show ginkgo has no significant impact on warfarin.[1] Monitor closely.
4	19	Inhibits platelet aggregation in in vitro and in vivo tests.[1] A report suggests it can lower INR in a previously stabilised patient.[7] Monitor closely.
4	22	Case report suggested increase in INR.[5] Avoid high doses of the herb.
4	23	Grapeseed is rich in polyphenolics and has the ability to inhibit platelet aggregation Caution with high doses of the herb. Interaction is theoretical and of uncertain clinical significance.
4	24	In vitro and in vivo antiplatelet activity has been established.[1,7] Interaction is of uncertain clinical significance.
4	25	In vitro and clinical data suggest that guggul increased coagulation and prothrombin time, decreased platelet adhesiveness, increased fibrinolytic activity and inhibited platelet aggregation.[6]
4	29	In vitro and in vivo tests suggest glycyrrhizin inhibits prothrombin and isoliquiritigenin inhibits platelet aggregation.[1] Interaction is of uncertain clinical significance.
4	42	Reduced blood levels of warfarin have been noted in case reports from concurrent administration of *Hypericum* preparations.[1,2,4,5] St John's wort is a known inducer of cytochrome P450 enzymes, causing increased drug metabolism. Avoid concurrent use.
4	43	Due to St Mary's thistle having inhibitive effects on the cytochrome P450 system, a potential increase in drug levels is possible.[1] Interaction is of uncertain clinical significance.
4	44	Curcumin, a key constituent of turmeric, has been shown to inhibit platelet aggregation in vitro.[11] Caution with doses greater than 15 g/day.[5]
4	46	Clinical study observed willow to have antiplatelet activity.[5] Higher doses than 240 mg of salicin per day may have a more significant effect.[1] Monitor patient closely in higher dosage.
5	9	In vivo test on rats found that celery juice prolonged the action of phenobarbitone.[1] Interaction is of uncertain clinical significance.
5	18	In vivo animal studies and two case reports suggest a potential interaction is possible with concurrent use of ginkgo, causing reduced drug effects.[5] Interaction is of uncertain clinical significance.
5	28	Isolated methysticin reversibly blocked epileptiform activity in various in vitro seizure models, showing anticonvulsant activity.[2] Interaction is of uncertain clinical significance.
5	42	St John's wort is known to induce the cytochrome P450 system, resulting in the increased metabolism of multiple drugs.[1] Avoid concurrent use.
5	43	St Mary's thistle has been shown to inhibit cytochrome P450 3A4, therefore reducing drug metabolism. This may lead to increased blood levels of carbamazepine and associated adverse effects.[1]
6	42	Potential for serotonergic syndrome with concurrent use.[1,2,5] St John's wort may decrease tricyclic drug plasma levels, and also may increase available serotonin. Avoid if possible, or use only under close medical supervision.
7	42	A clinical study demonstrated the potential for St John's wort to decrease drug levels.[5] Monitor patient.
8	29	High-dose administration for longer than six weeks may result in pseudoaldosteronism and blood pressure increase.[5] Avoid long-term use at doses > 100 mg/day of glycyrrhizin.[5]
8	36	Animal studies have shown the oil of peppermint to increase felodipine bioavailability.[1] Monitor patient as drug dosage requirement may need modification.
9	14	Case reports suggest that evening primrose oil may reduce seizure threshold and reduce drug effectiveness in patients with schizophrenia being administered phenothiazines.[1] Avoid concurrent use until safety profile is established.[1]
10	16	Garlic has been demonstrated in a clinical study to reduce serum levels of saquinivir and drug effectiveness, resulting in poor clinical outcomes.[1] Avoid concurrent use.
10	42	St John's wort is known to reduce drug levels via the cytochrome P450 and P-gp systems, resulting in reduced drug effectiveness and poor clinical outcomes.[1,5] Avoid concurrent use.

Drug	Herb	Drug–herb interaction (continued)
11	1	In vivo studies demonstrated a potentiation of phenobarbitone-induced sleeping time.[1] Interaction may be beneficial but is of uncertain clinical significance and requires medical supervision. Use caution.
11	28	Potential to increase sedative effects.[1] Interaction may be beneficial but is of uncertain clinical significance and requires medical supervision. Drug dosage modification may be required.
11	34	Potential to increase sedative effects.[1] Interaction may be beneficial but is of uncertain clinical significance and requires medical supervision.
11	42	St John's wort is known to induce the cytochrome P450 system and P-gp, resulting in reduced drug levels and poor clinical outcomes.[1] Avoid concurrent use
11	45	Potential to increase sedative effects.[1] Interaction may be beneficial but is of uncertain clinical significance and requires medical supervision.
12	28	Kava can be used to ease the symptoms of benzodiazepine withdrawal if done under medical supervision.[1] Drug dosage modification may be required.
12	34	Potential to increase sedative effects. Interaction may be beneficial, but is of uncertain clinical significance and requires medical supervision.[1]
12	42	A clinical study demonstrated reduced drug levels with concurrent midazolam and St John's wort use.[5] Avoid concurrent use unless under medical supervision. Drug dosage modification may be required.
13	42	St John's wort is known to induce the cytochrome P450 system and P-gp. Case reports show herb can decrease serum levels.[1,2,4,5] Avoid concurrent use.
14	2	Oral use of aloe long-term may deplete potassium levels, which lower the threshold for digoxin toxicity.[1,5] Avoid concurrent long-term use unless under medical supervision.
14	7	Avoid excessive use of laxative herbs as enhanced digoxin toxicity caused by lowered potassium levels is possible.[5] Avoid concurrent long-term use unless under medical supervision.
14	20	Siberian ginseng has the potential to interfere with digoxin assay,[5] and may produce false positive test results.[1]
14	24	Long-term use of high-dose guarana can deplete potassium levels, which lowers the threshold for digoxin toxicity.[1] Avoid concurrent long-term use unless under medical supervision.
14	27	In vitro and in vivo studies demonstrate hawthorn as having a positively inotropic and chronotropic activity.[1] Interaction may be beneficial, but is of uncertain clinical significance.
14	29	Long-term use of high-dose licorice can deplete potassium levels, which lowers the threshold for digoxin toxicity.[1,5] Avoid concurrent use.
14	30	Concurrent administration of digoxin and *Convallaria* may enhance drug effects and side effects.[7] Avoid concurrent use.
14	40	Avoid excessive use of laxative herbs as enhanced digoxin toxicity caused by lowered potassium levels is possible.[5] Avoid concurrent long-term use unless under medical supervision.
14	42	St John's wort is known to induce the cytochrome P450 system and P-gp,[1] resulting in the increased metabolism of digoxin. A clinical study demonstrated that St John's wort significantly decreased serum levels of digoxin within 10 days of concurrent use.[1] Avoid concurrent use.[2,4,7]
15	20	Co-administration may increase drug tolerance and improve patient immune function.[1] Interaction may be beneficial but is of uncertain clinical significance and requires medical supervision.
15	39	Rosemary inhibits P-glycoprotein so may affect the bioavailability of P-gp substrates.
15	42	Clinical studies have shown St John's wort may decrease drug levels resulting in poor clinical outcomes.[5] Avoid concurrent use.
15	43	Research suggests that St Mary's thistle may reduce toxic effects[1] and may reduce drug efficacy. Interaction may be beneficial and requires medical supervision.
16	19	Based on the pharmacological activity of Korean ginseng, the potential to increase stimulating effects exists. Interaction is of uncertain clinical significance.
16	24	Based on the pharmacological activity of guarana, the potential to increase stimulating effects exists.
17	42	Breakthrough bleeding has been reported in 12 cases: this is suggestive of reduced drug effectiveness.[1] Reports from Britain and Sweden suggest unwanted pregnancies have occurred with concurrent use.[8] Avoid use with low-dose oral contraceptive pill (OCP) (< 50 mcg of oestrogen) if possible.[1,2]
18	29	Concurrent use of licorice preparations has been shown to increase the effects of both topical and oral corticosteroids.[1]
19	29	Concurrent use of licorice preparations has been shown to increase the effects of both topical and oral corticosteroids.[1]
20	2	Oral use of aloe long term may deplete potassium levels.[5] Monitor patient.
20	7	Oral use of cascara long term may deplete potassium levels.[5] Monitor patient.
20	24	Guarana may theoretically increase diuresis while also decreasing hyptotensive activity.[1] Interaction is of uncertain clinical significance.
20	29	Long-term use of high dose licorice can deplete potassium levels.[1,5] Avoid doses > 100 mg/day glycyrrhizin for periods more than two weeks.[1] Monitor patient.
20	40	Oral use of senna long term may deplete potassium levels.[5] Monitor patient.
21	28	Dopamine antagonistic effects have been reported.[1] Avoid concurrent use unless under medical supervision.
22	28	Based on the pharmacological activity of kava, concurrent use may theoretically increase sedation.[1] Interaction is theoretical and of uncertain clinical significance.
22	42	St John's wort may decrease serum levels of methadone.[1] Avoid concurrent use.
23	42	St John's wort is known to induce the cytochrome P450 system and P-gp,[1] resulting in the increased metabolism of medications. Decrease drug efficacy of hormone replacement therapy or OCP is possible.
24	5	Based on the pharmacological activity of bladderwrack, the potential to interact with preparations containing thyroid hormones exists.[8]
24	6	Based on the pharmacological activity of bugleweed, the potential to interact with preparations containing thyroid hormones exists.[8] Avoid concurrent use. Bugleweed may also interfere with thyroid diagnostic procedures that utilise radioactive isotopes.[8]
24	32	Based on the pharmacological activity of motherwort, the potential to interact with preparations containing thyroid hormones exists.[8] Avoid concurrent use.

Drug	Herb	Drug–herb interaction (continued)
25	3	Andrographis has shown hypoglycaemic activity in vivo comparable to metformin.[1] Interaction is theoretical and of uncertain clinical significance. Monitor patient's blood sugar level (BSL).
25	15	Fenugreek reduces BSL but the exact mechanism of action is unclear.[7] Monitor patient's BSL. Drug dose modification may be required.
25	21	Galegine, an alkaloid from goat's rue, has been shown to have hypoglycaemic properties. Use cautiously and monitor patient's BSL regularly.[5] Drug dose modification may be required.
25	26	Gymnema has a well-documented hypoglycaemic activity causing the enhanced reduction of blood glucose. Use cautiously and monitor patient's BSL regularly.[5] Drug dose modification may be required.
25	33	Two furanosesquiterpenes isolated from myrrh exhibited hypoglycaemic activity in vivo in normal and diabetic models.[8] Interaction is theoretical and of uncertain clinical significance. Monitor patient's BSL.
26	42	St John's wort increases the metabolism of simvastatin, and therefore drug dosage modification may be required.[1]
27	3	Due to the known immunostimulant activity of andrographis, a theoretical potential for reduced drug effectiveness exists. Interaction is of uncertain clinical significance.
27	4	Due to the known immunostimulant activity of astragalus, a theoretical potential for reduced drug effectiveness exists. Interaction is of uncertain clinical significance.
27	8	Due to the known immunostimulant activity of cat's claw, a theoretical potential for reduced drug effectiveness exists. The manufacturers of products standardised to pentacyclic oxindole alkaloids (POAs) warn against the use of cat's claw in patients receiving immunosuppressive medications.[5] Interaction is of uncertain clinical significance.
27	13	Due to the known immunostimulant activity of echinacea, a theoretical potential for reduced drug effectiveness exists.[5] Interaction is of uncertain clinical significance.
27	16	Due to the known immunostimulant activity of garlic,[1] a theoretical potential for reduced drug effectiveness exists. Interaction is of uncertain clinical significance.
27	19	Due to the known immunostimulant activity of Korean ginseng, a theoretical potential for reduced drug effectiveness exists. Interaction is of uncertain clinical significance.
27	20	Due to the known immunostimulant activity of Siberian ginseng, a theoretical potential for reduced drug effectiveness exists. Interaction is of uncertain clinical significance.
27	35	Due to the known immunostimulant activity of pau d'arco, a theoretical potential for reduced drug effectiveness exists. Interaction is of uncertain clinical significance.
27	36	Peppermint oil has been shown in animal studies to increase the oral bioavailability of cyclosporine.[1] Interaction is of uncertain clinical significance.
27	37	Due to the known immunostimulant activity of pokeroot a theoretical potential for reduced drug effectiveness exists. Interaction is of uncertain clinical significance.
27	42	St John's wort is known to induce the cytochrome P450 system and P-gp. Case reports suggest it may reduce drug effectiveness.[5] Avoid concurrent use.
27	43	Research suggests that St Mary's thistle and cisplatin may reduce toxicity effects.[1] Interaction may be beneficial and requires medical supervision.
28	27	Clinical studies have shown the ability for tannins and other polyphenolics to reduce iron absorption. Separate doses of iron by two hours. Caution in patients suffering from anaemia.
28	39	Clinical studies have shown the ability for tannins and other polyphenolics to reduce iron absorption. Separate doses of iron by two hours. Caution in patients suffering from anaemia.
29	38	A case report suggests decreased lithium concentrations with concurrent administration of psyllium,[5] resulting in reduced drug effectiveness. Ensure dosage is separated by a minimum of two hours.
30	9	Celery contains psoralens; however, it does not seem to be photosensitising even after large oral doses. May increase the risk of phototoxicity with concurrent PUVA (psoralen and ultraviolet A) therapy.[1] Interaction is of uncertain clinical significance.
30	42	Hypericin may increase sensitivity to ultraviolet radiation.[1] Use caution, especially in preparations containing high hypericin content. Interaction is of uncertain clinical significance.

REFERENCES

1. Braun L, Cohen M. Herbs and natural supplements: an evidence-based guide. Marrickville: Elsevier; 2005.
2. ESCOP Monographs. 2nd ed. Exeter European Scientific Cooperative on Phytotherapy; 2003.
3. Wilt T, Ishani A, Mac Donald R, et al. Pygeum africanum for benign prostatic hyperplasia. Cochrane Database Syst Rev 2008;3:1–20.
4. WHO monographs on selected medicinal plants. Geneva: World Health Organization; 2003.
5. Mills S, Bone K. The essential guide to herbal safety. St Louis, Missouri: Churchill Livingstone; 2005.
6. Bone K. Clinical applications of Ayurvedic and Chinese herbs: monographs for the Western herbal practitioner. Warwick: Phytotherapy Press; 1996.
7. Gruenwald J, Brendler T, Jaenicke C. Physicians desk reference for herbal medicines. 3rd ed. Montvale: Thomson PDR; 2004.
8. Bone K. A clinical guide to blending liquid herbs: herbal formulations for the individual patient. St Louis: Churchill Livingstone; 2003.
9. WHO monographs on selected medicinal plants. Geneva: World Health Organization; 1999.
10. Blumenthal M, Brinckmann J, Wollschlaeger B. The ABC clinical guide to herbs. 1st ed. Austin: American Botanical Council; 2003.
11. Mills S, Bone K. Principles and practice of phytotherapy. London: Churchill Livingstone; 2000.

APPENDIX **2**

Drug–nutrient interaction chart

Justin Sinclair
ND, MHerbMEd
Christine Sinclair
ND, MHSc

This chart is designed as a quick reference only. Further investigation may be required before making a clinical decision. This chart has been compiled using evidence-based texts, journal articles and monographs to give a current summary of known drug–nutrient interactions. Where applicable, supportive evidence has been referenced to allow for further investigation. The chart has been designed using a colour-coded system to highlight the different levels of supportive evidence and clinical significance. The table uses drug classes as major headings for ease of information retrieval, and provides a summary of important or clinically relevant information at the end of each heading.

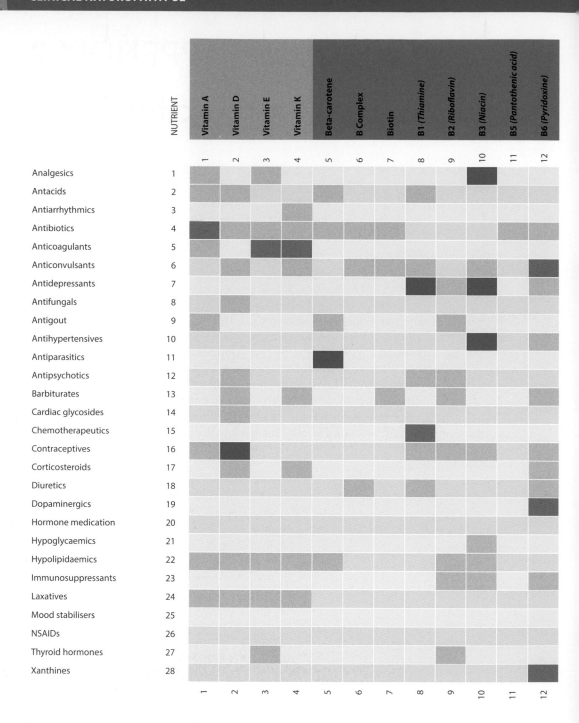

Nutrient columns: 1 Vitamin A, 2 Vitamin D, 3 Vitamin E, 4 Vitamin K, 5 Beta-carotene, 6 B Complex, 7 Biotin, 8 B1 (Thiamine), 9 B2 (Riboflavin), 10 B3 (Niacin), 11 B5 (Pantothenic acid), 12 B6 (Pyridoxine)

Drug rows: 1 Analgesics, 2 Antacids, 3 Antiarrhythmics, 4 Antibiotics, 5 Anticoagulants, 6 Anticonvulsants, 7 Antidepressants, 8 Antifungals, 9 Antigout, 10 Antihypertensives, 11 Antiparasitics, 12 Antipsychotics, 13 Barbiturates, 14 Cardiac glycosides, 15 Chemotherapeutics, 16 Contraceptives, 17 Corticosteroids, 18 Diuretics, 19 Dopaminergics, 20 Hormone medication, 21 Hypoglycaemics, 22 Hypolipidaemics, 23 Immunosuppressants, 24 Laxatives, 25 Mood stabilisers, 26 NSAIDs, 27 Thyroid hormones, 28 Xanthines

Legend

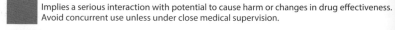 Implies a serious interaction with potential to cause harm or changes in drug effectiveness. Avoid concurrent use unless under close medical supervision.

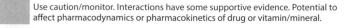 Use caution/monitor. Interactions have some supportive evidence. Potential to affect pharmacodynamics or pharmacokinetics of drug or vitamin/mineral.

 Potentially beneficial interaction.

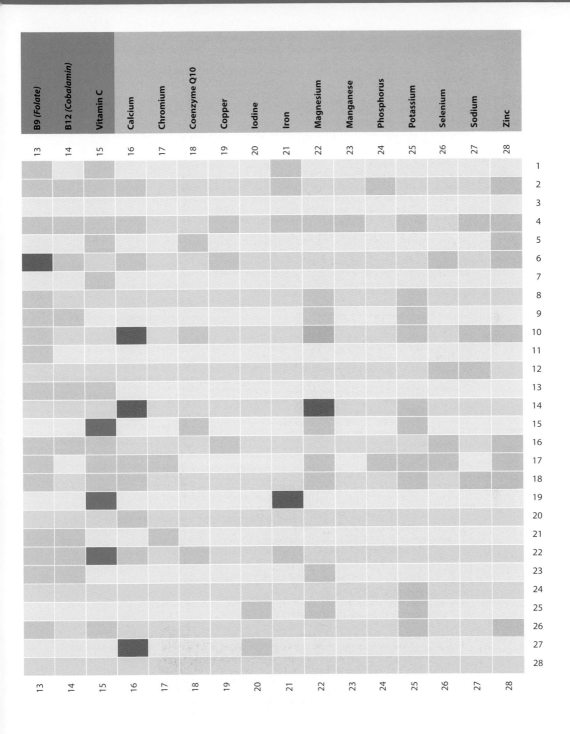

Drug	Nutrient	Drug–nutrient interaction
1	1	Salicylates reduce vitamin A clearance.[5]
1	3	Vitamin E can potentially have an additive effect (e.g. reducing platelet aggregation) with co-administration of aspirin.[6,7]
1	10	Aspirin may decrease high-dose nicotinic acid-induced flushing.[6]
1	13	Aspirin can inhibit folate-dependent enzymes, interfere with folate metabolism and increase urinary excretion. Supplement folic acid with high-dose or chronic aspirin use.[2,7]
1	15	Vitamin C decreases elimination of salicylates (i.e. aspirin); salicylates reduces vitamin C absorption.[3,5,6,8]
1	21	Salicylates increase iron losses from digestive tract. Chronic use or high dose of aspirin increases the risk of iron deficiency or anaemia due to gastrointestinal (GI) bleeding.[5,7]
2	1	Antacids potentially reduce vitamin A absorption.[5]
2	2	H₂ antagonists may inhibit action of vitamin D hydroxylase and could reduce hepatic activation of vitamin D, potentially causing deficiency.[7]
2	5	Proton-pump inhibitors may reduce absorption of beta-carotene by inhibiting gastric acid production.[7]
2	8	Antacids interfere with the absorption of thiamine. Separate intake of thiamine and antacids by a minimum of two hours.[7]
2	13	H₂ antagonists and other antacids that interfere with pH balance in the GI tract can impair folic acid absorption and availability.[7]
2	14	Proton-pump inhibitors may decrease absorption of B12. H₂ antagonists may deplete B12 stores.[2,5,6,7,8]
2	15	Antacids reduce vitamin C absorption. Vitamin C can increase the amount of aluminium absorbed in aluminium-based antacids (separate doses by a minimum of two hours).[5,8]
2	16	Proton-pump inhibitors and H₂ antagonists decrease absorption of calcium.[6,7]
2	21	H₂ antagonists and proton-pump inhibitors can reduce absorption and bioavailability of iron. Iron can bind cimetidine in the GI tract and reduce its absorption.[4,7,8]
2	24	Aluminium-containing antacids reduce phosphorus absorption.[5,6]
2	28	H₂ antagonists may deplete zinc absorption and availability; separate zinc administration from drug by a minimum of two hours.[2,7]
3	4	Quinidine impairs vitamin K status.[5]
4	1	Neomycin reduces absorption of vitamin A. Concurrent use of tetracycline antibiotics and vitamin A is associated with adverse effects such as headache and benign intracranial hypertension. Concurrent use is contraindicated, particularly at vitamin A doses over 10,000 IU per day.[5,7]
4	2	Rifampicin increases vitamin D turnover; neomycin can impair absorption of vitamin D. Supplement with vitamin D with extended antibiotic use.[1,5,7]
4	3	Neomycin can impair absorption/utilisation of Vitamin E.[5,6]
4	4	Tetracycline, chloramphenicol and neomycin reduces endogenous vitamin K production by colonic bacteria.[5,7]
4	5	Neomycin can impair absorption and increase elimination of beta-carotene.[5,7]
4	6	B vitamins may interfere with tetracycline pharmacokinetics; concomitant intake may significantly impair bioavailability.[7]
4	7	Neomycin and chloramphenicol reduce endogenous biotin production by colonic bacteria.[5,6]
4	11	Antibiotics can reduce endogenous production of vitamin B5 by GI flora.[8]
4	12	Chloramphenicol and cycloserine increases urinary vitamin B6 excretion; neomycin may interfere with activity of vitamin B6; gentamicin may interfere with vitamin B6 metabolism and contribute to its depletion. Simultaneous intake of pyridoxine with tetracyclines can reduce absorption and availability of both agents.[5,6,7]
4	13	Trimethoprim may cause folic acid depletion by reducing absorption and impairing metabolism; sulphonamide impairs folate metabolism; nitrofurantoin and neomycin reduces folate absorption; chloramphenicol increases folate requirements; cycloserine impairs folate metabolism.[2,5]
4	14	Chloramphenicol reduces B12 absorption; cycloserine impairs vitamin B12 metabolism; aminoglycoside antibiotics decrease vitamin B12 absorption and biosynthesis, interferes with metabolism and increases B12 elimination.[5,7]
4	15	Tetracycline impairs vitamin C metabolism and increases urinary excretion. Gentamicin efficacy may be decreased by vitamin C. Monitor closely.[2,5]
4	16	Aminoglycosides may increase calcium excretion; chelation may occur between calcium and tetracycline which can impair the absorption of both agents.[2,7,8]
4	19	Copper can bind to ciprofloxacin and reduce its absorption. Separate doses by a minimum of two hours.[7]
4	21	Tetracycline antibiotics, chloramphenicol and neomycin can decrease iron's effectiveness.[4]
4	22	Aminoglycosides increase urinary excretion of magnesium; tetracyclines form insoluble complexes with magnesium thereby reducing absorption of both. Separate doses by at least two hours.[2,8]
4	23	Tetracycline reduces absorption of manganese.[6]
4	25	Aminoglycosides increase urinary excretion of potassium; penicillin increases urinary potassium excretion.[2,5]
4	27	Aminoglycosides may deplete sodium stores.[2]
4	28	Chelation between tetracycline (other than doxycycline) and zinc can cause impaired absorption of both agents. Ciprofloxacin may bind with zinc, inhibiting absorption and availability of both agents.[2,5,7]
5	1	Large doses of vitamin A may enhance anticoagulant response and increase risk of bleeding. Monitor patient closely in higher dosage.[2]
5	3	High-dose vitamin E may enhance the effect of coumadin-derived anticoagulants by decreasing vitamin K levels and activity. Avoid concurrent use.[2,5,6,7]
5	4	High-dose vitamin K will interfere with the therapeutic action of warfarin. Avoid concurrent use.[2,5,7]
5	15	Vitamin C can shorten prothrombin time and antagonise warfarin response.[2,5]
5	18	Coenzyme Q10 may decrease the effectiveness of warfarin. Case reports have been documented of coenzyme Q10 decreasing INR in patients previously stabilised on anticoagulant therapy.[6,8]
5	28	Binding may occur with zinc and warfarin, inhibiting absorption and bioavailability of both. Separate doses to reduce likelihood of this occurring. Monitor patient closely.[7]

Drug	Nutrient	Drug–nutrient interaction (continued)
6	2	Phenytoin increases vitamin D metabolism in the liver and may reduce serum levels; primidone increases vitamin D breakdown and excretion. Monitor serum vitamin D levels and bone status.[5,7,8]
6	4	Phenytoin and phenobarbitone may increase the breakdown of vitamin K; primidone increases vitamin K breakdown and excretion.[5,6,7]
6	6	Dilantin may increase the risk of anaemia and nerve problems due to deficiency of B vitamins. Zonisamide may deplete stores of B1, B2, B3, B6, B12.[1,2]
6	7	Phenytoin, phenobarbitone, primidone and carbamazepine may decrease biotin levels.[6]
6	8	Phenytoin interferes with thiamine function causing thiamine levels to be depleted. Monitor for signs of deficiency.[7]
6	10	Niacinamide may potentiate action of anticonvulsants (primidone, carbamazepine) by decreasing drug clearance.[6,7]
6	12	High doses of B6 increase catabolism of phenytoin; primidone decreases serum B6 levels; valproic acid may decrease plasma B6 levels in chronic use; carbamazepine may decrease plasma B6 levels with chronic use. Anticonvulsants may increase the risk of hyperhomocysteinaemia.[5,6,7]
6	13	Folate reduces phenytoin bioavailability and may antagonise its anticonvulsant action. Primidone may cause folic acid deficiency leading to megaloblastic anaemia; valproic acid may decrease folate levels; carbamazepine may decrease folate levels. High doses of folic acid may decrease serum levels of those drugs listed here.[2,5,6]
6	14	Long-term carbamazepine usage led to a decrease in vitamin B12 levels in children; primidone decreases serum B12 levels. Monitor for B12 deficiency.[5,8]
6	16	Phenytoin and primidone reduces calcium absorption and can reduce serum levels of vitamin D. Monitor closely in those at risk of osteoporosis.[5,7]
6	19	Valproic acid may induce copper deficiency by increasing excretion into bile; phenytoin may increase serum copper levels. Clinical significance unknown.[5,7]
6	26	Valproic acid reduces selenium serum levels.[5,7]
6	28	Valproic acid reduces zinc serum levels; phenytoin increases zinc requirements.[5,7]
7	8	Co-administration of B vitamins (particularly thiamine) with tricyclic antidepressants such as nortriptyline have shown improved response.[7]
7	9	Tricyclic antidepressants inhibit riboflavin conversion of flavin mononucleotide (FMN) and flavin adenine dinucleotide (FAD), impairing riboflavin absorption and activity. Co-administration of B2 is advisable under medical supervision.[5,6,7,8]
7	10	Combination of imipramine, tryptophan and niacinamide has been shown to more effective for bipolar disorder than imipramine alone.[8]
7	12	Phenelzine may act as a pyridoxine antagonist and reduce levels of vitamin B6.[7]
7	19	Megadoses (> 2 g/d) may reduce therapeutic response of tricyclic antidepressants. Monitor patient closely in higher dosage.[2]
8	2	Ketoconazole may decrease serum 1,25 dihydroxyvitamin D levels. Monitor for vitamin D deficiency with long-term use.[6,7,8]
8	13	Pentamidine may impair folate metabolism.[5]
8	22	Magnesium may reduce absorption of ketoconazole; amphotericin B may increase urinary magnesium excretion.[5]
8	25	Fluconazole may cause hypokalaemia; amphotericin B may increase urinary potassium excretion.[2,5]
9	1	Colchicine may impair vitamin A absorption and interfere with retinol homoeostasis by blocking release of retinol-binding protein.[5,7]
9	5	Colchicine may induce intestinal malabsorption of beta-carotene and block hepatic release of retinol-binding protein.[5,7]
9	9	Probenecid impairs absorption of vitamin B2.[5,6,7]
9	13	Colchicine may decrease folate levels; however, major supportive evidence is lacking.[6,7]
9	14	Colchicine may interfere with vitamin B12 absorption and metabolism by reducing IF-B12 receptors. Monitor for B12 deficiency.[5,6,7]
9	22	Colchicine may impair absorption of magnesium; however, major supportive evidence is lacking. Consider separation of doses.[7]
9	25	Colchicine may impair absorption and increase loss of potassium.[7]
10	10	High doses of niacin may enhance the hypotensive action of alpha adrenergic blockers.[6]
10	12	Hydralazine increases urinary excretion of vitamin B6 and acts as a well-known B6 antagonist.[5,6,7]
10	13	Hydralazine may impair folate metabolism.[5]
10	16	Calcium may have an antagonistic effect on the therapeutic action of calcium channel blockers, potentially increasing risk of arrhythmias. Avoid high-dose supplements.[8]
10	18	Hydralazine may reduce coenzyme Q10 serum levels.[8]
10	22	Magnesium may enhance the hypotensive effect of calcium channel blockers.[8]
10	25	ACE inhibitors can elevate potassium levels in patients with impaired renal function; beta-blockers can elevate potassium levels and cause hyperkalaemia.[2,3,5,6,7]
10	27	ACE inhibitors may increase sodium excretion.[3]
10	28	ACE inhibitors may bind to zinc ions, depleting zinc tissue levels causing a possible deficiency.[7]
11	5	Combining anthelmintic agents with increased beta-carotene intake can reduce symptoms of intestinal parasites while supporting epithelial integrity and immune response.[7]
11	13	Pyrimethamine reduces folic acid levels in serum.[2,5]
12	2	Cholecalciferol may decrease metabolism of thioridazine, potentially increasing activity and adverse effects of the drug by inhibiting cytochrome P450 2D6.[7]
12	8	Neuroleptics may reduce thiamine absorption and increase excretion.[5]
12	9	Phenothiazine and chlorpromazine impair riboflavin metabolism. Simultaneous intake may impair activity of both drug and vitamin.[5,7]

Drug	Nutrient	Drug–nutrient interaction (continued)
12	26	Clozapine may decrease selenium levels.[7]
12	27	Increased sodium intake decreases lithium's effectiveness; decreased sodium intake may increase lithium toxicity.[2]
13	2	Phenobarbitone can interfere with vitamin D metabolism and decrease serum levels.[2,6]
13	4	Barbiturates may increase vitamin K breakdown and biliary excretion.[5]
13	7	Barbiturates may decrease plasma biotin levels.[5,6]
13	9	Barbiturates impair riboflavin metabolism and decrease serum levels.[5,7]
13	12	B6 may reduce barbiturate response. Monitor patient closely.[2]
13	13	High doses of folate may reverse the effects of barbiturates.[5]
13	14	Barbiturates may impair vitamin B12 metabolism and decrease serum levels.[5]
13	15	Phenobarbitone can decrease ascorbic acid absorption.[2]
14	2	Vitamin D may interact with digoxin causing hypercalcaemia leading to arrhythmias. Monitor patient closely.[2]
14	16	Administered concurrently, high-dose calcium supplements can act synergistically with cardiac glycosides, which may induce arrhythmias and potentiate their toxicity.[8]
14	22	Magnesium and digoxin may chelate reducing absorption and bioavailability of both agents.[2,7]
14	25	Hypokalaemia may enhance toxic effect of digoxin. Monitor potassium levels closely.[2,7]
15	8	Fluorouracil inhibits conversion of thiamine to thiamine pyrophosphatase. Thiamine restriction and depletion is considered essential. Close medical supervision advised.[2,7]
15	15	Vitamin C may potentiate antineoplastic activity of paclitaxel, cisplatin and adriamycin. Potential beneficial interaction but specialist monitoring and guidance is essential.[6,8]
15	18	Adriamycin increases coenzyme Q10 requirements.[5]
15	22	Cisplatin can deplete magnesium stores resulting in hypomagnesaemia.[2,5,7]
15	25	Cisplatin may increase potassium excretion via the urine.[5]
16	1	Oral contraceptives may increase serum vitamin A levels. Monitor patient.[2,5,6,8]
16	2	Vitamin D acts synergistically with oestrogen to prevent bone loss.[8]
16	8	Decreases in thiamine levels seen with oral contraceptive use.[7]
16	9	Oral contraceptives may increase demand for vitamin B2. Consider increasing intake with long-term use.[8]
16	10	Oral contraceptives may reduce vitamin B3 levels.[8]
16	12	Oral contraceptives may reduce the absorption of B6 and increase requirements. Monitor patient.[1]
16	13	Folic acid requirements are increased with concurrent use.[2,7,8]
16	14	Oral contraceptives may decrease vitamin B12 serum concentrations. Consider supplementation with long-term use.[4,7]
16	15	Intermittent use may cause contraceptive failure; oral contraceptives may cause increased ascorbic acid turnover in tissues and reduce plasma levels.[2,5,7]
16	19	Exogenous female hormones (particularly progestin) may enhance copper absorption and elevate levels.[5,7]
16	26	Oral contraceptives may decrease selenium levels.[7]
16	28	Oral contraceptives may decrease serum levels of zinc.[5,7]
17	2	Corticosteroids increase vitamin D requirements by reducing calcium uptake and depleting active vitamin D via unknown mechanisms.[5,7,8]
17	4	Corticosteroids can cause increased urinary loss of vitamin K.[7]
17	12	Corticosteroids may increase urinary excretion of vitamin B6.[5]
17	13	Corticosteroids may impair folate metabolism.[5]
17	15	Corticosteroids increase vitamin C requirements based on experimental data. Consider supplementation with long term drug therapy.[5,8]
17	16	Corticosteroids reduce calcium absorption and increase urinary excretion.[5,7]
17	17	Corticosteroids increase chromium excretion and may play a role in steroid-induced diabetes.[7,8]
17	22	Corticosteroids may reduce absorption of magnesium. Consider supplementation with long-term drug therapy.[5,7]
17	24	Corticosteroids reduce phosphorus absorption and increase urinary excretion.[5]
17	25	Corticosteroids may deplete potassium levels to a clinically significant degree.[5,7]
17	26	High-dose oral corticosteroids increase urinary selenium loss and may lower plasma selenium levels.[7]
17	28	Internal or exogenous glucocorticoids can affect zinc metabolism. Oral corticosteroids may increase urinary zinc excretion.[5,7]
18	6	Thiazides increase urinary excretion of B vitamins.[5]
18	8	Bumetanide and furosemide (loop diuretics) may cause thiamine deficiency with chronic use.[6,7]
18	12	Furosemide increases urinary excretion of vitamin B6 in chronic renal failure.[7]
18	13	Potassium sparing diuretics (triamterene) may cause folic acid depletion.[2,5,7]
18	15	Thiazides increase urinary excretion of vitamin C; ascorbic acid (co-administered) can increase the bioavailability of furosemide and enhance its diuretic and natriuretic effects.[5,7]
18	16	Thiazides increase calcium retention by decreasing urinary excretion of calcium.[5,7,8]
18	22	Diuretics may inhibit magnesium absorption and increase urinary excretion of magnesium, increasing potassium depletion.[5,7,8]
18	25	Potassium wasting diuretics may cause hypokalaemia. Monitor patient.[7]
18	27	Furosemide may deplete sodium and other electrolytes.[2]
18	28	Thiazides can increase urinary excretion of zinc; potassium sparing diuretics (amiloride) may cause zinc accumulation by reducing urinary excretion; triamterene may increase urinary zinc excretion in the short term and may cause depletion in extended use.[5,7,8]
19	12	High levels of pyridoxine may accelerate peripheral conversion of levodopa to dopamine, reduce the availability of dopa for conversion to dopamine and impair the therapeutic activity of levodopa. Avoid supplemental intake of vitamin B6 with levodopa monotherapy.[5,6,7]
19	15	A case report suggests levodopa co-administration with vitamin C may reduce drug side effects.[8]

Drug	Nutrient	Drug–nutrient interaction (continued)
19	21	Concurrent administration of iron with levodopa/carbidopa may reduce the bioavailability of both drugs. Separate doses by two hours.[6,7,8]
20	16	Oestrogen replacement therapy increases calcium absorption and decreases urinary excretion.[5]
21	10	Niacin may reduce the effectiveness of certain oral hypoglycaemic drugs.[5,8]
21	13	Metformin decreases serum folate levels; folic acid may reduce metformin-associated homocysteinaemia.[5,6]
21	14	Metformin reduces vitamin B12 absorption and lowers serum B12 levels.[5,6,7,8]
21	17	Chromium enhances hypoglycaemic action of insulin through multiple mechanisms. Both potentially beneficial and dangerous. Close patient monitoring advised.[5,7]
22	1	Cholestyramine and colestipol decreases vitamin A absorption; HMG-CoA reductase inhibitors increase serum levels of vitamin A; orlistat may decrease vitamin A absorption.[2,4,5,6,7,8]
22	2	Cholestyramine and colestipol decrease vitamin D absorption; orlistat may reduce vitamin D absorption.[2,5,6,7,8]
22	3	Cholestyramine and colestipol decrease vitamin E absorption; orlistat reduces vitamin E absorption.[2,5,6]
22	4	Cholestyramine and colestipol decrease vitamin K absorption.[2,5,7]
22	5	Cholestyramine and colestipol decrease beta-carotene absorption; orlistat may decrease absorption of beta-carotene.[5,6,7,8]
22	9	Cholestyramine and colestipol decrease absorption of riboflavin.[6]
22	10	Cholestyramine and colestipol may reduce nicotinic acid absorption and may have synergistic antihyperlipidaemic effects. Potentially beneficial interaction.[2,6]
22	13	Cholestyramine decreases folate absorption.[2,8]
22	14	Cholestyramine and colestipol may decrease enterohepatic reabsorption of vitamin B12.[6]
22	15	Vitamin C taken with chitosan may increase the cholesterol-lowering effect.[8]
22	16	Cholestyramine and colestipol decrease calcium absorption.[2,5,7]
22	18	HMG-CoA reductase inhibitors impair coenzyme Q10 metabolism.[5]
22	21	Bile acid sequestrants reduce iron absorption.[4,7,8]
23	9	Methotrexate impairs riboflavin metabolism.[5]
23	10	Azathioprine can deplete niacin.[7]
23	12	Azathioprine increases urinary vitamin B6 excretion.[5]
23	13	Methotrexate may cause folate deficiency; folate supplementation may decrease methotrexate effects. Closely monitor patient. Azathioprine impairs folate metabolism.[2,5,8]
23	14	Methotrexate may cause folate deficiency; folate supplementation may decrease methotrexate effects. Closely monitor patient. Azathioprine impairs folate metabolism.[2,5,8]
23	22	XCyclosporine may cause severe hypomagnesaemia.[7]
24	1	Overuse may cause a deficiency of vitamin A.[1]
24	2	Overuse may cause a deficiency of vitamin D.[1]
24	3	Overuse may cause a deficiency of vitamin E.[1]
24	4	Overuse may cause a deficiency of vitamin K.[1]
24	25	Laxatives may deplete potassium levels.[7]
25	20	Lithium may impair iodine metabolism.[5]
25	22	Lithium may increase blood levels of magnesium. Both lithium and magnesium may compete. Adverse effects unlikely; monitor patient.[5,7]
25	25	Lithium may increase blood levels of potassium.[5]
26	13	Frequent use of NSAIDs may lower the absorption of folate. Monitor patient.[1]
26	15	Frequent use of NSAIDs may lower the absorption of vitamin C. Monitor patient.[1]
26	25	NSAIDs may alter potassium metabolism through a range of mechanisms.[7]
26	28	NSAIDs may increase urinary zinc excretion and contribute to zinc depletion.[7]
27	3	Thyroxine may impair vitamin E metabolism.[5]
27	9	Thyroxine may reduce riboflavin absorption.[5]
27	16	Chelation between thyroid medications and calcium can impair the absorption of both, particularly with calcium carbonate. Thyroid hormones increase urinary calcium excretion.[6,7]
27	20	Due to the complex nature of thyroid disorders it is advised that iodine supplementation only be conducted under medical supervision.[8]
28	12	Theophylline impairs vitamin B6 metabolism; vitamin B6 may increase risk of theophylline-induced seizures.[5,6]

REFERENCES

1. Ismail M. Drug–food interactions and role of pharmacist. Asian J Pharm Clin Res 2009;2(4): 1–10.

2. Gura KM. Drug interactions. In: Hendricks KM, Duggan C, editors. Manual of pediatric nutrition. 4th ed. Hamilton: ON: BC Decker; 2005.

3. VanZyl M. The effects of drugs on nutrition. South Afr J Clin Nutr 2011;24(3).

4. Yetley EA. Multivitamin and multivitamin dietary supplements: definitions, characterisation, bioavailability and drug interactions. Am J Clin Nutr 2007;85(Suppl.): 269S–76S.

5. Zimmerman M. Handbook of nutrition. New York: Thieme; 2001.

6. Hendler SS, Rorvik D. PDR for nutritional supplements. 1st ed. Montvale New Jersey: Thomson; 2001.

7. Stargrove M, Treasure J, McKee D. Herb, nutrient and drug interactions. Missouri: Mosby Elsevier; 2008.

8. Braun L, Cohen M. Herbs and natural supplements: an evidence-based guide. 2nd ed. Marrickville: Elsevier; 2007.

APPENDIX **3**

Chemotherapy drugs and concurrent nutraceutical use

Janet Schloss
ND

Chemotherapy drug	Primary indications	Side effects and major toxicities	Nutrient/herbs	Action involved
Alkalising agents—substitute alkyl chemical structure for a hydrogen atom in DNA resulting in cross-linking of each strand of DNA and preventing cell division				
Nitrogen mustards				
Chlorambucil (Leukeran)	Chronic lymphocytic leukaemia (CLL), Hodgkin's and non-Hodgkin's lymphomas	Bone-marrow suppression, toxicity to mucous membranes	Avoid glutathione during actual treatment, but have on non-chemo days[1]	Increases cell resistance[2]
			Immune herbs (e.g. *Echinacea* spp., *Andrographis*, *Astragalus membranaceous*)	Reduces side effects, but could reduce drug effectiveness Use with caution[3]
Cyclophospha-mide (Cytoxan)	Acute and chronic leukaemias, ovary and breast cancer, neuroblastomas, retinoblastomas, lymphomas, multiple myeloma, mycosis fungoides	Bone-marrow suppression, haemorrhagic cystitis, nausea, vomiting, anorexia, darkening of skin and nails, diarrhoea, facial flushing, headache, increased sweating, swollen lips, rash, hair loss, gonadal suppression, no menstruation, leucopenia, dizziness, weakness, hyperglycaemia, cardiotoxicity	Avoid glutathione during actual treatment, but have on non-chemo days[1]	Increases cell resistance[4]
			Vitamin C	Enhances effectiveness, reduces side effects[5]
			Vitamin A	Improves effectiveness, reduces side effects[6]
			Folic acid	Improves survival, improves efficacy[7]
			Beta-carotene	Reduces toxicity, increases effectiveness[8]
			Genistein	Aids killing tumour cells[9,10]
			Withania somnifera	Reduces side effects, but may stimulate stem cell proliferation Use with caution[11]

Chemotherapy drug	Primary indications	Side effects and major toxicities	Nutrient/herbs	Action involved
Ifosfamide (Ifex)	Testicular tumours	Bone marrow suppression, nausea, vomiting, encephalopathy, mucous membrane toxicity	Avoid glutathione during actual treatment, but have on non-chemo days[1]	Increases cell resistance[4]
			Beta-carotene	Reduces toxicity, increases effectiveness[8]
			Taurine	Reduces renal toxicity[12]
Mechlorethamine (Mustargen)	Lung cancers, Hodgkin's and non-Hodgkin's lymphomas, chronic leukaemia, malignant effusions, mycosis fungoides, polycythemia vera	Bone-marrow suppression, severe nausea and vomiting, diarrhoea, anorexia, metallic taste, neurotoxicity, weakness, hair loss, leucopenia, hyperuricaemia, gonadal suppression or missing menstrual period, peptic ulcers	Avoid glutathione during actual treatment, but have on non-chemo days[13]	Increases cell resistance[4]
			Immune herbs (e.g. *Echinacea* spp., *Andrographis paniculata*, *Astragalus membranaceus*)	Reduces side effects, but could reduce drug effectiveness Use with caution[3,13]
Melphalan (Alkeran)	Multiple myeloma, ovarian cancer	Bone marrow suppression, allergic reactions, mucous membrane toxicity	Avoid glutathione during actual treatment, but have on non-chemo days[1]	Increases cell resistance[4]
			Vitamin E	Enhances inhibition of oestrogen-dependent tumour growth[14–16]
			Beta-carotene	Reduces toxicity, increases effectiveness[8]
Uracil mustard (Uracil)	CLL, chronic myeloid leukaemia (CML), non-Hodgkin's, mycosis fungoides	Leucopenia, thrombocytopenia, mucous membrane toxicity	Avoid glutathione during actual treatment, but have on non-chemo days[1]	Increases cell resistance[4]
Nitrosureas				
Carmustine (BiCNU)	Primary brain tumours, multiple myeloma	Bone marrow suppression, lung fibrosis, nephrotoxicity	Avoid glutathione during actual treatment, but have on non-chemo days[1]	Increases cell resistance[4]
			Vitamin C	Makes drug more effective through oxidative stress[16,17]
			Maitake mushroom (beta-glucan)	Aids in inducing apoptosis, making drug more effective[18]
			Vitamin E	Aids in protecting non-cancer cells in low glutathione levels with vitamin C[17]

Chemotherapy drug	Primary indications	Side effects and major toxicities	Nutrient/herbs	Action involved
Cisplatin (Platinol)	Bladder, ovarian and testicular carcinomas	Nephrotoxicity, severe nausea and vomiting, bone marrow suppression, neurotoxicity, blurred vision, dizziness, anorexia, depression, anaemia	Melatonin	Reverses adverse drug effects, especially myelosuppression, cachexia and neurotoxicity[19–21]
			Glutamine	Improves drug effectiveness, reduces mucosal injury in the gut and mouth: 4 g/day[22,23]
			Beta-carotene	Reduces toxicity, increases effectiveness[8,15]
			Magnesium	Reduces side effects of drug, and magnesium deficiency associated with drug[24,25]
			Potassium	Decreases deficiency associated with drug[26,27]
			Green tea	Reduces drug resistance by inhibiting P-glycoprotein, improves drug effectiveness[26]
			Carnitine	Reduces side effects, 4 g/day for seven days reduces fatigue[28]
			Selenium	Reduced side effects—nephrotoxicity, myeloid suppression and weight loss[28]
			Calcium	Increases effectiveness and decreases gastrointestinal toxicity[29]
			Vitamin D	Increases effectiveness and decreases gastrointestinal toxicity[29]
			Silybum marianum	Increased drug effectiveness, reduced side effects[27]
			Avoid vitamin B6	Although it decreases neurotoxicity, it decreases duration effect of drug[30]
Lomustine (CeeNU)	Primary brain tumours and Hodgkin's lymphomas	Bone marrow suppression, anorexia, nausea, vomiting, neurotoxicity, nephrotoxicity, hepatotoxicity, fibrosis	Avoid glutathione during actual treatment, but have on non-chemo days[1]	Increases cell resistance[4]
			Vitamin C	Decreases side effects[31]
			Vitamin A	Decreases side effects[31]
			Vitamin E	Aids in protecting non-cancer cells in low glutathione levels with vitamin C[17] Protects bacteria toxicity[32]

Chemotherapy drug	Primary indications	Side effects and major toxicities	Nutrient/herbs	Action involved
Streptozotocin (Zanosar)	Pancreatic cancer	Nephrotoxicity, nausea, vomiting	Avoid glutathione during actual treatment, but have on non-chemo days[1]	Increases cell resistance[4]
			Vitamin C	Decreases excessive oxidation[33]
			Vitamin E	Decreases excessive oxidation[4]
			Quercetin	Decreases oxidative damage[34]
			Lipoic acid	Increases reduced glutathione[35]
			Fish oils—docosahexaenoic acid (DHA), eicosapentaenoic acid (EPA)	Increases reduced glutathione[35]
Pipobroman (Vercyte)	Chronic granulocytic leukaemia	Bone marrow suppression, nausea, vomiting, diarrhoea	Avoid glutathione during actual treatment, but have on non-chemo days[1]	Increases cell resistance[4]
Thiotepa (Thioplex)	Breast, ovarian, bladder cancers, lymphomas, malignant effusions	Bone marrow suppression	Avoid glutathione during actual treatment, but have on non-chemo days[1]	Increases cell resistance[4]
			Calcium	Improves efficacy of drug[36]
			Vitamin D	Works synergistically with drug and improves efficacy[37–40]
			Vitamin A	Increases efficacy of drug via DNA replication[41]
			Vitamin E	Increases efficacy of drug via DNA replication, decreases side effects[41]
			Vitamin C	Increases cytotoxicity of drug[42]
Other				
Busulfan (Myleran)	CML	Bone marrow suppression, hyperpigmentation, gynaecomastia	Avoid glutathione during actual treatment, but have on non-chemo days[1]	Increases cell resistance[4] Note: Cysteine levels were not depleted and aided glutathione levels after[43]
			Quercetin	Aids antiproliferative action[44]
			Vitamin E	Stops depletion and cell damage during bone transplantation[43]
			Vitamin C	Stops depletion and cell damage during bone transplantation[43]
			Zinc	Stops depletion and cell damage during bone transplantation[43]
			Avoid iron	Overload levels can occur before and during bone transplantation[45]

Chemotherapy drug	Primary indications	Side effects and major toxicities	Nutrient/herbs	Action involved
Carboplatin (Paraplatin)	Ovarian carcinoma, prostate cancer, brain tumours, neuroblastomas	Bone marrow suppression, nausea, vomiting, neurotoxicity, neuropathies, ototoxicity	Avoid glutathione during actual treatment, but have on non-chemo days[1]	Increases cell resistance[4]
			Vitamin D	Works synergistically with drug and improves efficacy[37–40]
			Calcium	Improves efficacy of drug,[36] decreases gastrointestinal toxicity[29]
			Vitamin A	Decreases side effects[46]
			Melatonin	Reverses adverse drug effects, especially myelosuppression, cachexia and neurotoxicity[19,20,47]
Cisplatin (Platinol)	Bladder, ovarian and testicular carcinomas	Nephrotoxicity, severe nausea and vomiting, bone marrow suppression, neurotoxicity, blurred vision, dizziness, anorexia, depression, anaemia	Avoid glutathione during actual treatment, but have on non-chemo days[1]	Increases cell resistance[4]
			Vitamin C	Enhances effectiveness, reduces side effects[5,15,16,48]
			Vitamin E	Enhances drug, aids inhibition of oestrogen, 300 mg/day taken before treatment and continued for three months reduced the severity of neurotoxicity[15,16,28,49]
			Vitamin A	Improves effectiveness, reduces side effects[46,50,51]
			Lipoic acid	Inhibits nuclear factor kappa B cells (NF-κB), reduces drug resistance and side effects,[2] aids in reducing peripheral neuropathy[52]
			DHA/EPA	Reduces late radionecrosis, improves blood perfusion, increases cell-kill count[53]
			Quercetin	Potentiates drug activity, inhibits P-glycoprotein, reduces drug resistance[54, 55]
			Zinc	Chemopotentiating agent as it aids in DNA repair[56]

Chemotherapy drug	Primary indications	Side effects and major toxicities	Nutrient/herbs	Action involved
Antimetabolites—interfere with the synthesis of DNA and RNA, specifically S phase				

Chemotherapy drug	Primary indications	Side effects and major toxicities	Nutrient/herbs	Action involved
Antimetabolites—interfere with the synthesis of DNA and RNA, specifically S phase				
Cytarabine (Cytosar-U)	Acute myeloid leukaemia (AML), acute lymphocytic leukaemia (ALL)	Bone-marrow suppression, anorexia, oral and gastrointestinal (GI) ulceration, mucositis, conjunctivitis	Calcium	Improves efficacy of drug[57]
			Vitamin D	Improves drug efficacy[57–59]
			Vitamin A	Improves drug efficacy[58]
			Quercetin	Potentiates drug activity, inhibits P-glycoprotein, reduces drug resistance[55]
			Glutamine	Improves drug effectiveness, reduces mucosal injury in the gut and mouth: 4 g/day[22,23]
5-Fluorouracil (Adrucil, 5-FU)	Colon, rectum, breast, stomach, ovarian and pancreatic cancers, head and neck cancers	Diarrhoea, stomatitis, bone marrow suppression, oesophagopharyngitis, leucopenia, thrombo-cytopenia, GI ulceration, dermatitis, anorexia, alopecia, weakness, dry skin, diarrhoea, phlebitis, mucositis	Vitamin C	Enhances effectiveness, reduces side effects[9]
			Vitamin E	Enhances drug[16]
			Vitamin B6	Reduces pain in palms and feet,[60,61] may ↓ toxic side effect of palmar plantar erythrodysaesthesia (PPE)[62]
			Vitamin A	Reduces dose, improves anti-tumour effect,[63] reduces side effects[16]
			Bromelain	Can reduce dose of drug to result in cancer regression[64]
			Glutamine	Improves drug effectiveness, reduces mucosal injury in the gut and mouth: 4 g/day[22,23]
			Folic acid—use with caution Do not use on chemo days	Improves survival, improves efficacy[4] Drug can deplete folate levels and certain polymorphisms may affect treatment Only to be used in non-chemo weeks[65,66]
			Quercetin	Aids apoptosis[67,68]
Floxuridine (FUDR)	GI adenocarcinoma with liver metastasis	Bone-marrow suppression, stomatitis, anaphylaxis	Vitamin C	Aids drug efficacy[69]
Fludarabine (Fludara)	CLL	Bone-marrow suppression, fever, chills, nausea, vomiting, infection	Similar to 5-FU	No studies located
Mercaptopurine (Purinethol)	ALL, AML	Bone-marrow suppression, anorexia, cholestasis	Similar to 5-FU	No studies located

Chemotherapy drug	Primary indications	Side effects and major toxicities	Nutrient/herbs	Action involved
Methotrexate (Folex)	Breast, head and neck, lung, trophoblastic, renal, ovarian, bladder and testicular cancers, ALL, non-Hodgkin's lymphomas, meningeal leukaemia, mycosis fungoides, osteosarcoma	Bone-marrow suppression, diarrhoea, stomatitis, nausea, vomiting, anorexia, acne, boils, skin rash or itching, loss of hair, GI ulcers and bleeding, leucopenia, infections, thrombocytopenia, pharyngitis, liver toxicity, pneumonitis, pulmonary fibrosis, renal failure, hyperuricaemia, cutaneous vasculitis	Folic acid—use with extreme caution or avoid	Drug binds with dihydrofolate reductase to inhibit DNA and RNA synthesis[4]
			Vitamin A	Improves effectiveness, reduces side effects[16,70,71]
			Glutamine	Improves white blood cell (WBC) count, improves drug effectiveness, reduces mucosal injury in the gut and mouth: 4 g/day[22,23]
			Adenosine	Chemoprotective action, improves WBC recovery. Can be taken with chemotherapy[72,73]
			Green tea (EGCG and ECG)	Inhibits dihydrofolate reductase (DHFR), therefore increases efficacy of drug[74]
			Enterococcus faecium (probiotic bacteria)	Improves anti-inflammatory effects of drug[75]
			N-acetylcysteine	Decreases gastrotoxicity[75]
			Vitamin E	Decreases side effects[70,76]
Thioguanine	Acute nonlymphocytic leukaemia (ANLL)	Bone-marrow suppression		
Antibiotics—interfere with DNA functioning by blocking the transcription of new DNA or RNA (they delay or inhibit mitosis)				
Bleomycin (Blenoxane)	Squamous cell carcinoma, lymphomas, testicular cancer	Chills, fever, pneumonitis, mucositis, lung fibrosis, hyperpigmentation, pulmonary toxicity, hypersensitivity reactions	Vitamin C	Enhances effectiveness, reduces side effects[16]
			Vitamin E	Enhances drug[16]
			Beta-carotene	Reduces toxicity, aids effectiveness[8]
Dactinomycin (Cosmegen)	Wilm's tumour, Ewing's sarcoma, choriocarcinoma, rhabdomyosarcoma	Bone-marrow suppression	Similar to doxorubicin	No studies located
Liposomal daunorubicin (DaunoXome)	HIV, Kaposi's sarcoma	Bone-marrow suppression, cardiomyopathy, severe mucositis	Vitamin D	Improved drug efficacy[59]

Chemotherapy drug	Primary indications	Side effects and major toxicities	Nutrient/herbs	Action involved
Doxorubicin (Adriamycin)	Acute leukaemia, Wilm's tumour, soft tissue and bone sarcomas, Hodgkin's disease, lymphomas, breast and various other carcinomas	Bone-marrow suppression, cardiomyopathy, severe mucositis, darkening of soles, palms and nails, diarrhoea, red urine, loss of hair (alopecia), leucopenia, thrombocytopenia, stomatitis, oesophagitis, cellulitis, nephropathy, hyperuricaemia	Vitamin C	Enhances effectiveness, reduces side effects[16]
			Vitamin E	Enhances drug, decreases side effects, especially alopecia[77–80]
			Vitamin A	Improves effectiveness, reduces side effects[16,80]
			Selenium	Reduces lipid peroxide induced cardiotoxicity[80]
			Genistein	Aids killing tumour cells[9,81,82]
			Coenzyme Q10	Maintains cellular energetics,[9] decreases cardiotoxic side effects[83]
			Lipoic acid	Reduces side effects[84]
			DHA/EPA	Reduces late radionecrosis, improves blood perfusion, increases cell-kill count[52]
			Melatonin	Reverses adverse drug effects, especially mylosuppression, cachexia and neurotoxicity[19,20]
			Quercetin	Potentiates drug activity, inhibits P-glycoprotein, reduces drug resistance[55]
			Beta-carotene	Reduces toxicity, aids effectiveness[8]
			Carnitine	Reduced side effects, especially those cardiotoxic[85,86]
			Ginkgo biloba	Prevents cardiotoxicity (only animal studies)[87]
			Vitamin B6	May ↓ toxic side effect of palmar plantar erythrodysaesthesia (PPE)[62]
Idarubicin (Idamycin)	AML	Severe bone-marrow, suppression, infection, alopecia, nausea, vomiting, haemorrhage	No studies located	

Chemotherapy drug	Primary indications	Side effects and major toxicities	Nutrient/herbs	Action involved
Mitomycin (Mutamycin)	Disseminated adenocarcinomas of pancreas or stomach	Bone-marrow suppression	Selenium	Decreased chromosomal mutations from chemotherapy[88]
			Vitamin B2	Aids drug under radiation, having a radio-protective effect[89]
			Vitamin C	Aids drug under radiation having a radio-protective effect[89–91]
			Vitamin E	Potentiates drug under radiation[90]
			Beta-carotene	Potentiates drug under radiation[90]
			Quercetin	Protects non-cancer cells DNA from damage[92]
			Rutin	Protects non-cancer cells DNA from damage[92]
			Green tea	Increases efficacy of drug[93]
Mitoxantrone (Novantrone)	ANLL	Cardiotoxicity, severe myelosuppression	Melatonin	Decreases side effects and immunosuppression[19]
			Similar to doxorubicin	
Pentostatin (Nipent)	Hairy cell leukaemia	Bone-marrow suppression, renal toxicity, rash	Adenosine	Aids efficacy of the drug[94]
Plicamycin (Mithracin)	Testicular tumours, hypercalcaemia	Epistaxis, haemorrhage, nausea, bone-marrow suppression, stomatitis, vomiting, diarrhoea	No studies located	
Mitotic inhibitors—plant alkaloids that block cell division in metaphase				
Etoposide (VePesid)	Refractory testicular tumours, small cell lung cancer	Bone-marrow suppression, alopecia, hypotension with rapid infusion	Genistein	Aids killing, reduces multi-drug resistance[8,81]
			Beta-carotene	Reduces toxicity, aids effectiveness[8]
			Melatonin	Reverses adverse drug effects, especially myelosuppression, cachexia and neurotoxicity[19,20]
			Vitamin A	Improves effectiveness, reduces side effects[16,46]
			Vitamin D	Improved drug efficacy[59]
Teniposide (Vumon)	ALL	Bone-marrow suppression, mucositis, alopecia		
Vinblastine (Velban)	Breast and testicular cancer, Hodgkin's and non-Hodgkin's lymphomas, Kaposi's sarcoma, mycosis fungoides	Leucopenia, alopecia, muscle pain, hyperuricaemia, neurotoxicity, nausea, vomiting, hair loss, cellulitis, stomatitis, rectal bleeding, haemorrhagic colitis	Vitamin C	Enhances effectiveness, reduces side effects[16]
			Quercetin	Potentiates drug activity, inhibits P-glycoprotein, reduces drug resistance[55]
			Glycyrrhiza glabra	Additive effects[95]

Chemotherapy drug	Primary indications	Side effects and major toxicities	Nutrient/herbs	Action involved
Vincristine (Oncovin)	ALL, rhabdomyosarcoma, neuroblastoma, Wilm's tumour and various other carcinomas	Mild to severe paraesthesias, jaw pain, ataxia, muscle wasting, constipation, anorexia, nausea, vomiting, autonomic toxicity, neurotoxicity, painful urination, bed wetting, constipation, orthostatic hypotension, lack of sweating	Vitamin E	Enhances drug[16]
			Vitamin A	Improves effectiveness, reduces side effects[16]
			Lipoic acid	Inhibits NF-κB, reduces drug resistance and side effects[2,96]
			DHA/EPA	Reduces dose, reduces late radionecrosis, improves blood perfusion, increases cell-kill count[52]
			Bromelain	Can reduce dose of drug to result in cancer regression[64]
			Glutamine	Improves drug effectiveness, reduces mucosal injury in the gut and mouth: 4 g/day[22,23]
Vinorelbine (Navelbine)	Non-small cell lung cancer	Bone-marrow suppression, nausea, vomiting, asthenia	Resveratrol	Increases apoptosis and cell necrosis, decreases dose of drug[97]
			Propolis	Increases apoptosis and cell necrosis, decreases dose of drug[97]
			Gamma-linolenic acid (GLA)	Increases chemosensitivity[98]
Miscellaneous antineoplastic agents				
Hormones—used in neoplasms sensitive to hormonal growth controls in the body They reportedly interfere with the growth-stimulating receptors on target tissues				
Corticosteriods (e.g. prednisone, dexamethasone)	Lymphocytic leukaemias and lymphomas—both Hodgkin's and non-Hodgkin's, breast and brain cancer Also used in conjunction with radiotherapy to decrease oedema	Nausea, vomiting, anorexia, diarrhoea, gastric irritation, headaches, vertigo, insomnia, restlessness, ↑ sweating, ↑ bruising, purpura	Vitamin D	Works synergistically with drug and improves efficacy,[40] aids calcium absorption[99]
			Calcium	Minimises bone demineralisation from the drug,[99] reduces side effects[3]
			Vitamin C	Enhances drug efficacy and decreases dose of drug[100] Increases wound healing[100]
			Vitamin E	Enhances drug efficacy and decreases dose of drug[100]
			Selenium	Enhances drug efficacy and decreases dose of drug[100]
			Fibre (FOS)	Enhances drug efficacy and decreases dose of drug[100]
			Fish oils (DHA/EPA)	Enhances drug efficacy and decreases dose of drug[100]
			Chromium	Reduced side effects,[3] drug linked with increased urinary loss[101]
			Glycyrrhiza glabra	Potentiates drug effects[3]

Chemotherapy drug	Primary indications	Side effects and major toxicities	Nutrient/herbs	Action involved
Antiandrogens				
Bicalutamide (Casodex)—inhibits androgens from receptors binding to target tissues	Prostate cancer	Hot flushes, pruritus, breast tenderness, gynaecomastia, hepatic disturbances, depression, alopecia, ↓ libido, haematuria	Vitamin E	Aids drug efficacy[102]
			Zinc	May assist anti-androgen affect[103]
			Arginine	Aids presentation of cells for drug action,[104] aids androgen-receptor inhibition[105]
			Serine	Aids presentation of cells for drug action[104]
			Lysine	Aids presentation of cells for drug action[104]
			B12, B6, folate, S-adenosyl methionine (SAMe) or methionine	Aids in methylation of amino acids to assist drug's action[104]
Flutamide (Eulexin)—orally, inhibits the uptake or binding of androgens to target tissues	Ovarian cancer, testicular steroidogenesis, prostate cancer	Diarrhoea, impotency, hepatotoxicity, anorexia, insomnia, leucopenia, anaemia, thrombocytopenia, macrocytic anaemia, oedema, photosensitivity	I3C indole-3-carbinol	Potent chemotherapy agent that controls growth of prostate cells[106]
			Vitamin E	Decreases toxic effects of polychlorinated biphenyls (PCBs) on prostate cells, thus aiding drug's effect[107]
			Vitamin C	Depleted by drug[108]
			Vitamin D	Decreases bone demineralisation[109]
			Calcium	Decreases bone demineralisation[109]
Nilutamide (Nilandron)—blocks testosterone effects on androgen receptors	Metastatic prostatic cancer	Nausea, alcohol intolerance, dark/light adaptation problems, dizziness, impotence, ↓ libido, hot flushes, body hair loss, sweating, ↑ transaminases	L-cysteine (or glutathione)	Decreases toxicity of drug[110]
			Vitamin E	Aids in glutathione levels and decreasing toxicity of drug[110]
			Vitamin B3	No research but traditionally used to help with alcohol detoxification[3]
Goserelin (Zoladex)—inhibitor of pituitary gonadotrophins	Prostate carcinoma	Hot flushes, sexual dysfunction, decreased erections, fertility impairment, impotence, sweating, blood pressure changes, oedema, breast pain, temporary bone pain, ↓ bone mineral density (BMD), nausea	Vitamin E	May be low in prostate cancer patients, may aid drug efficacy[111]
			Vitamin D	Decreases bone demineralisation[109,112,113]
			Calcium	Decreases bone demineralisation[109,112,113]

Chemotherapy drug	Primary indications	Side effects and major toxicities	Nutrient/herbs	Action involved
Oestrogens (e.g. diethylstilboestrol [DES], polyoestradiol, ethinyl oestradiol, oestramustine)	Androgen sensitive prostatic cancer, advanced breast cancer in postmenopausal women	Inducing thrombosis	Quercetin	Reduces DNA damage[114, 115]
			Resveratrol	Acts as an agonist for the drugs, acts on NF-κB[116–118]
			Melatonin	Anti-proliferative affect[119]
Anti-oestrogens				
Tamoxifen— synthetic antioestrogen that binds to receptors	Breast cancer	Nausea, vomiting, headaches, hot flushes, weight gain, impotency, endometrial cancer, thromboembolism, ocular toxicity, hepatotoxicity	Avoid genistein	Interacts with drug's action[4,120–124]
			Avoid red clover	Interacts with drug's action[125]
			Daidzein	Aids drug in decreasing carcinogenesis[126]
			Vitamin C (also works with other antioxidants)[15]	Enhances effectiveness, reduces side effects[16]
			Melatonin	Reverses adverse drug effects, especially cachexia and neurotoxicity[19,20]
			Resveratrol	Anti-inflammatory aids drug effectiveness[122,127]
			Quercetin	Anti-inflammatory effect aids drug effectiveness,[122,127] potentiates drug by anticell proliferation and prevention of angiogenesis[128]
			Green tea	Aids in cancer prevention, aids apoptosis[129–131]
			Coenzyme Q10	Increases antioxidant activity, decreases carcinogenesis[132,133]
			Niacin (B3)	Increases antioxidant activity[133]
			Riboflavin (B2)	Increases antioxidant activity[133]
			Folate, vitamin B12, methionine	Methylation helps to decrease homocysteine levels linked with ↑ cardiovascular disease[135]
			Actaea racemosa	May work synergistically to have a cytotoxic affect against cancerous cell growth[136]

Chemotherapy drug	Primary indications	Side effects and major toxicities	Nutrient/herbs	Action involved
Raloxifene (Evista)	Breast cancer	Hot flushes, leg cramps, thromboembolism, headaches, nausea, diarrhoea, oedema, arthralgia, sinus, rhinitis, weight gain	Genistein	Decreases bone demineralisation[137, 138]
			Vitamin D	Decreases bone demineralisation[139]
			Calcium	Decreases bone demineralisation[139]
			Resveratrol	Decreases vaginal stratification, preserves neuronal function while on drug[140,141]
			Quercetin	Aids in inhibition of aromatase[124,142]
			Folate, vitamin B12, methionine	Methylation helps to decrease homocysteine levels linked with ↑ cardiovascular disease[134, 135]
Toremifene (Fareston)— similar to tamoxifen	Metastatic breast cancer in postmenopausal women	Hypocholesterolaemic, thromboembolism (possible), hypercalcaemia, hot flushes, sweating, dizziness, GI upset, leucorrhoea, vaginal bleeding, oedema, pain, endometrial hypotrophy	Same as tamoxifen	
Anastrozole (Arimidex)— inhibits steroid aromatase, reducing oestrone synthesis in the adrenal glands	Palliative therapy of advanced breast cancer in post menopausal women	Hot flushes, vaginal dryness, bleeding, hair thinning, joint pain, stiffness, back and breast pain, peripheral oedema, cough, pharyngitis, asthenia, somnolence, insomnia, headache, rash, GI upset, ↑ cholesterol, weight gain, depression	Calcium	Increases bone mineral density[142]
			Vitamin D	Increases bone mineral density[142]
Testolactone (Teslac)— aromatase inhibitor	Premenopausal women with non-terminated or terminated ovarian function	Hot flushes, decreased bone mineral density	Relatively new drug; no studies of interactions with vitamins or herbs have been conducted as of yet	
Progestins (e.g. Medroxy-progesterone [Depo-Provera] and megestrol [Megace])	Advanced endometrial cancer, advanced carcinoma of the breast, advanced renal carcinoma	Menstrual irregularities, ↓ BMD, anaphylaxis, thromboembolism, ocular effects, adrenal disturbances, abscesses, urticaria, pruritus, rash, acne, hirsutism, alopecia, sweating, nausea, breast tenderness, cervical changes, weight gain, abdominal pain	Calcium	Decreases risk of oesteoporosis[143]
			Vitamin D	Decreases risk of oesteoporosis[144]
			Genistein—avoid high doses	High doses may have detrimental effects in stimulating tumour growth[145]
			Vitamin E	Protective effect against endometrial cell wall damage[146]
			Vitamin B12	Drug reduces levels so corrects deficiency[147]
			Vitamin A	Protective effect[148]

Chemotherapy drug	Primary indications	Side effects and major toxicities	Nutrient/herbs	Action involved
Other agents				
Altretamine (Hexalen)	Palliative treatment of persistent or recurrent ovarian cancer	Nausea, vomiting, neurotoxicity, myelosuppression, central nervous system (CNS) changes—ataxia, dizziness, mood alterations	Avoid vitamin B6	Although decreases neurotoxicity, it decreases duration effect of drug[30]
			Zinc	Drug depletes zinc stores, so aids mineral deficiency[30]
Topotecan (Hycamtin)— topoisomerase inhibitor	Multiple myeloma, relapsed or refractory metastatic carcinoma of the ovary after failure of other therapies	Neutropenia, leucopenia, thrombocytopenia, anaemia, headache, diarrhoea, stomach pain, nausea, vomiting, alopecia, tiredness, dyspnoea, neuromuscular pain	Quercetin	Sensitiser to chemo drug, aids effect[149]
VEGF inhibitor (vascular endothelial growth factor—anti-angiogenesis)—interferes with the growth of cancer by blocking the formation and growth of new blood vessels in the tumour				
Avastin (Bevacizumab)— recombinant humanised monoclonal IgG$_1$ antibody	Colon, rectum, lung or breast cancer	Reaction to injection, bleeding, GI tract perforations, haemorrhage, hypertension, fistula formation, proteinuria, epistaxis, headache, rhinitis, taste alteration, dry skin, rectal haemorrhage, lacrimation disorder, exfoliative dermatitis	No studies located	
Erbitux (Cetuximab)— recombinant humanised monoclonal IgG$_1$ antibody	Colon and rectum cancer, sometimes head and neck cancers	Reaction to injection, acne-like skin rash, severe skin rash, slow heart rate, weak pulse, fainting, slow breathing, chest pain, heavy feeling, fever, chills, flu symptoms, easy bruising, bleeding, hot dry skin, white patches or sores in mouth, headaches, dryness	No studies located	
Miscellaneous agents				
Asparaginase (Elspar, Kidrolase)— reduces asparagines to aspartic acid	ALL	Hyperammonaemia, headaches, anorexia, nausea, vomiting, abdominal cramps, decreases blood clotting factors, allergic reactions, liver toxicity, pancreatitis and anaphylaxis	Glutamine—use with caution	Deamination of glutamine assists drug's action[150,151]
Caelyx (contains doxorubicin)	Ovarian cancer, Kaposi's sarcoma	See doxorubicin	See doxorubicin	

Chemotherapy drug	Primary indications	Side effects and major toxicities	Nutrient/herbs	Action involved
Cladribine (Leustatin)	Hairy cell leukaemia	Severe anaemia, infection, skin rash, bleeding or bruising, anorexia, headache, nausea, vomiting, fatigue	Glucosamine hydrochloride	Increases B-cell apoptosis[152]
Dacarbazine (DTIC-Dome)	Malignant melanoma, Hodgkin's disease	Flu-like syndrome, anorexia, nausea, vomiting, diarrhoea, cardiotoxicity, alopecia	Green tea	Inhibits melanoma growth and metatasis[153]
			Vitamin C	Aids growth inhibitory effect[15]
			Vitamin E	Aids growth inhibitory effect in combination with other antioxidants[15]
			Beta-carotene	Aids growth inhibitory effect in combination with other antioxidants[15]
			Vitamin A	Aids growth inhibitory effect in combination with other antioxidants[15]
			Quercetin—avoid	Inhibits liver enzyme P450 (CYP1A2), which helps make the drug active[154]
Docetaxel (Taxotere)	Advanced breast cancer	Bone-marrow suppression, nausea, diarrhoea, stomatitis, fever, skin reactions, myalgia, fluid retention neurotoxicity, alopecia	GLA	If given together for 24–48 hours before and during drug treatment, it works in synergy with drug[155]
			Vitamin E	Prevents oxidisation of GLA to assist synergy with drug[155]
			Vitamin B6	May ↓ toxic side effect of PPE[62]
			Vitamin D	Aids anti-neoplastic effect[156–158]
Gemcitabine (Gemzar)— pyrimidine nucleoside antimetabolite	Adenocarcinoma of the pancreas, kidney and bladder cancers, non-small cell lung cancer	Dyspnoea, peripheral oedema, a flu-like syndrome, nausea, vomiting, diarrhoea, rash, paraesthesia, stomatitis, myelosuppression	DHA/EPA	Doesn't interfere and may potentiate drug[159]
			Quercetin	Sensitiser for chemo drug[149]
Hydroxyurea (Hydrea)	Head, neck, ovarian carcinoma, chronic myelocytic leukaemia, malignant melanoma	Bone-marrow suppression, diarrhoea, anorexia, nausea, vomiting, drowsiness	Vitamin D	Improved drug efficacy[59]
			Calcium	Improves efficacy of drug[57]
			Vitamin E	Aids in increasing low vitamin E levels in CML patients after treatment,[160] decreases toxicity damage[161]
			Vitamin C	Decreases toxic side effects with vitamin E[162]
			Zinc	Enhances drug's effect[163,164]
			Quercetin	Aids drug in DNA synthesis inhibition[165]

Chemotherapy drug	Primary indications	Side effects and major toxicities	Nutrient/herbs	Action involved
Irinotecan (Camptosar)— topoisomerase I inhibitor	Metastatic colorectal cancer, rectal cancer	Severe diarrhoea, myelosuppression, nausea, vomiting	Zinc	Chemopotentiating agent as it aids in DNA repair[56,166]
			Selenium	Decreases side effects and toxicity[167,168]
			Quercetin	Aids action of drug[169]
			Glutamine	Decreases diarrhoea side effect[22]
Levamisole (Ergamisol)— anthelmintic	Colorectal cancer	Bone-marrow suppression, nausea, diarrhoea, metallic taste, arthralgia, flu-like syndrome	Selenium—113 mg	Prevents weight loss and increased glutathione levels[170]
			Cobalt—72 mg	Prevents weight loss[170]
Mitotane (Lysodren)	Inoperable adrenal cortex cancer	Adrenal gland insufficiency, dark skin, diarrhoea, anorexia, depression, nausea, vomiting, weakness, drowsiness, light headedness	No studies located	
Paclitaxel (Taxol)	Metastatic ovarian cancer, metastatic breast cancer	Severe allergic reactions, bone-marrow suppression, peripheral neuropathy, muscle pain, alopecia, gastric distress	Vitamin C	Enhances effectiveness, reduces side effects[16,171]
			Glycyrrhiza glabra	Potentiates the effects of paclitaxel[95]
			Vitamin D	Works synergistically with drug and improves efficacy[29,40]
			Calcium	Increases effectiveness and decreases GI toxicity[29]
			Glutamine	Decreases side effects[22,23]
			Vitamin E	Enhances drug absorption and utilisation, decreases neurotoxicity[171–174]
			Beta-carotene	Decreases side effects[8,171]
			Quercetin	Aids drug absorption and plasma concentrations[175]
			Andrographis paniculata, Astragalus membranaceus, Scutellaria baicalensis, Allium spp., *Panax ginseng, Eleutherococcus senticosus, Echinacea* spp.	Reduces side effects Use with caution[3,176]
			Lipoic acid	Aids in reducing peripheral neuropathy[52]
Aldesleukin (Proleukin)	Renal cell carcinoma	Oedema, anaemia, thrombocytopenia, hypotension	No studies located	

Chemotherapy drug	Primary indications	Side effects and major toxicities	Nutrient/herbs	Action involved
Epirubicin (Ellence)	Metastatic breast cancer, mesothelioma	Cardiotoxicity, dehydration, alopecia, transient ECG changes, nausea, vomiting, diarrhoea, mucositis, myelosuppression, mild anaemia	Melatonin	Decreases toxicity and increases efficacy of drug[19,20,177]
			Avoid glutathione	Increases drug resistance[178,179]
			Coenzyme Q10	Protective effect against cadiotoxicity[180,181]
G-CSF (Neupogen)	Used to decrease the potential for infection in people receiving myelosuppressive agents	Nausea, vomiting, hair loss, diarrhoea, fevers, mucositis, anorexia, fatigue, bone pain	Vitamin C	Works in synergy to increase vitamin C uptake[182,183]
			Vitamin A	Works in synergy with drug[184,185]
			Vitamin E	Works with drug and vitamin A to normalise neutrophils, improve platelets and red blood cells[186,187]
Granulocyte-macrophage colony-stimulating factor (pro-inflammatory cytokine)	Acute lymphoblastic anaemia, Hodgkin's disease, non-Hodgkin's lymphoma	Redness/pain at the site of injection, fever, rapid or irregular heartbeat, sores on skin, wheezing, chest pain	Vitamin C	Decreases reactive oxygen species (ROS) produced from the drug[188,189]
			Vitamin A	Inhibited the differentiation and maturation of cord blood dendritic cells in bone marrow[190,191]
			Adenosine	Increases granulocyte-macrophage colony-stimulating factor (GM-CSF) in bone marrow[192]
Imatinib (Gleevec)—phosphotyrosine kinase inhibitor	GI cancers, glioblastomas, adenoid cystic cancers, prostate cancers, leukaemia	Myelosuppression, hepatotoxicity, oedema, bleeding	Vitamin C	Restores sensitivity to drug[182]
			Flavonoids (e.g. quercetin)	Aids drug in inhibiting cyclin-dependent kinases, inhibits angiogenic mediators and induces apoptosis[193]
			Vitamin D	Effects cytokines in leukaemic cells and aids in control of apoptotic-gene expression in synergy with drug and vitamin A[194]
			Vitamin A	Effects cytokines in leukaemic cells and aids in control of apoptotic-gene expression in synergy with drug and vitamin E[194]

Chemotherapy drug	Primary indications	Side effects and major toxicities	Nutrient/herbs	Action involved
Interferon	Hairy cell leukaemia, genital warts, AIDS, Kaposi's sarcoma, bladder cancer, chronic active hepatitis	Flu-like syndrome, fever, chills, muscle pain, loss of appetite, lethargy, myelosuppression, nausea, vomiting, neurotoxicity, cardiotoxicity	Carnitine	Reduces fatigue associated with treatment: 2 g/day[195]
			Scutellaria baicalensis	Use with caution: reports of acute pneumonitis due to allergic-immunological mechanism[3]
			Vitamin C	Aids growth inhibitory effect[15,16]
			Vitamin E	Aids growth inhibitory effect in combination with other antioxidants[15,16]
			Beta-carotene	Aids growth inhibitory effect in combination with other antioxidants[15,16]
			Vitamin A	Aids growth inhibitory effect in combination with other antioxidants[15,16]
Oxaliplatin (Eloxatin)	Colorectal cancer	Neurological toxicity, myelosuppression	Lipoic acid	Aids efficacy of drug[196]
Pegaspargase (Oncasper)	ALL	Hypersensitivity reactions, hepatotoxicity, coagulopathies, cardiotoxicity	No studies located	
Pemetrexed (Alimta)—inhibits several folate-dependent enzymes that play roles in purine and pyrimidine synthesis	Lung cancer, mesothelioma	Neutropenia, diarrhoea, nausea/vomiting, mucositis, skin rash, spermatoxicity	Folic acid	Decreases side effects[197–200]
			Vitamin B12	Decreases side effects[197–200]
Procarbazine (Matulane)—alkylating and weak monoamine oxidase inhibitors (MAOIs)	Hodgkin's disease	Bone-marrow suppression, pneumonitis, nausea, vomiting, weakness, drowsiness, myalgia, muscle twitching, insomnia, nightmares, increased nervousness	Vitamin C	Enhances effectiveness, reduces side effects[16]
			Vitamin C	Decrease spermatoxicity of drug[201]
			N-acetylcysteine	Decrease spermatoxicity of drug[201]
Rituximab (Rituxan)	B-cell non-Hodgkin's lymphoma	Fever, chills, weakness, headache, angio-oedema, hypotension, myalgia, nausea, vomiting, leucopenia, pruritus, rash	No studies located	

Chemotherapy drug	Primary indications	Side effects and major toxicities	Nutrient/herbs	Action involved
Temozolomide (Temodar)	Melanoma, intermediate-grade gliomas	Myelosuppression, GI upset, thrombocytopenia, infertility, fatigue, headache, nausea, vomiting, constipation, anorexia, rash, alopecia	Resveratrol	Aids in apoptosis in the S phase of cell mitosis[202]
			Zinc	Chemopotentiating agent as it aids in DNA repair[56, 66]
Tretinoin (Vesanoid)—a retinoid	Acute promyelocytic leukaemia	Headaches, fever, increased weakness, malaise, shivering, infections, haemorrhage, peripheral oedema	No studies located	
Combination therapy				
Folfox— combination name for treatment with folinic acid, fluorouracil and oxaliplatin	Colon cancer	Increased risk of infection, headaches, aching muscles, cough, sore throat, tiredness, breathlessness, bruising more easily than normal, anaemia	Calcium and magnesium	Decreases neurotoxicity[203]
			Lipoic acid	Decreases neurotoxicity[203]
			Glutathione	Aids in decreasing neurotoxicity[203]

General supplementation for chemotherapy

Drug	Nutrient/herb	Potential outcome	Recommendation	Evidence/comments
Chemotherapy in general	*Eleutherococcus senticosus*	Improved treatment tolerance	Use with caution; however, possible beneficial interaction	Co-administration may increase drug tolerance and improve immune function[3]
	Withania somnifera	Reduced side effects	Observe: beneficial interaction	May prevent drug-induced bone-marrow suppression[3]
	Adenosine	Increases WBC	Use in conjunction with treatment and up to one month after chemo	Acts as a chemoprotective agent[2]
	Ganoderma spp./ *Lentinula* spp.	Increases WBC	Use in conjunction with treatment and up to three months after chemo	Increase or support immune response[2]
	Selenium	Chemoprotective	Used mainly in breast, prostate, colon and lung cancer	Has protective effects from various sources of chemo and has a variety of effects[204]
	Digestive enzymes	Increased absorption of nutrients	Decreased GI tract function and GI tract toxicity is common during chemotherapy	Aids absorption of nutrients[2]
	Liver support	Decreased systemic damage from drugs	During chemotherapy use low dose as you don't want to increase clearance of drug too soon Increase dose for liver protection and function	Decreases liver toxicity and congestion plus increases liver function[2]

REFERENCES

1. Frischer H, Ahmad T. Severe generalized glutathione reductase deficiency after antitumour chemotherapy with BCNU″[1,3-bis(chloroethyl)-1-nitrosourea]. J Lab Clin Med 1977;89(5):1080–91.

2. Osiecki H. Cancer: a nutritional/biochemical approach. 2nd ed. Brisbane: BioConcepts Publishing; 2003.

3. Braun L, Cohen M. Herbs and natural supplements, an evidence-based guide. 3rd ed. Sydney: Elsevier; 2005.

4. Salerno E. Pharmacology for health professionals. St Louis: Mosby; 1999.

5. Kurbacher CM, et al. Ascorbic acid (vitamin C) improves the antineoplastic activity of doxorubicin, cisplatin, and paclitaxel in human breast carcinoma cells in vitro. Cancer Lett 1996;103(2):183–9.

6. Tsutani H, et al. Pharmacological studies of retinol palmitate and its clinical effect in patients with acute non-lymphocytic leukemia. Leuk Res 1991;15(6):463–71.

7. Branda RF, et al. Nutritional folate status influences the efficacy and toxicity of chemotherapy in rats. Blood 1998;92(7):2471–6.

8. Teicher BA, et al. In vivo modulation of several anticancer agents by beta-carotene. Cancer Chemother Pharmacol 1994;34(3):235–41.

9. Conklin A. Dietary antioxidants during cancer chemotherapy: impact on chemotherapeutic effectiveness and development of side effects. Nutr Cancer 2000;37(1):1–18.

10. Wietrzyk J, et al. Antiangiogenic and antitumour effects in vivo of genistein applied alone or combined with cyclophosphamide. Anticancer Res 2001;21(6A):3893–6.

11. Davis L, Kuttan G. Effect of Withania somnifera on cyclophosphamide-induced urotoxicity. Cancer Lett 2000;148(1):9–17.

12. Badary OA. Taurine attenuates Fanconi syndrome induced by ifosfamide without compromising its anti-tumour activity. Oncol Res 1998;10(7):355–60.

13. Mills S, Bone K. The essential guide to herbal safety. St Louis: Churchill Livingstone; 2005.

14. Heisler T, et al. Peptide YY and vitamin E inhibit hormone-sensitive and -insensitive breast cancer cells. J Surg Res 2000;91(1):9–14.

15. Prasad KN, et al. Modification of the effect of tamoxifen, cis-platin, DTIC, and interferon-alpha 2b on human melanoma cells in culture by a mixture of vitamins. Nutr Cancer 1994;22(3):233–45.

16. Prasad KN, et al. High doses of multiple antioxidant vitamins: essential ingredients in improving the efficacy of standard cancer therapy. J Am Coll Nutr 1999;18(1):13–25.

17. Nakagawa Y, et al. Relationship between ascorbic acid and alpha-tocopherol during diquat-induced redox cycling in isolated rat hepatocytes. Biochem Pharmacol 1991;42(4):883–8.

18. Fullerton SA, et al. Induction of apoptosis in human prostatic cancer cells with beta-glucan (maitake mushroom polysaccharide). Mol Urol 2000;4(1):7–13.

19. Lissoni P, et al. Treatment of cancer chemotherapy-induced toxicity with the pineal hormone melatonin. Support Care Cancer 1997;5(2):126–9.

20. Jung B, Ahmad N. Melatonin in cancer management: progress and promise. Cancer Res 2006;66(20):9789–93.

21. Lissoni P, et al. A randomized study of chemotherapy with cisplatin plus etoposide versus chemo-endocrine therapy with cisplatin, etoposide and the pineal hormone melatonin as a first-line treatment of advanced non-small cell lung cancer in patients in a poor clinical state. J Pineal Res 1999;23(1):15–19.

22. Savarese DM, et al. Prevention of chemotherapy and radiation toxicity with glutamine. Cancer Treat Rev 2003;29(6):501–13.

23. Anderson PM, et al. Oral glutamine reduces the duration and severity of stomatitis after cancer chemotherapy. Cancer 1998;83:1433–9.

24. Buckley JE, et al. Hypomagnesemia after cisplatin combination therapy. Arch Intern Med 1982;144:2347.

25. Van de Loosdrecht AA, et al. Seizures in a patient with disseminated testicular cancer due to cisplatin-induced hypomagnesaemia. Acta Oncol 2000;39:239–40.

26. Sadzuka Y, et al. Modulation of cancer chemotherapy by green tea. Clin Cancer Res 1998;4(1):153–6.

27. Sonnenbichler J, et al. Stimulatory effects of silibinin and silicristin from the milk thistle Silybum marianum on kidney cells. J Pharmacol Exp Ther 1999;290(3):1375–83.

28. Ali BH, Al Moundhri MS. Agents ameliorating or augmenting the nephrotoxicity of cisplatin and other platinum compounds: some recent research. Food Chem Toxicol 2006;44(8):1173–83.

29. Meara DJ, et al. Role of calcium in modulation of toxicities due to cisplatin and its analogs: a histochemical approach. Anticancer Drugs 1997;8(10):988–99.

30. Slavik M, et al. Changes in serum copper and zinc during treatment with anticancer drugs interfering with pyridoxal phosphate. Adv Exp Med Biol 1989;258:235–42.

31. Georgian L, et al. The protective effect of vitamin A and vitamin C on the chromosome-damaging activity of CCNU. Morphol Embryol (Bucur) 1986;32(4):241–5.

32. Gadjeva V, et al. Spin labeled antioxidants protect bacteria against the toxicity of alkylating antitumor drug CCNU. Toxicol Lett 2003;144(3):289–94.

33. Blasiak J, et al. Genotoxicity of streptozotocin in normal and cancer cells and its modulation by free radical scavengers. Cell Biol Toxicol 2004;20(2):83–96.

34. Mahesh T, Menon VP. Quercetin allievates oxidative stress in streptozotocin-induced diabetic rats. Phytother Res 2004;18(2):123–7.

35. Yilmaz O, et al. Effects of alpha lipoic acid, ascorbic acid-6-palmitate, and fish oil on the gluthione, malonaldehyde, and fatty acid levels in erythrocytes of streptozotocin induced diabetic male rats. J Cell Biochem 2002;86(3):530–9.

36. Saunders DE, et al. Additive inhibition of RL95–2 endometrial carcinoma cell growth by carboplatin and 1,25 dihydroxyvitamin D3. Gynecol Oncol 1993;51(2):155–9.

37. Beer TM, et al. High-dose calcitriol and carboplatin in metastatic androgen-independent prostate cancer. Am J Clin Oncol 2004;27(5):535–41.

38. Wigington DP, et al. Combination study of 1,24(S)-dihydroxyvitamin D2 and chemotherapeutic agents on human breast and prostate cancer cell lines. Anticancer Res 2004;24(5A):2905–12.

39. Trump DL, et al. Anti-tumor activity of calcitriol: pre-clinical and clinical studies. J Steroid Biochem Mol Biol 2004;89–90(1–5):519–26.

40. Johnson CS, et al. Vitamin D-related therapies in prostate cancer. Cancer Metastasis Rev 2002;21(2):147–58.

41. Radu L, et al. The combined action of thiotepa and lomustine cytostatics, of estradiol hormone and of vitamins E and A on Walker tumor chromatin structure. Rom J Endocrinol 1993;31(3–4):149–53.

42. Lialiaris T, et al. Enhancement and attenuation of cytogenetic damage by vitamin C in cultured human lymphocytes exposed to thiotepa or L-ethionine. Cytogenet Cell Genet 1987;44(4):209–14.

43. Jonas CR, et al. Plasma antioxidant status after high dose chemotherapy: a randomised trial of parenteral nutrition in bone marrow transplantation patients. Am J Clin Nutr 2000;72(1):181–9.

44. Hoffman R, et al. Enhanced anti-proliferative action of busulphan by quercetin on the human leukaemia cell line K562. Br J Cancer 1989;59(3):347–8.

45. Durken M, et al. Deteriorating free radical-trapping capacity and antioxidant status in plasma during bone marrow transplantation. Bone Marrow Transplant 1995;15(5):757–62.

46. Lovat PE, et al. Synergistic induction of apoptosis of neuroblastoma by fenretinide or CD437 in combination with chemotherapeutic drugs. Int J Cancer 2000;88(6):977–85.

47. Ghielmini M, et al. Double-blind randomized study on the myeloprotective effect of melatonin in combination with carboplatin and etoposide in advanced lung cancer. Br J Cancer 1999;80(7):1058–61.

48. Antunes LM, et al. Protective effects of vitamin C against cisplatin-induced nephrotoxicity and lipid peroxidation in adult rats: a dose dependent study. Pharmacol Res 2000;41(4):405–11.

49. Pace A, et al. Neuroprotective effect of vitamin E supplementation in patients treated with cisplatin chemotherapy. J Clin Oncol 2003;21(5):927–31.

50. Weisman RA, et al. Phase I trial of retinoic acid and cis-platinum for advanced squamous cell cancer of the head and neck based on experimental evidence of drug synergism. Otolaryngol Head Neck Surg 1998;118(5):597–602.

51. Kalemkerian GP, et al. A phase II study of all-trans-retinoic acid plus cisplatin and etoposide in patients with extensive stage small cell lung carcinoma: an Eastern Cooperative Oncology Group Study. Cancer 1998;83(6):1102–8.

52. Melli G, et al. Alpha-lipoic acid prevents mitochondrial damage and neurotoxicity in experimental chemotherapy neuropathy. Exp Neurol 2008;214(2):276–84.

53. Bougnoux P. n-3 polyunsaturated fatty acids and cancer. Curr Opin Clin Nutr Metab Care 1999;2(2):121–6.

54. Jakubowicz-Gil J, et al. The effect of quercetin on pro-apoptotic activity of cisplatin in HeLa cells. Biochem Pharmacol 2005;69(9):1343–50.

55. Francescato HD, et al. Protective effect of quercetin on the evolution of cisplatin-induced acute tubular necrosis. Kidney Blood Press Res 2004;27(3):148–58.

56. Sliwinski T, et al. Zinc salts differentially modulate DNA damage in normal and cancer cells. Cell Biol Int 2009;33(4):542–7.

57. Studzinski GP, et al. Potentiation by 1-alpha, 25 dihydroxyvitamin D3 of cytotoxicity to HL-60 cells produced by cytarabine and hydroxyurea. J Natl Cancer Inst 1986;76(4):641–8.

58. Kim CH. Increased expression of N-acetylglucosaminyltransferase-V in human hepatoma cells by retinoic acid and 1alpha,25-dihydroxyvitamin D3. Int J Biochem Cell Biol 2004;36(11):2307–19.

59. Makishima M, et al. Growth inhibition and differentiation induction in human monoblastic leukaemia cells by 1alpha-hydroxyvitamin D derivatives and their enhancement by combination with hydroxyurea. Br J Cancer 1998;77(1):33–9.

60. Vukelja SJ, et al. Pyridoxine for the palmar-plantar erythrodysesthesia syndrome. Ann Intern Med 1989;111(8):688–9.

61. Fabian CJ, et al. Pyridoxine therapy for palmar-plantar erythrodysesthesia associated with continuous 5-fluorouracil infusion. Invest New Drugs 1990;8(1):57–63.

62. Nagore E, et al. Antineoplastic therapy-induced palmar plantar erythrodysesthesia ('hand-foot') syndrome. Incidence, recognition and management. Am J Clin Dermatol 2000;1(4):225–34.

63. Nakashima T, et al. Phase 1 study of concurrent radiotherapy with TS-1 and vitamin A (TAR therapy) for head and neck cancer. Gan To Kagaku Ryoho 2005;32(6):803–7.

64. Lotz-Winter H. On the pharmacology of bromelain: an update with special regard to animal studies on dose-dependent effects. Planta Med 1990;56(3):249–53.

65. Toffoli G, Cecchin E. Uridine diphosphoglucuronosyl transferase and methylenetetrahydrofolate reductase polymorphisms as genomic predictors of toxicity and response to irinotecan-, antifolate- and fluoropyrimidine-based chemotherapy. J Chemother 2004;16(Suppl. 4):31–5. [Review].

66. Etienne MC, et al. Thymidylate synthase and methylenetetrahydrofolate reductase gene polymorphisms: relationships with 5-fluorouracil sensitivity. Br J Cancer 2004;90(2):526–34.

67. Zhong X, et al. Effects of quercetin on the proliferation and apoptosis in transplantation tumor of breast cancer in nude mice. Sichuan Da Xue Xue Bao Yi Xue Ban 2003;34(3):439–42.

68. Koide T, et al. Influence of flavonoids on cell cycle phase as analyzed by flow-cytometry. Cancer Biother Radiopharm 1997;12(2):111–15.

69. Yuan H, Zhang Z. Some factors affecting sister-chromatid differentiation (SCD) and sister-chromatid exchange (SCE) in Hordeum vulgare. Mutat Res 1992;272(2):125–31.

70. Pyrhonen S, et al. Randomised comparison of fluorouracil, epidoxorubicin and methotrexate (FEMTX) plus supportive care with supportive care alone in patients with non-resectable gastric cancer. Br J Cancer 1995;71(3):587–91.

71. Nagai Y, et al. Vitamin A, a useful biochemical modulator capable of preventing methotrexate damage during methotrexate treatment. Pharmacol Toxicol 1993;73:69–74.

72. Fishman P, et al. Adenosine acts as a chemoprotective agent by stimulating G-CSF production: a role for A1 and A3 adenosine receptors. J Cell Physiol 2000;183(3):393–8.

73. Ohana G, et al. Differential effect of adenosine on tumour and normal cell growth: focus on the A3 adenosine receptor. J Cell Physiol 2001;186(1):19–23.

74. Navarro-Peran E, et al. Kinetics of the inhibition of bovine liver dihydrofolate reductase by tea catechins: origin of slow-binding inhibition and pH studies. Biochemistry 2005;44(20):7512–25.

75. Rovensky J, et al. The effects of Enterococcus faecium and selenium on methotrexate treatment in rat adjuvant-induced arthritis. Clin Dev Immunol 2004;11(3–4):267–73.

76. Mivazono Y, et al. Oxidative stress contributes to methotrexate-induced small intestinal toxicity in rats. Scand J Gastroenterol 2004;39(11):1119–27.

77. Perez JE, et al. High-dose alpha-tocopherol as a preventive of doxorubicin-induced alopecia. Cancer Treat Rep 1986;70(10):1213–14.

78. Shinozawa S, et al. Effect of high dose alpha-tocopherol and alpha-tocopherol pretreatment on adriamycin (doxocurbicin) induced toxicity and tissue distribution. Physiol Chem Phys Med NMR 1988;20(4):329–35.

79. Ripoll EA, et al. Vitamin E enhances the chemotherapeutic effects of adriamycin on human prostatic carcinoma cells in vitro. J Urol 1986;136(2):529–31.

80. Quiles JL, et al. Antioxidant nutrients and adriamycin toxicity. Toxicology 2002;180(1):79–95.

81. Versantvoort CH, et al. Genistein modulates the decreased drug accumulation in non-P-glycoprotein mediated multidrug resistant tumour cells. Br J Cancer 1993;68(5):939–46.

82. Monti E, Sinha BK. Antiproliferative effect of genistein and adriamycin against estrogen-dependent and -independent human breast cell carcinoma lines. Anticancer Res 1994;14(3):1221–3.

83. Conklin KA. Coenzyme Q10 for prevention of anthracycline-induced cardiotoxicity. Integr Cancer Ther 2005;4(2):110–30.

84. Dovinova I, et al. Combined effect of lipoic acid and doxorubicin in murine leukaemia. Neoplasma 1999;46(4):237–41.

85. Mijares A, Lopez JR. L-carnitine prevents increase in diastolic [Ca²⁺] induced by doxocurbicin in cardiac cells. Eur J Pharmacol 2001;425(2):117–20.

86. Waldner R, et al. Effects of doxoibicin-containing chemotherapy and a combination with L-carnitine on oxidative metabolism in patients with non-Hodgkin lymphoma. J Cancer Res Clin Oncol 2006;132(2):121–8.

87. Yeh YC, et al. A standardized extract of Ginkgo biloba suppresses doxorubicin-induced oxidative stress and p53-mediated mitochondrial apoptosis in rat testes. Br J Pharmacol 2009;156(1):48–61.

88. Hu Q, et al. Antimutagenicity of selenium-enriched rice on mice exposure to cyclophosphamide and mitomycin C. Cancer Lett 2005;220(1):29–35.

89. Fuga L, et al. Vitamin B2 (riboflavin) and a mixture of vitamin B2 and C affects MMC efficiency in aerated media under irradiation. Anticancer Res 2004;24(6):4031–4.

90. Kammerer C, Getoff N. Synergistic effect of dehydroascorbic acid and mixtures with vitamin E and beta-carotene on mitomycin C efficiency under irradiation in vitro. In Vivo 2004;18(6):795–8.

91. Krishnaia AP, Sharma NK. Ascorbic acid potentiates mitomycin C-induced micronuclei and sister chromatid exchanges in human peripheral blood lymphocytes in vitro. Teratog Carcinog Mutagen 2003;(Suppl. 1):99–112.

92. Undeger U, et al. The modulating effects of quercetin and rutin on the mitomycin C induced DNA damage. Toxicol Lett 2004;151(1):143–9.

93. Kurita T, et al. A dosage design of mitomycin C tablets containing finely powdered green tea. Int J Pharm 2004;275(1–2):279–83.

94. Niitsu N, Homma Y. Adenosine analogs as possible differentiation-inducing agents against acute myeloid leukemia. Leuk Lymphoma 1999;34(3–4):261–71. [Review].

95. Rafi MM, et al. Modulation of bcl-2 and cytotoxicity by licochalcone-A, a novel estrogenic flavonoid. Anticancer Res 2000;20(4):2653–8.

96. Berger M, et al. Effect of thioctic acid (alpha-lipoic acid) on the chemotherapeutic efficacy of cyclophosphamide and vincristine sulphate. Arzneimittelforschung 1983;33(9):1286–8.

97. Scifo C, et al. Resveratrol and propolis as necrosis or apoptosis inducers in human prostate carcinoma cells. Oncol Res 2004;14(9):415–26.

98. Menendez JA, et al. Synergistic interaction between vinorelbine and gamma-linolenic acid in breast cancer cells. Breast Cancer Res Treat 2002;72(3):203–19.

99. Nesbitt LT. Minimizing complications from systemic glucocorticosteroid use. Dermatol Clin 1995;13(4):925–39.

100. Seidner DL, et al. An oral supplement enriched with fish oil, soluble fiber, and antioxidants for corticosteroid sparing in ulcerative colitis: a randomized, controlled trial. Clin Gastroenterol Hepatol 2005;3(4):358–69.

101. Ravina A, et al. Reversal of corticosteroid-induced diabetes mellitus with supplemental chromium. Diabet Med 1999;16(2):164–7.

102. Thompson TA, Wilding G. Androgen antagonist activity by the antioxidant moiety of vitamin E, 2,2,5,7,8-pentamethyl-6-chromanol in human prostate carcinoma cells. Mol Cancer Ther 2003;2(8):797–803.

103. Jiang F, Wang Z. Identification and characterization of PLZF as a prostatic androgen-responsive gene. Prostate 2004;59(4):426–35.

104. Kang Z, et al. Coregulator recruitment and histone modifications in transcriptional regulation by the androgen receptor. Mol Endocrinol 2004;18(11):2633–48.

105. Juniewicz PE, et al. Effects of androgen and antiandrogen treatment on canine prostatic arginine esterase. Prostate 1990;17(2):101–11.

106. Zhang J, et al. Indole-3-carbinol induces a G1 cell cycle arrest and inhibits prostate-specific antigen production in human LNCaP prostate carcinoma cells. Cancer 2003;98(11):2511–20.

107. Mi Y, Zhang C. Toxic and hormonal effects of polychlorinated biphenyls on cultured testicular germ cells of embryonic chickens. Toxicol Lett 2005;155(2):297–305.

108. Mathur PP, Chattopadhyay S. Involvement of lysosomal enzymes in flutamide-induced stimulation of rat testis. Andrologia 1982;14(2):171–6.

109. Diamond T, et al. The effect of combined androgen blockade on bone turnover and bone mineral densities in men treated for prostate carcinoma: longitudinal evaluation and response to intermittent cyclic etidronate therapy. Cancer 1998;83(8):1561–6.

110. Fau D, et al. Mechanism for the hepatotoxicity of the antiandrogen, nilutamide. Evidence suggesting that redox cycling of this nitroaromatic drug leads to oxidative stress in isolated hepatocytes. J Pharmacol Exp Ther 1992;263(1):69–77.

111. Iynem AH, et al. The effect of prostate cancer and antiandrogenic therapy on lipid peroxidation and antioxidant systems. Int Urol Nephrol 2004;36(1):57–62.

112. Diamond TH, et al. Osteoporosis and spinal fractures in men with prostate cancer: risk factors and effects of androgen deprivation therapy. J Urol 2004;172(2):529–32.

113. Hatano T, et al. Incidence of bone fracture in patients receiving luteinizing hormone-releasing hormone agonists for prostate cancer. BJU Int 2000;86(4):449–52.

114. Cemeli E, et al. Modulation by flavonoids of DNA damage induced by estrogen-like compounds. Environ Mol Mutagen 2004;44(5):420–6.

115. Kitson TM, et al. Interaction of sheep liver cytosolic aldehyde dehydrogenase with quercetin, resveratrol and diethylstilbestrol. Chem Biol Interact 2001;130–132(1–3):57–69.

116. Gehm BD, et al. Estrogenic effects of resveratrol in breast cancer cells expressing mutant and wild-type estrogen receptors: role of AF-1 and AF-2. J Steroid Biochem Mol Biol 2004;88(3):223–34.

117. Morris GZ, et al. Resveratrol induces apoptosis in LNCaP cells and requires hydroxyl groups to decrease viability in LNCaP and DU 145 cells. Prostate 2002;52(4):319–29.

118. Cho DI, et al. Effects of resveratrol-related hydroxystilbenes on the nitric oxide production in macrophage cells: structural requirements and mechanism of action. Life Sci 2002;71(17):2071–82.

119. Karasek M, et al. Melatonin inhibits growth of diethylstilbestrol-induced prolactin-secreting pituitary

909

tumor in vitro: possible involvement of nuclear RZR/ROR receptors. J Pineal Res 2003;34(4):294–6.

120. Jones JL, et al. Genistein inhibits tamoxifen effects on cell proliferation and cell cycle arrest in T47D breast cancer cells. Am Surg 2002;68(6):575–7, discussion 577–8.

121. Ju YH, et al. Dietary genistein negates the inhibitory effect of tamoxifen on growth of estrogen-dependent human breast cancer (MCF-7) cells implanted in athymic mice. Cancer Res 2002;62(9):2474–7.

122. Ravindranath MH, et al. Anticancer therapeutic potential of soy isoflavone, genistein. Adv Exp Med Biol 2004;546:121–65. [Review].

123. Liu B, et al. Low-dose dietary phytoestrogen abrogates tamoxifen-associated mammary tumour prevention. Cancer Res 2005;65(3):879–86.

124. Fiorelli G, et al. Estrogen synthesis in human colon cancer epithelial cells. J Steroid Biochem Mol Biol 1999;71(5–6):223–30.

125. Herbal Medicine Research and Education Centre. Herbs used in menopause. Comp Med 2005;4(4):51.

126. Constantinou AL, et al. The soy isoflavone daidzein improves the capacity of tamoxifen to prevent mammary tumours. Eur J Cancer 2005;41(4):647–54.

127. Donnelly LE, et al. Anti-inflammatory effects of resveratrol in lung epithelial cells: molecular mechanisms. Am J Physiol Lung Cell Mol Physiol 2004;287(4):L774–83.

128. Ma ZS, et al. Reduction of CWR22 prostate tumor xenograft growth by combined tamoxifen-quercetin treatment is associated with inhibition of angiogenesis and cellular proliferation. Int J Oncol 2004;24(5):1297–304.

129. Fujiki H, et al. Cancer prevention with green tea and monitoring by a new biomarker, hnRNP B1. Mutat Res 2001;480–481:299–304. [Review].

130. Suganuma M, et al. Mechanisms of cancer prevention by tea polyphenols based on inhibition of TNF-alpha expression. Biofactors 2000;13(1–4):67–72.

131. Suganuma M, et al. Combination cancer chemoprevention with green tea extract and sulindac shown in intestinal tumor formation in Min mice. J Cancer Res Clin Oncol 2001;127(1):69–72.

132. Perumal SS, et al. Combined efficacy of tamoxifen and coenzyme Q10 on the status of lipid peroxidation and antioxidants in DMBA induced breast cancer. Mol Cell Biochem 2005;273(1–2):151–60.

133. Perumal SS, et al. Augmented efficacy of tamoxifen in rat breast tumorigenesis when gavaged along with riboflavin, niacin, and CoQ10: effects on lipid peroxidation and antioxidants in mitochondria. Chem Biol Interact 2005;152(1):49–58.

134. De Leo V, et al. Menopause, the cardiovascular risk factor homocysteine, and the effects of treatment. Treat Endocrinol 2004;3(6):393–400. [Review].

135. Palomba S, et al. Lipid, glucose and homocysteine metabolism in women treated with a GnRH agonist with or without raloxifene. Hum Reprod 2004;19(2):415–21.

136. Al Akoum M, et al. Synergistic cytotoxic effect of tamoxifen and black cohosh on MCF-7 and MDA-MB-231 human breast cancer cells: an in vitro study. Can J Physiol Pharmacol 2007;85(11):1153–9.

137. Rickard DJ, et al. Phytoestrogen genistein acts as an estrogen agonist on human osteoblastic cells through estrogen receptors alpha and beta. J Cell Biochem 2003;89(3):633–46.

138. Rliwinski L, et al. Differential effects of genistein, estradiol and raloxifene on rat osteoclasts in vitro. Pharmacol Rep 2005;57(3):352–9.

139. Antoniucci DM, et al. Vitamin D insufficiency does not affect bone mineral density response to raloxifene. J Clin Endocrinol Metab 2005;90(8):4566–72.

140. Hascalik S, et al. Effects of resveratrol, raloxifene, tibolone and conjugated equine estrogen on vaginal squamous cell maturation of ovariectomized rats. Gynecol Obstet Invest 2005;60(4):186–91.

141. Celik O, et al. Magnetic resonance spectroscopic comparison of the effects of resveratrol (3,4′,5-trihydroxy stilbene) to conjugated equine estrogen, tibolone and raloxifene on ovariectomized rat brains. Eur J Obstet Gynecol Reprod Biol 2005;120(1):73–9.

142. Paterson AH. Evaluating bone mass and bone quality in patients with breast cancer. Clin Breast Cancer 2005;5(Suppl. 2):S41–5.

143. Lindsay R, et al. Bone response to treatment with lower doses of conjugated estrogens with and without medroxyprogesterone acetate in early postmenopausal women. Osteoporos Int 2005;16(4):372–9.

144. Brodowska A. The influence of hormonal replacement therapy on bone density in postmenopausal women depending on polymorphism of vitamin D receptor (VDR) and estrogen receptor (ER) genes. Ann Acad Med Stetin 2003;49:111–30.

145. Day JK, et al. Dietary genistein increased DMBA-induced mammary adenocarcinoma in wild-type, but not ER alpha KO, mice. Nutr Cancer 2001;39(2):226–32.

146. Subakir SB, et al. Oxidative stress, vitamin E and progestin breakthrough bleeding. Hum Reprod 2000;15(Suppl. 3):18–23.

147. Barnes JF, et al. Effects of two continuous hormone therapy regimens on C-reactive protein and homocysteine. Menopause 2005;12(1):92–8.

148. Meram I, et al. Trace elements and vitamin levels in menopausal women receiving hormone replacement therapy. Clin Exp Obstet Gynecol 2003;30(1):32–4.

149. Sliutz G, et al. Drug resistance against gemcitabine and topotecan mediated by constitutive hsp70 overexpression in vitro: implication of quercetin as sensitiser in chemotherapy. Br J Cancer 1996;74(2):172–7.

150. Panosyan EH, et al. Deamination of glutamine is a prerequisite for optimal asparagines deamination by asparaginases in vivo (CCG-1961). Anticancer Res 2004;24(2C):1121–5.

151. Rotoli BM, et al. Inhibition of glutamine synthetase triggers apoptosis in asparaginase-resistant cells. Cell Physiol Biochem 2005;15(6):281–92.

152. Myszka H, et al. Synthesis and induction of apoptosis in B cell chronic leukemia by diosgenyl 2-amino-2-deoxy-beta-D-glucopyranoside hydrochloride and its derivatives. Carbohydr Res 2003;338(2):133–41.

153. Liu JD, et al. Inhibition of melanoma growth and metastasis by combination with (-)-epigallocatechin-3-gallate and dacarbazine in mice. J Cell Biochem 2001;83(4):631–42.

154. Reid JM, et al. Metabolic activation of dacarbazine by human cytochromes P450: the role of CYP1A1, CYP1A2, and CYP2E1. Clin Cancer Res 1999;5(8):2192–7.

155. Menendez JA, et al. Omega-6 polyunsaturated fatty acid gamma-linolenic acid (18:3n-6) enhances docetaxel (Taxotere) cytotoxicity in human breast carcinoma cells: relationship to lipid peroxidation and HER-2/neu expression. Oncol Rep 2004;11(6):1241–52.

156. Beer TM, et al. Rationale for the development and current status of calcitriol in androgen-independent prostate cancer. World J Urol 2005;23(1):28–32. [Review].

157. Beer TM, Myrthue A. Calcitriol in cancer treatment: from the lab to the clinic. Mol Cancer Ther 2004;3(3):373–81. [Review].

158. Beer TM, et al. Quality of life and pain relief during treatment with calcitriol and docetaxel in symptomatic

metastatic androgen-independent prostate carcinoma. Cancer 2004;100(4):758–63.

159. Wynter MP, et al. Effect of n-3 fatty acids on the antitumour effects of cytotoxic drugs. In Vivo 2004;18(5):543–7.

160. Ghalaut PS, et al. Serum vitamin E levels in patients of chronic myeloid leukaemia. J Assoc Physicians India 1999;47(7):703–4.

161. Przybyszewski WM, et al. Protection of L5178Y cells by vitamin E against acute hydroxyurea toxicity does not change the efficiency of ribonucleotide reductase-mediated hydroxyurea-induced cytotoxic events. Cancer Lett 1987;34(3):337–44.

162. Malec J, et al. Hydroxyurea-induced toxic side-effects in animals and an attempt at reducing them with vitamins E and C. Neoplasma 1989;36(4):427–35.

163. Makaroy AA, et al. Zinc(II)-mediated inhibition of ribonuclease Sa by an N-hydroxyurea nucleotide and its basis. Biochem Biophys Res Commun 2004;319(1):152–6.

164. Higgin JJ, et al. Zinc(II)-mediated inhibition of a ribonuclease by an N-hydroxyurea nucleotide. Bioorg Med Chem Lett 2003;13(3):409–12.

165. Wong WS, McLean AE. Effects of phenolic antioxidants and flavonoids on DNA synthesis in rat liver, spleen, and testis in vitro. Toxicology 1999;139(3):243–53.

166. Miknyoczki SJ, et al. Chemopotentiation of temozolomide, irinotecan, and cisplatin activity by CEP-6800, a poly(ADP-ribose) polymerase inhibitor. Mol Cancer Ther 2003;2(4):371–82.

167. Fakih M, et al. Selenium protects against toxicity induced by anticancer drugs and augments antitumor activity: a highly selective, new, and novel approach for the treatment of solid tumors. Clin Colorectal Cancer 2005;5(2):132–5.

168. Cao S, et al. Selective modulation of the therapeutic efficacy of anticancer drugs by selenium containing compounds against human tumor xenografts. Clin Cancer Res 2004;10(7):2561–9.

169. Yoshikawa M, et al. Transport of SN-38 by the wild type of human ABC transporter ABCG2 and its inhibition by quercetin, a natural flavonoid. J Exp Ther Oncol 2004;4(1):25–35.

170. Bremner I, et al. Control of selenium and cobalt deficiency in lambs by supplementation of oral anthelmintics. Vet Rec 1988;123(9):217–18.

171. Pathak AK, et al. Chemotherapy alone vs chemotherapy plus high dose multiple antioxidants in patients with advanced non small cell lung cancer. J Am Coll Nutr 2005;24(1):16–21.

172. Varma MV, Panchagnula R. Enhanced oral paclitaxel absorption with vitamin E-TPGS: effect on solubility and permeability in vitro, in situ and in vivo. Eur J Pharm Sci 2005;25(4–5):445–53.

173. Siewinski M, et al. Determination of cysteine peptidases-like activity and their inhibitors in the serum of patients with ovarian cancer treated by conventional chemotherapy and vitamin E. J Exp Ther Oncol 2004;4(3):189–93.

174. Argyriou AA, et al. Vitamin E for prophylaxis against chemotherapy-induced neuropathy: a randomized controlled trial. Neurology 2005;64(1):26–31.

175. Choi JS, et al. Enhanced paclitaxel bioavailability after oral administration of paclitaxel or prodrug to rats pretreated with quercetin. Eur J Pharm Biopharm 2004;57(2):313–18.

176. Taixiang W, et al. Chinese medical herbs for chemotherapy side effects in colorectal cancer patients. Cochrane Database Syst Rev 2005;(1):CD004540.

177. Reiter RJ, et al. Melatonin: reducing the toxicity and increasing the efficacy of drugs. J Pharm Pharmacol 2002;54(10):1299–321.

178. Kinnula K, et al. Endogenous antioxidant enzymes and glutathione S-transferase in protection of mesothelioma cells against hydrogen peroxide and epirubicin toxicity. Br J Cancer 1998;77(7):1097–102.

179. Jarvinen K, et al. Antioxidant defense mechanisms of human mesothelioma and lung adenocarcinoma cells. Am J Physiol Lung Cell Mol Physiol 2000;278(4):L696–702.

180. Shinozawa S, et al. Protective effects of various drugs on adriamycin (doxorubicin)-induced toxicity and microsomal lipid peroxidation in mice and rats. Biol Pharm Bull 1993;16(11):1114–17.

181. Solaini G, et al. Inhibitory effects of several anthracyclines on mitochondrial respiration and coenzyme Q10 protection. Drugs Exp Clin Res 1985;11(8):533–7.

182. Tarumoto T, et al. Ascorbic acid restores sensitivity to imatinib via suppression of Nrf2-dependent gene expression in the imatinib-resistant cell line. Exp Hematol 2004;32(4):375–81.

183. Vera JC, et al. Colony-stimulating factors signal for increased transport of vitamin C in human host defense cells. Blood 1998;91(7):2536–46.

184. Higucki T, et al. Induction of differentiation of retinoic acid-resistant acute promyelocytic leukemia cells by the combination of all-trans retinoic acid and granulocyte colony-stimulating factor. Leuk Res 2004;28(5):525–32.

185. Matsui W, et al. Requirement for myeloid growth factors in the differentiation of acute promyelocytic leukaemia. Br J Haematol 2005;128(6):853–62.

186. Ganser A, et al. Improved multilineage response of hematopoiesis in patients with myelodysplastic syndromes to a combination therapy with all-trans-retinoic acid, granulocyte colony-stimulating factor, erythropoietin and alpha-tocopherol. Ann Hematol 1996;72(4):237–44.

187. Maurer AB, et al. Changes in erythroid progenitor cell and accessory cell compartments in patients with myelodysplastic syndromes during treatment with all-trans retinoic acid and haemopoietic growth factors. Br J Haematol 1995;89(3):449–56.

188. Carcamo JM, et al. Vitamin C inhibits granulocyte macrophage-colony-stimulating factor-inducing signaling pathways. Blood 2002;99(9):3205–12.

189. Vera JC, et al. Colony-stimulating factors signal for increased transport of vitamin C in human host defense cells. Blood 1998;91(7):2536–46.

190. Tao YH, Yang Y. Effects of vitamin A on the differentiation, maturation and functions of dendritic cells from cord blood. Zhonghua Er Ke Za Zhi 2004;42(5):340–3.

191. Hengesbach LM, Hoag KA. Physiological concentrations of retinoic acid favor myeloid dendritic cell development over granulocyte development in cultures of bone marrow cells from mice. J Nutr 2004;134(10):2653–9.

192. Fishman P, et al. The A3 adenosine receptor as a new target for cancer therapy and chemoprotection. Exp Cell Res 2001;269(2):230–6.

193. Faderl S, Estrov Z. Commentary: effect of flavonoids on normal and leukemic cells. Leuk Res 2003;27(6):471–3.

194. Mogattash S, Lutton JD. Leukemia cells and the cytokine network: therapeutic prospects. Exp Biol Med 2004;229(2):121–37.

195. Neri S, et al. L-carnitine decreases severity and type of fatigue induced by interferon-alpha in the treatment of patients with hepatitis C. Neuropsychobiology 2003;47(2):94–7.

196. Gedlicka C, et al. Effective treatment of oxaliplatin-induced cumulative polyneuropathy with alpha-lipoic acid. J Clin Oncol 2002;20(15):3359–61.

197. Socinski MA, et al. The evolving role of pemetrexed (Alimta) in lung cancer. Semin Oncol 2005;32(2 Suppl. 2):S16–22. [Review].

198. Buddle LS, Hanna NH. Antimetabolites in the management of non-small cell lung cancer. Curr Treat Options Oncol 2005;6(1):83–93. [Review].

199. Adjei AA. Pharmacology and mechanism of action of pemetrexed. Clin Lung Cancer 2004;5(Suppl. 2):S51–5. [Review].

200. Fossella FV. Pemetrexed for treatment of advanced non-small cell lung cancer. Semin Oncol 2004;31(1 Suppl. 1): 100–5. [Review].

201. Horstman MG, et al. Separate mechanisms for procarbazine spermatotoxicity and anticancer activity. Cancer Res 1987;47(6):1547–50.

202. Fuggetta MP, et al. In vitro antitumour activity of resveratrol in human melanoma cells sensitive or resistant to temozolomide. Melanoma Res 2004;14(3):189–96.

203. Grothey A. Clinical management of oxaliplatin-associated neurotoxicity. Clin Colorectal Cancer 2005;5(Suppl. 1): S38–48.

204. El-Bayoumy K, Sinha R. Molecular chemoprevention by selenium: a genomic approach. Mutat Res 2005;591(1–2): 224–36.

APPENDIX 4

Food sources of nutrients

Order is approximately indicative of ranking of content.

Nutrient	Common food source
Vitamins	
A	Liver, sweet potato, carrots, spinach, butternut pumpkin, dandelion greens, butter, eggs
B1	Whole grains, pork, sunflower seeds, nuts, legumes
B2	Liver, other organ meats, mushrooms, ricotta cheese, milk, meats, eggs, cheese, whole grains, oysters
B3	Tuna, liver, chicken, beef, halibut, mushrooms, nuts, whole grains
B5	Egg yolk, liver, kidney, brewer's yeast—widespread in most foods
B6	Steak, legumes, potato, salmon, bananas, whole grains, other meats and fish
B12	Meat, fish, shellfish, eggs, cheese, milk, oysters, fermented foods
Folate	Brewer's yeast, leafy greens, asparagus, wholegrain cereals, legumes, nuts, liver
C	Pawpaw, oranges, rockmelon, broccoli, brussels sprouts, tomatoes, grapefruit, cabbage, strawberries
D	Fatty and canned fish, butter, margarine, cream, cheese, eggs—also synthesised in skin upon exposure to sunlight
E	Vegetable oils, nuts, olive oil, wheat germ, avocado, egg, fatty fish and small amounts in wholegrain cereals and green vegetables
K	Green vegetables, cheese, soy, butter, pork, eggs—also synthesised by healthy intestinal microflora
Biotin	Brewer's yeast, liver, kidney, legumes, eggs, chard, bitter greens—also synthesised by healthy intestinal microflora
Minerals	
Boron	Legumes, nuts, whole grains, fruits and vegetables, beer, wine, cider
Calcium	Yoghurts and cheeses, sesame seeds (tahini), milk, bony fish (particularly sardines), clams, oysters, broccoli, nuts, dried fruit

Nutrient	Common food source
Chromium	Brewer's yeast, mushrooms, prunes, asparagus, organ meats, whole grains, tea, cheese
Copper	Liver, shellfish, whole grains, legumes, eggs, meats, fish
Fluoride	Tea, bony fish—very small amounts in most food sources
Iodine	Seafood, sea vegetables, iodised table salt, sunflower seeds, liver, mushrooms—nutrient soil-dependent in other sources
Iron	Organ meats, other meats, oysters, nuts, legumes, leafy greens, whole grains, eggs
Magnesium	Nuts, legumes, whole grains, soy, parsnips, molasses, cocoa mass, corn, peas, leafy greens
Manganese	Whole grains, nuts, leafy greens, tea, blueberries, pineapple
Molybdenum	Soy, legumes, buckwheat, oats, whole grains, nuts, meat
Phosphorus	Meats, fish, poultry, eggs, milk, cheese, nuts, legumes, whole grains
Potassium	Avocadoes, bananas, dried fruits, oranges, peaches, potatoes, legumes, tomatoes, wheat bran, eggs, apricots, nuts
Selenium	Brazil nuts, kidney, tuna, crab, lobster—nutrient particularly soil-dependent
Sulfur	Most protein foods
Zinc	Oysters, wheat germ, meats, liver, whole grains, pumpkin seeds, nuts
Phytonutrients	
Anthocyanins	Red, blue and purple berries, red and purple grapes, red wine
Carotenoids	Carrots, pumpkin, butternut pumpkin, sweet potato, pawpaw, red and yellow capsicum, corn, kale, leafy greens, tomatoes, rockmelon, paprika, peas
Chlorophyll	Spinach, parsley, watercress, beans, rocket, leeks
Cruciferous indoles	Cruciferous vegetables (broccoli, brussels sprouts, cabbage, kale, turnip, radish, swedes, horseradish, watercress)
Flavanols	Tea, cocoa, berries, grapes, apples
Hesperidin and rutin	Citrus fruits and juices (especially grapefruit and blood oranges)
Isoflavones	Soy, legumes
Isothiocyanates	Cruciferous vegetables, garlic
Lignans	Linseed, sesame seeds, kale, broccoli, apricots, cabbage
Lutein and zeaxanthin	Spinach, kale, leafy greens, peas, squash, butternut pumpkin, broccoli, brussels sprouts, corn
Luteolin and other flavones	Parsley, thyme, celery, chillies
Lycopene	Tomato paste, tomato puree, watermelon, tomatoes, pink grapefruit
Quercetin and other flavonols	Onions, shallots, kale, broccoli, apples, berries, tea
Fats	
Omega-3	Oily fish, oysters, linseed, walnuts

APPENDIX **5**

Laboratory reference values

The reference values and ranges for these blood tests are given in the system of international units (SI) and are based on guidelines from the Royal College of Pathologists of Australasia. They may vary from laboratory to laboratory. When paediatric reference ranges may differ from adult ranges they are indicated by an asterisk (*). Further information and resources can be found at the online manual of the Royal College of Pathologists of Australasia at www.rcpamanual.edu.au.

Investigation/application	Reference value	Potential increased level	Potential decreased level
Electrolytes			
Potassium			
Monitoring status with diuretic usage, acid–base balance or mineralocorticoid status*	3.5–5.0 mmol/L	Acidosis, tissue damage, renal failure and mineralocorticoid deficiency Drugs such as ACE inhibitors, NSAIDs, diuretics	Alkalosis, vomiting or diarrhoea, mineralocorticoid excess Drugs such as insulin, diuretics, salbutamol
Sodium			
Monitoring fluid and electrolyte status	135–145 mmol/L	Dehydration, vomiting or diarrhoea, kidney disease, excess mineralocorticoids, excess salt intake or retention	Low salt intake, high blood glucose, mineralocorticoid or thyroid deficiency Excess water intake Kidney, heart or liver failure
Sodium:potassium ratio	28–34	> 34 + raised sodium → potassium deficiency	< 28 → sodium deficiency, also low magnesium and vitamin E
Chloride			
Assess cause of acid–base imbalance	95–107 mmol/L	High sodium and metabolic acidosis	Low sodium and metabolic alkalosis
Bicarbonate			
Acid–base imbalance and metabolic abnormalities	23–32 mmol/L	Metabolic alkalosis, compensated respiratory acidosis, potassium deficiency, excess laxatives or vomiting	Metabolic or diabetic acidosis, excess lactic acid, alcohol or aspirin, fasting

Investigation/application	Reference value	Potential increased level	Potential decreased level
Kidney function			
Urea			
Renal function	3.0–8.0 mmol/L	Excess protein, renal failure, kidney stones, congestive heart failure, enlarged prostate, gastrointestinal bleeding, diarrhoea or vomiting, dehydration or sweating	Low protein intake, water retention, urea cycle defects, poisoning or severe liver damage < 5.0 → dietary protein deprivation
Urate			
Gout, pregnancy-induced hypertension*	M 0.17–0.45 mmol/L F 0.12–0.40 mmol/L	Gout, pregnancy-induced hypertension, renal failure, fasting, excess lactate or ketones Drugs such as diuretics, low-dose salicylates	Protein insufficiency and poor nucleotide synthesis
Creatinine			
Glomerular filtration	M 0.04–0.13 mmol/L F 0.04–0.10 mmol/L	Conditions of decreased filtration (hypovolaemia, hypotension), renal or postrenal obstruction	Low muscle mass, pregnancy < 0.06 → poor protein tissue bulk
Urea:creatinine ratio	70–90	> 90 → excess protein tissue breakdown	< 70 → dietary protein deprivation
Calcium			
Hypo- or hyperparathyroidism, malignancy*	2.10–2.60 mmol/L	Hyperparathyroidism, malignancy, sarcoidosis, vitamin A or D toxicity	Hypoparathyroidism, renal failure, osteomalacia, rickets, thyroid or parathyroid surgery Calcium < 2.3 + phosphate < 1.0 → calcium and phosphate deficiency
Phosphate			
Renal failure, hyper- or hypoparathyroidism, metabolic bone disease	0.90–1.35 mmol/L	Hypoparathyroidism, hypercalcaemia due to malignancy, renal failure	Hyperparathyroidism, use of magnesium or aluminium-containing antacids
Calcium:phosphate ratio	1.0–2.4	> 2.4 + phosphate < 1.0 → calcium deficiency	< 2.2 with phosphate > 1.0 → phosphate deficiency
Proteins			
Amount of albumin and immunoglobulins present in serum	60–80 g/L	Increased immunoglobulins, dehydration	Low albumin, reduced immunoglobulins
Albumin			
Hydration, nutritional status, liver disease, catabolic disorders	38–50 g/L	Dehydration, level may be overestimated in severe deficiency depending on analysis method	Acute phase response, impaired protein synthesis < 35 g/L → severe protein deprivation

Investigation/application	Reference value	Potential increased level	Potential decreased level
Globulins			
Hypo- and hypergamma-globulinaemia	Consult pathologist	Chronic inflammation, infection, autoimmune disease	Catabolic enteropathy, humoral immunodeficiency
Liver function			
Bilirubin			
Hepatobiliary disease, haemolysis*	Total: < 20 µmol/L Direct: < 3 µmol/L	Gilbert's syndrome, hepatobiliary disease, megaloblastic anaemia, fasting or insulin resistance, lack of cofactors B3, B6, magnesium, iron or glutamine	
Alkaline phosphatase (ALP)			
Hepatobiliary or bone disease*	< 120 U/L	Paget's disease, liver damage, excess bone activity, tissue repair	Zinc deficiency, abnormal dentition and fragile bones
Gamma-glutamyl transferase (GGT)			
Liver disease*	M < 65 U/L F < 45 U/L	Liver dysfunction with cholestasis, diabetes, excess alcohol, pancreatitis, prostatitis, acute liver damage	Impaired protein synthesis, vitamin B6 deficiency
Alanine aminotransferase (ALT)			
Liver cell damage*	< 35 U/L	Hepatocellular damage	Vitamin B6, B1 or zinc deficiency
Aspartate aminotransferase (AST)			
Liver cell damage*	< 40 U/L	Hepatocellular damage, haemolysis during collection, muscle tissue breakdown, copper toxicosis	Vitamin B6, B1 or zinc deficiency
Lactate dehydrogenase (LD) Liver disease, malignancy, skeletal muscle damage	110–230 U/L	Myocardial infarction, liver disease, haemolysis, ineffective erythropoiesis, muscle disease and tissue damage, some malignancies	
Blood cells			
Red cell count (RCC)*	M 4.5–6.5 × 10^{12}/L F 3.8–5.8 × 10^{12}/L Reticulocytes: 0.5–2.0%	Polycythaemia, dehydration, in response to low oxygen levels (smoking, high altitude, chronic diseases)	Anaemia, haemorrhage, chronic infection or renal failure, pregnancy, over-hydration, leukaemia, multiple myelomas

Investigation/application	Reference value	Potential increased level	Potential decreased level
Haemoglobin			
Anaemia*	M 130–180 g/L F 115–165 g/L	Anaemia	
Mean cell volume (MCV)			
Macro- or microcytic anaemia*	81–98 fL	Macrocytic anaemia, vitamin B12 or folate deficiency, hypothyroidism, chronic liver disease Drugs that affect B12 status (anticonvulsants, antimetabolics)	Microcytic anaemia, iron deficiency, malignancy, rheumatoid arthritis, haemoglobinopathies, radiation or lead poisoning
White cell count (WCC)			
Infection, inflammation, bone marrow failure*	4.0–11.0 × 10⁹/L	Acute infection, tissue necrosis, leukaemias, collagen diseases, sickle cell anaemia, parasites, stress Drugs such as aspirin, heparin, digoxin, lithium	Viral infections, malaria, haematopoietic diseases, alcoholism, systemic lupus erythematosus (SLE), rheumatoid arthritis Drugs such as antibiotics, paracetamol, sulfanomides, diuretics, indomethacin, oral hypoglycaemic agents
Neutrophils*	Band: 0.05 × 10⁹/L Mature: 2.0–7.5 × 10⁹/L	Acute bacterial infections, inflammation, tissue damage, solid tumours, excessive exercise, allergies, pregnancy and labour	Viral infections, overwhelming bacterial infection, aplastic anaemia, acute leukaemia, vitamin B12 or folate deficiency, malnutrition, SLE
Lymphocytes*	1.0–4.0 × 10⁹/L	Stress, uraemia, neoplasia, infections, rickets, ulcerative colitis, Addison's disease	Aplastic and pernicious anaemia, burns, protein malnutrition, toxic chemical exposure, pneumonia, high-dose adrenocorticosteroids
Eosinophils*	0.0–0.4 × 10⁹/L	Parasitic worm infections, allergic diseases, Hodgkin's lymphoma	
Basophils*	0.01–0.1 × 10⁹/L	Chronic myeloid leukaemia	
Monocytes*	0.2–0.8 × 10⁹/L	Chronic bacterial infections, tuberculosis, subacute bacterial endocarditis, ulcerative colitis, cirrhosis, haemolytic anaemias, SLE	
Platelet count*	150–400 × 10⁹/L	Acute illness, chronic inflammation, splenectomy, thrombocythaemia	Increased tendency to bleed and bruise
Cholesterol			
Total cholesterol*	< 5.5 mmol/L	Cardiovascular disease risk	

Investigation/application	Reference value	Potential increased level	Potential decreased level
High-density lipoprotein (HDL)	> 1.00 mmol/L		Cardiovascular disease risk
Low-density lipoprotein (LDL)	< 3.5 mmol/L	Cardiovascular disease risk	Acute illness
Triglycerides*	< 2.0 mmol/L	Secondary to nephrotic syndrome, hypothyroidism, pancreatitis, insulin resistance or diabetes, alcoholism, ocular cicatricial pemphigoid (OCP) or steroid medication	Chronic disease
Homocysteine	5–15 μmol/L	Lack of methylation cofactors vitamin B12, folate, methionine	
Thyroid function			
Thyroid stimulating hormone (TSH)*	0.3–5.0 mU/L	Hypothyroidism, elevated mercury levels	
T4	10.0–20.0 pmol/L	Hyperthyroidism	Hypothyroidism
T3	3.3–8.2 pmol/L		With low T4 → low thyroxine activity secondary to nutrient deficiency such as iodine or autoimmune disease With normal T4 → impaired conversion due to nutrient deficiency such as selenium, hyperinsulinaemia
Thyroid antibodies	Consult pathologist	Hashimoto's thyroiditis, other autoimmune thyroid dysfunctions, other tissue specific autoimmune disorders	
Food allergies—refer to Chapter 6 on food sensitivity			
IgA		Chronic infections, inflammatory bowel disease	Recurrent intestinal infection, dairy protein intolerance, other food sensitivities
IgE	Varies with age—consult pathologist	Allergic reactions	
IgG		Chronic infections, intestinal parasites, food sensitivities	Malnutrition
IgM		Viral infections, hepatobiliary disease, food sensitivities	Immune suppression, protein loss from bowel
Antigliadin antibodies		Gluten intolerance or coeliac disease	

919

Investigation/application	Reference value	Potential increased level	Potential decreased level
Tumour markers			
PSA (prostate-specific antigen)	0–4.0 µg/L	Benign prostatic hypertrophy Marked elevation is indicative of prostate cancer, but normal or slightly raised levels do not exclude it	
CEA (carcinoembryonic antigen)	< 7.5 µg/L	Recurrence of colonic adenocarcinoma and breast carcinoma following resection	
AFP (alpha fetoprotein)	< 10 µg/mL	Detection and monitoring of hepatocellular carcinoma and germ cell tumours Assessment of risk for neural tube and other defects in utero, including Down syndrome (one of the components of the 'triple test')	
CA-125	< 35 U/mL	Marker for serous carcinoma, especially ovarian	
Glucose			
Glucose (fasting)	3.5–6.0 mmol/L	Diabetes mellitus	Hypoglycaemia
Glucose (random)	3.5–9.0 mmol/L	Diabetes mellitus	Hypoglycaemia
HbA$_{1c}$	4.7–6.1%	Diabetes mellitus (indicative of levels over past three months)	
Other endocrine tests			
Cortisol 8 a.m.	130–700 nmol/L	Stress, OCP use, adrenal or adrenocorticotrophic hormone (ACTH)-producing tumours, Cushing's syndrome	Addison's disease, hypopituitarism
Cortisol 4 p.m.	80–350 nmol/L	Stress, OCP use, adrenal or ACTH-producing tumours, Cushing's syndrome	Addison's disease, hypopituitarism
FSH adult	1.9 IU/L	Various interpretations—see Chapter 34 on fertility	
FSH ovulation	10–30 IU/L		
FSH postmenopausal	4–200 IU/L		
Oestradiol menopausal	< 200 pmol/L		
Testosterone	M 10–35 nmol/L F < 3.5 nmol/L		

Markers of inflammation: erythrocyte sedimentation rate (ESR) and C-reactive protein (CRP)

Comparison between ESR and CRP

- Both investigations are markers of inflammation and there tends to be a broad correlation between them.
- The CRP levels rise faster than the ESR.
- The levels are similar after 24 hours or so.
- CRP levels fall faster than the ESR.
- CRP levels (unlike ESR) are not affected by pregnancy.
- ESR may be very high with a normal CRP in giant cell arteritis and polymyalgia rheumatica.
- CRP costs more.

Relative values (mm/hour) of typical examples of ESR readings

Very high (over 80 mm/hour)	High (40–80 mm/hour)	Moderate to low elevation (20–40 mm/hour)	Low (< 1 mm/hour)
Giant cell arteritis (temporal arteritis) and polymyalgia rheumatica Multiple myeloma Tuberculosis Deep abscess Bacterial endocarditis Acute osteomyelitis	Rheumatic fever Pyelonephritis Other bacterial infections Viral infections with cold agglutinins Collagen disorders (e.g. rheumatoid arthritis, SLE) Solid tumours, especially metastases Leukaemia/lymphomas Myocardial infarction Inflammation of healing	Most acute and chronic infections (e.g. recent viral) Severe other illness Anaemia Pregnancy Drugs, especially contraceptives Elevated serum cholesterol level Laboratory error (e.g. tilted tube) Idiopathic—normal	Idiopathic—normal Sickle-cell anaemia Polycythaemia NSAIDs Old specimen

There is a lag phase of 24–48 hours between the onset of inflammatory stimulation and the production of inflammatory proteins that increase in the ESR. There is also a delay in the fall of the ESR after resolution of the inflammation because the fibrinogen levels can remain elevated for six days or so after acute tissue damage—this can take four to eight weeks to return to normal.

A normal value of < 20 mm/hour generally excludes inflammation. The OCP can push the level to 20–25 mm/hour.

Normal values of ESR—reference interval

Child	
	2–15 mm/hour
Adult male	
17–50 years	1–10 mm/hour
> 50 years	2–15 mm/hour
Adult female	
17–50 years	3–12 mm/hour
> 50 years	5–20 mm/hour

C-reactive protein levels (normal value < 10 mg/L)

Marked elevation > 40 mg/L	Normal to mild elevation
Bacterial infection Abscess Crohn's disease Active rheumatic disease: – rheumatic fever Connective tissue disorders: – rheumatoid arthritis – vasculitis Malignant disease Trauma/tissue injury	Viral infection Ulcerative colitis SLE Atherosclerosis Steroid/oestrogen therapy

Interpretation of iron studies

Condition	Serum iron	Total iron binding capacity	% transferrin saturation	Ferritin
	14–30 (µmol/L)*	45–80 (µmol/L)*	F 20–55% M 20–60% (transferrin 2–3.5 g/L)*	20–250 (µg/L)*
Iron deficiency	↓	N or ↑	↓	↓↓
Thalassaemia	N or ↑	N	N or ↑	↑
Anaemia of chronic disease	↓	N or ↓	↓	N or ↑
Sideroblastic anaemia	N or ↑	N	N or ↑	↑
Haemochromatosis	↑	↓	↑↑	↑↑

N = normal
*Reference range

APPENDIX 6

Taxonomic cross-reference of major herbs

Botanical name	Common name
Achillea millefolium	Yarrow
Aesculus hippocastanum	Horse chestnut
Agathosma betulina	Buchu
Agropyron repens	Couchgrass
Albizia lebbeck	Albizia
Alchemillia vulgaris	Lady's mantle
Aloe spp.	Aloe vera
Althaea officinalis	Marshmallow
Andrographis paniculata	Andrographis
Anemone pulsatilla	Pasque flower, pulsatilla
Angelica sinensis	Dong quai
Apium graveolens	Celery seed
Arctium lappa	Burdock
Arctostaphylos uva-ursi	Uva ursi, bearberry
Arnica montana	Arnica
Artemisia absinthium	Wormwood
Asclepias tuberosa	Pleurisy root
Asparagus racemosus	Shatavari
Astragalus membranaceus	Astragalus
Avena sativa	Oats
Azadirachta indica	Neem
Bacopa monnieri	Bacopa, brahmi
Baptisia tinctoria	Baptisia
Berberis aquifolium	Oregon grape
Berberis aristata	Indian barberry
Berberis vulgaris	Barberry
Bupleurum falcatum	Bupleurum
Calendula officinalis	Calendula, marigold
Capsella bursa-pastoris	Shepherd's purse
Caulophyllum thalictroides	Blue cohosh

Botanical name	Common name
Centella asiatica	Gotu kola
Chamaelirium luteum	False unicorn root
Chelidonium majus	Greater celandine
Chionanthus virginicus	Fringe tree
Actaea racemosa	Black cohosh
Cinnamomum zeylanicum	Cinnamon
Codonopsis pilosula	Codonopsis
Coleus forskohlii	Coleus
Commiphora molmol	Myrrh
Crataegus monogyna	Hawthorn
Crataeva nurvala	Crataeva
Curcuma longa	Turmeric
Cynara scolymus	Globe artichoke
Dioscorea villosa	Wild Yam
Echinacea angustifolia Echinacea purpurea	Echinacea
Eleutherococcus senticosus	Siberian ginseng, eleutherococcus
Epilobium parviflorum	Willow herb
Equisetum arvense	Horsetail
Eschscholzia californica	Californian poppy
Euphorbia hirta	Euphorbia
Euphrasia officinalis	Eyebright
Filipendula ulmaria	Meadowsweet
Foeniculum vulgare	Fennel
Fucus vesicolus	Bladderwrack
Galega officinalis	Goat's rue
Galium aparine	Cleavers, clivers
Gentiana lutea	Gentian
Geranium maculatum	Cranesbill
Ginkgo biloba	Ginkgo
Glycyrrhiza glabra	Liquorice
Grindelia camporum	Grindelia
Gymnema sylvestre	Gymnema
Hamamelis vulgaris	Witch hazel
Harpagophytum procumbens	Devil's claw
Hemidesmus indicus	Hemisdesmus
Humulus lupulus	Hops
Hydrastis canadensis	Goldenseal
Hypericum perforatum	St John's wort

Botanical name	Common name
Hyssopus officinalis	Hyssop
Iberis amara	Bitter candytuft
Inula helenium	Elecampane
Iris versicolor	Blue flag
Lavandula spp.	Lavender
Leonurus cardiaca	Motherwort
Lycopus virginicus	Bugleweed
Marrubium vulgare	White horehound
Matricaria recutita	Chamomile
Melissa officinalis	Lemon balm
Mentha piperita	Peppermint
Mentha spicata	Spearmint
Paeonia lactiflora	White peony, peony
Panax ginseng	Korean ginseng
Panax notoginseng	Tienchi ginseng
Passiflora incarnata	Passionflower
Peumus boldo	Boldo
Phytolacca decandra	Poke root
Piper methysticum	Kava
Piscidia erythrina	Jamaica dogwood
Plantago ovata	Psyllium
Prunus serotina	Wild cherry
Rehmannia glutinosa	Rehmannia
Rhamnus purshiana	Cascara
Rosmarinus officinalis	Rosemary
Rubus idaeus	Red raspberry leaf
Rumex crispus	Yellow dock
Ruscus aculeatus	Butcher's broom
Salvia officinalis	Sage
Sambucus nigra	Elder flower
Schisandra chinensis	Schisandra
Scutellaria baicalensis	Baical skullcap
Scutellaria lateriflora	Skullcap
Serenoa repens	Saw palmetto
Silybum marianum	Milk thistle, St Mary's thistle
Smilax ornata	Sarsaparilla
Solidago virgaurea	Goldenrod
Stellaria media	Chickweed
Symphytum officinale	Comfrey

Botanical name	Common name
Tabebuia avellanedae	Pau d'arco
Tanacetum parthenium	Feverfew
Taraxacum officinale	Dandelion
Thuja occidentalis	Thuja
Thymus vulgaris	Thyme
Tilia spp.	Linden, lime flowers
Trifolium pratense	Red clover
Trigonella foenum-graecum	Fenugreek
Turnera diffusa	Damiana
Tylophora indica	Tylophora
Ulmus fulva	Slippery elm
Uncaria tomentosa	Cat's claw
Urtica dioica	Nettle, stinging nettle
Vaccinum prunifolium	Bilberry
Valeriana edulis	Mexican valerian
Valeriana officinalis	Valerian
Verbascum thapsus	Mullein
Verbena officinalis	Vervain
Viburnum opulus	Cramp bark
Viburnum prunifolium	Black haw
Viscum album	Mistletoe
Vitex agnus-castus	Chaste tree
Withania somnifera	Withania, ashwaganda
Zanthoxylum clava-herculis	Prickly ash
Zea mays	Cornsilk
Zingiber officinale	Ginger
Ziziphus spinosa	Spiny jujube

Common name	Botanical name
Albizia	*Albizia lebbeck*
Aloe vera	*Aloe* spp.
Andrographis	*Andrographis paniculata*
Arnica	*Arnica montana*
Astragalus	*Astragalus membranaceus*
Bacopa, brahmi	*Bacopa monnieri*
Baical skullcap	*Scutellaria baicalensis*
Baptisia	*Baptisia tinctoria*
Barberry	*Berberis vulgaris*
Bearberry	*Arctostaphylus uva-ursi*

Common name	Botanical name
Bilberry	*Vaccinum prunifolium*
Bitter candytuft	*Iberis amara*
Black cohosh	*Actaea racemosa*
Black haw	*Viburnum prunifolium*
Bladderwrack	*Fucus vesicolus*
Blue cohosh	*Caulophyllum thalictroides*
Blue flag	*Iris versicolor*
Boldo	*Peumus boldo*
Buchu	*Agathosma betulina*
Bugleweed	*Lycopus virginicus*
Bupleurum	*Bupleurum falcatum*
Burdock	*Arctium lappa*
Butcher's broom	*Ruscus aculeatus*
Calendula, marigold	*Calendula officinalis*
Californian poppy	*Eschscholzia californica*
Cascara	*Rhamnus purshiana*
Cat's claw	*Uncaria tomentosa*
Celery seed	*Apium graveolens*
Chamomile	*Matricaria recutita*
Chaste tree	*Vitex agnus-castus*
Chickweed	*Stellaria media*
Cinnamon	*Cinnamomum zeylanicum*
Cleavers, clivers	*Galium aparine*
Codonopsis	*Codonopsis pilosula*
Coleus	*Coleus forskohlii*
Comfrey	*Symphytum officinale*
Cornsilk	*Zea mays*
Couchgrass	*Agropyron repens*
Cramp bark	*Viburnum opulus*
Cranesbill	*Geranium maculatum*
Crataeva	*Crataeva nurvala*
Damiana	*Turnera diffusa*
Dandelion	*Taraxacum officinale*
Devil's claw	*Harpagophytum procumbens*
Dong quai	*Angelica sinensis*
Echinacea	*Echinacea angustifolia* *Echinacea purpurea*
Elder flower	*Sambucus nigra*
Elecampane	*Inula helenium*
Euphorbia	*Euphorbia hirta*

Common name	Botanical name
Eyebright	*Euphrasia officinalis*
False unicorn root	*Chamaelirium luteum*
Fennel	*Foeniculum vulgare*
Fenugreek	*Trigonella foenum-graecum*
Feverfew	*Tanacetum parthenium*
Fringe tree	*Chionanthus virginicus*
Gentian	*Gentiana lutea*
Ginger	*Zingiber officinale*
Ginkgo	*Ginkgo biloba*
Globe artichoke	*Cynara scolymus*
Goat's rue	*Galega officinalis*
Goldenrod	*Solidago virgaurea*
Goldenseal	*Hydrastis canadensis*
Gotu kola	*Centella asiatica*
Greater celandine	*Chelidonium majus*
Grindelia	*Grindelia camporum*
Gymnema	*Gymnema sylvestre*
Hawthorn	*Crataegus monogyna*
Hemisdesmus	*Hemidesmus indicus*
Hops	*Humulus lupulus*
Horse chestnut	*Aesculus hippocastanum*
Horsetail	*Equisetum arvense*
Hyssop	*Hyssopus officinalis*
Indian barberry	*Berberis aristata*
Jamaica dogwood	*Piscidia erythrina*
Kava	*Piper methysticum*
Korean ginseng	*Panax ginseng*
Lady's mantle	*Alchemillia vulgaris*
Lavender	*Lavandula officinalis*
Lemon balm	*Melissa officinalis*
Liquorice	*Glycyrrhiza glabra*
Linden, lime flowers	*Tilia* spp.
Marshmallow	*Althaea officinalis*
Meadowsweet	*Filipendula ulmaria*
Mexican valerian	*Valeriana edulis*
Milk thistle, St Mary's thistle	*Silybum marianum*
Mistletoe	*Viscum album*
Motherwort	*Leonurus cardiaca*
Mullein	*Verbascum thapsus*

Common name	Botanical name
Myrrh	*Commiphora molmol*
Neem	*Azadirachta indica*
Nettle, stinging nettle	*Urtica dioica*
Oats	*Avena sativa*
Oregon grape	*Berberis aquifolium*
Pasque flower, pulsatilla	*Anemone pulsatilla*
Passionflower	*Passiflora incarnata*
Pau d'arco	*Tabebuia avellanedae*
Peppermint	*Mentha piperita*
Pleurisy root	*Asclepias tuberosa*
Poke root	*Phytolacca decandra*
Prickly ash	*Zanthoxylum clava-herculis*
Psyllium	*Plantago ovata*
Red clover	*Trifolium pratense*
Red rasberry leaf	*Rubus idaeus*
Rehmannia	*Rehmannia glutinosa*
Rosemary	*Rosmarinus officinalis*
Sage	*Salvia officinalis*
Sarsaparilla	*Smilax ornata*
Saw palmetto	*Serenoa repens*
Schisandra	*Schisandra chinensis*
Shatavari	*Asparagus racemosus*
Shepherd's purse	*Capsella bursa-pastoris*
Siberian ginseng, eleutherococcus	*Eleutherococcus senticosus*
Skullcap	*Scutellaria lateriflora*
Slippery elm	*Ulmus fulva*
Spearmint	*Mentha spicata*
Spiny jujube	*Ziziphus spinosa*
St John's wort	*Hypericum perforatum*
Thuja	*Thuja occidentalis*
Thyme	*Thymus vulgaris*
Tienchi ginseng	*Panax notoginseng*
Turmeric	*Curcuma longa*
Tylophora	*Tylophora indica*
Uva ursi	*Arctostaphylos uva-ursi*
Valerian	*Valeriana officinalis*
Vervain	*Verbena officinalis*
White horehound	*Marrubium vulgare*
White peony, peony	*Paeonia lactiflora*

Common name	Botanical name
Wild cherry	*Prunus serotina*
Wild yam	*Dioscorea villosa*
Willow herb	*Epilobium parviflorum*
Witch hazel	*Hamamelis vulgaris*
Withania, ashwaganda	*Withania somnifera*
Wormwood	*Artemisia absinthium*
Yarrow	*Achillea millefolium*
Yellow dock	*Rumex crispus*

Index

Page numbers followed by '*f*' indicate figures, '*t*' indicate tables, and '*b*' indicate boxes.